Manual of Spine Surgery

Uwe Vieweg · Frank Grochulla

Editors

Manual of Spine Surgery

Second Edition

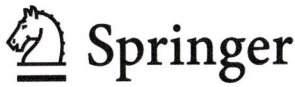
Springer

Editors
Uwe Vieweg
Surgical and Conservative Spine Therapy
Hospital Rummelsberg
Schwarzenbruck, Germany

Frank Grochulla
Metropol Medical Center
Center for Orthopaedics, Neurosurgery and
Traumatology, Nuremberg
Germany

ISBN 978-3-662-64060-9   ISBN 978-3-662-64062-3   (eBook)
https://doi.org/10.1007/978-3-662-64062-3

This Springer imprint is published by the registered company Springer-Verlag GmbH, DE part of Springer Nature.
The registered company address is: Heidelberger Platz 3, 14197 Berlin, Germany

Preface

The second edition of *Manual of Spine Surgery* has become necessary as a consequence of the rapid expansion of spine surgery using different minimally invasive and non-fusion techniques. To do justice to this development, the second edition of *Manual of Spine Surgery* aims to present the different techniques to spinal surgeons in a clear and instructive way using detailed illustrations. Its coverage of different principles and techniques of contemporary spine surgery, including anatomy, pathology, procedures, and instrumentations, makes it highly useful as a refresher before surgery, an easily digestible study guide. The success of any spinal operation depends on good definition of the indications, consideration of the contraindications, technical and organizational factors, correct preoperative preparation, and positioning of the patient and good operating technique. The description of different open, less invasive or minimally invasive techniques with more than 700 illustrations will provide the spinal surgeon useful guidelines for their use. The *Manual of Spine Surgery, Second Edition* is authoritative, concise, and portable, designed for use in a fast-paced clinical setting. The book is a daily companion for spinal surgeons and spinal therapeutics caring for patients with spinal disorders.

Uwe Vieweg
Frank Grochulla

Contents

Contributors

Sashin Ahuja University Hospital of Wales, Cardiff, UK

Florian Maria Alfen Orthopaedic Spine Center Dr. Alfen, Würzburg, Germany

Wilson T. Asfora Department of Neurosurgery, Sanford School of Medicine, Sanford Neurosurgery and Spine, University of South Dakota, Sioux Falls, SD, USA

Edward Bayle Department of Spinal Surgery, The Centre for Spinal Studies and Surgery, Queens Medical Centre, University Hospital NHS Trust, Nottingham, UK

Jörg Böhme Department of Trauma Surgery, Orthopaedics and Specialist Septic Surgery, St. Georg Hospital Leipzig, Leipzig, Germany

Pia Borgas Faculty of Medical Sciences, University College London, London, UK

Bronek Boszczyk The Centre for Spinal Studies and Surgery, Queens Medical Centre, University Hospital NHS Trust, Nottingham, UK

Torsten Bräuer Spine Section of the Orthopedic Department Norwegian University of Science and Technology (NTNU), Trondheim, Norway

Paulo Tadeu Maia Cavali Department of Scoliosis os Hospital AACD-Sao Paulo, Sao Paulo, Brazil

Grégoire P. Chatain Department of Neurosurgery, School of Medicine, University of Colorado, Aurora, CO, USA

Bruno Domokos Orthopaedic Spine Center Dr. Alfen, Würzburg, Germany

Jörg Drumm Center for Spine Surgery, SRH Klinikum Karlsbad-Langensteinbach, Karlsbad, Germany

Stefan Endres Department for Orthopedic Surgery, Kreiskrankenhaus Rheinfelden/Baden, Baden, Germany

Michael A. Finn Department of Neurosurgery, School of Medicine, University of Colorado, Aurora, CO, USA

Guilherme Augusto Foizer Department of Orthopedic Surgery, Unicamp, Campinas, Brazil

Spine Surgery at Hospital Adventista de São Paulo, São Paulo, Brazil

Volker Fuchs Department of Orthopedics, AMEOS Hospital Halberstadt, Halberstadt, Germany

Oliver Gonschorek Department of Spine Surgery, BGU Trauma Center Murnau, Murnau, Germany

Frank Grochulla Metropol Medical Center, Clinic for Orthopedics, Trauma Surgery and Spinal Surgery, Nuremberg, Germany

Ulrich Hahn Department for Trauma and Orthopedic Surgery, Medical Center Geldern, Geldern, Germany

Stefan Hellinger OOCC München MVZ, Munich, Germany

Christian Hohaus Department of Neurosurgery, BG Klinikum Bergmannstrost, Halle, Germany

Johannes Keck Clinic for Surgical and Conservative Spinal Therapy with Interdisciplinar Spinal Deformities Centre and Rummelsberg Sectional Center, Hospital Rummelsberg, Schwarzenbruck, Germany

Annette Kienle Mechanical Implant Testing, SpineServ GmbH & Co. KG, Ulm, Germany

Philipp Kobbe Department of Trauma and Reconstructive Surgery, University Clinic RWTH Aachen, Aachen, Germany

Stefan Kroppenstedt Department of Spinal Surgery, Center of Orthopedic Surgery, Sana Hospital Sommerfeld, Kremmen, Germany

Theophilo Asfora Lins Clínica Phitris, Sãu Paulo, Brazil

Departamento de Ortopedia e Traumatologia, Escola Paulista de Medicina - UNIFESP, Sãu Paulo, Brazil

Hans Jörg Meisel Department of Neurosurgery, BG Klinikum Bergmannstrost, Halle, Germany

Markus Melloh Institute of Health Sciences, Zurich University of Applied Sciences, Winterthur, Switzerland

UWA Medical School, The University of Western Australia, Nedlands, Western Australia, Australia

Kiril Mladenov Department of Pediatric Orthopedic Surgery, AKK Altonaer Children's Hospital, Hamburg, Germany

Robert Morrison Spine & Scoliosis Center, Asklepios Klinik Bad Abbach, Germany

Samuel Morris Centre for Spinal Studies and Surgery, Queen's Medical Centre, Stockport, UK

Hannes Moritz Clinic for Surgical and Conservative Spinal Therapy with Interdisciplinar Spinal Deformities Centre and Rummelsberg Sectional Center, Rummelsberg Hospital, Schwarzenbruck, Germany

Jacques D. Müller-Broich Department of Orthopedics (Friedrichsheim), University Hospital Frankfurt am Main, Frankfurt am Main, Germany

Everard Munting Clinique Saint Pierre, Ottignies, Belgium

Jürgen Nothwang Rems-Murr-Klinik Schorndorf, Department for Trauma Surgery and Orthopedics, Schorndorf, Germany

Gregor Ostrowski Center for Spine Surgery, SRH Klinikum Karlsbad-Langensteinbach, Karlsbad, Germany

Palaniappan Lakshmanan Sunderland Royal Hospital, Sunderland, UK

Luca Papavero Clinic for Spine Surgery, Schoen Clinic Hamburg, Hamburg, Germany

J. Petrovics Center for Spine Surgery, Orthopedics, and Traumatology, SRH Klinikum Karlsbad-Langensteinbach, Karlsbad, Germany

Tobias Pitzen Center for Spine Surgery, Orthopedics, and Traumatology, SRH Klinikum Karlsbad-Langensteinbach, Karlsbad, Germany

Valentin Quack Department of Trauma and Reconstructive Surgery, University Clinic RWTH Aachen, Aachen, Germany

Christoph Röder Institute for Evaluative Research in Medicine, University of Bern, Bern, Switzerland

Sebastian Ruetten Department of Orthopädic Surgery, Center for Spine Surgery and Pain Therapy, Center for Orthopaedics and Traumatology, St. Anna-Hospital, Herne, Germany

Michael Ruf Center for Spine Surgery, SRH Klinikum Karlsbad-Langensteinbach, Karlsbad, Germany

Khalid Saeed Department of Spinal Surgery, New Cross Hospital, The Royal Wolverhampton Hospitals NHS Trust, Wolverhampton, UK

Fabio Dos Santos Neurosurgery, ColunaRS—Clínica de Cirurgia da Coluna Vertebral, Porto Alegre RS, Brazil

Stefan Schären Department of Orthopaedic Surgery/Spine, University Hospital, Basel, Switzerland

Meic H. Schmidt Department of Neurosurgery, University of New Mexico, Albuquerque, NM, USA

Kirsten Schmieder Department of Neurosurgery, University Hospital Knappschaftskrankenhaus Bochum, Bochum, Germany

Werner Schmoelz Department of Orthopaedics and Traumatology - Biomechanics, Medical University of Innsbruck, Innsbruck, Austria

Christian Schultz Augsburg, Germany

Christoph J. Siepe Schön Klinik München Harlaching, Spine Center, Academic Teaching Hospital and Spine Research Institute of the Paracelsus Medical University (PMU, Salzburg, AU), Munich, Germany

Steffen Sola Department of Neurosurgery, University of Rostock, Rostock, Germany

Christoph Spang Orthopaedic Spine Center Dr. Alfen, Würzburg, Germany

Marco Teli The Walton Centre for Neurology and Neurosurgery, Liverpool, UK

Per Trobisch Eifelklinik St. Brigida, Department of Spine Surgery, Simmerath, Germany

Sven Y. Vetter Division of Spinal Surgery at BG Trauma Center Ludwigshafen at Heidelberg University Hospital, Ludwigshafen, Germany

Uwe Vieweg Department of Conservative and Surgical Spine Therapy with Interdisciplinary Spinal Deformities Centre and Rummelsberg Sectional Center, Hospital Rummelsberg, Schwarzenbruck, Germany

Karsten Wiechert Schön Klinik Munich Harlaching, Spine Center "Am Michel", Hamburg, Germany

Cornelius Wimmer Department of Spine Surgery, Trauma Center, Trostberg, Germany

Department of Orthopaedic Surgery, University of Innsbruck, Innsbruck, Austria

Michael Winking ZW-O Spine Center, Klinikum Osnabrück, Osnabrück, Germany

Mehmet Zileli Neurosurgery Department, Sanko University, Gaziantep, Türkiye

Thomas Zweig Spine in the Center, Bern/Langenthal, Switzerland

Part I

General Aspects of Spinal Surgery

Definition and Trends of Modern Spinal Surgery

Uwe Vieweg

1.1 Introduction and Core Messages

Spine surgery is a field of operative medicine. The spine calls for a variety of different surgical access techniques because of its elongated shape and the varying anatomic situations in its different regions. Pathologies and their localisation, and also technological development, have given rise to numerous surgical procedures, for example, microscopic and endoscopic discectomy, percutaneous instrumentation, endoscopically guided instrumentation, complex anterior–posterior spinal reconstruction, dynamic procedures (disc and nucleus replacement) and also procedures incorporating biological processes (stem cell therapy, growth factors, etc.). Spine surgery is a unique surgical speciality typically involving both orthopaedic and neurosurgical specialists. Rather than developing still further as a separate, highly specialised, surgical discipline, spine surgery should be seen within the overall therapeutic context and should join forces with other areas of therapy to provide interdisciplinary treatment of the spine for the benefit of patients.

1.2 Definition

Spine surgery refers to the area of surgery concerned with the diagnosis and treatment of spinal disorders. This surgical subspeciality is concerned with the management of disorders of the spine, employing both operative and non-operative forms of treatment to preserve and restore function. Spine surgery is used to treat diseases and injuries affecting different structures in the spinal column and may therefore be indicated for a variety of spine problems. Generally, surgery may be performed for degenerative disorders, trauma, instability, deformities, infections and tumours. With regard to epidemiology and health economics, these problems affecting the body's central structural axis, particularly the degenerative disorders, are among the major challenges facing the health systems of modern industrialised countries. Spine surgery is thus crucially important. In most cases, it is performed with the purpose of correcting an anatomical lesion or stabilising the spine, if the patient has not shown significant improvement with conservative treatments. Spine surgery is performed by neurosurgeons and by orthopaedic and trauma surgeons. Operations involving the spine may also be carried out by radiologists (vertebroplasty, kyphoplasty) or general surgeons. Recent advances have led to a number of technical developments which are now employed to aid spine surgery, including the following:

- Spinal navigation and spinal robotics
- Fluoroscopy
- Spinal implants
- Bone substitutes, stem cells and growth factors
- Endoscopy
- Microscopy
- Neurophysiological monitoring
- Improved instruments and retractors
- High-frequency surgery

In the USA, back pain is the most common cause of activity limitation in people younger than 45 years. Back pain is the fifth-ranking cause of admission to hospital and the third most common reason for surgery [1–3]. The USA has the highest rate of spine surgery in the world, but spine surgery shows wider geographic variations than most other procedures [1, 2].

U. Vieweg (✉)
Department of Conservative and Surgical Spine Therapy with Interdisciplinary Spinal Deformities Centre and Rummelsberg Sectional Center, Hospital Rummelsberg,
Schwarzenbruck, Germany
e-mail: uwe.vieweg@sana.de

1.2.1 Spine Organisations and Societies

In recent years, a number of scientific associations and societies have been founded by different surgeons to encourage applied research in the area of spine surgery (see Table 1.1). Germany's first such organisation was founded in 1955 under the name Deutsche Gesellschaft für Wirbelsäulenforschung (German Society for Spine Research). In 2006, in Munich, this society amalgamated with its sister organisation, the Deutsche Gesellschaft für

Table 1.1 Some major national and international spine organisations

Name of society	Abbreviation	Founded	Administrative office	Number of members	Specialties	WWW	Journal publications
North American Spine Society	NASS	1984	Burr Ridge/Washington, USA	>5000	Orthopaedic surgery, neurosurgery, neurology, radiology, research	Spine.org	*The Spine Journal, The Spine Line*
AANS/CNS-Joint Neurosurgical Committee on Spine	AANS/CNS	2003	Washington, USA	>1430	Neurosurgery	Spinesection.org	
American Board of Spine Surgery	ABSS	1997	New York, USA	–	Neurosurgery, orthopaedic surgery	American Board of SpineSurgery.org	*Journal of American Board of Spine Surgery*
EuroSpine—Spine Society of Europe	EuroSpine	1998	Zürich, Ulster, Switzerland	530	Neurosurgery, orthopaedic surgery	Eurospine.org	*European Spine Journal*
Deutsche Wirbelsäulengesellschaft	DWG	2005	Ulm, Germany	7 > 1000	Orthopaedics, traumatology, spinal surgery, neurosurgery, physical medicine, rehabilitation, research, anaesthesiology, pain management, others	DWG.org	*European Spine Journal*
AO Spine	AO Spine	2003	Duebendorf, Switzerland	>4500	Orthopaedics, neurosurgery research	AOSpine.org	*InSpine Evidence-Based Spine Surgery*
Cervical Spine Research Society	CSRS	1973	Rosemont, IL, USA	>200	Biomechanical engineering, neurology, neurosurgery, radiology, orthopaedic surgery	CSRS.org	*The Cervical Spine.* Lippincott Raven
International Society for the Study of the Lumbar Spine	ISSLS	1998	Gothenburg, Sweden	>380	Orthopaedics, neurosurgery, radiology, neurology	ISSLS.org	*The Lumbar Spine,* Lippincott Williams & Wilkins
Scoliosis Research Society	SRS	1966	Milwaukee, USA	>1000	Orthopaedics, neurosurgery, others	srs.org	
Association of European Research Groups for Spinal Osteosynthesis	ARGOS	1996	Strasbourg, France	–	Orthopaedics, neurosurgery, radiology, neurology, anatomy	Argospine.org	*ARGO Spine News and Journal EJOST*
The Spine Arthroplasty Society	SAS	1999	Aurora, IL, USA	1400	Orthopaedics, neurosurgery, research, others	SpineArthroplasty.org	*SAS Journal*

Wirbelsäulenchirurgie (German Society for Spine Surgery), to form the Deutsche Wirbelsäulengesellschaft (DWG, German Spine Society). The North American Spine Society (NASS) (founded in 1984) is one of the largest scientific organisations concerned with the diagnosis and treatment of spine diseases. NASS is a multidisciplinary medical organisation dedicated to fostering evidence-based ethical spine care by promoting education, research and advocacy. NASS has more than 5000 members from many different disciplines including orthopaedic surgery, neurosurgery, physiatry, neurology, radiology, anaesthesiology, research, physical therapy and other spine care professions. The EuroSpine (former European Spine Society (ESS), European Spinal Deformity Society (ESDS)) was founded in 1998 in Innsbruck, Austria. The aims of EuroSpine, the Spine Society of Europe (ES), are to stimulate the exchange of knowledge and ideas in the field of research, prevention and treatment of spine diseases and related problems and to coordinate efforts undertaken in European countries for further development in this field. The ES with the support of the EuroSpine Foundation introduces a European education plan for spine specialists to foster excellence in spinal care (see EuroSpine courses, www.Eurospine.org).

The AO Foundation (Arbeitsgemeinschaft für Osteosynthesefragen—Association for the Study of Internal Fixation—commonly called AO) was established in 1958 by a group of Swiss surgeons to address diseases and injuries to the musculoskeletal system and has now grown to become a highly influential worldwide organisation. Distribution and sales of all AO products are done through Synthes via a subsidiary! From March 2006, Synthes acquired existing Synthes-branded products from the AO Foundation. Within the AO Foundation, a group of spine surgeons led by John Webb, Max Aebi and Paul Pavlov supported by the AO's industrial partners pushed for greater autonomy for the spine surgeons within the AO. As a consequence of this development, the AO Spine International was established in June 2003. Today, the AO Spine has a membership of around 4500 surgeons, researchers and allied spine professionals. The American Board of Spine Surgery (ABSS) and the American board of spinesurgery.org were established in 1997 and 1999, respectively. The ABSS sets standards for professional training and certification in spine surgery, promoting quality assurance, while the American College of Spine Surgery encourages sponsors and accredits suitable training programmes. Its primary goal is to assist the public and the medical profession by setting educational and postgraduate training requirements for spine surgeons and by promoting continuing quality assurance programmes. As the list in Table 1.1 demonstrates, a great many organisations have come into being, sometimes in competition with one another. They include purely scientific non-profit organisations and scientific societies allowing links with industry and bodies representing particular professional interests (boards and academies). For some of these organisations,

where the profiles are similar, fusion may be an interesting option for the future to enable resources to be employed more effectively.

1.3 Trends of Spinal Surgery

In recent years, two trends have developed in spine surgery. These are *minimally invasive and/or less invasive spine surgery (MISS and LISS)* and *non-fusion technology*. In the future developments in regenerative medicine, using a variety of biological processes such as stem cell applications for improved bone fusion, growth factors and replacement of disc tissue may become spine surgery's next trend (Table 1.2).

1.3.1 Minimally Invasive and Less Invasive Spine Surgery

Minimally invasive techniques have given rise to a whole new range of technologies aimed at reducing surgical trauma. Minimally invasive procedures such as percutaneous treatments in outpatient settings are becoming more and more popular. The techniques of minimally invasive and less invasive spinal surgery have earned a permanent place in the operative treatment of the spine. In essence, minimally invasive spine surgery involves operating through small incisions, usually with the aid of endoscopic or microscopic visualisation. These procedures provide surgical options that address pathological conditions in the spinal column without producing the types of morbidity commonly seen in open surgical procedures. MISS and LISS are gentle, quick, efficient and economical. The advantages are low blood loss, small skin incisions, reduced post-operative pain, minimal damage to the skin and muscles, faster and better rehabilitation and a more rapid return to normal activities. The ventral spine can be treated with the aid of special retractor systems and modern implants, surgically addressed operating with endoscopic assistance or entirely endoscopically. The dorsal spine can be accessed from the dorsal side, either percutaneously or with the aid of special retractor systems.

1.3.2 Non-fusion Techniques

Non-fusion techniques aim to provide stabilisation while maintaining the mobility and function of the spine and eliminating the pain caused by the damaged spinal disc. Individuals who have already undergone spinal fusion may develop problems in the vertebrae and discs next to the fusion site (so-called adjacent level degeneration) even when the fusion itself has been entirely successful. These problems tend to develop several years after initial surgery. When segments of the spine are fused together, the segments next to the fusion are subjected to increased forces. This is one reason why spi-

Table 1.2 Simplified list of approaches and available operating techniques (decompression, fusion, non-fusion) for different spinal levels

Level	Anterior approaches				Posterior approaches			
		Decompression	Fusion	Non-fusion		Decompression	Fusion	Non-fusion
C0–C2	Transoral	Resection of the odontoid	Plate	No	Midline	Laminectomy and	Rod-screw	No
	Extraoral	Resection of the vertebral body	Plate	No	Posterolateral	Hemilaminectomy	Screw plate	No
			Transarticular screw				Transarticular screw	
							Wiring	
C3–C7	Anterolateral	Discectomy	Plating	Artificial disc	Midline	Laminectomy and	Rod-screw	Laminoplasty
		Uncoforaminotomy	Cage/spacer implantation		Posterolateral	Hemilaminectomy	Screw plate	
		Resection of the vertebral body	Vertebral body replacement			Foraminotomy		
T1–T12	Sternotomy	Discectomy	Plate	No	Midline	Laminectomy and	Rod-hook	No
	Thoracotomy	Resection of the vertebral body	Cage/spacer implantation			Costotransversectomy	Rod-screw	
	– Classic		Vertebral body replacement			Hemilaminectomy		
	– Mini-open							
	– Endoscopic							
L1–S1	Anterior	Discectomy	Plating	Artificial disc	Midline	Laminectomy	Rod-screw system	Interspinous spacer
		Resection of the vertebral body	Cage	Nucleus replacement	Posterolateral	Hemilaminectomy	Screws	Pedicle screw-based systems
			Vertebral body replacement			Foraminotomy	Screw plate system	Facet replacement systems
	Anterolateral	Resection of the vertebral body	Plating	Nucleus replacement				
		Discectomy	Cage					
			Vertebral body replacement					

nal disc or nucleus replacement and dynamic stabilisation are being developed. Total disc replacement in the lumbar spine, using an artificial disc, is the most advanced non-fusion technique currently in use, but other procedures such as nucleus replacement, posterior dynamic stabilisation and interspinal distraction are also used. The aim of total disc replacement is to relieve low back and leg pain due to disc degeneration and restore the motion of the spine. The artificial disc is a device made of two base plates connected with or without a pivot. This structure allows a different wide range of movements. The new motion preservation technologies of spine arthroplasty could offer significant advantages, including the maintenance of range of motion and mechanical characteristics, restoration of natural disc height and spinal alignment, significant pain reduction and prevention of adjacent segment degeneration [4]. Dynamic stabilisation describes the treatment method of achieving stabilisation by maintaining the disc with a controlled motion segment [5]. Dynamic stabilisation can be achieved using graft ligament systems, pedicle screw-based systems, facet replacement systems and interspinous process spacers.

1.3.3 Outlook

The future of spine surgery will be determined by further developments in spinal navigation and by the introduction of various minimally invasive, partially percutaneous, techniques and new implants. Fusion techniques and fusion materials will change considerably. The implants will increasingly be made of various partially absorbable biomaterials. Microelectromechanical systems and the use of growth factors or genetic techniques will be part of daily practice. In the more distant future, the solutions will probably lie more in disc repair by cell biology than in replacement with mechanical hardware. The future will show whether disc regeneration by injected chondrocytes or application of molecules such as anticatabolics, non-chondrogenic mitogens, chondrogenic morphogens and intracellular regulators is a real option for early tissue repair surgery, as is currently being considered for more disabling and advanced degenerative disc disease [6–8]. New techniques are being developed to fight the degenerative process itself. Among these is gene therapy, which could provide long-term delivery of molecules to retard or even reverse degenerative processes. All these developments will mean that the various pathological processes in the spine can be treated on a much more individual basis. There will be individualised spinal surgery, in some cases rigid and in others dynamic and function preserving or a combination of the two. In order to prepare the surgeons of the future, medical training will have to include a subspecialisation in spinal surgery. A higher level of training in general and specialised spinal surgery must be guaranteed [7]. The ever-growing socioeconomic pressure resulting from the increasing frequency of spinal diseases and their consequences is driving forward the development of differential diagnostic procedures and efficient targeted treatment. This pressure will become more acute in the coming years as the average age of the population increases and the financial resources of health systems decrease. The future of spine surgery must also lie in interdisciplinary efforts to prevent spinal disease. Over the coming decades, the subspecialisation of this area will progress almost by law, starting with professional subspecialisation and working towards developing spine surgery as a separate speciality. However, the future of spine surgery must also lie in interdisciplinary efforts to prevent spinal disease. Rather than developing still further as a separate, highly specialised, surgical discipline, spine surgery should be seen within the overall therapeutic context and should join forces with other areas of therapy to provide interdisciplinary treatment of the spine for the benefit of patients.

References

1. Praemer A, Furnes S, Rice DP. Musculoskeletal conditions in the United States. Rosemont: AAUS; 1992. p. 1–99.
2. Taylor VM, Deyo R, Cherkin DC, Kreuter W. Low-back pain hospitalization: recent United States trends and regional variations. Spine. 1994;19:1207–13.
3. Debure A. Modern trends in spinal surgery. J Bone Joint Surg Br. 1992;74:6–8.
4. Shibata KM, Kim DH. Historical review of spinal arthroplasty and dynamic stabilizations. In: Kim DH, Cammisa FP, Fessler RG, editors. Dynamic reconstruction of the spine. New York/Stuttgart: Thieme; 2006. p. 1–16.
5. Freudiger S, Dubois G, Lorrain M. Dynamic neutralisation of the lumbar spine confirmed on a new lumbar spine stimulator in vitro. Arch Orthop Trauma Surg. 1992;119:127–32.
6. Kaech D. Future perspectives in spine surgery. ArgoSpine News J. 2008;19:77.
7. Vieweg U. Stabilization in spine surgery-past, present, and future. BackUp. 2005;1:1–2.
8. Deyo RA, Mirza SK. Trends and variations in the use of spine surgery. Clin Orthop Relat Res. 2006;443:139–46.

Principles of Surgical Stabilisation of the Spine

Tobias Pitzen, Jörg Drumm, Gregor Ostrowski, and Michael Ruf

2

2.1 Introduction and Core Messages

The human spine is a complex structure, consisting of "rigid" bodies (vertebrae), connected by flexible components (ligaments and discs). The main functions of the human spine are the following:

1. To maintain an upright posture under a huge variety of loading mechanisms and situations
2. To protect the neural elements (nerve roots, spinal cord)

According to White and Panjabi, spinal stability is defined as "the ability of the spine under physiological loads to limit patterns of displacement so as not to damage or irritate the spinal cord band nerve roots and to prevent incapacitating deformity, pain or deficits due to structural changes" [1]. Conversely, spinal instability may be defined as the absence of spinal stability. Consequently, spinal instability may result in the loss of normal posture (Figs. 2.1, 2.2 and 2.3) and second in pain, next in damage to the neural structures. To prevent or treat these, spinal instability calls for spinal stabilisation. If performed correctly, spinal stabilisation will transfer the unstable spine into a stable spine. Within this chapter, the main principles (also to the authors' opinion) for spinal stabilisation will be illuminated.

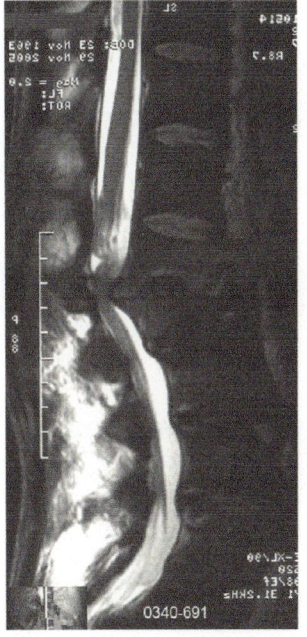

Fig. 2.1 MRI of the lumbar spine of a 42-year-old butcher, suffering from low back pain and fever at night. Kyphotic deformity of the spine due to a large defect (spondylodiszitis) within the L1/L2 disc and L1 and L2 bodies and—consequently—disruption of the posterior ligaments

2.2 How to Diagnose "Spinal Instability"?

Although the above definition on spinal instability is probably the best ever given, it is difficult to translate into measurable distances and angles. Especially in degenerative diseases, it may be more than even difficult to judge segmental instability. In, however, tumour or trauma spine conditions, it is at least more obvious if a spinal segment is unstable as shown as follows:

- Large defects within the vertebral body (Figs. 2.1 and 2.2).
- Wedge-shaped vertebral bodies, affection of two or three "columns" as described by Denis [2].

T. Pitzen (✉)
Center for Spine Surgery, Orthopedics, and Traumatology, SRH Klinikum Karlsbad-Langensteinbach, Karlsbad, Germany
e-mail: tobias.pitzen@srh.de

J. Drumm · G. Ostrowski · M. Ruf
Center for Spine Surgery, SRH Klinikum Karlsbad-Langensteinbach, Karlsbad, Germany

© Springer-Verlag GmbH Germany 2023
U. Vieweg, F. Grochulla (eds.), *Manual of Spine Surgery*, https://doi.org/10.1007/978-3-662-64062-3_2

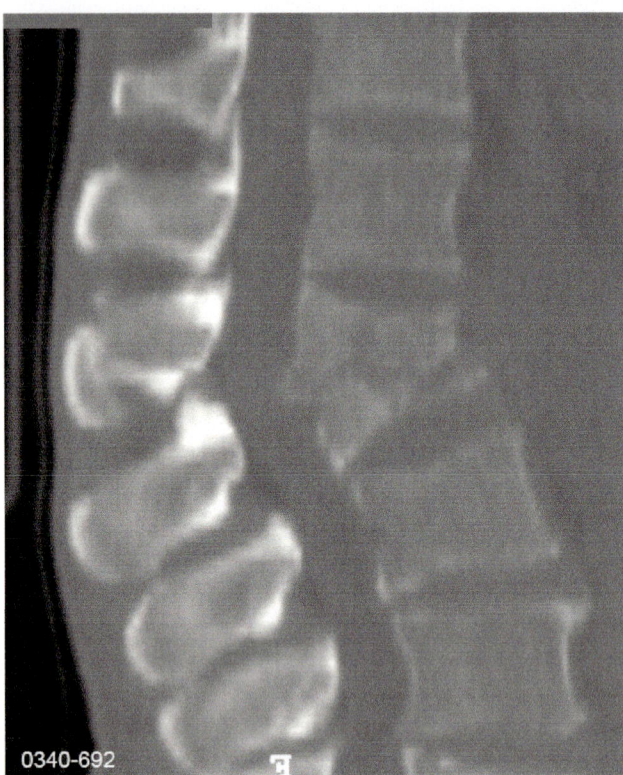

Fig. 2.2 Corresponding CAT scan, midline reconstruction

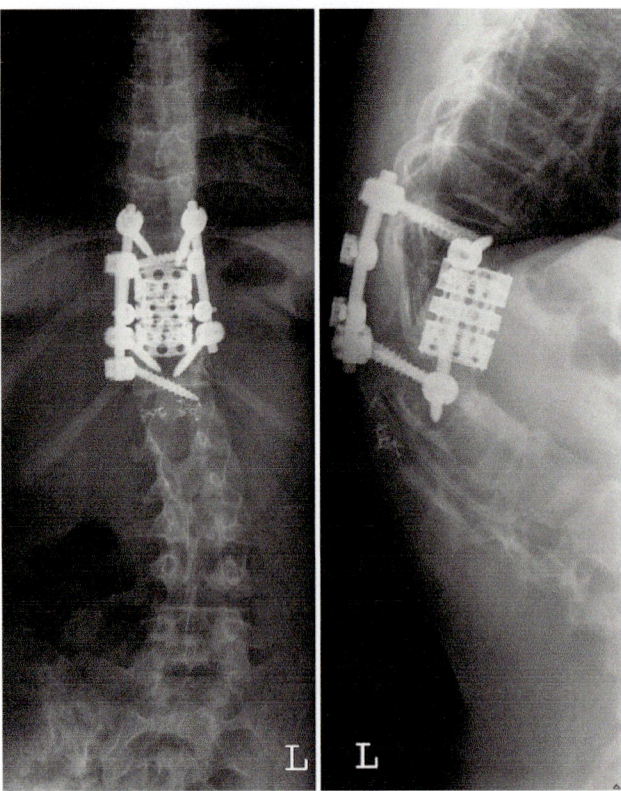

Fig. 2.3 Lateral and AP x-ray of the thoracolumbar spine region of a 12-year-old girl having undergone a spondylectomy of the 11th thoracic vertebra. As a result of a short segment stabilisation within the TL junctional region using a cage, lateral screw rod fixation and posterior screw rod fixation, both sagittal and coronal profile of the spine, could not permanently be stabilised

- Horizontal translation of more than 3–5 mm and/or angulation of more than 11 deg (Figs. 2.1, 2.2 and 2.3).
- Disruption of the disc and the ligaments as diagnosed by MRI scans (Fig. 2.4) may indicate spinal instability, especially if combined with local pain and neurological deficits.

2.2.1 Spinal Stabilisation with Respect to the Localisation of Pathology

As rule of thumb, any kind of anterior pathology (Figs. 2.1, 2.2 and 2.4) is probably treated in the best way by anterior approach, decompression and fixation, and any kind of posterior pathology (Figs. 2.1 and 2.2) by posterior approach, decompression and fixation. Combined instability due to combined pathology usually calls for combined AP fixation (Fig. 2.5).

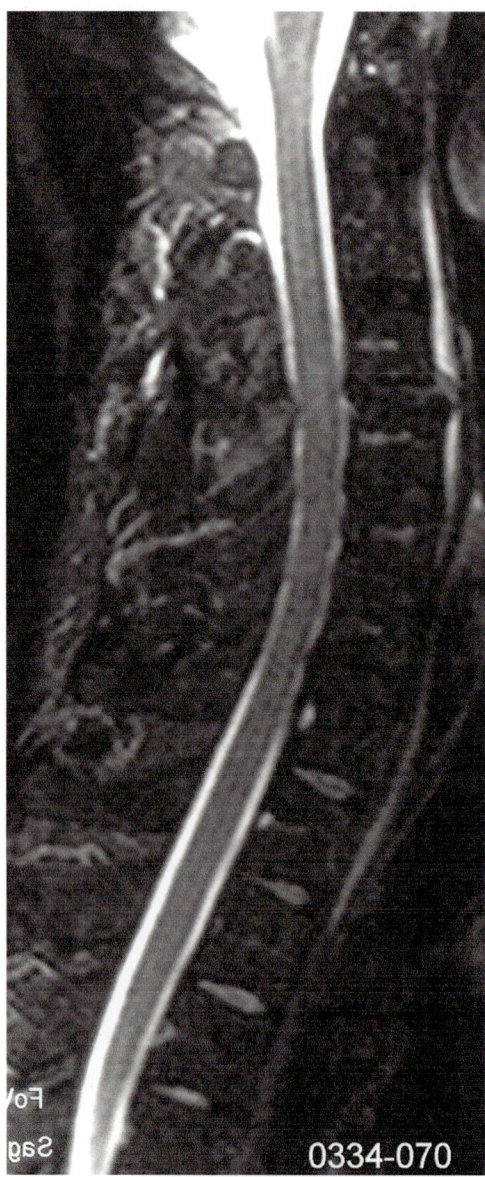

Fig. 2.4 MRI of the cervical spine of the patient mentioned within the text. Destruction of the anterior longitudinal ligament and the disc C3-C4

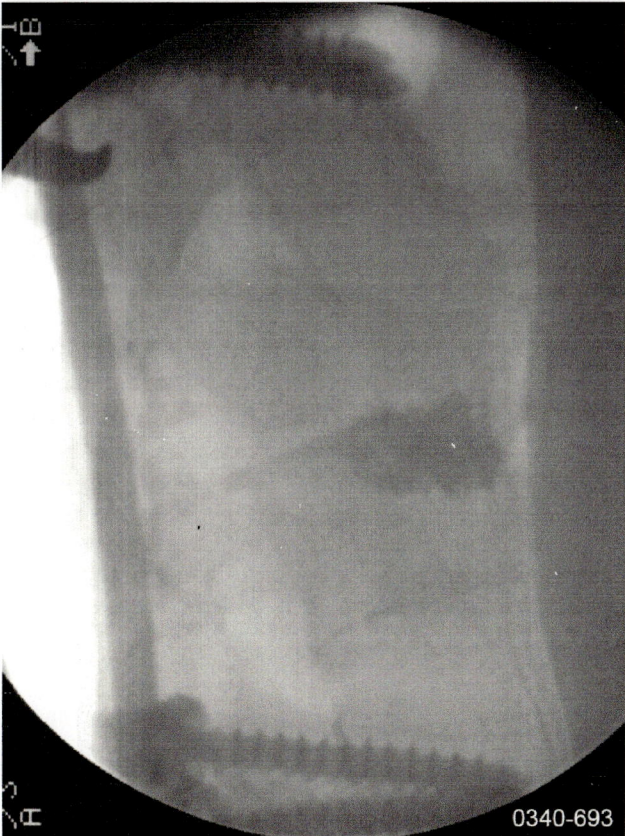

Fig. 2.5 Following posterior pedicle screw rod fixation, the spine is realigned and—at least temporarily—able to resist bending moments against flexion-extension, lateral bending and axial rotation. However, due to the anterior defect indicated by contrast dye, axial loading (lifting the patient up) should *not* be performed

2.3 First Steps in Spinal Stabilisation Procedures (External Stabilisation, Realignment, Decompression)

For external stabilisation, the patient's spine must be immobilised (first by external means, that is, immobilisation mattress and orthesis) as soon as severe instability is suspected or diagnosed. However, please keep in mind that any kind of external fixation—even a halo body jacket—allows some degree of motility within the cervical spine [3]. Everybody involved in the patient's treatment must be familiar with the fact that his/her spine is considered to be unstable. Care must be taken, if the patient is transported, for example, to the operating room or intubated for surgery.

Realignment may be performed as closed or open procedure. Closed procedures usually include traction on the cervical spine, applied by external force, brought to the head by a fixed clamp [4]. In addition, manoeuvres including some degree of re-inclination or inclination or rotation may be added according to the patient's individual trauma mecha-

nism. There is, however, always the risk of dislocation of bone or disc fragments that may compress the spinal cord. Thus, closed reduction is *not* recommended by the author, even if not accompanied by neuro-monitoring. To the authors' opinion, it is safer to perform an open reduction after decompression of the neural structures.

2.4 Internal Stabilisation of the Spine

Following decompression and realignment of the spine, several implants may be used to stabilise the spine. It is, however, difficult to select the appropriate type of instrumentation. The following aspects may help to select the appropriate type of implant(s) for internal stabilisation of the spine.

2.4.1 The Preferred Implants for Posterior Spine Stabilisation

There are lateral mass screws (within the cervical spine between C3 and C6 and for the atlas) or pedicle screws (for C2 and C7 in the cervical spine and all over the thoracic and lumbar spine), connected by rods (and there is a possibility to use cross connectors to fix both rods with each other). There are different pros and cons for both types of screws: pedicle screws have a higher pull-out force and give a better three-dimensional fixation than facet screws, meaning that a pedicle screw rod fixation usually resists higher loading forces than a facet screw rod fixation [5]. However, the mechanical strength of facet screw rod fixation is usually sufficient for cervical spine stabilisation. The complication rate of pedicle screws is much higher than for facet screws [6, 7]. As an alternative to screw rod constructs, different types of hooks or wires may be used to fix a segment, but the mechanical superiority of modern screw rod constructs is undebatable. Whatever has been used for posterior stabilisation procedure, the final construct must stabilise the spine against flexion-extension, lateral bending and axial rotation and distraction. Posterior instrumentation systems, however, are usually not performed to stabilise against axial loading or compression.

2.4.2 The Preferred Implants for Anterior Spine Stabilisation

If anterior decompression was necessary, anterior stabilisation must follow. In case of disc excision, the disc may be replaced by a piece of tricortical bone graft, by a cage or—in case of degenerative instability—by a disc prosthesis. In case of vertebral body resection, this may be replaced again by piece of tricortical bone graft, by a cage, usually filled with bone graft or bone substitute. Such cage or bone graft mainly stabilises against compression and does stabilise against flexion and to some smaller degree to lateral bending and rotation—but never against loading the spine in extension if the anterior longitudinal ligament has been cut. Adding an anterior plate (or an anterior screw—rod fixation within the thoracolumbar spine) to this construct, however, adds stability in extension. The combination of cage, anterior plate and monosegmental posterior fixation by facet screw rod systems usually immobilises a spinal segment even if all ligaments are destroyed [8]. Keep, however, in mind the so-called junctional regions (especially cervico-thoracic or thoracolumbar) of the spine usually require longer constructs (Figs. 2.3 and 2.6).

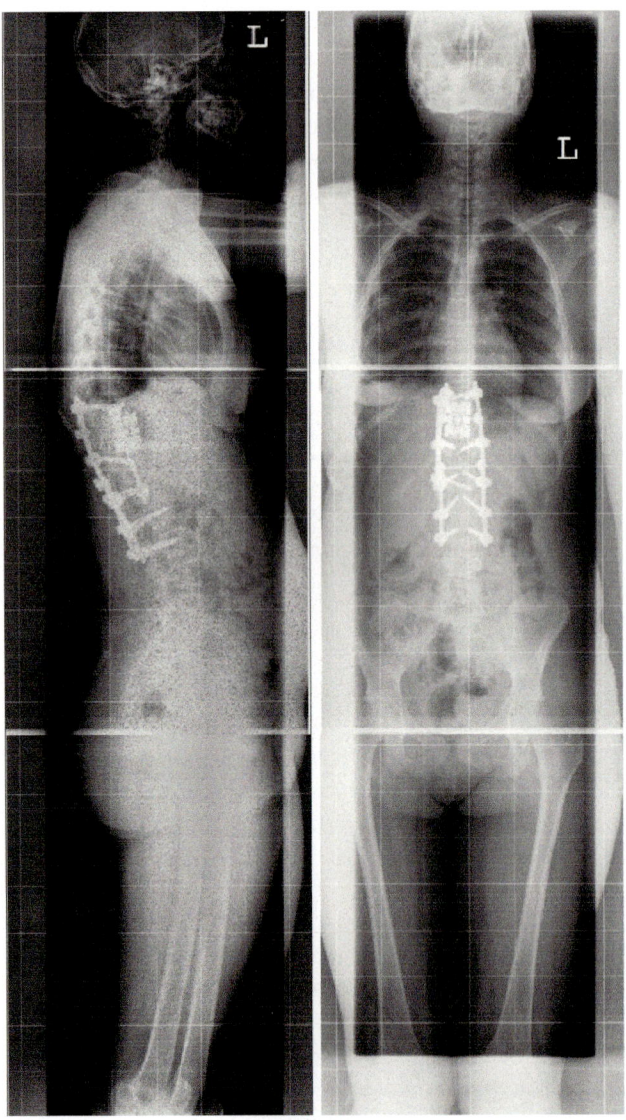

Fig. 2.6 Lateral and AP view of the whole spine following anterior-posterior revision of the above case with an additional cage and longer screw rod construct. Perfect AP and lateral profile of the spine

2.5   Posterior vs Anterior Stabilisation

As a rule of thumb, posterior stabilisation of the spine is usually indicated if the posterior aspects of the spine are destroyed (Figs. 2.1, 2.2 and 2.3). It is obvious from Figs. 2.1 and 2.2 that the posterior stabilisation is—at least temporarily—sufficient to fix the spine after realignment. However, anterior stabilisation using a cage or bone graft is usually—and also in this case—required, if the anterior aspect of the spine is affected, which is also obvious from Figs. 2.1 and 2.2. The large defect as indicated by contrast dye must be bridged by an implant to carry the axial compression load applied to the spine (Fig. 2.5). Again, there is no doubt that posterior instrumentation systems like facet screw rod or—even more pronounced—pedicle screw rod fixation provide much more three-dimensional stability (stability in flexion-extension, lateral bending and axial rotation) than anterior stabilisation [9]. Thus, if there is an extremely unstable situation, a posterior instrumentation usually provides better fixation. That is why posterior stabilisation is usually the first step in fixing an extremely unstable spine. However, anterior interbody stabilisation (using any type of a cage or even a bone graft) provides much more stability against axial loading or compression. This will result in a very stable construct, able to resist almost any kind of loading. Within the cervical spine, anterior plating provides three-dimensional stability and is especially useful if additional stability vs extension loading (reclination of the head) is required. Thus, if stabilisation against compression is needed, a cage or bone graft should be inserted, and a plate is helpful to provide stability against extension.

2.6   How Implants Work

Posterior stabilisation systems (such as pedicle screw rod systems or facet screw rod systems) are performed
- to stabilise the segment(s) in all directions (flexion-extension, rotation, lateral bending),
- but *not* to stabilise against compression loading.
  Anterior interbody systems (cages, disc prosthesis) are performed as follows:
- To transfer axial compression load between two vertebral bodies
- To restore height within one or more segments
- To prevent kyphotic angulation
- To stabilise the segment(s) in flexion, rotation and lateral bending (not in extension in case of the ant-long ligament resected)

Anterior plates and anterior screw rod systems are performed as follows:

- To add additional stabilisation to a cage construct, especially in extension after resection of the resected anterior longitudinal ligament, thus preventing a cage from dislocation

2.6.1 Should a Rigid (Constrained), Semi-Rigid or Dynamic Implant Be Used?

Within a rigid implant construct, there is no motility between the components of the construct, that is, between screws and plate of an anterior cervical plate system. Conversely, there is some motility between the components of a semi-constrained or even dynamic system. As a consequence, some surgeons may prefer rigid implants in patients suffering from extremely unstable spine segments. There is, however, some evidence that, for example, in a cervical spine trauma model, dynamic plates are at least equal to rigid ones with respect to three-dimensional stabilisation [10]. Moreover, speed of fusion is significantly higher, and rate of implant complication is significantly lower in the presence of a dynamic plate. Conversely, loss of correction is more pronounced if dynamic plates are used [11].

2.7 Temporary vs Permanent Stabilisation

So far, principles of temporary stabilisation of the spine have been described. However, keep in mind that these implants will fail (break, dislocate) if there is no bony heal-ing between the adjacent vertebral bodies. Only bony bridging between the fixed vertebrae will result in permanent stability (Fig. 2.7). Thus, autologous bone graft should be harvested from the iliac crest or elsewhere and transplanted at the posterior and anterior site—whatever has been exposed, both anterior and posterior if possible. If no autograft is available, use some kind of bone substitute. Note that the graft is in contact with the patient's bone and avoid non-steroidal anti-inflammatory drugs, steroids and smoking for the time of bone healing.

2.8 Mechanism of Trauma

To analyse the mechanism of trauma may also help to select the appropriate type of instrumentation. The appropriate instrumentation will stabilise the spine by acting against the forces and moments that have caused the injury. This means, however, that we must illuminate this mechanism of trauma. The following example may help:

A 38-year-old male was involved into a traffic accident. He complained about severe neck pain. A small wound was seen at his forehead. CAT (computer-assisted tomography) scans (sagittal reconstruction, Fig. 2.8) did not show any dislocation or fracture. A lesion with the anterior longitudi-

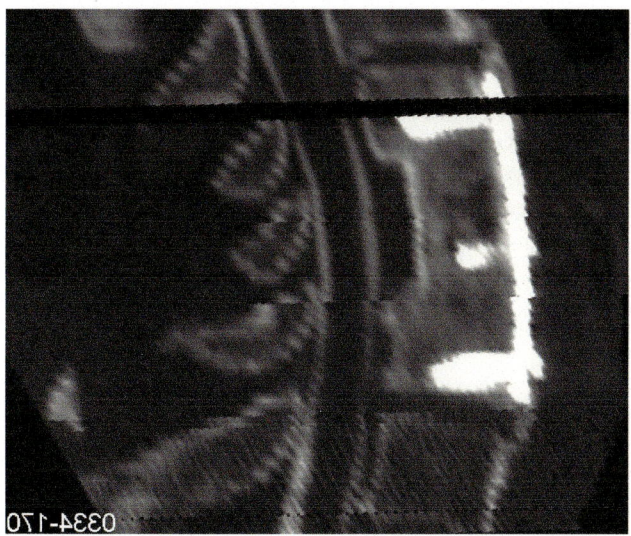

Fig. 2.7 Bone bridging C4-C6 following replacement of the C5 vertebral body using a tricortical iliac crest graft. A permanent stabilisation is achieved by bony bridging

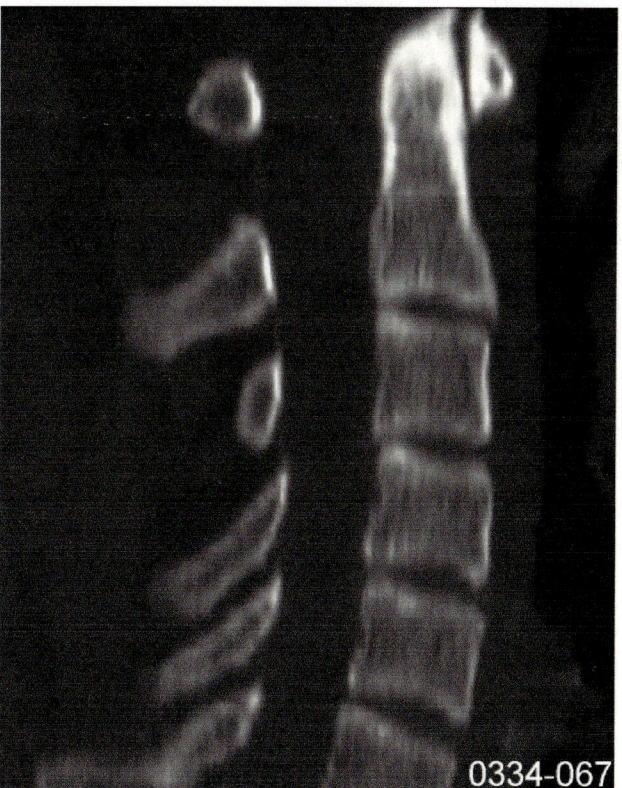

Fig. 2.8 CAT scan of the cervical spine of the patient described within the text. No bony destruction

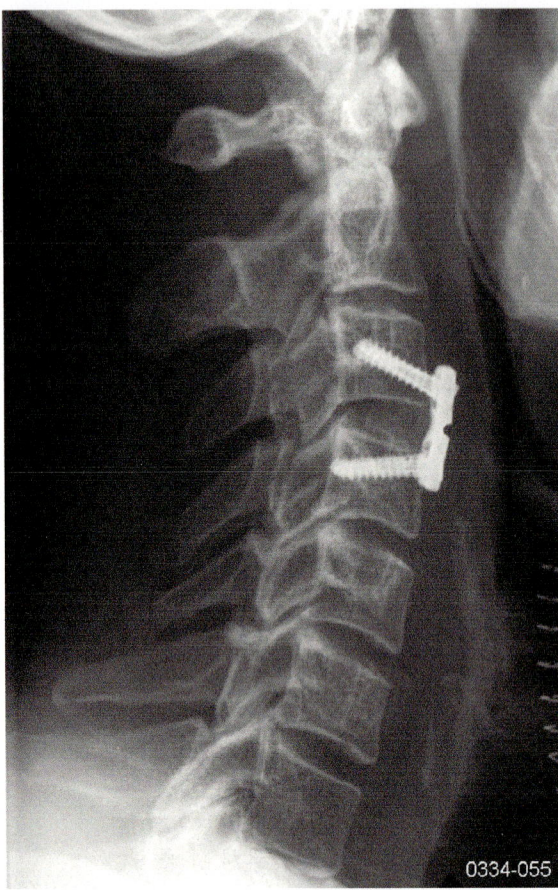

0334-055

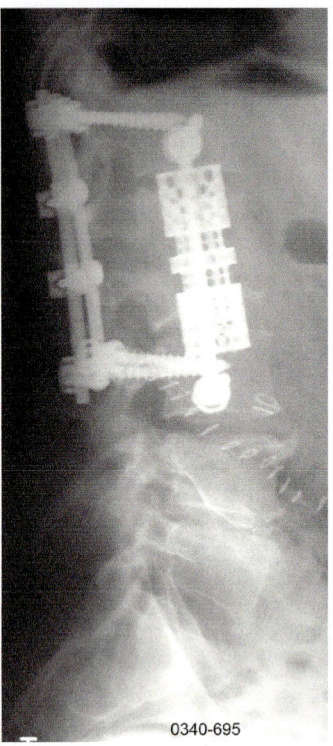

0340-695

Fig. 2.10 After cage insertion and lateral screw rod fixation, the spine now resists loading in axial compression. This is an example for combined, anterior posterior stabilisation due to a combined anterior-posterior instability

Fig. 2.9 Lateral x-ray of the cervical spine of the above-mentioned patient

nal ligament and the disc, however, was seen in the MRI (Fig. 2.4). As a summary from this short—but very important—information, it may be concluded that hyperextension (wound at the forehead) was the main injury vector to resulting in destruction of the disc and the anterior longitudinal ligament. Thus, the disc must be excised and replaced by a bone graft or cage. As a further consequence, the ideal fixation must be able to work against extension—which is an anterior plate. Due to the fact that the disc must be replaced, the complete type of instrumentation is a cage/bone graft and an additional anterior plate (Fig. 2.9).

2.8.1 Loading the Construct After Surgery

As long as no bony fusion is apparent via computer-assisted tomography, we must be careful when mobilising the patient. Mechanics of the implants/the construct may give valuable information concerning "what is allowed and what forbidden". The following two examples may help:

1. A patient, in who a cervical vertebral body (one-level) reconstruction has been performed using a cage, may be loaded in compression. If all the posterior ligaments are intact, flexion, lateral bending and rotation may be without major danger. There is, however, limited stability in extension! Adding a plate enlarges stability in extension.
2. A patient, in who a spondylitis destructed a disc and major parts of the adjacent vertebral bodies, underwent posterior instrumentation using a pedicle screw rod system (Figs. 2.1, 2.2 and 2.5). Although such instrumentation will result in three-dimensional stability and stability against distraction, there is no stability in compression. Thus, this patient should not walk around or sit; however, he/she may be rotated. After anterior reconstruction using a cage, the construct will be able to resist also axial compression loading (Fig. 2.10).

Thus, be familiar with the biomechanics of the implants.

References

1. White AA III, Panjabi MM. Clinical biomechanics of the spine. 2nd ed. Philiadelphia, PA: JB Lippincott; 1990.
2. Denis F. The three column spine and its significance in the classification of acute thoracolumbar injuries. Spine. 1995;20:1122–7.
3. Dickmann CA, Crawford NA. Biomechanics of the craniovertebral junction. In: Dickmann CA, Spetzler RF, Sonntag VKH, editors. Surgery of the craniovertebral junction. New York: Thieme; 1998. p. 59–80.

4. Sutton DC, Silveri CP, Cotler JM. Initial evaluation and management of the spinal injury patient. In: Cotler J, Simpson J, An H, Silveri C, editors. Surgery of spinal trauma. Philadelphia, PA: Lippincott Williams and Wilkins; 2000. p. 113–27.

5. Kothe R, Rüther W, Schneider E, et al. Biomechanical analysis of transpedicular screw fixation in the subaxial spine. Spine. 2004;29:1869–75.

6. Kast E, Mohr K, Richter HP, et al. Complications of transpedicular screw fixation in the cervical spine. Eur Spine J. 2006;15:327–34.

7. Sekhon LH. Posterior cervical lateral mass screw fixation: analysis of 1026 consecutive screws in 143 patients. J Spinal Disord Tech. 2005;18:297–303.

8. Pitzen T, Lane C, Goertzen D, et al. Anterior cervical plate fixation: biomechanical effectiveness as a function of posterior element injury. J Neurosurg. 2003;99:84–90.

9. Schmidt R, Wilke HJ, Claes L, et al. Pedicle screws enhance primary stability in multilevel cervical corpectomies: biomechanical in vitro comparison of different implants including constrained and nonconstrained posterior instrumentations. Spine. 2003;28:1821–8.

10. Dvorak MF, Pitzen T, Zhu Q. Anterior cervical plate fixation: a biomechanical study to evaluate the effects of plate design, endplate preparation, and bone mineral density. Spine. 2005;30:294–301.

11. Pitzen TR, Chrobok J, Stulik J, et al. Implant complications, fusion, loss of lordosis, and outcome after anterior cervical plating with dynamic or rigid plates: two-year results of a multi-centric, randomized, controlled study. Spine. 2009;34:641–6.

Implant Materials in Spinal Surgery

3

Werner Schmoelz

3.1 Introduction and Core Messages

Generally, biomaterials used in orthopaedic surgery can be classified in three groups: metals, ceramics and polymers. Ideally, material properties of orthopaedic implants should have a low elastic modulus close to the cortical bone, high wear resistance, high strength, high corrosion resistance, high fracture toughness and high ductility. Unfortunately, no material is standing out in all desirable properties, and some of the characteristics such as low elastic modulus and high strength are even opposing. Therefore, the material chosen for any kind of implant is depending on its specific requirements which are most important and necessary for the particular function of the implant. This may lead to different components of one implant being manufactured of different materials to best suit its intended application. In the last century, spinal implants were mainly manufactured of metal alloys such as stainless steel, pure titanium and titanium-aluminium-vanadium. In recent years, developments in the field of non-metallic biomaterials lead to the application of new materials such as PEEK and composite materials.

3.2 Definition

Orthopaedic implant materials can be grouped to the more general description of biomaterials. A consensus of experts in biomaterial science defined the term biomaterial as a non-viable material used in a medical device, intended to interact with biological systems [1].

Generally, biomaterials used in orthopaedic surgery can be classified in three groups: metals, ceramics and polymers. Ideally, material properties of orthopaedic implants should have a low elastic modulus close to the cortical bone, high wear resistance, high strength, high corrosion resistance, high fracture toughness and high ductility. Unfortunately, no material is standing out in all desirable properties, and some of the characteristics such as low elastic modulus and high strength are even opposing. Therefore, the material chosen for any kind of implant is depending on its specific requirements which are most important and necessary for the particular function of the implant. This may lead to different components of one implant being manufactured of different materials to best suit its intended application. In the last century, spinal implants were mainly manufactured of metal alloys such as stainless steel, pure titanium and titanium-aluminium-vanadium. In recent years, developments in the field of non-metallic biomaterials lead to the application of new materials such as PEEK and composite materials.

3.3 Physical Characteristics

3.3.1 Strength

The ability of a material to withstand an applied stress is called strength. Yield strength refers to the point in the stress strain curve after which plastic deformation occurs. Strength of a material may vary with the stress (compressive, tensile or shear) applied. For most orthopaedic implants, fatigue strength is the most relevant criterion, as it refers to the material's ability to withstand alternating stresses under cyclic

W. Schmoelz (✉)
Department of Orthopaedics and Traumatology - Biomechanics,
Medical University of Innsbruck, Innsbruck, Austria
e-mail: werner.schmoelz@i-med.ac.at

© Springer-Verlag GmbH Germany 2023
U. Vieweg, F. Grochulla (eds.), *Manual of Spine Surgery*, https://doi.org/10.1007/978-3-662-64062-3_3

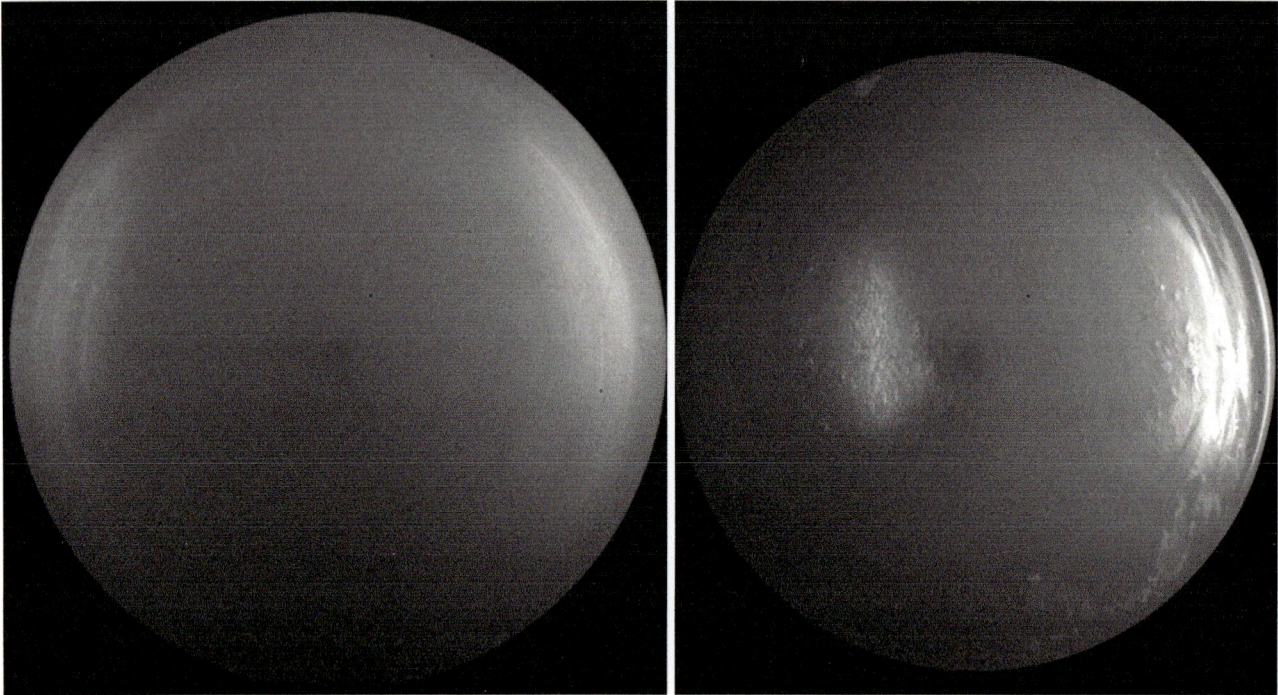

Fig. 3.1 PE (polyethylene) core of a total disc replacement after test in a wear simulator. *Left*: unloaded control specimen. *Right*: loaded test specimen showing circular wear at the *right-hand side*

loading. This is especially important during the daily routine of the patient. Strength of a metallic material is depending on its microstructure and can be altered in the fabrication process (casting, forging, annealing, etc.)

3.3.2 Flexibility: Elastic Modulus

The elastic modulus describes the magnitude at which a material deforms when subjected to stress. It is determined from the linear slope of a stress versus strain curve. In order to minimize stress shielding, the elastic modulus of implants should be in the range of cortical bones.

3.3.3 Corrosion Resistance

Degradation of materials into its constituent atoms caused by electrochemical reactions with its surroundings is called corrosion. The human body fluids present a very hostile environment to metals making corrosion resistance an important aspect in the biocompatibility of a material. The occurrence of small holes in the surface due to break-up of the corrosion-resistant oxide film is called pitting corrosion. Crevice corrosion can occur in rod/screw or plate/screw connections of spinal instrumentation through development of a local chemistry causing corrosion [2], while galvanic corrosion results

from two different metals with different electrode potentials and the body fluid forming a voltage cell.

3.3.4 Wear Resistance

Relative motion between two surfaces in contact causes erosion of the material called wear. In contrast to corrosion, wear is produced by a mechanical action in the form of contact and motion causing the removal of small particles from a surface (see Fig. 3.1). Wear debris can induce inflammatory reactions causing local bone loss and threatening implant fixation (see Fig. 3.2). Generally, the amount of wear increases with the applied load and decreases with the hardness of the worn surface.

3.3.5 Biocompatibility

Generally, biocompatibility is defined as the ability of a material to perform with an appropriate host response in a specific application [1]. For orthopaedic implants, this can be interpreted as the property of being biologically compatible by not producing a toxic, injurious or immunological response in the human body. However, it should be considered that biocompatibility refers to a specific material and not to a device, which is often composed of more than one material.

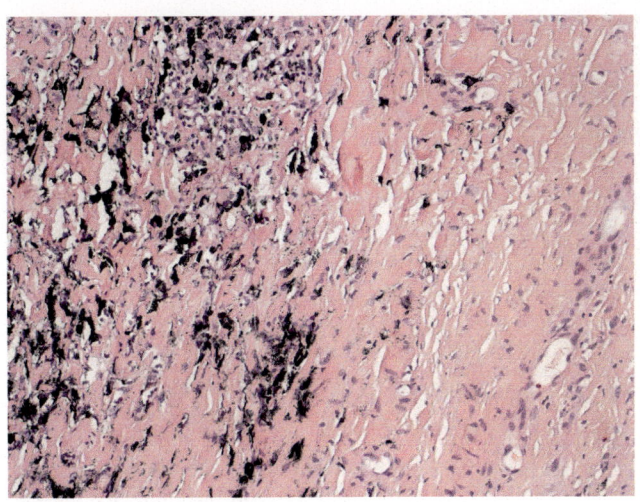

Fig. 3.2 Tissue responses to metal wear particles next to an implant

3.4   Commonly Applied Implant Materials

The bulk of orthopaedic implants used for skeletal reconstructions (e.g. plates, screws, rods and joint replacements) are manufactured of metallic biomaterials. This is due to their ability to withstand high and also dynamic loads. In order to improve implant fixation and/or cell ingrowth, the anchoring surfaces can be roughened, precoated or refined with porous coatings.

An excerpt of material properties of commonly used implant materials and its comparison to the cortical bone is listed in Table 3.1. Further information on chemical composition and additional material properties can be found in the references.

3.5   Metals

The majority of implants used in spinal instrumentation (screws, rods, hooks, vertebral body replacements, etc.) are manufactured of metallic materials. They provide high tensile, compressive, shear and fatigue strength, biocompatibility, corrosion and wear resistance required in the application of load-bearing implants in orthopaedic surgery. Flexibility and strength of a metallic alloy also depend on the fabrication processes (casting, cold and hot forging). After fabrication, the material properties can be enhanced by heat treatment (annealing). Wear resistance of metals can be further improved by processes such as nitriding and ion implantation.

3.5.1   Stainless Steel

The most commonly used stainless steel is 316L (ASTM F138, F139). It is composed of iron, carbon, chromium, nickel and molybdenum. While the carbon content is kept low, the alloying additions improve the corrosion resistance. While stainless steel has been and is used in fracture plates, pedicle instrumentation and screws, a trend towards titanium (Ti)-based implants due to the superior biocompatibility was seen in recent years. However, stainless steel implants still gain a worldwide popularity due to its cost-effectiveness compared to Ti-based alloys.

3.5.2   Cobalt-Chromium Alloys

The most commonly used cobalt-chromium alloys are cobalt-nickel-chromium-molybdenum (CoNiCrMo, ASTM F562) and cobalt-chromium-molybdenum (CoCrMo, ASTM

Table 3.1 Mechanical material properties of implant materials

Material	ASTM designation	Elastic modulus in GPa	Yield strength in MPa	Ultimate strength in MPa
Metals				
Stainless steel [3]	F55, F56, F138, F139	190	331–1213	586–1350
CoCr alloys [3]	F75, F562	210–232	448–1500	951–1795
Ti alloys				
CPTi [4]	F67	110	485	760
Ti-6Al-4V [3]	F136	116	896–1034	965–1103
Ti-35Nb-7Zr-5Ta [5]	–	55	596	
Polymers				
PMMA [6]	F451–99	1.8–3.3	35–70	38–80
PEEK [7, 8]	F2026–02	3.6–13	12–60	70–208
UHMWPE [9]	F648	0.5–1.3	20–30	30–40
Ceramics				
Alumina [10]	F603–83	380	310–3790	310–3790
Zirconia [7]	F1873–98	201	420–7500	420–7500
Cortical bone [11, 12]	–	12–20	114	133–205

F75). While chromium improves the corrosion resistance, molybdenum increases the strength and makes it strong, hard, biocompatible and corrosion resistant. Due to these characteristics, it is used in joint replacements and fracture stabilisations requiring a long service life. However, the high percentage of nickel in CoNiCrMo raises concerns of possible toxicity by wear particles.

3.5.3 Titanium Alloys

First attempts to use titanium as orthopaedic implant material date back to the late 1930s. Commercially pure titanium (CPTi, ASTM F67) and the titanium alloy (Ti-6Al-4V, ASTM F136) are among the most common applied titanium-based materials. The increased biocompatibility and corrosion resistance of titanium alloys compared to stainless steel and CoCr alloys are attributed to a stable oxide film protecting it from corrosion. The elastic modulus of titanium alloys is closer to the bone and approximately half of stainless steel and CoCr alloys, while their strength generally exceeds that of stainless steel. Due to the lower resistance to wear compared to CoCr alloys, Ti alloys are hardly applied as bearing material.

An advantage of Ti-based alloys is their feature to produce fewer artefacts in computer tomography (CT) and magnetic resonance imaging (MRI) scans. Currently, attempts in material research are being made to reduce the elastic modulus of Ti-based alloys to further approximate that of the cortical bone.

3.6 Ceramics

Ceramics are characterized by a high wear resistance, low friction and good biocompatibility but also reduced fracture toughness. Therefore, they are mainly used for bearing surfaces in joint replacements. The most commonly used ceramics in total hip arthroplasty are zirconia (ZrO_2) and alumina (Al_2O_3). Other forms of ceramics used in orthopaedics are hydroxyapatite and glass ceramics in the form of implant coatings.

3.7 Polymers

Generally, considering all types of medical applications, polymers form the largest group of biomaterials. For polymers used in orthopaedic implants, the most important characteristics for choosing a specific polymer are yield stress, wear rate and creep resistance.

3.7.1 Polyethylene (PE)

Low friction coefficient, low wear rate and resistance to creep of PE in the form of ultra-high molecular weight polyethylene (UHMWPE) are the reasons for PE being the most common bearing material in total joint arthroplasty (TJA). It was initially introduced in total hip replacements by Sir J. Charnley, later adopted for total knee replacements and recently for total disc replacements.

3.7.2 Polymethyl Methacrylate (PMMA)

Plexiglas is the trade name of another, to the general population's more known form of PMMA. For orthopaedic application, PMMA was first applied in the fixation of the hip stems and acetabular components in hip arthroplasty. Nowadays, injectable PMMA cements are available with varying viscosities, depending on their application. They are characterized by a high resistance to creep, sufficient yield strength and their capability to form a structural interface with surrounding bones. In spinal surgery, they are applied in vertebroplasty and kyphoplasty procedures and, in selected cases, for implant fixation of pedicle screws in patients suffering from osteoporosis.

3.7.3 Polyether Ether Ketone (PEEK)

Initially developed for demanding engineering application and widely used in aerospace and automotive industries, PEEK was commercially available as biomaterial at the end of the last century. Mechanical properties of PEEK composites can be adapted to its desired application by addition of carbon fibres and even exceed those of titanium alloys. In spinal instrumentation, PEEK and PEEK composites are commonly applied in fusion cages and in some designs for pedicle screws and internal fixator rods. Its radiolucency allows the assessment of bony fusion without typical artefacts seen caused by metallic implants.

References

1. Williams DF. Definitions in biomaterials. In: Proceedings of a consensus conference of the European Society for Biomaterials, Chester, 3–5 March 1986. New York: Elsevier; 1986.
2. Vieweg U, van Roost D, Wolf HK, et al. Corrosion on an internal spinal fixator system. Spine. 1999;24:946–51.
3. Brunski JB. Classes of material used in medicine. In: Rater BD, Hoffmann AS, Schoen FJ, Lemons JE, editors. Biomaterials science: an introduction to materials in medicine. London: Elsevier/Academic; 2004. p. 137–53.

4. Breme J, Biehl V. Metallic biomaterials. In: Black J, Hastings G, editors. Handbook of biomaterial properties. London: Chapman & Hall; 1998. p. 135–213.

5. Geetha M, Singh AK, Asokamani R, et al. Ti based biomaterials, the ultimate choice for orthopaedic implants – a review. Prog Mater Sci. 2009;54:397–425.

6. Polymers: a property database. 2010. http://www.polymersdatabase.com/. Accessed 2010.

7. Hallab NJ, Wimmer M, Jacobs JJ. Material properties and wear analysis. In: Yue JJ, Bertangnoli R, McAfee PC, An HS, editors. Motion preservation surgery of the spine. Philadelphia: Saunders/Elsevier; 2008. p. 52–62.

8. Kurtz SM, Devine JN. PEEK biomaterials in trauma, orthopedic, and spinal implants. Biomaterials. 2007;28(32):4845–69.

9. Park J, Lakes RS. Biomaterials – an introduction. 3rd ed. New York: Springer Science + Business Media; 2007.

10. Li J, Hastings G. Oxide bioceramics: inert ceramic materials in medicine and dentistry. In: Black J, Hastings G, editors. Handbook of material properties. London: Chapman & Hall; 1998. p. 340–54.

11. Ashman RB, Cowin SC, Van Buskirk WC, et al. A continuous wave technique for the measurement of the elastic properties of cortical bone. J Biomech. 1984;17:349–61.

12. Reilly DT, Burstein AH. Review article. The mechanical properties of cortical bone. J Bone Joint Surg Am. 1974;56:1001–22.

Mechanical and Biomechanical Testing of Spinal Implants

4

Werner Schmoelz and Annette Kienle

4.1 Introduction and Core Messages

Mechanical and biomechanical testing provides crucial information about the safety, effectiveness and function of spinal implants. Mainly static and dynamic tests are carried out. While mechanical tests may be carried out according to testing standards or in some cases to individual testing procedures, biomechanical tests should be conducted according to published recommendations or in case of dynamic testing, as individual test procedures. In order to allow for direct comparison between testing laboratories, it should be strived for standardised testing. However, as standardised loading often simplifies the in vivo occurring conditions, more physiological testing can be carried out additionally and may become the next improved testing standard. Mechanical testing focuses mainly on the safety issue, while effectiveness and function of an implant can be tested in a biomechanical setup. Each type of implant generally requires specific mechanical and biomechanical tests depending on its design, material, indication and function. In general, mechanical testing can be subdivided in static and dynamic fatigue testing as well as special types of testing such as wear or corrosion testing. Biomechanical testing concentrates on quasi-static and short-term dynamic testing mostly in interaction with the biological tissue.

4.2 Mechanical Testing

4.2.1 Static Testing

Almost all new implants require static mechanical testing. A spinal artificial disc, for example, will probably not receive clearance without static compression, subsidence, creep, luxation and expulsion testing. While compression and subsidence testing are well prescribed in ASTM (American Society for Testing and Materials) standards [1, 2], creep, luxation and expulsion need to be investigated according to individual testing protocols. The ASTM F 2077 and ASTM F 2346 standards propose static axial compression until failure to test a spinal intervertebral implant's strength [2] (see Fig. 4.1). This standardised loading protocol allows for comparison between testing laboratories. However, the test results are difficult to interpret since uniaxial loading does not represent the normal, multiaxial loading of the spine. Objective safety requirements are non-existent, and therefore results have to be compared with those from competitive implants. Unfortunately, such data is scarce in the scientific literature, and the databases used by regulatory authorities are mostly non-public. Therefore, new implants are often directly compared with an already approved predicate device, which is similar in shape, materials and indications. If there is no predicate device available, the results may also be interpreted based on the scientific literature. This, however, requires a scientific background of the testing laboratory.

ASTM or ISO (International Organization for Standardization) standards do not cover all testing procedures needed to characterise the implant's safety. Expulsion tests with artificial discs, for example, are among these tests. In these cases, individual testing procedures have to be developed, resulting in different designs from testing laboratory to testing laboratory. This complicates comparisons between results. On the other hand, non-standardised procedures can be adapted to the individual needs of the implant and to the physiological loading of the spine, which facilitates interpretation of the results.

W. Schmoelz (✉)
Department of Orthopaedics and Traumatology - Biomechanics, Medical University of Innsbruck, Innsbruck, Austria
e-mail: werner.schmoelz@i-med.ac.at

A. Kienle
Mechanical Implant Testing, SpineServ GmbH & Co. KG, Ulm, Germany
e-mail: annette.kienle@spineserv.de

© Springer-Verlag GmbH Germany 2023
U. Vieweg, F. Grochulla (eds.), *Manual of Spine Surgery*, https://doi.org/10.1007/978-3-662-64062-3_4

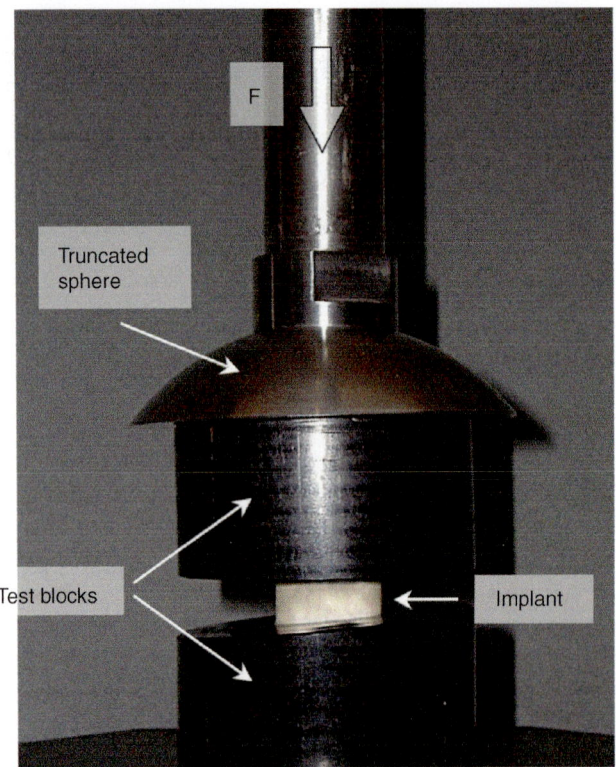

Fig. 4.1 Test setup for axial compression testing according to ASTM F 2077 [3]. An uniaxial load is applied to the implant through a truncated sphere and two test blocks, which represent the adjacent vertebral bodies

4.2.2 Dynamic Fatigue Testing

Dynamic testing is relevant to characterise the implant's risk of failure due to repetitive cyclic loading. A new posterior stabilisation device, for example, is commonly tested in a vertebrectomy model according to ASTM F 1717 [4] (see Fig. 4.2). Two "vertebral bodies" made of ultra-high molecular weight polyethylene positioned with a large gap in between represent a bisegmental spinal segment after complete resection of the middle vertebral body. The implant spans this gap and transfers all loads between both "vertebral bodies", which is an extreme "worst case". Therefore, the run-out loads, that is, the maximum loads tolerated without implant failure, are small compared to the in vivo loads. Thus, similar to static testing, comparative data are essential. The vertebrectomy model is well established for anterior and posterior stabilisation systems of the spine; however, semi-rigid fixation devices, such as an internal fixator, which allows some movement, cannot be tested in this model since these implants rely on anterior support. A new ISO standard addresses this requirement [5]. Anterior support is simulated using springs (see Fig. 4.2). This also helps in interpreting the results since the loading conditions become more physiological. Such improvements of testing standards are under development also for other types of

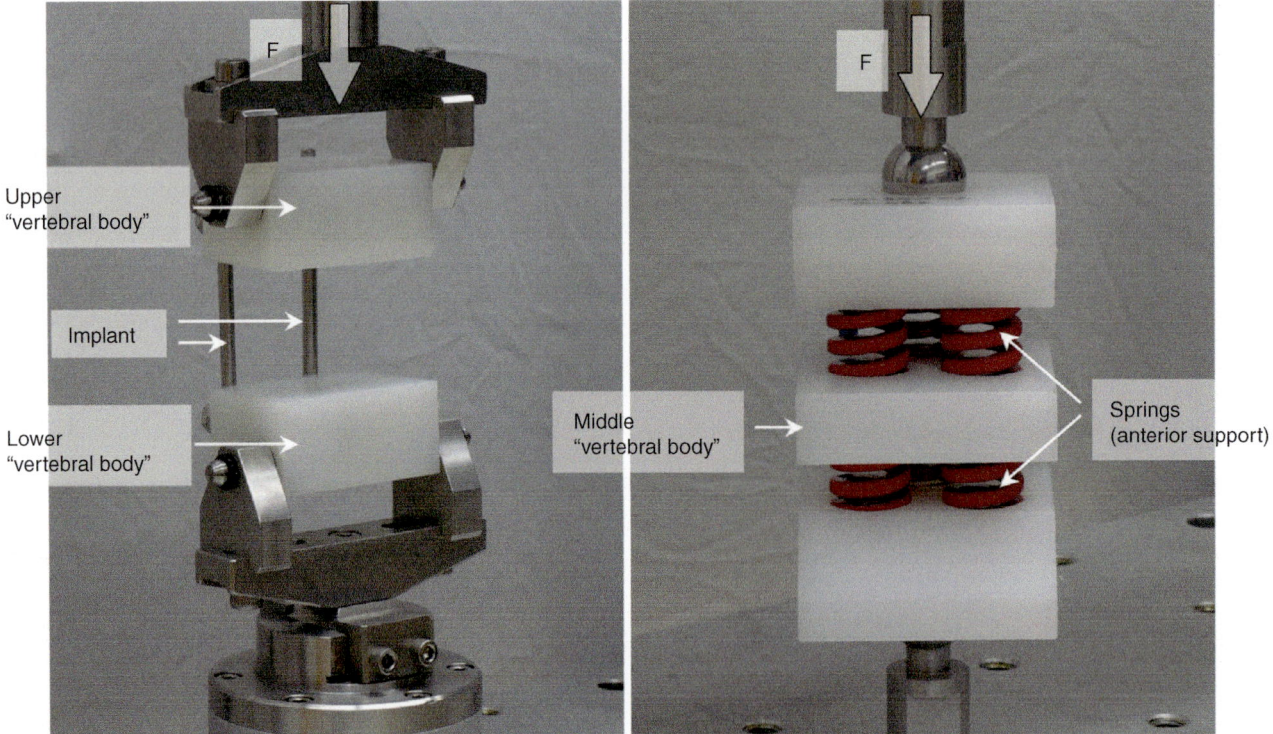

Fig. 4.2 *Left*: "Vertebrectomy model" according to ASTM F 1717 [4]. The implant spans a gap (vertebrectomy) between two "vertebral bodies". *Right*: Testing according to ISO/FDIS 12189 [5]. The middle ver-

tebral body is not removed. Springs assure for anterior support (on this photograph, the implant itself cannot be seen since it is mounted to the posterior side of the construct)

motion preserving implants such as facet joint or nucleus replacements.

Besides the test setup, the number of loading cycles also needs to be adapted to the in vivo situation. The number of loading cycles usually ranges between 2.5 and 10 millions. Two and a half million cycles are used for implants, which are implanted into the human body only for a few weeks or months, while 10 million loading cycles are generally used for "permanent" implants such as artificial discs. It is stated that five million loading cycles represent about 2–2.5 years in a patient's life [3, 4]. Ten million cycles of "extreme" loading, as applied for wear testing, are said to represent 80 years [6]. Unfortunately, scientific data are scarce on this topic.

4.3 Biomechanical Testing

4.3.1 Quasi-Static Flexibility Testing

Biomechanical in vitro testing assessing the immediate post-implantational effectiveness and function of spinal instrumentation in a treated segment should be carried out using pure bending moments according to the recommendations of spinal implant testing [7, 8]. Several research groups implemented the concept of pure moment loading in different setups. The concept induces rotational motion in one of the main motion planes (lateral bending, flexion/extension and axial rotation), while the remaining five degrees of freedom are allowed to move freely (see Fig. 4.3). During loading, the bending moment and the intersegmental motion are recorded continuously using a six-component load cell and a three-dimensional motion analysis system. The standard outcome parameters to evaluate biomechanical effects of the applied instrumentation are the range of motion (RoM) and the neutral zone (NZ). The load transfer or the change of load transfer of an instrumented segment compared to the intact motion segment can be assessed by measurements of the intradiscal pressure [9, 10] or instrumented internal fixator rods [11, 12]. For more physiological loading of the spine, an axial preload induced by the upper body mass and/or muscle forces acting on the spine may be included in the test setup [13]. Upon its introduction, this was named "follower load". However, the application of a follower load also has some drawbacks, as shear forces due to the subjective placement of the follower load can be induced. Additionally, experiments carried out with and without a follower load generally reported the same effects of spinal instrumentation on RoM and NZ for both test setups, except for different absolute magnitudes [14]. Therefore, in order to allow comparison of test results obtained in different laboratories for different spinal instrumentations, loading protocols other than pure moment should be carried out in addition and

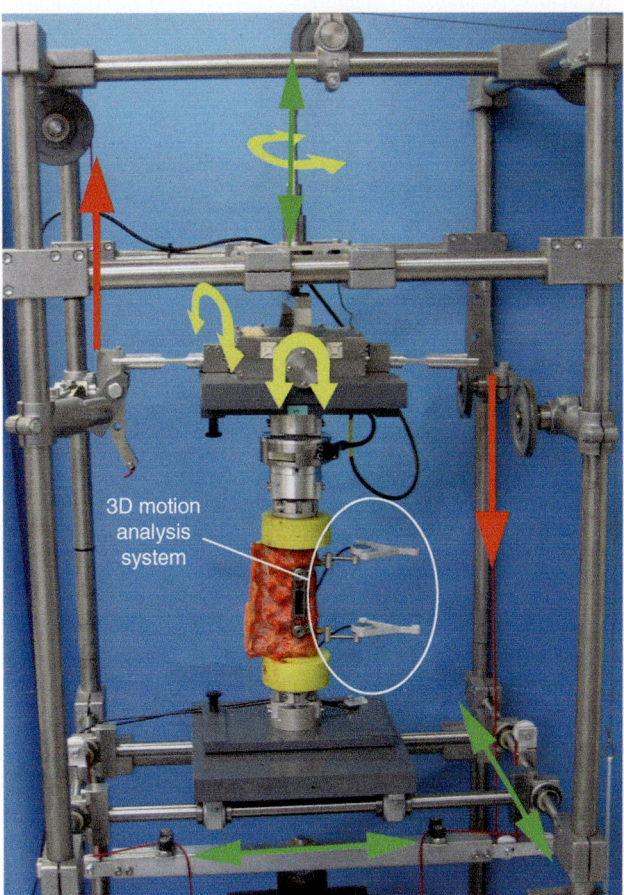

Fig. 4.3 Custom-built test bench to apply pure moments. *Green arrows* show translational degrees of freedom, *yellow arrows* show rotational degrees of freedom and *red arrows* show force couple to induce pure moments

not instead. A common method to compensate for inter-specimen variation and to highlight the effect of instrumentation on the RoM of a treated segment is normalisation, in which the RoM of a treated segment is reported as percentage of the native untreated motion segment.

4.3.2 Dynamic Loosening of Implants

To investigate long-term effectiveness and function of spinal instrumentation, various custom-built test setups in servohydraulic material testing machines have been developed and applied (see Fig. 4.4). These setups are intended to investigate implant anchorage and to provoke loosening at the implant–bone interface by repetitive loading, which can be of particular interest in the treatment of patients suffering from reduced bone quality. Generally, biomechanical tests intending to provoke implant failure or loosening apply a cyclic force-controlled loading protocol simulating from a few days up to

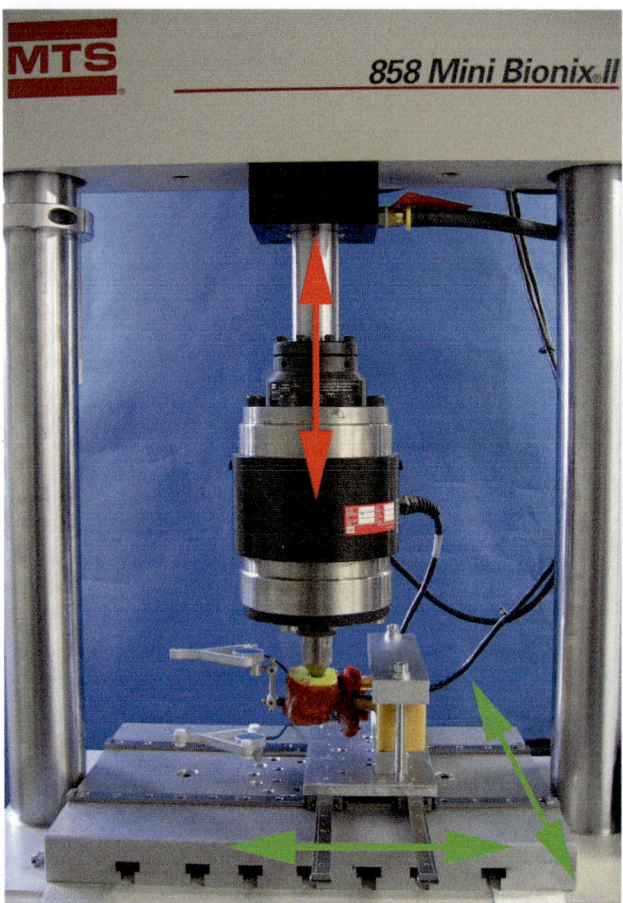

Fig. 4.4 Experimental test setup to provoke loosening of pedicle screws. *Green arrows* show translational degree of freedom, and *red arrows* show load application

several months of in vivo loading. In order to accelerate the in vivo occurring loosening/failure of the implant–bone interface, different loading protocols can be applied. A constant force, while the location of load application is varied [15], and a stepwise increasing load protocol, with a fixed point of load application [16], are often used. To provoke loosening and show a correlation of the number of load cycles to failure and the bone mineral density, a continuously increasing force-controlled loading protocol [17] is best suited to show differences in implant anchorage of various fixation and screw designs.

Test setups for implant loosening can encompass either the full assembly of the instrumentation [16, 18, 19] or only single screws of an assembly [20–22]. While single screw

testing allows a comparison of screw anchorage in the left and right pedicle of one vertebra with comparable bone quality and pedicle morphology, it does not give any information on the performance of the full assembly. However, because of anatomical variations of specimens from different donors, differences in screw design or augmentation technique/material can be better shown in a left-right paired test setup.

References

1. ASTM F 2267-04. Standard test methods for measuring load induced subsidence of intervertebral body fusion device under static axial compression. Current edition approved Dec. 1, 2011. Published January 2012; Reapproved 2011. p. 1–7.
2. ASTM F 2346-05. Standard test methods for static and dynamic characterization of spinal artificial discs. Current edition approved Dec. 1, 2011. Published January 2012; Reapproved 2011. p. 1–10.
3. ASTM F 2077-11. Test methods for intervertebral body fusion devices. Current edition approved July 15, 2011; 2011. p. 1–9.
4. ASTM F 1717-11A. Standard test methods for spinal implant constructs in a vertebrectomy model. Current edition approved July 1, 2011; 2011. p. 1–20.
5. ISO/FDIS 12189: 2008(E). Implants for surgery - mechanical testings of implantable spinal devices - fatigue test method for spinal implant assemblies using an anterior support. Published 2008-02-29; 2008.
6. ASTM F 2423-11. Standard guide for functional, kinematic and wear assessment of total disc prostheses. Current edition approved July 1, 2011. Published August 2011; 2011. p. 1–9.
7. Panjabi MM. Biomechanical evaluation of spinal fixation devices: I. a conceptual framework. Spine (Phila Pa 1976). 1988;13(10):1129–34.
8. Wilke HJ, Wenger K, Claes L. Testing criteria for spinal implants: recommendations for the standardization of in vitro stability testing of spinal implants. Eur Spine J. 1998;7(2):148–54.
9. Schmoelz W, Huber JF, Nydegger T, et al. Influence of a dynamic stabilisation system on load bearing of a bridged disc: an in vitro study of intradiscal pressure. Eur Spine J. 2006;15:1–10.
10. Wilke HJ, Neef P, Caimi M, et al. New in vivo measurements of pressures in the intervertebral disc in daily life. Spine. 1999;24(8):755–62.
11. Cripton PA, Jain GM, Wittenberg RH, et al. Load-sharing characteristics of stabilized lumbar spine segments. Spine. 2000;25(2):170–9.
12. Rohlmann A, Bergmann G, Graichen F, et al. Comparison of loads on internal spinal fixation devices measured in vitro and in vivo. Med Eng Phys. 1997;19(6):539–46.
13. Patwardhan AG, Havey RM, Carandang G, et al. Effect of compressive follower preload on the flexion-extension response of the human lumbar spine. J Orthop Res. 2003;21(3):540–6.
14. Niosi CA, Zhu QA, Wilson DC, et al. Biomechanical characterization of the three-dimensional kinematic behaviour of the Dynesys dynamic stabilization system: an in vitro study. Eur Spine J. 2006;15(6):913–22.
15. Kettler A, Schmoelz W, Shezifi Y, et al. Biomechanical performance of the new BeadEx implant in the treatment of osteoporotic

vertebral body compression fractures: restoration and maintenance of height and stability. Clin Biomech. 2006;21(7):676–82.

16. Disch AC, Knop C, Schaser KD, et al. Angular stable anterior plating following thoracolumbar corpectomy reveals superior segmental stability compared to conventional polyaxial plate fixation. Spine (Phila Pa 1976). 2008;33(13):1429–37.

17. Ferguson SJ, Winkler F, Nolte LP. Anterior fixation in the osteoporotic spine: cut-out and pullout characteristics of implants. Eur Spine J. 2002;11(6):527–34.

18. Schulze M, Gehweiler D, Riesenbeck O, et al. Biomechanical characteristics of pedicle screws in osteoporotic vertebrae-comparing a new cadaver corpectomy model and pure pull-out testing. J Orthop Res. 2017;35(1):167–74.

19. Wilke HJ, Kaiser D, Volkheimer D, et al. A pedicle screw system and a lamina hook system provide similar primary and long-term stability: a biomechanical in vitro study with quasi-static and dynamic loading conditions. Eur Spine J. 2016;25(9):2919–28.

20. Bostelmann R, Keiler A, Steiger HJ, et al. Effect of augmentation techniques on the failure of pedicle screws under cranio-caudal cyclic loading. Eur Spine J. 2017;26(1):181–8.

21. Lindtner RA, Schmid R, Nydegger T, et al. Pedicle screw anchorage of carbon fiber-reinforced PEEK screws under cyclic loading. Eur Spine J. 2018;27(8):1775–84.

22. Weiser L, Huber G, Sellenschloh K, et al. Time to augment?! Impact of cement augmentation on pedicle screw fixation strength depending on bone mineral density. Eur Spine J. 2018;27(8):1964–71.

Spinal Retractors

5

Luca Papavero

5.1 Introduction and Core Messages

Open surgical retractors provide continuous, unobstructed access to surgical sites. They unavoidably push the retracted tissue increasing intra-tissue pressure and reducing perfusion.

The ischemic damage tends to increase as time and amount of retraction increase. The resultant ischemia can damage the compressed tissues if perfusion is not restored within reasonable time periods ranging, depending on the tissue types and their locations, from tens of seconds (brain) to several minutes or longer (muscle). Unless the surgeon provides for repetitive removal or reduction of retraction, there is no available option for preventing this problem. Tubular retractors inserted via a transmuscular route cause less increase of the intramuscular pressure, less postoperative muscular damage seen on the MRI (magnetic resonance imaging), and less postoperative analgesic consumption. They seem to provide a valuable alternative in certain spinal surgeries. Radiolucent retractor blades allow for an unobstructed view of the surgical target area. Furthermore, bony anatomy is visualized more detailed because it becomes the most dense structure in the X-ray beam.

5.2 Definition

Most self-retaining retractors have an elongated rack bar and two retracting arms: a fixed retracting arm and a movable retracting arm. Both arms typically extend in a direction normal to the rack bar. The movable arm can be displaced along the rack bar using a crank, which also acts as a torque lever, to activate a pinion mechanism. Two blades are provided, usually below the retractor arms. The basic design and mechanism for separating the two or more spreader or retractor arms have remained relatively unchanged since the first introduction of retractors. The relationship between increased intramuscular pressure (IMP), reduced intramuscular blood flow (BF), and low back pain (LBP) has been shown in a rat model where a balloon increased IMP of the lumbar paraspinal muscles and decreased intramuscular BF [1]. Compared to sham groups, at one day after balloon insertion, IMP for the balloon group was significantly higher while intramuscular BF was lower. Expression of pain mediating substance P in the L1 DRG was also significantly greater for the balloon group. Furthermore, compared to normal lumbar paraspinal muscles, at 1 h after insertion, muscles of the balloon group showed edematous fibers. At 1, 7, and 28 days after insertion, muscle fibers displayed edema, inflammatory cell infiltration, and clear atrophy. Prolonged use of self-retaining retractors causes reduction in muscle function and is suspected to increase scar tissue generation and postoperative spinal muscle dysfunction [2]. For thoracic and lumbar pedicle screwing, we have abandoned the practice of Adson retractors inserted during the whole procedure. With the help of a handheld retractor, each single entry point is visualized. The advantages are the considerably reduced overall retraction time and the only intermittent ischemia of the paravertebral muscles [3]. Furthermore, the convergent direction of the screw insertion is more easily achieved (Fig. 5.6).

L. Papavero (✉)
Clinic for Spine Surgery, Schoen Clinic Hamburg, Hamburg, Germany
e-mail: luca.papavero@yahoo.de

© Springer-Verlag GmbH Germany 2023
U. Vieweg, F. Grochulla (eds.), *Manual of Spine Surgery*, https://doi.org/10.1007/978-3-662-64062-3_5

Muscle injury is closely related to muscle retraction and relaxation during lumbar disk surgery [4]. After lumbar laminectomy, total duration of muscle retraction greater than 60 min is associated with significant worse VAS (visual analog scale) scores for back pain and ODI and SF-36 scores for disability at 6 months after surgery. However, no relationship between outcome parameters and retractor type, operating surgeon, and wound length has been demonstrated [5]. The reported data refer to standard retractors. The insertion of open retractors via a subperiosteal approach has been compared in cadaver and clinical studies with the transmuscular insertion of tubular retractors. The latter showed a significantly lower increase of IMP in lumbar paraspinal muscles. Furthermore, significantly less muscle edema was seen on MRI in the minimally invasive group 6 months after surgery [6]. The analgesic consumption after lumbar microdiscectomy was less when the disk herniation had been removed via a transmuscular approach by tubular retractor than via the subperiosteal route by an open retractor [7].

5.3 Classification of Retractors

Due to the myriad of retractors and their modifications used in spinal surgery, any classification must be necessarily incomplete. Therefore, the criteria presented in the following are tentative:

(a) *Holding mechanism*
1. Handheld
2. Self-retaining
3. Table-fixed
(b) *X-ray imaging*
1. Opaque (stainless steel)
2. Semilucent (titanium, aluminum)
3. Lucent (PEEK, carbon)
(c) *Muscle/bone contact*
1. Subperiosteal
2. Transmuscular
(d) *Anatomical region*
1. Cervical
2. Thoracic
3. Lumbosacral
(e) *Approach to the spine*
1. Anterior
2. Lateral
3. Posterior

Of course, a retractor may be defined by several parameters crossing the various criteria of classification. Furthermore, the individual surgical experience may favor the use of a spreader designed, for example, for the anterior cervical approach in dorsal lumbar transmuscular pedicle screw insertion. On the other hand, a tubular retractor originally designed for lumbar disk herniation surgery may be fruitfully used for minimally invasive anterior odontoid screwing [8].

5.4 Clinical Examples

A very limited selection of retractors is presented with keywords highlighting the most interesting features of their application. The examples represent an author's choice which reflects necessarily only a fragment of the experience of the spine community.

The author is well aware of the fact that many readers will miss their workhorses and apologizes in advance. However, an exhaustive presentation of retractors would be beyond the scope of this chapter.

5.5 Cervical Spine

Transoral approach: self-retaining; ring-type with independent blades (Fig. 5.1)

Anterior subaxial approach: table-fixed miniaturized retractor with half-shell blades (Fig. 5.2)

Posterior subaxial approach: self-retaining (Adson, Gelpi) for conventional open approach. Frequent release of the retractor (e.g., sharp Gelpi) performing cervical laminoplasty has been demonstrated to reduce significantly postoperative axial neck pain ($P < 0.025$) and hypotrophy of the neck muscles ($P < 0.001$) compared to continuous opening of retractor (e.g., blunt Adson) (Fig. 5.3a) [9]. Table-fixed tubular retractor for transmuscular approach (dorsolateral foraminotomy, lateral mass screw insertion, Fig. 5.3b).

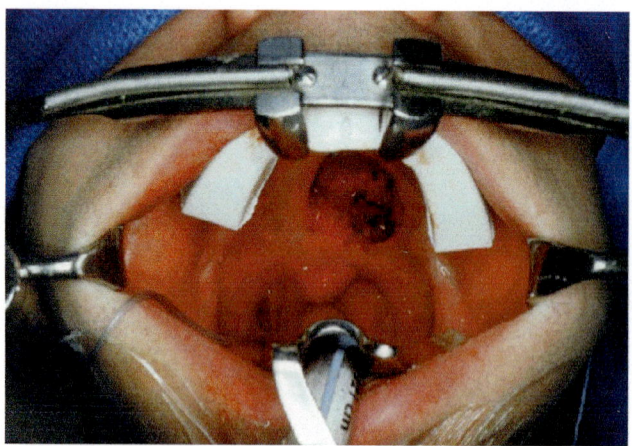

Fig. 5.1 Oral intubation with a flexometallic tube positioned at the *bottom* of the mouth. Furthermore, the tube is protected by the half-shell-shaped tongue retracting blade. The mouth is kept open with a gag that rests against the upper dental arch (rubber protection) and depresses the tongue (avoid squeezing between the tongue blade and the teeth). Examples: Crockard (Codman, USA), Spetzler-Sonntag (Aesculap, Germany) (Courtesy of img.medscape.com)

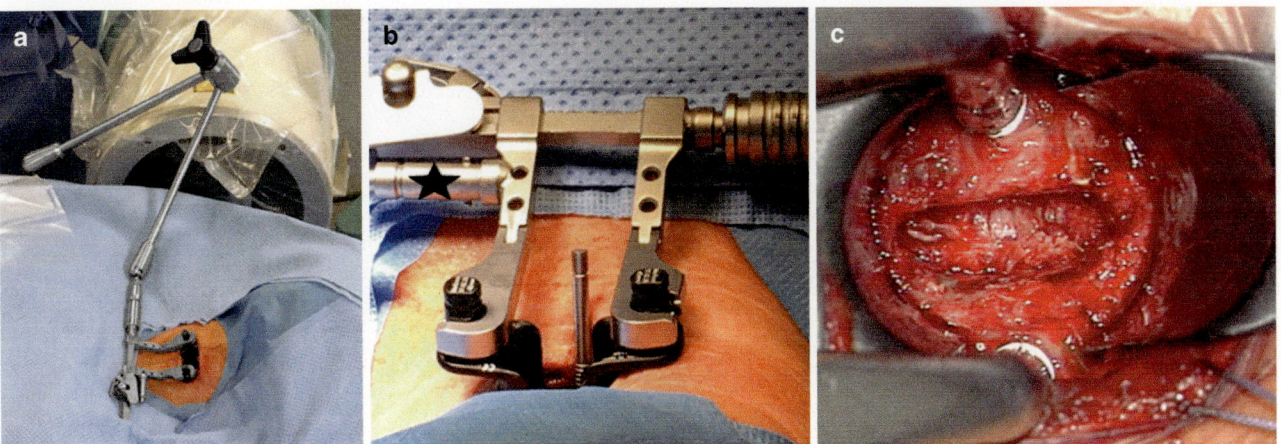

Fig. 5.2 (**a**) The conventional self-retaining cervical spreader has been substituted with a table-fixed one to prevent slippage of the blades from underneath the m. longus colli. (**b**) The retractor has been downsized by 50% compared with a conventional one and features a bilateral quick-lock (black star) for the table-fixed arm. (**c**) The half-shell blades (20 mm width) reduce the blood flow of the esophageal wall following a 30 mm wide opening by 17.4% compared with 48% by a 12 mm flat blade [9] (manufacturer: Medicon eG, Germany)

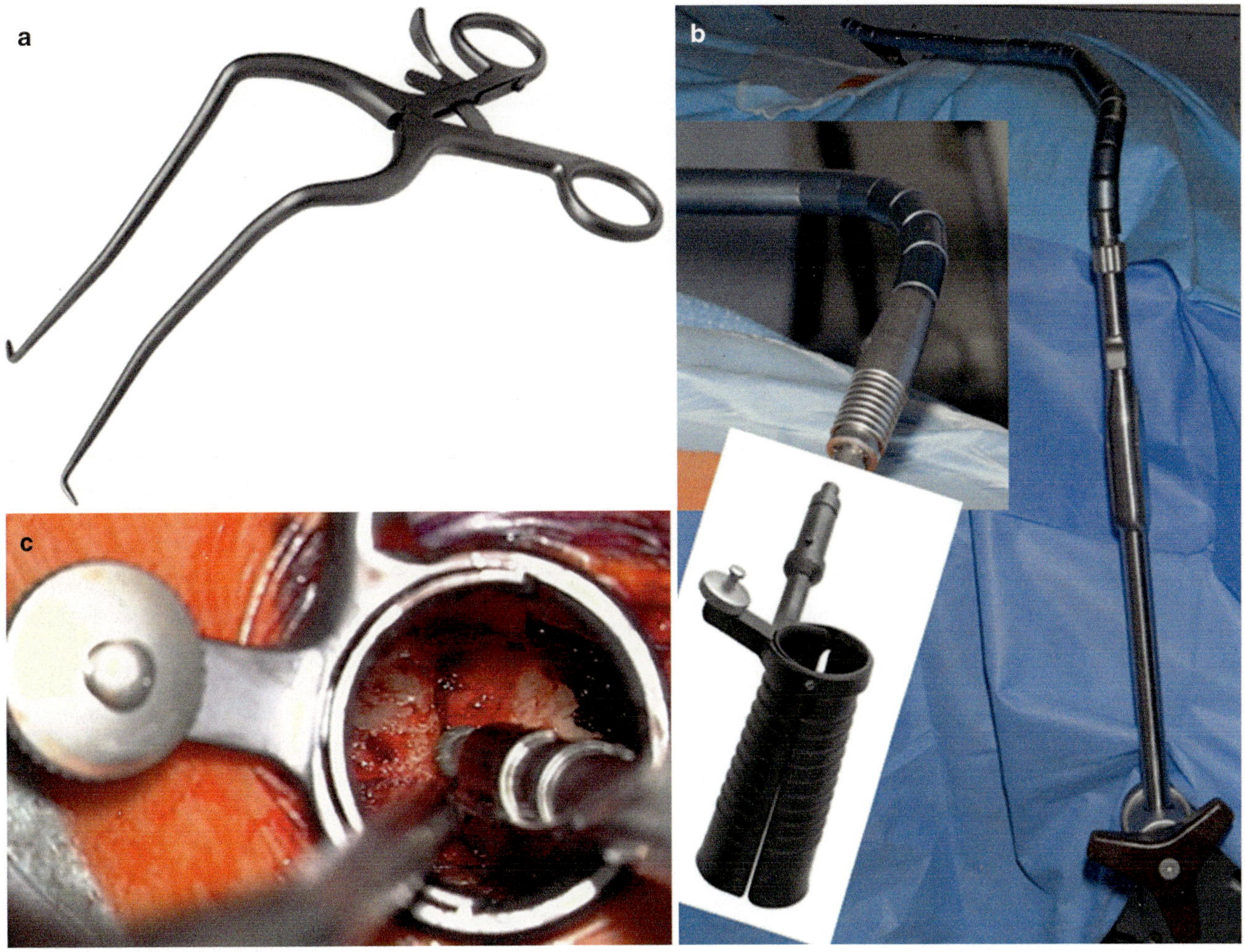

Fig. 5.3 (**a**) Deep Gelpi retractor (with permission of Aesculap AG, Tuttlingen, Germany). (**b**) The table-fixed adjustable holding arm, "the snake," holds an expandable tubular retractor in situ. Usually, the cylindrical retractor is inserted by blunt splitting of the paravertebral cervical or lumbar muscles (manufacturer: Medicon eG, Germany). (**c**) Expanded tubular retractor at the cervical level: In the depth the "V-Shaped" yellow ligament is shown. The drill starts with shaping the keyhole

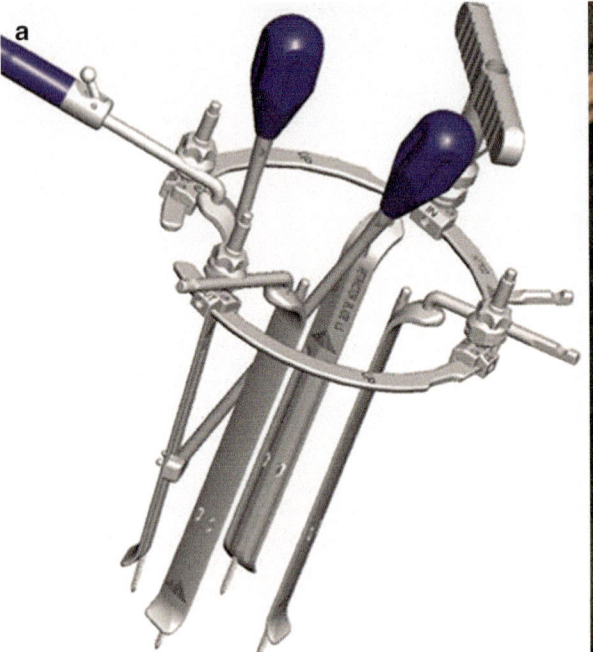
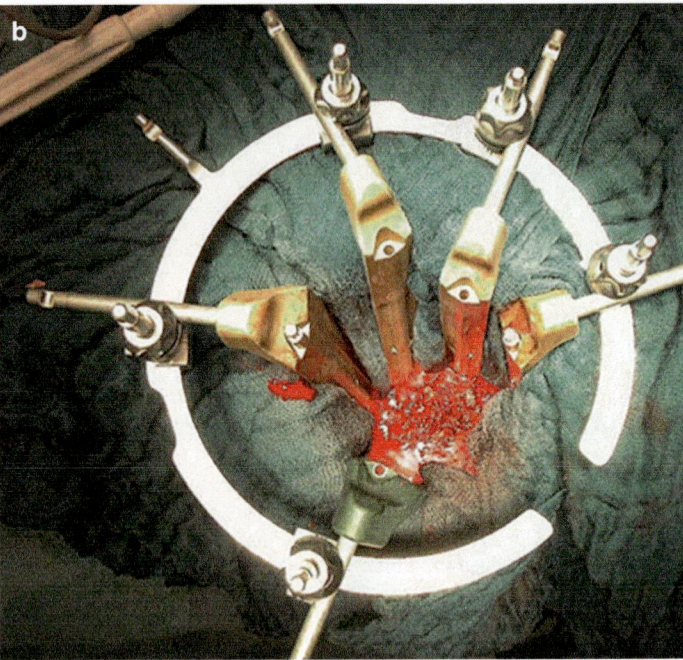

Fig. 5.4 The EndoRing (Medtronic, USA) may be used as a self-retaining, pin-based system or may be attached to existing table-based systems. The blade pusher allows the surgeon to safely manipulate the retractor blade(s), while surrounding anatomy is protected behind the blade: (**a**) illustration and (**b**) intraoperative view (with permission from the Medtronic International Trading Sarl ©02/12/2010 Medtronic International Trading Sarl)

5.6 Thoracic Spine

Lateral approach: table-fixed ring-type retractor, blades of aluminum, pins for blade fixation into the vertebral bodies (Fig. 5.4)

   Posterior approach: *see lumbosacral spine*.

5.7 Lumbosacral Spine

Anterior approach: a table-fixed ring-type is frequently used (see thoracic spine) (Fig. 5.5). An alternative is the self-retaining retractor anchored to the vertebral bodies.

   Posterior approach: Until 10 years ago, decompression and stabilization have been mostly performed via a subperiosteal bilateral open route. The surgical target area is approached with the aid of familiar bony landmarks. The advantage of this technique is the excellent anatomical view. Disadvantages are the denervation and the postoperative hypotrophy of the paravertebral muscles with functional impairment (Figs. 5.6a and 5.7).

5.8 Conclusions

- The review of the literature indicates that a lot of efforts are being made to minimize the tissue ischemia related to retraction.
- Experimental surgical retractors with integrated force and oxygenation sensors monitor or report real-time data to the surgeon. They quantify better the retraction damage, so "safe" thresholds of magnitude and duration can be defined [10].
- A further promising investigation is the "perfusion stimulating retractor." On this principle, when the capillary blood flow is interrupted for an acceptably short time, perfusion is partially or fully restored shortly after retraction is removed. The cyclic application and reduction of pressure enable sufficient perfusion to be maintained over the course of the surgical procedure.

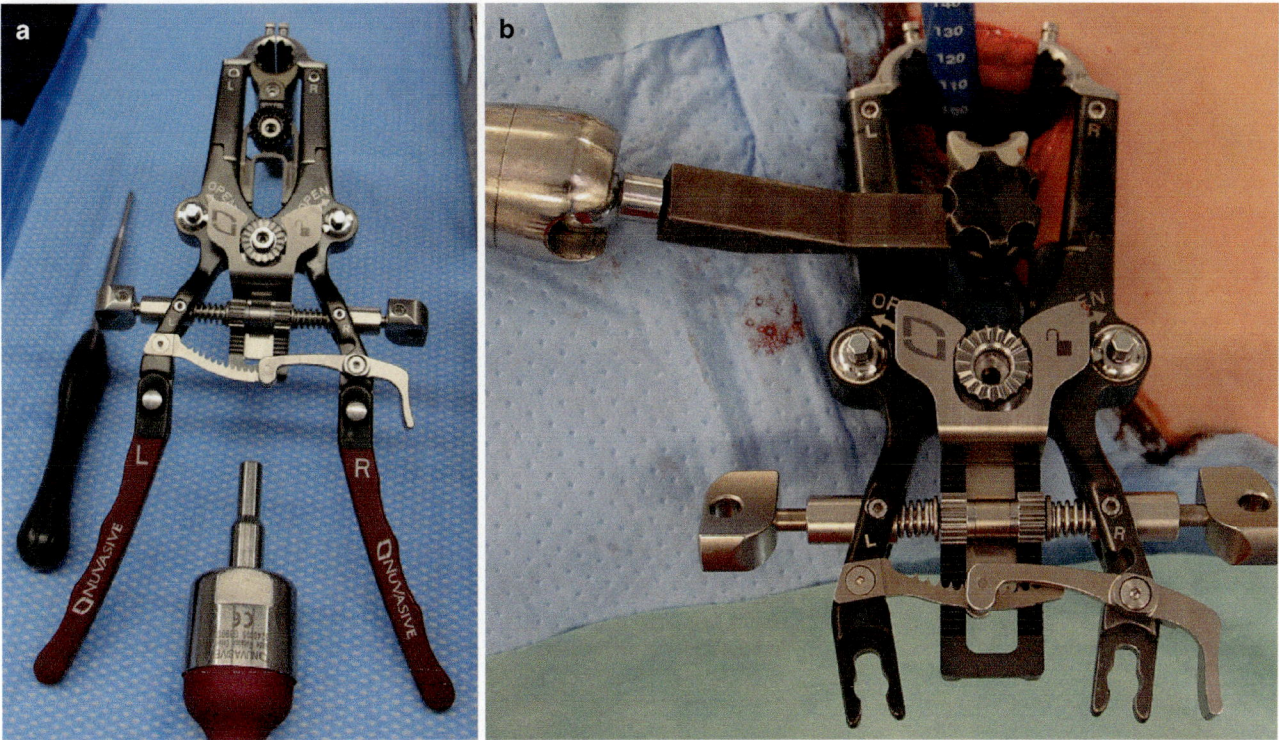

Fig. 5.5 Option for the lateral mini-open approach to the lumbar/thoracic spine: (**a**) table-anchored speculum-type retractor with counter-blade (XLIF, NuVasive); (**b**) in situ (with permission from NuVasive Germany GmbH, Bremen, Germany)

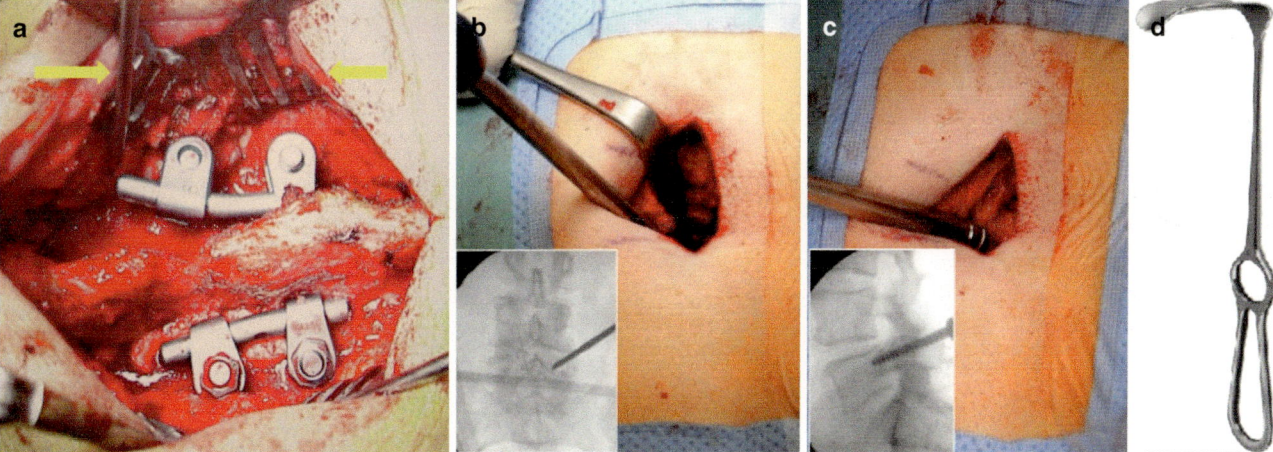

Fig. 5.6 (**a**) Conventional lumbar monosegmental fixation. (**a**) Two Adson retractors (yellow arrows) provide the exposure by permanent retraction. (**b**) Via a much smaller approach, the temporary retraction of a part of the paravertebral muscles enables the insertion of the pedicle awl. (**c**) The screw is inserted without any retraction device. (**d**) Slim designed handheld muscle retractor

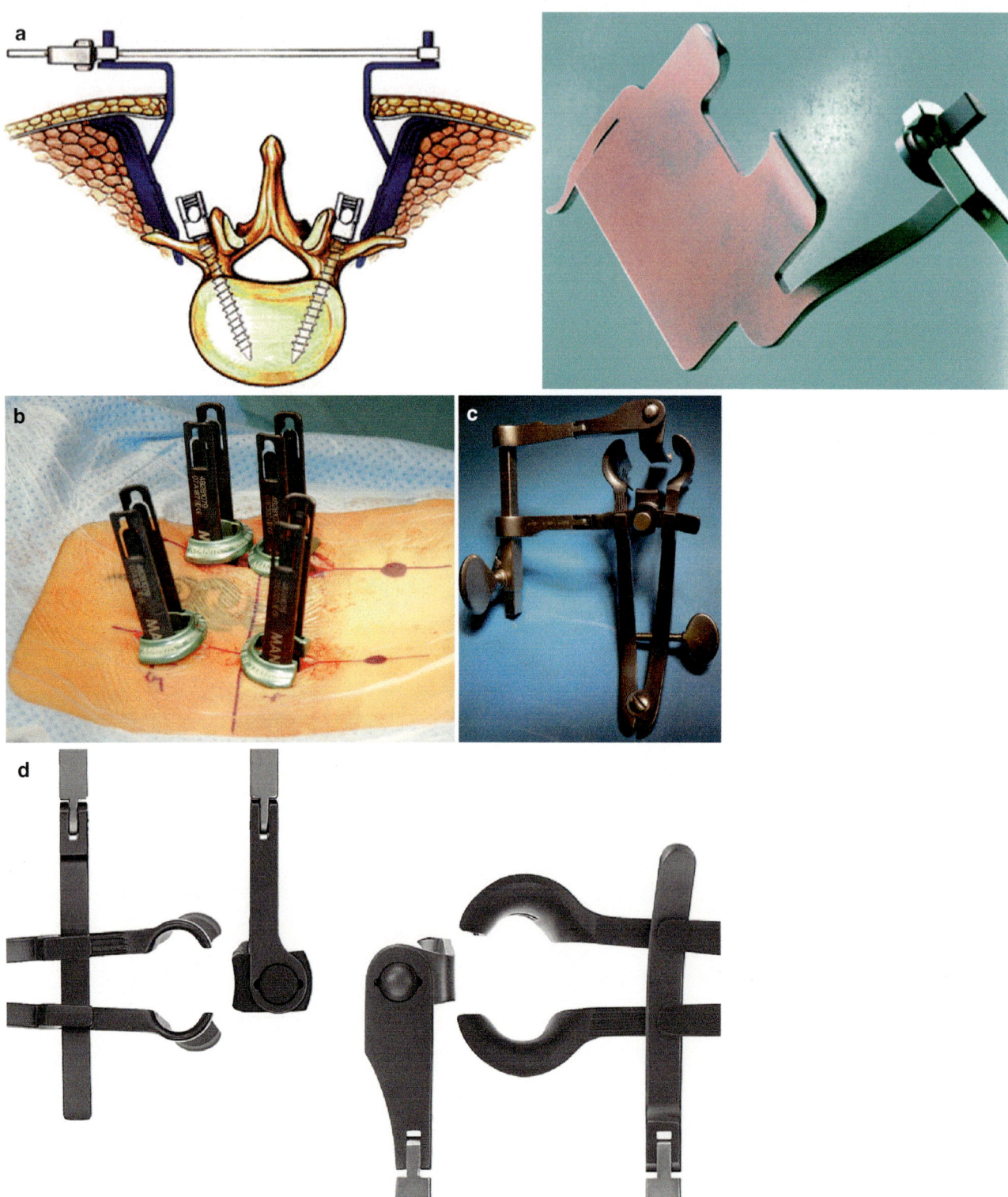

Fig. 5.7 (**a**) The uncommon design of the retractor aims to reduce the skin incision and, at the same time, to maximize the retraction of the muscle tissue in order to allow unobstructed introduction of pedicle screws (SLR, Aesculap) (with permission from Aesculap AG, Germany). (**b**) Following the percutaneous, transmuscular, fluoroscopy-aided insertion of the pedicle screw, slim titanium blades are docked into the screw head in order to retract the muscle and to allow the insertion of the rod (Stryker, USA). (**c**) The Caspar-type retractor has been developed in the 1970s and is still one of the most popular retractors in spinal microsurgery (Aesculap AG, Germany). (**d**) The miniaturized Caspar-type retractor (*left*) reduces the length of the skin incision and the amount of muscle dissection and facilitates lateral fluoroscopy because of the blades made of aluminum (Medicon eG, Germany)

References

1. Kobayashi Y, Kikuchi S, Konno S, et al. Increased intramuscular pressure in lumbar paraspinal muscle and low back pain. Poster 101 at EuroSpine, 25–28 Oct 2007, Brussells; 2007.

2. Taylor H, McGregor A, Medhi-Zadeh S, et al. The impact of self-retaining retractors on the paraspinal muscles during posterior spinal surgery. Spine. 2002;27:2758–62.

3. Yokohama T. Release of the muscle retractors can reduce axial symptoms after cervical laminoplasty. Poster presented at the 31st annual meeting cervical spine research society, CSRS, 11–13 Dec 2003, Scottsdale; 2003.

4. Kotil K, Tunckale T, Tatar Z, et al. Serum creatine phosphokinase activity and histological changes in the multifidus muscle: a prospective randomized controlled comparative study of discectomy with and without retraction. J Neurosurg Spine. 2007;6:121–5.

5. Datta G, Gnanalingham K, Peterson D, et al. Back pain and disability after lumbar laminectomy: is there a relationship to muscle retraction? Neurosurgery. 2004;54:1413–20.

6. Stevens K, Spenciner D, Griffiths K, et al. Comparison of minimally invasive and conventional open posterolateral lumbar fusion using magnetic resonance imaging and retraction pressure studies. J Spinal Disord Tech. 2006;19:77–86.

7. Brock M, Kunkel P, Papavero L. Lumbar microdiscectomy: subperiosteal vs. transmuscular approach and influence on the early postoperative analgesic consumption. Eur Spine J. 2008;17:518–22.

8. Hott JS, Henn JS, Sonntag VK. A new table-fixed retractor for anterior odontoid screw fixation: technical note. J Neurosurg. 2003;98(Suppl 3):294–6.

9. Kieslich S. Anteriore cervikale Dekompression und Fusion: Der Einfluss von unterschiedlich konfigurierten Retraktorvalven auf die postoperative Dysphagie. Dissertation. Universitätsklinikum Hamburg Eppendorf; 2015.

10. Fischer G, Saha S, Horwat J et al. Intra-operative ischemia sensing surgical instruments. Poster at complex medical engineering, 15–18 May 2005, Takamatsu; 2005.

Fluoroscopy and Spinal Navigation

6

Stefan Kroppenstedt

6.1 Introduction and Core Messages

Standard fluoroscopy is familiar to most spine surgeons because it provides real-time intraoperative visualization of spinal anatomy. The major limitations of fluoroscopy are occupational radiation exposure and the fact that the images can only be obtained in one plane at a time. Image-guided spinal navigation has evolved as a spinal surgical tool overcoming the limitations of standard fluoroscopy. It has been proven to be a versatile and effective tool for facilitating complex surgical procedures. However, image guidance has its limitations and does not replace the surgeon's own experience and judgment. There are several modalities of spinal image guidance (such as CT-based, fluoroscopy-based, three-dimensional C-arm fluoroscopy), and each has its own advantages and limitations. Pitfalls and errors are related to issues of the accuracy, technique, and overall ease of use of the technology during surgery. A thorough understanding of these problems is required to ensure an effective use of image-guided navigation for spinal surgery.

S. Kroppenstedt (✉)
Department of Spinal Surgery, Center of Orthopedic Surgery, Sana Hospital Sommerfeld, Kremmen, Germany
e-mail: s.kroppenstedt@sana-hu.de

6.2 Fluoroscopy

Fluoroscopy is an X-ray procedure that produces real-time moving images of internal structures through the use of a fluoroscope. Standard fluoroscopy is familiar to most spine surgeons because it provides immediate intraoperative visualization of spinal anatomy. A modern surgical image intensifier (also called C-arm because of its shape) consists of a generator (radiation source), an image receiver (intensifier with camera), and a monitor unit (containing an image memory and processing unit) (Fig. 6.1). Today, two monitors are mandatory for surgical machines. The C-arm is fixed on a mobile stand in such a way that it can be moved and turned to all sides (transverse and longitudinal to the patient, orbital movement around the patient, rotation and adjustment of height).

6.2.1 Radiation Protection

Besides the fact that the images can only be obtained in one plane at a time, a further major limitation of fluoroscopy is occupational radiation exposure. Thus, radiation protection is a very important issue. When using X-rays on a patient, a differentiation is made between effective radiation and scattered radiation. Part of the effective radiation is scattered by the patient's body and leaves the body as lower-energy scatter radiation in all directions. In order to protect the user and the parts of the patient's body not being

Fig. 6.1 Surgical image intensifier (C-arm) consisting of a generator (**a**), an image receiver (**b**), and a monitor unit (**c**) (with permission of Siemens)

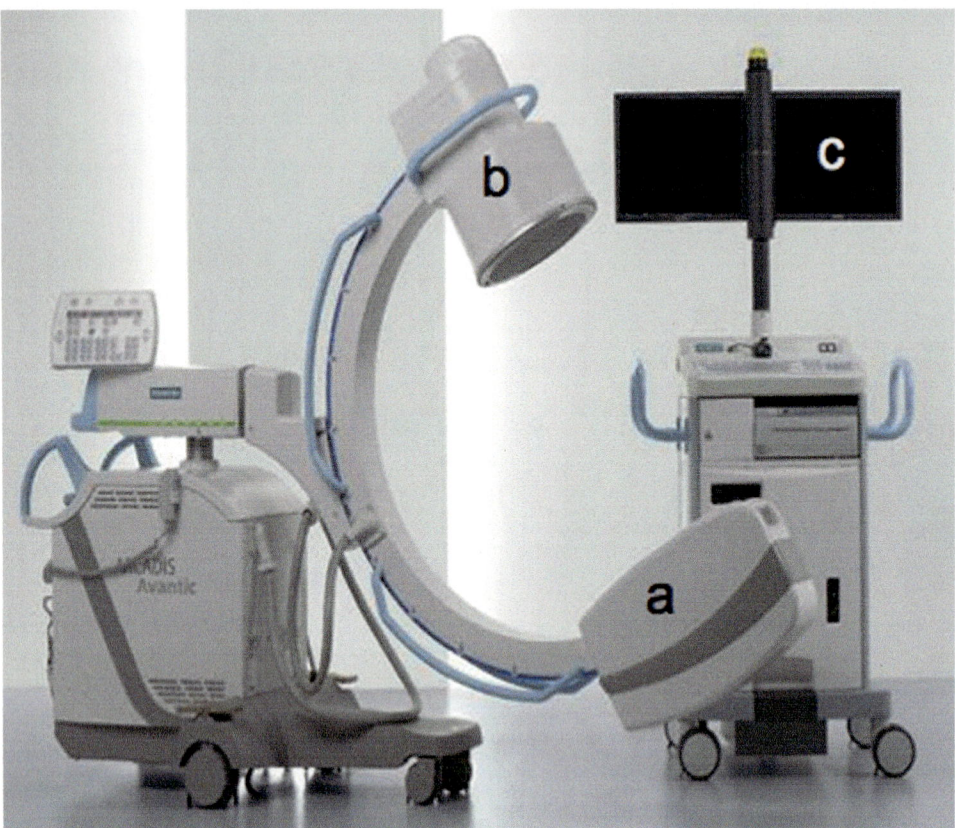

examined from this scattered radiation, the following rules should be observed:

(a) Prevention of scattered radiation:
- Keep the radiation times as short as possible.
- Do not start radiation until the emitter and image receiver system are correctly positioned. A laser light visor makes it easier to position the machine without radiation.
- Use pulse techniques for procedures with movement.
- As far as possible, always work with the lowest dose (half-dose program).
- Use the slot or iris diaphragm for gating because the amount of scattered radiation is directly related to the patient volume through which radiation has passed.

(b) Protection from scattered radiation:
- Distance is the best radiation protection because radiation decreases by the square of the distance.
- Use radiation protection clothing.
- Cover those parts of the patient's body which are not being examined.

In addition, positioning the image receiver system as close as possible to the patient's body (Focal spot/skin distance is thereby enlarged.) does not only improve the physical image quality but also considerably reduce radiation exposure for the patient [1].

6.3 Tips and Tricks

- Check before every operation that the machine is fully functional.
- After the patient has been positioned (before washing and covering), ensure that a trouble-free use of the C-arm during the operation will be possible.
- Everyone in the room must wear protective clothing.
- Prevent of and protect from scattered radiation.
- Store images with important interim results so that they are available later on for documentation.
- Whenever an image has to be compared with another one, transfer one image to the auxiliary monitor.
- After the operation, save/document the necessary images.

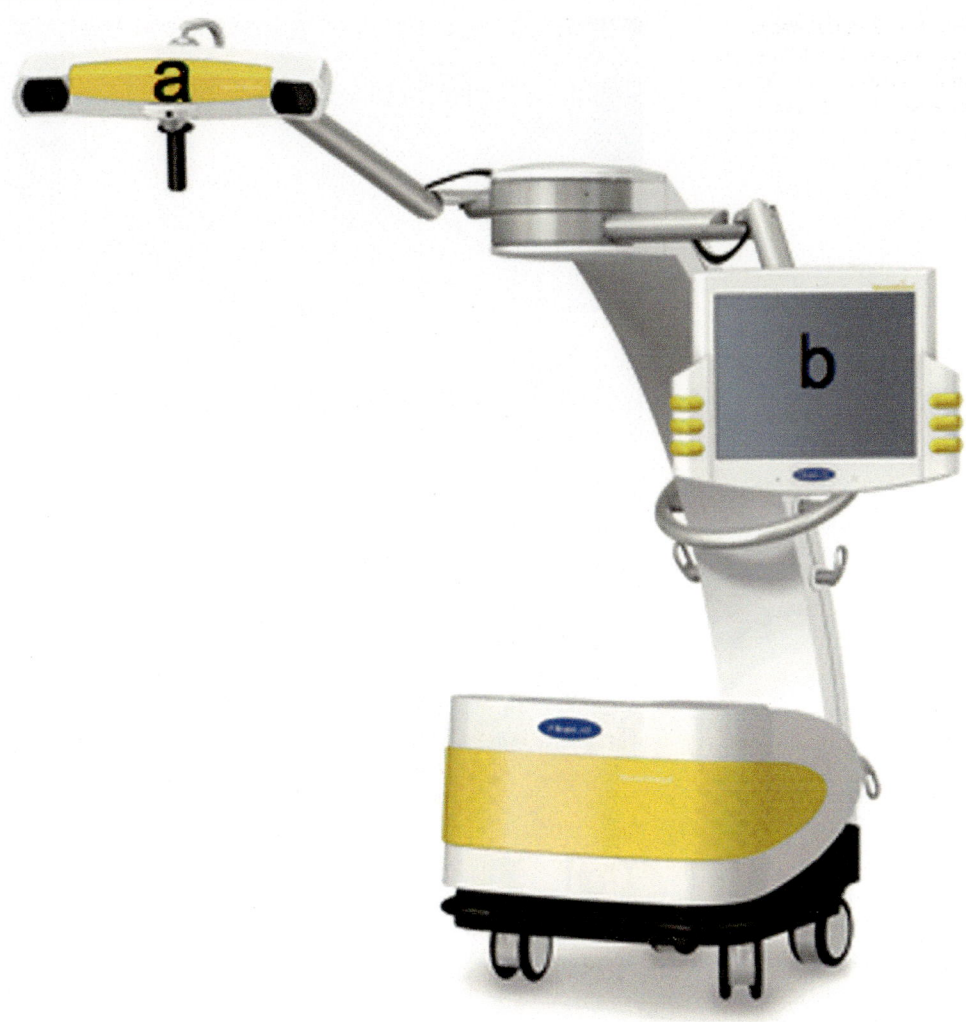

6.4 Spinal Navigation

Using spinal navigation technology, a three-dimensional model of the patient's spine appears on a computer screen with virtual representations of real surgical instruments that the surgeons have in their hand. A variety of spinal navigational systems are available on the market using different imaging modalities for navigation. The common components of most of these systems include an image-processing computer workstation interfaced with two-camera optical localizer (Fig. 6.2); a dynamic reference base (DRB), which is fixed at the patient; and navigated instruments. The camera transmits and tracks infrared light, which is continuously reflected back to the camera by passive reflectors attached to the DRB and the navigated instruments (Fig. 6.3). Alternatively, the infrared light is emitted by a series of LEDs mounted on the DRB and navigated instruments. The tracked infrared light is relayed to

the computer workstation. After registration process, the computer workstation provides simultaneous, multiplanar visualization of the spinal anatomy and allows virtually any dedicated or manual calibrated surgical instrument to be tracked in relation to the displayed anatomy in real time (Fig. 6.4) [2]. At present, the various different imaging modalities in use for spinal navigation include CT, fluoroscopy, the combination of both (CT-fluoro matching), and three-dimensional fluoroscopy [3, 4].

6.4.1 Preoperative CT-Based Image Guidance

CT-based navigation systems use a preoperatively acquired CT data set, which has to be transferred to the computer workstation. The computer reconstructs the data into different views. Thus, preoperative surgical planning is possible. Intraoperatively, after surgical exposure, the image-

Fig. 6.3 Reference frame
(**a**) attached to a spinous
process C2 and navigated drill
bit (**b**)

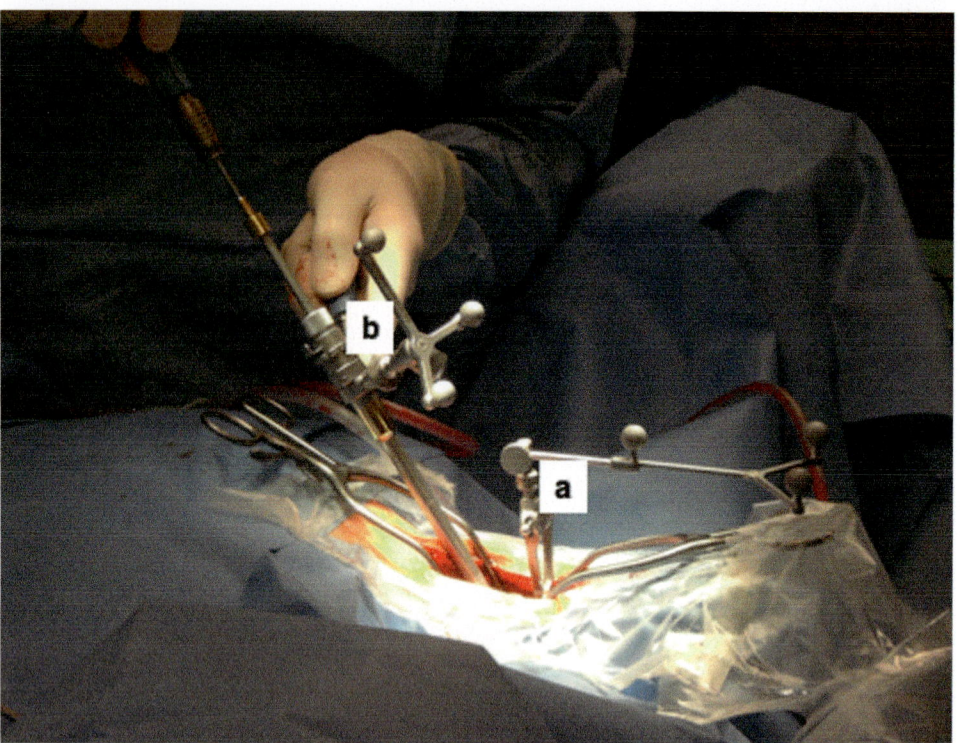

guided procedure begins with the patient registration. The DRB is attached firmly to the spine. The electrooptical camera tracks the spatial position of the patient by way of signals from DRB. The surface of the vertebral level of interest is touched/scanned with a registration probe (matching Fig. 6.5). This information allows the computer to create a contour map of the vertebra, which is then automatically mapped to CT data. Finally, the accuracy of the system needs to be verified. The probe tip is placed on several anatomic landmarks within the operative field, and the computer workstation monitor displays the virtual probe. The positions of the real and virtual probes had to correspond.

6.4.1.1 Advantages

- Preoperative surgical planning is possible.
- No occupational radiation exposure.
- Radiolucent table is not a must.

6.4.1.2 Disadvantages

- It requires a special CT protocol preoperatively.
- Registration process can be difficult and time-consuming.
- Because the CT images are acquired preoperatively with the patient in a different position than at the time of sur-

gery, the preoperative data set may not reflect the intraoperative anatomy on others and then the registered level.

6.4.2 Fluoroscopy-Based Image Guidance

Fluoroscopy-based image guidance uses intraoperative fluoroscopic images gained with a C-arm on which a calibration target is attached or temporarily hold into the beam. The images (at least one projection) are automatically transferred to the computer workstation for processing. The computer shows the saved fluoroscopic images that allow for the superimposition of the tracked surgical instruments. In contrast to CT-based navigation, no manual registration (matching) is necessary. Software programs exist that can match a preoperative CT scan with intraoperatively acquired fluoroscopic data (CT-fluoro matching).

6.4.2.1 Advantages

- It provides real-time intraoperative visualization of the spinal anatomy.
- It is suited for minimal access applications.

Fig. 6.4 Workstation screen demonstrating a trajectory for the insertion of a C1–C2 transarticular screw (*upper screen*) and a C5 facet screw (*lower screen*)

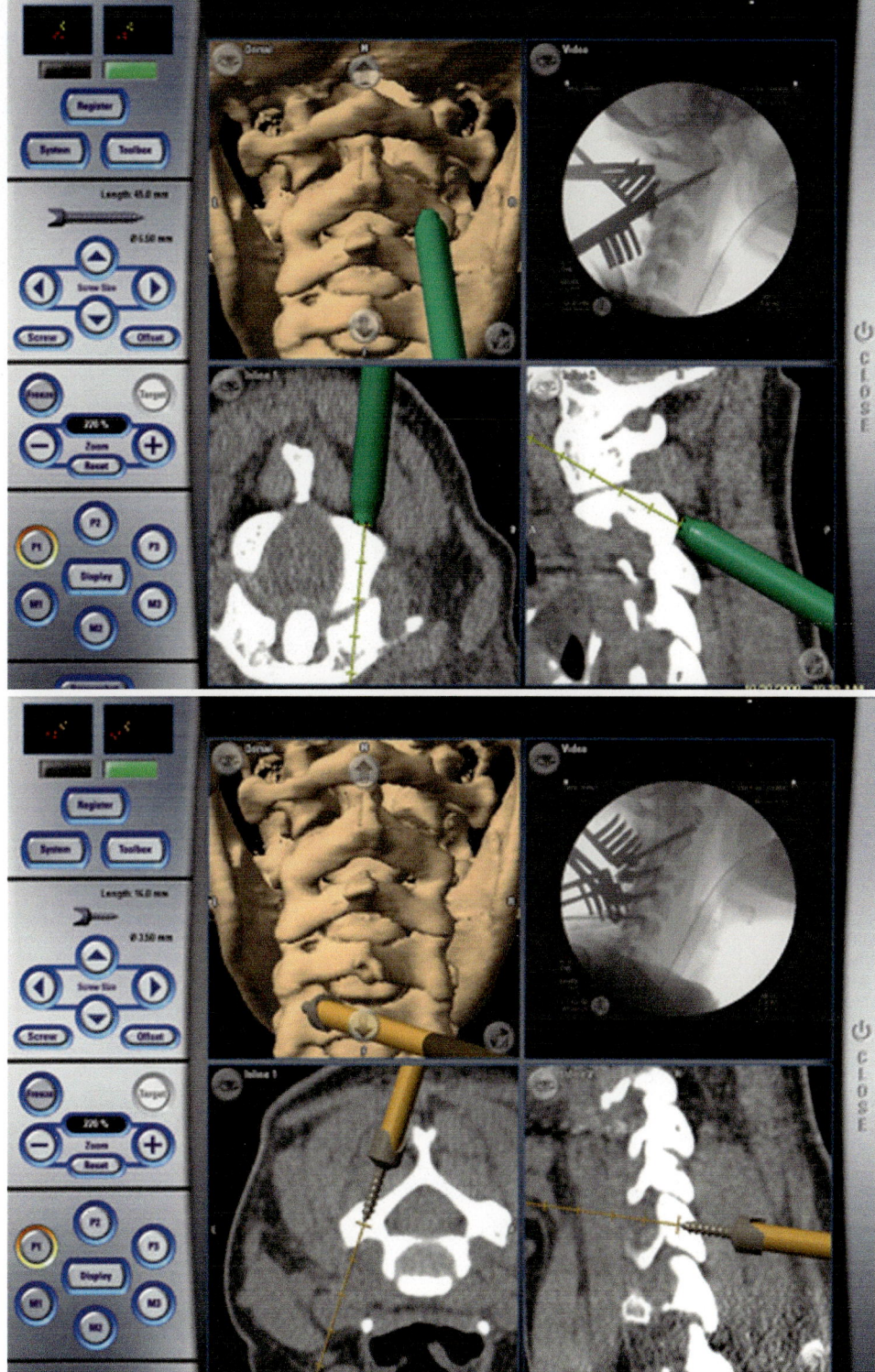

Fig. 6.5 Navigational workstation screen demonstrating a region matching for C2 vertebra

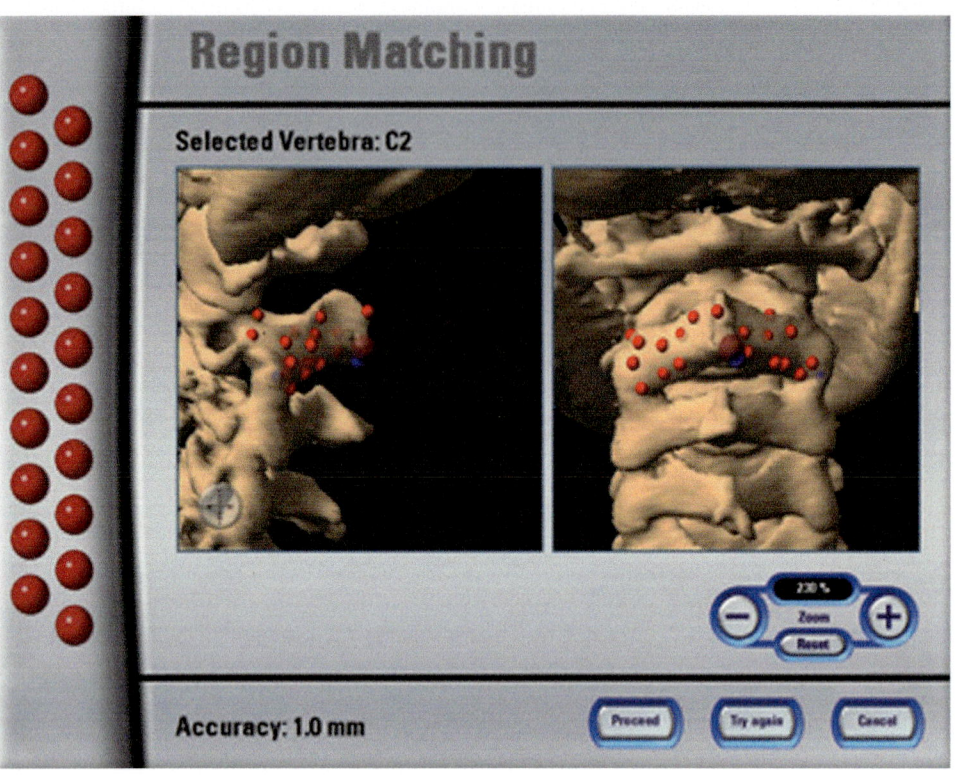

Fig. 6.6 Three-dimensional C-arm fluoroscopy. The isocentric C-arm rotates automatically 190 deg around the patient (with permission of Siemens)

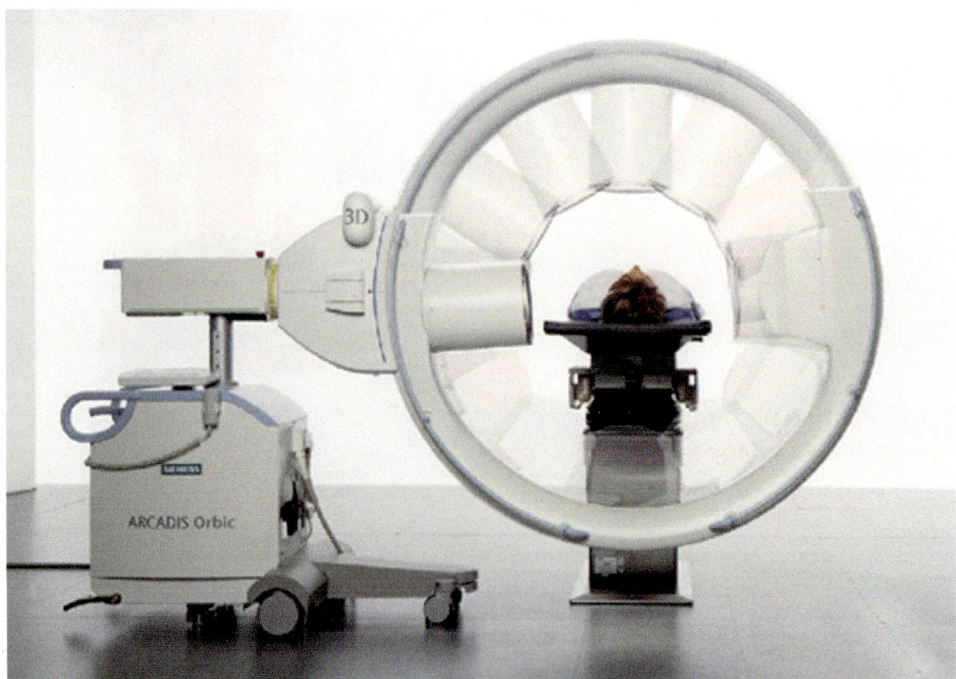

6.4.2.2 Disadvantages

- It does not offer the axial images that are helpful during CT-based navigation.
- Impaired image quality in certain areas of the spine like the lower cervical or upper thoracic spine and under certain conditions like in patients who are obese and osteopenic or have spinal deformity.

6.4.3 Preoperative CT-Based Image Guidance, Registered with Fluoroscopy (CT-Fluoro Matching)

The minimally invasive CT-fluoro matching method uses two intraoperatively acquired fluoroscopy images to register a preoperatively acquired CT data set. For this registration, the level of interest in the fluoroscopy image and in the CT is fused by the system after a manual prepositioning workflow.

6.4.3.1 Advantages

- Minimally invasive registration
- Full CT image quality, three-dimensional reconstructions, and axial views

6.4.3.2 Disadvantages

- Extra time for pre-positioning steps
- Final verification of the registration accuracy demanding for minimally invasive cases

6.4.4 Three-Dimensional C-Arm Fluoroscopy-Based Image Guidance

Three-dimensional C-arm fluoroscopy uses a rotating C-arm fluoroscope fitted with a calibration target. An isocentric C-arm is capable of obtaining multiple successive images during an automated partial rotation around the patient while maintaining the relevant spinal anatomy in the center of the field (Fig. 6.6). Specialized software allows the fluoroscopic images to be reconstructed into axial, sagittal, and coronal views, and the unit can effectively function as a CT scanner.

6.4.4.1 Advantages

- It reduces X-ray exposure to surgical team.
- It is well suited for minimal access applications.

- The three-dimensional C-arm provides three-dimensional reconstructed views of the patient as currently positioned on the operating room table.
- The surgeon-dependent registration step is eliminated.
- As many as three adjacent lumbar levels can be imaged and navigated during each cycle.
- It offers the ability to obtain a postoperative scan while still in the operating room.

6.4.4.2 Disadvantages

- High radiation exposure to the patient
- High initial costs

6.5 Indications

- The following spinal fixation procedures are especially useful:
    - Upper cervical and cervicothoracic junction
    - Deformities
    - Less invasive/percutaneous approaches
- En bloc tumor resection
- Biopsy

6.6 Contraindications

- Insufficient image quality.
- Verification of the system accuracy fails.
- Lack of experience in spinal navigation.
- Surgeon is not able to perform the surgical procedure without navigation.

6.7 Technical Prerequisites

- Complete spinal navigation system
- Carbon table and carbon head clamp/fixation (exception: CT-based navigation)

6.8 Tips and Tricks

- Put the monitor of the C-arm in an ergonomic position directly next to the monitor of the workstation. The surgeon must be allowed to look at the monitors easily during the operation.
- Using (*three-dimensional*) *C-arm*: Before the operation, check if images can be gained without artifacts, and position the camera to allow for unimpaired line of sight for registration during scan.
- Using *CT-based navigation*: Check if preoperatively acquired CT data can be used for navigation (e.g., no arti-

facts due to CT table); additional use of a standard C-arm can be very helpful.

- DRB has to be fixed tightly to avoid relative movements causing inaccuracies. If the DRB gets loose after registration, registration must be repeated.
- It is strongly recommended to repeat regularly the verification of the system accuracy, especially before inserting a new screw.
- Position the camera to allow for unimpaired communication between the components (DRB and navigated instruments), while the surgeon can keep his ergonomic position.
- For MIS surgeries: Consider placing all relevant wires first, and then continue with screw hole preparation since inserting the k-wires will have less negative influence on the registration accuracy on adjacent levels.

References

1. Kreienfeld H, Klimpel H, Bottcher V. Use of X-rays in the operating suite. In: Aschemann D, Krettek C, editors. Positioning techniques in surgical applications, vol. 4.2. Berlin: Springer; 2006. p. 37–9.
2. Holly LT, Foley KT. Image guidance in spine surgery. Orthop Clin N Am. 2007;38:451–61.
3. Gebhard F, Weidner A, Liener UC, et al. Navigation at the spine. Injury. 2004;35(Suppl 1):35–45.
4. Holly LT, Foley KT. Intraoperative spinal navigation. Spine. 2003;28:54–61.

Surgical Microscopy in Spinal Surgery

7

Frank Grochulla

7.1 Introduction and Core Messages

Minimally invasive spinal surgery aims to achieve good clinical outcomes, comparable to those of conventional open surgery, while minimising the risk of iatrogenic trauma resulting from the surgical procedure. Surgical microscopes are one of the most exciting advances in the surgical field. The use of the microscope as a surgical tool was pioneered by Carl Zeiss, a leading German company in the optical and optoelectronic industry. The surgical microscope was first used for ENT surgery in the middle of the 1950s. In the mid-1970s, it was used in spine surgery. Pioneers such as Caspar, Yasargil and Williams were the first spine surgeons to perform microsurgical procedures for the treatment of lumbar disc diseases [1–4]. Since then, the surgical microscope has become an important tool in the field of spinal surgery.

7.2 Definition

The operating microscope used in minimally invasive and microsurgery is a stereoscopic binocular microscope with different magnification levels, giving an upright three-dimensional image. The microscope is used to obtain good visualisation of fine structures in the operating field. In the standing type of microscope, a motorised zoom lens system operated by hand or foot controls provides an adjustable working distance. In head-mounted models, interchangeable eyepieces provide the magnification needed. The surgical microscope brings the deep anatomical structures into

sharp and brilliant magnified detail, enabling surgeons to perform minimally invasive procedures. It also helps them to preserve important deeper structures and thus to reduce tissue trauma and blood loss (see advantages and disadvantages of loupes and surgical microscopes, Table 7.1). In summary, the microscope is a very helpful tool, enabling the surgeon to perform microsurgical procedures in spinal surgery. Different types of surgical microscope are available. Stand-/floor-type and table-type models are the most common. Wall- and ceiling-mounted surgical microscopes are also available. The two most widely used surgical microscope systems in spine surgery are manufactured by Zeiss and Leica (see Fig. 7.1).

7.3 Advantages

- Simultaneous magnification and illumination of the surgical field
- Three-dimensional magnification
- Coaxial illumination
- Comfortable standing or sitting position for surgeon and assistant (Fig. 7.2), independent of line of sight
- Shared viewing for assistant (teaching)
- Short learning curve
- Smaller skin incisions and less traumatic approaches
- Reduced tissue trauma and blood loss
- Video recording (see Fig. 7.3) for medico-legal and scientific reasons and for teaching

7.4 Disadvantages

Using a surgical microscope has no real disadvantages. However, some aspects that should be kept in mind are the following:

- Some "disadvantages" (e.g. hand-eye coordination) are associated with the learning curve of the surgeon and can be avoided by continuous microsurgical education.

F. Grochulla (✉)
Metropol Medical Center, Clinic for Orthopedics, Trauma Surgery and Spinal Surgery, Nuremberg, Germany
e-mail: frank.grochulla@mmc-nuernberg.de

© Springer-Verlag GmbH Germany 2023
U. Vieweg, F. Grochulla (eds.), *Manual of Spine Surgery*, https://doi.org/10.1007/978-3-662-64062-3_7

Table 7.1 Advantages and disadvantages of loupes and surgical microscopes

	Loupes	Microscopes
Magnification	Limited range and fixed	Greater range and changeable during surgery
Motion	Long surgery causes neck fatigue and movement of loupes	No movement of microscope
Focus	Refocusing is necessary to restart surgery	Microscope in constant focus regardless of surgeon's attention
Illumination	Not parallel to line of vision	Parallel to line of vision and stronger
Deep three-dimensional vision	Limited with smaller skin incisions (<65 mm)	Maintained with even a 25-mm incision
Teaching	Assistants excluded	Assistants included
Surgeon's neck	Fixed in flexion and requiring repositioning. Fatigue during long surgery	Spared, inclinable binocular head can be adjusted

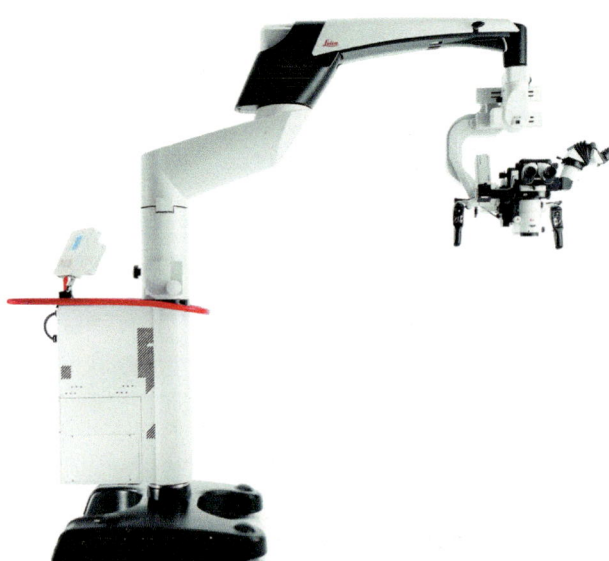

Fig. 7.1 Surgical microscope M525 MS3 (Leica)

- Specially designed retractor systems and instruments are necessary for microsurgery with small skin incisions.
- The visual field is limited. Microsurgery therefore requires meticulous preoperative planning and detailed knowledge of anatomical topography.

7.5 Components of a Surgical Microscope System

7.5.1 Optical System

The optical system of a modern microscope for spine surgery should have the following features:
- At least two tiltable binocular heads for the surgeon and assistant
- Eyepiece tubes with adjustable distance (see Figs. 7.4, 7.5 and 7.6)
- Objective lenses are available with focal lengths from 150 to 400 mm. For spine surgery, 300–400-mm lenses are usual.

7.5.2 Illumination System

The best source of illumination for spinal microsurgery is a xenon light source. This gives a higher light intensity than halogen light sources.

7.5.3 Control System

Surgical microscopes are available with foot or hand controls to adjust magnification, zoom, focus and positioning. Most higher-end equipment comes with motorised foot-controlled focusing as standard, allowing hands-free focusing. Some units also have motorised controls, allowing the surgeon to centre the field of view and tilt the angle of the head assembly via servo motors.

7.5.4 Coupling and Stands

The most advanced principle is the electromagnetic coupling of the microscope to its stand (see Fig. 7.1). This kind of coupling provides comfortable and easy (free floating) controlled movement of the microscope along all axes.

7.5.5 Video Systems and Recording

These are necessary for medico-legal and scientific reasons. High-resolution three-chip digital cameras are used in combination with professional video recording systems.

7.6 Microscope Adjustability

The following features of the surgical microscope can be adjusted:
- Tilt of eyepiece
- Interocular distance
- Eyepiece length
- Focus

Fig. 7.2 Spinal microsurgery in face-to-face position allows the surgeon and assistant to switch position without either sacrificing comfort

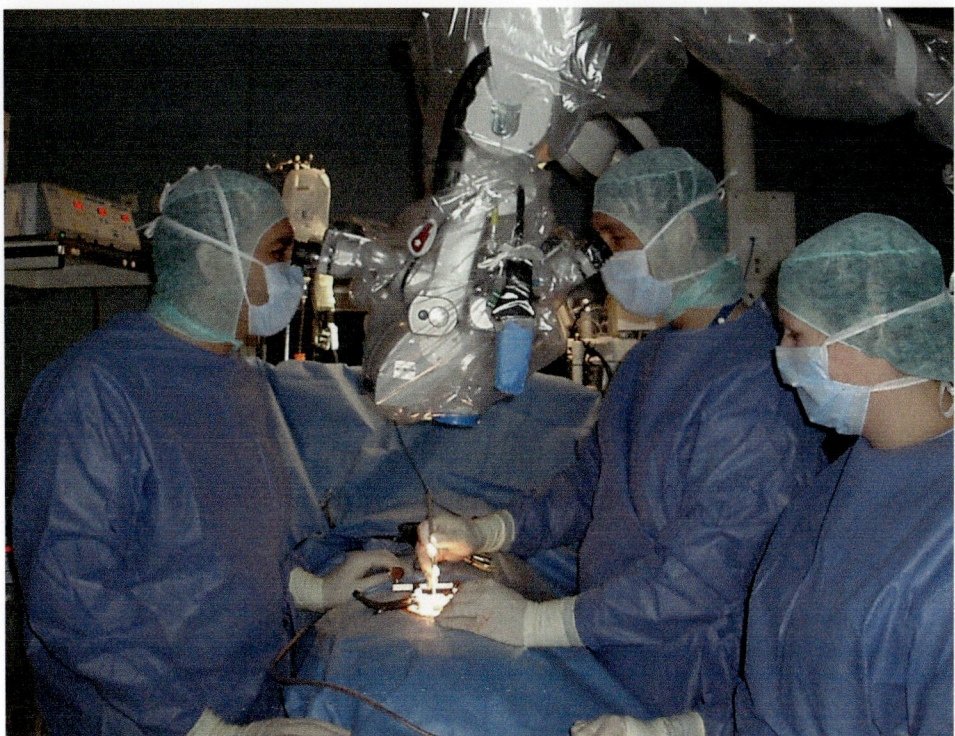

Fig. 7.3 Video- and computer-based recording system

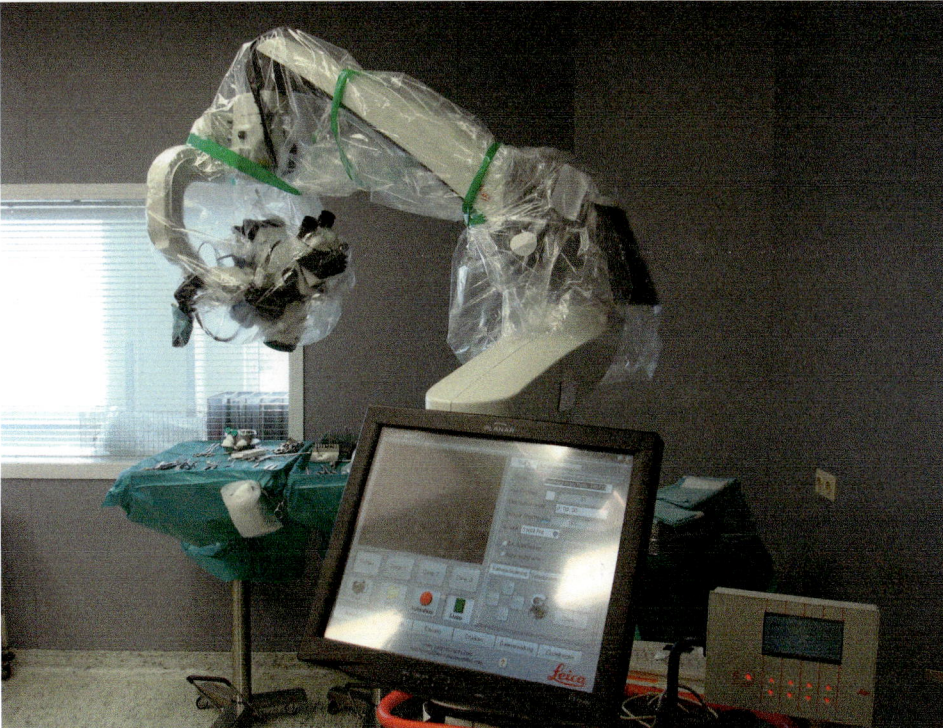

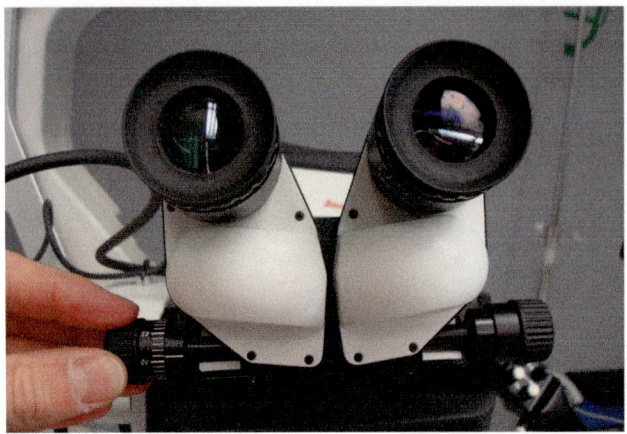

Fig. 7.4 Binocular tubes with adjustable interpupillary distance

- Field and location of autofocus if available
- Zoom/magnification
- Light focus
- Light intensity
- Distance between lens and surgical field
- Degrees of freedom for movement

7.7 Microsurgical Applications

Spinal microsurgery encompasses a wide variety of applications [5] (as listed below):

(a) *Cervical spine*
- Anterior cervical decompression and fusion
- Uncoforaminotomy
- Total disc replacement
- Vertebral artery decompression
- Foraminotomy posterior
- Laminoplasty

(b) *Thoracic spine*
- Anterior transthoracic approaches (discectomy, fractures)
- Costotransversectomy
- Discectomy

(c) *Lumbar spine*
- Disc herniations
- Spinal stenosis
- Foraminal stenosis
- Synovial cysts
- Posterior lumbar interbody and transforaminal lumbar interbody fusion preparation
- Minimally invasive anterior approaches

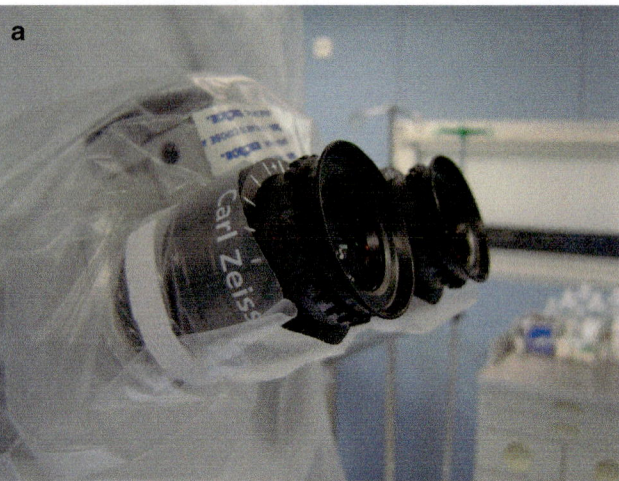

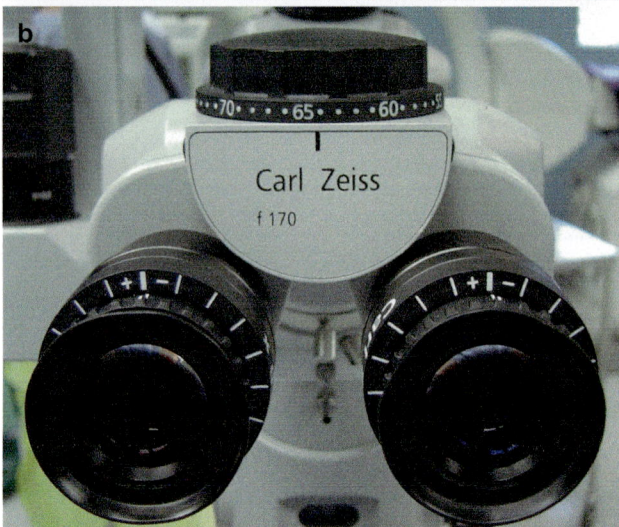

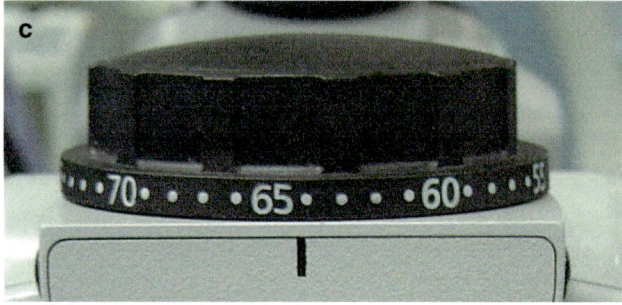

Fig. 7.5 (**a–c**) Sterile adjustment of interocular distance. Adjustments are possible to give the most comfortable position

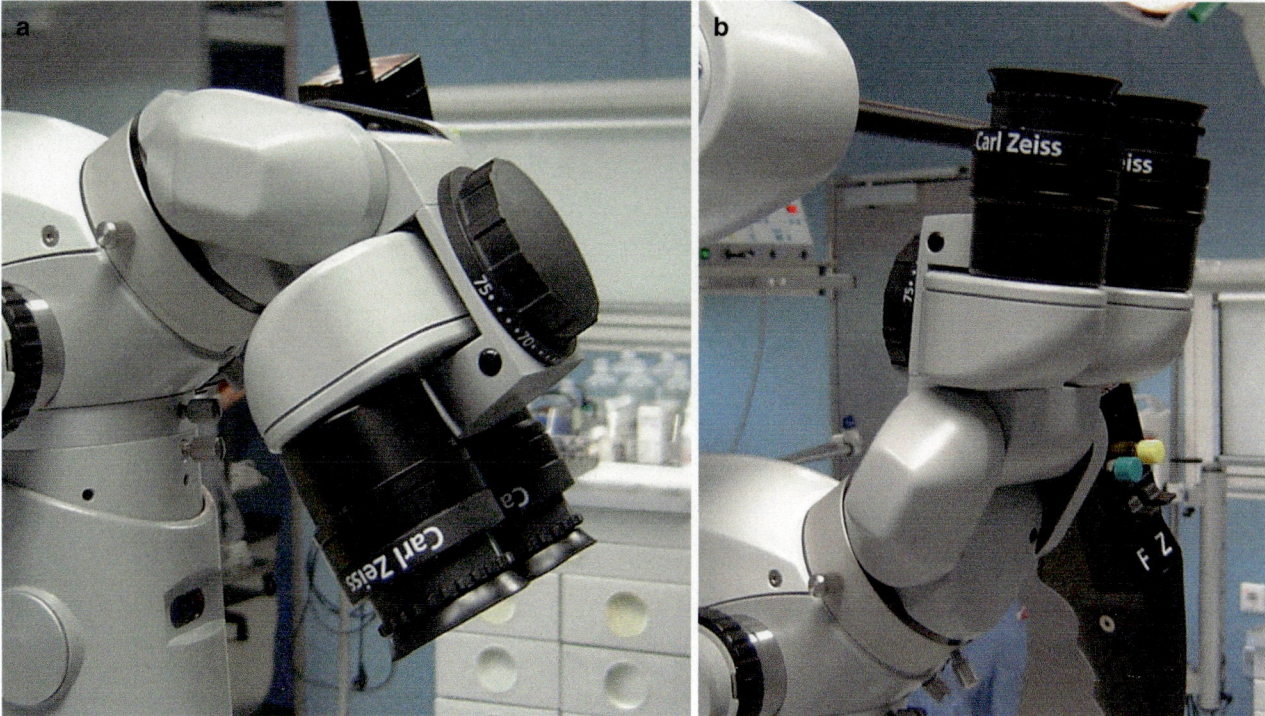

Fig. 7.6 (**a, b**) Adjustment of tilt of binocular head depending on the height of the operating field, the height of the surgeon and the tilt of the microscope

References

1. Caspar W. A new surgical procedure for lumbar disc herniation causing less tissue damage through a microsurgical approach. Adv Neurosurg. 1977;4:74–7.
2. Mayer HM. Spinal microsurgery. In: Mayer HM, editor. Minimally invasive spine surgery. Berlin: Springer; 2006.
3. McCulloch JA, Young PA. The microscope as a surgical aid. In: McCulloch JA, Young PA, editors. Essentials of spinal microsurgery. Philadelphia: Lippincott – Raven; 1998.
4. Williams RW. Microlumbar discectomy: a conservative surgical approach to the virgin herniated lumbar disc. Spine. 1978;3:175–82.
5. Yasargil MG. Microsurgical operation of herniated lumbar disc. Adv Neurosurg. 1977;7:81.

Endoscopy in Spinal Surgery

8

Uwe Vieweg

8.1 Introduction and Core Messages

An endoscope (from the Greek *éndon*, meaning inside, and *skopein*, meaning to observe) is a device with which it is possible to look at or carry out manipulations within a living organism. Endoscopes may be flexible or rigid. In spine surgery, endoscopes are used both in purely percutaneous applications and with assistance via various minimalized posterior and anterior access routes. For example, they are used with a posterior lumbar access route for endoscopic disc surgery and with anterior thoracic access. The use of endoscopes allows for surgical manoeuvres to be performed through small incisions. The benefits of endoscopic surgery are threefold. Since the incisions are smaller, the recovery from surgery is much quicker. There is also less pain, and there is less damage to the surrounding tissues.

8.2 Definition

Endoscopy is a minimally invasive medical procedure that is used to access the interior surfaces of an organ or preforming spaces by inserting a tube (endoscope) into the body. In the late 1970s and early 1980s, endoscopic techniques were advanced so that they could be used in both diagnosis and treatment of disease. The endoscopic techniques used in other surgical disciplines have now been applied in the treatment of spinal disorders. Improved fibre-optic light sources and the advent of the three-chip camera have resulted in improvements in visualization of the structures surrounding the spine. By using special endoscopes, instruments and implants, spinal surgeons have been enabled to treat some spinal column disorders with less injury to surrounding tissues. The endoscopic techniques minimize post-operative pain. Thoracoscopes and laparoscopes have been used to perform anterior release of scoliotic or kyphotic deformities and to perform transthoracic microsurgical discectomies. The role of spinal thoracoscopy has expanded to include corpectomy, vertebral reconstruction with internal fixation, hardware application and resection of neurogenic, spinal and paraspinal tumours [1–5]. Advances in interbody fusion cage technology have generated a great deal of interest in laparoscopic techniques [2]. The summary of the most compelling advantages of endoscopic procedures over open surgery is the following:

- Smaller incisions.
- Less tissue trauma.
- Minimal blood loss.
- Earlier return to activities and work.
- Easier operative approach in obese patients.
- Local or regional anaesthesia can be used in combination with conscious sedation.
- Less post-operative pain medication is required.
- Outpatient surgery is possible.

An endoscope usually consists of the following:

- *A rigid or flexible optical system* (see Figs. 8.1, 8.2, 8.3c and 8.4a, b).

  A rigid endoscope transmits images of the object or area being examined through a system of lenses in the endoscope stem to the eyepiece. In flexible endoscopes, the light is usually carried by glass fibres. Such a system may consist of up to 42,000 individual fibres, each of which has a diameter of 7–10 µm.

- *An illumination system*

  The light source is normally outside the body, and the light is typically directed via an optical system. A cold

U. Vieweg (✉)
Department of Conservative and Surgical Spine Therapy with Interdisciplinary Spinal Deformities Centre and Rummelsberg Sectional Center, Hospital Rummelsberg, Schwarzenbruck, Germany
e-mail: uwe.vieweg@sana.de

Fig. 8.1 Schematic representation of a flexible endoscope

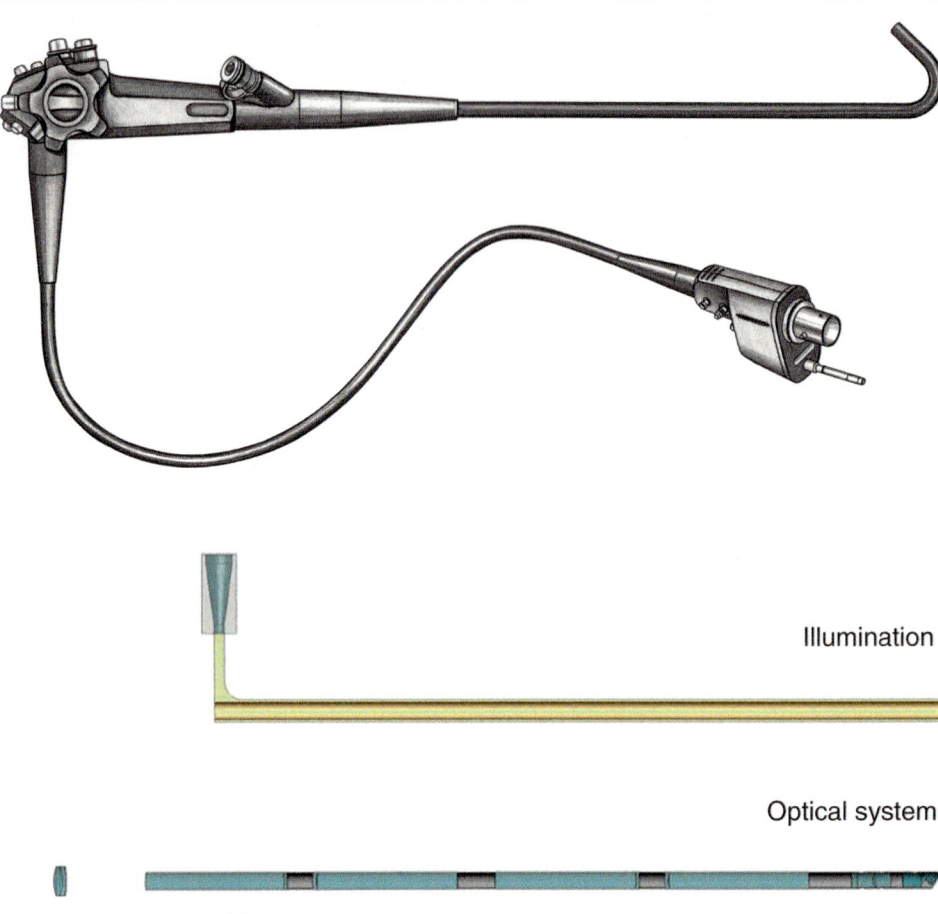

Fig. 8.2 Schematic representation of a rigid endoscope

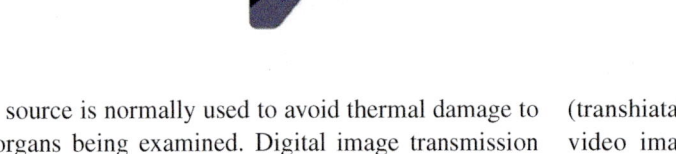

Illumination

Optical system

Mechanical housing

light source is normally used to avoid thermal damage to the organs being examined. Digital image transmission techniques (video endoscopy) may be employed.

- *A lens system*
  This system transmits the image to the viewer from the fibrescope. It allows the surgeon to look both straight ahead and at an angle.
- *A working channel*
  This allows medical instruments or manipulators to be introduced.
- Endoscopes may also be equipped with *suction and irrigation*.

Spinal endoscopy is a procedure in which a small endoscope is passed up through the tailbone into the epidural space (transhiatal or through the sacral hiatus). This allows direct video imaging of the inside of the spinal canal. Spinal endoscopy is also known as epiduroscopy because the endoscope is looking into the epidural space (see Fig. 8.4a, b). During a spinal endoscopy, an attempt may be made to remove some of the scar tissues or adhesions from around trapped nerves.

Endoscopic spine surgery utilizes dilatation technology to achieve surgical access through the soft tissue (including the skin, subcutaneous fat and muscle/fascia) instead of cutting in order to minimize tissue trauma. Beyond the reduced access trauma, the main differences between the endoscopic and the microsurgical microscopic techniques are in the image dimensionality (two-dimensional with endoscopy

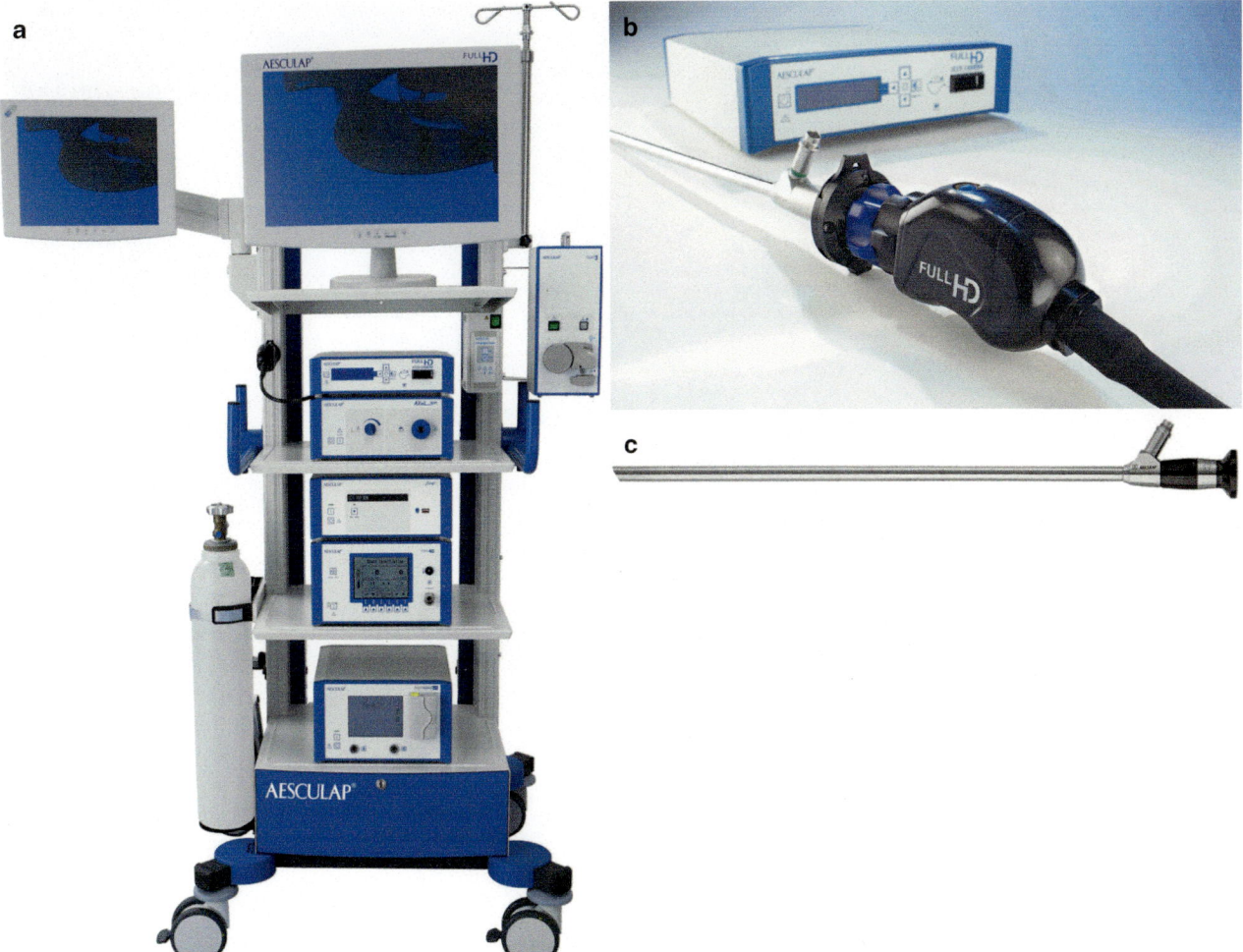

Fig. 8.3 (**a–c**) Video transmission sequence involving a three-chip camera, rigid endoscope with 30 deg eyepiece, xenon light source, two monitors for surgeon and assistants, video recorder and printer and suction and irrigation unit (with permission of Aesculap AG, Tuttlingen, Germany)

versus three-dimensional in microsurgery). Other differences are employing an angulated and close-up perspective and a straight but remote optical perspective, respectively. A number of instrument sets for endoscopic spine surgery are available on the market. They vary considerably in their technical specifications and in the indications they are designed to treat. It is each individual surgeon's responsibility to ascertain that she or he is using an instrument set that is well suited for the planned procedure. While an endoscopic approach to the spine reduces the (visible) trauma of the surgical approach, this minimal invasiveness comes at a price—reduced and two-dimensional visibility in, and limited expandability of, the surgical field. To a large extent, the entry route into the spinal canal or the foramen is dictated by the approach and trajectory chosen and by the local anatomy. Anatomical limitations are set mostly by osseous structures, such as the facet joints, the pedicles and the laminae, but also by the exiting nerve root for foraminal approaches and the vertebral arteries for cervical approaches. In combination with the characteristics of the optical system (angle of view, magnification, etc.), the size of the working channel and the tools available, the anatomy places clear limitations on which areas can be viewed and which lesions can be treated safely. There are burrs, trephines and rongeurs available that allow for the endoscopic resection of the bone in order to expand the operative field and enlarge access. However, whenever repositioning of instruments through additional access portals, blind reaming with trephines and excessive bony resection are necessary; the advantages of the minimally invasive procedure over a traditional microsurgical approach are reduced and in some cases may even become a disadvantage. Biplanar fluoroscopy is essential for accurate planning of the approach and for intraoperative control and recording of instrument position.

Fig. 8.4 Epiduroskop
(KARL STORZ Endoskope)
(**a**, **b**)

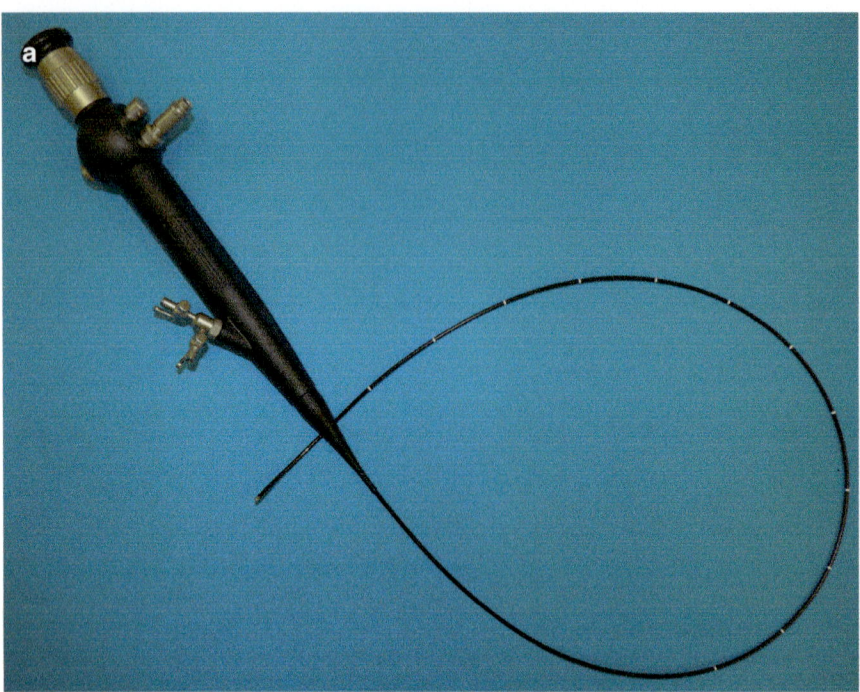

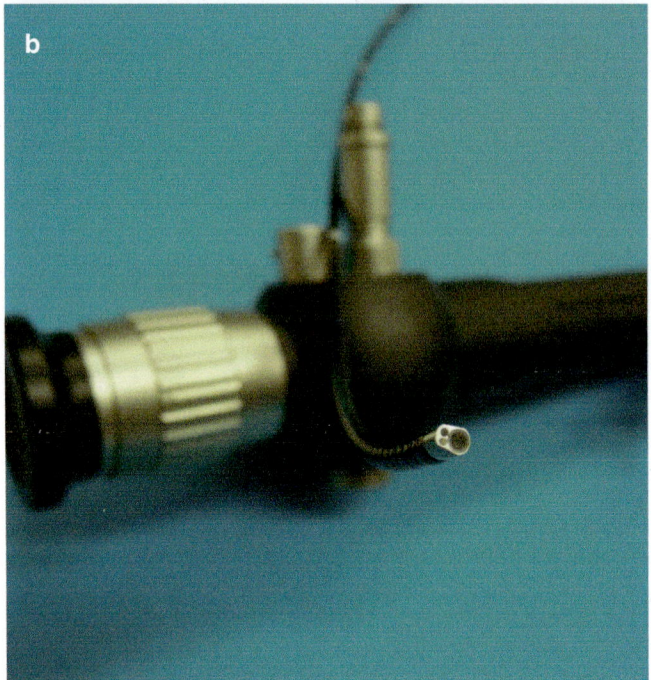

8.3 Types

Endoscopes differ both in their optical systems and in the particular applications for which they are appropriate as follows:

- *Rigid endoscope*
  In a rigid endoscope, the optical system is made up of a series of prisms and lenses arranged in sequence (see Fig. 8.2).

- *Fibre endoscope*
  A fibre endoscope is a flexible endoscope. In this case, the optical system consists of glass fibre bundles. It allows a greater area to be observed and gives a brighter image (see Fig. 8.1).

- *Electronic endoscope*
  The electronic endoscope is a further development of the fibre endoscope. A CCD chip acting as a miniaturized

television camera is mounted at its tip and allows an image to be transmitted to a monitor.

- *Chromoendoscope and zoom endoscope*
  A chromoendoscope allows cells to be stained. In gastroenterology, for example, areas of mucous membranes can be sprayed with a harmless pigment such as indigo carmine. This is actually not relevant for spine surgery.

Endoscopic spinal surgery requires coordination of the following:

- *Endoscopic surgical access*
  Using different thoracoscopic or laparoscopic portals or serial tubular dilators
- *Operative guidance*
  Intraoperative fluoroscopy is essential to confirm the working level.
- *Endoscopic visualization*
  Digital imaging, endoscopic considerations and illumination
- *Endoscopic surgical instruments*
  Dissection tools, retractors, irrigation, suction, haemostasis, cautery and endoscopic drills
- *Spine implants for endoscopic use*

8.4   Endoscopy in Spine Surgery

8.4.1   Anterior Cervical Spine

Endoscopically assisted transoral surgery represents an alternative to standard microsurgical techniques for transoral approaches to the anterior cervicomedullary junction [6].

The anterior approach is very similar to the traditional microsurgical approach, with the neurovascular sheath being positioned lateral to the working channel and the visceral structures medial to the working channel. The tip of the working sleeve is positioned against the anterior longitudinal ligament and the edge of the anterior part of the adjacent vertebral bodies. The disc space can then be passed without performing a discectomy, which is not possible with traditional microsurgery. Herniectomy and, if necessary, removal of osteophytes are carried out with suitable instruments including burrs, trephines, microresectors, various types of forceps, drills, hooks and bipolar microelectrodes. Using this approach, the foraminal areas and the spinal canal can be reached with excellent control of the operating field, but the interpedicular space is not accessible. In the cervical spine—more than in the other segments of the spine—an anterior endoscopic approach facilitates the effective anatomical decompression of the spinal canal and/or the nerve roots (plus in select cases, even the vertebral artery) without requiring replacement of the disc by fusion or arthroplasty.

There is usually no need for a drain or for post-operative immobilization.

8.4.2   Posterior Cervical Spine

The approach and the surgical technique are similar to traditional surgery but are performed using a working tube of varying diameters and the typical endoscopic instruments mentioned for the anterior approach. Fessler and Khoo [7] have reported on minimally invasive cervical microendoscopic foraminotomy in 25 patients.

8.4.3   Anterior Thoracic Spine

With the aid of thoracoscopy and mediastinoscopy, and using specially adapted trocars and instruments, spine operations can be carried out either entirely endoscopically or with endoscopic assistance. Using thoracoscopy, for example, it is possible to carry out decompression in cases of thoracic disc prolapse or instrumented procedures with additional ventrolateral plating. In 1994, Rosenthal et al. [3] reported the first excision of a herniated thoracic disc by thoracoscopic surgery. Video-assisted thoracoscopic surgery can be used for a variety of spinal indications [8, 9]. The nerve roots and the spinal cord can be decompressed, bone grafts can be placed for interbody fusion and vertebral body reconstruction and internal fixation can be applied to stabilize the thoracic spine [10] (Figs. 8.5 and 8.6).

8.4.4   Posterior Lumbar Spine

Interlaminar Approach

This approach is very similar to the traditional microsurgical approach. Access to the spinal canal is via a limited flavotomy, and the risks of damaging the dura or neural structures are similar to those applying to the microsurgical approach. Depending on the angle of entry into the interlaminar window in the sagittal plane and the level treated, it may be easy or difficult to actually reach the posterior aspect of the disc. The interpedicular region is very difficult to reach if at all, as is the contralateral side of the ventral epidural space. If the interlaminar window is very small, this approach may not be feasible without resection of the laminar edge and/or the medial aspect of the facet joint, especially with some of the more modern endoscopes that have a larger working channel but also a larger outer diameter.

One clear advantage is the easy convertibility to an open approach.

Posterolateral Approach

This is the best known foraminal approach to the lumbar spine and can be used for foraminal and extraforaminal disc herniations as well as for intradiscal procedures. It uses an angle of about 60 deg to the sagittal plane and approaches the

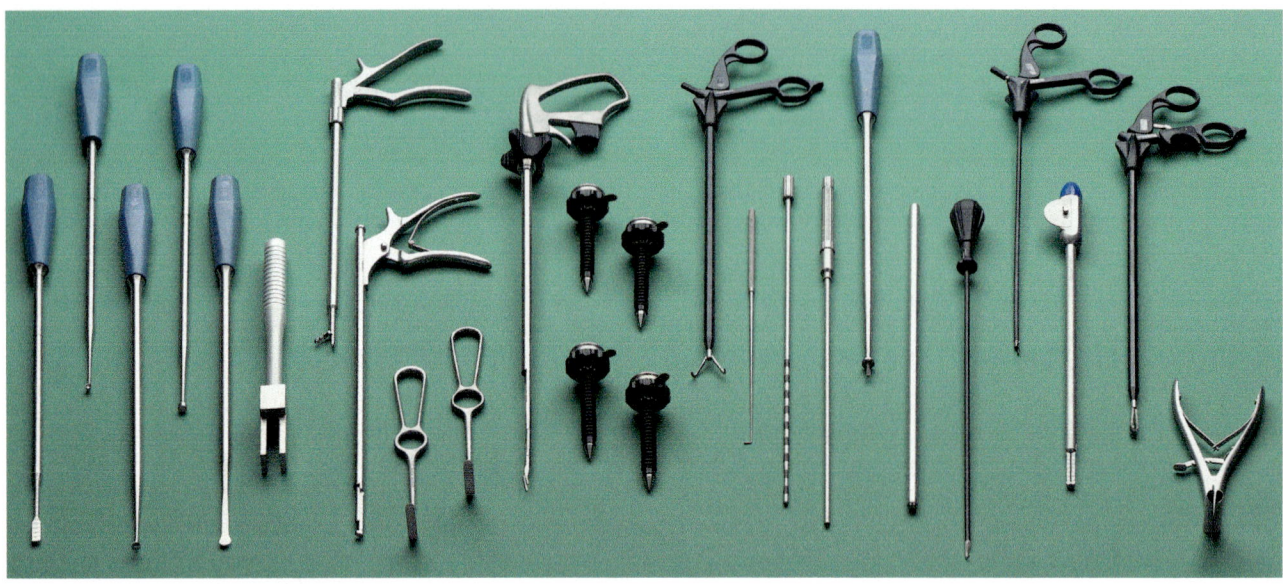

Fig. 8.5 Special long-stemmed instruments for the thoracoscopic preparation of prevertebral structures, discs and the bone (Miaspas TL, Aesculap) (with permission of Aesculap AG, Tuttlingen, Germany)

Fig. 8.6 Operating room set-up for endoscopic spine surgery with arrangement commonly used for thoracoscopy. The video monitors are in the surgeon's direct line of sight (with permission of Aesculap AG, Tuttlingen, Germany)

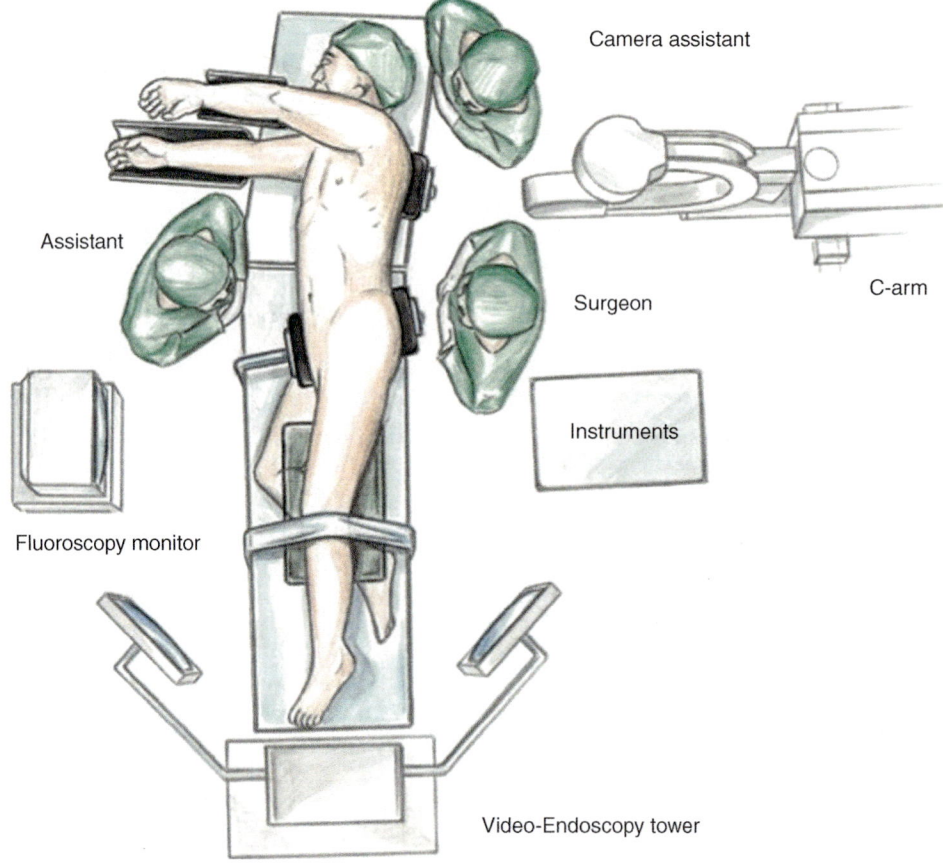

Fig. 8.7 Selective percutaneous endoscopic cervical decompression (PECD) by Dr. Hellinger (with permission of KARL STORZ Endoskope, Germany)

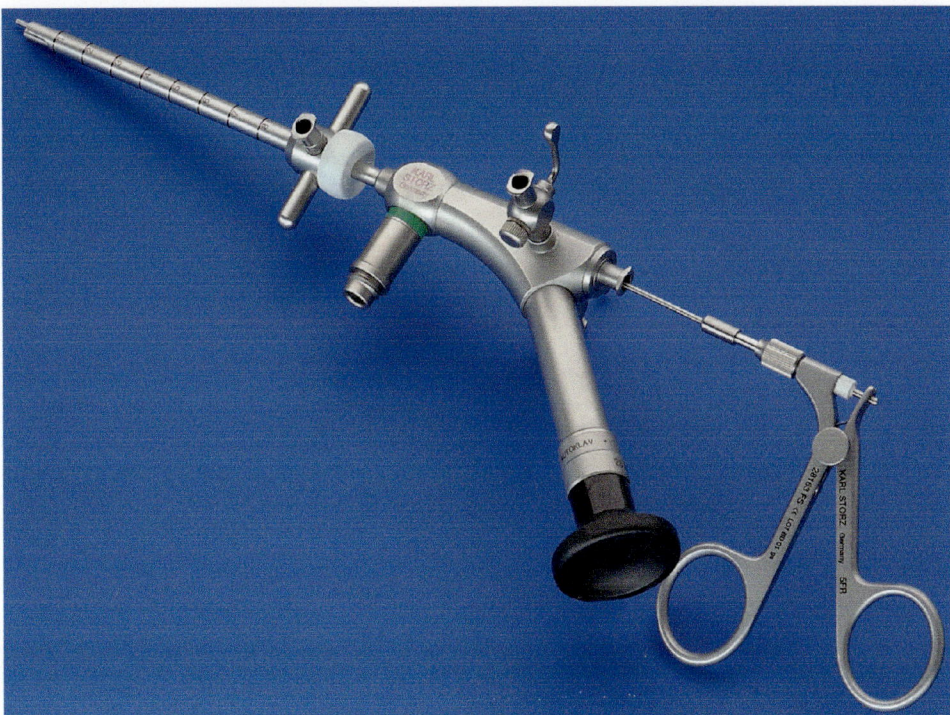

foramen at the level of the disc. It can be performed with the patient either prone or in a lateral decubitus position. The main intraoperative risks are damage to the exiting nerve root (especially where there is advanced loss of disc height) and to blood vessels. To gain adequate access, it is often necessary to ream the lateral aspect of the superior articular process, especially in patients with short pedicles and even without the presence of osteophytes at the facet joint. The ventral epidural space can only be reached in its lateral aspect.

Far or Extreme Lateral Approach

This approach is a more recent development and has largely been pioneered by Ruetten et al. [4]. Using this approach, it is possible to reach the ventral epidural space (with the exception of the interpedicular area) and the foraminal and extraforaminal areas. The foramen is approached at an angle of slightly less than 90 deg to the sagittal plane. The skin is penetrated at about the level of the facet joints in the coronal plane. The patient should be placed in a prone position. This ensures that there is less interference with the facet joint that occurs with the posterolateral approach, but short pedicles and a large bulging disc can still make it difficult to reach the ventral epidural space. The operative risks are much the same as those applying to the posterolateral approach. There is a higher risk of injury to the dura and the added risk of injury to retroperitoneal organs at the upper lumbar levels. The retroperitoneal anatomy at the level of interest therefore needs to be examined using CT or MRI prior to performing this approach at higher lumbar levels.

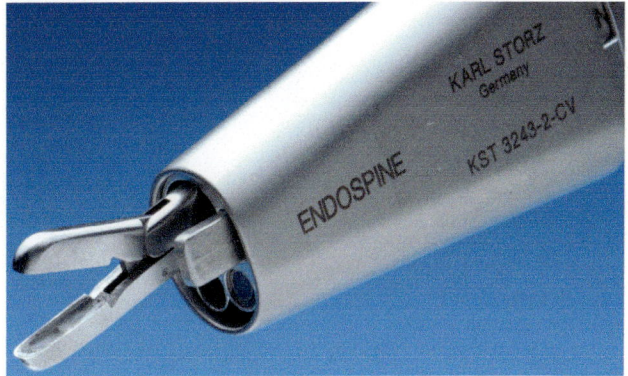

Fig. 8.8 ENDOSPINE operating tube (with permission of KARL STORZ Endoskope, Germany)

8.4.5   Anterior Lumbar Spine

Laparoscopy makes it possible to carry out various surgical procedures on the ventral spine. In 1991, Obenchaim [11] performed a laparoscopic L5–S1 discectomy followed, in 1992, by Bohlmann and Zdeblick's [2] L5–S1 fusion with laparoscopic placement of an interbody cage. Anterior arthrodesis has been performed by laparoscopic insertion of cages at the L4/L5 and L5/S1 levels [10]. Laparoscopic retroperitoneal techniques have been used for anterior plating to fixate the anterior column rigidly to restore stability [12].

The spinal endoscopy can be divided in percutaneous- (see Figs. 8.7, 8.8, 8.9 and 8.10, selective percutaneous endo-

Fig. 8.9 Thoracoscopic spine surgery—set according to Rosenthal (with permission of KARL STORZ Endoskope, Germany)

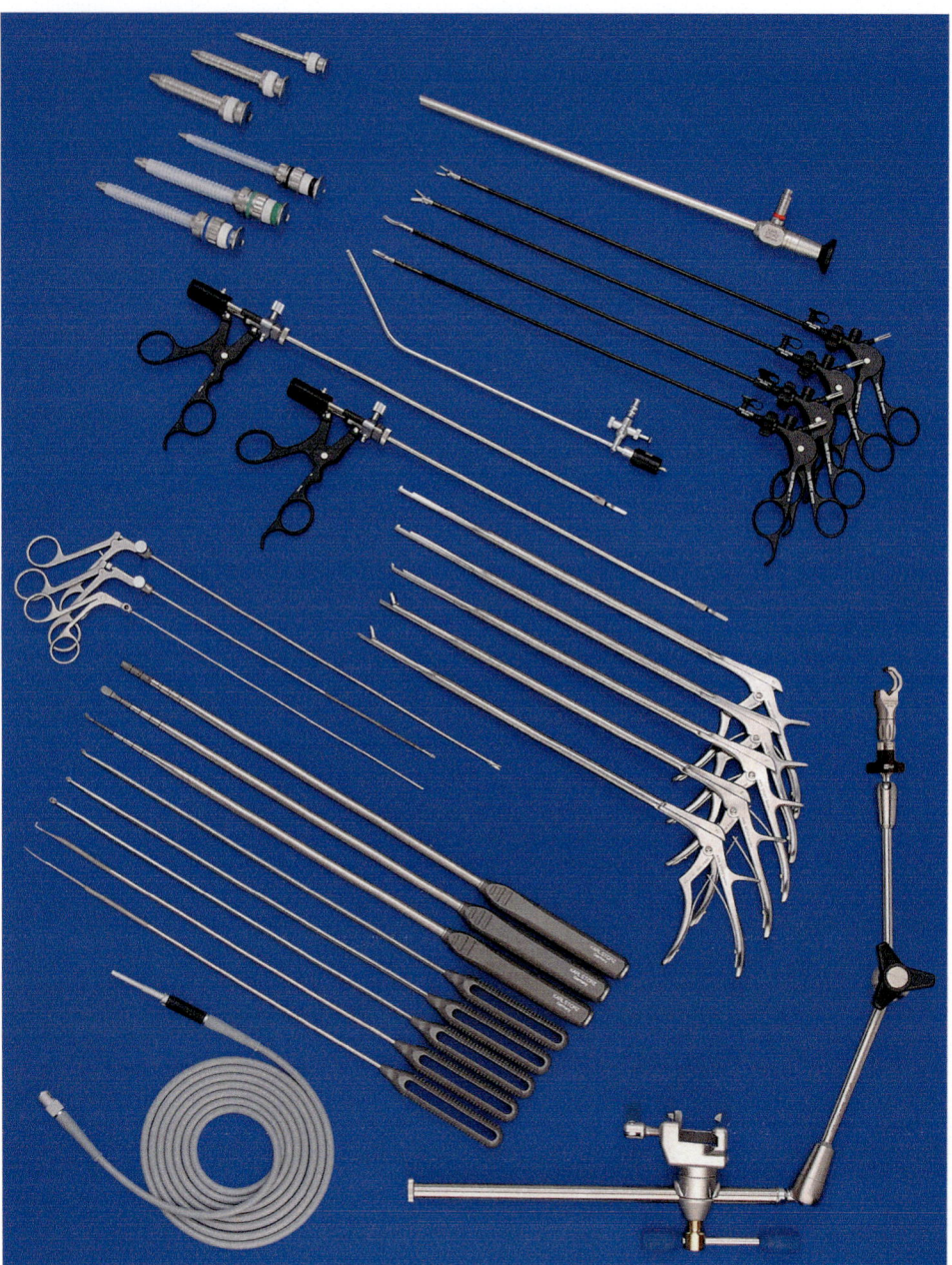

scopic cervical decompression (PECD); ENDOSPINE operating tube; thoracoscopic spine surgery, set according to Rosenthal; percutaneous lumbar transforaminal endoscopy, KARL STORZ Endoskope) or endoscopic-assisted (EASYGO!, KARL STORZ Endoskope) techniques.

8.5   Tips and Tricks

- Endoscopes are precision instruments and must be handled with care. Any damage to the shaft or excessively hard knocks can cause the lenses to become loose or slip inside the instrument. A typical sign of this is clouding of the eyepiece which can lead to a

complete breakdown if the endoscope is subjected to further damage.

- The end of the shaft containing the prism must be protected from high temperatures. All manufacturers give their own recommendations, but an upper limit between +65°C and +70°C is common. Some manufacturers achieve upper limits between +150°C and +200°C.
- If the glass fibres in a flexible endoscope are damaged or subjected to extreme bending, the individual glass fibres may break. This causes small black dots to appear in the endoscopic image.
- To learn these techniques, it is essential that surgeons receive adequate training. This includes practice with cadaver and in vivo models, preceptorships and proctor-

Fig. 8.10 Percutaneous lumbar transforaminal endoscopy (with permission of KARL STORZ Endoskope, Germany)

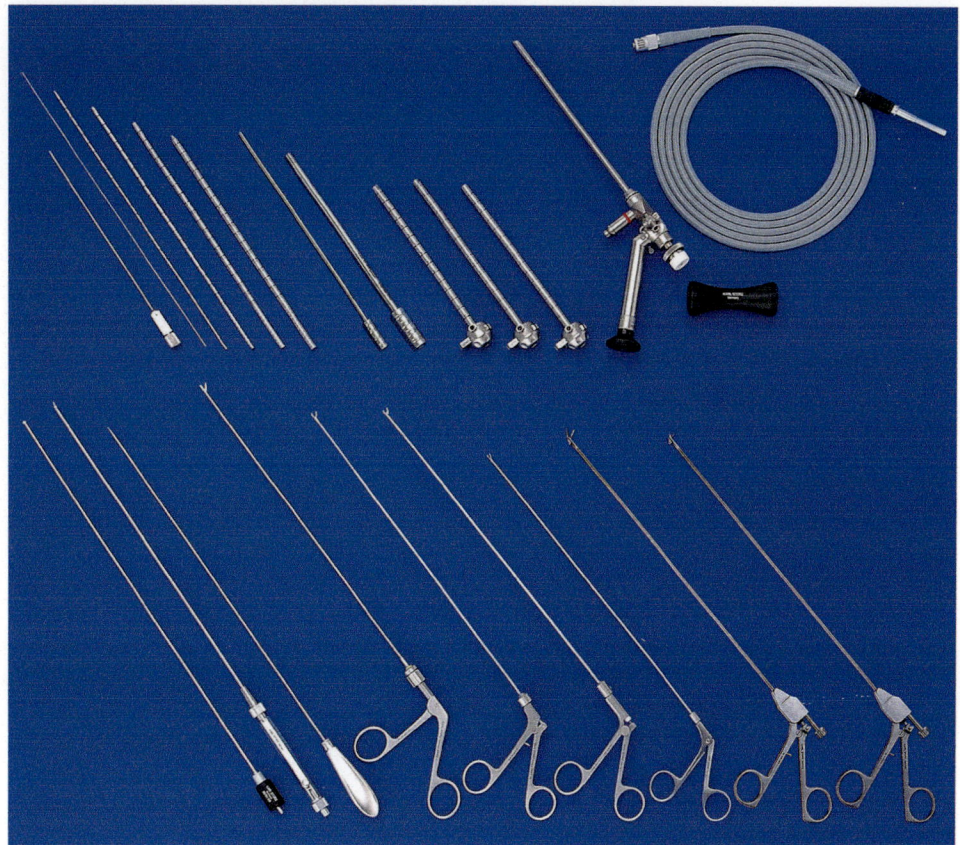

ship training and, ultimately, teaching in residency and spinal fellowship programmes.

References

1. Beisse R, Potulski M, Beger J, et al. Entwicklung und klinischer Einsatz einer thorakoskopisch implantierbaren Rahmenplatte zur Behandlung thorakolumbaler Frakturen und Instabilitäten. Orthopade. 2002;31:413–22.
2. Bohlmann H, Zdeblick T. Anterior excision of herniated thoracic discs. J Bone Joint Surg Am. 1988;70:1038–47.
3. Rosenthal D, Rosenthal R, De Simone A. Removal of protruded thoracic disc using microsurgical endoscopy. Spine. 1994;19: 1087–91.
4. Ruetten S, Komp M, Merk H, et al. Full-endoscopic interlaminar and transforaminal lumbar discectomy versus conventional microsurgical technique: a prospective, randomized, controlled study. Spine. 2008;33:931–9.
5. Ruetten S, Meyer O, Godolias G. Endoscopic surgery of the lumbar epidural space (epiduroscopy): results of therapeutic intervention in 93 patients. Minim Invasive Neurosurg. 2003;46:1–4.
6. Frempong-Boadu A, Faunce W, Fessler R. Endoscopically assisted transoral-transpharyngeal approach to the craniovertebral junction. Neurosurgery. 2002;51:60–6.
7. Fessler RG, Khoo LT. Minimally invasive cervical microendoscopic foraminotomy: an initial clinical experience. Neurosurgery. 2002;51:37–45.
8. Raju S, Balabhadra V, Kim DH, et al. Thoracoscopic decompression and fixation (MACS-TL). In: Kim DH, Fessler RG, Regan JJ, editors. Endoscopic spine surgery and instrumentation. New York: Thieme; 2005.
9. Waisman M, Saute M. Thoracoscopic spine release before posterior instrumentation in scoliosis. Clin Orthop. 1997;336:130–6.
10. Kim DH, Jaikumar S, Kam AC. Minimally invasive spine instrumentation. Neurosurgery. 2002;5:15–25.
11. Obenchaim TG. Laparoscopic discectomy: case report. J Laparoendosc Surg. 1991;1:145–9.
12. Mack MJ, Regan JJ, Bobechko WP. Application of thoracoscopy for diseases of the spine. Ann Thorac Surg. 1993;56:736–8.

Equipment for Full Endoscopic Spinal Surgery

9

Sebastian Ruetten

9.1 Introduction and Core Messages

Minimally invasive techniques can reduce tissue damage. Endoscopic operations have advantages which have raised these procedures to the standard in various areas. In arthroscopy, working with rod-lens optics under continuous fluid irrigation has proven valuable. In addition to reduced traumatization, improved visual and light conditions are achieved. Full endoscopic operations on the lumbar spine can usually be performed uniportal via trans-/extraforaminal or interlaminar approaches. Analogous to the arthroscopy, there is a continuous intraoperative irrigation. Since usually only one access is used, the instruments must be inserted through an intraendoscopic working canal. These days, the equipment available offers operation technical possibilities comparable to those known from microscope-assisted surgery.

9.2 Definition of Spinal Endoscopy

Full endoscopic technique is the term for a relatively newly developed method for endoscopic uniportal operations of the lumbar spinal canal and adjacent structures under constant visual control and continuous intraoperative irrigation via a minimally traumatizing access using rod-lens optics with an intraendoscopic working canal. On the lumbar spine, there are existing two different surgical approaches: the trans-/extraforaminal approach through or outside the intervertebral foramen and the interlaminar approach through the interlaminar window.

S. Ruetten (✉)
Department of Orthopädic Surgery, Center for Spine Surgery and Pain Therapy, Center for Orthopaedics and Traumatology, St. Anna-Hospital, Herne, Germany
e-mail: spine-pain@annahospital.de

9.3 Basic Equipment of Spinal Endoscopy

In addition to standard surgical accessories and small parts, the following basic equipment of the instruments we use (Richard Wolf GmbH, Knittlingen, Germany) are necessary for full endoscopic operations of the lumbar spine:

- *Rod-lens optics*
  The oval rod-lens optics have an outer diameter of maximal 6.9 mm and contain an eccentric working canal with a diameter of 4.1 mm. Moreover, the light source system and an irrigation canal are in the optics unit. The visual angle is 25 deg. The optics for trans-/extraforaminal and interlaminar accesses differ in their usable length (Fig. 9.1).

- *Access instruments*
  Access is made bluntly in the dilator technique.
  For the trans-/extraforaminal approach, the following instruments are necessary:
  - Spinal needle: for puncture of the target area in or outside the spinal canal
  - Target wire: for subsequent control of the dilators after removal of the spinal needle
  - Dilator creates the access for the final operation sheath
  - Operation sheath: for insertion of the optics after removal of the dilators

  For the interlaminar approach, the following instruments are necessary:
  - Dilator creates the access for the final operation sheath.
  - Operation sheath: to insert the optics after removal of the dilators.

  The operation sheaths have a beveled opening which creates a field of vision and work area in an area without clear anatomically preformed hollows. The irrigation fluid is drained off between the oval optics and round operation sheath. The operation sheaths for trans-/extraforaminal and interlaminar accesses differ in their usable length (Fig. 9.2).

U. Vieweg, F. Grochulla (eds.), *Manual of Spine Surgery*, https://doi.org/10.1007/978-3-662-64062-3_9

Fig. 9.1 Rod-lens optics with intraendoscopic working canal (with permission from Wolf Endoscope, Knittlingen, Germany)

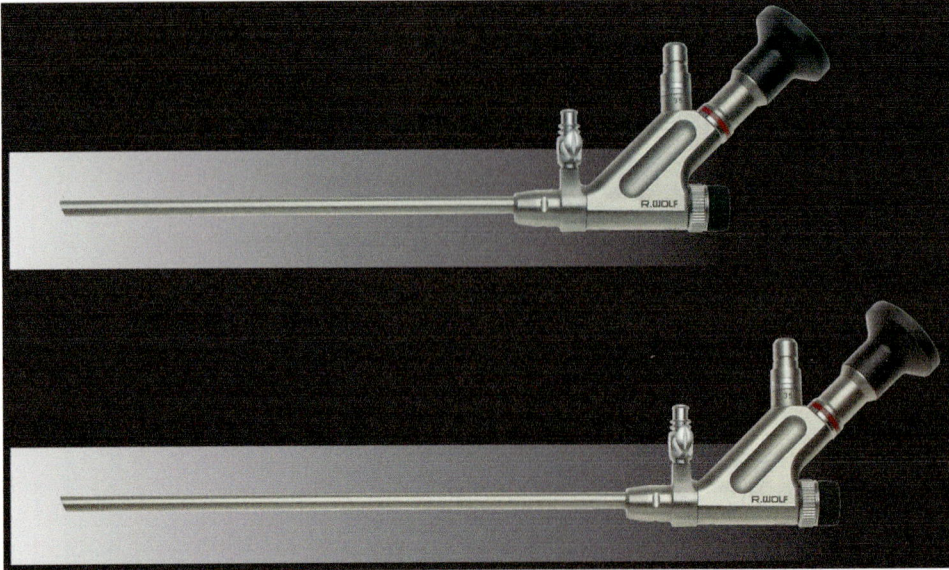

Fig. 9.2 Dilator and operation sheath (with permission from Wolf Endoscope, Knittlingen, Germany)

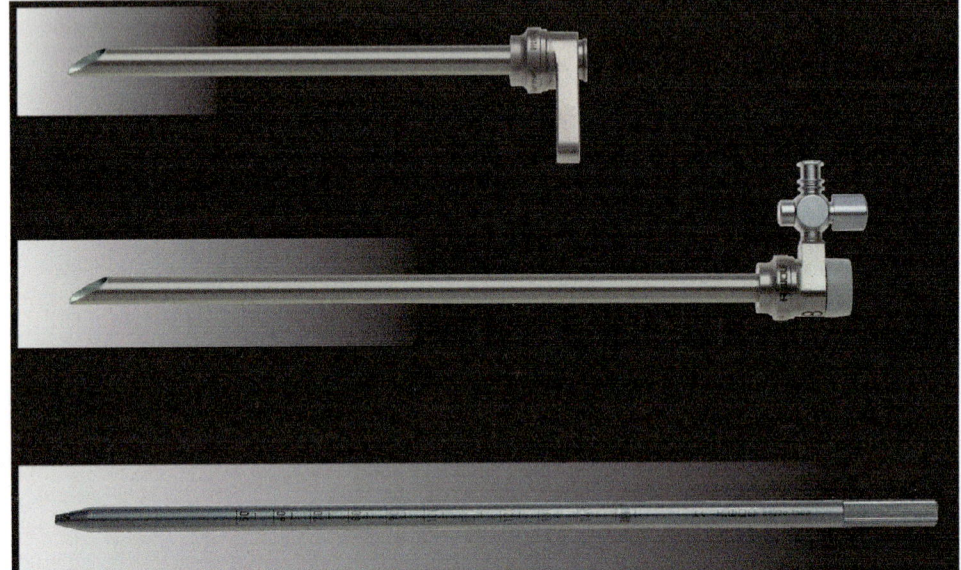

- *Manual instruments*
  The instruments are inserted through the intraendoscopic working canal of the optics. There is a wide variety of punches, shears, rongeurs, and other supplies with diameters from 2.5 to 4 mm. The manual instruments for the trans-/extraforaminal and interlaminar approach differ in their usable length (Fig. 9.3).
- *Motor-driven burrs and shavers*
  The burrs and shavers are also inserted via the working canal so that visualization is guaranteed at all times. For bone resection, there are various diamond and normal burrs in ball or oval shapes with various soft tissue protec-

tors. The diameter ranges from 2.5 to 4 mm. The shavers for nucleus resection have a diameter of 4 mm (Fig. 9.3).
- *Bipolar coagulation and preparation*
  For intraoperative coagulation and soft tissue preparation, there are semiactive flexible, bipolar ball electrodes. They are used with radiofrequency current which can reduce tissue damage in the immediate vicinity of neural structures.
- *Basic unit for endoscopic operations*
  In addition to the operation instruments and the optics, general instruments for endoscopic operations under fluid flow are needed, such as monitor, camera unit, light

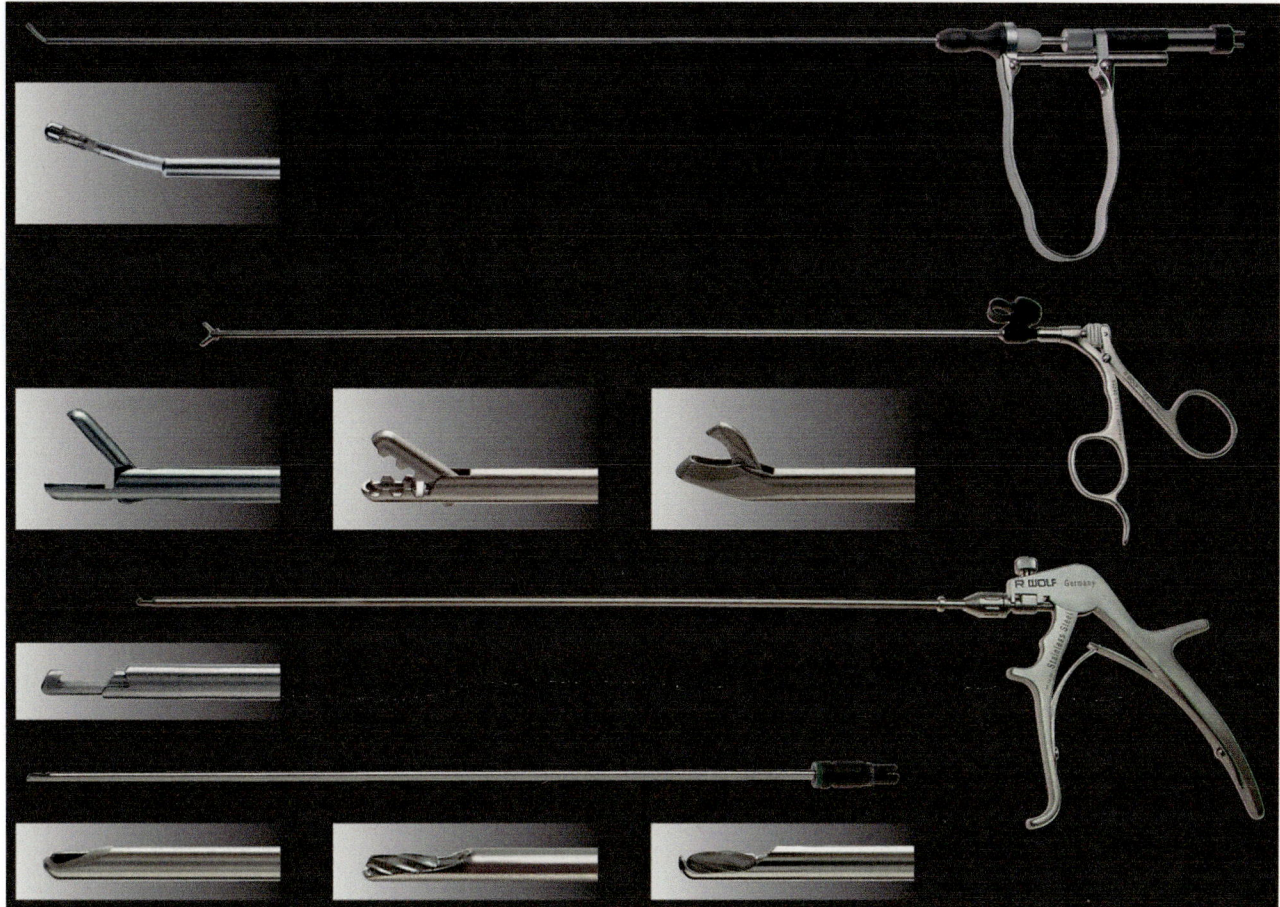

Fig. 9.3 Instruments and burrs (with permission from Wolf Endoscope, Knittlingen, Germany)

source, documentation system, fluid pump, shaver system, and radiofrequency generator. Some of the instruments available for arthroscopy or endoscopy can be used (Fig. 9.4).

- *Technical setup in the operating theater*
  An X-ray permeable, electrically adjustable operating table and a C-arm are needed. Positioning of the basic units and instruments is made individually and corresponding to the procedure in arthroscopy or endoscopy.

9.4 Tips and Tricks

- Observance of the general indications for the surgical procedure (decompression due to radicular or neurogenic symptoms)
- Observance of the specific indication criteria for the utilization of each approach (trans-/extraforaminal or interlaminar)

Transforaminal [1–4]
- In consideration of abdominal structure performance of a lateral approach to reach the spinal canal sufficiently under constant visualization
- Performance of the approach strictly to the caudal part of the disc level to avoid damaging of the exiting nerve root
- Performance of the extraforaminal approach in cases of intra-/extraforaminal disc herniations or foraminal stenosis
- In cases of insufficient mobility in the spinal canal resection of the ventral bony aspect of the ascending facet

Interlaminar [2–5]
- Performance of the skin incision as medial as possible to facilitate introducing of the endoscope in the spinal canal
- Preparation and identification of the lateral margin of the neural structures before mobilization to avoid damaging of the dura

Fig. 9.4 Endoscopy tower with basic equipment (with permission from Wolf Endoscope, Knittlingen, Germany)

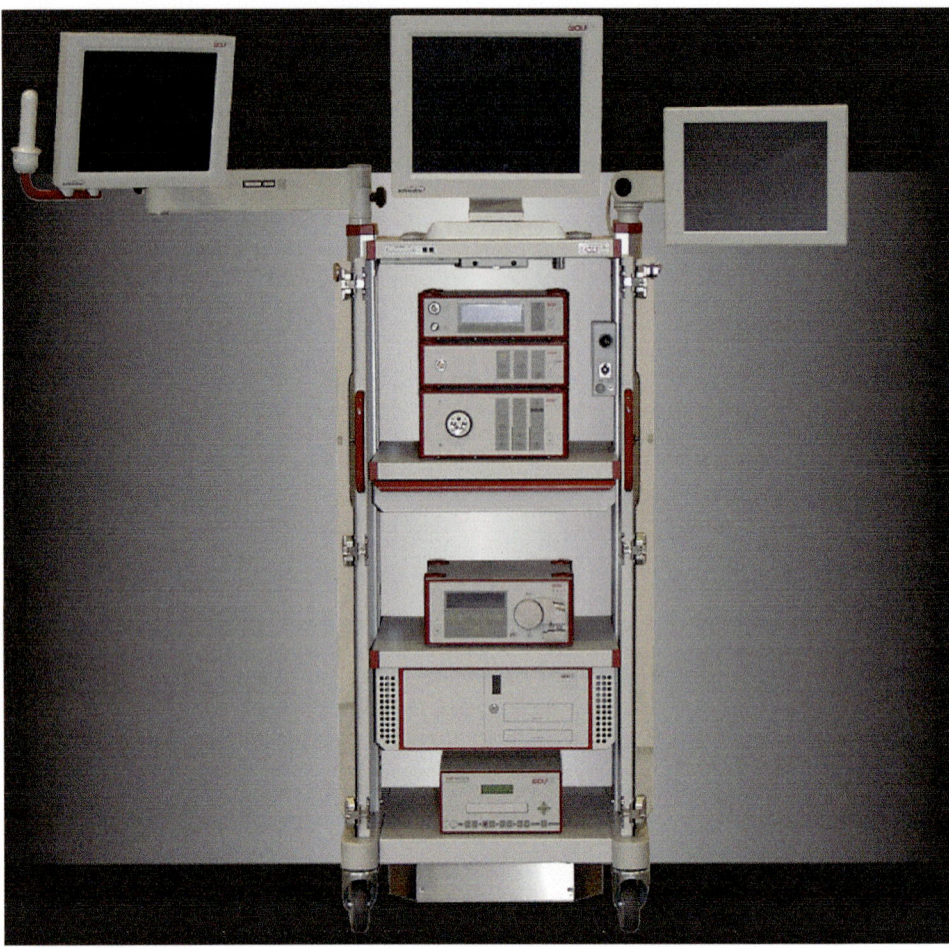

– Avoidance of immoderate retraction for a long time of the neural structures
– In cases of insufficient mobility in the spinal canal or during the approach resection of bony aspect

References

1. Ruetten S, Komp M, Godolias G. An extreme lateral access for the surgery of lumbar disc herniations inside the spinal canal using the full-endoscopic uniportal transforaminal approach. Technique and prospective results of 463 patients. Spine. 2005;30:2570–8.
2. Ruetten S, Komp M, Merk H, Godolias G. Use of newly developed instruments and endoscopes: full-endoscopic resection of lumbar disc herniations via the interlaminar and lateral transforaminal approach. J Neurosurg Spine. 2007;6:521–30.
3. Ruetten S, Komp M, Merk H, Godolias G. Full-endoscopic interlaminar and transforaminal lumbar discectomy versus conventional microsurgical technique: a prospective, randomized, controlled study. Spine. 2008;33:931–9.
4. Ruetten S, Komp M, Merk H, Godolias G. Recurrent lumbar disc herniation following conventional discectomy: a prospective, randomized study comparing full-endoscopic interlaminar and transforaminal versus microsurgical revision. J Spinal Disord Tech. 2009;22:122–9.
5. Ruetten S, Komp M, Merk H, Godolias G. Surgical treatment for lumbar lateral recess stenosis with the full-endoscopic interlaminar approach versus conventional microsurgical technique: a prospective, randomized, controlled study. J Neurosurg Spine. 2009;10:476–85.

Electrosurgery

10

Uwe Vieweg

10.1 Introduction and Core Messages

In electrosurgery, a high-frequency electric current is applied to the biological tissue as a means to cut, coagulate, desiccate or fulgurate the tissue. When a current is passed through the tissue, the cell liquid expands and evaporates, and the cell explodes, which causes the cutting or coagulation effect. This technique underlies many modern surgical procedures. It is therefore important for spine surgeons to be familiar with its basic physical principles and safety measures.

10.2 Definition

Electrosurgery uses high-frequency energy for cutting, cutting with simultaneous coagulation and coagulation procedures on the human tissue (synonyms: HF surgery, diathermia, electrocauterisation, electrosurgery). Today, high-frequency surgery or electrosurgery is an established feature in the different surgical disciplines. Most high-frequency surgical devices now work with frequencies of about 300–600 kHz (see Fig. 10.1). The advantages of high-frequency surgery are that bleeding is minimal, the high working temperature prevents contamination with microorganisms and the surgical procedure requires only a small skin incision.

10.3 Procedures and Devices

- Haemostasis and tissue cutting with high-frequency currents alone (e.g. MBC 200 Söring GmbH)
- Haemostasis and tissue cutting with high-frequency currents and additional helium gas as a carrier for the electric current (e.g. CPC 1000–1500–3000 cold plasma coagulation, Söring GmbH)
- Haemostasis and devitalisation of the tissue with high-frequency currents and additional ionised argon gas (e.g. VIO-APC 2 argon plasma coagulation, Erbe Elektro medizin GmbH)
- High-frequency-induced thermotherapy (tissue ablation) with high-frequency currents and hollow insulated shaft

U. Vieweg (✉)
Department of Conservative and Surgical Spine Therapy with Interdisciplinary Spinal Deformities Centre and Rummelsberg Sectional Center, Hospital Rummelsberg, Schwarzenbruck, Germany
e-mail: uwe.vieweg@sana.de

Fig. 10.1 Frequency range
for most high-frequency
electrosurgical devices

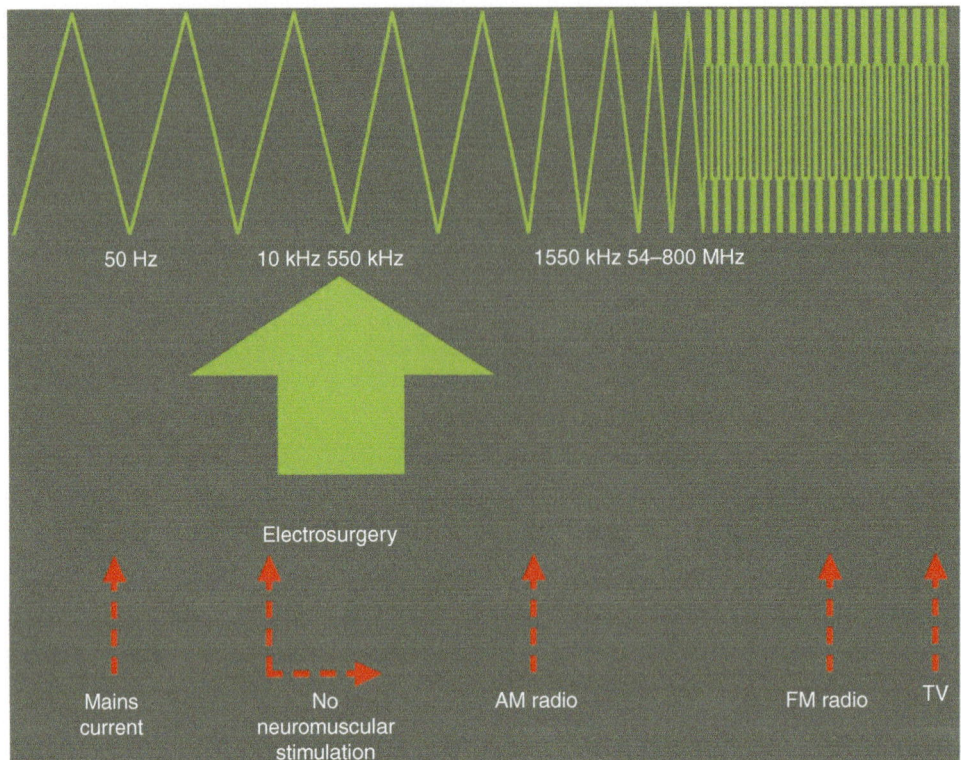

needle electrodes perfused with saline solution (e.g. Elektrotom HITT 106, Integra LifeSciences)

- High-frequency-induced thermotherapy of facet joints, for example, with high-frequency currents supplied through insulated needles specially positioned within the tissue (e.g. MultiGen RF generator, Stryker)

10.4 Manufacturers of High-Frequency Electrosurgical Generators

The manufacturers of high-frequency electrosurgical generators are the Aaron Medical Industries, adeor Medical Technologies GmbH, Aesculap AG, Elliquence, Ellman International, Erbe Elektromedizin GmbH, Gyrus ENT, Integra LifeSciences, MEGADYNE Medical Products, Naeem Jee Corporation, PEAK Surgical, Schuco, Söring GmbH and Stryker Valleylab.

10.5 Basic Physical Principles [1–5]

When a current is passed through the tissue, the cell liquid expands, and the cell explodes and evaporates, which causes the cutting or coagulation effect. Three effects are important when the body is subjected to an electric current: the Faraday effect, the electrolytic effect and the thermal effect. Nerve and muscle cells can be stimulated electrically. In the human

tissue, the stimulation effect is greatest with an alternating current of approximately 100 Hz. This effect decreases with increasing frequency, thus losing its damaging, or even life-threatening, action.

With high-frequency alternating currents, electrolysis and nerve stimulation occur only to a very small extent. According to Joule's law, the heat ΔQ produced per tissue volume ΔV is directly proportional to the resistivity ρ of the tissue and the square of the current density j, $\Delta Q = \rho \cdot j^2 \cdot \Delta V \cdot \Delta t$. Current densities of $j = 1$–6 A/cm² are usual. The body tissue has a higher electrical resistance than the metal cutting electrode. The flow of current therefore heats up the surrounding tissue but not the electrode. The effect is particularly strong close to the operating electrode because the whole current flows through a very small cross-sectional area of the tissue. At the neutral electrode, the returning current is spread out over a large area and thus causes only slight heating of the tissue. The degree of tissue heating caused by an electric current depends on the following factors: the current density, the resistivity of the tissue and the length of time for which current is applied.

The following variables influence the effect exerted on the tissue: power setting, size of electrode, time, manipulation of electrode, type of the tissue, waveform and eschar. The smaller the electrode, the greater is the current density. Consequently, the same tissue effect can be achieved with a smaller electrode, even though the power setting is reduced. At any given setting, the longer the generator is activated, the

Fig. 10.2 Illustration of the effects of the two electrosurgical processes—coagulation and incision—on the tissue (coagulation: energy dried out by heat-coagulated cell; incision: high energy density, fluid evaporates, cell expands, cell explodes) [6]

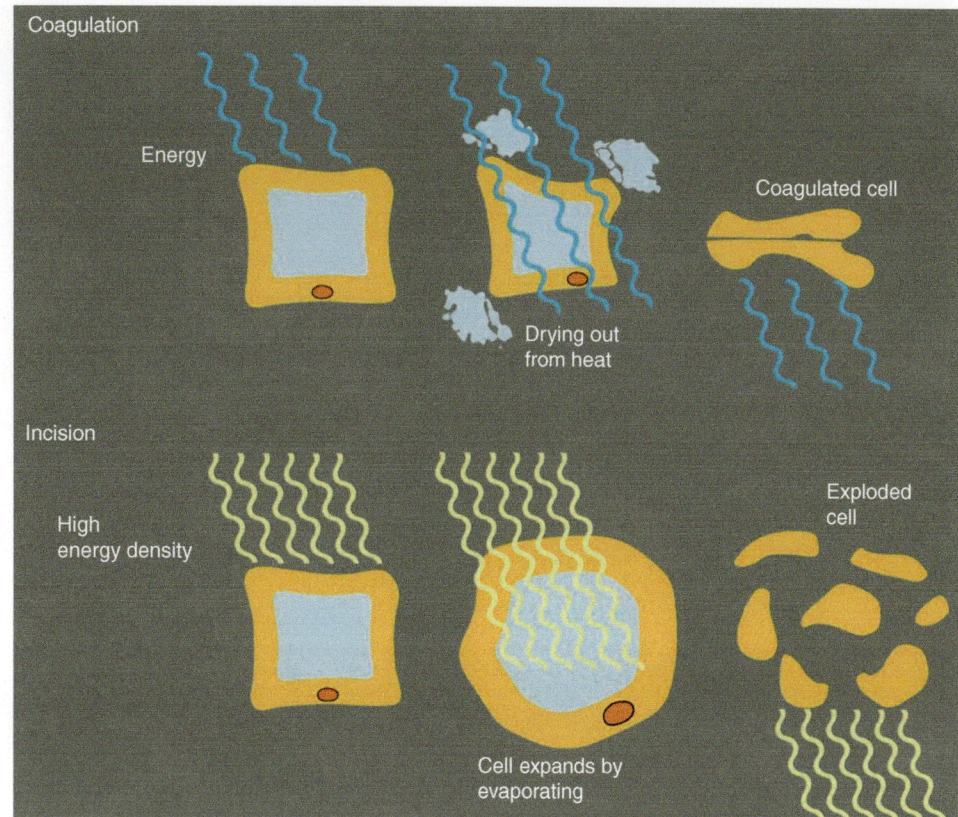

more heat is produced. The greater the heat, the farther it will travel to the adjacent tissue (thermal spread). Tissues vary widely in resistance. Eschar is relatively high in resistance to current. Keeping electrodes clean and free of eschar will enhance performance by maintaining lower resistance within the surgical circuit.

10.6 Effect of High-Frequency Current

The surgical effects of high-frequency currents can be divided into two main groups: cutting and coagulation [1, 3, 5–7]. Cutting severs the tissue, while coagulation dries the tissue out.

- Coagulation is the clotting of protein with reduction of volume and loss of water (see Fig. 10.2). Coagulation can be divided into deep and surface coagulation or into desiccation and fulguration (see Fig. 10.3). Desiccation refers to coagulation induced using an inserted needle electrode (contact coagulation). Fulguration or spray coagulation refers to surface carbonisation or surface coagulation caused by spark discharge from an electrode held close to the tissue (non-contact coagulation). The intra- and extracellular fluid is evaporated by sparks emitted from the tip of the electrode which is held a few millimetres from the tissue and moved over it. The main

difference between fulguration and desiccation is that fulguration does not involve contact between the tissue and the electrode. This effect is primarily used when sealing the tissue over a large surface. The depth of coagulation depends on the strength of the current used. If a large current is used, carbonisation occurs, and eschar forms which inhibits the spread of the heat to a greater depth. When the electrode is subsequently removed, the burnt tissue is removed as well because it sticks to the electrode tip. However, if a small current and a long duration of action are selected, the tissue around the electrode, down to a depth slightly greater than the diameter of the electrode, is vaporised. Coagulation can also be divided into the following categories depending on the qualities of the current used:

Soft coagulation (<190 V): In this case, no spark or arc of light occurs, and no unwanted cutting is caused. Carbonisation is prevented.

Forced coagulation (*up to* 2.35 kV *peak*): Arcs of light are produced in order to reach a greater coagulation depth. In the process, carbonisation cannot be avoided. Ball electrodes with a small surface area are usually used for this purpose.

Spray coagulation (*up to* 8 kV *peak*): In spray coagulation, long and powerful arcs of light are produced which heat the tissue both exogenously and endogenously. In

Fig. 10.3 Illustration of the effects of the two electrosurgical processes—coagulation and incision—and their subgroups (pure cut, blend cut, desiccation, fulguration) [6]

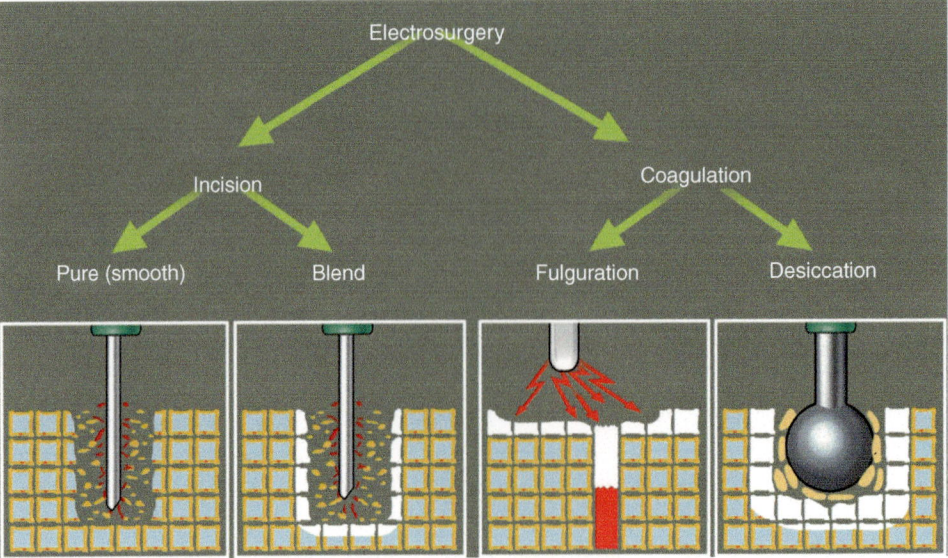

this process, no spark or arc of light occurs, and no unwanted cutting is caused.

- Incision involves cutting of the tissue with high-frequency current and electrodes with a small surface area. Explosive evaporation of cellular fluids at the site of the cut severs the tissue and coagulates it at the cut edges (see Fig. 10.2). Incisions are divided into pure cuts and blend cuts (see Fig. 10.3). A pure or smooth incision (cut) exerts as little lateral haemostatic effect as possible.

10.7 Electrode Configurations

Modern, high-frequency electrosurgical devices transfer electrical energy to the human tissue via a treatment electrode (in a bipolar or monopolar configuration) that remains cool (see Table 10.1). In the bipolar configuration, the voltage is applied to the tissue using special forceps of which one tine is connected to one pole of the generator and the other tine is connected to the other pole of the generator. When a piece of tissue is held with the forceps, a high-frequency electric current flows between the tines, heating the intervening tissue. In monopolar electrosurgery, the active electrode is in the surgical site. The patient's return electrode is attached somewhere else on the patient. The current must flow through the patient to the patient's return electrode. In the monopolar configuration, the patient is in contact with the return electrode, a relatively large or a flexible metallised plastic pad which is connected to the generator. The surgeon uses a pointed electrode to make contact with the tissue. The electric current flows from the electrical tip through the body to the return electrode and then back to the electrosurgical generator.

10.8 Safety Measures

- Insulation
  The patient must lie fully insulated on the operating table (dry drapes, plastic mats, etc.). He/she must also be insulated from all metal items and any tubes capable of conducting electricity. Dry cellulose pads are necessary in skinfolds, breastfolds and between extremities. For high-power surgical uses under anaesthesia, the monopolar modality relies on good electrical contact between return electrode and the body. If contact with the return electrode is insufficient, severe burns (third-degree) can occur in areas of poor contact with the return electrode or where contact is made with grounded metal objects serving as an unintended return path.

- Position and type of neutral electrode
  The neutral electrode should be placed as close to the operating area as possible and should have good contact with the patient tissue. So-called split return electrodes should always be used. These monitor the contact quality of the return electrode to the patient. The so-called return electrode monitoring (CQM) system (safety system) was developed to avoid burns under the return electrodes. This system measures the contact quality of the surface between the return electrode and the patient all the time, also while the generator is activated, and monitors every change during the entire surgical procedure.

- Anaesthesia equipment
  For preoperative monitoring, only ECG cables with high resistance inputs or HF choke may be used. Before the operation, it is important to ensure that the current from the active electrode to the return electrode is not conducted through the heart area or that any such conduction is minimised.

Table 10.1 Differences between the monopolar and bipolar configurations in electrosurgery

	Monopolar	Bipolar
Poles	Electrodes with small surface area in operating region, return via large area neutral electrode	Both poles are held directly over the tissue with forceps whose tines are insulated against each other. Current flows between the two poles only
Action	Strong local heating of the tissue at the electrode tissue junction (coagulation) and sparking and fulguration at high voltages	Local heating of the tissue only between the electrodes; coagulation as a result
Uses	Coagulation; desiccation; fulguration; tissue cutting, sometimes with sloughing/scab formation; blood vessel closure	Coagulation, good closure of blood vessels
Advantages	Many different applications possible with change of electrodes; rapid haemostasis	Small currents required (only about 20–30% of that needed for monopolar HF), route followed by current can be calculated, risk of burns
Disadvantages	Neutral electrode needs to be fixed, risk of burns if neutral electrode comes unstuck, current flow through the body cannot be precisely controlled, short circuiting possible via contact with earthed metal items	Tissue cutting, fulguration

10.9 Tips and Tricks

- Correct positioning (dry and insulated)
- No contact with grounded objects
- No skin-to-skin contact (between individual parts of the patient's body)
- Short cables, no contact to grounded metal parts
- No looping of cables and no fixation with metal brackets
- Cautious handling of disinfectants (the alcohol contained can be ignited by electric sparks)
- Return electrode monitoring (CQM) system (safety system)

10.10 Current Trends

Further developments in electrosurgery involve the use of helium gas (cold plasma coagulation) or ionised argon gas (argon plasma coagulation) which allows current flow without contact between electrode and the tissue. Both plasma coagulation techniques require no return electrode and do not involve current flow through the body or areas of vaporisation within the tissue. It therefore permits rapid and controlled haemostasis without major tissue damage.

References

1. Hainer BL. Fundamentals of electrosurgery. J Am Board Fam Pract. 1991;4:419–26.
2. Arnold P, Advincula WK. The evolutionary state of electrosurgery: where are we now? Curr Opin Obstet Gynecol. 2008;20:353–8.
3. Boughton RS, Spencer SK. Electrosurgical fundamentals. J Am Acad Dermatol. 1987;16:862–7.
4. Elliott-Lewis EW, Mason AM, Barrow DL. Evaluation of a new bipolar coagulation forceps in a new bipolar coagulation forceps in a thermal damage assessment. Neurosurgery. 2009;65(6):1182–7.
5. Vellimana AK, Sciubba DM, Noggle JC, et al. Current technological advantages of bipolar coagulation. Neurosurgery. 2009;64:11–9.
6. Hausmann V. High-frequency surgery. In: Krettek C, Aschemann D, editors. Positioning techniques in surgical applications. Heidelberg: Springer; 2006. p. 41–54.
7. Reidenbach HD. Fundamentals of bipolar high-frequency surgery. Endosc Surg Allied Technol. 1993;1:85–90.

Surgical Motor Systems in Spinal Surgery

11

Frank Grochulla and Uwe Vieweg

11.1 Introduction and Core Messages

Surgical motor systems are important power tools in microsurgical procedures at the cervical, thoracic and lumbar spine, whenever preparation and removal of the bone become necessary.

Motor systems are surgical instruments, which are divided in high- and low-speed systems. The motor systems are operating with electrical, pneumatic or Akku power source controlled by foot pedal or hand tip. Common power tools in spinal surgery are drill systems, bone saws and burrs. Especially high-speed drill systems are important tools for opening procedures of the spinal canal.

11.2 History

Important milestones were the invention of the first electric surgical motor in 1935 by Aesculap, the introduction of pneumatic power systems in the 1960s, the pioneering work with flexible cable motors in the 1970s, the battery-powered motor systems in the 1980s and the incorporation of pneumatic and electric high-speed systems in the 1990s. Power tools have undergone many improvisations and modifications in the past two decades and have improved tremendously in their functionality and versatility [1–4].

F. Grochulla (✉)
Metropol Medical Center, Clinic for Orthopedics, Trauma Surgery and Spinal Surgery, Nuremberg, Germany
e-mail: frank.grochulla@mmc-nuernberg.de

U. Vieweg
Department of Conservative and Surgical Spine Therapy with Interdisciplinary Spinal Deformities Centre and Rummelsberg Sectional Center, Hospital Rummelsberg, Schwarzenbruck, Germany
e-mail: uwe.vieweg@sana.de

11.3 Components and Technical Details

There are a number of surgical motor systems on the market. Differences exist in the source of power, the revolutions per minute (rpm) ranging from 10,000 rpm up to 90,000 rpm and more and the activation of the motor system (by hand or by foot).

11.3.1 Power Systems

- *Pneumatic high-speed power system* (HiLAN® XS, ComPact Air Drive II, Air Pen Drive, Synthes)
  The sterilisable coaxial flexible hose connects the pneumatic motor with a foot pedal.
- *Electric power system* (microspeed® uni Aesculap; Servotronic EC I/II 100, Medicon Instruments; Linotec E9000, Stryker; Zimmer surgical motor systems, Electric Pen Drive, Synthes) (Fig. 11.1)

The differences between electric and pneumatic power systems are in respect to personal preference and electric instead of pressured air.

Personal preference	Electric instead of pressured air
Noise level	Pneumatic systems generate a higher noise level than electric motor systems
Handling	Electric systems is easier to set up (no need for pressured air)
	Cable is more flexible and lighter than air hoses
Versatility	Electric system can usually cover more indication fields (low speed, high speed, pistol, shave in one system)
Individuality	Individual settings and acceleration/stopping characteristics
	Oscillation angle, etc., can be adjusted via the control unit to individual preferences
Price	Electric systems tend to be more expensive than pneumatic ones

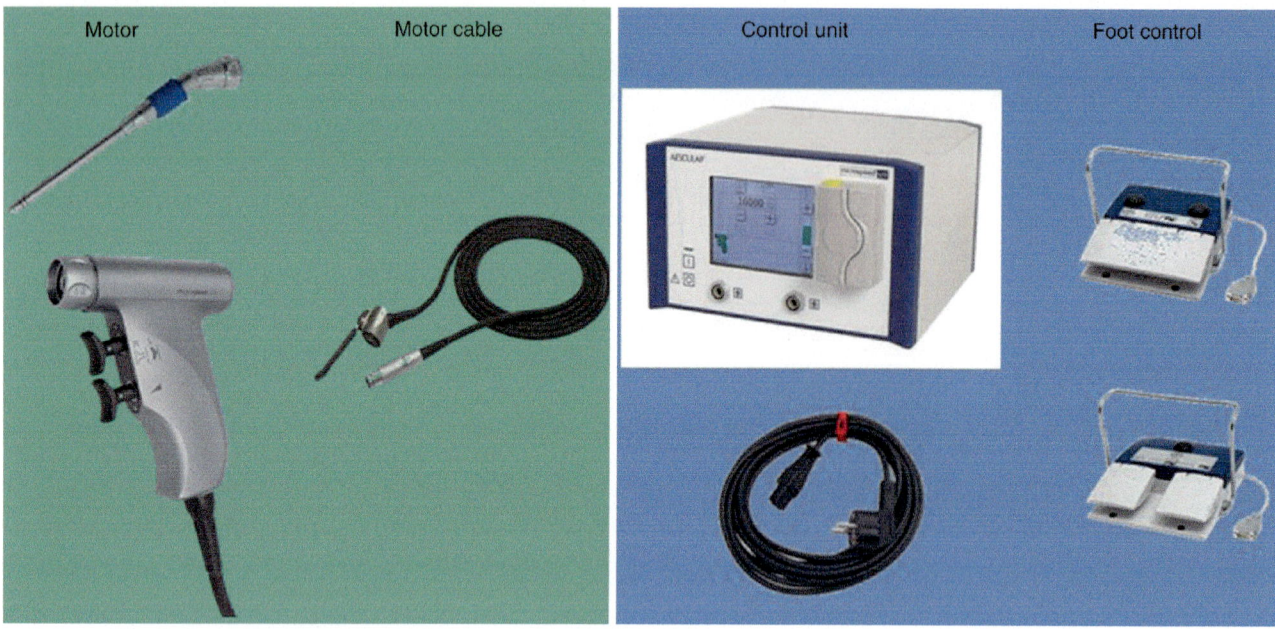

Fig. 11.1 Components of surgical motor systems (motor unit, handpiece, control unit, connecting cable, foot control) (with permission of Aesculap AG, Tuttlingen, Germany)

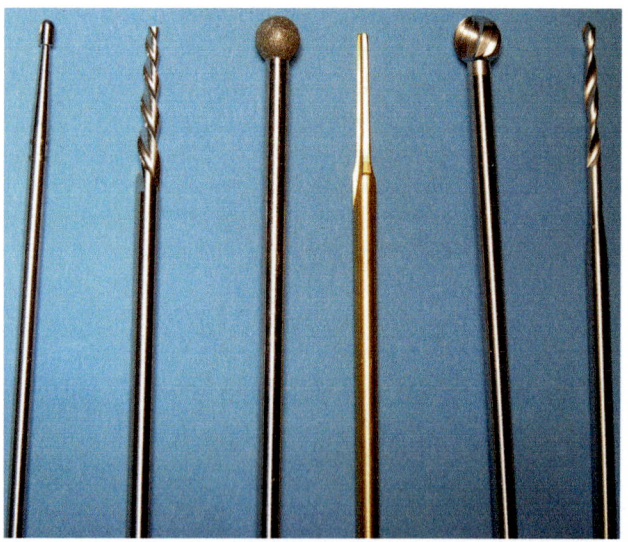

Fig. 11.2 Cutting and diamond burrs, Rosen burr and diamond burr

11.3.2 Accessories

The motor systems consist of various *attachments* (burrs, drills, saws). Burrs and drills are available in different sizes and shapes (Fig. 11.2). The more aggressive cutting burrs (cylindrical burr, Rosen burr) are applicable to remove the hard cortical and cancellous bone. These cutting burrs should not be used in the spinal canal because of the risk of tearing the soft tissue (dura, neural structures). Less aggressive burrs such as diamond burrs are more applicable for preparing in the near of important soft tissue structures such as vessels, nerves and dura.

The *handpieces* are available in angulated or straight designed shape. Angulated handpieces are more useful in microsurgical procedures. *Irrigation* is always necessary when using a high-speed motor system in order to avoid local hyperthermic reactions. Continuous irrigation should

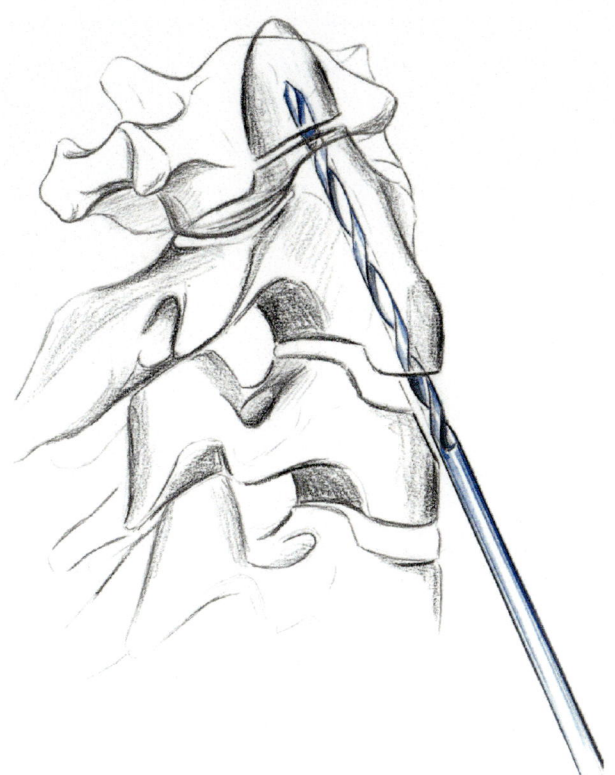

Fig. 11.3 Pre-drilling for osteosynthesis screws (with permission of Aesculap AG, Tuttlingen, Germany)

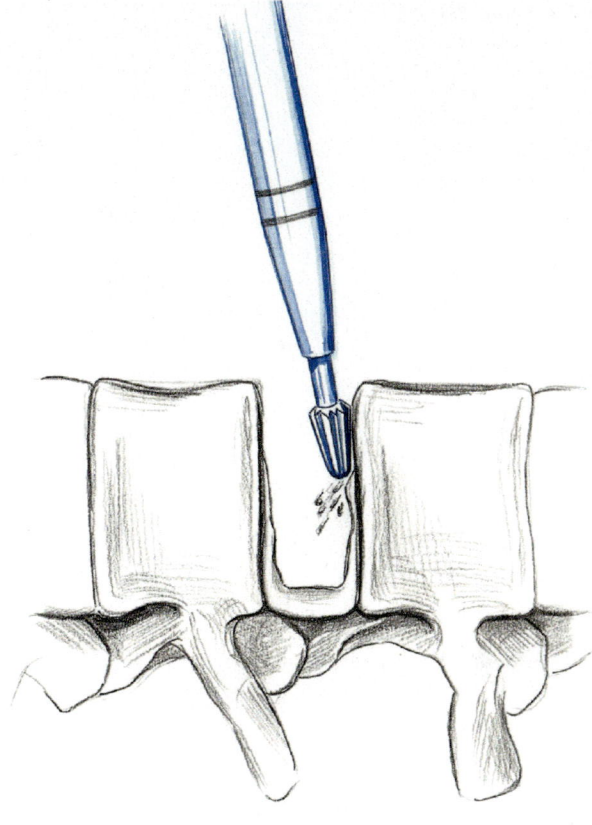

Fig. 11.5 Preparation of implant bed for corpectomies or interbody fusions (with permission of Aesculap AG, Tuttlingen, Germany)

be used with an integrated irrigation system which provides an electronically controlled permanent irrigation. If not available, a simple irrigation by using a syringe is possible.

11.4 Indications

All the different systems available for varied indications on the spine are the following:

- Decortications/pre-drilling for distraction, pedicle or osteosynthesis screws with a high-speed burr or high-speed drill (see Figs. 11.2 and 11.3)
- Preparation of implant bed for corpectomies or interbody fusions (see Fig. 11.4)
- Harvesting and modelling of autologous bone graft with saws/high-speed or low-speed burrs (see Figs. 11.5 and 11.6)
- Decompression/access preparation (laminoplasty, laminotomy, laminectomy, facetectomy, foraminotomy) with a high-speed or low-speed burr or laminectomy drill/craniectomy (see Figs. 11.7, 11.8, 11.9, 11.10 and 11.11)

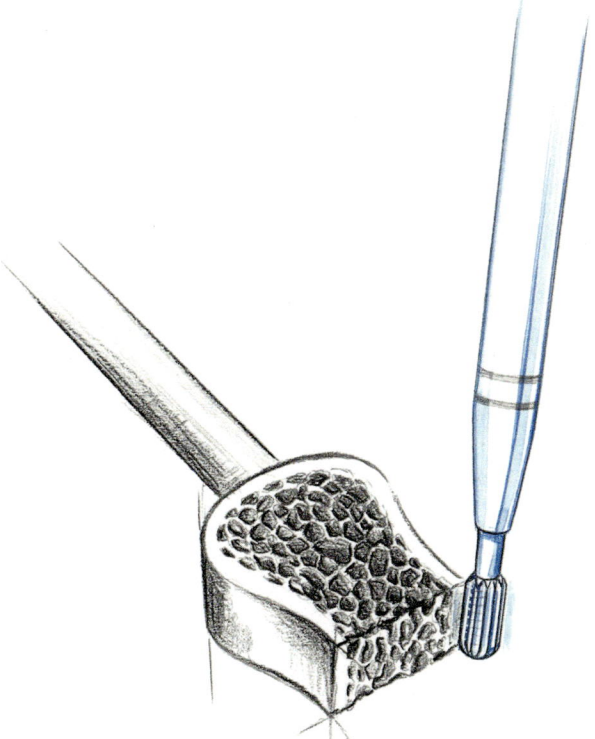

Fig. 11.4 Decortications/pre-drilling for distraction, pedicle or osteosynthesis screws with a high-speed burr or high-speed drill (with permission of Aesculap AG, Tuttlingen, Germany)

Figs. 11.6 and 11.7 Harvesting and modelling of autologous bone graft with saws/high-speed or low-speed burrs (with permission of Aesculap AG, Tuttlingen, Germany)

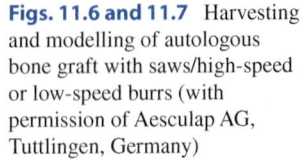

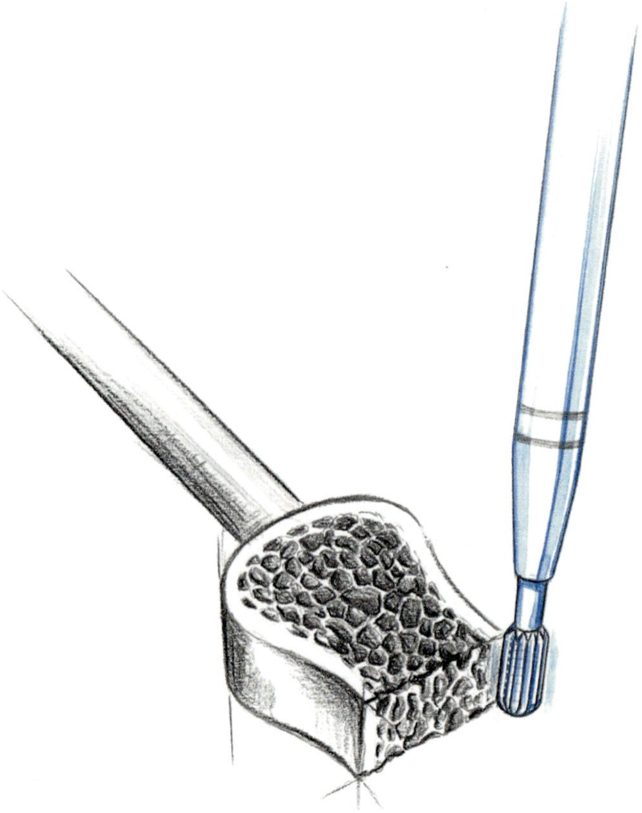

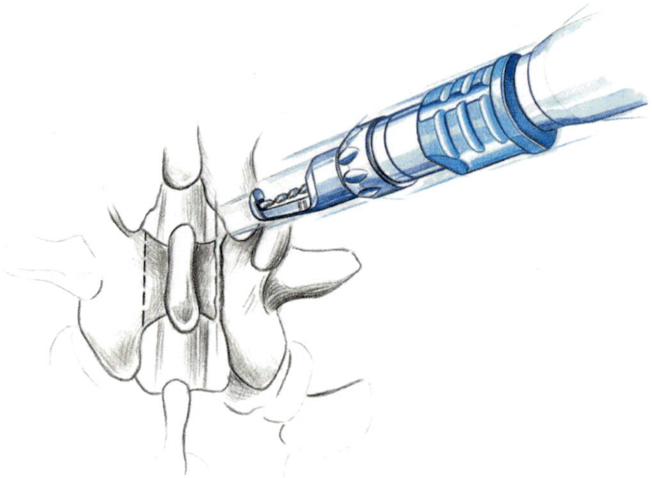

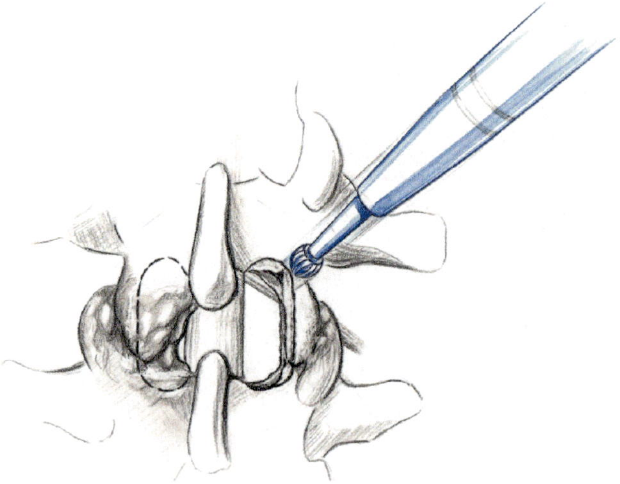

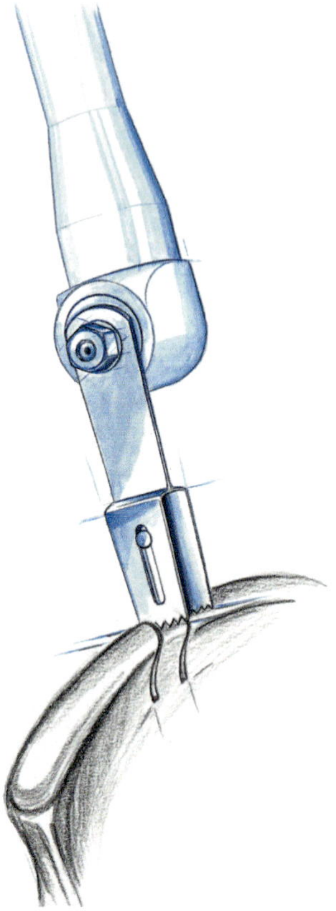

Figs. 11.8 and 11.9 Access preparation (laminoplasty, laminotomy, laminectomy facetectomy, foraminotomy) with a high-speed or low-speed burr or laminectomy craniectomy drill (with permission of Aesculap AG, Tuttlingen, Germany)

Fig. 11.10 Vertebral body resection with a long handpiece over a mini-thoracotomy (with permission of Aesculap AG, Tuttlingen, Germany)

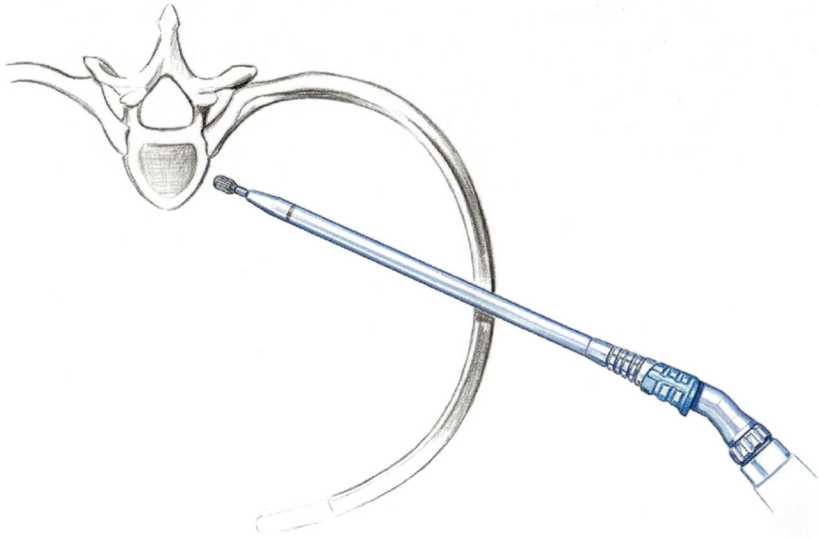

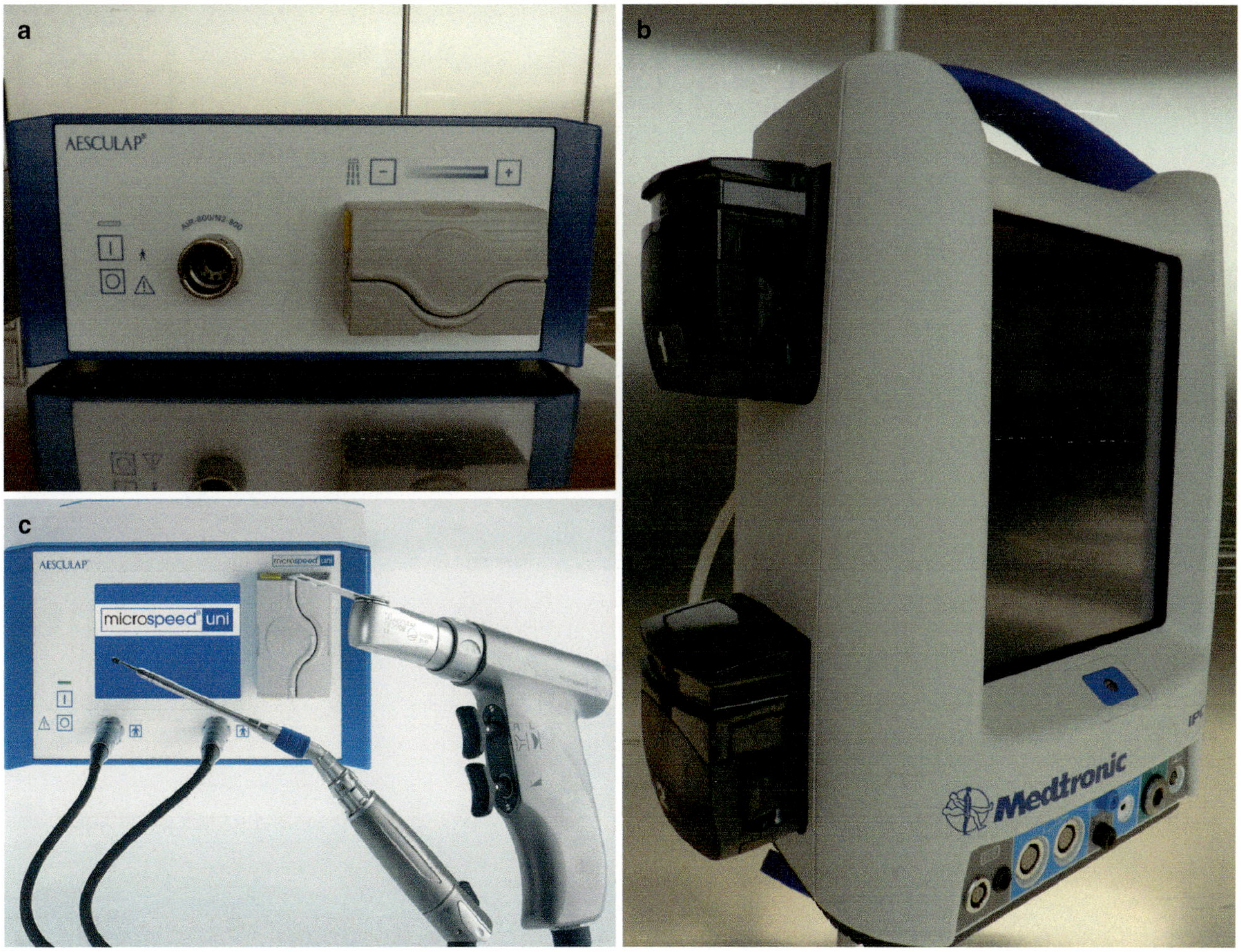

Fig. 11.11 (**a**) Pneumatic motor (HiLAN, Aesculap), (**b**) electric motor system (Midas Rex Legend, Medtronic) and (**c**) electric motor system with different handpieces (HiLAN, Aesculap) (with permission of Aesculap AG, Tuttlingen, Germany)

11.5   Tips and Tricks

- Lubricating the power systems is a simple and safe affair. The motor and handpieces are sprayed with special oil spray before sterilisation cycle.
- Complete lubrication of the motor and handpieces is ensured, making permanent intraoperative lubrication unnecessary.
- Before use, the instrument should be completely checked by the surgeon.
- A high-speed burr with foot pedal should be controlled by the surgeon only.
- Always work with intact and sharp tools (drills) to avoid damage or overheating of the motor system.

References

1. Albee FH. Some scientific aspects of orthopaedic surgery. J Bone Joint Surg Am. 1929;XI:696.
2. Beer RR, et al. Biorobotic approaches to the study of motor systems. Curr Opin Neurobiol. 1998;8(6):777–82.
3. Dyas FG. The treatment of acute osteomyelitis of the long bones by means of the dental engine and a large burr: preliminary report. JAMA. 1914;LXII(1):216.
4. Kale S. Power tools in orthopaedic surgery – an update. Orthop Prod News. 2008;48:56–62.

Bone Grafts and Bone Graft Substitutes

12

Robert Morrison

12.1 Introduction and Core Messages

Bone grafts or substitutes are used in spinal surgery to fill defects, to bridge defects or to promote spondylodesis. The physiological process is similar to that of fracture healing and incorporates the same spatial and temporal factors. The ideal material should provide osteogenetic, osteoinductive and osteoconductive properties. The traditional autologous bone grafts are probably still considered the "golden standard", but the problems associated with them bring up the need for substitutes. One alternative is the acquirance of allogenic or xenogenic bone grafts, which have specific problems of their own, which limit their use. The other aspect is the use of bone substitutes, which come in a growing variety of materials, shapes and application forms. Currently, none of these substitutes unite all of the prerequisites shown above, but they have the advantage of unlimited supply without causing additional problems such as donor site morbidity. And the combination of such substitutes as scaffold with the utilization of growth factors and mesenchymal stem cells brings with them a completely new array of possibilities.

12.2 Definition

12.2.1 Bone Graft

The bone is harvested from different parts of the patient. It is most commonly from the iliac crest but also from the vertebral structures, the ribs, the tibia as well as the fibula [1].

R. Morrison (✉)
Spine & Scoliosis Center, Asklepios Klinik Bad Abbach, Germany
e-mail: dr.morrison@web.de

12.2.2 Bone Graft Substitute

It replaces the autologous bone in order to achieve defect filling and bridging and also fusion [2]. It provides unlimited supply and eliminates donor site morbidity. But no substitute provides the combination of osteoinductive, osteoconductive and osteogenetic properties [1].

12.3 Physiology of Bone Regeneration

The bone is one of the few organs that retains the potential for regeneration throughout life. In contrast to other organs, the bone does not repair defects with scar material of poor quality but rather reinstates its original values. But fracture healing and therefore also bone regeneration are complex physiological processes.

Two basic principles of bone healing are described in literature [3] as follows:

- Primary bone healing ("direct healing") is very rare and not the usual form of healing achieved in spinal surgery.
- Secondary bone healing involves intramembranous and endochondral ossification and leads to callus formation. Callus formation is achieved through undifferentiated multipotent mesenchymal stem cells (MSCs) and requires cell vitality and blood supply.

In this cascade of bone regeneration, certain prerequisites are known. Most importantly, a vital cell population has to be present. MSCs have to be either present or transferred to the site via blood supply. These cells are transferred to a cell population with osteoblastic phenotypes.

In addition, the fracture haematoma offers a vast supply of signalling molecules (ILs, TNFs, TGFs, VEGF) to induce healing. Within the group of TGFs, the so-called bone morphogenetic proteins (BMP-2, BMP-7) have been extensively studied and shown to play a decisive role in the healing process [4]. The third important element is the extracellular matrix, providing a natural scaffold for the cellular interactions. This

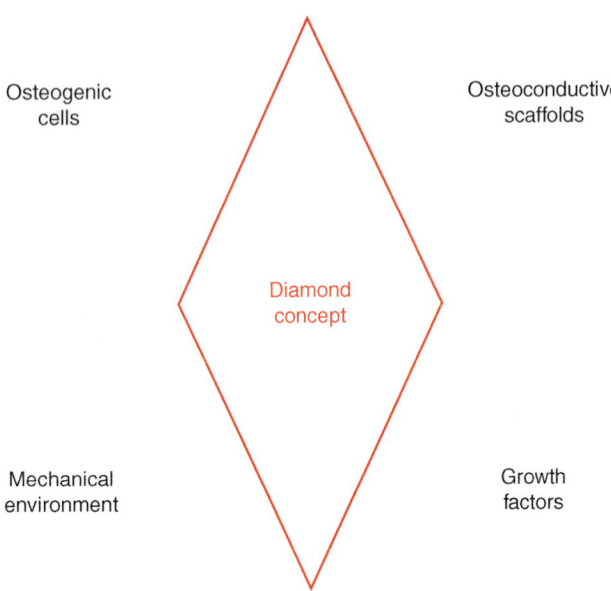

Osteogenic cells

Osteoconductive scaffolds

Diamond concept

Mechanical environment

Growth factors

Fig. 12.1 "Diamond concept" regarding bone healing [5]

can be replaced by an immense number of osteoconductive materials such as allografts, demineralized bone matrix (DBM), hydroxyapatite and calcium-based ceramics, among others. These scaffolds have been shown to have an optimal pore size of 150–500 µm. The last important factor, important for fracture healing and bone formation, is the mechanical stability. All four components combined are described as the "diamond concept" (Fig. 12.1). It is well described in extremity fractures and of equal importance in spinal surgery [5].

12.4 Clinical Application

Therefore, bone or bone substitutes should preferably have the three properties mentioned above. **Osteogenicity** refers to the fact that they contain osteoblastic cells and are thereby capable of directly forming the bone. **Osteoconductivity** refers to the situation in which they provide a structure along which osteoblasts can attach and thereby the bone can grow. **Osteoinductivity** is the ability to induce nondifferentiated stem cells or osteoprogenitor cells to differentiate into osteoblasts. A "perfect" bone graft substitute would incorporate all three characteristics.

12.5 Autologous Bone Grafts

The "golden standard" of bone grafts is the autologous bone, although it is an area of growing controversy [1]. It is mostly harvested from the iliac crest, depending upon positioning of the patient. This donor site has the advantage of having a

supply of the cancellous as well as cortical bone (tricortical graft) (Figs. 12.2 and 12.3).

Advantages
• Osteogenetic
• Osteoconductive
• Osteoinductive

Disadvantages
• Limited supply.
• High failure rate is reported.
• Risk of iliac crest fracture (Fig. 12.4).
• Correctional loss due to remodelling [6].
• Donor site morbidity (limited with correct utilization).
• Additional operation time.

Harvest sites
• Iliac crest (anterior, posterior)
• Locally (vertebral body, spinous process, lamina, etc.)
• Rib portion (in transthoracic approaches)
• Tibia/fibula

12.6 Surgical Technique of Iliac Crest Graft Harvesting

The bone from the iliac crest can be easily harvested. When choosing the anterior crest, one must be aware of the lateral femoral cutaneous nerve. On the other hand, a safety margin of at least 3 cm should be left from the anterior superior crest, where the hip flexion muscles derive from. We recommend harvesting the graft using a double-blade oscillating saw. The desired depth can also be harvested using a "graft cutter". This way a defined cortical graft is obtained, leaving room for additional harvesting of cancellous bone chips using a spoon. The defect is filled using a haemostatic pad, the fascia is closed and a drain should be placed to prevent a painful haematoma. Alternatively, according to the clinical application, "bone plugs" can also be harvested using special instruments (Fig. 12.5). This leaves less defect and can also be harvested in other locations.

12.7 Bone Graft Substitutes

These materials should ideally have the osteogenetic, osteoconductive and osteoinductive characteristics of an autograft without the substantial side effects. Most of these materials only provide osteoconductivity. Their integration into the bone substance can take place in different ways [7]. One way is the direct integration or resorption followed by conversion into the bone. The other way would be some kind of "graft-versus-host reaction" resulting in a self-contained graft or even a (partial) loss of graft substance without integration [8].

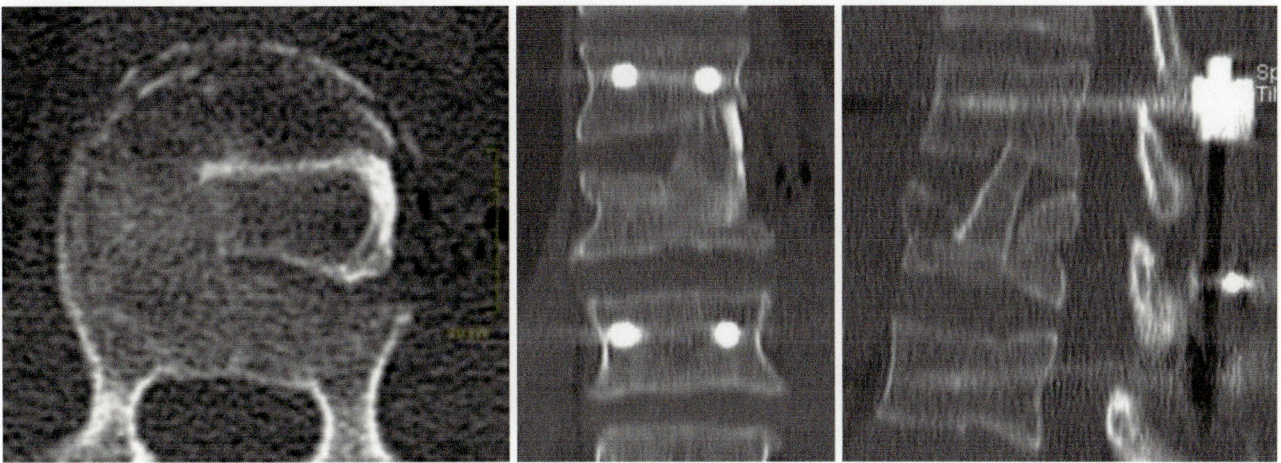

Fig. 12.2   CT scans in three planes documenting the correct size and positioning of a tricortical autograft

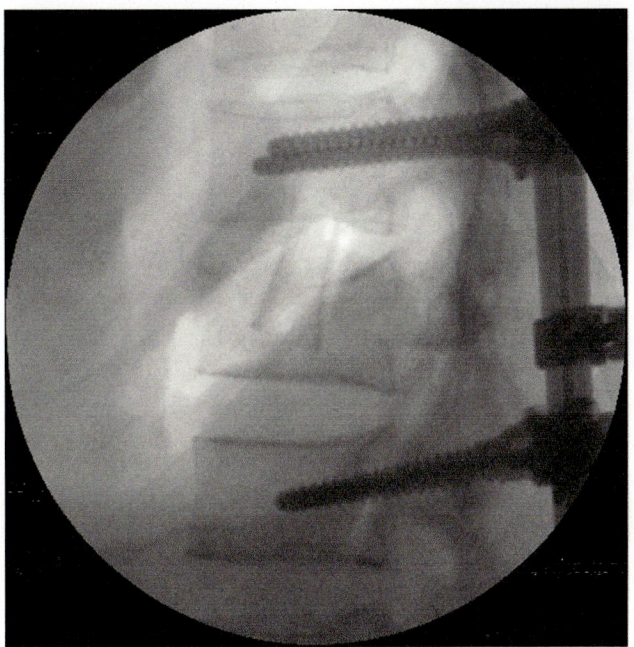

Fig. 12.3   Plain radiograph of a monosegmental, anterior spondylodesis with a tricortical iliac crest autograft following bisegmental, posterior stabilization

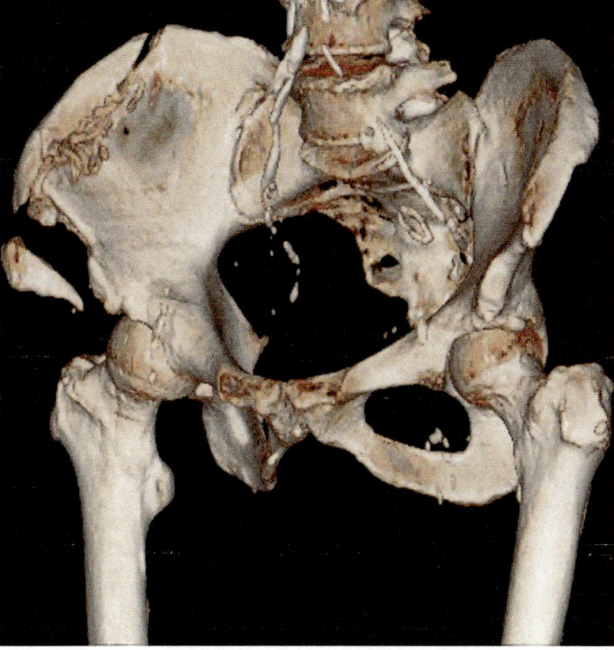

Fig. 12.4   Iliac crest fracture following bone harvest from the anterior iliac crest in the right side

12.8   Allografts

This relates to the tissue taken from one person for transplantation into another. This type of treatment has spread due to recent improvements in procurement, preparation and storage. Clinics with a high turnover of allografts have their own storage areas. This concept of bone banking is connected to a great deal of legal issues, showing great variations in different countries [9]. They are useful however to enlarge the volume of the autologous bone.

Advantages
- Osteoconductive
- Unlimited supply
- Multiple shapes and sizes
- No donor site morbidity

Disadvantages
- Not osteogenic (due to chemical processes in the making)
- Weak osteoinductive properties
- Possibility of infectious disease transmission

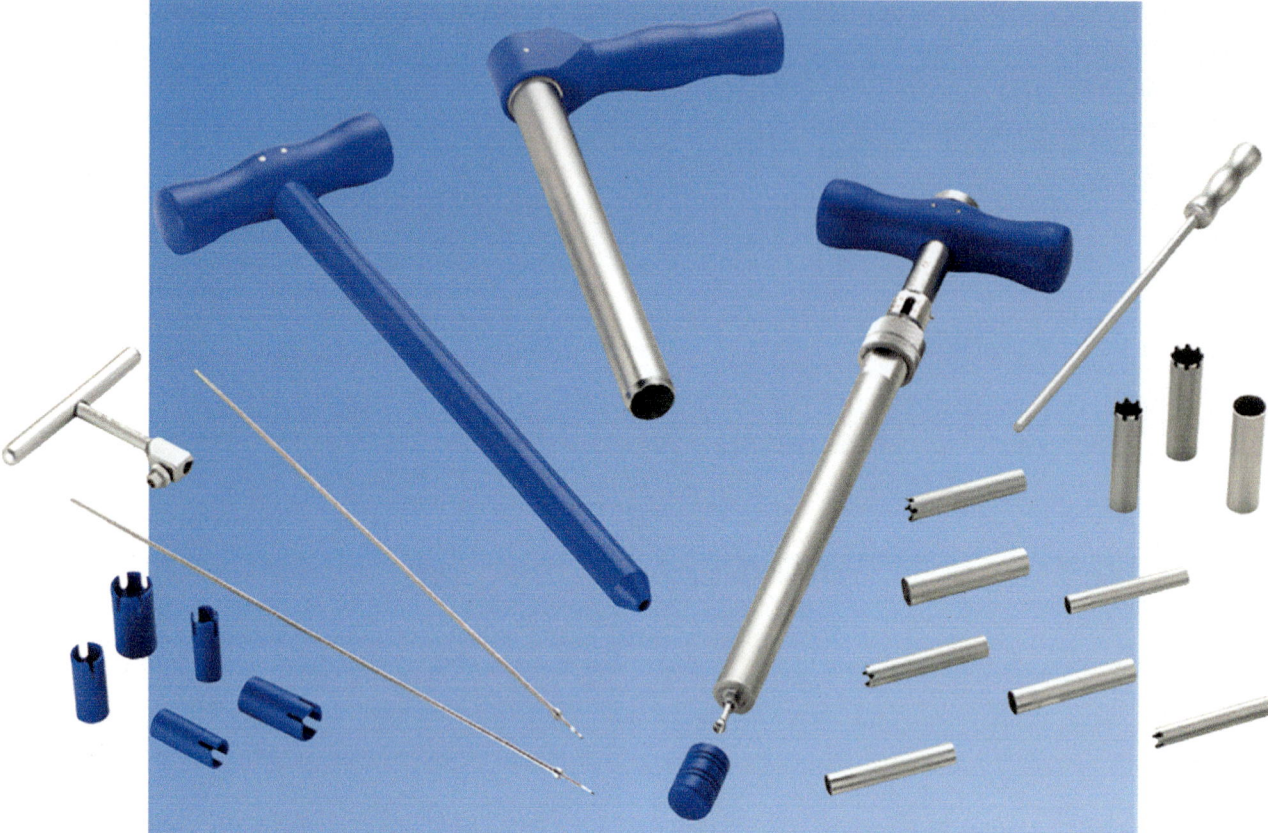

Fig. 12.5 Bone graft harvesting set (Synthes) used for different sizes of "plugs" (© by Synthes)

12.9 Demineralized Bone Matrix (DBM) and Bone Morphogenetic Protein (BMP)

DBM is a demineralized allograft bone with osteoinductive activity [10]. Demineralized bone matrixes are prepared by acid extraction of the allograft bone, resulting in loss of most of the mineralized components but retention of collagen and noncollagenous proteins, including growth factors. The efficacy of a demineralized bone matrix (DBM) as a bone graft substitute or extender may be related to the total amount of bone morphogenetic protein (BMP) present and the ratios of the different BMPs present. The multitude of different BMPs are all capable of recruiting bone-forming cells and encouraging local cells to aid in the bone formation process. There are up to now over 20 different BMPs known, but the clinical research is currently limited to BMP-2 and BMP-7. The different types of BMPs seem to show substantial variations in their osteogenetic potency. Recently, BMP has been associated with cancer, but further studies have found no correlation [11].

Advantages
- Osteoinductive with promoted bone formation [12].
- Osteoinductive potency is very variable in different products [4].

- Graft extender (in combination with autografts).

Disadvantages
- Poor structural integrity
- BMP alone not osteoconductive

12.10 Hydroxyapatite (Ca$_{10}$(PO$_4$)$_6$(OH)$_2$) and Tricalcium Phosphate (Ca$_3$(PO$_4$)$_2$)

These substitutes are mainly known as bone void fillers. Taking into account their specific strengths (e.g. fast curing, fluid injection, etc.) and their weaknesses (low shear stress, poor biodegradability, etc.), new applications have arisen. These materials come in a wide array of different application forms (Fig. 12.6).

Advantages
- Osteoconductive (Fig. 12.7)
- Lasting stability
- Availability

Disadvantages
- Not osteoinductive
- Not osteogenic

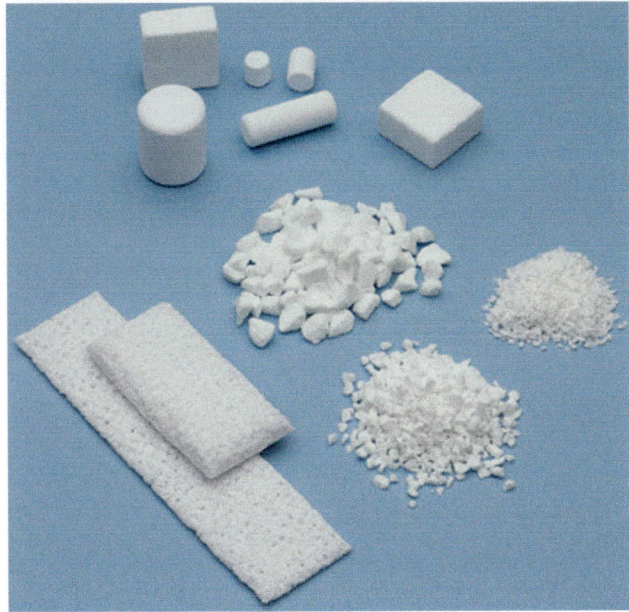

Fig. 12.6 An array of different forms and shapes used in calcium phosphate bone substitutes (© by Synthes)

Table 12.1 Exemplary list of calcium phosphate products on the market (among others)

Product	Company	Type
Nanostim	Medtronic	Synthetic tricalcium
BoneSource	Howmedica	CaP cement
Alpha-BSM	DePuy	CaP cement
Calcibon	Biomet/Merck	CaP putty
MIMIX	Biomet	Synthetic tricalcium phosphate
Cerasorb	Curasan	Beta-tricalcium phosphate
ChronOS	Synthes	Beta-tricalcium phosphate
Vitoss	Orthovita	Beta-tricalcium phosphate
Pro osteon	Interpore cross	Coralline hydroxyapatite
Endobon	Biomet/Merck	Cancellous hydroxyapatite
BioFuse	Corin	Hydroxyapatite/CaP
Actifuse	ApaTech	Silicated calcium phosphate

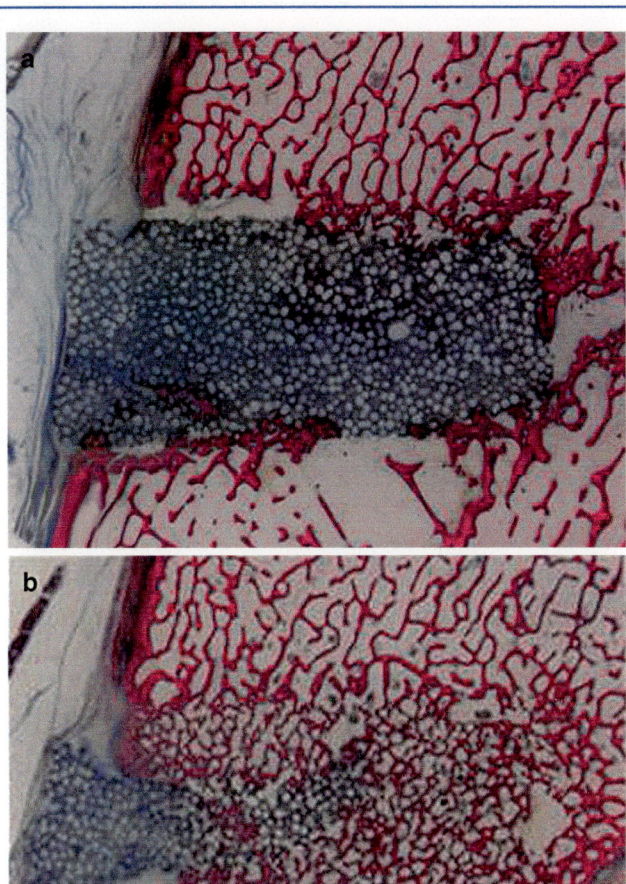

Fig. 12.7 (**a, b**) Histological findings using chronOS mixed with blood 6 weeks (**a**) and 12 weeks postoperatively (© by Synthes)

12.11 Clinical Application

Current evolutions within this field, such as biphasic, injectable CaP and silicated CaP, widen the array of applications, offering a good supplement in achieving spinal fusion [13] (filling cages, lining cages, extending grafts, etc.) (Table 12.1). These substances should be rehydrated using the patients' blood before applying (Fig. 12.8).

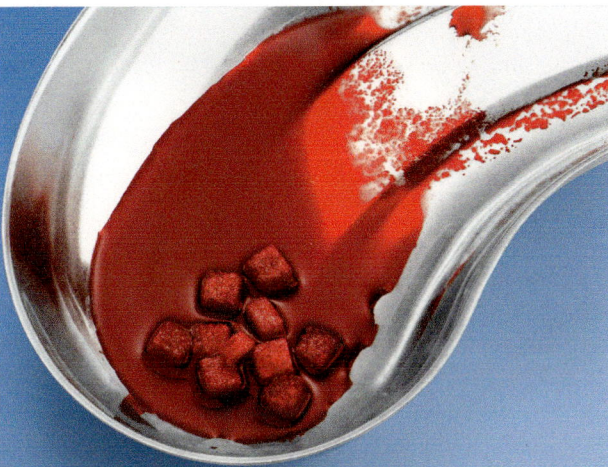

Fig. 12.8 ChronOS blocs mixed with blood (© by Synthes)

12.12 Other Ceramics (Sea Corals, Calcium Sulphate)

These substances are currently researched to evaluate their usefulness to supplement or even replace the ceramics in use today.

12.13 Outlook

Tissue engineering and the further development of growth factors offer great potential for the future of fusion and bone substitutes. Materials will evolve and offer "ideal" and individual solutions for specific indications [14]. But currently, the autologous bone is still the golden standard [15]. The diversity of current substitutes will make further comparative studies quite difficult.

References

1. Sen MK, Miclau T. Autologous iliac crest bone graft: should it still be the gold standard for treating nonunions? Injury. 2007;38(Suppl 1):S75–80.
2. Bone Graft Alternatives (according to the North American Spine Society). http://www.spine.org/Documents/bone_grafts_2006.pdf
3. Phillips AM. Overview of the fracture healing cascade. Injury. 2005;36(Suppl 3):S5–7.
4. Papakostidis C, Kontakis D, Bhandari M, et al. Efficacy of autologeous iliac crest bone graft and bone morphologic proteins for posterolateral fusion of lumbar spine – a metaanalysis of the results. Spine. 2008;33(19):E680–92.
5. Giannoudis PV, Einhorn TA, Marsh D. Fracture healing: the diamond concept. Injury. 2007;38(Suppl 4):S3–6.
6. Morrison RH, Thierolf A, Weckbach A. Volumetric changes of iliac crest autografts used to reconstruct the anterior column in thoracolumbar fractures: a follow-up using CT scans. Spine. 2007;32(26):3030–5.
7. Berven S, Tay BK, Kleinstueck FS, et al. Clinical applications of bone graft substitutes in spine surgery: consideration of mineralized and demineralized preparations and growth factor supplementation. Eur Spine J. 2001;10(Suppl 2):S169–77.
8. Schimandle JH, Boden SD. Bone substitutes for lumbar fusion: present and future. Oper Tech Orthop. 1997;7:60–7.
9. Friedlaender GE. Bone-banking. J Bone Joint Surg Am. 1982;64:307–11.
10. Petersen B, Whang PG, Iglesias R, et al. Osteoinductivity of commercially available demineralized bone matrix. Preparations in a spine fusion model. J Bone Joint Surg Am. 2004;86-A(10):2243–50.
11. Cooper GS, Kou TD. Risk of cancer following lumbar fusion surgery with recombinant human bone morphogenic protein-2 (rhBMP-2): an analysis using a commercially insured patient population. Int J Spine Surg. 2018;12(2):260–8.
12. Kwong FN, Harris MB. Recent developments in the biology of fracture repair. J Am Acad Orthop Surg. 2008;16(11):619–25.
13. Becker S, Maissen O, Ponomarev I, et al. Osteopromotion by a beta-tricalcium phosphate/bone marrow hybrid implant for use in spine surgery. Spine. 2006;31(1):11–7.
14. Giannoudis PV, Tzioupis CC, Tsirids E. Gene therapy in orthopaedics. Injury. 2006;37(Suppl 1):S30–40.
15. Morris MT, Tarpada SP, Cho W. Bone graft materials for posterolateral fusion made simple: a systematic review. Eur Spine J. 2018;27:1856–67.

On- and Offline Documentation of Spine Procedures: Spine Tango

Thomas Zweig, Marco Teli, Everard Munting, Samuel Morris, and Markus Melloh

13.1 Introduction and Core Messages

Today, quality assurance and systematic data collections are finally becoming more commonplace; however, they are often independent undertakings of surgeons or hospitals. As a result, the isolated use of databases and content to study smaller groups makes data pooling and harmonisation difficult and impedes important quality assurance processes, particularly benchmarking. In 2000, EuroSpine, the Spine Society of Europe, at the initiative of Dieter Grob and Max Aebi and with the help of Chris Röder, launched Spine Tango, an on- and offline registry of spinal interventions (surgical and conservative) aimed at assuring quality in outcome research and enabling national and international benchmarking. A scientific clinical fellowship was introduced to support the distribution on every layer. Spine Tango later evolved to include postmarket surveillance of surgical implants. Information on Spine Tango and a battery of recommended physician and patient-based instruments can be found under www.eurospine.org—Spine Tango.

T. Zweig (✉)
Spine in the Center, Bern/Langenthal, Switzerland
e-mail: spine@hin.ch

M. Teli
The Walton Centre for Neurology and Neurosurgery, Liverpool, UK

E. Munting
Clinique Saint Pierre, Ottignies, Belgium

S. Morris
Centre for Spinal Studies and Surgery, Queen's Medical Centre, Stockport, UK

M. Melloh
Institute of Health Sciences, Zurich University of Applied Sciences, Winterthur, Switzerland

UWA Medical School, The University of Western Australia, Nedlands, Western Australia, Australia

13.2 Definition of Quality in Health Care

To those not involved in quality improvement in a professional capacity, it might appear a relatively simple task to define "quality"; however, more than 2000 years after Plato invented this term, there is still great debate regarding the meaning of the word [1]. The American Society for Quality (ASQ) defines quality as "a subjective term for which each person has his or her own definition" [2]. According to a user-based approach, quality can be defined as "meeting or exceeding customer satisfaction" [3]. Quality is a multidimensional construct, and the dimensions are specific to each category. The US Agency for Healthcare Research and Quality defines quality in health care as "doing the right thing, at the right time, in the right way, for the right person, and having the best possible results" [4].

The quality measures in health care assess the following three components:
- Structure (resources such as staff and equipment)
- Process (therapeutic interventions, prescribing, interactions with patients)
- Outcomes (end results of health care such as mortality and attainment of patient's expectations) [4, 5]

Wensing and Elwyn [6] defined preferences as patient's ideas about what should occur in health-care systems. Evaluations are patient's "reactions" to their experience of health care, and reports are objective observations (e.g. how long the patients had to spend in the waiting room).

The measures used to obtain the patients' view can be classified into the following three categories:
- Preferences
- Evaluations
- Reports

Naturally, the scope and utility of a quality measurement process will depend on the choices made when selecting measurement tools. The choice of the type of measure depends on the aspect being assessed and the purpose of the evaluation (educational, certification, accreditation, quality control or quality improvement) [7]. One of the most widespread means of measuring processes and outcomes is the assessment of patient satisfaction (evaluation category). Outcome satisfaction is also one of the criteria for assessing the validity of process measures. Indeed, according to Chassin [8], a measure of process is valid when it is related to health outcomes (mortality, patient satisfaction, etc.). Hence, the responses to questions concerning satisfaction with treatment, typically used in treatment outcome studies, can also be seen as outcome measures in the quality control and improvement context.

13.2.1 Overlap of Outcome Research and Quality Control

Medical disciplines have adopted the practice of quality control through data collection and measurement tools, but there is often less enthusiasm among medical institutions to be guided by data and implement findings in a rigorous or systematic fashion. The growing emphasis on an evidence-based approach in the medical setting has led to a corresponding increase in the number and quality of studies in the twenty-first century, examining the efficacy of surgical and non-surgical treatments. These studies are usually conducted in university hospitals and clinics that have an in-house research staff or that cooperate with academic research institutions. The studies are not commonly perceived by the care provider (hospitals and clinics) as being something from which they can benefit from an economical point of view; in contrast, carrying out such research can sometimes be seen as a drain of resources. The research activities on treatment outcomes are merely seen as something that may indirectly benefit the institution in terms of prestige and corporate social responsibility. However, the possibility of economic benefit from corporate social responsibility activities is not a sufficiently persuasive argument for increasing investment in research—otherwise, all the public and private hospitals and clinics would likely have their own research departments or research staff. Significantly, in all of this, one important factor is typically overlooked: research projects in the field of treatment outcomes and their predictors can be useful to the provider in a much more direct way in terms of quality improvement and the control of service performance [9].

13.3 EuroSpine "Spine Tango": An International Spine Registry for Quality Assurance, Outcome Research, Postmarket Surveillance of Implants and Conservative Interventions

13.3.1 History and Objectives

All over the world, efforts are being made to set up surgical registries on regional, state or even national levels. Spine surgery represents a challenge for all registry endeavours. The variety of levels, pathologies, accesses and surgical techniques confounds all attempts to formulate a concise yet comprehensive questionnaire. Under the auspices of EuroSpine, the Spine Society of Europe, a project was launched for the design and implementation of a documentation system for spinal surgery in 2000. This effort was introduced as "Spine Tango" and was conducted in collaboration with the Institute for Evaluative Research in Orthopaedic Surgery at the University of Bern, Switzerland.

Goals of Spine Tango were the following:

- Presentation of *state-of-the-art* European spine surgery, including all pathologies, levels, accesses and single- as well as multiple-staged surgeries
- *Outcome research* and *prospective observational evaluation* of different surgical techniques as an alternative to randomised controlled trials
- *Benchmarking* on national and international levels
- *Quality assurance and quality improvement*

Spine Tango was probably the first international spine registry initiative to face the challenge of developing a comprehensive questionnaire covering all major spine pathologies and interventions, as well as spanning all anatomical levels. To accomplish this task, a technically demanding computer application was a prerequisite. The consensus and piloting process for the Spine Tango surgical questionnaires "surgery" and "follow-up" took about 5 years and required around 4000 completed forms. The results are two double-sided A4 questionnaires (surgery, staged surgery) and one single-sided questionnaire for follow-up, all of which can be completed online or using scannable paper questionnaires. At the same time that the physician-based content was finalised, a working group at the Schulthess Hospital in Zurich, Switzerland, had developed and validated the COMI (Core Outcome Measures Index) instruments for neck and low back pain which became the officially recommended patient-based documentation instruments in the framework of the Spine Tango registry [10]. To date, the Spine Tango database has grown to over 750,000 cases, and currently, about 40 hospitals participate from 5 continents and will become the mandatory register in Switzerland and Germany while in the pilot phase in Belgium [11].

13.3.2 Content: Physician Based

The refined set of questions still allows documentation of the broad spectrum of pathologies and treatments in spine surgery. This is made possible by means of a list of main pathologies and their specifications and the so-called surgical matrix, a terminology system reducing the interventions to their basic principles—decompression, fusion, stabilisation rigid, stabilisation motion preserving, percutaneous procedures and others. The duplication and, hence, separation of these principles into anterior and posterior ones completes the matrix.

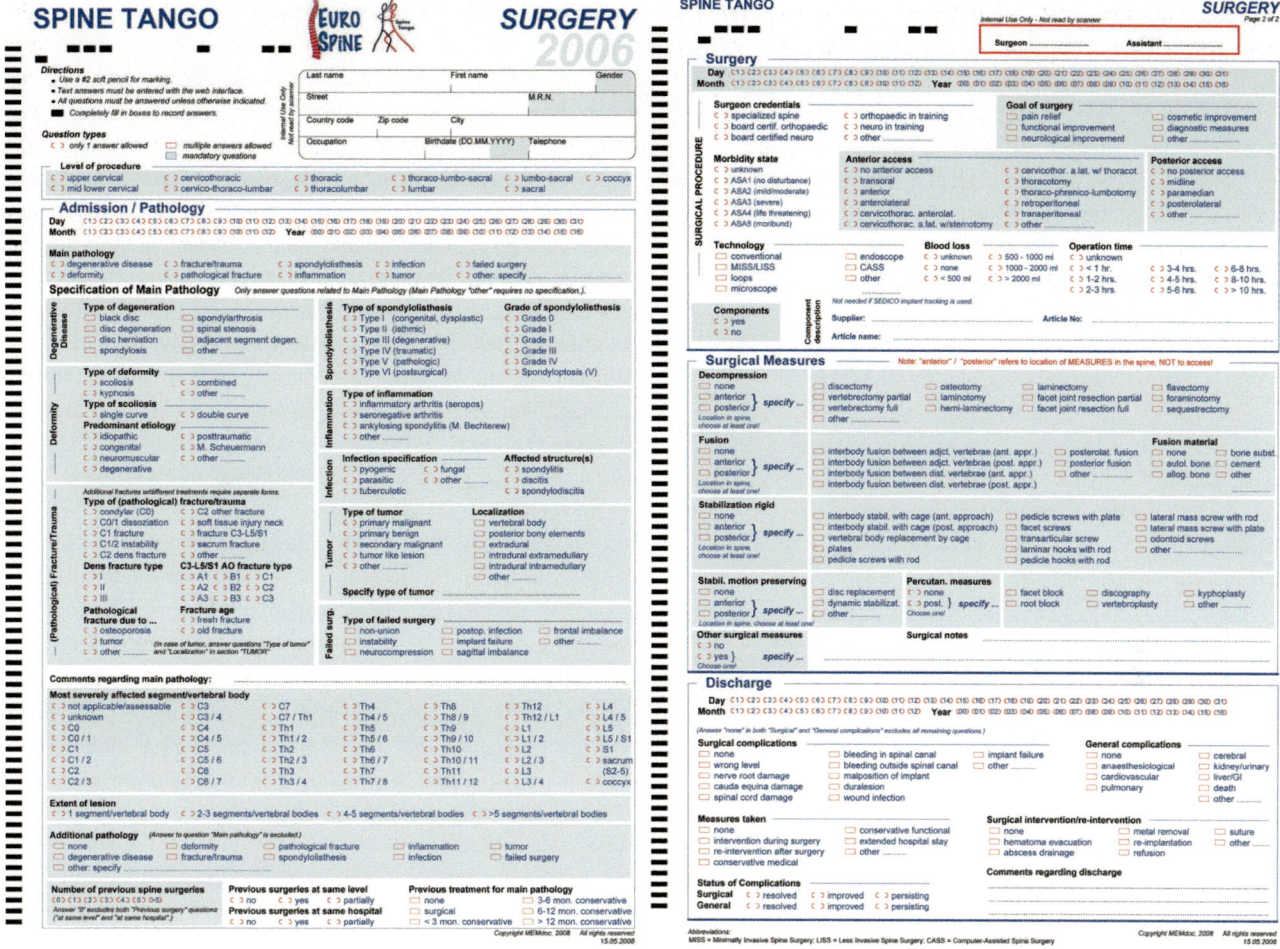

Fig. 13.1   SSE Spine Tango surgery form (front and back side). All questions with *blue* background are mandatory

13.3.3 Surgery Form

The first half of the front page of the "surgery" form serves to specify the level of the procedure, admission date, case history (previous conservative and surgical treatments), main and additional pathology, most severely affected segment and extent of lesion. This information is grouped into the "admission" subform. The "specification of main pathology" subform makes up the second part of page one and comprises one to three questions per "main pathology" category. These serve to provide more information about the main pathology. On the reverse side of the sheet are the "surgery", "surgical measures" and "discharge" subforms. The "surgery" subform is the largest (12 questions) and inquires about surgery date, implants used, goals of surgery, the surgical matrix, surgeon credentials, access and technology, operation time, morbidity state and blood loss. The "surgical measures" subform applies the same principle as the "specification of main pathology" subform—only the items relevant to the information given for

the matrix questions need to be completed. Typically, this can be done with two to four questions. Finally, the "discharge" subform inquires about the discharge date, surgical and general in-hospital complications, measures taken and status of complications upon discharge. It makes up between three and seven questions (Fig. 13.1).

13.3.4 Staged Surgery Form

In addition to the surgery form, there is also a so-called staged form and a follow-up form. The staged form serves to document the second part of a planned two-stage procedures, that is, procedures where the patient remains in the hospital between the first and the second interventions. If the patient is discharged, a new surgery form must be completed. Also, if an early revision is carried out, the correct way to document this is with a new surgery form with the diagnosis "failed surgery".

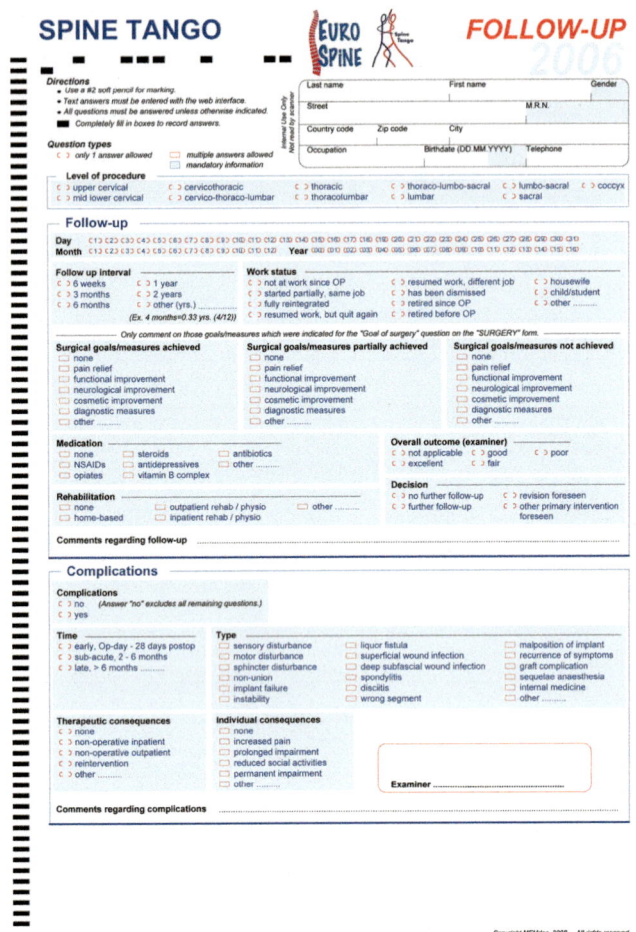

Fig. 13.2 SSE Spine Tango follow-up form (one page only)

13.3.5 Follow-Up Form

The follow-up form is just one side of the A4 sheet and consists of a "follow-up" subform and a "complications" subform. In its paper format, it can be completed in less than 1 min. After the date of follow-up and the follow-up interval have been completed, the patient's work status is documented, and the surgical goals that were achieved, partially achieved or not achieved at all are indicated. Only the surgical goals that are indicated on the surgery form are to be considered. Current medication, rehabilitation and the surgeon's rating of the outcome are then recorded. The last question in the "follow-up" subform inquires about the need (or not) for further follow-up, revision surgery or another primary intervention.

In the absence of complications, the "complications" subform can be completed with just one answer "no" to the "complications" question. Where complications have arisen, the point of time at which they occurred, the type of complications and the therapeutic and individual consequences are inquired about (Fig. 13.2). All forms can be found as PDF files under www.eurospine.org—Spine Tango—forms.

13.3.6 Content: Patient Based

The proportion of positive outcomes after spinal surgery depends to a large extent on the manner in which outcome is assessed [12], and there is no single, universally accepted method. In the past, clinicians typically judged the outcome from their own perspective, using simple rating schemes such as "excellent, good, moderate and poor". The technical success of the operation also lent itself to evaluation by means of sophisticated imaging at follow-up. However, most of the time, these measures proved to be only weakly associated with outcomes of relevance to the patient and to society [13]. It is now widely accepted that the focus should be placed on patient-orientated measures and that the patient should be the main judge of outcome, with the result that clinician-based methods have been complemented by a diverse range of patient self-assessment questionnaires. A standardised set of outcome measures for use with back patients were proposed in 1998 by a multinational group of experts [13]. There was general consensus that the most appropriate core outcome measures should include the following domains: pain, back-specific function, generic health status (well-being), work disability, social disability and patient satisfaction [13, 14]. Accordingly, the group proposed a parsimonious set of seven preoperative questions that would cover each of these domains, yet be brief enough to alleviate the respondent's burden, and hence be practical for routine clinical use and quality management. At the time of follow-up, information about occurrence of complications and their bothersomeness from the patient's perspective, reoperations, satisfaction with overall medical care in the hospital and extent to which surgery helped are inquired with four additional questions. The satisfaction question may, for example, be used to evaluate the patient's perception of the "process performance" in a six-sigma quality improvement initiative [8, 9]. Sufficient clinical research has meanwhile been conducted with the COMI score outcome forms for providing details about their application and administration and about clinically and statistically important facts like the minimum clinically relevant score improvement, standardised response mean values (effect sizes) and dichotomisation of outcomes into "good" and "poor" results [15] (Fig. 13.3). All COMI forms can be found as PDF files under www. eurospine.org—Spine Tango—forms.

13.3.7 Content: Conservative Form

It took more than a decade from the launch of Spine Tango in 2000 before the need for a documentation form for non-surgical treatments of the spine led to the development of a "Spine Tango Conservative" form (Kessler et al. Eur Spine J 2011). Shortly afterwards followed patient-based forms for the non-surgical treatment of the back and neck (COMI back conservative/COMI neck conservative). Implementation of the Spine Tango Conservative 2011 form has been reported in a UK, secondary care setting [11, 16]. In 2018, an interna-

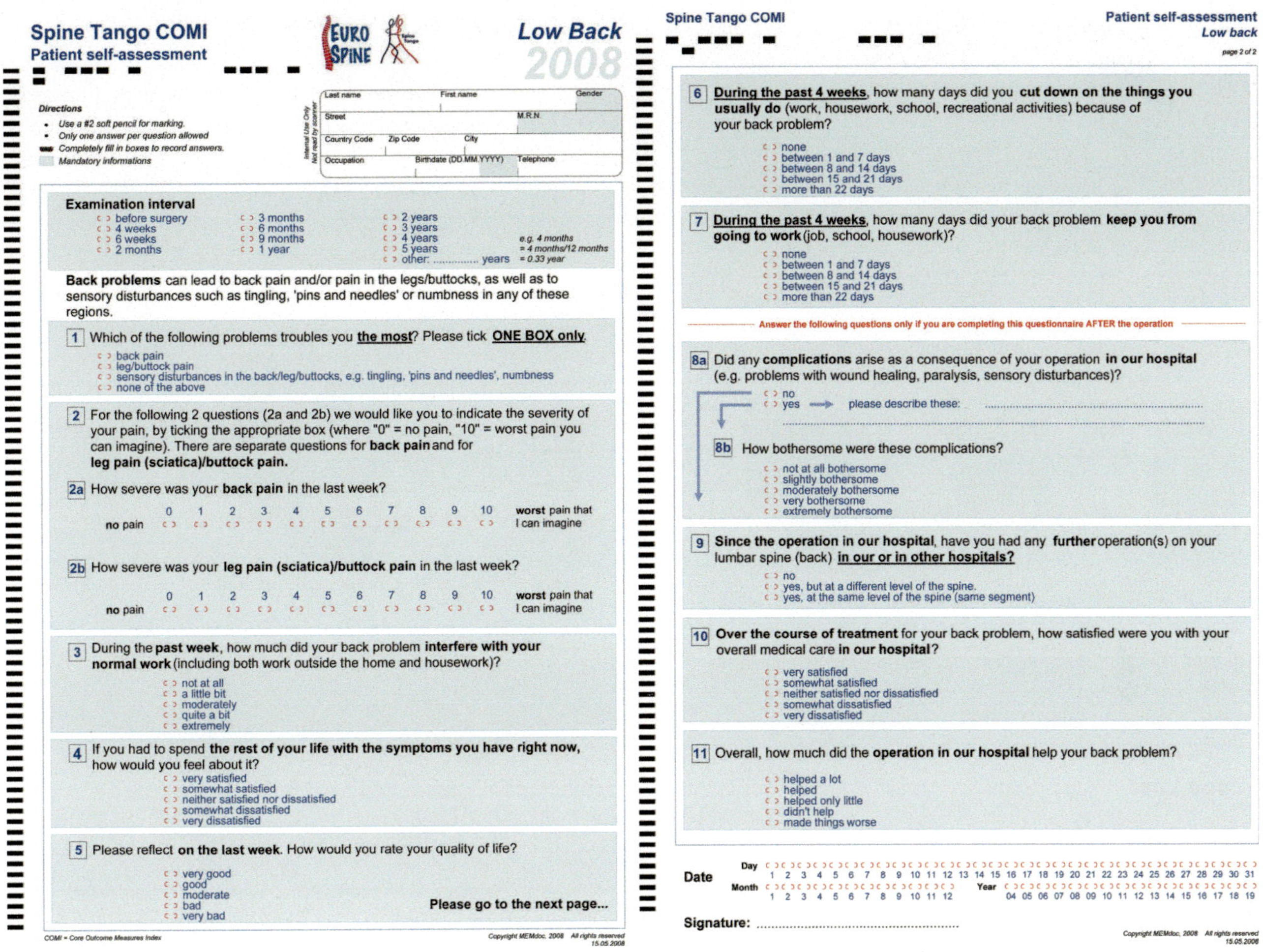
Spine Tango COMI
Patient self-assessment
EURO SPINE
Low Back
2008

Directions
- Use a #2 soft pencil for marking.
- Only one answer per question allowed
- Completely fill in boxes to record answers.
- Mandatory informations

Internal Use Only
Not read by scanner

Last name | First name | Gender
Street | M.R.N.
Country Code | Zip Code | City
Occupation | Birthdate (DD.MM.YYYY) | Telephone

Examination interval
- before surgery
- 4 weeks
- 6 weeks
- 2 months
- 3 months
- 6 months
- 9 months
- 1 year
- 2 years
- 3 years
- 4 years
- 5 years
- other: .... years

e.g. 4 months = 4 months/12 months = 0.33 year

Back problems can lead to back pain and/or pain in the legs/buttocks, as well as to sensory disturbances such as tingling, 'pins and needles' or numbness in any of these regions.

1 Which of the following problems troubles you the most? Please tick ONE BOX only.
- back pain
- leg/buttock pain
- sensory disturbances in the back/leg/buttocks, e.g. tingling, 'pins and needles', numbness
- none of the above

2 For the following 2 questions (2a and 2b) we would like you to indicate the severity of your pain, by ticking the appropriate box (where "0" = no pain, "10" = worst pain you can imagine). There are separate questions for **back pain** and for **leg pain (sciatica)/buttock pain.**

2a How severe was your **back pain** in the last week?

no pain 0 1 2 3 4 5 6 7 8 9 10 **worst** pain that I can imagine

2b How severe was your **leg pain (sciatica)/buttock pain** in the last week?

no pain 0 1 2 3 4 5 6 7 8 9 10 **worst** pain that I can imagine

3 During the **past week**, how much did your back problem **interfere with your normal work** (including both work outside the home and housework)?
- not at all
- a little bit
- moderately
- quite a bit
- extremely

4 If you had to spend **the rest of your life with the symptoms you have right now,** how would you feel about it?
- very satisfied
- somewhat satisfied
- neither satisfied nor dissatisfied
- somewhat dissatisfied
- very dissatisfied

5 Please reflect **on the last week**. How would you rate your quality of life?
- very good
- good
- moderate
- bad
- very bad

Please go to the next page...

COMI = Core Outcome Measures Index
Copyright MEMdoc 2008 All rights reserved 15.05.2008

Spine Tango COMI
Patient self-assessment
Low back
page 2 of 2

6 During the past 4 weeks, how many days did you **cut down on the things you usually do** (work, housework, school, recreational activities) because of your back problem?
- none
- between 1 and 7 days
- between 8 and 14 days
- between 15 and 21 days
- more than 22 days

7 During the past 4 weeks, how many days did your back problem **keep you from going to work** (job, school, housework)?
- none
- between 1 and 7 days
- between 8 and 14 days
- between 15 and 21 days
- more than 22 days

Answer the following questions only if you are completing this questionnaire AFTER the operation

8a Did any **complications** arise as a consequence of your operation **in our hospital** (e.g. problems with wound healing, paralysis, sensory disturbances)?
- no
- yes → please describe these: ....

8b How bothersome were these complications?
- not at all bothersome
- slightly bothersome
- moderately bothersome
- very bothersome
- extremely bothersome

9 **Since the operation in our hospital**, have you had any **further** operation(s) on your lumbar spine (back) in our or in other hospitals?
- no
- yes, but at a different level of the spine.
- yes, at the same level of the spine (same segment)

10 **Over the course of treatment** for your back problem, how satisfied were you with your overall medical care **in our hospital**?
- very satisfied
- somewhat satisfied
- neither satisfied nor dissatisfied
- somewhat dissatisfied
- very dissatisfied

11 Overall, how much did the **operation in our hospital** help your back problem?
- helped a lot
- helped
- helped only little
- didn't help
- made things worse

Date
Day 1 2 3 4 5 6 7 8 9 10 11 12 13 14 15 16 17 18 19 20 21 22 23 24 25 26 27 28 29 30 31
Month 1 2 3 4 5 6 7 8 9 10 11 12
Year 04 05 06 07 08 09 10 11 12 13 14 15 16 17 18 19

Signature: ....

Copyright MEMdoc 2008 All rights reserved 15.05.2008

Fig. 13.3 COMI patient assessment form for low back pain

tional consensus meeting was held in Zurich, involving clinicians from medical, surgical and conservative therapy disciplines as well as researchers with data registry expertise. The purpose was to redevelop the Spine Tango Conservative form to improve capture of the complexities of single and multidisciplinary conservative spinal care and to enable direct comparison of conservative interventions with surgery. In the following 12 months, the Spine Tango Conservative 2018 form was further refined, and it is now available on the EuroSpine website. Although more detailed than its predecessor, it is similarly quick to complete and allows data analysis that is tailored to the needs of conservative clinicians and services and allows comparison with the surgical treatment of similar pathologies.

13.3.8 Technology

Spine Tango has long left the early stage of a simple web page for data entry and has grown into an international project with a sophisticated information technology structure and a multitude of clinical and scientific experts serving the user community and developing the registry further. The central database is now part of a documentation portal hosted by the Northgate Public Services, UK; it offers various methods for clinical, implant and radiographic data collection and a multitude of possibilities for data downloads and online statistical queries. An important step was the implementation of the so-called modules and national satellite servers that anonymise data for protecting user's and patient's privacy in the respective country before sending the clinical data set to the central server in the UK (Fig. 13.4). Such modules are meanwhile installed in Germany, Austria, Belgium, Italy, the UK, Australia, the USA, Mexico and Brazil. Users whose country does not yet have such a national filter server may use the Swiss/international module under www.spinetango.org. Access to the servers is centrally routed via the EuroSpine home page under www.eurospine.org—Spine Tango—access registry.

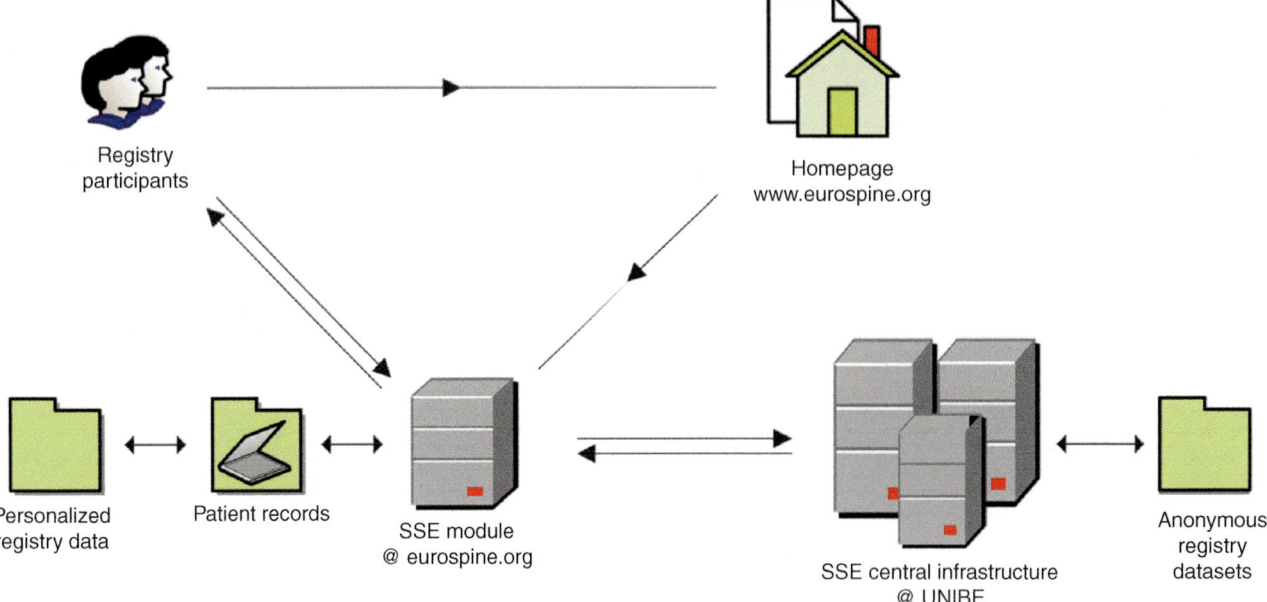

Fig. 13.4 Spine user routing and data segregation in the national modules

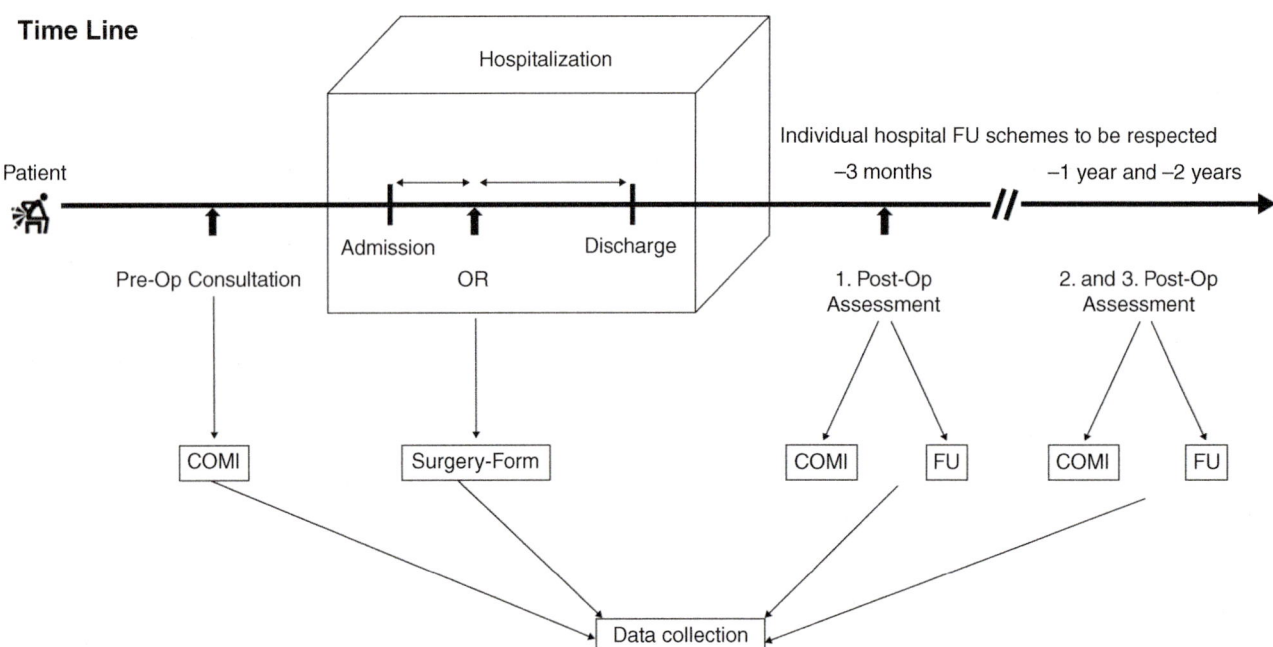

Fig. 13.5 Spine Tango pre- and postoperative physician- and patient-based data collection

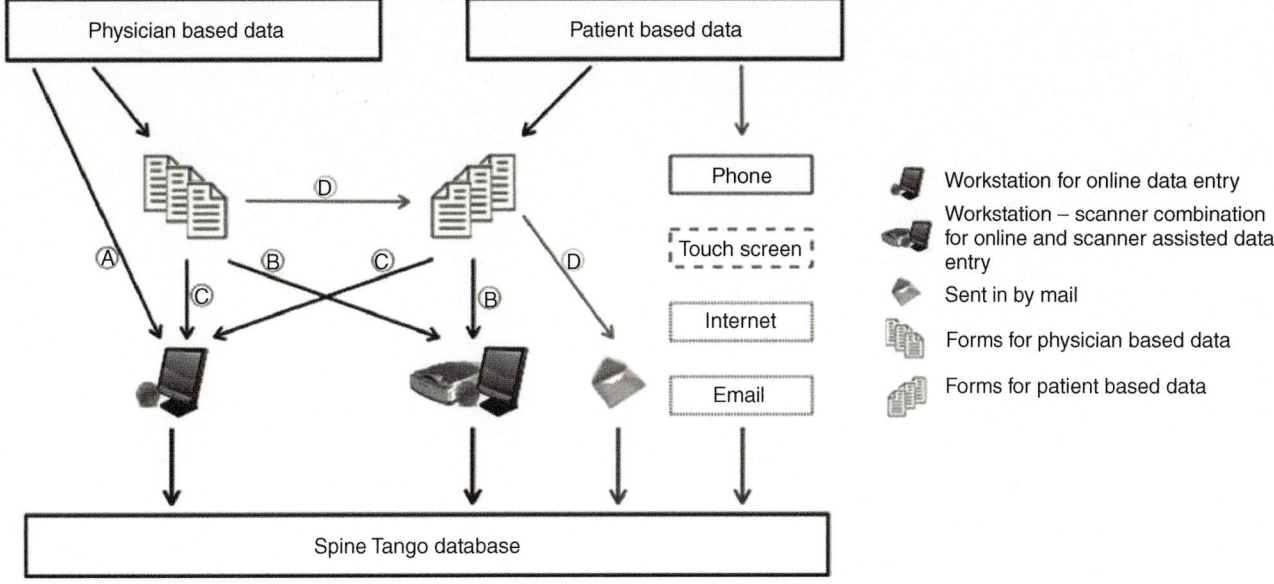

Fig. 13.6 Possible modes of data collection with Spine Tango

13.3.9 Workflow

A generic application which serves a multitude of hospitals with different sizes, structures and staff coverage can only be customised to a certain extent to the individual expectations and needs of a user, that is, a single surgeon or a department. Therefore, an intelligent and creative integration of the Tango project and its processes into the day-to-day workflows is key for success and a sustainable future of the data collection efforts [17]. Direct online data entry, paper-based data collection with OMR (optical mark reader) compatible paper forms and simple PDFs for later data punching are options which mainly depend on factors like web access and number of web terminals in the OR, wards and outpatient clinic; pre- and postoperative administration of patient questionnaires by face-to-face interview, mail or telephone interview in addition to the surgeon-based data collection represents additional efforts that need the respective financial and human resources (Fig. 13.5). There are currently five possible ways by which forms and questionnaires can be transferred to the database (Fig. 13.6): online data entry (A), paper-based data capture with OMR scanner-assisted entry of data (B), paper-based data capture with data punching using the online interface (C), paper-based data capture with mailing of the forms to the IEFO or other partner institutions for OMR scanner-assisted entry of data (D) and finally a hybrid method of direct online entry of surgical data (A) and OMR scanner-assisted entry of patient questionnaires (B) or direct online entry of surgical data (A) and delayed online entry of questionnaires that were completed on paper by the patients (C).

13.3.10   Spine Tango Publications

Up to date (July 2020), there have been 68 peer-reviewed papers published on Spine Tango. In the first decade of Spine Tango's existence, there were 12 papers published, which mainly focused on set-up, rationale and handling of the Spine Tango database. In the second decade, papers predominantly focused on outcomes (Yagdiran et al. Eur Spine J 2020), comparative analyses (Zweig et al. 2017, Sabou et al. J Z Spine 2019) and prediction models (Aghayev et al. World Neurosurg 2020). However, one topic has remained highly popular over all this time: low back pain (Sethi et al. J Orthop 2019).

References

1. Röder C, El-Kerdi A, Grob D, et al. A European spine registry. Eur Spine J. 2002;11:303–7.
2. American Society for Quality. Quality glossary. Qual Prog. 2002;35:43–61.
3. Garvin D. What does product quality really mean? Sloan Manag Rev. 1984;26:25–43.
4. Röder C, Chavanne A, Mannion AF, et al. SSE Spine Tango–content, workflow, set-up. Eur Spine J. 2005;14:920–4.
5. Campbell SM, Braspenning J, Hutchinson A, et al. Research methods used in developing and applying quality indicators in primary care. BMJ. 2003;326:816–9.
6. Wensing M, Elwyn G. Methods for incorporating patients' views in health care. BMJ. 2003;326:877–9.
7. Sower S, Fair F. There is more to quality than continuous improvement: listening to Plato. Qual Manag J. 2005;12:8–20.
8. Chassin MR. Is health care ready for six sigma quality? Milbank Q. 1998;76:565–91.

9. Impellizzeri FM, Bizini M, Leunig M, et al. Money matters: exploiting the data from outcomes research for quality improvement initiatives. Eur Spine J. 2009;3:348–59.

10. Mannion AF, Elfering A, Staerkle AR, et al. Outcome assessment in low back pain: how low can you go? Eur Spine J. 2005;14:1014–26.

11. Morris S, Booth J. Shaping conservative spinal services with the Spine Tango Registry. Eur Spine J. 2018;27(3):543–55.

12. Mannion AF, Elfering A. Predictors of surgical outcome and their assessment. Eur Spine J. 2006;1:93–108.

13. Deyo RA, Battie M, Boerskens AJ, et al. Outcome measures for low back pain research. A proposal for standardized use. Spine. 1998;23(2):2003–13.

14. Bombardier C. Outcome assessments in the evaluation of treatment of spinal disorders: summary and general recommendations. Spine. 2000;25:3100–3.

15. Mannion AF, Porchet F, Kleinstück FS, et al. The quality of spine surgery from the patient's perspective. Part 1: the core outcome measures index in clinical practice. Eur Spine J. 2009;3:367–73.

16. Morris S, Booth J, Hegarty J. Spine Tango registry data collection in a conservative spinal service: a feasibility study. Eur Spine J. 2016;25(9):2984–92.

17. Müller ME, Allgöwer M, Willenegger H. Die Gemeinschaftserhebung der Arbeitsgemeinschaft für Osteosynthesefragen. Arch klin Chir. 1963;304:808–17.

Spinal Orthoses

14

Uwe Vieweg

14.1 Introduction and Core Messages [1–3]

The first evidence of the use of spinal orthoses can be traced back to Galen (131–201 AD). Primitive orthotic devices were made of items that were readily available during this period: leather, whalebone and tree bark. Technology has revamped the field of orthotics, with new stronger and lighter materials. Although materials available for orthotic construction have changed, the types of pathologic conditions treated have remained virtually constant for years. The primary goal of modem orthoses is to aid a weakened muscle group or correct a deformed body part. The clinician's priority should be to determine which spinal motion to control, prefabricated versus custom orthoses. The availability of prefabricated orthoses today presents the rehabilitation team with a variety of choices and some challenges. Many of the prefabricated orthoses come in various sizes and can be fitted to patients often with little or no adjustment. While this can be a benefit to the patient and the team in terms of time, care should be taken to ensure that the design and function of these orthoses are appropriate for the patient's condition and not used purely for convenience. Custom orthoses, in most cases, provide a more comfortable fit with a higher degree of control and can be designed to accommodate a patient's unique body shape or deformities. Computer-aided design (CAD) and computer-aided manufacturing (CAM) technology is available to help the practitioner improve efficiency in design and fabrication, as well as reducing the invasiveness of orthotic measurement of the patients. The development of computer-aided design (CAD) and computer-aided manufacturing (CAM) has allowed the fabrication of orthoses today in less time than it took only a few years ago. The BioScanner is one of the CAD-CAM systems available.

14.2 Definition and Classification [1, 4–6]

An orthosis is a singular device used to aid or align a weakened body part. Orthoses are made of elastic or solid plastic materials or a combination of both, as well as drill and elastic fabric. Reinforcements made of aluminium or steel are used for elastic fabrics. Aluminium is preferred for its better X-ray transparency and lighter weight. In terms of manufacturing, supports can be categorized into bespoke body-surrounding orthoses made of fabric, bodices or bandages and corsets or trunk orthoses. Orthoses can also be active, with dynamic muscle use, partially active, with the use of muscle power via static mechanical influences, and passive with a static mechanical protection. Internationally, spinal orthoses are classified according to the location of the spinal segments (International Summary Description of Orthosis Types or Orthoses for the Trunk and Pelvic Areas [6]). Some acronym examples of spinal orthoses are the following:

CO: cervical orthosis
CTO: cervicothoracic orthosis
CTLSO: cervicothoracolumbosacral orthosis
TLSO: thoracolumbosacral orthosis
LSO: lumbosacral orthosis
SO: sacral orthosis

U. Vieweg (✉)
Department of Conservative and Surgical Spine Therapy with Interdisciplinary Spinal Deformities Centre and Rummelsberg Sectional Center, Hospital Rummelsberg, Schwarzenbruck, Germany
e-mail: uwe.vieweg@sana.de

© Springer-Verlag GmbH Germany 2023
U. Vieweg, F. Grochulla (eds.), *Manual of Spine Surgery*, https://doi.org/10.1007/978-3-662-64062-3_14

14.3   Biomechanic

Orthoses perform the following main functions:

- *Kinetic memory*
  The pressure of the orthoses stimulates the sensory system and provides a "reminder" to the patient of the correct posture (the so-called reminder effect).
- *Increased intra-abdominal pressure*
  Due to the increased intra-abdominal pressure, the so-called toothpaste tube effect on the bone corrects the spinal posture (see Fig. 14.1).
- *Three-point support*
  A number of orthoses use the three-point principle to achieve correction and immobilization (lordosis, kyphosis, derotation)
- *Extension*
  Vertebral segments are erected across to fix bone points.
- *Endpoint control*
  Depending on its design, the orthoses restrict movement at the endpoints.
- *Activating erecting function (reminding orthoses)*
  In the cervical region, axial rotation occurs at the specialized atlantoaxial joint. At the lower cervical levels, flexion, extension and lateral flexion occur freely. However, the articular processes, which face anteriorly or posteriorly, limit rotation. In the thoracic region, movement in all planes is possible, although to a lesser degree. In the lumbar region, flexion, extension and lateral flexion occur, but rotation is limited because of the inwardly facing articular facets. An understanding of the three-column concept of spine stability is helpful to ensure that the proper orthosis is prescribed. The anterior column consists of the anterior longitudinal ligament, the annulus fibrosus and the anterior half of the vertebral body. The middle column consists of the posterior longitudinal ligament, the annulus fibrosus and the posterior half of the vertebral body. The posterior column consists of the interspinous and supraspinous ligaments, the facet joints, the lamina, the pedicles and the spinous processes. The loss of normal spinal anatomy can affect the stability of the spine. Spine motion can be classified with reference to horizontal (transverse), frontal (coronal) and sagittal planes. The spinal motion can shift the centre of gravity, which is normally located approximately 2–3 cm anterior to the S1. In the cervical region, axial rotation occurs at the specialized atlantoaxial joint. At the lower cervical levels, flexion, extension and lateral flexion occur freely. However, the articular processes face anteriorly or posteriorly. In the cervical spine, extension occurs predominantly at the occipital C1 junction. Lateral bending occurs mainly at the C3-C4 and C4-C5 levels. Axial rotation occurs mostly at the C1-C2 levels. In the thoracic spine, flexion and extension occur primarily at the T11-T12 and T12-L1 levels. Lateral bending is fairly evenly distributed throughout the thoracic levels. Axial rotation occurs mostly at the T1-T2 level, with a gradual decrease towards the lumbar spine. The thoracic spine is the least mobile because of the restrictive nature of the rib cage. In the lumbar spinal segment, movement in the sagittal plane occurs more at the distal segment, with lateral bending predominantly at the L3-L4 level. Knowledge of the normal spinal range of motion helps in understanding how the various cervical orthoses (CO) can limit that range.

14.4   Cervical Orthoses (CO) [1, 2, 4]

The *halo orthoses* provide flexion, extension and rotational control of the cervical region. Pressure systems are used for control of motion, as well as to provide slight distraction for immobilization of the cervical spine. This orthosis provides maximum restriction in motion of all the cervical orthoses. It is the most stable orthosis, especially in the superior cervical spine segment. A halo is used for approximately 10–12 weeks to ensure healing of a fracture or of a spinal fusion. Usually a cervical collar is indicated after the halo is removed, because the muscles and ligaments supporting the head become weak after disuse. All pins on the halo ring should be checked to ensure tightness 24–48 h after application.

Cervical orthoses Philadelphia or Miami (see Fig. 14.2) provide some control of flexion, extension and lateral bending and minimal rotational control of the cervical region. Pressure systems are used for control of motion, as well as to

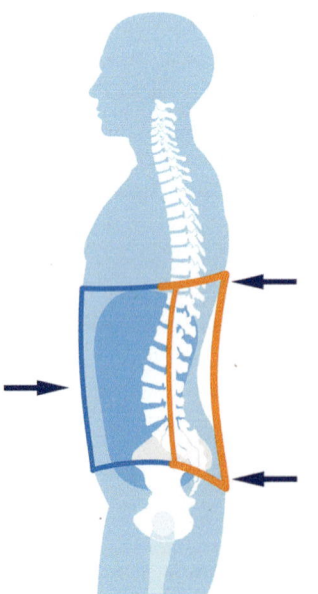

Fig. 14.1 The *toothpaste tube effect* on the bone corrects the spinal posture (reproduced with permission from Bauerfeind AG, Germany [2])

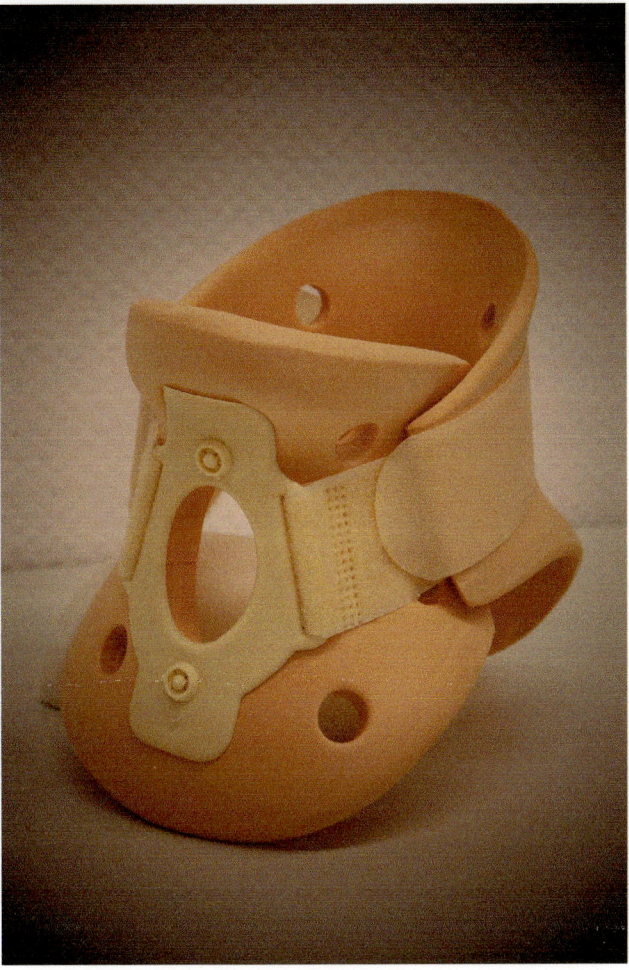

Fig. 14.2 Cervical orthoses—Philadelphia

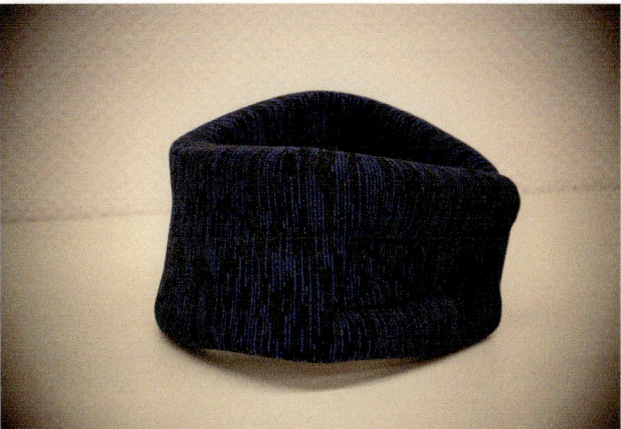

Fig. 14.3 Soft cervical orthoses

provide slight distraction for immobilization of the cervical spine. Circumferential pressure is also intended to provide warmth and as a kinaesthetic reminder for the patient. These orthoses are prefabricated, consisting of one or two pieces that are usually attached with Velcro straps. Other options include a Schanz compression collar (tricoprene elastic bandage) or a soft cervical support (see Fig. 14.3).

14.5 Cervicothoracic Orthosis (CTO)

14.5.1 Sternal Occipital Mandibular Immobilizer (SOMI)

The biomechanics provide control of flexion, extension, lateral bending and rotation of the cervical spine. Pressure systems are used for control of motion, as well as to provide slight distraction for immobilization of the spine. A benefit of the SOMI orthosis is that it can be done while the patient is in the supine position. The SOMI is a good choice for patients who are restricted to bed, because there are no posterior rods to interfere with comfort of the patient. A headband can be added so that the chin piece can be removed. This maintains stability but improves accessibility for daily hygiene and eating. The SOMI is prefabricated, consisting of a cervical portion with removable chin piece and bars that curve over the shoulders. Also used are posts that fixate the cervical portion to the sternal portion of the orthosis. The anterior section supports the mandible and rests on the superior edge of the sternum, with the inferior anterior edge terminating at the level of the xiphoid. The posterior aspect of the orthosis supports the head at the occipital level. Indications are cervical sprains, strains, stable fracture protection and limited mobility during the healing process in the postoperative patient. Contraindications are unstable fractures with ligament instability. The *Yale orthosis* consists of chin and occipital pieces that extend higher on the skull in the posterior region; this increases comfort. The Yale orthosis is a modified Philadelphia collar with a thoracic extension. The extension consists of fibreglass that extends both anteriorly and posteriorly and has thoracic straps that hold the sections together. The thoracic extension to the orthosis helps to stabilize injuries at the vertebral levels of C6-T2. The four-poster is a rigid cervical orthosis with anterior and posterior sections consisting of pads that lie on the chest and are connected by leather straps.

14.6 Cervicothoracolumbosacral Orthoses (CTLSO)

The *Milwaukee orthosis* is used for scoliosis management and provides control of flexion, extension and lateral bending of the cervical, thoracic and lumber spine.

The Milwaukee *orthosis* is a good choice for patients who need correction in the higher thoracic region of the spine.

Indication is the scoliotic management of the high thoracic curves. Contraindications are lower thoracic and lumbar curves.

14.7 Thoracolumbosacral Orthoses (TLSO)

14.7.1 Torso Orthoses

Torso orthoses are mainly used for conditions affecting the lumbar spine or the thoracolumbar junction. Orthoses should always be regarded as just one element of a multimodal reactivating treatment concept. The aim of the treatment should always be to develop the body's own supportive "corset" of muscles. A common indication for prescribing an orthosis for this part of the body is lumbago which is proving resistant to therapy; in this case, the orthosis is used to complement the existing therapy. It is important that there is a clear indication for use of a particular type of orthosis, that is, the physician responsible for the patient's treatment must have a clear idea about the aims of the orthosis therapy. Lumbar supports (Fig. 14.4a–c) can be used for acute lumbar spine syndrome and mild degeneration of the spine. These products are made from breathable, elastic fabric, and they support and relieve the lumbar spine. An integral pad in the lumbar area can help to relieve tension and pain. The *lumbar corset* is a support for the spine which is used for patients with lumbago and pain in the lumbar region. There is an integral pad in this region to relieve pain and support the lumbar area. The corset can be prescribed as a ready-made product, or a custom-made solution can be produced. However, the orthosis is contraindicated for obese patients. The length and height of the pad must be selected to suit the region where relief is required. It is important to establish whether the pad needs to be adjusted to provide support or to reduce the lordosis of the spine. The *Lindemann corset* based on a grid of stays has a more complex design and is used to relieve, support and restrict the movement of the lumbar spine and thoracolumbar junction. The corset can be used temporarily, for long-term treatment, or post-operatively, and it is indicated for static muscular insufficiency, mild osteoporosis, lumbago, degenerative changes in the lumbar spine, Baastrup's disease and grade 1 spondylolisthesis. The traditional Lindemann corset/corset based on a grid of stays consists of an elastic, raised, 2/3 corset with a circular pelvic frame and tensioning strap system. Eight to ten plastic or spring band steel back stays, which are connected together without elasticity of extension, are integrated into the corset to provide additional stabilization for the relevant section of the spine. The main effect is achieved through compression of the soft tissues and the lordosing effect of the orthosis. As well as made-to-measure products, prefabricated lumbar orthoses made from modern knitted fabrics and strap systems are increasingly used nowadays. The *flexion orthosis* is indicated for dorsal vertebral joint syndromes in particular, with indications including facet syndrome, lumbar syndrome, lumbar spinal stenosis and sciatica. It is also suitable for postoperative care following intervertebral disc prolapse surgery. This type of orthosis consists of a ready-made corset with an integrated raised pad or bridging frame. This bridging frame distributes forces away from the lumbar spine out towards the thoracic spine, pelvis and sacrum. This effect can be further supported by means of an abdominal pad which compresses the abdominal cavity and straightens the spine. In this case too, it is generally industrially manufactured products that are used. If greater restriction of movement is needed, for example, for a more pronounced diagnosis, the rigid *Hohmann bridging corset* can be prescribed. The corset is designed to bridge the lordosis and is therefore able to compensate for the increased lordosis and, at the same time, to immobilize the painful section of the spine. The extensive immobilization of the lumbar spine is effected by means of a

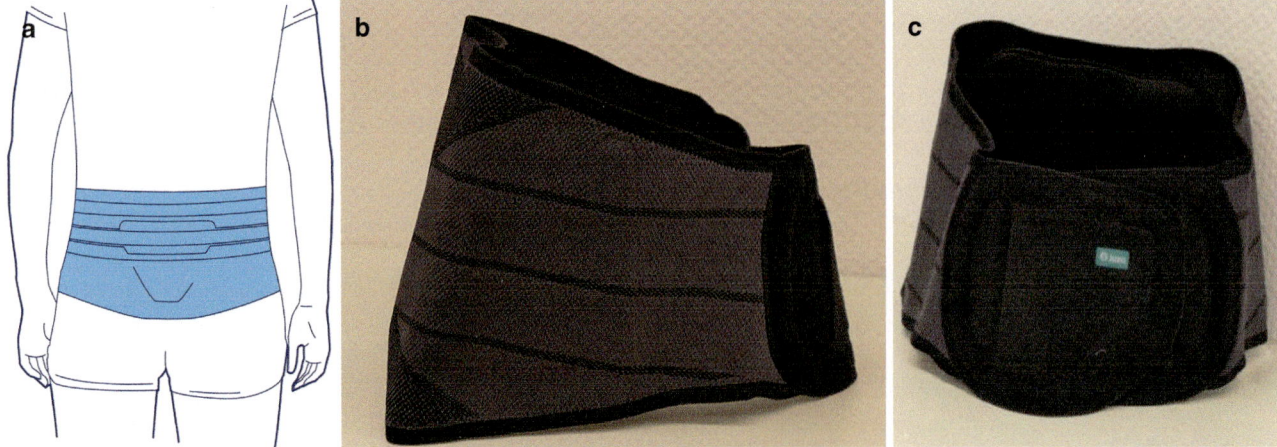

Fig. 14.4 Lumbar support corset: (**a**) illustration (reproduced with permission from Bauerfeind AG, Germany [2]), (**b**) side view, (**c**) front view

rigid drill fabric corset. There are dorsolateral aluminium braces, connected by rigid rods, which encompass the pelvis and torso and provide a frame structure to stabilize the bridging corset at the torso. Extension and flexion movements as well as tilting to the side are all largely prevented. The bridging corset is indicated for intervertebral disc conditions with severe pain, paralytic scoliosis in the lumbar region, tumour metastasis, osteoporosis and post-operative segmentary instability and for follow-up treatment for fractures as well as for discitis. The *thoracolumbar orthosis* can be used for senile osteoporosis and degenerative changes of the thoracic and lumbar spine and for stable fractures. This orthosis, which extends up into the thoracic region, consists of a semi-elastic corset, a pelvic harness, two paravertebral longitudinal rods and two shoulder loops for straightening purposes. The orthosis straightens, stretches and supports the spine. Overall, mobility is not restricted as much as it is with a framed support corset. As a result of the shoulder strap arrangement, no pressure is exerted on the thoracic region, so there is a very good acceptance of this orthosis. The *framed support corset* (see Fig. 14.5a, b) offers maximum immobilization of the torso, and it is only indicated for severe pain. Indications are inflammatory and destructive processes of the lumbar spine and of the lower to middle thoracic spine (but not above this level), severe osteoporosis with vertebral fractures and unstable fractures in the thoracic spine (not above the level of the middle thoracic spine). The aim of the orthosis therapy is to immobilize the lumbar and thoracic segments of the spine and to prevent inclination, rotation and lateral movement to the side. The bridging corset has a frame

design with torso braces which encompass the thoracic region or reclination pads which are positioned below the claviculae. The pelvis is immobilized by means of a plastic pelvic cage.

The *three-point corset* (see Fig. 14.6a, b) is used in the conservative treatment of stable fractures of the lumbar and lower thoracic spine. However, the corset is contraindicated in the case of unstable vertebral fractures, which must be stabilized surgically. The aim of the orthosis therapy is to straighten and stabilize the lumbar and lower thoracic spine. The three-point corset connects the pubic bone, sternum and spine by means of a rigid pelvic ring. Nowadays, the orthoses are usually supplied as ready-made products in a range of sizes. It is important to ensure that the orthosis is sitting correctly and that there is good support at the sternum and pubic symphysis. Indications are traumatic or pathologic spinal fractures in the mid to lower thoracic region or lumbar region. Contraindications are obesity, excessive lordosis and a need for increased lateral stability. The *cruciform anterior spinal hyperextension (CASH)* orthosis controls the flexion for the lower thoracic and lumbar regions. The system consists of posteriorly directed forces through a sternal and suprapubic pad and an anteriorly directed force applied through a thoracolumbar pad attached to a strap that extends to the horizontal anterior bar. When properly fitted, the sternal pad is 1½ in. below the sternal notch, and the suprapubic pad is 1½ in. above the symphysis pubis. Indications are mild compression fractures of the lower thoracic and thoracolumbar regions. Contraindications are unstable fractures or burst fractures.

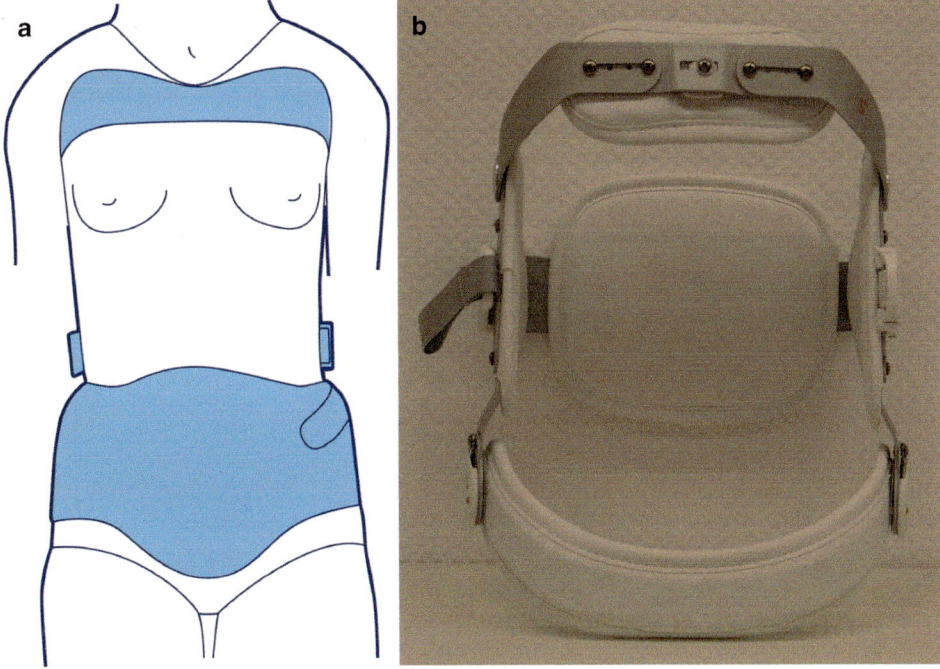

Fig. 14.5 Frame support corset: (**a**) illustration (reproduced with permission from Bauerfeind AG, Germany [2]), (**b**) ready-made frame support corset

Fig. 14.6 Three-point corset: (**a**) illustrations in (**a**) (front) and from (**b**) (back) (reproduced with permission from Bauerfeind AG, Germany [2])

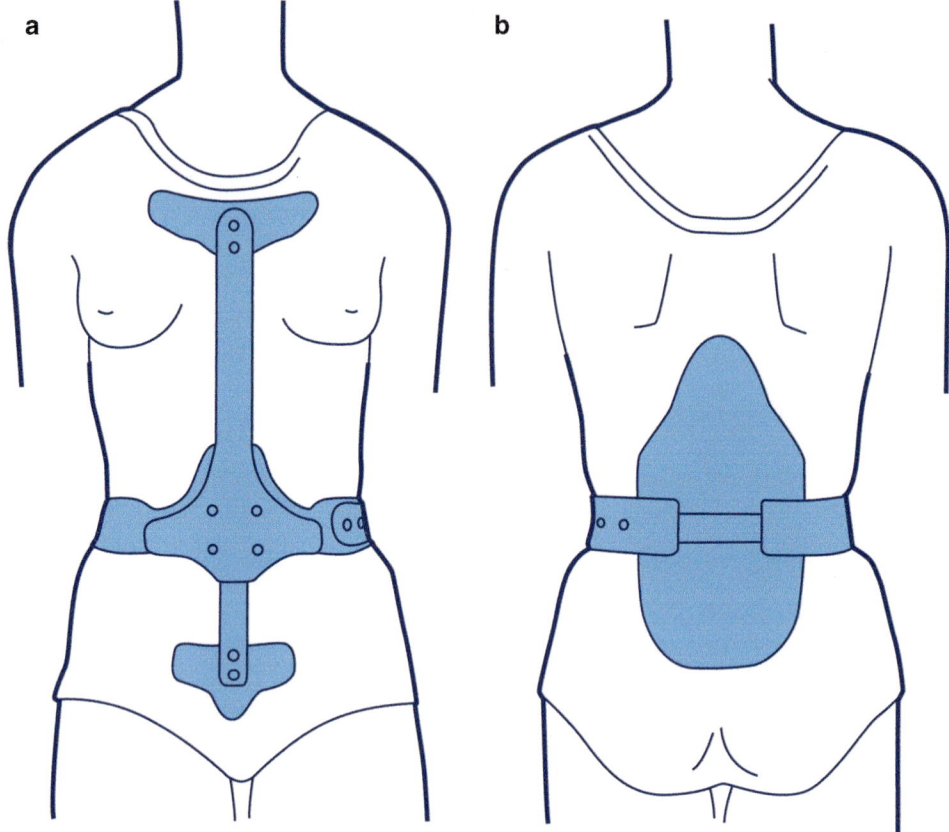

14.8 Lumbosacral Orthosis (LSO)

The biomechanics of the lumbosacral orthosis are the anterior and lateral trunk containments. The restriction of flexion and extension can be achieved with the addition of steel stays posteriorly. Design and fabrication are made from cloth that wraps around the torso and hips. Adjustments are done with laces on the sides, back or front. Closure can be with hook and loop or hook and eye fasteners or snaps. Many different styles are available in prefabricated sizes, usually in 2-in. increments, and are designed to fit the body circumference at the level of the hips. Indications are low back pain, herniated discs and lumbar muscle strain and to control gross trunk motion for pain control after single-column compression fractures with one-third or less anterior height loss. Contraindications are unstable fractures.

14.9 Sacral Orthosis (SO)

The biomechanics of sacroiliac orthosis or sacral orthosis are to provide anterior and lateral trunk containment and to assist in the restriction of some pelvic flexion and extension. It also

aids in compression of the pelvis. This orthosis is usually made from cloth that wraps around the pelvis and hips. Some models also include laces on the side in which adjustments can be made, whereas others use straps for adjusting. Indications are pelvic fractures or symphysis pubis fractures or strains. It is useful to control motion and for pain control. Contraindications are unstable fractures, as well as fractures or conditions in the lumbar region.

14.10 Specialized Orthosis

Specific indication points must be observed when dealing with scoliosis and/or kyphosis, as well as with osteoporotic fractures. Some of these have already been described.

14.10.1 Scoliosis [4, 7]

Idiopathic (infantile, juvenile, adolescent), congenital and neuromuscular scolioses have different aetiologies, treatment approaches and outcomes. With idiopathic scoliosis, the evaluation should reveal no anomalous vertebrae, spinal

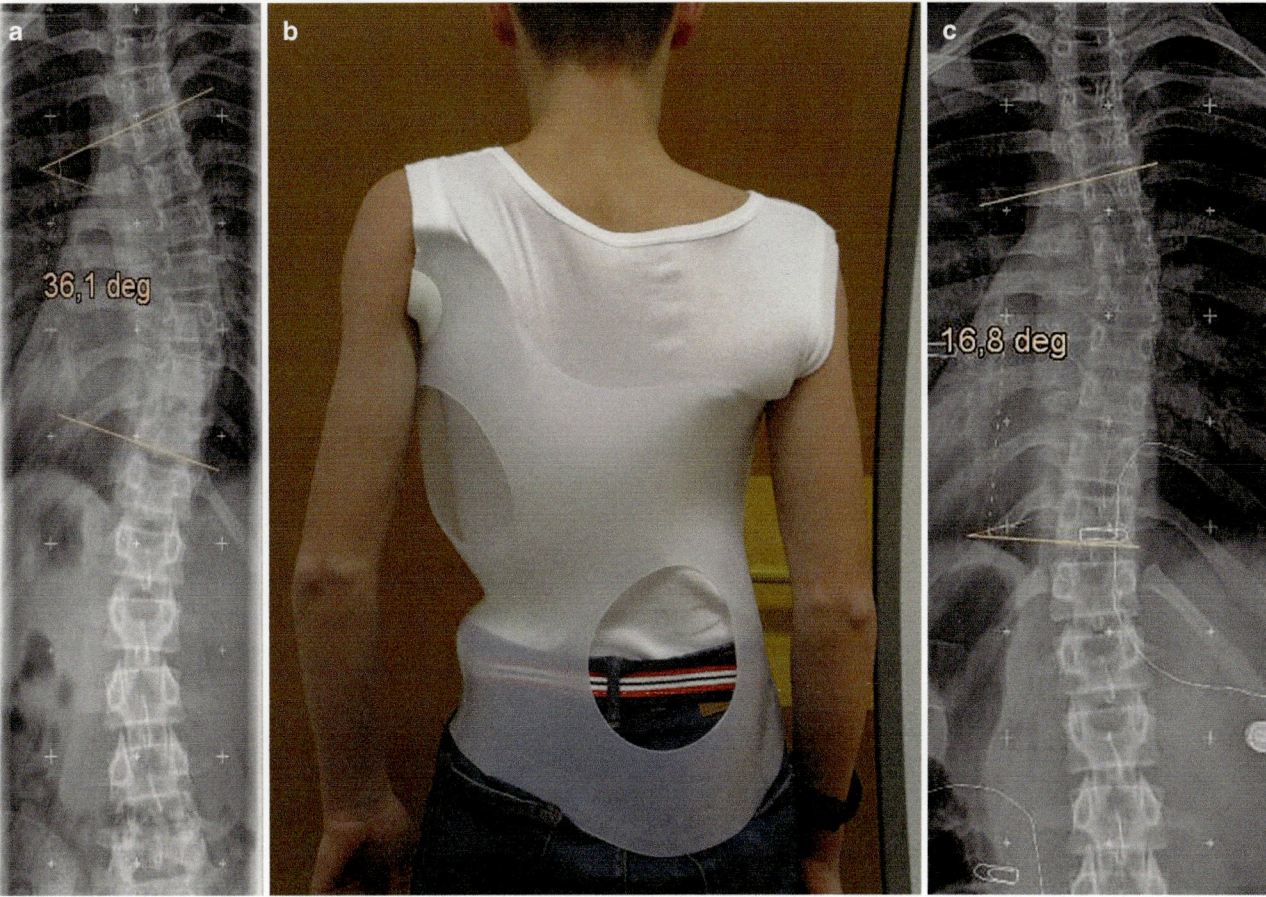

Fig. 14.7 (**a**) A 14-year-old patient with a idiopatic scoliosis. X-ray of the thoracic and lumbar spine pretreatment. (**b**) Patient in standing position from behind with a Chêneau brace. (**c**) X-ray with applied Chêneau brace

tumours or other neurologic abnormalities. Most cases remain stable for a long period and progress late in life when osteoporosis and degenerative spinal conditions normally have their onset. There is evidence to indicate that an orthosis can slow the progression of idiopathic scoliosis, and it is therefore the non-operative treatment of choice. Juvenile idiopathic scoliosis is more likely to be associated with adult corpulmonal and death. Treatment should begin when curves reach approximately 25 deg. Because thoracic curves predominate, the *Milwaukee brace* might be more effective than the *TLSO*. The *Milwaukee brace* is an externally applied *cervicothoracolumbosacral orthosis (CTLSO)* brace used in the treatment of adolescent scoliosis that is especially effective to correct kyphosis. Adolescent idiopathic scoliosis is the most common type for which an orthosis is indicated. Curves with an apex at T9 or lower can be managed with a TLSO (Cheneau) (see Fig. 14.7a–c).

14.10.2 Osteoporosis Orthosis [5, 6]

In the initial stages of osteoporosis, one of the aims of orthosis therapy is to remind the patient to straighten up. Although rigid orthoses were used in the past, the trend nowadays is for elastic orthoses, as these are more readily accepted by patients. In addition to the orthoses already mentioned, there are elastic straightening orthoses. Shoulder straps help to provide additional straightening of the shoulders. The orthosis consists of a bar over the spinous processes and straps. These are usually ready-made orthoses with a carbon or aluminium back splint to help with the straightening process. There are straps in the pelvic region and at the shoulders, and these provide extra postural support. These orthoses are sometimes supplied in combination with a bodysuit. They work primarily through the straightening function of the shoulder straps and remind patients to straighten up (Fig. 14.8).

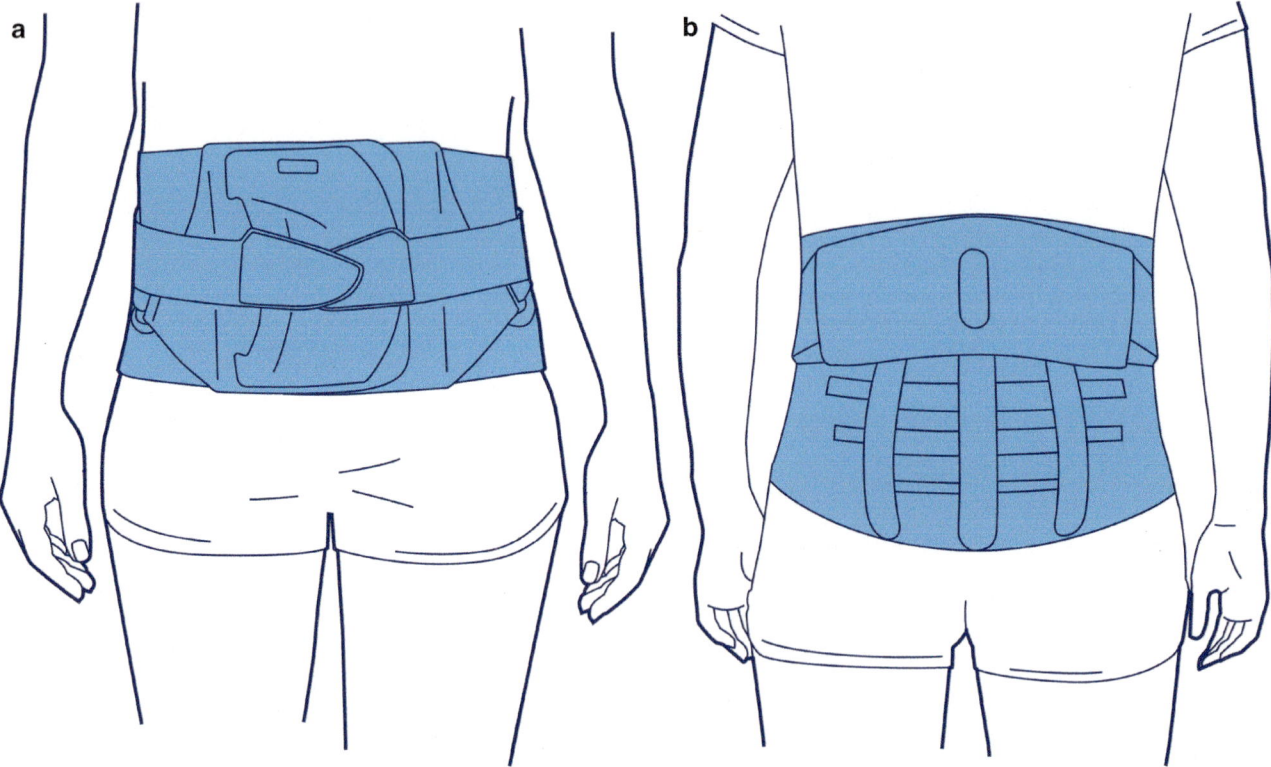

Fig. 14.8 (**a** and **b**) Cross support bodice front view and rear view

References

1. Agabegi SS, Asghar FA, Herkowitz HN. Spinal orthoses. J Am Acad Orthop Surg. 2010;18:657–67.
2. Greitemann B, Baumgartner R. Technische Orthopädie. Stuttgart: Thieme; 2017.
3. Valle-Jones JC, Walsh H, O'Hara J, et al. Controlled trial of a back support ('Lumbotrain') in patients with non-specific low back pain. Curr Med Res Opin. 1992;12:604–13.
4. Baumgartner B, Greitemann B. Grundkurs Technische Orthopädie. Stuttgart: Georg Thieme Verlag KG; 2007.
5. Namdar N, Arazpour M, Ahmadi BM. Comparison of the immediate efficacy of the Spinomed® back orthosis and posture training support on walking ability in elderly people with thoracic kyphosis. Disabil Rehabil Assist Technol. 2017;21:1–4.
6. Newman M, Minns Lowe C, Barker K. Spinal orthoses for vertebral osteoporosis and osteoporotic vertebral fracture: a systematic review. Arch Phys Med Rehabil. 2016;97:1013–25.
7. Climent JM, Sanchez J. Impact of the type of brace on the quality of life of adolescents with spine deformities. Spine. 1999;24:1903–8.

Biological Repair Options in Degenerative Disk Diseases

15

Christian Hohaus and Hans Jörg Meisel

15.1 Introduction and Core Messages

Biological repair for degenerative disk diseases has right now a very slide attention in the field of treatment for this very common disorder with a high impact in the public health community. Therapeutic options for biological repair include the substitution of growth factors, transplantation of cells, tissue engineering, and gene modification. The aim of the repair and regenerative treatment is to prevent further progression of disk degeneration, supplement tissue loss, and stabilizing anatomy that might diminish disk degeneration-associated symptoms. Among cell-based therapies, transplantation of autologous intervertebral disk cells harvested from herniated disk material seems to be a promising option [1, 2]. Harvesting the disk cell material is a standard procedure by performing a microsurgical sequestrectomy in cases of disk herniation. Cell separation, culture, and expansion, although not simple, are possible and should be done with appropriate expertise under GMP (good manufacturing practice) conditions. The proceeding for the transplantation is comparable to the former routinely performed discography.

Intervertebral disk degeneration is a common disorder that negatively impacts quality of life, affecting 40% of younger individuals and prevalent in more than 90% of individuals older than 50 years of age. Treatment options, either operative or conservative, fail to treat the underlying pathology of the degenerating disk. Degeneration of the disk is a multifactorial process; among those, age and genetic loading [3], biomechanical forces [4], and environmental factors such as immobilization, trauma, and application of nicotine [5] are the most important. Age-related diseases such as diabetes, arterial hypertension, and complications associated with vascular diseases have been defined as relevant factors as well [6]. The level of disk degeneration can be graded from early stage which still has a higher number of viable cells and less structural damage through an intermediate to an advanced degenerative stage at which viable disk cells are depleted and structural damage of the disk anatomy is conspicuously abnormal. Biological repair options that supplement tissue loss buffer the inflammatory milieu of the degenerating disk, offering a feasible strategy to treat the underlying pathology depending on the stage of degeneration [7] (Fig. 15.1). This knowledge has led to regenerative therapeutic options for degenerated disk diseases which includes substituting growth factors, transplanting cells, engineering tissue, and modifying genes. Some preclinical efforts have been successful suggesting that proteoglycan synthesis increases in a canine model after direct injection of recombinant TGF-beta in combination with epidermal growth factor [8]. Similarly, direct stimulation of cells with osteogenic protein-1 or BMP-7 in rabbit intervertebral disks resulted in an increase in proteoglycan synthesis as well as restoration of disk height [9–11]. Intradiskal delivery of BMP-7 for regeneration of inter-

C. Hohaus (✉)
Department of Neurosurgery, Städtisches Klinikum Dessau, Dessau-Roßlau, Germany
e-mail: christian.hohaus@klinikum-dessau.de

H. J. Meisel
Department of Neurosurgery, BG Klinikum Bergmannstrost, Halle, Germany

vertebral disk degeneration in a non-chondrodystrophic canine model however did not promote disk regeneration but instead resulted in the formation of the extradiskal bone [12]. In a first clinical study combined matrix components and growth factors that were directly injected into degenerated disks. Over the course of a 12-month follow-up, an improvement in function and pain in patients was measured as probably the effect of stimulation of the intervertebral disk regeneration [13]. Despite the success achieved, the concern for therapeutic support for such techniques seemed severely limited due to the availability of viable cells and limitation in application to only early stages of disk degeneration [14]. Disk herniation is thought to be an extension of progressive disk degeneration and is the most common reason for radicular symptoms in the lumbar spine leading to an operative treatment. As a potential source of compatible biologic material, the herniated material from the degenerated disk has been considered as a potential donor for both nucleus pulposus cells and chondrocytes because of inherent viability and autologous compatibility [15]. Culturing and expanding these cells, although not simple, are possible, and following successful transplantation, cells produce both type II collagen and appropriate proteoglycans [1]. Transplantation of these expanded cultured cells would afford an option to expand the viable cell content in the degenerated disk, reduce pro-inflammatory cytokines, and contribute potentially in increasing the extracellular matrix which is critical to mechanical damping and anatomical restoration. In a canine study, the hypothesis is that restoration of intervertebral disk morphology by transplantation of cultured autologous chondrocytes into the nucleus pulposus could be validated [16]. Autologous disk cell transplantation in lumbar disk degeneration disease was established initially in a prospective randomized controlled clinical trial in 2002—the EuroDisc Study. After the first promising results published in 2007 and 2008 [2, 17], the routine treatment in selected cases with monosegmental degeneration in the lumbar spine and requiring an operative treatment of disk herniation started. Until now, more than 150 patients have been treated with this promising regenerative treatment option.

15.2 Indication

The autologous disk cell transplantation is a therapeutic option to prevent further disk degeneration for patients undergoing a microsurgical sequestrectomy where in addition to the surgery, cells are harvested from the disk material and cultured for transplantation.

The indication for the microsurgical sequestrectomy is usually lumbar disk degeneration with herniated disk material resulting in a root nerve compression with radicular and lumbar back pain, neurological deficits, and reduced life quality. Patients from 18 up to 65 years of age with monosegmental disk degeneration could be treated with body mass index that has to be below 28.

Conservative treatment should be ineffective over more than 3 weeks or the neurological deficits were pronounced.

An MRI of the lumbar spine with sagittal and axial T1 and T2 sequences was mandatory. The initial degeneration was graduated with the Modic score [18, 19]. Only patients with Modic grade 1 or below and a disk height at the minimum of two-thirds of the adjacent disks were included into the trial to be sure that the degeneration is still in the intermediate phase [7] and the environment in the disk is stable enough for the integration of the cells after transplantation.

15.3 Contraindication

Patients with previous surgery in the affected motion segment were excluded as well as patients with Modic grade 2 and higher in the preoperative MRI.

Patients with spondylolisthesis were excluded as well as patients with sclerotic changes or a progressive degenerative spinal disorder.

Pregnant women and patients with progressive neurological deficits or with generalized diseases and inflammatory diseases, acute or chronic, were contraindications for cell transplantation as well. Patients with progressive loss of disk height after the microscopic sequestrectomy in the MRI before transplantation or with ongoing disk degeneration using MRI criteria should not be transplanted, estimating a decreased effect of cell viability in these cases.

Recurrent disk herniation in the MRI pretransplantation is another exclusion criterion.

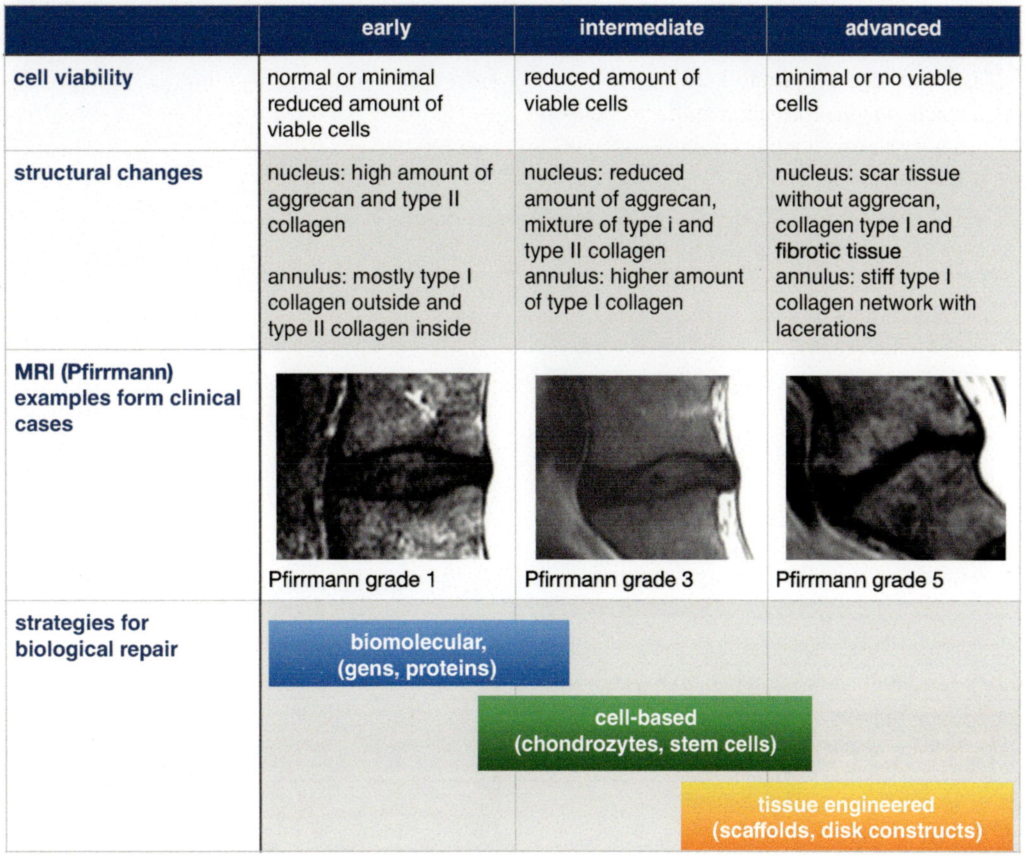

	early	intermediate	advanced
cell viability	normal or minimal reduced amount of viable cells	reduced amount of viable cells	minimal or no viable cells
structural changes	nucleus: high amount of aggrecan and type II collagen annulus: mostly type I collagen outside and type II collagen inside	nucleus: reduced amount of aggrecan, mixture of type i and type II collagen annulus: higher amount of type I collagen	nucleus: scar tissue without aggrecan, collagen type I and fibrotic tissue annulus: stiff type I collagen network with lacerations
MRI (Pfirrmann) examples form clinical cases	Pfirrmann grade 1	Pfirrmann grade 3	Pfirrmann grade 5
strategies for biological repair	biomolecular, (gens, proteins)	cell-based (chondrozytes, stem cells)	tissue engineered (scaffolds, disk constructs)

Fig. 15.1 Degeneration of the intervertebral disk and options for the biological repair. Comparison of MRI classification (Pfirrmann), schematic graduation of intervertebral changes and therapeutic strategies

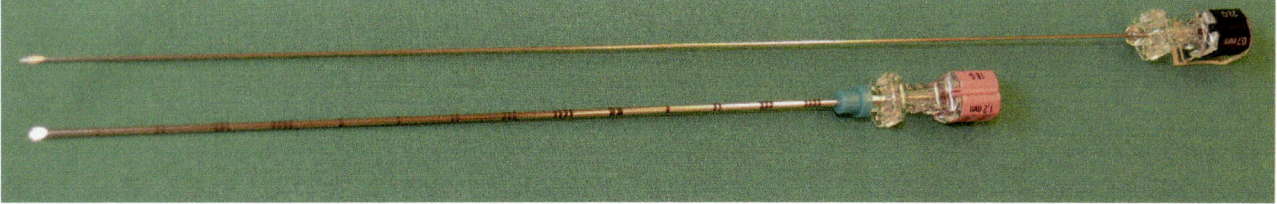

Fig. 15.2 An 18G cannula for puncturing the outer rim of the annulus fibrosus and a 22G cannula to puncture the inner annulus

15.4 Technical Requirements

Necessary requirements for the microscopic sequestrectomy are C-arm, microscope, and the usual microsurgical instruments. For the transplantation, a C-arm, a tool to measure the intradiskal pressure (ICP device or a hydrostatic pressure device), and two needles for the punction of the affected intervertebral disk are required. An 18G cannula is recommended for puncturing the outer rim of the annulus fibrosus and a 22G cannula to puncture the inner annulus and applicate the cells into the nucleus (Fig. 15.2).

15.5 Operative Treatment

The necessary surgical intervention to perform the decompression of the root nerve caused by disk herniation was done by an experienced neurosurgeon trained in performing microsurgical microscopic sequestrectomy procedure, under general anesthesia. The herniated disk material was detached and removed. The intervertebral disk was not opened actively.

The preserved herniated disk material was cultured under GMP conditions (co.don AG, Teltow, Germany). The chon-

Fig. 15.3 Fluoroscopic view of the disk after puncture with needle-in-needle technique

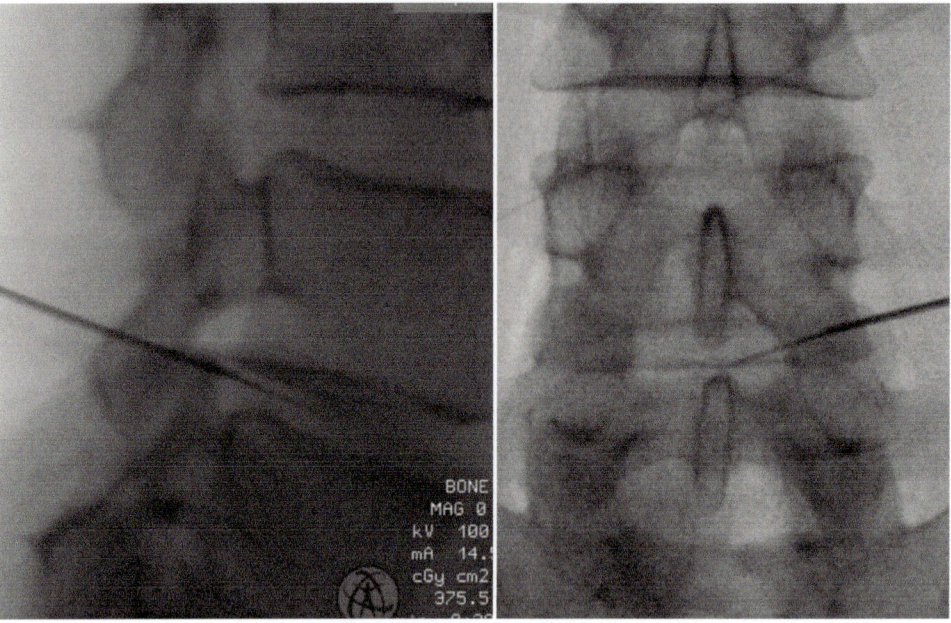

drocytes were separated and cultured in patient's serum until reaching the necessary amount of cells for transplantation. These cultured cells were stored under GMP conditions until the time point of transplantation.

15.6 Cell Transplantation

The cell transplantation was planned within 12 weeks after the initial operative treatment. From the previous animal studies, we know that the annulus fibrosus will be healed after this time and will be able to contain the added volume of implanted cells [1]. Normal clinical and neurological examination and MRI of the lumbar spine excluding any recurrent disk herniation or other progressive disk degenerations were mandatory before planning the transplantation. The intervention was performed in prone position under local anesthesia and fluoroscopic control (Fig. 15.3). The affected intervertebral disk was punctured with two atraumatic cannulas using a needle-in-needle technique (Fig. 15.4). To prevent an injury of the initial affected root nerve, the puncture was done from the opposite side. To be sure that the annulus fibrosus is intact, a pressure volume test [20] was carried out using a high precision probe used for measuring the intracranial pressure (Fig. 15.5). The test was successful in all cases. The prepared solution contained more than five million living disk cells in 0.5 mL physiological sodium solution. This volume was inserted into the intervertebral disk over the time of 3 min (Fig. 15.6).

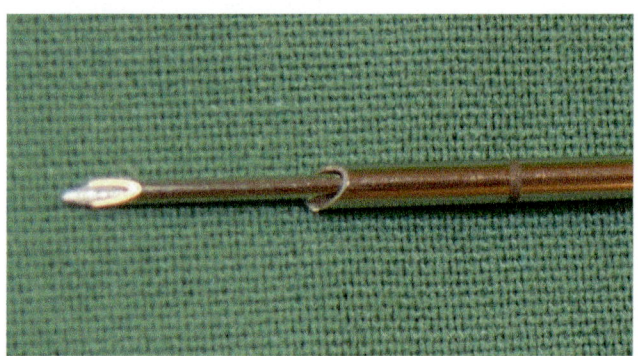

Fig. 15.4 The needle-in-needle technique using an 18G cannula to puncture the annulus fibrosus and a 22G cannula to puncture the inner annulus and applicate the cells into the nucleus

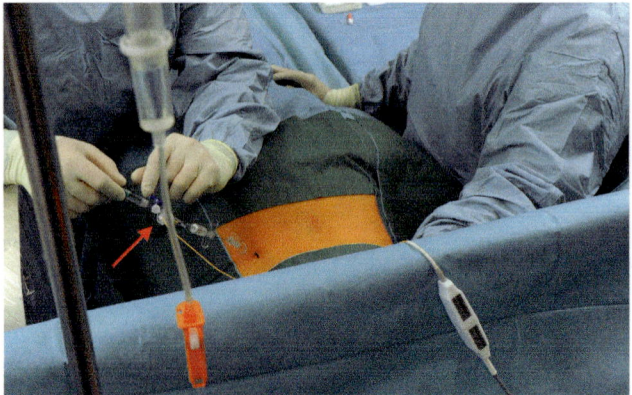

Fig. 15.5 Pressure-volume-test using an ICP-probe (red arrow) to measure the pressure in the intervertebral disk to detect a leakage in the annulus fibrosous

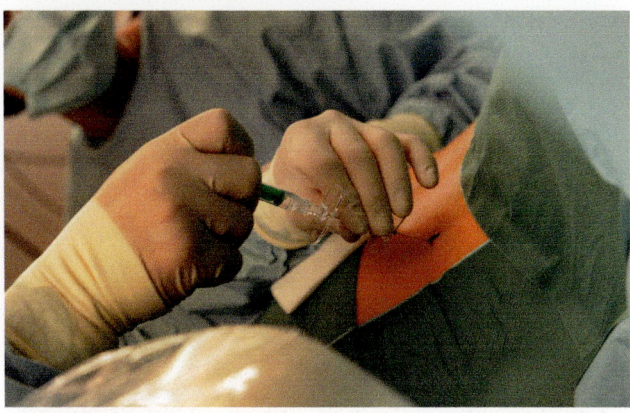

Fig. 15.6 Cell transplantation in 0.5 mL fluid

15.7 Postoperative Procedures

A lying position is endorsed for the patients after cell transplantation for 1 day. The remobilization is allowed wearing a lumbar orthosis for the next 3 weeks. This should provide an auxiliary stabilization for the treated segments and prevent strong movements to facilitate implanted cell integration into the affected intervertebral disk.

15.8 Conclusion

Autologous disk cell transplantation comes out as a treatment option for patients suffering from degenerative disk disease (DDD) with the need of an operative intervention for disk herniation. This will be promoted from the results of our clinical study and our experience with more than 150 transplantations of autologous disk cells in affected disks in the last 15 years. A clear reduction in pain and an increase in life quality were seen in all treated patients in the EuroDisc study (Fig. 15.7). The return to work rate was 100% after cell transplantation. There was no evidence of local reaction after the cell transplantation. Inflammatory complications like spondylodiscitis did not appear after transplantation. In the clinical setting, the stable disk height assessed in the MR images over 2 years in the transplantation group and a definite reduction in the reherniation rate are signs for the stabilization and the decrease in degenerative process in the intervertebral disk.

A complete regeneration of degenerated intervertebral disks is currently not a therapeutic option for the high number of affected patients. The prevention of further progression of the disk degeneration process and its associated symptoms is the goal of regenerative medicine at this time.

A therapeutic option, for patients without herniated disk material and for that reason without an indication for an operative procedure to harvest disk material, is the ongoing evaluation of transplanting bone marrow stem cells into

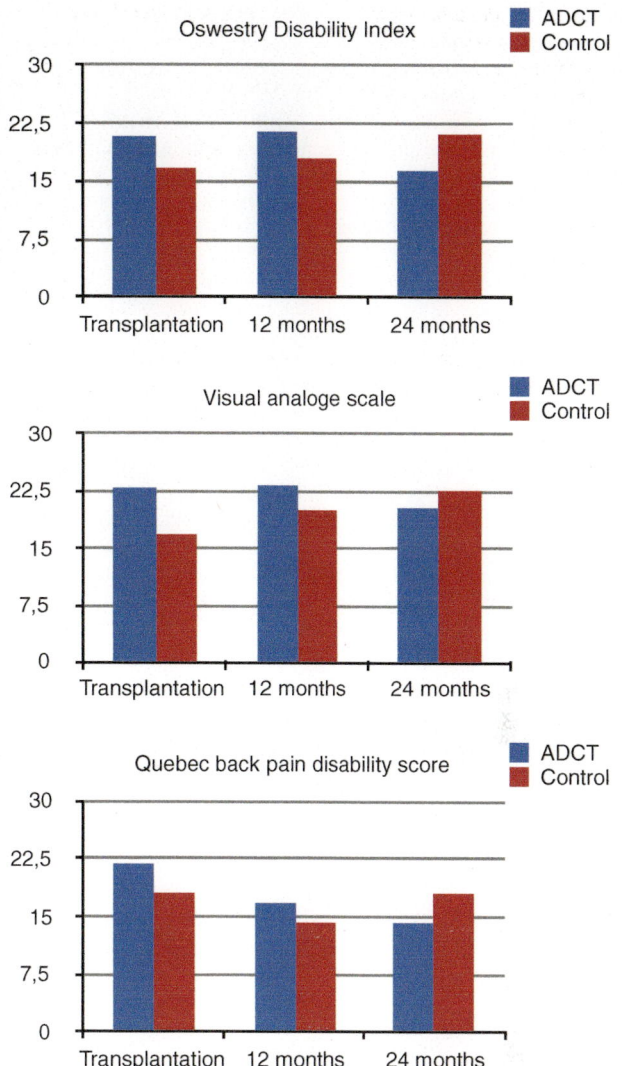

Fig. 15.7 Descriptive analysis of efficacy after 24 months for the Oswestry disability index, Quebec back pain disability score and Visual analoge scale (back pain) shows a clear benefit for the treatment group

early-stage degenerated disks. A prospective, multicenter randomized, double-blind trial, comparing intradiskal allogeneic adult BM-MSC therapy and sham-treated controls in subjects with chronic low back pain due to lumbar degenerative disk disease (DDD) unresponsive to conventional therapy, is recruiting patients since summer 2019.

References

1. Ganey TM, Meisel HJ. A potential role for cell-based therapeutics in the treatment of intervertebral disc herniation. Eur Spine J. 2002;11(Suppl 2):S206–14.
2. Hohaus C, Ganey TM, Minkus Y, Meisel HJ. Cell transplantation in lumbar spine disc degeneration disease. Eur Spine J. 2008;17(Suppl 4):492–503.

3. Battie MC, Videman T, Gibbons LE, et al. Volvo award in clinical sciences. Determinants of lumbar disc degeneration. A study relating lifetime exposures and magnetic resonance imaging findings in identical twins. Spine. 1995;20(24):2601–12.

4. Lotz JC, Staples A, Walsh A, Hsieh AH. Mechanobiology in intervertebral disc degeneration and regeneration. Conference Proceedings: Annual International Conference of the IEEE Engineering in Medicine and Biology Society IEEE Engineering in Medicine and Biology Society Annual Conference (vol. 7); 2004. p. 5459.

5. Pye SR, Reid DM, Adams JE, et al. Influence of weight, body mass index and lifestyle factors on radiographic features of lumbar disc degeneration. Ann Rheum Dis. 2007;66(3):426–7.

6. Anderson DG, Tannoury C. Molecular pathogenic factors in symptomatic disc degeneration. Spine J. 2005;5(6 Suppl):260s–6s.

7. Moriguchi Y, Alimi M, Khair T, et al. Biological treatment approaches for degenerative disk disease: a literature review of in vivo animal and clinical data. Global Spine J. 2016;6(5):497–518.

8. Thompson JP, Oegema TR Jr, Bradford DS. Stimulation of mature canine intervertebral disc by growth factors. Spine. 1991;16(3):253–60.

9. An HS, Takegami K, Kamada H, et al. Intradiscal administration of osteogenic protein-1 increases intervertebral disc height and proteoglycan content in the nucleus pulposus in normal adolescent rabbits. Spine. 2005;30(1):25–31.

10. Masuda K, Imai Y, Okuma M, et al. Osteogenic protein-1 injection into a degenerated disc induces the restoration of disc height and structural changes in the rabbit anular puncture model. Spine. 2006;31(7):742–54.

11. Chaofeng W, Chao Z, Deli W, et al. Nucleus pulposus cells expressing hBMP7 can prevent the degeneration of allogenic IVD in a canine transplantation model. J Orthop Res. 2013;31(9):1366–73.

12. Willems N, Bach FC, Plomp SG, et al. Intradiscal application of rhBMP-7 does not induce regeneration in a canine model of spontaneous intervertebral disc degeneration. Arthritis Res Ther. 2015;17:137.

13. Klein RG, Eek BC, O'Neill CW, et al. Biochemical injection treatment for discogenic low back pain: a pilot study. Spine J. 2003;3(3):220–6.

14. Sakai D, Mochida J, Iwashina T, et al. Differentiation of mesenchymal stem cells transplanted to a rabbit degenerative disc model: potential and limitations for stem cell therapy in disc regeneration. Spine. 2005;30(21):2379–87.

15. Gorensek M, Jaksimovic C, Kregar-Velikonja N, et al. Nucleus pulposus repair with cultured autologous elastic cartilage derived chondrocytes. Cell Mol Biol Lett. 2004;9(2):363–73.

16. Ganey T, Libera J, Moos V, et al. Disc chondrocyte transplantation in a canine model: a treatment for degenerated or damaged intervertebral disc. Spine. 2003;28(23):2609–20.

17. Meisel HJ, Siodla V, Ganey T, et al. Clinical experience in cell-based therapeutics: disc chondrocyte transplantation A treatment for degenerated or damaged intervertebral disc. Biomol Eng. 2007;24(1):5–21.

18. Modic MT, Ross JS. Magnetic resonance imaging in the evaluation of low back pain. Orthop Clin North Am. 1991;22(2):283–301.

19. Modic MT. Degenerative disc disease: genotyping, MR imaging and phenotyping. Skelet Radiol. 2007;36(2):91–3.

20. Brock M, Gorge HH, Curio G. Intradiscal pressure-volume response: a methodological contribution to chemonucleolysis. Preliminary results. J Neurosurg. 1984;60(5):1029–32.

Medical Strengthening Therapy for Treatment of Back Pain

16

Christoph Spang, Bruno Domokos,
and Florian Maria Alfen

16.1 Introduction and Core Messages

16.1.1 The Association Between Chronic Back Pain and Deconditioning of Deep Paraspinal Muscles

Despite extensive research, the neurophysiological mechanisms and morphological changes associated with acute and chronic low back pain have not yet been fully understood. However, it is well established that deconditioning of the deep paraspinal back extensor muscles is a major factor in this process [1] and that conditioning of these muscles can significantly decrease the pain condition [2]. Often discussed in this context is the function and structure of the multifidus [3], the most medially located back muscle and the largest one that spans the lumbosacral junction. It primarily serves to maintain the erector posture of the trunk and to abduct and rotate the trunk [4, 5]. Furthermore, it is important for stabilizing the "neutral zone" range of motion of the back and is thus essential for maintaining back health [3]. Reduced lumbar extension strength/endurance, atrophy, and excessive fatigability are shown to be associated with low back pain [1]. Exercises that specifically strengthen these muscles have shown to recover patients from back pain and to maintain back health [2, 6].

Morphological and imaging studies have revealed that patients with low back pain exhibit significant atrophies in the paraspinal back muscles compared to healthy individuals (Fig. 16.1) [7–11]. Apart from muscle size, distinct fat infiltration in the paraspinal muscles (Fig. 16.1) has been associated with low back pain, disability, low muscle function, and pain intensity [12–14]. This correlation was mainly found in adults and older individuals, and is more pronounced in chronic patients [15–17]. Other features observed in low back pain are the conversion of muscle fiber I into II leading to less adaption to aerobic exertion [18] and impairment of corticomotor control of the lumbar multifidus muscles [19]. Analyses of multifidus muscle biopsies have also measured elevated inflammatory processes, decreased vascularity, and active degeneration in back pain patients [20].

Impairment of paraspinal muscle size and function results in a lack of spine stability and can potentially facilitate the development of pathological changes such as spine degeneration and disc herniation. In fact, several MRI studies have shown that more severe and extensive multifidus atrophy was present in low back pain patients with radiculopathy and disc herniation than in those without [15, 21]. Furthermore, an association of high degrees of fat infiltration in the multifidus and the erector spinae muscles with decreased disc height and advanced Modic changes has been observed [14]. Additionally, a correlation between disc degeneration, paraspinal atrophy, fat infiltration, and facet joint degeneration in patients with disc herniation has been found [22]. Even in degenerative conditions like lumbar spinal stenosis, lumbar kyphosis, and spondylolisthesis, impairment of paraspinal muscle structure and function has been suggested to contribute [11, 23–25]. Thus, strong paraspinal back muscles are required for maintaining and regaining spine health. Impairment on the other hand is associated with spine disease and back pain conditions.

16.1.2 Analogy to Pain Conditions in the Neck Region

The results of studies investigating neck pain suggest similar mechanisms to occur, namely, a deconditioning of the cervical paraspinal extensor muscles. Patients with chronic neck pain exhibit a smaller cross-sectional area (CSA) of the cervical multifidus and the semispinalis capitis muscle com-

C. Spang (✉) · F. M. Alfen
Orthopaedic Spine Center Dr. Alfen, Würzburg, Germany
e-mail: christoph.spang@dr-alfen.de

B. Domokos
Orthopaedic Spine Center Dr. Alfen, Würzburg, Germany

Institute of Sports Sciene, University of Würzburg, Würzburg, Germany

pared to healthy individuals [26–28]. Cervical myelopathy has been found to be associated with increased fat infiltration and CSA asymmetry at the level below the compression [29]. Even patients with chronic whiplash syndrome, cervicogenic headache and cervical radicular pain exhibit atrophies in several local muscles [30–32]. It can be summarized that deconditioning processes seem to be strongly associated with pain conditions in the neck region.

16.1.3 Physical Loading for Maintaining and Regaining Spinal Health

Numerous studies have proven the benefits of physical activity for spinal health. In contrast, physical inactivity is associated with narrower lumbar intervertebral discs, high paraspinal fat content, and the occurrence of chronic low back pain [33]. Studies on astronauts have shown that chronic unloading of the spine may disrupt stability [34]. Reduced disc height and increased disc degeneration also correlate with obesity and age [35, 36]. Fat replacement and atrophy in the paraspinal muscles increase with age and are more progressive compared to other muscles in the human body [37]. Thus, appropriate physical loading is required for maintaining and regaining spinal health during life span. In an MRI study on Olympic high-level athletes, 52% of the examined patients showed moderate to severe spine degeneration and disc pathologies [38]. Furthermore, multifidus muscle atrophy together with low back pain is often found in elite athletes [39]. These observations indicate that a key contribution to optimal spinal health can only be made with the right type and dose of physical activity. Based on this knowledge, new types of medical strengthening therapies have been developed involving machine based isolated training of the deep lumbar and cervical extensor muscles.

16.2 Methods

16.2.1 ILEX: Isolated Lumbar Extension Resistance Exercise

16.2.1.1 Selective Conditioning of the Paraspinal and Lumbar Extensor Muscles

Based on the results of multiple studies, specific conditioning of the deep lumbar extensors is a key strategy for optimal treatment of back pain conditions [1]. In fact, exercise programs causing hypertrophy of the multifidus muscle lead to pain relief in patients with chronic back pain [39]. However, selective strengthening of these muscles is challenging as the hip extensor muscles (e.g., gluteus maximus, ischiocrural muscles) may contribute to a greater degree of measured torque and influence muscle fatigue [6, 40]. For this purpose, several training devices have been developed over the years. According to Steele and colleagues, superior clinical outcomes are achieved by using a restraint system in which the pelvis is stabilized and the patient is seated in semi-sitting position [6] (Fig. 16.2). Posterior pelvis stabilization has shown to enhance the recruitment of lumbar extensor muscles during dynamic extension. Semi-sitting position minimizes the activity of hip extensors compared to seated position [41–43]. With these additives, fatigue in the muscles of the lower back can be achieved effectively. For quantification of lumbar extension strength, repeated measures of isometric lumbar extension strength can be performed [44, 45]. For effective assessment, the following requirements need to be fulfilled: pelvic stabilization, standardization of testing positioning, and correction of body weight [45, 46]. Furthermore, these machines (e.g. Powerspine Back/Neck, MedX LE/CE) and the restraint system have been adopted and implemented by the *Society for Medical Strengthening Therapy* (German original: "Gesellschaft für Medizinische

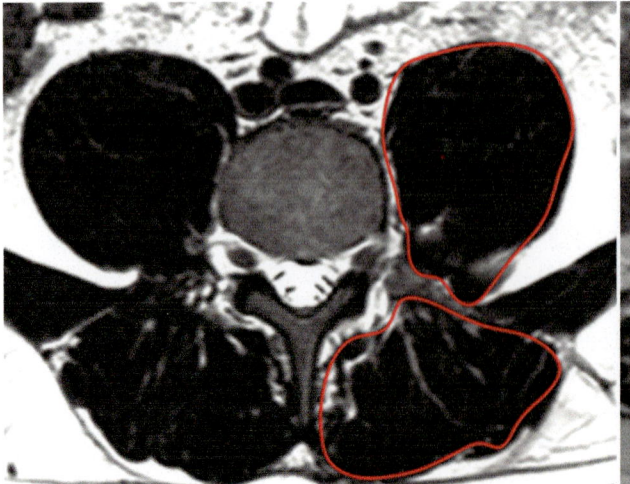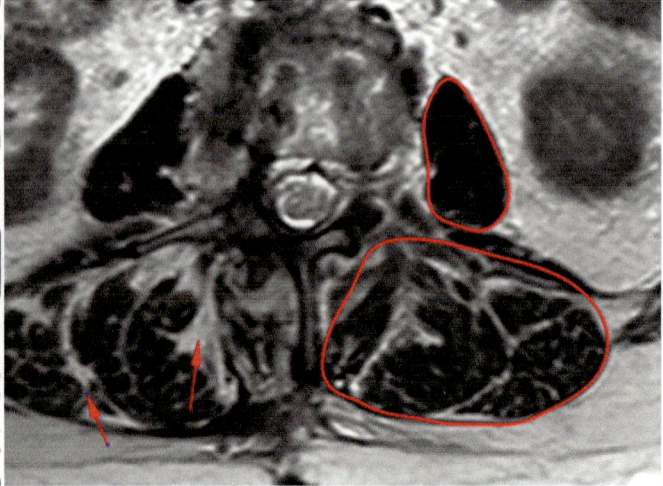

Fig. 16.1 Cross section of the lumbar spine and its surrounding muscles of a healthy individual (left) and one with back pain (right). Patient's paraspinal back muscles exhibiting atrophy and high degrees of local fat infiltration (arrows)

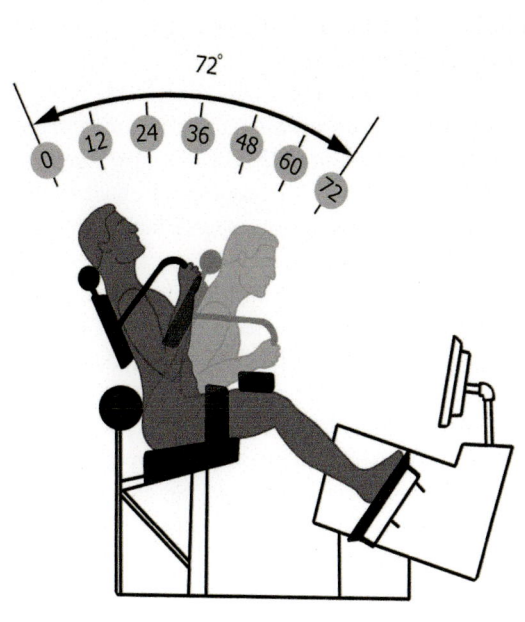

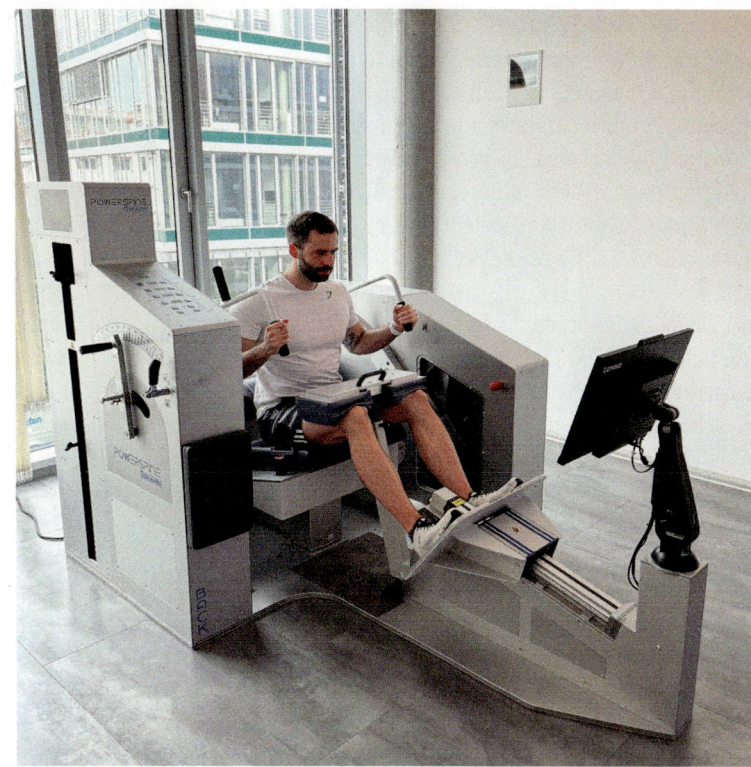

Fig. 16.2 Lumbar extension machine with restraint system

Kräftigungstherapie", GMKT) into their guidelines for medical strengthening therapy.

16.2.1.2   Adjustments to the Patient's Anthropometric Properties

To start the medical strengthening therapy, the patient's anthropometric properties need to be adjusted to the lumbar extension machine. At first, the patient is seated, and the knees are positioned in a way to align the thighs parallel with the seat (Fig. 16.2). A lap belt is placed over the top of the thighs, just below the waist (thigh restraint), and tightened. Furthermore, a knee/femur restraint is applied. This arrangement provides for the stabilization of the pelvis during the training by pushing the femurs down- and backward, fixing the pelvis in place against the restraint pad [47]. With the support of a foot board, pressure is applied to the bottom of the feet with the legs positioned at 60° of knee flexion (Fig. 16.2). With these systems, any vertical movement of the thighs or pelvis is restricted [47]. After the position is standardized and the pelvic restraints tightened to stabilize the pelvis, the patient is moved to a neutral, upright position to determine the center line of the torso mass. This position is influenced mainly by the current shape of the spine and the spine disorder the patient is specifically suffering from. At this point, a counterweight is locked into place to neutralize the gravitational forces of the head, torso and upper extremities. For this purpose, the subject needs to rest at the back pad at 0° of flexion if the condition allows [45]. Furthermore, subjects are also tested for any limitations in range of lumbar motion between 0° and 72° to enable the maximum safety during the exercise. Since many acute patients report pain or discomfort in maximal flexion and extension, the range of motion needs to be adjusted based on the individual's reported pain and pathology. Interestingly, exercising in a limited range of motion has been found to be sufficient to increase lumbar extension torque in full range of motion [48, 49]. With this in mind, exercise protocols can be customized for different spinal disorders by limiting the ROM without subverting efficiency. Patients with disc herniations mainly benefit from a restriction in flexion, whereas stenosis patients and those with spondylolisthesis should have a more comprehensive limitation in extension. Our clinical experience has shown that choosing optimal, pathology-specific ROM is essential for the clinical outcome. For most patients, smaller ROM should be sufficient at the beginning and can then be increased progressively during the therapy, preferably within the first 12 sessions (usually around 6 weeks after session 1). Advanced devices (e.g., using Alflexus Software) may support the therapist in decision-making by providing ROM recommendations based on the patient's pathology.

16.2.1.3 Test Procedure for Isometric Strength Assessment

After the apparatus has been adjusted to the patient's anthropometric properties, an isometric extension strength test is commonly performed. Exceptions apply for patients suffering from one of the following contraindications: acute disc herniation, severe pain, osteoporosis, tumors, heart issues, and problems with eye pressure. For determining the isometric extension strength, at least four positions within the chosen ROM should be tested. The movement arm of the machine is locked into the respective position before subjects are instructed to extend their back against the upper back pad by gradually building tension over a 2–3 s period [47]. The generated isomeric torque is then displayed on the screen. Once maximal tension is reached, the patient is instructed to maintain the contraction for 1 s before relaxing. Between each isometric contraction, a rest period of about 10 s is provided while the patient is moved softly between flexion and extension several times. The isometric torque values generated during this procedure can then be compared to normative data from healthy individuals. Thus, muscle atrophies and imbalances can be detected and interpreted. For purposes of formative and summative evaluation, the isometric strength test should be repeated at least once during the rehabilitation program as well as at the end.

16.2.1.4 Exercise Protocol: Training Characteristics and Optimal Adjustment During the Therapy

The actual training consists of a dynamic lumbar extension resistance exercise. To this date, there have been different opinions about optimal load intensity and repetitions. The following descriptions are primarily based on a protocol evolved from the experience in our spine center and based on recent research data (see below). In general, studies on the efficiency have mostly revealed that 1–2 exercise sessions per week with high intensities targeting momentary muscular failure provide sufficient training stimulus for the development of lumbar extension strength [2, 6, 44, 50]. Interestingly, the outcome was found to be unaffected by the set volume [51]. Thus, one set leading to momentary muscle failure is sufficient. For optimal results, we recommend 18–25 exercise sessions (1–2 times per week). As described above, the ROM should be adjusted to the patient's pathology. We claim that this differentiation is crucial for successful rehabilitation, particularly in severe cases. Each flexion-extension cycle should last for around 10 s (4 s extension, 2 s holding in maximal extension, 4 s flexion) providing for a sustained time under tension of the muscles aimed to fatigue with this exercise. Apparently, most patients must not train to muscular exhaustion during the first six training sessions. The first training sessions are characterized by a gradual adaption of the spine to higher loads. This approach has proven to be a particularly safe and therefore beneficial strategy for acute patients. It is not until after 8–12 sessions when patients should aim for total muscle fatigue after 12–15 repetitions. In order to avoid fast and swinging movements, the speed of each flexion-extension cycle is guided by a benchmark on the screen. The increase of training weights and the modifications of the ROM are based in accordance with the patient's current pain status and well-being.

Furthermore, it is important that the process is monitored by regular clinical examinations of a medical doctor. We recommend having these appointments after sessions 6, 12, and 18. In severe cases, a higher frequency may be favorable. Before the first and after the last training session, pain scores (e.g., VAS, Oswestry Disability Index) should be taken. If a patient after 18 sessions (twice per week) has not achieved the desired outcome, 7 extra sessions with longer recovery periods in between (usually one session per week) have proven to be beneficial in many instances. Besides, in order to sustain the intervention outcome in the long term, one exercise session every 2–4 weeks is recommended. According to our experience, this low-frequent stimulus is sufficient for maintaining restored functionality of the lumbar paraspinal extensor muscles in the vast majority of patients. Despite the high number of successful therapy responders, there is a considerable variance depending on the severity of the disorder and factors such as the patient's lifestyle. If pain/condition improvement was inadequate after 25 sessions, other treatment options (e.g., surgery) have to be discussed (see below).

16.2.1.5 Clinical Outcome

Recent studies on the clinical value have shown that isolated extension resistance training provides very good results for rehabilitating patients with different kinds of back pain conditions [2], thus representing a highly promising treatment option. It appears to be sufficient and effective for significant and meaningful improvements in perceived pain and disability [2, 52, 53], a clinical outcome that is associated with increased isometric lumbar extension strength during therapy [53]. Further findings from Steele et al. describe that intervertebral discs can potentially heal and regenerate when applied to appropriate loading but also degenerate after chronic overload [52]. This highlights the importance of standardized protocols and highly educated therapists, especially for the treatment of patients with advanced stages of spine degeneration. Despite convincing clinical results, the effect on muscle and spine structure as well as the underlying mechanisms responsible for these results has yet to be investigated in more depth [1, 6]. Considering the biopsychosocial nature of back pain, deconditioning of the multifidus and the lumbar extensor muscles must not be treated as the only relevant factor. Steele et al. have shown that there is a degree of variability in response to exercise between different patients [40]. According to this research, psychosocial aspects are associated with high-intensity low back pain [54]. To deal with this circumstance, the relationship between the patient and the therapist should be highlighted, focusing on building a trustful and optimistic attitude towards the intervention. Furthermore, in several cases (particularly in the acute phase), it might also be helpful to include manual therapy or osteopathic treatment to resolve functional imbalances and relax potential muscle hardening [55].

16.2.2 ICEX: Isolated Cervical Extension Resistance Exercise

For the conditioning of the paraspinal neck muscles, the same principles as for the lumbar spine should be applied. Through the application of several restraint systems, neck extensor muscle activity is increased. The patient is restrained via seat belt, shoulder harness, and torso restraint to inhibit any additive strength effect from trunk musculature during the testing and training procedure [56–58] (Fig. 16.3). Most importantly, the resistance head pad needs to be adjusted by the therapist with caution at the appropriate segmental level of the cervical spine (C7 processus spinosus). The procedure for determining range of motion (0°–126°) and adjusting the counterweight is similar to ILEX. However, it is generally recommended that the intensity of exercise should be lower than for patients with low back pain. Especially patients suffering from headache and high muscle tension may not tolerate high intensities. Studies have shown that cervical extension training enhances isometric strength and that repeated measures can be used for quantification [57]. As described above, the association between deconditioning and structural changes in the deep cervical extensor with neck pain and related disorders is well known [56]. Specific isolated cervical extension exercise has shown the potential to increase isometric neck strength [58, 59] decreasing neck pain symptoms [60]. Even patients with migraine and headache may respond positively to this treatment option.

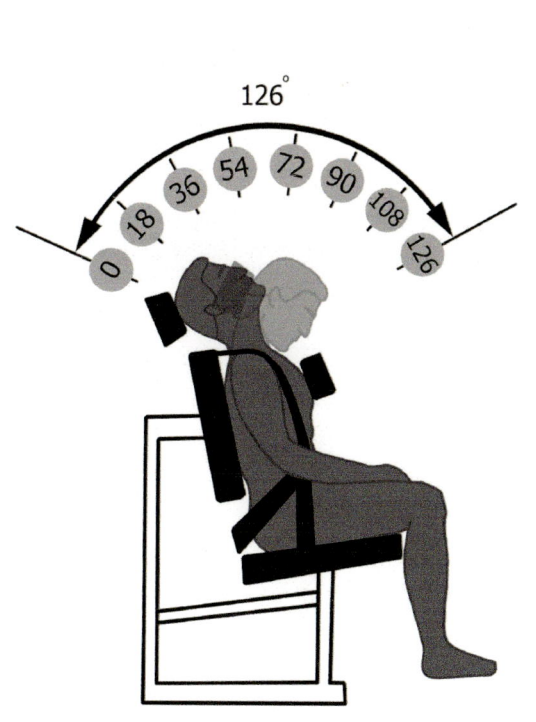

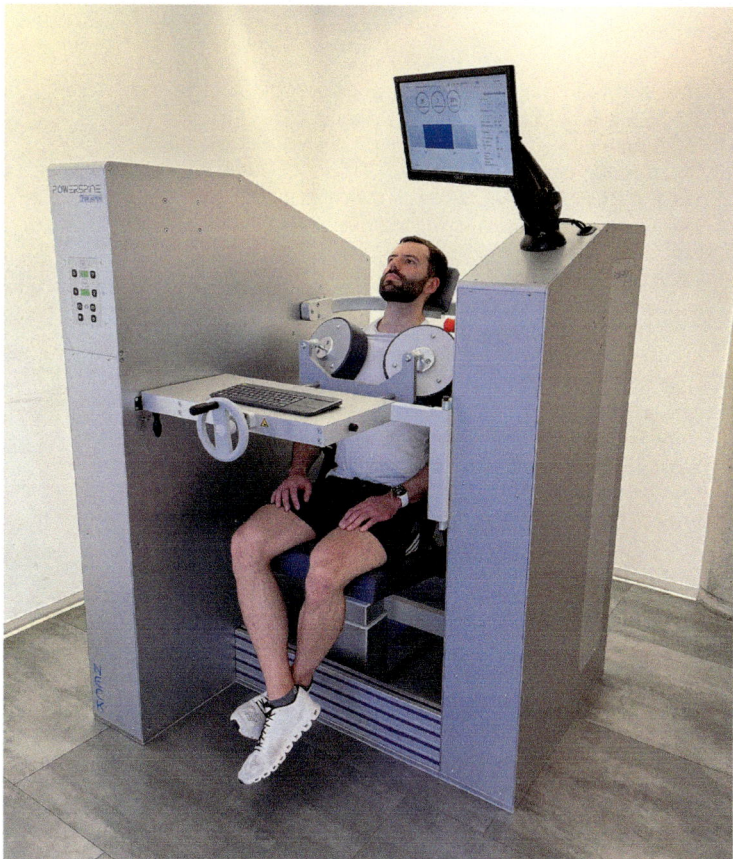

Fig. 16.3 Cervical extension machine with restraint system

16.3 Outlook

It can be summarized that medical strengthening therapy using the described machines (e.g. Powerspine Back/Neck, MedX LE/CE) including restraint systems is a very useful method for the prevention and rehabilitation of chronic back pain. However, despite positive clinical outcome, surgery may be the only effective option remaining in some patients, especially for those exhibiting advanced forms of structural changes and spine degeneration. In fact, for patients suffering from neurological deficits, persisting high pain and bladder dysfunction, surgery is still considered to be the first option. Nonetheless, if surgery was applied, medical strengthening therapy can be considered as part of the postoperative rehabilitation program in order to maintain surgical outcome and restore muscular function quickly. For optimal spine health, it is essential to condition the paraspinal muscles in order to prevent spine diseases and chronic pain.

Acknowledgment The authors would like to thank radiologist Dr. Heiko Braun for providing MRI images.

References

1. Steele J, Bruce-Low S, Smith D. A reappraisal of the deconditioning hypothesis in low back pain: review of evidence from a triumvirate of research methods on specific lumbar extensor deconditioning. Curr Med Res Opin. 2014;30(5):865–911.
2. Steele J, Bruce-Low S, Smith D. A review of the clinical value of isolated lumbar extension resistance training for chronic low back pain. PM R. 2015;7(2):169–87.
3. Freeman MD, Woodham MA, Woodham AW. The role of the lumbar multifidus in chronic low back pain: a review. PM R. 2010;2(2):142–6.
4. Macintosh JE, Valencia F, Bogduk N, et al. The morphology of the human lumbar multifidus. Clin Biomech. 1986;1(4):196–204.
5. Macintosh JE, Bogduk N. The biomechanics of the lumbar multifidus. Clin Biomech. 1986;1(4):205–13.
6. Steele J, Bruce-Low S, Smith D. A review of the specificity of exercises designed for conditioning the lumbar extensors. Br J Sports Med. 2015;49(5):291–7.
7. Barker KL, Shamley DR, Jackson D. Changes in the cross-sectional area of multifidus and psoas in patients with unilateral back pain: the relationship to pain and disability. Spine. 2004;29(22):E515–9.
8. Beneck GJ, Kulig K. Multifidus atrophy is localized and bilateral in active persons with chronic unilateral low back pain. Arch Phys Med Rehabil. 2012;93(2):300–6.
9. Goubert D, De Pauw R, Meeus M, et al. Lumbar muscle structure and function in chronic versus recurrent low back pain: a cross-sectional study. Spine J. 2017;17(9):1285–96.
10. Wan Q, Lin C, Li X, Zeng W, Ma C. MRI assessment of paraspinal muscles in patients with acute and chronic unilateral low back pain. Br J Radiol. 2015;88:20140546.
11. Yarjanian JA, Fetzer A, Yamakawa KS, et al. Correlation of paraspinal atrophy and denervation in back pain and spinal stenosis relative to asymptomatic controls. PM R. 2013;5(1):39–44.
12. Le Cara EC, Marcus RL, Dempsey AR, et al. Morphology versus function: the relationship between lumbar multifidus intramuscular adipose tissue and muscle function among patients with low back pain. Arch Phys Med Rehabil. 2014;95(10):1846–52.
13. Takashima H, Takebayashi T, Ogon I, et al. Analysis of intra and extramyocellular lipids in the multifidus muscle in patients with chronic low back pain using MR spectroscopy. Br J Radiol. 2018;91(1083):20170536.
14. Teichtahl AJ, Urquhart DM, Wang Y, et al. Fat infiltration of paraspinal muscles is associated with low back pain, disability, and structural abnormalities in community-based adults. Spine J. 2015;15(7):1593–601.
15. Ekin EE, Kurtul Yildiz H, Mutlu H. Age and sex-based distribution of lumbar multifidus muscle atrophy and coexistence of disc hernia: an MRI study of 2028 patients. Diagn Interv Radiol. 2016;22(3):273–6.
16. Kjaer P, Bendix T, Sorensen JS, et al. Are MRI-defined fat infiltrations in the multifidus muscles associated with low back pain? BMC Med. 2007;5:2.
17. Sions JM, Coyle PC, Velasco TO, et al. Multifidi muscle characteristics and physical function among older adults with and without chronic low back pain. Arch Phys Med Rehabil. 2017;98(1):51–7.
18. Demoulin C, Crielaard JM, Vanderthommen M. Spinal muscle evaluation in healthy individuals and low-back-pain patients: a literature review. Joint Bone Spine. 2007;74(1):9–13.
19. Masse-Alarie H, Beaulieu LD, Preuss R, Schneider C. Corticomotor control of lumbar multifidus muscles is impaired in chronic low back pain: concurrent evidence from ultrasound imaging and double-pulse transcranial magnetic stimulation. Exp Brain Res. 2016;234(4):1033–45.
20. Shahidi B, Hubbard JC, Gibbons MC, et al. Lumbar multifidus muscle degenerates in individuals with chronic degenerative lumbar spine pathology. J Orthop Res. 2017;35(12):2700–6.
21. Min JH, Choi HS, Ihl Rhee W, Lee JI. Association between radiculopathy and lumbar multifidus atrophy in magnetic resonance imaging. J Back Musculoskelet Rehabil. 2013;26(2):175–81.
22. Sun D, Liu P, Cheng J, et al. Correlation between intervertebral disc degeneration, paraspinal muscle atrophy, and lumbar facet joints degeneration in patients with lumbar disc herniation. BMC Musculoskelet Disord. 2017;18(1):167.
23. Fortin M, Lazary A, Varga PP, Battie MC. Association between paraspinal muscle morphology, clinical symptoms and functional status in patients with lumbar spinal stenosis. Eur Spine J. 2017;26(10):2543–51.
24. Kang CH, Shin MJ, Kim SM, et al. MRI of paraspinal muscles in lumbar degenerative kyphosis patients and control patients with chronic low back pain. Clin Radiol. 2007;62(5):479–86.
25. Nava-Bringas TI, Ramirez-Mora I, Coronado-Zarco R, et al. Association of strength, muscle balance, and atrophy with pain and function in patients with degenerative spondylolisthesis. J Back Musculoskelet Rehabil. 2014;27(3):371–6.
26. Fernandez-de-las-Penas C, Albert-Sanchis JC, Buil M, et al. Cross-sectional area of cervical multifidus muscle in females with chronic bilateral neck pain compared to controls. J Orthop Sports Phys Ther. 2008;38(4):175–80.
27. Rezasoltani A, Ahmadipoor A, Khademi-Kalantari K, Javanshir K. The sign of unilateral neck semispinalis capitis muscle atrophy in patients with chronic non-specific neck pain. J Back Musculoskelet Rehabil. 2012;25(1):67–72.
28. Rezasoltani A, Ali-Reza A, Khosro KK, Abbass R. Preliminary study of neck muscle size and strength measurements in females with chronic non-specific neck pain and healthy control subjects. Man Ther. 2010;15(4):400–3.
29. Fortin M, Dobrescu O, Courtemanche M, et al. Association between paraspinal muscle morphology, clinical symptoms, and functional

status in patients with degenerative cervical myelopathy. Spine. 2017;42(4):232–9.

30. Elliott JM, Pedler AR, Jull GA, et al. Differential changes in muscle composition exist in traumatic and nontraumatic neck pain. Spine. 2014;39(1):39–47.

31. Noormohammadpour P, Dehghani-Firouzabadi A, Mansournia MA, et al. Comparison of the cross-sectional area of longus colli muscle between patients with cervical radicular pain and healthy controls. PM R. 2017;9(2):120–6.

32. Uthaikhup S, Assapun J, Kothan S, et al. Structural changes of the cervical muscles in elder women with cervicogenic headache. Musculoskelet Sci Pract. 2017;29:1–6.

33. Teichtahl AJ, Urquhart DM, Wang Y, et al. Physical inactivity is associated with narrower lumbar intervertebral discs, high fat content of paraspinal muscles and low back pain and disability. Arthritis Res Ther. 2015;17:114.

34. Bailey JF, Miller SL, Khieu K, et al. From the international space station to the clinic: how prolonged unloading may disrupt lumbar spine stability. Spine J. 2018;18(1):7–14.

35. Hicks GE, Morone N, Weiner DK. Degenerative lumbar disc and facet disease in older adults: prevalence and clinical correlates. Spine. 2009;34(12):1301–6.

36. Urquhart DM, Kurniadi I, Triangto K, et al. Obesity is associated with reduced disc height in the lumbar spine but not at the lumbosacral junction. Spine. 2014;39(16):E962–6.

37. Dahlqvist JR, Vissing CR, Hedermann G, et al. Replacement of paraspinal muscles with aging in healthy adults. Med Sci Sports Exerc. 2017;49(3):595–601.

38. Wasserman MS, Guermazi A, Jarraya M, et al. Evaluation of spine MRIs in athletes participating in the Rio de Janeiro 2016 Summer Olympic Games. BMJ Open Sport Exerc Med. 2018;4: e000335.

39. Hides JA, Stanton WR, McMahon S, et al. Effect of stabilization training on multifidus muscle cross-sectional area among young elite cricketers with low back pain. J Orthop Sports Phys Ther. 2008;38(3):101–8.

40. Steele J, Fisher J, Bruce-Low S, Smith D, Osborne N, Newell D. Variability in strength, pain, and disability changes in response to an isolated lumbar extension resistance training intervention in participants with chronic low back pain. Healthcare. 2017; 5(4):75.

41. da Silva RA, Larivière C, Arsenault AB, et al. Pelvic stabilization and semisitting position increase the specificity of back exercises. Med Sci Sports Exerc. 2009;41(2):435–43.

42. Larivière C, da Silva RA, Arsenault AB, et al. Specificity of a back muscle exercise machine in healthy and low back pain subjects. Med Sci Sports Exerc. 2010;42(3):592–9.

43. San Juan JG, Yaggie JA, Levy SS, et al. Effects of pelvic stabilization on lumbar muscle activity during dynamic exercise. J Strength Cond Res. 2005;19(4):903–7.

44. Graves JE, Pollock ML, Foster D, et al. Effect of training frequency and specificity on isometric lumbar extension strength. Spine. 1990;15(6):504–9.

45. Robinson ME, Greene AF, O'Connor P, et al. Reliability of lumbar isometric torque in patients with chronic low back pain. Phys Ther. 1992;72(3):186–90.

46. Graves JE, Pollock ML, Carpenter DM, et al. Quantitative assessment of full range-of-motion isometric lumbar extension strength. Spine. 1990;15(4):289–94.

47. Graves JE, Fix CK, Pollock ML, et al. Comparison of two restraint systems for pelvic stabilization during isometric lumbar extension strength testing. J Orthop Sports Phys Ther. 1992;15(1):37–42.

48. Graves JE, Pollock ML, Leggett SH, et al. Limited range-of-motion lumbar extension strength training. Med Sci Sports Exerc. 1992;24(1):128–33.

49. Steele J, Bruce-Low S, Smith D, Jessop D, Osborne N. A randomized controlled trial of limited range of motion lumbar extension exercise in chronic low back pain. Spine (Phila Pa 1976). 2013;38(15):1245–52.

50. Pollock ML, Leggett SH, Graves JE, et al. Effect of resistance training on lumbar extension strength. Am J Sports Med. 1989;17(5):624–9.

51. Steele J, Fitzpatrick A, Bruce-Low S, Fisher J. The effects of set volume during isolated lumbar extension resistance training in recreationally trained males. PeerJ. 2015;3:e878.

52. Steele J, Bruce-Low S, Smith D, et al. Can specific loading through exercise impart healing or regeneration of the intervertebral disc? Spine J. 2014;15(10):2117–21.

53. Steele J, Fisher J, Perrin C, et al. Does change in isolated lumbar extensor muscle function correlate with good clinical outcome? A secondary analysis of data on change in isolated lumbar extension strength, pain, and disability in chronic low back pain. Disabil Rehabil. 2019;41(11):1287–95.

54. Ng SK, Cicuttini FM, Wang Y, et al. Negative beliefs about low back pain are associated with persistent high intensity low back pain. Psychol Health Med. 2017;22(7):790–9.

55. Ranger TA, Teichtahl AJ, Cicuttini FM, et al. Shorter lumbar paraspinal fascia is associated with high intensityl low back pain and disability. Spine. 2016;41(8):E489–93.

56. Schomacher J, Falla D. Function and structure of the deep cervical extensor muscles in patients with neck pain. Man Ther. 2013;18(5):360–6.

57. Pollock ML, Graves JE, Bamman MM, et al. Frequency and volume of resistance training: effect on cervical extension strength. Arch Phys Med Rehabil. 1993;74(10):1080–6.

58. Leggett SH, Graves JE, Pollock ML, Shank M, Carpenter DM, Holmes B, et al. Quantitative assessment and training of isometric cervical extension strength. Am J Sports Med. 1991;19(6):653–9.

59. Highland TR, Dreisinger TE, Vie LL, Russell GS. Changes in isometric strength and range of motion of the isolated cervical spine after eight weeks of clinical rehabilitation. Spine. 1992;17(6 Suppl):S77–82.

60. Evans R, Bronfort G, Nelson B, Goldsmith CH. Two-year follow-up of a randomized clinical trial of spinal manipulation and two types of exercise for patients with chronic neck pain. Spine. 2002;27(21):2383–9.

Haemostasis in Spinal Surgery: An Overview

Fabio Dos Santos

17.1 Introduction and Core Messages

Management of haemostasis during surgery has many components that start with good surgical technique, good preoperative planning and anaesthetic support [1]. Spine surgery implies in some specific aspects: bone surface exposure can be a very significant source of bleeding [2]; some spine tumours (e.g. renal cancer metastasis) are well known from its potential bleeding. Revision surgical cases, platelet dysfunction and coagulopathies are also factors that have been considered. Retroperitoneal spine surgery can create significant source of bleeding during exposure or accidental vascular lesion of tumour, deformity and degenerative and trauma causes. The choice and the proper positioning of the patient in the surgical table will also prevent additional risk of bleeding. In posterior spinal surgery, there are two specific requirements: adequate position of the spine and an unrestricted abdomen with reduction of bleeding from epidural venous system.

Table 17.1 Factors contributing to intraoperative bleeding [3]

- Exposed bone (spine osteotomy, osteoporotic fracture, tumour, etc.).
- Diffused capillaries (e.g. large surfaces).
- Unseen sources of bleeding (e.g. retroperitoneal spaces).
- Surgical incisions.
- Tissues not amenable to suturing.
- Low-pressure suture lines.
- Stripped adhesions.
- Positioning on surgical table.
- Coagulopathies and platelet dysfunction.

17.2 Definition and Pathophysiology

Several factors can contribute to the occurrence of intraoperative bleeding related to the surgical procedure itself (Table 17.1). Spine surgery implies in some specific aspects: bone surface exposure can be a very significant source of bleeding [2]; some spine tumours (e.g. renal cancer metastasis) are well known from its potential bleeding. Revision surgical cases, platelet dysfunction and coagulopathies are also factors that have been considered. Retroperitoneal spine surgery can create significant source of bleeding during exposure or accidental vascular lesion of tumour, deformity and degenerative and trauma causes. The choice and the proper positioning of the patient in the surgical table will also prevent additional risk of bleeding. In posterior spinal surgery, there are two specific requirements: adequate position of the spine and an unrestricted abdomen with reduction of bleeding from epidural venous system. Intraoperative blood loss is a common problem that can be encountered especially in multilevel spine fusion procedures. Currently, in the literature, there is no clear definition for significant haemorrhage in spine surgery, and there are no exact reports on consequences associated with major blood loss under these circumstances [4]. Major blood loss may lead to blood, platelet and factor transfusions. Although blood screening has improved the safety considerably over the years, there are still known risks of transfusion, including potential transfusion reactions and alloimmunization as well as infectious risks, such as hepatitis, human immunodeficiency virus, cytomegalovirus and transfusion-associated bacterial sepsis. Furthermore, there is emerging data suggesting that blood transfusion may be associated with an increased risk of postoperative infections. Additionally, the costs of blood replacement must be considered.

Spinal surgery can include now a great number of different scenarios with patient- and procedure-related aspects (Table 17.2) [5]. Spine surgeon must adopt effective surgical techniques that reduce the amount of the exposed, bleeding tissue during surgery to decrease blood loss and avoid the risks and costs associated with transfusion.

F. Dos Santos (✉)
Neurosurgery, ColunaRS—Clínica de Cirurgia da Coluna Vertebral, Porto Alegre RS, Brazil
e-mail: fstneuro@gmail.com

© Springer-Verlag GmbH Germany 2023
U. Vieweg, F. Grochulla (eds.), *Manual of Spine Surgery*, https://doi.org/10.1007/978-3-662-64062-3_17

Table 17.2 Patient and procedure aspects

- **Adult patients**
  1. Thin periosteum
  2. Stiffer spines than children
  3. Arthritic facet joints
  4. Comorbidities: Hypertension, heart disease, lung disease, diabetes, vascular disease, previous spine surgery, allergies, previous blood transfusion, cigarette smoking, cancer, anaemia, high body mass index
  5. Surgery-related aspects: Emergency of elective cases—Tumour, traumatic cases, deformity, infection, revision cases, fusion, single or combined approaches (anterior and posterior)
  6. Medications: Anti-depressive drugs, anticoagulant treatment, non-steroidal anti-inflammatories, herbal and naturalistic supplements
  7. Estimated blood loss: [3]
     (a) Non-instrumented fusions 800 mL
     (b) Instrumented fusions 1517 mL
     (c) Deformities 1000–3000 mL
     (d) Osteotomies 325–4700 mL
- **Paediatric patients**
  1. Thick periosteum
  2. More flexible spines than adults
  3. Comorbidities: Heart disease, lung disease, cerebral palsy, mielomeningocele, neurogenic bladder, neuromuscular disease, poor nutrition status, epilepsy
  4. Surgery-related aspects: Emergency or elective cases—Tumour, traumatic cases, deformity, revision cases, multiple-level fusion, single or combined approaches (anterior and posterior), harvesting autogenous iliac crest bone
  5. Medications: Antiepileptic drugs. Estimated blood loss (EBL) methods: [3]
     (a) EBV = 70 mL/kg [3]
     (b) Idiopathic scoliosis 9.8 mL/kg
     (c) Secondary scoliosis 14.1 mL/kg
     (d) Muscular dystrophy 29.3 mL/kg [3]
     (e) EBL per level—Anterior approaches, 60–135 mL/level; posterior approaches, 65–150 mL/level

17.3 Haemostasis in Adult Patients

Adult patients can have thin periosteum bones with wider vascular channels. Epidural venous bleeding can be very significant in obese patients. The spine in adult cases can be stiffer than adolescents; facet joints can have degenerative deformation that may require extensive bone resection. Osteotomies are a source of bleeding irrespective of the surgeon's choice especially in cases that required sagittal balance correction. Adult patients with medical comorbidities cannot tolerate hypotension or controlled hypotension because of risk damage caused by decreased perfusion to critical organs. Adult patients have frequent use of different types of medications and herbal supplements that can increase bleeding. Patients sometimes forget or miss to tell medical staff about these habits. Some values of estimated blood loss (EBL) are listed from current literature, but good rule is always control blood losses during the surgery and made the correct replacement therapy.

17.4 Haemostasis in Paediatric Patients

Paediatric patients can comprise a very heterogeneous group of patients. Paediatric spine pathology can be flexible or rigid ones as seen in some congenital malformations. Comorbidities present in the paediatric group can pose other specific management. In the paediatric group, all preoperative estimates cannot be exact; therefore in all cases, volume of blood suctioned from the operative field, blood collected on sponges (determined from weighing by operating room nurses), drapes, gowns and sometimes on the floor can be of utmost importance on this matter.

Paediatric patients can tolerate controlled hypotension better than adult patients. The length of time of surgery and extra loss with harvesting autogenous iliac crest bone are other factors increasing blood loss in these patients. Some studies about EBL in specific surgical treatment of some paediatric spine pathologies are listed in Table 17.2 for reference. Effective haemostasis in surgery can offer various advantages to the patient, surgeon and health-care facility. As a result of intraoperative blood loss, the need for allogenic or autologous blood transfusions and the risks associated with blood transfusions are increased [6, 7]. Reduced length of stay in the intensive care unit (ICU) and overall length of hospital stay have been related to reductions in the amount of blood transfused. Excessive intraoperative blood loss also has been shown to significantly increase the risk of major perioperative complications [8, 9].

17.5 Techniques for Maintaining Haemostasis in Surgery

Surgeons have an array of options to control bleeding, including mechanical and thermal techniques and devices as well as pharmacotherapies and topical agents which are listed in Table 17.3.

17.5.1 Mechanical Techniques

Application of direct pressure or compression at a bleeding site is often the surgeon's first choice to assist in the control of bleeding. Other mechanical methods, including sutures, staples and ligating clips, are useful if the source of bleeding is easily identifiable and able to be sealed. Compression or other mechanical methods, however, may not be appropriate during all surgical procedures, for example, if the source of bleeding is diffuse or hard to identify or the patient has an inherent or surgery-induced coagulopathy resulting from the type of surgical procedure (e.g. hemodilution, hypothermia) or prior administration of antiplatelet or anticoagulant medications [10]. One of the earliest topical haemostatic agents was *cotton*, in the form of gauze sponges. Although such

Table 17.3 Techniques for maintaining haemostasis in surgery [3]

- **Mechanical techniques**
  - Direct pressure
  - Sutures
  - Staples
  - Ligating clips
  - Fabric pads
  - Gauzes
  - Sponges
  - Preoperative autologous blood donation (AUT)
  - Intraoperative cell salvage (ICS)
  - Postoperative autologous transfusion (PAT)
  - Bone wax
  - Preoperative embolization
- **Thermal techniques**
  - Cryotherapy
  - Electrocautery
  - Harmonic scalpel
  - Laser
  - Ultrasonic osteotome
- **Chemical techniques**
  - Neuraxial blockade
  - Controlled hypotensive anaesthesia
  - Local vasoconstrictors
  - Aprotinin
  - Aminocaproic acid
  - Tranexamic acid
  - Erythropoietin (EPO)
  - Desmopressin
  - Collagen
  - Cellulose
  - Gelatines
  - Thrombins
  - Fibrin sealants
  - Haemostatic matrices

materials concentrate blood and coagulation products via physical adsorption, they are not absorbed by the body, and upon removal, the clot may be dislodged, leading to further bleeding. *Autologous blood donation (AUT)* has emerged as one of the principal means to avoid or reduce allogeneic blood transfusion. These techniques involve collection and reinfusion of the patient's own blood, preoperative acute normovolemic hemodilution, intraoperative salvage of blood from surgical field and post-operative blood salvage (collected and reinfused within first 6–8 post-operative hours) [11]. AUT has some other advantages, for example, in patients with rare blood groups, with multiple alloantibodies. It can be used safely and effectively in adult but also in adolescents. García-Erce et al. [12] showed in their study that preoperative blood autologous donation needs to be associated with other blood-saving methods (haemostatic drugs, for example, EPO and perioperative blood salvage) in some specific scoliosis patients for better results. In addition, blood retrieval is not recommended in patients with haemoglobin (Hb) levels lower than 11 g/dL [13]. By maintaining adequate haemoglobin concentrations during repeated blood collection, it is possible to reduce the interval between donations and retrieve a larger number of autologous blood units, thereby covering the predicted requirements. A meta-analysis study published by Henry et al. concluded that preoperative donation of autologous blood reduces exposure to allogeneic blood transfusion by 68% [14]. However, for those patients who donated autologous blood, the risk of receiving any transfusion (allogeneic and/or autologous) was increased by 24%. The increased rate of exposure to any transfusion may be attributed to two factors: (1) patients who donate autologous blood in general have lower preoperative haemoglobin levels than those patients who do not predonate autologous blood and therefore have an increased probability of requiring an intraoperative and/or post-operative blood transfusion; (2) the availability of predonated autologous blood engenders a more liberal transfusion policy. An analysis we performed of 35 non-randomized studies of AUT showed that the overall transfusion rate (allogeneic and/or autologous) was 67% in patients allocated to AUT [15]. This result is similar to what was seen in this meta-analysis of randomized controlled trials, which showed an overall transfusion rate (allogeneic and/or autologous) of 78% in those patients randomized to AUT. On the basis of the current evidence, AUT appears effective in reducing exposure to allogeneic blood. However, preoperative autologous donation exposes patients to other potential risks associated with blood donation and blood transfusion. As reported, the incidence of reactions occurring at the time of donation is similar for allogeneic and autologous donors (between 2% and 5%), with most reactions being mild and of a vasovagal origin [16]. Autologous blood can become contaminated with bacteria and can cause circulatory overload, particularly in elderly patients if used in a liberal fashion without a transfusion protocol. As with any transfusion, there is the ever-present risk of transfusing the wrong blood due to clerical, laboratory or ward error [17]. The overall benefits of AUT probably outweigh the harms for some groups, for instance, those who have been alloimmunized through repeated transfusion and are contemplating elective surgery. However, a full assessment of the balance of benefit and harm requires a better understanding of the clinical value of legitimate indications for red cell transfusion. *Intraoperative cell salvage (ICS) and post-operative autologous transfusion (PAT)* seem to avoid some of the problems of blood storage. During surgery, the intraoperatively salvaged blood can be processed to obtain a red cell concentrate ready for transfusion [18]. This procedure has few complications, the most normal being dilution coagulopathy when a large volume of processed blood is being transfused. However, in spine surgery, the effectiveness of ICS (inhaled corticosteroid) is controversial, and its selective use for operations with high intraoperative blood loss is recommended [19]. Finally, in a retrospective study by Reitman et al. [20], the USB (unwashed filtered shed blood) group required fewer post-operative transfusions (1 U to 36% of patients in the US group versus 1 U to 50% of patients in the control group). However, the authors concluded that the difference was less than expected and that the use of USB was not cost-effective during most elective lumbar procedures. PAT consists of recuperation and reinfusion of shed blood from post-operative draining, total knee arthroplasty being the operation where it has been used the most. There are now in the market a number of devices for collecting post-operative shed blood, the principal differentiating characteristic being the existence or not of a washing process for the salvaged blood. When the ICS is not used, PAT is normally performed by using devices that recuperate and retransfuse shed blood to the patient as unwashed filtered shed blood (USB). USB contains certain activated coagulation factors as well as degrading products of the fibrinogen so that its reinfusion could lead to a coagulopathy. When analysing the evolution of the levels of these proteins in samples obtained from the patients at 1 and 24 h after reinfusion, a trend to normalization was seen, and no alterations were detected in standard coagulation times [21]. In 13 studies, nearly 700 patients undergoing surgery who received a reinfusion of an average of 560 mL of USB did not experience clinically significant coagulopathy or increase in postoperative bleeding [22]. *Bone wax* is a well-known topical haemostatic agent composed of beeswax and baseline. It allows clot formation by stopping blood flow from damaged vessels into the bone [23]. Bone wax is known to inhibit osteogenesis and bone healing in some animal studies [24, 25]. It should never be left in fusion sites and within the spinal canal. It must never be used also in contaminated fields [26]. *Preoperative embolization of spinal lesions* of great bleeding potential seems to be a rational surgical strategy when it is available and the lesion is reachable by endovascular selective catheterization [27]. Vertebral metastases are responsible for 30–70% of spinal tumours [28]. The most highly vascular metastases are from thyroid and renal cell carcinoma [29]. Some publications in the literature clearly showed that preoperative endovascular embolization reduced intraoperative blood loss [30, 31]. This procedure has been described as beneficial in cases of vertebral aneurysmal bone cysts [32], vertebral haemangiomas [33], osteoblastoma, chondroma, chondrosarcoma [34] and many types of vertebral metastases [35]. The embolization procedure is more frequently performed in lumbar and thoracic spine tumours than in cervical spine lesions. The reason is that in cervical spine lesions, one can see frequent anastomoses between carotid, vertebral and subclavian arteries. The risk of cerebral or spinal cord embolization in these cases is increased [36]. The protocol must include the correct vascular anatomy of the region of interest, the identification of blush pattern of the lesion and the selection of the specific material for embo-

lization (e.g. coils, polyvinyl alcohol (PVA) particles). All endovascular procedures should precede in 20 days at least the surgical treatment of the lesion. Partial embolization cases seem to not reduce the amount of bleeding during the surgery, so it must be informed to the surgical team for proper or adjusted measures at the time of surgery.

17.5.2 Thermal Techniques

Thermal techniques, such as cryotherapy, harmonic scalpels, lasers and ultrasonic osteotome, also have become viable surgical options to reduce bleeding. In spinal tumour surgery, preoperative embolization procedure sometimes cannot be enough to reduce the blood flow or cannot be accomplished for anatomical limitations. *Cryocoagulation* can be performed intraoperatively after adequate exposure of the tumour. The system uses liquid nitrogen as the circulating agent with which freezing is induced. Probe temperatures can reach a nadir of $-180\,°C$. Probe sizes used on this purpose are in 3 and 5 mm diameter. Straight- and flat-head probes can be used on this technique. These can be inserted eccentrically in the tumour and gradually moved towards its centre and towards the spinal cord and canal. Ultrasonography is used to monitor the ice ball of the cryotherapy, as well as to ensure that the spinal cord or spinal nerves are not affected. Cryotherapy treatment times varies from 5 to 10 min. Somatosensory-evoked potentials must be monitored during the procedure. The spinal cord and spinal nerves should be protected at all times from the probe. The extent of cryocoagulation is controlled using intraoperative ultrasonography (with a 12-mHz transducer) or by establishing physical separation of the spinal cord from the tumour. The echogenicity of the frozen tissue differs distinctly from that of the unfrozen tissue such that the extent of freezing is visible on the ultrasound and controlled accordingly. Following freezing of the tumour, the probe can be removed, and resection of the tumour is then conducted. The other advantages of this method besides the reduction of intraoperative bleeding are that it allows a more radical tumour excision, prevents intraoperative spillage from tumour content and therefore permits a better spinal reconstruction [37]. *Harmonic scalpel (HS)* is an ultrasonically activated coagulator which generates less heat and minimal smoke during surgery compared to electrocauterization (EC). The lower degree of heat generation causes less thermal injury to the tissue than regular EC. The outstanding quality of the HS is its ability to coagulate and cut vessels. Cakir et al. [38] made a cost-effective study with two matched blinded posterior spine surgery groups. The author concluded that the use of HS resulted in statistically significantly less intraoperative and post-operative less blood loss and less operating times than EC. Although the HS is an expensive device, the personnel costs for autologous blood predonation were not taken into consideration. This device was considered cost neutral in cases with major anticipated blood loss. *The ultrasonic BoneScalpel™* (Bone Scalpel, Misonix, USA) is a tissue-specific device that allows to the surgeon to make precise osteotomies while protecting collateral or adjacent soft tissue structures. The device is comprised of a blunt ultrasonic blade that oscillates at over 22,500 cycles with an imperceptible microscopic amplitude. The recurring impacts pulverize the non-compliant crystalline structure resulting in a precise cut. The more compliant adjacent soft tissue is not affected by the ultrasonic oscillation. One recent paper reported an experience with 128 consecutive spine surgeries with the use of the ultrasonic scalpel [39]. The majority of the patients had previous spine surgeries and/or spinal deformity. In all cases, the ultrasonic scalpel was successfully used to create the needed osteotomies with high precision to facilitate the surgical procedure without percussion on the spinal column or injury to the underlying nerves. The major advantage (although difficult to objectively quantify) of this ultrasonic device is the reduction of bleeding which helps to create and maintain visibility in the surgical field. The authors have noticed that by virtue of the precision and ease of control (oscillation versus rotation), the efficiency of the surgery has improved. As a result, those often technically challenging osteotomy procedures can now be performed in less time with the ultrasonic scalpel. The ultrasonic scalpel uses a narrow blade with a self-irrigating system that provides lubrication and cooling into the cutting cavity and limits the risk of mechanical and thermal injury [40]. However, they reported one incident of dural tear from the overheating of the local tissue by the scalpel blade sitting in one position. It is imperative that the surgeon continues to move the device and not let it bind in one position. A total of 11 dural injuries (8.6%) occurred in their case series. Since majority of the patients had previous spine surgery and/or spinal deformity, this dural injury rate is comparable with previous reports [41].

17.5.3 Chemical Techniques

Depending on the procedure and location of the bleeding tissue, it may be impractical or impossible to effectively stop blood loss via mechanical or thermal haemostatic techniques. For example, in bony surfaces, parenchymal tissues, inflamed or friable vessels or tissues containing multiple and diffused capillaries, it is extremely difficult to maintain haemostasis with these methods. The use of effective pharmacological methods during surgery can be a useful option or an adjunct to other methods in these situations. The pharmacological methods seek to augment surgical haemostasis by enhancing the natural coagulative mechanisms or in reduction of bleeding by indirect effects as in case of specific anaesthesiology

techniques. *Neuraxial blockade* is the term for central blocks involving the spinal, epidural and caudal spaces. While it is now an invaluable adjunct and even occasionally an alternative to general anaesthesia, its use is not a new phenomenon [42]. Regardless of the class of local anaesthetic, these drugs can be divided into ones that are short, intermediate or long acting. Lidocaine has traditionally been the agent of choice or slightly longer surgical procedures that require an intermediate-acting local anaesthetic. Some centres have also adopted the use of mepivacaine for its longer length of action with a similar onset profile. Of note is the potential for an increased incidence of hypotension due to venous pooling from the beta effects of epinephrine-containing solutions. This phenomenon seems to be especially true to patients receiving lumbar epidural anaesthesia. Hypotension can also occur which is attributed to the reduction of sympathetic outflow via opioid receptors in the sympathetic ganglia. Longer-acting local anaesthetics used for epidural anaesthesia typically consist of either bupivacaine or ropivacaine in varying concentrations.

Another class of analgesic adjuvants includes alpha-adrenergic agonists. Clonidine is the main drug used in this class due to its production as a preservative-free preparation. The effects of epidurally administered clonidine are seen as early as 20 min after injection, with peak effects occurring in 1 h. The analgesic potency has been described as being comparable to epidurally administered morphine [43]. Adding clonidine to opioids in the epidural space has an additive effect, which results in a lower dose of narcotic necessary for optimal pain control. This as a consequence diminishes the incidence of respiratory depression that potentially occurs with neuraxial opioids. Clonidine is lipophilic and as a result is quickly redistributed systemically despite neuraxial injection. It therefore has both central and peripheral effects. At lower doses, the central effects cause sympatholysis leading to hypotension, while the peripheral effects at higher doses cause vasoconstriction. Clonidine administered in the low thoracic or lumbar region typically produces blood pressure effects similar to that seen with intravenous administration [44]. When given in the mid or upper thoracic regions, epidurally administered clonidine causes an even greater decrease in blood pressure [45]. This more substantial drop in blood pressure is attributed to blocking thoracic dermatomes that contribute to sympathetic fibres innervating the heart. In addition to the hypotensive potential of clonidine, bradycardia and nausea with or without vomiting are also potential side effects. *Controlled hypotensive anaesthesia (CHA)* has been used for many years as a means of reducing intraoperative blood loss and facilitating surgical exposure. Reduced intraoperative blood pressure leads to a direct reduction in bleeding from surgically injured arteries and arterioles. Venous dilation, in turn, decreases venous bleeding, especially from cancellous bony sinuses that do not collapse when transected [46]. There have been a number of prospective trials demonstrating the efficacy of controlled hypotension, alone or in combination with other techniques, at reducing the blood loss and transfusion requirement of major spinal surgery [47, 48]. However, other studies showed that CHA does not decrease transfusion requirements compared with normotensive anaesthesia in scoliosis surgery [49]. Anaesthetic agents used to induce deliberate hypotension in current practice include the volatile gases (isoflurane, desflurane and sevoflurane) and intravenous sedative medications (thiopental and propofol). Interference with the ability to measure and compare somatosensory- or motor-evoked potentials is the principal limitation to using any anaesthetic agents to produce hypotension. Concerns about hypotension are addressed during spine surgeries. Hypotension makes the patient more susceptible to cardiac arrest if a sudden surgical catastrophe or if a massive haemorrhage or tension pneumothorax occurs. In adult or critically ill patients, the ischaemic threshold of individual organs is impossible to estimate, and because monitoring of perfusion is indirect at best, there have been occasional case reports of complications noted following uneventful anaesthetics [50]. New onset or worsening of neurologic deficit below the level of surgery may result from direct injury or overdistraction of the spinal cord, hypoperfusion or a combination of the two. Continuous electrophysiologic monitoring of either the anterior spinal cord (motor-evoked potentials) or posterior cord (somatosensory-evoked potentials) is the standard of care for most complex spinal surgeries. Electrical evidence of decreased spinal cord function should lead the provider to abandon the hypotensive technique, accepting the potential for increased haemorrhage in exchange for maximizing perfusion. Myocardial ischaemia or infarct is rare following hypotensive anaesthesia and is usually the result of unrecognized hypovolaemia and vasoconstriction, anaemia, occult coronary disease or a combination. Sudden desaturation has been described during controlled hypotension, which may put vulnerable patients at risk [51]. Risk factors for decreased myocardial reserve, such as advanced age, diabetes, atherosclerosis or resting hypertension, are all relative contraindications to controlled hypotension. These patients may already have flow-limited myocardial perfusion, as well as altered autoregulatory thresholds in other organ systems. Another possible side effect of hypotension is the development of perioperative ischaemic optic neuropathy (POION) during surgery. Although this complication is very rare in spinal surgery, with previous studies citing incidence rates between 0% and 0.12%, the condition is debilitating and is still a cause for concern [52]. These patients can complain loss of vision in one eye—characterized by loss of colour vision, visual field defect and relative afferent pupillary defect. Although the cause of POION is unclear, it is thought to be related to compromised blood flow to the optic nerve. The Johns Hopkins study reported that the four affected patients by POION experienced anaemia, hypotension or both, during surgery. Other possible risk factors were prone position, long procedure times and significant intraoperative hydration. It is generally accepted that surgeons and anaesthesiologists should aim for mean arterial blood pressure of 50–60 mmHg to provide safe and adequate hypotension during spinal surgery in healthy patients [53]. In 1999, in a randomized trial performed on 235 elderly patients, the mean intraoperative arterial blood pressure reduced to as low as 45–55 mmHg was equally as safe as the less hypotensive group's mean pressure of 55–70 mmHg with respect to short- and long-term risks [54]. Local vasoconstrictors are used by infiltration of paraspinal muscles with epinephrine and ornipressin to reduce bleeding in many spine procedures [55]. However, no relation between intraoperative blood loss and the amount of injected epinephrine was observed [56]. The literature in this matter is scarce. Some reports of epinephrine usage in hypotensive epidural anaesthesia result in a reduced intraoperative bleeding in orthopaedic procedures [57]. Aprotinin, tranexamic acid (TXA) and epsilon aminocaproic acid (EACA) are drugs widely used in many types of surgeries as cardiac surgery, orthopaedic surgery and vascular surgery. Aprotinin is a non-specific, serine protease inhibitor, derived from the bovine lung, with antifibrinolytic properties. It acts as an inhibitor of several serine proteases, including trypsin, plasmin, plasma kallikrein and tissue kallikrein. Aprotinin also inhibits the contact phase activation of coagulation that both initiates coagulation and promotes fibrinolysis [58]. Drug regimen will not be given (see text below). *TXA and EACA* are synthetic lysine analogues (synthetic derivatives of the amino acid lysine) that act as effective inhibitors of fibrinolysis. TXA and EACA act principally by blocking the lysine binding sites on plasminogen molecules, inhibiting the formation of plasmin and therefore inhibiting fibrinolysis. Tranexamic acid is about 10 times more potent than aminocaproic acid and binds much more strongly to both the strong and weak sites of the plasminogen molecule than EACA [17]. TXA drug regimen usually given in patients with congenital bleeding disorders is 10 mg/kg and is suggested also for cardiac and major orthopaedic surgery. For complex procedures taking many hours, this could be followed by a maintenance infusion of 1 mg/kg/h. TXA is contraindicated in patients with renal and urethral pathologies because of the risk of clot formation and hydronephrosis [59]. EACA drug regimen usually given is 75–150 mg/kg followed by 12.5–30 mg/kg/h. EACA has been associated with hypotension, cardiac arrhythmias, myopathy and rhabdomyolysis but is the only available antifibrinolytic agent in some places. In 2013, the Cochrane Database of Systematic Reviews published a specific and a very comprehensive meta-analysis study with specific objective to assess all randomized controlled trials (RCTs) studying these drugs in respect of blood loss during surgery in adult patients, who need for red blood cell (RBC) transfusion, and adverse events, particularly vascular occlusion, renal dysfunction and death [60]. This review summarizes data from 252 RCTs that recruited over 25,000 participants. Of the 252 included trials, 173 were conducted in cardiac surgery, 53 trials were in orthopaedic surgery, 14 involved liver surgery, 5 were conducted in vascular surgery, 4 involved thoracic surgery, 1 involved gynaecological surgery, 1 involved neurosurgery and 1 trial was in orthognathic surgery.

Twenty trials of TXA versus control involving orthopaedic surgery reported total blood loss data (intraoperative and post-operative blood loss combined). These trials included a total of 1201 patients, of whom 605 were randomized to TXA and 596 were randomized to a control group. The use of TXA in orthopaedic surgery significantly reduced the total amount of blood lost during the perioperative period (*MD −446.19 mls, 95% CI −554.61 to −337.78 mls*). Heterogeneity between these trials was statistically significant (Chi^2 = 85.30, df = 19, *P* < 0.00001; *I^2* = 78%). *The use of TXA was not associated with an increased risk of myocardial infarction stroke, DVT renal failure or renal dysfunction*. Of the 65 trials of TXA that provided data on the number of patients exposed to allogeneic blood transfusion, 28 were assessed as having adequate allocation concealment of treatment schedule. For these 28 trials, the use of TXA reduced the rate of allogeneic blood transfusion by a relative 41% (RR 0.59, 95% CI 0.51–0.69). The use of EACA in orthopaedic surgery reduced blood loss during the perioperative period by around 300 mls per patient (MD −299.69 mls, 95% CI −522.54 to −76.84 mls). Heterogeneity between these trials was not statistically significant (Chi^2 = 0.73, df = 1, *P* = 0.39; *I^2* = 0%). The use of EACA was not associated with an increased risk of myocardial infarction, stroke, DVT, pulmonary embolism or renal failure/dysfunction. Of the 16 trials that provided data on the number of patients exposed to allogeneic blood transfusion, 5 were assessed as having adequate allocation concealment of treatment schedule. For these trials, the use of EACA did not statistically significantly reduce the rate of allogeneic blood transfusion (RR 0.82, 95% CI 0.58–1.16). Data from the head-to-head trials suggest an advantage of aprotinin over the lysine analogues TXA and EACA in terms of reducing perioperative blood loss, but the differences were small. In 2008, a large pharmacoepidemiological study by Schneeweiss et al. [61] confirmed the increased risk of death with aprotinin. After adjustment, the estimated risk of death was 64% higher in the aprotinin group than in the aminocaproic acid group (relative risk, 1.64; 95% confidence interval [CI], 1.50–1.78). This difference remained statistically significant after a range of analytical procedures including a propensity score-matched analysis and an instrumental variable analysis. Consequently, the balance of benefit and harm favours the use of the lysine analogues over aprotinin and

justifies the regulatory action that resulted in the withdrawal of aprotinin from international markets in 2008 [62]. This study concluded that tranexamic acid and epsilon aminocaproic acid provide worthwhile reductions in blood loss and the need for allogeneic red cell transfusion in adult surgical patients. Based on the results of randomized trials, their efficacy does not appear to be offset by serious adverse effects. The evidence is stronger for tranexamic acid than for epsilon aminocaproic acid. Another study published on the Cochrane Database of Systematic Reviews assess the efficacy and safety of aprotinin, tranexamic acid and aminocaproic acid in reducing blood loss and transfusion requirements in children undergoing scoliosis surgery including children and patients under 18 years of age [63]. The total number of participants in the included studies was 254, of whom 127 received placebo and 127 received antifibrinolytic drugs. Antifibrinolytic drugs decreased the amount of blood transfused by 327 mL and the amount of blood loss by 427 mL. However, the actual need of transfusion was not significantly decreased. Although no deaths or adverse events were noted with the use of these antifibrinolytic drugs, the number of children evaluated was too small and the duration of follow-up too short to draw any conclusion on their safety. The risk of being transfused was 13% lower in patients receiving antifibrinolytic drugs; however, the difference was not statistically significant (95% confidence interval (CI), 0.67–1.12). The authors concluded that antifibrinolytic drugs decrease blood loss in children undergoing scoliosis surgery and, therefore, could be added to the armamentarium of available techniques to reduce bleeding. Although the decrease in blood loss can be considered clinically important, whether antifibrinolytic drugs reduce the need for transfusions remains unclear. Further studies will be needed to clarify the efficacy of this class of drugs on this purpose. Erythropoietin (EPO) is a hormone that regulates erythropoiesis, acting on erythroid colony-forming units by stimulating progenitor cell differentiation in the bone marrow. EPO accelerates maturation of proerythroblasts to reticulocytes, stimulates the synthesis of haemoglobin (Hb) and promotes the release of reticulocytes to the circulation and their differentiation into mature red blood cells [64]. Recombinant human erythropoietin (rHuEPO) is a biosynthetic form of the natural hormone having the same biochemical structure and biological effect [65]. There are two types of rHuEPO: the alpha type and the beta type, presented in lyophilized form and reconstituted with saline solution [66]. Recombinant human erythropoietin can be administered intravenously or subcutaneously. It reaches peak plasma concentration faster by the intravenous route, although the half-life is shorter (5–10 h) [67]. Availability is lower with subcutaneous administration, but the half-life is longer (12–18 h), and this route is usually recommended for the management of perioperative anaemia [68]. Initially, the recommended dose was

300 IU/kg/day during 15 days [15, 69]. However, Goldberg demonstrated that a weekly dose of 600 IU/kg starting 3 weeks before the procedure achieved a higher increase in haemoglobin (1.44 g/dL versus 0.73 g/dL) with comparable safety and efficacy and lower cost [70]. Current recommended dosage is 600 IU/kg of subcutaneous rHuEPO weekly, given over 3 weeks (days 21, 14 and 7 before the surgical procedure) and on the day of surgery. In practice, administration of a 40,000 IU vial weekly is recommended in adults with a mean weight of around 65 kg. The 40,000 IU dose is authorized exclusively for preoperative rHuEPO treatment. When haemoglobin levels reach 15 g/dL at any of the preoperative analyses, rHuEPO administration is interrupted indefinitely [71]. Blood management is most difficult in adult patients with complex deformities requiring very aggressive surgery with circumferential approaches and long spinal instrumentation. Colomina et al. made a specific study in spine surgery and divided their patients in three groups, one who did not received EPO (degenerative and deformity cases) and other two groups who received EPO (degenerative (>2 levels) and adult deformity cases, respectively). Two groups received rHuEPO based on their protocol: the adult deformity patients, 98% complied with AUT estimations and only 14.6% required allogenic blood transfusion. In patients with degenerative cases (>2 levels) of surgery and a predicted blood loss of around 50% of total volume, nearly 97% did not require allogenic transfusions when rHuEPO treatment was associated with the AUT programme [72]. The authors conclude that surgery involving blood losses under 30% of the patient's total volume can be accomplished without the need for allogenic transfusion, if the baseline haemoglobin level is greater than 13 g/dL. Recombinant human erythropoietin administration is very effective for attaining this level and can be used as the only blood-sparing technique in these patients. When the expected blood loss is around 50% of the total volume, AUT is the standard technique applied. Addition of rHuEPO to AUT in these patients improves haemoglobin levels and facilitates retrieval of the autologous blood units required. This combination can avoid allogenic transfusion in 95% of the patients. When surgery is associated with a predicted blood loss close to the patient's total blood volume, the combined blood-sparing technique should always be used. Despite the complexity and aggressiveness of the procedure, with the combination of AUT and rHuEPO, more than 80% of the patients operated will not require allogenic transfusions. The disadvantages of rHuEPO therapy include side effects and cost. Side effects may include hypertension, myocardial infarction, angina and deep venous thrombosis, though previous literature showed that these effects were not increased compared with control groups [73]. The cost of the epoetin alfa dose regimen, a specific type of rHuEPO, is approximately US$400 per injection, or a total of US$1600 in the USA [74]. *Desmopressin*:

Deamino-8-D-arginin vasopressin (DDVAP or desmopressin) is an analogue of the natural hormone vasopressin or antidiuretic hormone (ADH). It increases the release of factor VIIc and von Willebrand factor (vWF) from endothelial cells, along with a paradoxical increase of plasminogen activator and prostaglandins. DDAVP, originally developed and licensed for the treatment of inherited defects of haemostasis, given by slow intravenous infusion at a dose of 0.3 µg/kg, acts by releasing ultralarge von Willebrand factor multimers from endothelial cells, leading to an enhancement of primary haemostasis [75]. Despite the successful use of DDAVP in patients with von Willebrand disease, congenital platelet disorders, renal failure, cirrhosis and long-term salicylate treatment, its effectiveness during spinal surgery has been controversial, as it is based on a small number of experimental studies [76]. Carless et al. published a systematic review about desmopressin use for minimizing allogenic blood transfusion in patients without congenital bleeding disorders failing to show any real and effective efficacy on this matter [77]. However, in patients with spinal disorders with von Willebrand disease requiring surgical treatment, a very specific and detailed preoperative surgical strategy will be needed using this drug for successful treatment [78]. Absorbable topical haemostatic agents have since been developed and provide useful adjunctive therapy when conventional methods of haemostasis are ineffective or impractical. Topical haemostatic agents can be applied directly to the bleeding site and may prevent continuous unrelenting bleeding throughout the entire procedure and into the postoperative recovery period. They are in the market in multiple types and options.

Collagen-based products: The efficacy of collagen-derived haemostatic agents has been established in standardized animal studies and clinically in man [79, 80]. They lead to thrombocyte adhesion and activation of coagulation factor XII (Hageman factor). Like gelatin products, collagen-based haemostatics can be of bovine, porcine or equine origin and are available in different forms, such as sheets, powder or aggregates. As they can cause adhesion formation and immune reactions, they should not be left in the spinal canal. They can interfere with bone healing and cause allergic reactions and infection. This should be applied dry with clean and dry instruments, and pressure with gloved fingers should never be placed, as the collagen-based products would adhere to the glove more than on the haemorrhage site. Postoperative adhesion of the haemostatic agent to neural structures is possible. Therefore, it is recommended to tease way the excess of product after 5–10 min. Swelling occurs, although less so than with other products, and surgeons should be aware of this when these products are left in place in rigid compartments [23]. *Oxidized cellulose* presents multiple mechanisms of action, including physical and mechanical actions in tamponade, blood absorption, swelling and gel formation and then surface interactions with proteins, platelets and intrinsic and extrinsic pathway activation. One major advantage of oxidized cellulose is its definite and potent action against a wide variety of pathogenic organisms, both in vivo and in vitro. This beneficial effect is immediate and is exerted by a low pH effect. The current theory is that this chemical haemostatic reduces the effective initial inoculum with an acid hostile ambient, allowing the host's natural defences to overcome the organism [81]. Activation of the initial coagulation phase is caused by their surface effect. They also induce a moderate acceleration of fibrinogen polymerization and seem to act as a caustic haemostat by decreasing pH [82]. Bacteriostatic properties of this product should be preferred in particularly contaminated fields. Obviously, should this event occur, the use of no agent at all is always better. Wadding or packing in rigid cavities (neural foramina) should be avoided, due to risks related to swelling phenomena. *Gelatin-based*: Absorbable gelatin sponges are available in multiple formulations (sheds, powder, foam). Except for thrombin-soaked formulations, their haemostatic effect appears to be a physical effect rather than a "surface effect". When compared with collagen-based products, gelatin sponges have been reported to form a better quality clot [83]. During spine procedures, attention should be paid to remove the excess, and the surgeon should be aware that gelatin can interfere with bone healing. In infected spaces, its use is contraindicated, because it may enhance the infectious process. It could be suggested placing it dry with moderate pressure on the bleeding site. This agent can double in volume by swelling and can also cause compressive complications. If soaked in thrombin, GF has an increased haemostatic action. *Thrombin*: The active topical haemostatic agent thrombin has been widely used in surgery for years. The agent has had a long history of clinical efficacy and safety in many surgical procedures [84]. Unlike passive agents, which rely on the presence of normal clotting processes, however, the active agent thrombin acts at the end of the clotting cascade, rendering its action less susceptible to coagulopathies caused by clotting factor deficiencies or platelet malfunction [85]. Thrombin can provide a logical and useful choice in patients receiving antiplatelet and/or anticoagulation agents, which is occurring in an increasing proportion of surgical cases [10]. Thrombin relies on the presence of fibrinogen in the patient's blood; however, it is ineffective in patients who have afibrinogenaemia, a rare condition reported to affect one in one million people. Additionally, thrombin itself does not need to be removed from the site of bleeding before wound closure, unlike many of the passive topical haemostatic agents, and degeneration and reabsorption of the resulting fibrin clot are achieved during normal wound healing [86]. The sprayable formulation of thrombin offers potential advantages in the surgical setting because wide surfaces can be treated instantaneously without the need for tamponade. Awareness of the potential of bovine thrombin products to induce antibodies has been raised; however, the clinical implications are still largely unclear [87]. Although many patients will demonstrate no clinical or laboratory abnormalities after the development of antibodies to thrombin preparations, abnormalities in blood coagulation tests are occasionally reported and have rarely been fatal [88]. *Fibrin sealants* are sterile, virally inactivated preparation of purified human fibrinogen and thrombin. Fibrin glue bypasses the clotting cascade by catalysing the conversion of fibrinogen into fibrin to immediately produce activated clotting factors [89]. Stimulating the formation of a fibrin clot, fibrin "glues" initiate the final stage of the clotting cascade. Two major families can be distinguished: the combination of a fibrinogen component together with a thrombin/Ca solution and, more recently, a collagen/thrombin component that uses the endogenous fibrinogen of the bleeding source. There are several concerning issues regarding the use of fibrin glue in the setting of lumbar spine surgery. From a practical standpoint, the approximate 20-min preparation time can be relatively significant when approaching the end of an operation. Once applied, the coagulum needs 3–5 min to attain optimal adherence and 2 h to reach its ultimate strength. The feasibility of providing appropriate setting conditions during bleeding, irrigation, building intradural pressure and movement remains questionable. There is also concern regarding the effect of fibrin glue on bone formation. Although some studies have shown fibrin glue to be a successful scaffold for bone growth when combined with osteoinductive or osteoconductive substances, multiple animal studies have raised concern that fibrin glue may inhibit bony fusion, even when using recombinant bone morphogenetic proteins [90, 91]. A Cochrane review on the use of fibrin sealants in surgery suggests efficacy, but this conclusion is hampered by the small number of trials and limitations in the methodology. Fibrin sealants have been reported to be effective in spine surgery and to diminish scar formation [92, 93].

Haemostatic matrices: The bicomponent medium of the second family of fibrin glues contains thrombin and a gelatin matrix. A tamponade effect of the swelling collagen granules restricts bleeding, while the gelatin matrix provides the structural integrity required to remain in situ. Its main advantage is that it can easily be used on wet and bleeding tissues, and favourable results have been reported in spinal procedures [10].

17.6 Assessing the Risk of Blood Transfusions in Spine Surgery

Many researches on literature discuss and try to define predictors that can be used to estimate the risk or probability of blood transfusion in elective spine procedures. Nuttall et al.

made a retrospective analysis of 244 patients who have submitted to spine procedures and after statistical linear multiple regression modelling concluded that low preoperative haemoglobin concentration, tumour surgery, increased number of posterior levels surgically fused, history of pulmonary disease, less amount of autologous blood available and no use of the Jackson table were significant determinants of the number of allogeneic RBC units transfused on the day of surgery. In the current study, idiopathic scoliosis was not found to be a predictor of increased RBC or coagulation product transfusions. A benefit from the use of hypotensive anaesthesia technique was not found in their study [94]. In another retrospective study, Lenoir et al. analysed 230 patients who were submitted to spine procedures [95]. Patients' data were analysed in a retrospective study trying to identify an individual probability of allogeneic transfusion in adult patients undergoing elective thoracolumbar spine surgery. These patients were submitted in a specific anaesthesia and transfusion protocols, and all patients received tranexamic acid in a continuous intravenous infusion until the skin closed. Different factors collected were tested in statistic techniques. The authors created a specific score including age, preoperative haemoglobin level, number of spine fusion levels and osteotomy as follows (PMTSS (predictive model of transfusion in spine surgery) score calculation, see Table 17.4).

Predictive model of transfusion in spine surgery (PMTSS) is calculated as the arithmetic sum of points assigned to each item, except in case of osteotomy, where the maximum number of points [4] is allocated in any case. When age <50 years, fusion level <2, haemoglobin (Hb) >14 or no osteotomy is planned, 0 points are, respectively, allocated for each item. The score is then comprised between 0 and 4 and defined five distinct levels of allogeneic transfusion risk.

Patients with score total above two points should be screened to preoperative blood-sparing techniques to reduce allogeneic blood transfusion. However, this study has some specific limitations recognized by the own authors; perhaps, this scale nowadays cannot be so precise because some new recent minimal invasive techniques used in spine surgery today that can be an effective treat to many spinal pathologies without no such bleeding were used before. Studied relationship between preoperative levels of fibrinogen,

bleeding and transfusion requirements in 82 consecutive adolescent idiopathic scoliosis patients. They analysed specific factors, all patients were submitted again a specific anaesthetic protocol and all cases received tranexamic acid intravenously at the initiation of all procedures. Intraoperative and post-operative blood volumes were recorded. In their study, when the predictive values of a fibrinogen concentration in the lower quartile (<2.8 g/L) on extensive bleeding and transfusions were calculated, high negative predictive values were obtained (94% and 88%, respectively), while the positive predictive values were low (47% and 30%, respectively). This means that for an individual patient with a fibrinogen value above 2.8 g/L, it is unlikely that the patient will bleed extensively during or after the procedure. Lower fibrinogen concentrations on the other hand do not necessarily result in a high bleeding volume or transfusion rate but provide information that these patients have an increased risk for these events. One may speculate if patients with high risk for bleeding complications and preoperative fibrinogen levels in the lower normal range may benefit from prophylactic fibrinogen administration. Fibrinogen concentrations obtained from human plasma are commercially available and currently used to treat inherited and acquired fibrinogen deficiency [96]. In a recent pilot study in cardiac surgery, patients who received prophylactic treatment with 2 g fibrinogen had a reduction in post-operative bleeding with 32% [3]. As seen in other studies, the authors also suggest that other studies will be needed to answer the significance of their results. As we can see, there are a growing number of tools and different strategies that can be used to avoid or lower the amount of allogeneic blood transfusion. These strategies must be organized and fashioned in specific situations to accomplish this objective. In a near future, other drugs and solutions will be part of our everyday routine.

References

1. Lawson JH. The clinical use and immunologic impact of thrombin in surgery. Semin Thromb Hemost. 2006;32(Suppl 1):98–110.
2. Samudrala S. Topical hemostatic agents is surgery: a Surgeon's perspective. AORN J. 2008;88:S1–11.
3. Karlsson M, Ternstrom L, Hyllner M, et al. Prophylactic fibrinogen infusion reduces bleeding after coronary artery bypass surgery. A prospective randomised pilot study. Thromb Haemost. 2009;102:137–44.
4. Elgafy H, Bransford RJ, McGuire R, Dettori J, Fischer D. Are there effective measures to decrease massive hemorrhage in major spine fusion surgery. Spine. 2010;35(95):S47–56.
5. Hu SS. Blood loss in adult spinal surgery. Eur Spine J. 2004;13(Suppl 1):S3–5.
6. Block JE. Severe blood loss during spinal reconstructive procedures: the potential usefulness of topical hemostatic agents. Med Hypotheses. 2005;65(3):617–21.
7. Bochicchio G, Dunne J, Bochicchio K, Scalea T. The combination of platelet-enriched autologous plasma with bovine

Table 17.4 *PMTSS score calculation*, parameter (allogeneic assigned points, transfusion predictor)

According to item	
Age > 50 years	1
Preoperative Hb	
Hb < 12 g/dL	2
12 < Hb < 14 g/dL	1
Spine fusion levels (n) > 2	1
Transpedicular osteotomy	4

collagen and thrombin decreases the need for multiple blood transfusions in trauma patients with retroperitoneal bleeding. J Trauma. 2004;56(1):76–9.

8. Carreon LY, Puno RM, Dimar JR 2nd, Glassman SD, Johnson JR. Perioperative complications of posterior lumbar decompression and arthrodesis in older adults. J Bone Joint Surg Am. 2003;85(11):2089–92.

9. McDonnell MF, Glassman SD, Dimar JR 2nd, Puno RM, Johnson JR. Perioperative complications of anterior procedures on the spine. J Bone Joint Surg Am. 1996;78(6):839–47.

10. Renkens KL Jr, Payner TD, Leipzig TJ, et al. A multicenter, prospective, randomized trial evaluating a new hemostatic agent for spinal surgery. Spine. 2001;26(15):1645–50.

11. Ridgeway S, Tai C, Alton P, Barnardo P, Harrison DJ. Pre-donated autologous blood transfusion in scoliosis surgery. J Bone Joint Surg Br. 2003;85:1032–6.

12. García-Erce J, Muñoz M, Bisbe E, Sáez M, Solano VM, Beltrán S, Ruiz A, Cuenca J, Vicente-Thomas J. Predeposit autologous donation in spinal surgery: a multicenter study. Eur Spine J. 2004;13(Suppl 1):S34–9.

13. Keating EM, Meding JB. Perioperative blood management practices in elective orthopaedic surgery. J Am Acad Orthop Surg. 2002;10:393–400.

14. Henry D A, Carless P A, Moxey A J, O'Connell D, Ker K, Fergusson DA. Pre-operative autologous donation for minimising perioperative allogeneic blood transfusion. Cochrane Database Syst Rev. 2001;(5):CD003602. https://doi.org/10.1002/14651858. CD003602.pub2.

15. Carless P, Moxey AJ, O'Connell D, Henry D. Autologous transfusion techniques: a systematic review of their efficacy. Transfus Med. 2004;14:123–44.

16. McVay PA, Andrews A, Hoag MS, Polan D, Skettino S, Stehling LC. Moderate and severe reactions during autologous blood donations are no more frequent than during homologous blood donations. Vox Sang. 1990;59:70–2.

17. Faught C, Wells P, Fergusson D, Laupacis A. Adverse effects of methods for minimizing perioperative allogeneic transfusion: a critical review of the literature. Transfus Med Rev. 1998;12:206–25.

18. Muñoz M, García-Vallejo JJ, Ruiz MD, Romero R, Olalla E, Sebastían C. Transfusion of post-operative shed blood: laboratory characteristics and clinical utility. Eur Spine J. 2004;13(Suppl 1):S107–13.

19. Chanda A, Smith DR, Nanda A. Autotransfusion by cell saver technique in surgery of lumbar and thoracic spinal fusion with instrumentation. J Neurosurg. 2002;96(Suppl 3):298–303.

20. Reitman CA, Watters WC 3rd, Sassard WR. The CS in adult lumbar fusion surgery: a cost-benefit outcomes study. Spine. 2004;29:1580–1583. discussion on p. 1584.

21. Sebastián C, Romero R, Olalla E, Ferrer C, García-Vallejo JJ, Muñoz M. Postoperative blood salvage and reinfusion in spinal surgery. Blood quality, effectiveness and impact on patient blood parameters. Eur Spine J. 2000;9:458–65.

22. Muñoz M, Sánchez-Arrieta Y, García-Vallejo JJ, Mérida FJ, Ruiz MD, Maldonado J. Autotransfusión pre y posoperatoria. Estudio comparativo de la hematología, bioquímica y metabolism eritrocitário en sangre predonada y sangre de drenaje postoperatorio. Sangre (Bar). 1999;44:433–50.

23. Schonauer C, Tessitore E, Barbagallo G, Albanese V, Moraci A. The use of local agents: bone wax, gelatin, collagen, oxidized cellulose. Eur Spine J. 2004;13(Suppl 1):S89–96.

24. Howard TC, Kelley RR. The effect of bone wax on the healing of experimental rat tibial lesions. Clin Orthop. 1969;63:226–32.

25. Geary JR, Frantz VK. New absorbable hemostatic bone wax. Experimental and clinical studies. Ann Surg. 1950;132:1128–37.

26. Johnson P, Fromm D. Effects of bone wax on bacterial clearance. Surgery. 1981;89(2):206–9.

27. Guzman R, Dubach-Schwizer S, Heini P, Lovblad K, Kalbermatten D, Schroth G, Remonda L. Preoperative transarterial embolization of vertebral metastases. Eur Spine J. 2005;14:263–8.

28. Boland PJ, Lene JM, Sundersen N. Metastatic disease of spine. Clin Orthop. 1982;1169:95–102.

29. Shi HB, Suh DC, Lee HK, Lim SM, Kim DH, Choi CG, Lee CS, Rhim SC. Preoperative transarterial embolization of spinal tumors: embolization techniques and results. AJNR Am J Neuradiol. 1999;20:2009–15.

30. Görich J, Solymosi L, Hasan I, Sittek H, Majdali R, Reiser M. Embolisation von Knochenmetastasen. Radiologie. 1995;35:55–9.

31. Manke C, Bretschneider T, Lenhart M, Strotzer M, Neumann C, Gmeinwieser J, Feuerbach S. Spinal metastases from renal cell carcinoma: effect of preopertative embolization on intraoperative blood loss. AJNR Am J Neuroradiol. 2001;22:997–1003.

32. Cory DA, Fritsch SA, Cohen MD, et al. Aneurysmal bone cysts: imaging findings and embolotherapy. Am J Roentgenol. 1989;153:369–73.

33. Esparza J, Castro S, Portillo JM, et al. Vertebral hemangiomas: spinal angiography and preoperative embolization. Surg Neurol. 1978;10:171–3.

34. Chiras J, Gaston A, Gaveau T et al. [Preoperative embolization in spinal pathology. Apropos of 21 cases]. J Radiol. 1983;64:397-403 (Fr).

35. Gellad FE, Sadato N, Numaguchi Y, et al. Vascular metastatic lesions of the spine: preoperative embolization. Radiology. 1990;176:683–6.

36. Vetter SC, Strecker EP, Ackermann LW, Harms J. Preoperative embolization of cervical spine tumors. Cardiovasc Intervent Radiol. 1997;20:343–7.

37. Nader R, Brent T, Nauta HJW, Crow W, vanSonnenberg E, Hadjipavlou A. Preoperative embolization and intraoperative cryocoagulation as adjuncts in resection of hypervascular lesions of the thoracolumbar spine. J Neurosurg Spine. 2002;97:294–300.

38. Cakir B, Ulmar B, Schmidt R, Kelsch G, Geiger P, Mehrkens H, Puhl W, Richter M. Efficacy and cost effectiveness of harmonic scalpel compared with electrocautery in posterior instrumentation of the spine. Eur Spine J. 2006;15:48–54.

39. Hu X, Ohmiess D, Lieberman I. Use of an ultrasonic osteotome device in spine surgery: experience from the first 128 patients. Eur Spine J. 2013;22(12):2845–9. https://doi.org/10.1007/s00586-013-2780-y.

40. Sanborn MR, Balzer J, Gerszten PC, Karausky P, Cheng BC, Welch WC. Safety and efficacy of a novel ultrasonic osteotome device in a ovine model. J Clin Neurosci. 2011;18:1528–33.

41. McMahon P, Dididze M, Levi AD. Incidental durotomy after spinal surgery: a prospective study in an academic institution. J Neurosurg. 2012;17:30–6.

42. Corning J. Spinal anesthesia and local medications of the cord. N Y J Med. 1885;42:483–5.

43. Tamsen A, Gordh T. Epidural clonidine produces analgesia. Lancet. 1984;2(8396):231–2.

44. De Kock M, Crochet B, Morimont C, Scholtes JL. Intravenous or epidural clonidine for intra- and postoperative analgesia. Anesthesiology. 1993;79(3):525–31.

45. De Kock M. Site of hemodynamic effects of alpha sub 2-adrenergic agonists. Anesthesiology. 1991;75:715–6.

46. Dutton RP. Controlled hypotension for spinal surgery. Eur Spine J. 2004;13(Suppl 1):S66–71.

47. Malcolm-Smith NA, McMaster MJ. The use of induced hypotension to control bleeding during posterior fusion for scoliosis. J Bone Joint Surg Br. 1983;65:255–8.

48. Mandel RJ, Brown MD, McCullough NC, et al. Hypotensive anesthesia and autotransfusion in spinal surgery. Clin Orthop. 1981;154:27.

49. Lennon RL, Hosking MP, Gray JR, et al. The effects of intraoperative blood salvage and induced hypotension on transfusion requirements during spinal surgical procedures. Mayo Clin Proc. 1987;62:1090–4.

50. Murphy MA. Bilateral posterior ischemic optic neuropathy after lumbar spine surgery. Ophthalmology. 2003;110:1454–7.

51. Bernard JM, Le Penven-Henninger C, Passuti N. Sudden decreases in mixed venous oxygen saturation during posterior spinal fusion. Anesth Analg. 1995;80:1038–41.

52. Chang SH, Miller NR. The incidence of vision loss due to perioperative ischemic optic neuropathy associated with spine surgery: the Johns Hopkins Hospital experience. Spine. 2005;30(11):1299–302.

53. Urmey WF. Combined regional and general anesthesia for orthopedic spine fusion surgery. Tech Reg Anesth Pain Manag. 2000;4(2):101–5.

54. Williams-Russo P, Sharrock NE, Mattis S, et al. Randomized trial of hypotensive epidural anesthesia in older adults. Anesthesiology. 1999;91(4):926–35.

55. Szpalski M, Gunzburg R. Management of haemostasis in spine surgery (touch breefings). Eur Musc Rev. 2008:53–7.

56. Guay J, Haig M, Lortie L, et al. Predicting blood loss in surgery for idiopathic scoliosis. Can J Anaesth. 1994;41:775–81.

57. Kiss H, Raffl M, Neumann D, et al. Epinephrine-augmented hypotensive epidural anesthesia replaces tourniquet use in total knee replacement. Clin Orthop Relat Res. 2005:184–9.

58. Fritz H, Wunderer G. Biochemistry and applications of aprotinin, the kallikrein inhibitor from bovine organs. Arzneimittelforschung. 1983;33:479–94.

59. Schulman S. Pharmacologic tools to reduce bleeding in surgery. Hematology. 2012;2012:517–21.

60. Henry DA, Carless PA, Moxey AJ, O'Connell D, Stokes BJ, Fergusson DA, Ker K. Anti-fibrinolytic use for minimising perioperative allogeneic blood transfusion. Cochrane Database Syst Rev. 2011;(5):CD001886. DOI: https://doi.org/10.1002/14651858. CD001886.pub1.

61. Schneeweiss S, Seeger JD, Landon J, Walker AM. Aprotinin during coronary-artery bypass grafting and risk of death. N Engl J Med. 2008;358:771–83.

62. Manufacturer removes remaining stocks of Trasylol [press release]. Silver Spring, MD: US Food and Drug Administration; 2008. http://www.fda.gov/NewsEvents/Newsroom/PressAnnouncements/2008/ucm116895.htm

63. A T, Cepeda MS, Schumann R, Carr DB. Antifibrinolytic agents for reducing blood loss in scoliosis surgery in children. Cochrane Database Syst Rev. 2008;(5):CD006883. https://doi.org/10.1002/14651858.CD006883.pub3.

64. Browne JK, Cohen AM, Egrie JC, Lai PH, Lin FK, Strickland T, Watson E, Stebbing N. Erythropoietin: gene cloning, protein structure, and biological properties. Cold Spring Harb Symp Quant Biol. 1986;51(1):693–702.

65. Cheung W, Minton N, Gunawardena K. Pharmacokinetics and pharmacodynamics of epoetin alfa once weekly and three times weekly. Eur J Clin Pharmacol. 2001;57:411–8.

66. Rosencher N, Ozier Y. Peri-operative use of EPO. Transfus Clin Biol. 2003;10:159–64.

67. Rosencher N, Woimant G, Ozier Y, Conseiller C. Preoperative strategy for homologous blood salvage and peri-operative erythropoietin. Transfus Clin Biol. 1999;6:370–9.

68. Goodnough LT, Monk TG, Andriole GL. Erythropoietin therapy. N Engl J Med. 1997;336:933–8.

69. de Andrade JR, Jove M, Landon G, Frei D, Guilfoyle M, Young DC. Baseline hemoglobin as a predictor of risk of transfusion and response to epoetin alfa in orthopedic surgery patients. Am J Orthop. 1996;25:533–42.

70. Goldberg MA. Perioperative epoetin alfa increases red blood cell mass and reduces exposure to transfusions: results of randomized clinical trials. Semin Hematol. 1997;34:41–7.

71. Stowell CP, Chandler H, Jove M, Guilfoyle M, Wacholtz MC. An open-label, randomized study to compare the safety and efficacy of perioperative epoetin alfa with preoperative autologous blood donation in total joint arthroplasty. Orthopedics. 1999;22:s105–12.

72. Colomina M, Bagó J, Pellsé F, Godet C, Villanueva C. Preoperative erythropoietin in spine surgery. Eur Spine J. 2004;13(Suppl 1):S40–9.

73. de Andrade JR, Frei D, Guilfoyle M. Integrated analysis of thrombotic/vascular event occurrence in epoetin alfa–treated patients undergoing major, elective orthopedic surgery. Orthopedics. 1999;22(1 Suppl):S113–8.

74. Shapiro GS, Boachi-Adjei O, Dhawlikar SH, Maier LS. The use of epoetin alfa in complex spine deformity surgery. Spine. 2002;27(18):2067–71.

75. Ruggeri ZM, Mannucci PM, Lombardi R, Federici AB, Zimmerman TS. Multimeric composition of factor VIII/von Willebrand factor following administration of DDAVP: implications for pathophysiology and therapy of von Willebrand's disease subtypes. Blood. 1982;59:1272–8.

76. Kovesi T, Royston D. Pharmacological approaches to reducing allogeneic blood exposure. Vox Sang. 2003;84:2–10.

77. Carless P A, Stokes B J, Moxey A J, Henry DA. Desmopressin use for minimising perioperative allogeneic blood transfusion. Cochrane Database Syst Rev. 2004;(5):CD001884. https://doi.org/10.1002/14651858.CD001884.pub2.

78. Bolan C, Rick M, Polly D Jr. Transfusion medicine management for reconstructive spinal repair in a patient with von Willebrand's disease and a history of heavy surgical bleeding. Spine. 2001;26(23):E552–6.

79. Orgill DP, Ehret FW, Regan JF, et al. Polyethylene glycol/microfibrillar collagen composite as a new resorbable hemostatic bone wax. J Biomed Mater Res. 1998;39:358–63.

80. Kruger J. Blutstillung bei neurochirurgischen Operationen. Eine Vergleichsstudie zwischen einem Kollagenvlies (LyostyptR) und einem Gelatine-Schwammchen (MarbagelanR). Zentralbl Neurochir. 1992;53:33–6.

81. Wagner WR, Pachence JM, Ristich J, Johnson PC. Comparative in vitro analysis of topical hemostatic agents. J Surg Res. 1996;66:100–8.

82. Levy ML, Day DJ, Fukushima T. Surgicel fibrillar absorbable oxidized regenerated cellulose. Neurosurgery. 1997;41:701–2.

83. Dehen M, Niederdellmann H, Lachner J. Mechanical properties of collagen or gelatine-stabilized blood clots. Dtsch Zahnarztl Z. 1990;45:553–6.

84. Lundblad RL, Bradshaw RA, Gabriel D, Ortel TL, Lawson J, Mann KG. A review of the therapeutic uses of thrombin. Thromb Haemost. 2004;91(5):851–60.

85. Oz MC, Rondinone JF, Shargill NS. FloSeal Matrix: new generation topical hemostatic sealant. J Card Surg. 2003;18(6):486–93.

86. Morikawa T. Tissue sealing. Am J Surg. 2001;182(2 Suppl):29S–35S.

87. Ortel TL, Charles LA, Keller FG, et al. Topical thrombin and acquired coagulation factor inhibitors: clinical spectrum and laboratory diagnosis. Am J Hematol. 1994;45(2):128–35.

88. Winterbottom N, Kuo JM, Nguyen K, et al. Antigenic responses to bovine thrombin exposure during surgery: a prospective study of 309 patients. J Appl Res. 2002;2(1) http://jrnlappliedresearch.com/articles/Vol2Iss1/winterbottom.htm

89. Weinstein JN, Tosteson TD, Lurie JD, Tosteson AN, Hanscom B, Skinner JS, et al. Surgical vs nonoperative treatment for lumbar disk herniation: the Spine Patient Outcomes Research Trial (SPORT): a randomized trial. JAMA. 2006;296:2441–50.

90. Turgut M, Erkus M, Tavus N. The effect of fibrin adhesive (Tisseel) on interbody allograft fusion: an experimental study with cats. Acta Neurochir. 1999;141:273–8.

91. Zarate-Kalfopulos B, Estrada-Villasenor E, Lecona-Buitron H, Arenas-Sordo Mde L, Garza-Hernandez AC, Reyes-Sanches A. Use of fibrin glue in combination with autologous bone graft as bone enhancer in posterolateral spinal fusion. An experimental study in New Zealand rabbits. Cir Cir. 2007;75:201–5.

92. Tredwell SJ, Sawatzky B. The use of fibrin sealant to reduce blood loss during Cotrel-Dubousset instrumentation for idiopathic scoliosis. Spine. 1990;15:913–5.

93. Carless PA, Anthony DM, Henry DA. Systematic review of the use of fibrin sealant to minimize perioperative allogeneic blood transfusion. Br J Surg. 2002;89:695–703.

94. Nuttall G, Horlocker T, Santrach P, Oliver W, Dekutoski M, Bryant S. Predictors of blood transfusions in spinal instrumentation and fusion surgery. Spine. 2000;25(5):596–601.

95. Lenoir B, Merckx P, Paugam-Burtz C, Dauzac C, Agostini M, Guigui P, Mantz J. Individual probability of allogeneic erythrocyte transfusion in elective spine surgery. Anesthesiology. 2009;110:105–1060.

96. Fenger-Eriksen C, Lindberg-Larsen M, Christensen AQ, et al. Fibrinogen concentrate substitution therapy in patients with massive haemorrhage and low plasma fibrinogen concentrations. Br J Anaesth. 2008;101:769–73.

Prophylaxis Against Thromboembolism in Spinal Surgery

18

Uwe Vieweg

18.1 Introduction and Core Messages

Venous thromboembolism (VTE) is a common and clinically serious event, with an age-related incidence that increases from circa 1 case per 1000 person-years at age 50 years to circa 5 cases per 1000 person-years at age 75 years [1].

The rationale for prophylaxis of venous thromboembolism is based on the clinically silent nature of the disease, the relatively high prevalence among hospitalized patients, and the potentially tragic consequences of a missed diagnosis [2].

18.2 Venous Thrombosis and Pulmonary Embolism (PE) [3–5]

Superficial venous thromboses cause discomfort but generally not serious consequences, as do the deep venous thromboses (DVTs) that form in the deep veins of the legs or in the pelvic veins. Nevertheless, they can progress to the deep veins through the perforator veins, or they can be responsible for a lung embolism mainly if the head of the clot is poorly attached to the vein wall and is situated near the saphenofemoral junction. Complications can arise when a venous thromboembolism lodges in the lung as a pulmonary embo-

lism [6]. Mortality from untreated PEs was said to be 26%. Deaths that are a result of VTE/PE were shown to be the most common cause of preventable hospital deaths. Autopsy results show that as many as 60% of patients dying in the hospital have had a PE, but the diagnosis has been missed in about 70% of the cases [6]. Hospitalized patients have between a 10% and 48% chance of developing a VTE [7]. 762,000 PEs/DVTs were reported in EU in 2004 [8, 2]. The incidence of a DVT in a hospital lies between 10% and 40% for medical or general surgical patients and 40% and60% following major orthopedic surgeries [2, 8, 9].

18.2.1 Diagnostics

The diagnostics of venous thrombosis due to clinical signs and symptoms is unreliable. Therefore, instrument-based diagnostics should be carried out immediately in the case of a suspected thrombosis or embolism, in order to objectively confirm or rule out this suspicion. Depending on the issue and the assumed localization of the thrombosis (pelvis, thighs, or lower legs), these diagnostic measures include the Duplex sonography, phlebography, perfusion scintigraphy, or CT and MR procedures.

18.3 Frequency of Occurrence of the Venous Thrombosis without Medication-Based Prophylaxis and Risk Factors [5, 2–10]

In the assessment of risk factors for specific procedure or injuries, it is important to remember the multifactorial etiology of venous thromboembolism. The frequency of occurrence of a deep vein thrombosis (DVT) in the cases

U. Vieweg (✉)
Department of Conservative and Surgical Spine Therapy with Interdisciplinary Spinal Deformities Centre and Rummelsberg Sectional Center, Hospital Rummelsberg, Schwarzenbruck, Germany
e-mail: uwe.vieweg@sana.de

© Springer-Verlag GmbH Germany 2023
U. Vieweg, F. Grochulla (eds.), *Manual of Spine Surgery*, https://doi.org/10.1007/978-3-662-64062-3_18

where no prophylactic treatment is performed may be low, medium, or high, depending on the scope of the medical operation, the extent of the injury, and the factors of disposition. The patients at greatest risk for VTE are those undergoing major lower extremity orthopedic surgery and those who have experienced major trauma or spinal cord injury [9, 11, 12]. The definition of risk groups for determining an indication for thromboembolism prophylaxis is crucial, taking the benefit-risk assessment into account. In addition to the risks of thrombosis due to an operation, injury, and/or immobility (expositional risks), the risk factors brought about by the patient's disposition are to be taken into consideration in order to decide whether or not measures of thromboembolism prophylaxis are required (at all) and if so which type and intensity of such measures are to be implemented. Venous thromboembolisms that have occurred previously in the patient's own medical history or in the patient's medical family history as well as the previous exposure to antithrombotic agents including possible reactions to these are of particular importance. If the patient's medical history displays a positive result with regard to the aforementioned factors, an increased dispositional risk has to be assumed, and a laboratory analysis should be considered to clarify a coagulation disorder. The dispositional risk factors for venous thromboembolism may be venous thromboembolism in the patient's medical history, congenital or acquired thrombophilic coagulation defects, malignant tumors, a pregnancy and postpartum period, advanced age, a therapy where sex hormones are either administered or blocked, chronic venous insufficiency, a severe systemic infection, overweight (body mass index <30), cardiac insufficiency, or a nephrotic syndrome. Together with the expositional risk factors, the dispositional risk factors define a patient's individual risk of thrombosis. If we take into account the previous frequency of occurrence of thromboses of patients who have been operated and/or who are traumatized, which has been determined by means of objective detection techniques, plus the additional risk constellation that is not procedure-related, patients can be classified by a low, medium, and high risk of thrombosis. Risk factors for venous thromboembolism are patient-related factors (age, previous thromboembolism, obesity, hormonal treatment, varicose veins, etc.) and procedure-related factors (total hip arthroplasty, total knee arthroplasty, plaster cast immobilization, spinal trauma, etc.). The levels of thromboembolism risk in surgical patients without prophylaxis are [2, 9] the following:

- **Low risk**: Minor surgery in patients aged <40 years with no additional risk factors
- **Moderate risk**: Minor surgery in patients with additional risk factors, non-major surgery in patients aged 40–60 years with no additional risk factors, and major surgery in patients aged <40 years with no additional risk factors
- **High risk**: Non-major surgery in patients aged >60 years or with additional risk factors; major surgery in patients aged >40 years or with additional risk factors
- **Highest risk**: Major surgery in patients aged >40 years plus prior VTE, cancer, or molecular hypercoagulable state, hip or knee arthroplasty and hip fracture surgery, major trauma, and spinal cord injury

18.4 Incidence of DVT and PE in the Population of Patients Undergoing Spinal Surgery [11, 13]

There are no accepted guidelines recommending a specific protocol for VTE prevention. It is difficult to determine the incidence of postoperative VTE in these different types of spinal surgeries. On the other side, the North American Spine Society (NASS) published an evidence-based clinical guideline on antithrombotic therapies in spine surgery. The guideline addresses key clinical questions surrounding the use of antithrombotic therapies in spine surgery [2]. The guideline does not represent a "standard of care" nor is intended as a fixed treatment protocol (Table 18.1).

In contrast to other orthopedic surgeries, in spine surgery, there is no manipulation of the limbs, where thrombosis usually originates. Major surgery or trauma of the lower extremities triggers the coagulation cascade. In these patients, a reduced venous flow and impaired endothelial function further increase the risk of developing deep vein thrombosis and pulmonary embolism [14]. Minimally invasive spinal surgery procedures, but also spinal reconstructions that are complex to some extent, possibly may have a different impact on the development of a thromboembolic occurrence. Patients who undergo spinal surgery are generally at low risk for VTE compared with craniotomy patients (Royston). Almost half of all thromboembolic events in spinal surgery occur after hospital discharge. In a study conducted by Fang et al., in 27,730 patients undergoing spinal surgery and included in the 2005–2011 ACS-NSQIP database, DVT was reported on 0.7% and pulmonary embolism in only 0.4% at 30 days postoperatively

Table 18.1 Risk factors for a DVT and PE

- Previous episode of thromboembolism.
- Prolonged immobility.
- Cancer.
- Obesity
- Pregnancy
- Oral estrogen
- Fever
- Atrial fibrillation
- CHF, shock
- Varicose veins
- Over 60 years old
- Hematologic disorders
- Trauma
- Central lines
- Dehydration
- Hypovolemia
- Surgical patients

[15]. The figures relating to the prevalence of a deep vein thrombosis or pulmonary embolism in the context of spinal operations vary between 0.63% and 33%. A clinically manifest thromboembolic complication does not seem to be common with spinal operations. Most of the prospective observational studies use an ultrasound screening with incidences between 2% and 14% of asymptomatic deep vein thrombosis in the context of different spinal surgery procedures. Since most studies were either carried out on a retrospective basis or showed a low methodological quality, risk factors can only be specified with reservations. Localization of the procedure, in particular an operation on the lumbar spine, still is the most reliably proved predictor of an asymptomatic DVT. The data with regard to the relevance of age are contradictory. Overweight, the duration of the medical procedure, the sex, and the number of days of bed rest have not shown any significant impact in the studies published so far. Although the increased thrombosis rate in the case of spinal cord injuries is well supported, no studies on spinal surgery itemizing motor deficits as a risk factor can be found. Corresponding to the inhomogeneous epidemiological data situation, there are contradictory studies relating to the benefit of thromboembolism prophylaxis. Only one relatively small randomized study compares mechanical prophylaxis to a control group without any prophylactic treatment for 50 different spinal operations. The results do not show any significant reduction of the asymptomatic rate of venous thrombosis from 25% to 8.5%. The rate of symptomatic thromboembolism did not show any significant difference. There are no meaningful studies relating to the risk of thromboembolism following spinal injuries. Nevertheless, thromboembolic complications must be taken into account, depending on the type and extent of the injury and the degree of immobility. In a prospective randomized study, in spite of prophylactic treatment with LMWH (low-molecular-weight heparin) vs. UFH (unfractionated heparin) in combination with IPC, phlebographically proven thromboses exceeding 60% in each case were reported. A combination of prophylactic treatment with physical measures seems advisable. Spinal injuries with damage to the spinal cord are listed as a contraindication for the administration of heparins by most manufacturers. This, however, is not to be considered as a prohibition. If it is possible to apply physical treatment, a decision on additional medicinal VTE prophylaxis must be made on a case-by-case basis. In the case of complete or incomplete paraplegic syndromes as a result of a spinal paralysis, a strongly increased VTE risk has to be assumed. In particular, in the case of incomplete and progressive lesions of the spinal cord and a proven intraspinal hematoma, the risk of bleeding has to be taken into consideration. TED stocking in combination with acetylsalicylic acid (SA) is an option in elective spinal surgery to decrease the incidence of thromboembolic complications [8]. Most elective spinal surgeries done through a posterior approach are associated with a low risk of VTE. Chemoprophylaxis may not be warranted as it is accompanied by a risk of serious wound and bleeding complications. In combined anterior posterior spinal surgery, LMWH or low-dose warfarin may be used postoperatively. Lee et al. [16] published a prospective study to determinate the rate of DVT following major spinal surgery without antithrombotic therapy. All 313 patients were analyzed with duplex ultrasonography. Lee et al. reported a 1.3% incidence of a DVT, with a clinically symptomatic presentation in 0.3% of patients. When interpreting the figures, it has to be regarded critically that the statistics do not include an exact figure relating to children. On the other side, Oda et al. reported a prospective study that analyzed the prevalence of DVT after posterior spinal surgery without antithrombotic therapy. He found an incidence of 15.5% DVD (lumbar 26.5%, thoracic 14.3%, cervical 5.6%) but without clinical magnification. A risk factor in the population was the period of bed rest. Patients with a spinal cord injury represent another dignity with regard to risk for VTE which is among the highest among all hospital admissions [17]. The incidence of DVT and PE within 3 months is 38% and approximately 5%, respectively [18]. The hypercoagulability state induced by traumatic injury, together with other

Table 18.2 Incidence of symptomatic deep vein thrombosis in the general population

Author	Population	Type of study	TVL/LE rate
Glynn et al., 2007 [6]	39,876 women, >45 years	Randomized, controlled study	TVL-0.12%
Naess et al., 2007 [22]	94,194 Norwegians, >18 years	Population-based, retrospective cohort study	TVT-0.093%; LE-0.050%
White et al., 2005 [23]	23.3 m, >18 years	Population-based, retrospective cohort study	TVT-0.093%
Oger et al., 2000 [14]	342,000 Frenchmen/Frenchwomen, >18 years	Population-based, retrospective cohort study	TVT/LE-0.124%
Silverstein et al., 1998 [24]	106,470 Americans, >18 years (1966–1990)	Population-based, retrospective cohort study	TVT/LE-0.117%
Nordström et al., 1992 [19]	366 Swedes, >18 years	Population-based, prospective cohort study	TVT-0.16%
Anderson et al., 1991 [25]	379,953 Americans, >18 years (1985–1986)	Population-based, prospective cohort study	TVT/LE-0.107%

factors such as obesity and prolonged immobilization, increases the VTE risk in patients with spine injuries [19] (Table 18.2).

The European guidelines on perioperative venous thromboembolism prophylaxis (ESA VTE Guidelines Task Force [20]) suggest for patients undergoing spinal surgery with no additional risk factors and no active thromboprophylaxis intervention apart from early mobilization. For patients undergoing spinal surgery with additional risk factors, the group recommends mechanical thromboprophylaxis, and the group suggests the addition of LMWH postoperatively when the risk of bleeding is presumed to be decreased [4].

18.5 Thromboembolism Prophylaxis

Thromboembolism prophylaxis may be provided by basic measures, based on physical and medication therapy.

18.5.1 Basic Measures and Physical Thromboembolism Prophylaxis

Basic measures are early mobilization; the provision of a critical diagnostic evaluation of measures that are immobilizing the patient, in particular with regard to the ankle and knee joint and to the pelvic region; requesting and instructing the patient to do exercises on his/her own muscle pump; reduction of the period of immobility; early operation, in particular in the case of injuries of the lower extremities, the pelvis and the thoracic spine and lumbar spine; and cardiovascular and respiratory therapy.

Some mechanical methods such as graduated stockings, foot pumps, and calf compressors have a good evidence base with studies showing a consist reduction in thrombosis. The ideal role is in conjunction with, rather than in competition with, chemical methods.

Physiotherapy, compression stockings, and early mobilization provide the basic measures which, however, cannot replace an indicated medication-based thromboprophylaxis. On the other hand, the basic measures are always additionally required if a medication-based thromboprophylactic treatment is performed. Both procedures complement each other to form an effective prophylaxis. Measures to prevent thromboses are active and passive movement exercises such as a bed pedal exerciser, a continuous passive motion device for mobilizing the ankle joint, and carefully fitted compression stockings (thigh-length/half stockings). Mechanical compression devices in the lower extremities are suggested in elective spinal surgery to decrease the incidence of thromboembolic complications.

18.5.2 Medication-Based Thromboembolism Prophylaxis [21]

The world of antithrombotic prophylaxis is a revolutionary phase due to the introduction of numerous compounds in the daily practice. Heparins are pharmaceutical products for medication-based thromboembolism prophylaxis (unfractionated heparin (UFH), low-molecular-weight heparins (LMWHs)), but also with a sufficient or insufficient impact on thromboprophylaxis, and substances such as danaparoid, fondaparinux, thrombin inhibitors, hirudin, vitamin K antagonists (coumarins), and platelet inhibitors. These drugs, however, may involve increased bleeding complication following medical measures and in particular after surgery. When bleeding complications occur while medication-based thromboembolism

Table 18.3 Frequency of occurrence of deep vein thrombosis in operative medicine without medication-based prophylaxis in compliance with the International Consensus, 2001

	Studies, n	Patients, n	TVT, %	95% CI, %
Abdominal surgery	54	4310	25	24–26
Retropubic prostatectomy	8	335	32	27–37
Transurethral prostatectomy	3	150	9	5–15
Gynecology				
Malignant tumor surgery	4	297	22	17–26
Benign disease	4	460	14	11–17
Elective hip replacement	17	851	51	48–54
Multiple traumas	4	536	50	46–55
Knee replacement	7	541	47	42–51
Hip fractures	16	836	45	41–48
Neurosurgery	5	280	22	17–27

prophylaxis is performed, apart from the possibility of a surgical bleeding, also a drug accumulation, for example, renal insufficiency or wrong dosage of drugs, must be taken into consideration and must be clarified by laboratory tests. In order to ensure expedient diagnostics, for unfractionated heparins and thrombin inhibitors, the measurement of the aPTT (activated partial thromboplastin time) and for low-molecular-weight heparins, danaparoid and fondaparinux, and determination of the anti-Xa activity or performance of the HEP test are required. The intensity of the anticoagulation with vitamin K antagonists is recorded by the determination of the INR. If serious bleeding complications occur while prophylactically dosed anticoagulants are administered, the dose of anticoagulants has to be reduced or the treatment has to be interrupted, and in the case of pathologically altered coagulation tests under UFH or LMWH, antagonization by means of protamine has to be taken into consideration (Table 18.3).

18.5.3 Heparins

Heparins are mucopolysaccharides, the anticoagulative potential of which is mainly unfolded by potentiating the antithrombin effect. They are extracted from the pig's intestine mucosa. Various fragmentation processes generate low-molecular-weight heparins.

18.5.3.1 Unfractionated Heparin (UFH)

The subcutaneous administration of UFH two or three times a day ("low-dose heparin": 2–3 × 5000 or 2 × 7500 IE/day) is effective for patients with a medium risk of thrombosis. This form of prophylaxis is to produce a thrombosis reduc-

tion in general surgery from approximately 30% to 5–15% and in trauma surgery from approximately 50% to 25–30%.

18.5.3.2 Low-Molecular-Weight Heparins (LMWHs)

Thanks to their improved pharmacological properties, a reduced incidence of undesirable effects compared to UFH, and their antithrombotic efficiency as well as a high practicability, LMWHs provide advantages compared to UFH. The low-molecular-weight heparins are not a homogeneous substance group. They feature different antithrombotic efficiencies and dosage recommendations. Low-molecular-weight heparins display a lower risk of heparin-induced thrombocytopenia (HIT) than unfractionated heparins. There are various undesired drug effects with the application of heparin. There are two forms of heparin-induced thrombocytopenia (HIT): heparin-induced thrombocytopenia type I (HIT I) and heparin-induced thrombocytopenia type II (HIT II). The thrombocyte decrease in the case of HIT I is low to medium, temporary in most cases, and clinically irrelevant. It occurs a few days (1–3) after the start of the treatment and only rarely reaches a value of <100,000/μL. With HIT I, an interruption of the heparin treatment is not necessary, as the number of thrombocytes will increase again during the next days, even if the treatment with heparin is continued. HIT II, an immunologically mediated form of thrombocytopenia, is a dangerous complication of the heparin application which may involve venous and/or arterial thromboembolism. With the administration of unfractionated heparin, in approximately 10% of the cases, patients undergoing extensive surgical and/or orthopedic procedures have the risk of antibodies; in up to 2–3%, they suffer the risk of thrombocytopenia (HIT II). When low-molecular-weight heparin is administered, these risks are much lower. With HIT II, the decrease in thrombocytes usually occurs between the 5th and the 14th days, more rarely up to the 21st day after the initial application. The numbers of thrombocytes often drop below 80,000/μL or below 50% of the initial value. Checking the characteristic of the number of thrombocytes, in particular between the 5th and the 21st days of the heparin administration, is recommended. With the long-term use of UFH at a dosage of 15,000–30,000 IE/day, more rarely in the case of LMWH, exceeding 4–6 months, it is known that osteopenia may occur.

18.5.3.3 Danaparoid

Danaparoid is a heparin-free heparinoid that is also extracted from the pig's intestine mucosa and that has an anticoagulatory effect. It is an effective form of the medication-based thromboembolism prophylaxis in situations in which the use of heparins is not permissible or not possible.

18.5.3.4 Fondaparinux

Fondaparinux is a pentasaccharide that is produced syntheti-cally, inhibiting antithrombin-mediated factor Xa. In the elective (hip replacement and knee replacement) and non-elective (hip fracture) high-risk surgery, in clinical studies at a dosage of 2.5 mg/day s.c., fondaparinux has proven to be antithrombotically superior compared to low-molecular-weight heparin. Prophylactic treatment with fondaparinux is started 6 h after the end of the operation. Under the influence of fondaparinux, neither heparin-induced thrombocytopenia (HIT II) was observed, nor a cross-reactivity with plasma of patients with HIT antibodies was proved.

18.5.3.5 Thrombin Inhibitors

In addition to the direct (i.e., effective without mediation by antithrombin) thrombin inhibitor hirudin, low-molecular-weight, also directly acting thrombin inhibitors are tested in clinical studies (e.g., melagatran/ximelagatran). They can also be administered orally. During hirudin treatment (2 × 15 mg/day s.c.), patients with an elective hip replace-ment showed substantially less deep vein thrombosis with a comparable risk of bleeding than under the influence of UFH or LMWH. Due to the missing cross-reaction with HIT type II antibodies, hirudin is used in particular for the medication-based thromboembolism prophylaxis for patients with HIT II.

Oral anticoagulants (vitamin K antagonists—couma-rins), warfarin, and other vitamin K antagonists of the cou-marin type are effective means for the perioperative prophylaxis of venous thromboembolism for patients with a medium or high risk. Due to the required laboratory tests (INR) and the increased risks of bleeding, in Europe, vita-min K antagonists are hardly used perioperatively; how-ever, they are occasionally used for long-term prophylaxis (INR 2.0–3.0). For patients with a low risk of thromboem-bolism, physical measures and measures to quickly mobi-lize the patients again can be considered sufficient. For patients with a medium risk and, in particular, with a high risk of thromboses, in addition to the physical measures and measures to quickly mobilize the patients, a medica-tion-based thromboprophylaxis is indicated. In contrast to North America, in Europe, the medication-based thrombo-embolism prophylaxis is usually started perioperatively or as soon as possible after a trauma. Fondaparinux is gener-ally only administered postoperatively. Today, patients are often discharged early from inpatient care after operations or after a trauma. If there are relevant risk factors of venous thromboembolism that are still remaining after the hospital discharge, a post-hospital prophylaxis should be taken into consideration. For patients with a total hip endoprosthesis and hip fracture and following extensive operation of malignant tumors in the field of abdominal surgery, clinical studies have shown the benefit of a 4–5-week medication-based thromboembolism prophylaxis, so that prophylactic treatment that has been started in the hospital should also be continued as outpatient treatment on a case-by-case basis. The doctor responsible for further treatment has to be informed about the necessity of the prophylactic treatment. The present results of the clinical studies are not sufficient yet to allow for a generally binding recommendation regarding the duration of the medication-based thrombo-embolism prophylaxis. This duration depends on additional dispositional risk factors, the surgical trauma, and the degree of immobility.

References

1. Nordstrom M, Lindblad B, Bergqvist D, et al. A prospective study of the incidence of deep-vein thrombosis within a defined urban population. J Intern Med. 1992;232:155–60.
2. Bono CM, Watters WC, Heggeness MH, et al. Antithrombotic therapies in spinal surgeries. Evidence-based clinical guidelines for multidisciplinary spine care. Spine J. 2009;9:1046–51.
3. Agnelli G. Prevention of venous thromboembolism in surgeries patients. Circualtion. 2004;110(24 Suppl 1):4–12.
4. Faraoni D, Ferrandis R, Geerts W, et al. European guidelines on perioperative venous thromboembolism prophylaxis. Eur J Anaesthesiol. 2017;34:1–6.
5. Goldhaber SZ. Pulmonary thromboembolism. In: Kasper DL, Braunwald E, Fauci AS, et al., editors. Harrison's principles of internal medicine (16th ed.). New York, NY: McGraw-Hill; 2005. p. 1561–5.
6. Eriksson BI, Wille-Jorgensen P, Kalebo P, et al. A comparison of recombinant hirudin with a low molecular weight heparin to pre-vent thromboembolic complications after total hip replacement. N Engl J Med. 1997;337:1329–35.
7. Cohen AT, Tapson VF, Bergmann JF, et al. Venous thrombo-embolism risk and prophylaxis in the acute hospital care setting (ENDORSE study): a multinational cross-sectional study. Lancet. 2008;371:387–94.
8. Anderson FA Jr, Wheeler HB, Goldberg RJ, et al. A population-based perspective of the hospital incidence and case-fatality rates of deep vein thrombosis and pulmonary embolism. The Worcester DVT Study. Arch Intern Med. 1991;151:933–8.
9. Brambilla S, Ruosi C, La Maida GA, et al. Prevention of venous thromboembolism in spinal surgery. Euro Spine J. 2004;13:1–8.
10. Knudson MM, Collins JA, Goodman SB, et al. Thromboembolism following multiple trauma. J Trauma. 1992;32:2–11.
11. Cohen AT, Agnelli G, Anderson FA, et al. Venous thromboembo-lism (VTE) in Europe. The number of VTE events and associated morbidity and mortality. Thromb Haemost. 2007;98(4):756–64.
12. Fang MC, Maselli J, Lurie JD, et al. Use and outcomes of venous thromboembolism prophylaxis after spinal fusion surgery. J Thromb Haemost. 2011;9:1318–25.
13. Gerlach R, et al. Postoperative nachroparin administration for prophylaxis of thromboembolic events is not associated with an increased risk of hemorrhage after spinal surgery. Eur Spine J. 2004;13:9–13.
14. Glynn RJ, Ridker PM, Goldhaber SZ, et al. Effects of random allocation to vitamin E supplementation on the occurrence of venous thromboembolism: report from the Women's Health Study. Circulation. 2007;116:1497–503.

15. Scottish Intercollegiate Guidelines Network (SIGN). Prophylaxis of venous thromboembolism. A national clinical guideline (SIGN Pub No. 62). Edinburgh: SIGN; 2002.

16. Lee HM, et al. Deep vein thrombosis after major spinal surgery: incidence in an East Asian population. Spine. 2000;25:1827–30.

17. Clagett GP, Anderson FA, Levine MN, Salzman EW, Wheeler HB. Prevention of venous thromboembolism. Chest. 1992;102(4 Suppl):391–407.

18. Sonaglia F, Rossi R, Agnelli G. End points in studies on the prevention of deep vein thrombosis. Semin Thromb Hemost. 2001;27:41–6.

19. International Consensus. Int Angiol. 2001;16:3–38.

20. Epstein NE. A review of the risk and benefits of differing prophylaxis regimens for the treatment of deep venous thrombosis and pulmonary embolism in neurosurgery. Surg Neurol. 2005;64:295–301.

21. Agnelli G, Mancini GB, Biagini D. The rationale for long-term prophylaxis of venous thromboembolism. Orthopedics. 2000;23(Suppl 6):643–6.

22. Geerts WH, Bergqvist D, Pineo GF, et al. Prevention of venous thromboembolism: American College of Chest Physicians evidence-based clinical practice guidelines (8th edition). Chest. 2008;133(6 Suppl):381S–453S.

23. Naess IA, Christiansen SC, Romundstad P, Cannegieter SC, Rosendaal FR, Hammerstrom J. Incidence and mortality of venous thrombosis: a population-based study. J Thromb Haemost. 2007;5(4):692–9.

24. Llau JV. Thrombembolism in orthopedic surgery. London: Springer; 2013.

25. Alban S. Pharmakologie der Heparine und der direkten Anti- koagulanzien. Haematologie. 2008;5:400–17.

Minimizing Human Error in Spinal Surgery

Uwe Vieweg and Robert Morrison

19.1 Introduction and Core Messages

The complication minimization or complication treat-ment can consist in the improve-ment of the treatment options, the improvement of the complication manage-ment, the improvement of the abilities, to remedy the complications, and the minimization of er-rors. The human-medical error represents an inappropriate treat-ment, administered for instance, not carefully, not cor-rectly, not in a timely manner. It can cover all areas of physician-related and medical activity with regard to prophylaxis, diagnosis, selection of the pla. We have different options to minimise errors (improvements of organization-al measures, management and policy (CIRS, checklists), technical competence and techni-cal skills "technical skills" (advanced training pro-grams, anatomical preparation training, simulation training on the model, live tissue training) and social competences "non-technical skills". These "non-tech-nical skills" are communication, appropriate at-ten-tion, leadership, decision-making and cooperation.

19.2 Complications and Medical Errors [1–4]

Complications could occur in any medical branch or any therapy. These complications are observed and perceived by doctors and patients in altogether different manner.

U. Vieweg
Department of Conservative and Surgical Spine Therapy with Interdisciplinary Spinal Deformities Centre and Rummelsberg Sectional Center, Hospital Rummelsberg, Schwarzenbruck, Germany
e-mail: uwe.vieweg@sana.de

R. Morrison (✉)
Spine & Scoliosis Center, Asklepios Klinik, Bad Abbach, Germany

Patients can view partial complications as an error. Doctors may similarly also interpret severe complications as a mis-take. However, while a complication cannot immediately be deemed a treatment error, a complication can result from an error. Complication is an undesirable consequence of a disease or an accident, or a therapy that is not part of the illness. Often this complication necessitates an additional or prolonged therapy. On the other hand, an error does not necessarily result in a complication. A complication based on an error would be termed an unforeseen occurrence (incident) (see Fig. 19.1). A critical incident is thus an error or event which could lead to an adverse event. The follow-ing example illustrates a so-called critical incident: A patient has a penicillin energy that is known to him. The anamnese does not address the history of the allergy, and therefore the patient's file does not contain a warning. A complication is thus also an adverse event. An adverse event is a harmful event that occurs as a result of the treat-ment rather than as a result of the disease itself. It is either avoidable (error) or unavoidable (classic complication). Subcategorizing the causes of a complication is important for later presenting and impacting the notion of holistic safety in medicine in general and particularly in the operat-ing room. The causes of a complication can be summarized as follows:

1. Accompanying symptoms (side effects) of a disease that cannot be avoided even in the best-case scenario
2. Adverse events or accompanying symptoms of therapy which also cannot always be circumvented (e.g. allergic skin reaction after the administration of antibiotics where the allergy was not known)
3. Consequences of inadequate diagnosis or therapy and related medical treatment problems (e.g. antibiotic administration in case of known allergy with resulting allergic skin reaction, adverse event)

The International Classification for Patient Safety describes five stages with or without an incident for the patient: normal functioning, event without risk, incident

© Springer-Verlag GmbH Germany 2023
U. Vieweg, F. Grochulla (eds.), *Manual of Spine Surgery*, https://doi.org/10.1007/978-3-662-64062-3_19

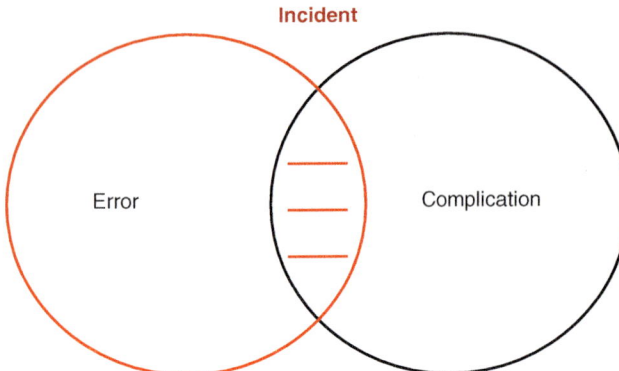

Fig. 19.1 Incident as an error-based complication

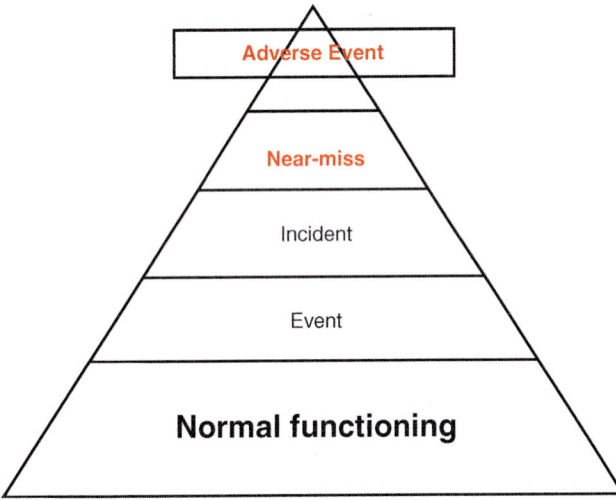

Fig. 19.2 Presentation of events and incidents according to the International Classification for Patient Safety

with risk, incident with no negative outcome (near miss) and incident with negative outcome (adverse event) (see Fig. 19.2). Patient safety is then defined as the absence of negative events. The complication minimization or complication treatment can consist in the improvement of the treatment options; the improvement of the complication management; the improvement of the abilities, to remedy the complications; and the minimization of errors. The human medical error represents an inappropriate treatment, administered, for instance, not carefully, not correctly and not in a timely manner. It can cover all areas of physician-related and medical activity with regard to prophylaxis, diagnosis, selection of the planning procedure, information and education and therapy and follow-up. The general error, on the contrary, can be defined as a deviation from an optimal or normalized state or method in a system determined in terms of its functions, or as a feature value accord-

ing to the German Institute for Standardization, which does not meet the predetermined requirements. These two definitions are important, because they are applied in the field of safety and/or in the industrial sector in general. The knowledge of the definitions of a complication and of a medical error opens the doors to the safety sciences. The experiences of the safety sciences contribute to the aerospace industry, to the industrial sector, but also to the energy industry, for example, in a nuclear power plant and increasingly also in medicine. In aviation, in particular, security sciences have clearly contributed to an error minimization. The number of deaths in aviation is estimated between 800 and 1200, but in medicine, for example, in the USA, it is possible to reckon with 100,000–200,000 deaths a year. The treatment must not harm the patients—this ancient principle of medical and nursing care has been redefined in the last 30 years under the heading of patient safety. The report of the Institute of Medicine (IOM), "To Err Is Human" [3], triggered an intensive debate worldwide about patient safety. Depending on the country and the study, up to 10% of all patients suffer from a "preventable adverse event" during the treatment. With these figures, it seems incomprehensible why the knowledge provided by the safety sciences in medicine is not implemented to the same extent as in aviation. In particular, this also takes into account the interrelationships between aviation and medicine, such as high-tech workplace, high-level teamwork, a high degree of physical and psychological stress, a frequently changing work intensity, the processing of high quantities of information and the confrontation with compelling decisions. Minor errors, whether in aviation or in medicine, can lead to fatal consequences for humans. There are many parallels between physicians and pilots. They belong to professions characterized by status consciousness and professional pride. The differences between aviation and medicine, however, explain why it is more likely to take into account the knowledge gained from the safety sciences in the aviation safety sciences. In aviation, the pilot himself or herself is affected by a particular fault. In aviation, the sum of money involved runs into millions, but if one were to take into account the entire company, the costs involved run into billions. An error that leads to a corresponding air crash becomes global headlines, and this puts pressure on the company. In the medical branch, mistakes always happen at the level of the individual patient. As these errors often occur in everyday medical practice, they are less likely to attract attention due to the complexity of the medical event, and mistakes can usually be covered up. Medical professionals perceive the complication as an adverse event. The advancement and development of the different therapy methods often aim at a minimization of complications. However, from the perspective of the medical practitioners, and more so from that of the patients, mistakes should not occur. A zero tolerance for errors seems to underlie any error denial. However, one must first be aware that it is human to err. This human potential for error is the basis for advancing the cause of humanity (Errare humanum est). This finding is the foundational motivation that fosters the science of patient safety. The physician is human and, therefore in his actions, is capable of committing errors. Human factors are a major cause of incidents through which patients are harmed. They are key to patient safety [5]. Mistakes may be covered up to protect personal reputation, owing to the threat of so-called medical malpractice litigations, because of the high expectations of the patients and the society, because of possible disciplinary procedures by employers and the fear of job loss. A bad culture of failures in the hospital could also be a reason for this. Mistakes are not deliberately concealed or hushed up by doctors with bad intent. This does not do justice to the medical profession. Already in the choice of a place of study, during study and as a young or experienced doctor, the professional ethos of "helping patients – curing patients – not harming patients" is all-pervasive. This complex could also be called: "A doctor does not make a mistake". Thus, there is likely to be a psychological barrier for confessing to mistakes. Perhaps this is also one of the reasons why the findings of the safety sciences are only slowly entering the daily clinical routine. Georg Ernst Stahl (1660–1734), the personal physician of Friedrich Wilhelm I, wrote several hundred years ago "It is not a mistake to make a mistake once, but it goes against the ethos of medical practice not to admit to or recognize one's own mistake, in order to make it possible to draw the necessary lessons for later". The classical as well as especially the modern principles of ethical action in medicine (Georgetown Mantra), such as the patient's right to self-determination (respect for autonomy), social justice (justice) and not least the well-being of the patient (benefice), and the principle of damage avoidance (non-maleficence) must necessarily motivate any medical practitioner to apply the knowledge of the safety sciences in medicine. Risk awareness and error prevention require the willingness and the ability to talk about risks and mistakes. Theoretical knowledge on this topic makes this easier. Theoretically, the concept of error is defined from different perspectives for all areas of our lives. Different models and terms define and describe errors, causes of errors or frequency of errors for all areas of everyday life.

19.3 Causes of Error [2, 4, 6, 7]

In the beginning, error research was mainly concerned with machines and devices, in order to minimize technical errors. This had practical consequences in the different industrial production processes. As a medical doctor, you may be confronted with the term "error rate" when collaborating with the implant manufacturer's industry. In the industry, it is possible to define this rate and even set the target of "zero error rate". However, since the overall work process is ultimately determined by humans, error research is now increasingly human-centred. Error research is therefore concerned with human beings in order to improve the error behaviour of the overall systems. This has been summarized under the human factors category. The procedures for general error research can also be used in medicine as follows:

1. Product quality—Is the operation successful?
2. Structural quality—Is the clinic modern and does the staff undergo regular training?
3. Process quality—Are operations management, as well as admission and release planned?
4. Expertise—Does the staff have the necessary knowledge?
5. Competence in methodology—Does the staff have specialized knowledge?

During the course of the error analysis, it is possible to notice that often several errors precede the occurrence of a serious incident. In this context, the so-called reason model [5, 8] offers a vivid representation of possible errors in the overall system, which are causally related to the environment (management, training, environment, workplace environment, individual, etc.) (see Fig. 19.3). A large number of studies show that a bad working environment has the same effect for errors as a turbocharger. There are various error possibilities with respect to the physician, for example, overload, training deficits, disease, incorrect indication, incorrect selection of a treatment method and a bad working environment. Psychological factors include lack of concentration, inability to respond, careless decisions, lightness, exuberance, stress, lack of knowledge and abilities and routine. Physical causes of defects include overload, fatigue, shock, injuries, illness including pain and influence of intoxicating or inhibiting factors (alcoholism, drug abuse, medication). Over 5 years, high-risk workplaces were analysed: the cockpit, the operating room and the control room of a nuclear reactor with regard to organization, behaviour, operating climate and communication style. The relationship between the workload and the type and amount of communication was established. When do the teams talk how much, and how

Fig. 19.3 Error chain based on reason, also Swiss Cheese Model [9]

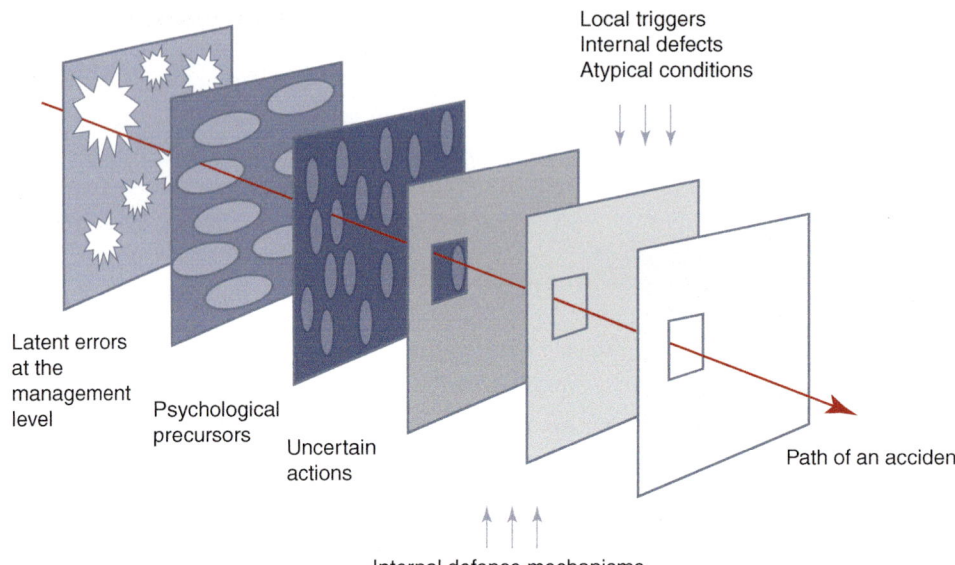

Local triggers
Internal defects
Atypical conditions

Latent errors at the management level

Psychological precursors

Uncertain actions

Internal defence mechanisms

Path of an accident

Table 19.1 Summary of important errors with keyword

"The dirty dozen" according to Gordon Dupont
– Lack of communication
– Lack of teamwork
– Pressure of social norms
– Overconfidence
– Lack of knowledge
– Lack of attention
– Lack of resources
– Distraction
– Lack of assertiveness
– Exhaustion
– Stress

does it impact on the tasks to be fulfilled? The results were summarized in the book *The Better the Team, the Safer the World*, which contains 20 concrete recommendations for dealing with difficult situations. Communication deficiencies are crucial factors in the emergence of faults in high-risk areas, such as control centres for nuclear reactors, cockpit and the operating room. For example, exhausted teams who know each other are better off than rested teams who do not know each other. Also hierarchy and fear of regression often prevent errors from being identified and named and are thus a cause of error. Gordon Dupont (Transport Canada) investigated 800 incidents in civilian and military aviation and identified the 12 most common causes of mistakes, incidents and accidents in aircraft maintenance. Using the catchphrase "the dirty dozen", he summarized the main causes of errors (ranging from lack of communication to distraction) (see Table 19.1). By knowing the main causes of errors, the so-called crisis resource management (CRM) in medicine is therefore aimed at improving patient safety; avoiding inci-

dents and complications (CRISIS) by using devices, methods and persons including oneself (resources); and taking cognitive, action-based and emotional influencing factors into account in crisis and routine management.

19.4 Error Minimizing

Error minimization is, in principle, possible using different approaches (see Table 19.2). On the one hand, the management must define the general conditions at the organizational level. Establishing a CIR system (CIRS) and working with checklists are two examples of how to influence the error rate through the management. But even the direct and indirect political influence forms a part of that. The patient safety alliance or the WHO-supported operation checklist must be mentioned. On the other hand, in medicine, the human being, the physician and thus the human factors occupy centre stage. The professionalism of a physician, meaning how well he is perceived as a physician by colleagues, but, of course, primarily by patients, is, however, dependent on his professional competence and his essential social competence. First, however, we judge a physician according to his technical and theoretical skills (so-called technical skills). It must be assumed that the better the technical and theoretical abilities of a physician, the lower the error rate. The "technical skills" can be learned through study, through advanced and further training. Modern concepts (advanced training concepts of the companies, training sessions carried out on anatomical preparation, live tissue training, simulation training on special models) help to raise the technical and professional skills to an even higher level. However, non-technical skills may have a much greater impact on error minimization.

Table 19.2 Overview of error minimization approaches

- Organizational measures, management and policy (CIRS, checklists, action alliance of patient safety)
- Technical competence and technical skills "technical skills" (advanced training programmes, anatomical preparation training, simulation training on the model, live tissue training)
- Social competence "non-technical skills"

Table 19.3 Summary of components of social competence (non-technical skills)

- Communication
- Leadership
- Situational attention
- Resolute decision-making
- Cooperation

These "non-technical skills" are communication, appropriate attention, leadership, decision-making and cooperation (see Table 19.3).

19.5 Organizational Framework Conditions, Management and Politics

19.5.1 Introduction of Preliminary and Follow-Up Discussions in the Operating Room

Conducting preliminary and follow-up discussions regarding an invasive surgery is one of the key pillars of patient safety in the operating room. The contents are based on the so-called WHO checklist. The patient is identified, for example, by the surgeon. The patient identifies the first and the last name, the date of birth, the location of the intervention and the type of intervention, and then the files and the pictures are compared, and any inconsistency must be clarified immediately. Secondly, the site of intervention is also marked by the surgeon or even outside the operating room when the patient is awake, again by comparing with the files and the patient again shows the location where the operation needs to be performed; the procedure is marked with a non-erasable pen, here, too; any inconsistency is clarified immediately. Thirdly, in the operating room, the assignment to the correct operating room is ensured, immediately preceding the anaesthesia, the patient's name is also again checked, type of surgery and site markings are checked, a room check is carried out and no anaesthesia is performed without the marking. And fourthly, the operation team checks the identification of the patient, the type of intervention and the appropriate imaging using the checklist. This is documented accordingly. The preliminary and follow-up discussions not only improve patient safety but also have a significant positive impact on the working environment.

19.5.2 Working with Checklists

Working with checklists offers an error-minimizing option. The checklists (also SOPs—standard operating procedures) originated in US aviation sector [10]. The field of anaesthesia has been using this checklist for more than 40 years [11]. The use of SOPs can significantly reduce mortality and morbidity. In clinical practice, these play a major role, for example, as surgical slip for surgical preparation, WHO checklists, surgical instrumentation lists, checklist of patient records, etc. The check-in and check-out can be carried out according to the recommendations of the WHO on the basis of the template/form and, preferably, using the hospital information system (HIS), whereby in the WHO checklist, "time out" and "sign out" play a big role. Time out, for instance, requires that the patient is clearly identified by name and date of birth, that the location of the operation is correctly marked or that the entire operating team is presented with name and function, etc.; sign out requires asking if the planned procedure was performed or the operation was fully documented, or if the instruments, compresses and needles were counted.

19.5.3 Introduction and Maintenance of a Critical Incident Reporting System (CIRS)

This is the beauty of a mistake: you do not have to make it twice (Thomas Alva Edison). If you make a mistake, you can only do three things (Paul Bryant): (1) admit it, (2) learn from it and (3) do not repeat it. These three points are ultimately practical in a CIRS. The establishment of a Critical Incident Reporting System (CIRS) is an important pillar for error detection and minimization in hospitals. The purpose of such an information system is to detect errors before they happen, namely, when there has been a "near-miss event". Such systems are long established in other industrial sectors [12, 13]. These are learning systems, which only work through the continuous, active cooperation of the employees, so as to ensure that potential sources of error are recognized and corrected. These "near-miss events" are reported anonymously to a specialized team, which processes the cases and analyses them in order to then identify effective ways to minimize the risk. Thus, events are diagnosed to avoid errors in the overall system. Here, a so-called learning without damage is possible, since only events are reported, in which no one has suffered any damage. This also explains the fact that a functioning CIRS is an important building block but can only function as a component of an integrative risk management (IRM). Thus, in the overall system, all cases can be analysed and processed accordingly. It is important to point out to the employees that they have the possibility to report errors anonymously without the fear of sanctions. It is important to realize that it is not a question of error, for an error is not caused intentionally, but is an expression of various latent problems contained in the system. But only if the employees are also ready to participate in a certain "error culture", it will be possible to successfully establish a CIRS in the hospital. No industrial sector that strives for high operational safety relinquishes the advantages of an incident reporting system. The most important criteria for a functioning operation are the following:

- Fullest support from the management and the will to implement
- Anonymity and guaranteed freedom from sanctions
- Notifications as free text
- Interdisciplinary analysis and processing of cases
- Prompt feedback to employees
  A CIRS is conducted as follows:
- Identifying (anomic reporting of "near-miss events")
- Analysing (what causes?)
- Evaluating
- Managing (corrective and preventive actions)
- Reporting (evaluating and deriving strategies)

A CIRS is part of an IRM, which also includes the complaints management.

19.6 Improvement of Non-technical Skills

Many airlines are interested in the personnel selection for the personality profile of their future personnel in the cockpit. In addition to cognitive and psychological criteria, complex requirements on personality are important. Personality-oriented behavioural analysis was developed in order to identify these characteristics. It is obvious that these selection criteria are also applicable in medicine. Unfortunately, however, some of the social skills are still not chosen as a selection criterion for medical studies. In the "Medical Studies (2020)" Master Plan, a project of the Union and the German political party SPD, these selection criteria had already been agreed upon in the 2013 Coalition Treaty. While the admission to universities is still dependent on the grade secured in the Abitur, or the school leaving examination, and is thus an important selection criterion, universities must, however, add on at least two new criteria (from such options as social and communicative skills, willingness to perform, previous work in a medical profession and voluntary commitment). In the aviation sector, there has been a long-standing demand that executives and flying and highly qualified technical personnel receive further and advanced training in the field of "human factors". The crew (cockpit) resource management (CRM) refer to NASA's workshop in 1979 after the catastrophic crash of Tenerife (1977) with a crash of Boeing 737-40 British Midland and the fall of the Boing 737-40 of the British Midland (1969). CRM training courses have been a prerequisite for FAA (USA) and JAA (Europe) pilots since these accidents. These courses address these findings with a view to increasing the awareness of the staff, with the following focus: increasing the professionalism of the individual by training the non-technical skills and improving the corporate and security culture. Since the situation in the team with regard to the workload and with regard to routine and habit as well as other organizational structures and as new employees are added to the team, this team training becomes necessary at regular intervals. An introduction of checklists and reliable work without an employee motivation and training makes no sense or can only be realized with an enormous organizational effort or with punished reprisals. Routine and increasing workload means updating the team training. The implementation is carried out in a one to three active team resource management courses that include all those involved in the process (surgeons, anaesthesiologists, surgical nurses), based on the aviation courses. Teamwork and leadership are an important part of team training. Now these courses are being offered by different providers in different formats. Table 4 presents three different courses (see Table 4).

References

1. Badke-Schaub P, Hofinger G, Lauche K. Human Factors. Psychologie sicheren Handelns in Risikobranchen. 2nd ed. Heidelberg: Springer; 2012.
2. Holzner E, Thomeczek C. Patientensicherheit. Wien: Facultas AG; 2005.
3. Kohn L, Corrigan JM, Donaldson MS; Committee on Quality of Health Care in America. Institute of Medicine. To err is human, building a safer health system. Washington DC: National Academy Press; 2001.
4. Leape LL. Error in medicine. JAMA. 1994;272:1851–7.
5. Reason J. Human error. Cambridge: Cambridge University Press; 1990.
6. Bogner MS. Human error in medicine. Hillsdale, NJ: Lawrence Erlbaum Associates; 1994. 411 pp.
7. Rall M, Dieckmann P, Stricker E; The Working Group Incident Reporting of the German Anesthesia Society DGAI and BDA. Das Patientensicherheits-Optimierungs-System PaSOS [Patient safety optimizing system PaSOS]. Anaesthesiol Intensivmed. 2006, 47:S20–S24.
8. Schmitt T. The better the team, the safer the world. Ladenburg: Gottlieb Daimler und Karl-Benz-Stiftung; 2007.

9. Pierre St M, Hofinger G, Buerschaper C. Notfallmanagement. Human Factors in der Akutmedizin. 2nd ed. Heidelberg: Springer; 2011.

10. Flanagan JC. The critical incident technique. Psychol Bull. 1954;51:327–58.

11. Cooper JB, et al. Preventable anesthesia mishaps. A study of human factors. Anesthesiology. 1978;49:399–406.

12. Möllemann A, et al. Clinical risk management. Implementation of an anonymous error registration system in the anesthesia department of a university hospital. Der Anaesthesist. 2005;54:377–84.

13. Rall M, Martin J, Geldner G, et al. Charakteristika effektiver Incident- Reporting-Systeme zur Erhöhung der Patientensicherheit [Characteristics of effective incident-reporting-systems for the increase of patient safety]. Anaesthesiol Intensivmed. 2006;47:S9–19.

Sagittal Balance Concept: Radiological Measurement Parameters

20

Theophilo Asfora Lins, Guilherme Augusto Foizer, and Wilson T. Asfora

20.1 Introduction and Core Messages

Over the last decades, there has been an increase in concern over quality of life issues, especially in the elderly patient. Spinal diseases are among the main factors that cause loss in quality of life in the elderly population because these diseases not only restrict independent mobility but also contribute to other mechanical, neurological, or chronic pain limitations [1]. In the large group of spinal diseases, deformities and degeneration with loss of sagittal balance are very prevalent, and the impact on daily activities is tremendous [2, 3]. In addition, studies have shown that the postoperative incidence of sagittal spinal imbalance, also known as flat back deformity, has increased [4–7], thus bringing greater significance to a fuller understanding of this theme in an attempt to mitigate or avoid unfavorable postoperative outcomes. To study conditions which involve deformities of the spine, it is necessary to establish what is considered "standard" for sagittal balance. Many authors have defined the ranges of spinopelvic parameters for specific populations. However, they stressed the fact that these anthropometrical parameters were very scattered as a result of human diversity, and therefore, it seemed difficult to define what is normal in the upright posture for a specific subject [1, 8]. Thus, it is believed that analyzing multiple parameters may lead to more consistently interpretable data. Many factors such as age, gender, weight, and morphology of the pelvis can cause variation of spinal and pelvic parameters, which in turn influences the ability to more accurately define what is an acceptable normal biometric standard for the aging spine.

20.2 Sagittal Balance

The spinal column consists of four main curves: cervical lordosis (CL), thoracic kyphosis (TK), lumbar lordosis (LL), and sacral kyphosis (SK). Between these curves, there are transition areas that may present some characteristics of both curves. These curvatures have mechanical functions to absorb loads applied to the spine in addition to allowing better utilization of muscle function, enhancing the movement through lever arms, and seeking a better erect posture [8], while always protecting the neurological structures. Moreover, due to an intimate relationship between the spine and the pelvis, upright posture also depends on spinopelvic relations and features that play a key role in this context. For a thorough evaluation of the spine, a lateral panoramic radiograph must be done using a vertical 30 × 90-cm film, maintaining a distance between the subject and the radiographic source, usually 250 cm. The subject should stand in a comfortable position with knees fully extended and arms, resting on supports, flexed forward to 45°. The radiograph is centered on the 12th thoracic vertebra and imaging taken during inhalation [8–14]. The most important sagittal spinal radiographic parameters for clinical and surgical practices are illustrated in Fig. 20.1.

Thoracic kyphosis (TK): This is an angle measured between the upper endplate of T4 and lower endplate of T12.

T. A. Lins (✉)
Clínica Phitris, São Paulo, Brazil

Departamento de Ortopedia e Traumatologia, Escola Paulista de Medicina - UNIFESP, São Paulo, Brazil
e-mail: theoasfora@gmail.com

G. A. Foizer
Department of Orthopedic Surgery, Unicamp, Campinas, Brazil

Spine Surgery at Hospital Adventista de São Paulo, São Paulo, Brazil

W. T. Asfora
Department of Neurosurgery, Sanford School of Medicine, Sanford Neurosurgery and Spine, University of South Dakota, Sioux Falls, SD, USA

© Springer-Verlag GmbH Germany 2023
U. Vieweg, F. Grochulla (eds.), *Manual of Spine Surgery*, https://doi.org/10.1007/978-3-662-64062-3_20

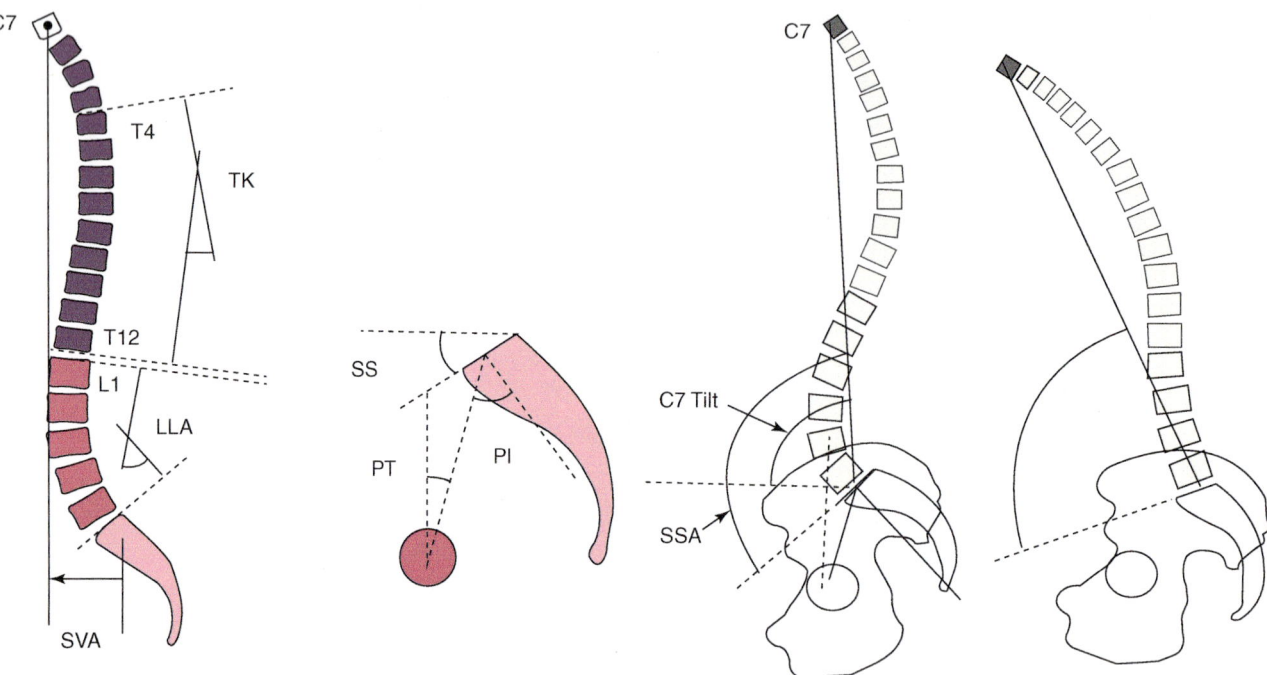

Fig. 20.1 Sagittal spinal radiologic parameters (original figure from Todd et al. [15]. Image reproduced with permission of the publisher)

Fig. 20.2 Positioning angles of C7; in case of severe kyphosis (*right*), SSA decreases strongly (original figure from Roussouly et al. [29]. Image reproduced with permission of the publisher)

Although there is great variation, normal values usually range between 20° and 50° [10, 13, 16, 17].

Lumbar lordosis (LL): This angle is formed between the upper endplate of L1 and the upper endplate of S1. It presents a wide variation, with values ranging from 30° to 79° in normal individuals. The lumbar lordosis is greatly influenced by the pelvic incidence (PI). Any increase in the pelvic incidence leads to increase of lumbar lordosis [3, 11, 13]. An adequate LL for the sagittal balance presents an estimated value of 80% of the sacral slope [17].

Sagittal vertical axis (SVA): This is used to document the location of the head with respect to the normal center of gravity (offset of the head from the sacral promontory). This is identified by a plumb line dropped from the center of the body of C7 to the sacral endplate. According to the Scoliosis Research Society guidance, sagittal balance occurs when the SVA lies within ±2 cm of the sacral promontory. There is controversy regarding the accuracy of the SVA as a measure of sagittal spine balance due to small changes in the position of lower extremity joints and segmental spine movement during radiographic imaging [18]. The C7 plumb line and center of gravity are not identical. Usually the center of gravity is located in front of the C7 plumb line and slightly behind the hip joints [19].

Spino-sacral angle (SSA): This is an angle formed between a line from the center of the C7 vertebra to the center of the vertebra of S1 and a horizontal line crossing the upper endplate of S1. It represents the overall orientation of the spine in the sagittal plane and the evaluation of how the

spinopelvic compensation is to keep C7 centered over the sacrum [13, 17, 20]. This is an angle that quantifies the global kyphosis of the whole spine. In a well-balanced spine, SSA remains proportional to sacral slope. In case of kyphosis, or loss of lumbar lordosis, SSA decreases. In severe kyphosis, SSA decreases strongly. These relations may provide a guide to evaluate the need of correction for the kyphosis. This parameter carries the advantage of being an angular measurement which avoids the error inherent in measuring offsets in noncalibrated radiographs (Fig. 20.2)

20.3 Anteroposterior Listhesis

It measures the linear displacement of one vertebra relative to another [17]. This is the distance in millimeters between the vertical line of the posterior wall of the upper vertebral body and the vertical line of the posterior wall of the inferior vertebral body.

20.4 Pelvic Parameters

Pelvic tilt (PT): The angle between the vertical and the line through the midpoint of the upper sacral endplate to the femoral head axis demonstrates the spatial orientation of the pelvis. Higher values represent retroversion of the pelvis or lower values of anteversion.

Sacral slope (SS): This is defined as the angle between the horizontal and the upper sacral endplates. A vertical sacrum is described by a low value and a horizontal sacrum by a high value.

Pelvic incidence (PI): This is defined as the angle between the perpendicular to the upper sacral endplates at its midpoint and the line connecting this point to the femoral head axis [11].

20.5   Interpretation of the Spinopelvic Parameters

It has recently been shown by different authors that the pelvic morphology can significantly influence the spinopelvic balance in normal and pathological conditions [21–23]. The ultimate goal of the spinopelvic balance is to maintain the head centered to the pelvis or, more precisely, to the center of gravity of the human body. To understand how this mechanism occurs, it is important to consider that the ideal spinal alignment allows an individual to assume standing posture with minimal muscular energy expenditure. This concept is reflected in the "cone of economy" or "cone of balance" principle conceptualized by Dubousset [24]. Within the center of the cone, the individual may remain in an ergonomically favorable erect position. However, larger deviations in the anterior-posterior or lateral plane will require greater energy use to maintain a standing position. Finally, progression outside of the "stable cone" results in a loss of postural control and the need for external supports. All adaptations of the spinopelvic parameters, therefore, aim to reestablish the sagittal balance. Many conditions may lead to sagittal imbalance. The most common are degenerative changes, such as hypertrophic facet joint arthritis, degenerative disc disease (DDD), bone remodeling, and atrophy of extensor muscles, resulting in a progressive kyphosis of the lumbar spine. There are other presentations such as individuals who had a long fusion for adolescent idiopathic scoliosis with subsequent degeneration distally, individuals with degenerative sagittal imbalance in whom fusions have initially been performed in the distal lumbar spine in a somewhat hypolordotic or kyphotic position with subsequent degeneration of segments above the fusion, and posttraumatic kyphosis and ankylosing spondylitis [25]. When the trunk is tilted anteriorly, the individual uses compensatory mechanisms in order to maintain the spinopelvic balance. The main compensatory mechanism are, from cranial to caudal, cervical hyperlordosis, reduction of thoracic kyphosis, increase of lordosis in the upper lumbar spine, retrolisthesis, retroversion of the pelvis, decrease of sacral slope, extension of the hips and flexion of the knees and ankle extension, as illustrated in Figs. 20.3, 20.4, 20.5. These mechanisms are rarely seen all together, but they are present in different degrees according to indi-

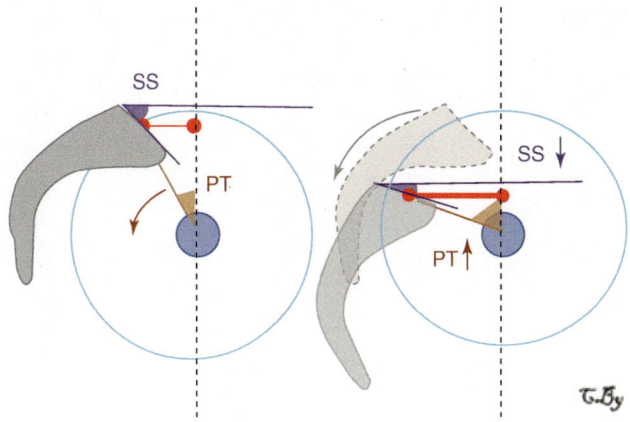

Fig. 20.3 Pelvis back tilt mechanism. Increase of pelvis tilt results in posterior placement of the sacrum related to the coxofemoral heads thus increasing the sacrofemoral distance (red line) (original figure from Barrey et al. [26]. Image reproduced with permission of the publisher)

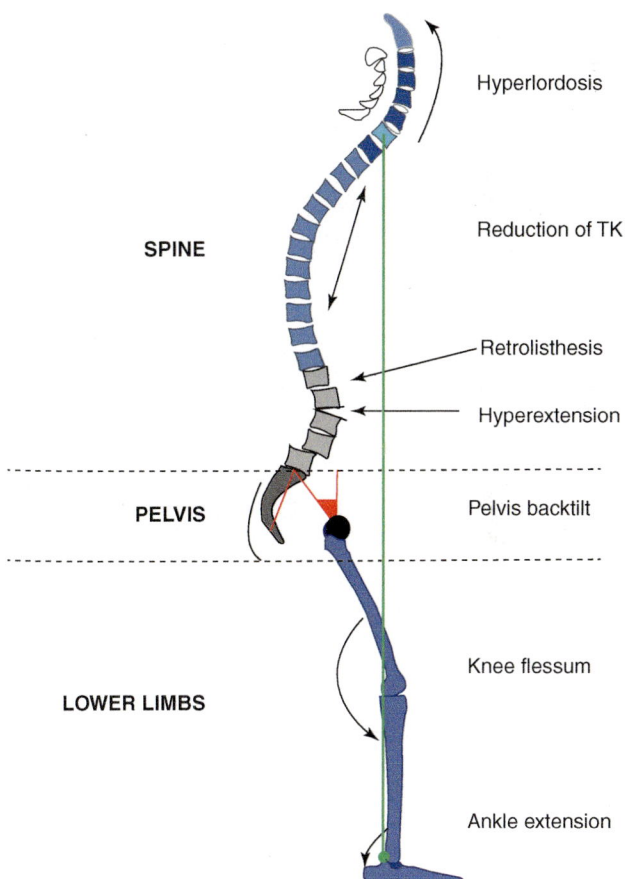

Fig. 20.4 Sagittal imbalance and the different compensatory mechanisms in the spine, pelvis, and lower limb areas (original figure from Barrey et al. [26]. Image reproduced with permission of the publisher)

vidual conditions: musculature status, arthrosis, stiffness of the spine, pain, and severity of the sagittal unbalance. Their basic concept is to extend adjacent segments of the kyphotic spine allowing for compensation of the elevated SVA but

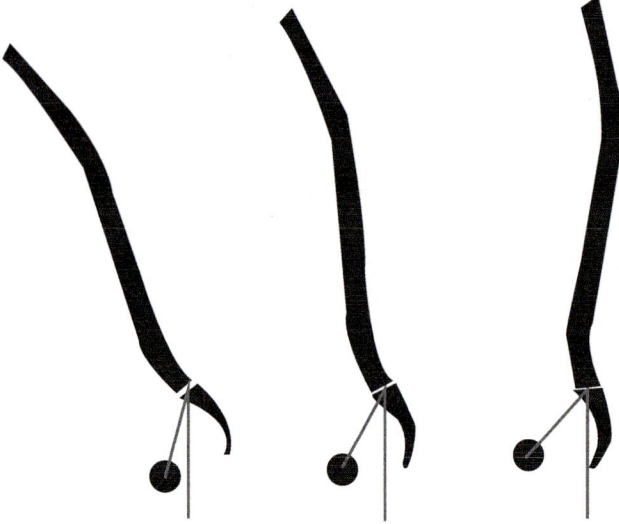

References

1. Garbossa D, et al. Pelvic parameters and global spine balance for spine degenerative disease: the importance of containing for the well being of content. Eur Spine J. 2014;23(Suppl 6):616–27.
2. Ismail AA, et al. Number and type of vertebral deformities: epidemiological characteristics and relation to back pain and height loss. European Vertebral Osteoporosis Study Group. Osteoporos Int. 1999;9(3):206–13.
3. DeWald CJ, Stanley T. Instrumentation-related complications of multilevel fusions for adult spinal deformity patients over age 65: surgical considerations and treatment options in patients with poor bone quality. Spine. 2006;31(19 Suppl):S144–51.
4. Krismer M. Comment to "Sagittal morphology and equilibrium of pelvis and spine" by G. Vaz et al. Eur Spine J. 2002;11(1):88.
5. Kumar MN, Baklanov A, Chopin D. Correlation between sagittal plane changes and adjacent segment degeneration following lumbar spine fusion. Eur Spine J. 2001;10(4):314–9.
6. Duval-Beaupère G, Robain G. Visualization on full spine radiographs of the anatomical connections of the centres of the segmental body mass supported by each vertebra and measured in vivo. Int Orthop. 1987;11(3):261–9.
7. Stagnara P, et al. Reciprocal angulation of vertebral bodies in a sagittal plane: approach to references for the evaluation of kyphosis and lordosis. Spine. 1982;7(4):335–42.
8. Vialle R, Levassor N, Rillardon L, Templier A, Skalli W, Guigui P. Radiographic analysis of the sagittal alignment and balance of the spine in asymptomatic subjects. J Bone Joint Surg Am. 2005;87(2):260–7.
9. Legaye J, Duval-Beaupère G, Hecquet J, Marty C. Pelvic incidence: a fundamental pelvic parameter for three-dimensional regulation of spinal sagittal curves. Eur Spine J. 1998;7(2):99–103.
10. Schwab F, Lafage V, Patel A, Farcy JP. Sagittal plane considerations and the pelvis in the adult patient. Spine. 2009;34:1828–33.
11. Schwab F, Patel A, Ungar B, Farcy JP, Lafage V. Adult spinal deformity-postoperative standing imbalance: how much can you tolerate? An overview of key parameters in assessing alignment and planning corrective surgery. Spine. 2010;35(25):2224–31.
12. Roussouly P, Gollogly S, Berthonnaud E, Dimnet J. Classification of the normal variation in the sagittal alignment of the human lumbar spine and pelvis in the standing position. Spine. 2005;30(3):346–53.
13. Kobayashi T, Atsuta Y, Matsuno T, Takeda N. A longitudinal study of congruent sagittal spinal alignment in an adult cohort. Spine. 2004;29(6):671–6.
14. Cavali PTM, et al. Correlation between symptoms and sagittal alignment parameters in patients with lumbar canal stenosis: a case-control study. Columna. 2012;11(4):302–9.
15. Todd C, Kovac P, Swärd A, et al. Comparison of radiological spinopelvic sagittal parameters in skiers and non-athletes. J Orthop Surg Res. 2015;10:162.
16. Lafage V, Schwab F, Patel A, Hawkinson N, Farcy JP. Pelvic tilt and truncal inclination: two key radiographic parameters in the setting of adults with spinal deformity. Spine. 2009;34(17):E599–606.
17. Pudles E, Defino HLA. A coluna vertebral: conceitos básicos. Porto Alegre: Artmed; 2014. p. 66–73.
18. Van Royen BJ, et al. Accuracy of the sagittal vertical axis in a standing lateral radiograph as a measurement of balance in spinal deformities. Eur Spine J. 1998;7(5):408–12.
19. Bridwell KH. Causes of sagittal spinal imbalance and assessment of the extent of needed correction. Instr Course Lect. 2006;55:567–75.
20. Berthonnaud E, Dimnet J, Roussouly P, Labelle H. Analysis of the sagittal balance of the spine and pelvis using shape and orientation parameters. J Spinal Disord Tech. 2005;18(1):40–7.
21. Jackson RP, Kanemura T, Kawakami N, Hales C. Lumbopelvic lordosis and pelvic balance on repeated standing lateral radiographs of

Fig. 20.5 For a given structural deformity, how pelvic retroversion compensates for spinal deformity. *Left*, no pelvic retroversion and high SVA; *middle*, moderate pelvic retroversion and SVA; *right*, high pelvic retroversion and no SVA [11]

may potentially result in adverse effects. It is believed that these compensatory mechanisms predispose patients to accelerate DDD, thus leading to an increase in preexisting sagittal imbalance [25]. In clinical practice, the angular values obtained in the radiograph help to identify regional angular alterations that may indicate imbalance. However, there is a certain difficulty in evaluating the absolute values of these angles, since the normal range for each of these parameters is wide [10]. For this reason, it is important to consider the harmony of the spinopelvic balance as a whole [27], and not just one of the parameters. In a simplified way, the harmonic balance consists of LL proportional to the PI, while the TK is proportional to the LL. Schwab et al. [11] suggested to maintain values of SVA <50 mm, PT <25°, and correction of LL such that LL = PI ± 9° in order to achieve good postoperative result. These parameters are of utmost importance to reestablish or maintain sagittal balance in spine surgery. Understanding the relationships between spinopelvic parameters allows the calculation of predicted lordosis for those who have altered parameters secondary to disease, which can then influence surgical planning for correction to pre-pathological lordosis:

PI = PT + SS

Rose et al. [30] also developed a formula for predicting the amount of lordosis needed to restore sagittal balance in preoperative planning, which takes into account PI and TK:

LL = PI + TK − 45

It is interesting to note that according to Lafage et al. [16], no parameters in the coronal plane seem to be related to pain and quality of life in the postoperative period. Sagittal balance, however, plays a vital role to achieve the best possible surgical outcome.

adult volunteers and untreated patients with constant low back pain. Spine. 2000;25:575–86.

22. Boulay C, Tardieu C, Hecquet J, et al. Sagittal alignment of spine and pelvis regulated by pelvic incidence: standard values and prediction of lordosis. Eur Spine J. 2006;15:415–22.

23. Roussouly P, Gollogly S, Noseda O, et al. The vertical projection of the sum of the ground reactive forces of a standing patient is not the same as the C7 plumb line: a radiographic study of the sagittal alignment of 153 asymptomatic volunteers. Spine. 2006;31:E320–5.

24. Dubousset J. Three-dimensional analysis of the scoliotic deformity. In: Weinstein SL, editor. Pediatric spine: principles and practice. New York: Raven Press; 1994.

25. Schwab F, Lafage V, Boyce R, et al. Gravity line analysis in adult volunteers: age-related correlation with spinal parameters, pelvic parameters, and foot position. Spine. 2006;31:E959–67.

26. Barrey C, Roussouly P, Le Huec JC, D'Acunzi G, Perrin G. Compensatory mechanisms contributing to keep the sagittal balance of the spine. Eur Spine J. 2013;22(Suppl 6):S834–41.

27. Barrey C, Roussouly P, Perrin G, Le Huec J-C. Sagittal balance disorders in severe degenerative spine. Can we identify the compensatory mechanisms? Eur Spine J. 2011;20(Suppl 5):626–33.

28. Merrill RK, et al. Incidence-lumbar lordosis mismatch: the importance of assessing the entire spine to achieve global sagittal alignment. Global Spine J. 2017;7(6):536–42.

29. Roussouly P, Pinheiro-Franco JL. Biomechanical analysis of the spino-pelvic organization and adaptation in pathology. Eur Spine J. 2011;20:609.

30. Rose PS, Bridwell KH, Lenke LG, Cronen GA, Mulconrey DS, Buchowski JM, Kim YJ. Role of pelvic incidence, thoracic kyphosis, and patient factors on sagittal plane correction following pedicle subtraction osteotomy. Spine (Phila Pa 1976). 2009;34(8):785–91.

Patient Positioning Techniques in Spinal Surgery

21

Sven Y. Vetter and Uwe Vieweg

21.1 Introduction and Core Messages

The objectives of correct patient positioning are to:

- Ensure access to patient´s airway, intravenous lines and monitor devices
- Prevent injury of anatomical structures
- Provide optimal surgical exposure
- Achieve stable positioning of the patient

The centrepiece of an operating theatre is the operating table. An operating table has the purpose to ensure a safe and stable positioning of the patient during surgery. Adjacent to the operating table are ceiling mounts for the anaesthetic and surgical equipment, as well as surgical room lights. In addition a C-arm image intensifier, a microscope or an endoscope tower system may be present in the operating theatre.

An operating table (Fig. 21.1a–f) should be mobile, radiolucent and adjustable in height, inclination and tilt. Special operating tables with different surgical frames and kneeling attachments have been designed over the years to realise adequate patient positioning and decrease intra-abdominal pressure to reduce perioperative bleeding.

S. Y. Vetter
Division of Spinal Surgery at BG Trauma Center Ludwigshafen at Heidelberg University Hospital, Ludwigshafen, Germany
e-mail: sven.vetter@bgu-ludwigshafen.de

U. Vieweg (✉)
Department of Conservative and Surgical Spine Therapy with Interdisciplinary Spinal Deformities Centre and Rummelsberg Sectional Center, Hospital Rummelsberg, Schwarzenbruck, Germany
e-mail: uwe.vieweg@sana.de

21.2 Factors Influencing Blood Loss During Positioning

The Batson venous plexus plays an important role with regard to blood loss during spinal surgery. The Batson plexus consists of three parts:

- An internal venous system
- An external venous system
- A complex network of connecting or anastomotic veins [1, 2]

The internal venous system (anterior internal veins, posterior internal veins, anastomotic veins) represents a continuous venous pathway from the sacrococcygeal region to the base of the skull [3]. The longitudinally travelling veins lie anterior to the vertebral bodies, on the outer aspect of the lamina and on the outer aspect of the transverse process. There is an extensive anastomotic system of veins connecting the internal and the external vertebral system and connecting both parts of the vertebral venous system to the systematic vena cava circulation. These anatomical features need to be taken into account when positioning patients undergoing spinal procedures. For example, placing obese patients in a prone position can result in an increase in intra-abdominal pressure, and thus increased intraoperative haemorrhage.

21.3 Methods of Reducing Blood Loss Without the Use of Frames

This can be achieved by means of various positioning techniques.

These include:

- The kneeling position
- The Mohammedan praying position
- The knee-chest position
- The Wayne tuck position [4–6]

© Springer-Verlag GmbH Germany 2023
U. Vieweg, F. Grochulla (eds.), *Manual of Spine Surgery*, https://doi.org/10.1007/978-3-662-64062-3_21

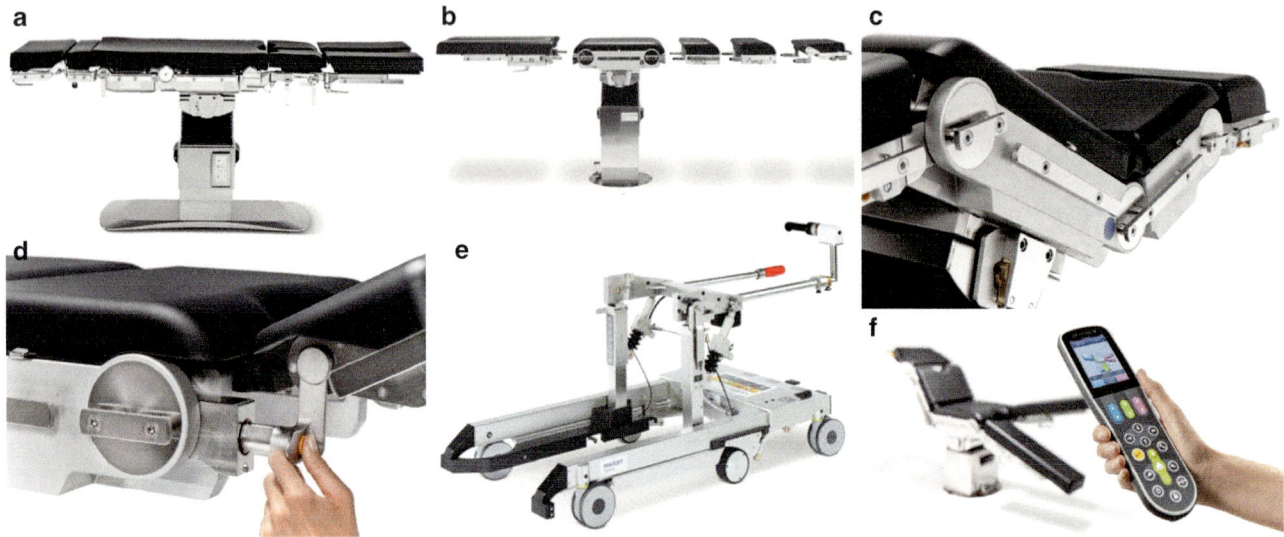

Fig. 21.1 (**a**–**f**) Operating table adjustment (height and longitudinal adjustment, inclination—Trendelenburg, reversed Trendelenburg—tilt right/left, flex position with key operation, beach chair position with key operation, adjustment range under back plate and leg plate, range for manual adjustment of upper plate)

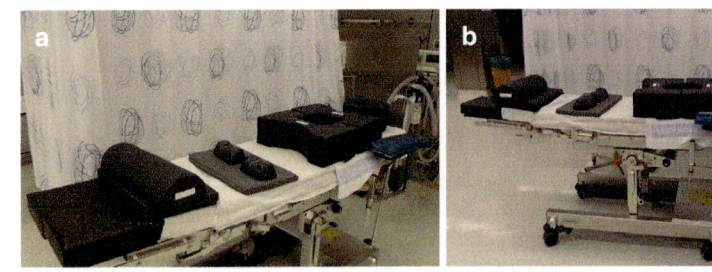
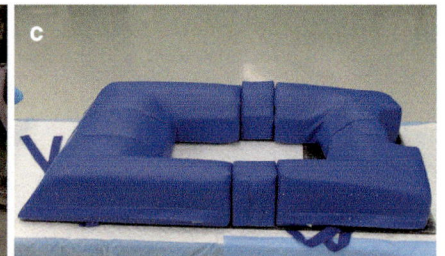

Fig. 21.2 (**a**–**c**) Operating table with back plate and head plate, various cushions and Wiltse frame© for surgery of the lumbar and thoracic spine in the prone position

Considerable flexion of the spine, hips and knees occur during such extreme tucked positions, and this may produce vascular and nerve compression in the popliteal compartment. An extreme flexed position may also tighten the posterior paraspinal muscle. Prolonged joint flexion is potentially harmful for patients with hip or knee disorders, joint degeneration or total joint replacement [7].

21.4 Methods of Reducing Blood Loss Using Frames

Positioning devices can be used to offset the abdominal decompression and preserve lordosis [8]. Many such devises are available (see Fig. 21.2a–c), including:
- The Relton-Hall frame
- The Canadian frame (Hastings)
- The Andrews frame
- The Wilson frame [8–10]

On the Andrews frame, patients are positioned in a modified knee-chest position with a chest pad and adjustable tibial support lowered to obtain 90° hip flexion. The tibial support may be adjusted to produce 60° hip flexion for spinal surgery. The frame allows the integration of the C-arm for intraoperative imaging. The usage of a Wilson frame (see Fig. 21.2a–c) is a convenient and stable method of maintaining patients in a flexed position for spinal surgery. It has two full-length curved pads, which provide continuous support for chest and pelvis. An alternative option is the Jackson surgical table. It can be rotated in an angle of 360°, allowing combined approaches.

21.5 The History of the Operating Table

The earliest operating furniture took into account the anatomical flexion points of the human body—in the hip and knee regions. The first operating tables were wooden and in some cases were particularly elaborately designed.

Subsequently developed operating tables were made out of metal and with mobile castors. Important features of these tables were that they allowed a Trendelenburg and reversed Trendelenburg positioning of patients. This was particularly important in the early days of surgery as there were very few other intensive care techniques that could be used to control circulation in the intraoperative situation. The so-called "large Heidelberg" operating table was the first that actually met all requirements for a system that could be used for general surgery. Contemporary mobile operating tables consist of a basis, an operating table column and the table top. Due to the provision of upper and lower backplates, seat plate, separate leg plates and hydraulic height adjustment systems, the ideal positioning of patients can be achieved for all sorts of surgical interventions. There were two versions of such operating tables that competed against each other: the Maquet 1120 system (originally designed in 1964) and the battery-powered hydraulic Heidelberger 1130 (1984–2003). The top was divided into eight segments and was radiolucent; the upper back section was motor-operated.

21.6 Positioning Equipment and Aids

There are various items of positioning equipment and aids available for supporting the positioning of patients for spinal surgical procedures (Fig. 21.2a–c):
- Pads with viscoelastic foam cores (such as head cushions, head rings, special cushions, wedge cushions, rolls and half-rolls, double-wedge cushions, knee positioning cushions, heel positioning cushions, etc.)
- Gel-filled pads
- Operating table overlays
- Universal positioning aids
- Universal frame system

21.7 Operating Table Accessories

The following accessories can be attached to an operating table:
- Head fixation piece
- Headrests
- Arm positioning devices
- Arm protectors
- Lateral support and multi-lateral support
- Anaesthesia screens
- Arm straps for anaesthesia screens
- Leg and body strap
- Armboards with clamps
- Radial setting clamps

- Humerus support plates
- Different clamps
- Head rest for neurosurgery
- Carbon fibre plate
- Thoracic supports
- Fixtures and head supports
- Ankle and knee cushion, tube pillow, wedge pillow
- Chest roll
- Closed and open head ring, gel-foam
- Operating table sections and different mattresses.

21.8 Special Equipment

For certain spinal surgical procedures, special equipment is required. This can include:
- Motor-operated headrest adjustors
- Spinal support systems/head extenders for intraoperative repositioning and fixation during surgery to the dorsal ventral spine in patients with a halo ring

21.9 Patient Warming Systems [11, 12]

There is the risk of the development of hypothermia in patients under anaesthesia, particularly during prolonged surgical procedures, which can have negative consequences for the cardiovascular system, wound healing and blood coagulation. The onset of hypothermia can occur within 60 min of the induction of anaesthesia. During this period, the body temperature of the patient is prone to decrease. If hypothermia is not prevented, the relative risk of serious complications increases by a factor of 3.25 for wound healing impairments, 4.49 for cardiac problems and 1.33 for increased haemorrhaging requiring blood transfusion in comparison to a situation in normothermia [11]. Modern body temperature management systems consist of a heat generator, warming blankets and warming underlays. These allow the body temperature of patients to be maintained in the normothermic range. In addition, there are various patient warming systems available from a range of manufacturers that include systems for warming blood and fluids for infusion.

21.10 Complications of Positioning in Spinal Surgery

The potential complications that can arise in connection with patient positioning for spinal surgery can be as follows:
- Injury to the lateral femoral cutaneous nerve
- Direct pressure on the eye

- Shoulder dislocation
- A common complication of the prone position is increased bleeding, mostly due to damage to engorged vertebral veins

21.11 Positioning in Spinal Surgery

The most common forms of positioning in spinal surgery are:

The Prone Position (see Fig. 21.3a–c)

- Used mainly for posterior procedures requiring access to the thoracic and lumbar spine.

The Lateral Position (see Fig. 21.4a, b)

- Used generally for anterior access to the thoracic and lumbar spine.

The Supine Position (see Fig. 21.5a, b)

- Used for procedures requiring access to the anterior cervical, thoracic and lumbar spine.

The da Vinci Position (see Fig. 21.6)

- Used for procedures requiring access to the anterior lower lumbar/sacral spine.

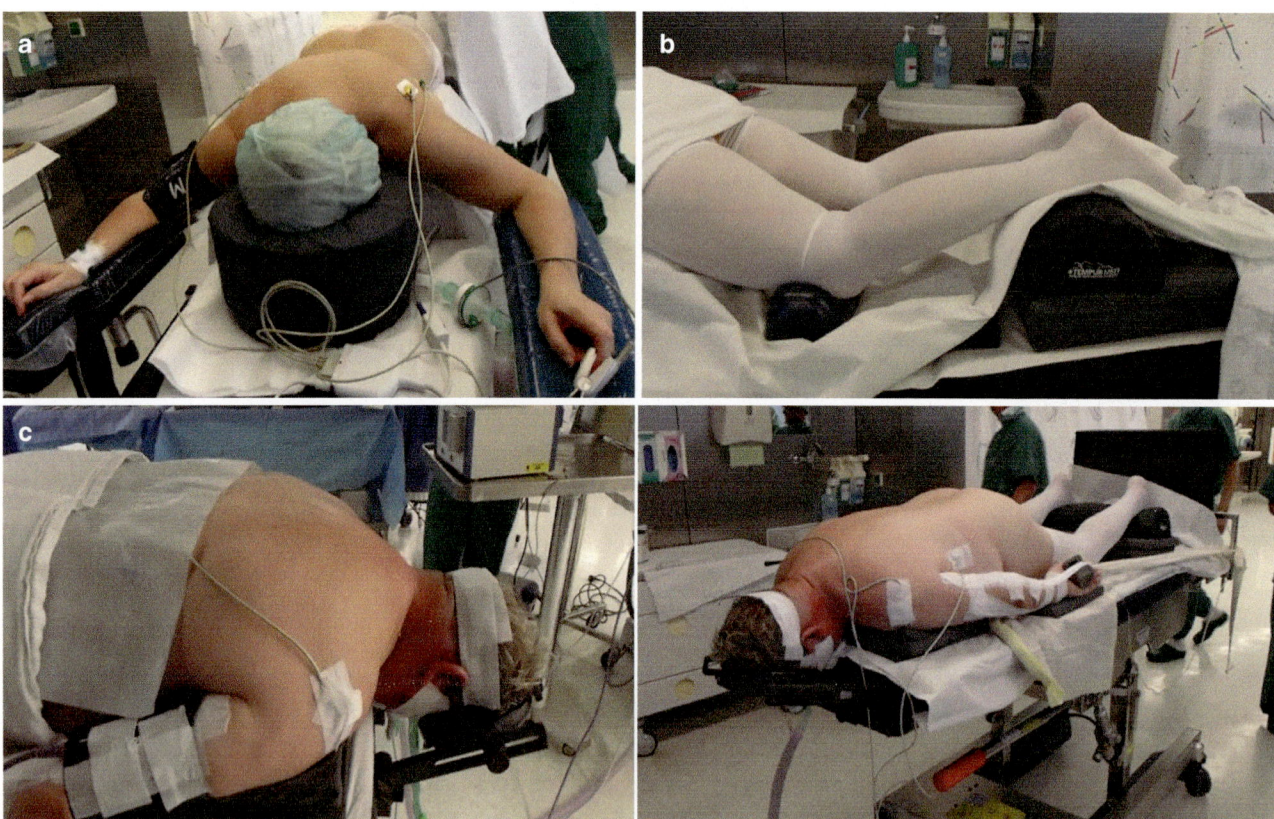

Fig. 21.3 (**a–c**) Patient in prone position on operating table with head ring (**a**) position of the legs (**b**) and (**c**) with horseshoe-shaped headrest

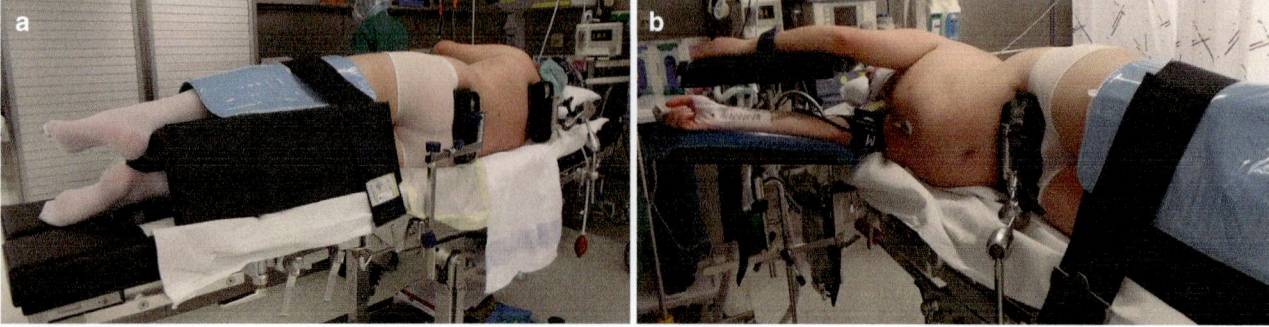

Fig. 21.4 (**a, b**) Patient in lateral position for anterior lumbar/thoracic procedure

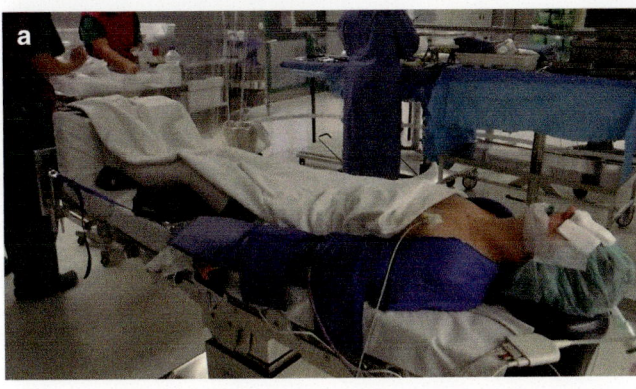
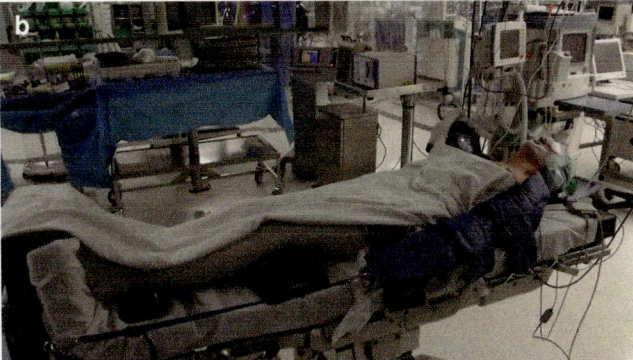

Fig. 21.5 (**a**, **b**) Patient in supine position for anterior cervical spine procedure

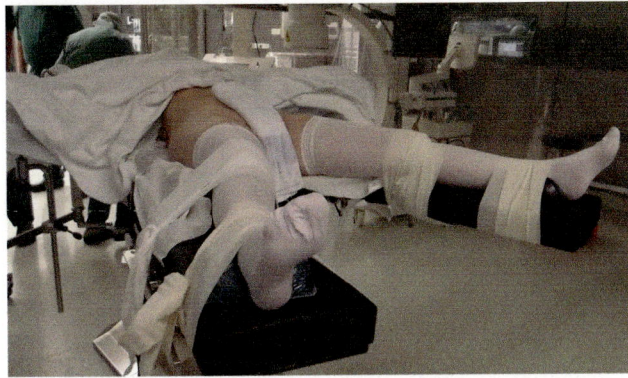

Fig. 21.6 da Vinci position for anterior lower lumbar procedure

21.11.1 The Prone Position

21.11.1.1 Surgery in the Thoracic and Lumbar Spine Areas in the Prone Position
(See Fig. 21.3a–c)

The prone position in which the patient is positioned head-first has traditionally been and remains the most common position used to access the posterior aspect of the thoracical, lumbar or sacral spine. The prone position is comfortable for surgeons, providing an adequate overview of both bone and neural structures in the treatment of fractures, deformities, tumours, spondylodiscitis, spondylolisthesis and degenerative disc disease. The patient may be at risk of the development of pressure ulcers and nerve damage. The position causes additional pressure for the skin and bony prominences. For this reason, positioning and, in particular, the aids employed must take these effects into account. The patient's arms should be tucked at the patient's sides with a bed-sheet and secured with arm guards to sleds.

Preparations:
- Arm positioning devices
- Special head positioning cushion for prone position
- Thorax, pelvic and wedge cushions, padded roll
- Special bolster for the prone position
  Positioning:
  Positioning on a standard operating table (Fig. 21.3a–c):
- Use adaptable arm positioning devices,
- Position the head on the special head positioning cushion, or skull-clamp
- Position the axillae freely with the thorax pad and ensure that the pelvic pad does not extend beyond the anterior superior iliac crest.

21.11.1.2 Checklist for Posterior Surgical Intervention to the Lumbar/Sacral and Thoracic Spine in the Prone Position

Operating table: Radiolucent modular operating table system

Positioning aids: Disposable sheet as underlay, towel as stretch cover, gel head cushion, white disposable head cushion, two-arm positioning devices with gel pads for arms, abdominal fixation belt, body warming blanket, surgical cotton sheet as top cover, horseshoe-shaped headrest (foam or silicone), silicone pads, half-roll, two to three tempur pillows.

Important: The positioning should minimize the restriction of the abdomen. Attach ECG leads to the back. Provide pressure ulcer prophylaxis, particularly in the region of the patellae, the heads of the fibulae, the toes, the iliac crest, the chin, the eyes, nose and arms. Do not flex arms significantly beyond 90° (risk of plexus damage); upper arms must not be constricted. Ensure male genitalia are not restricted and are not subjected to pressure. Mammae must also not be subjected to pressure. Ensure head and cervical vertebrae are in orthograde position. Use surgical site film in the sacral region to seal the anal cleft and prevent moisture collecting here, thus avoiding the risk of burns.

21.11.1.3 Checklist for Disc Surgery and Microsurgical Decompression of the Lumbar Spine in the Prone Position

Table: Radiolucent modular operating table system

Positioning aids: Sheet as underlay, towel as stretch cover, head gel cushion with surgical cap, white disposable head cushion, one arm positioning device with gel pads, Ulmer wheel, abdominal fixation belt, body warming blanket, surgical cotton sheet as top cover, two-arm positioning devices, gel cushions, gel mats, horseshoe-shaped headrest, silicon pads, half-roll, positioning frame, two to three cushioning pillows.

Important: Position iliac crest on the pelvic pad. Attach buttock supports to the upper gluteal fold. The thorax cushion should not touch the chin and should not extend beyond the lower end of the sternum. Patellae should not be restricted. The anal fold must be sealed with film to ensure that no moisture can penetrate. Provide for pressure ulcer prophylaxis, particularly in the region of the patellae, the heads of the fibulae, the toes, the iliac crest, the chin, the eyes, the nose and arms. Do not flex arms significantly beyond 90° (risk of plexus damage). Ensure male genitalia and Mammae are not restricted. Ensure head and cervical vertebrae are in orthograde position.

21.11.1.4 Posterior Access to the Cervical Spine with Horseshoe-Shaped Headrest (Skull Clamp) in the Prone Position

Indications are surgical procedures with posterior access to the upper and lower cervical spine. The options for intraoperative, external repositioning of the patient are limited.

Preparations:
- Arm positioning devices
- Horseshoe-shaped headrest or skull clamp

Positioning:
- Prone positioning of the operating table in the theatre.
- Fix and pre-position the horseshoe-shaped headrest to the head part of the operating table.
- Move the patient towards the head end until the shoulders are at the upper edge of the operating table with the scapulae still on the table.
- Position and fix the head in the horseshoe-shaped headrest.
- Position both arms along the body with arm protectors or secure the arms, fix in place with plasters if necessary.

21.11.1.5 Checklist for Surgery to the Posterior Cervical Spine in the Prone Position

Table: Extension table, carbon fibre-top table

Positioning aids: Half-roll, gel cushions, footrest, horseshoe-shaped headrest or skull clamp, arm extender, Fixomull tape, brown Leukoplast tape, sheet for arm fixation.

Important: Arm traction to improve lateral image quality may be considered but handled with caution due to nerval damage, especially of the C5 root. Cushioning in particular of the feet and the face are mandatory to avoid pressure caused ulcers (see Figs. 21.5 and 21.6).

21.11.2 Lateral Position

The indications for spinal surgery in the lateral position include procedures addressing the ventral column like interbody fusion or vertebral body replacement. For lateral positioning, the patient is placed either on the left or right side, depending on the side of the surgical access (Fig. 21.4a, b). The head should be placed in a pillow or head positioner and the positioning of the ear should be monitored. The patient's physiological spinal and neck alignment should be maintained during the procedure, and a safety restraint should be secured across the hips. Risks to a patient in the lateral position include pressure to points on the dependent side of the body, such as ears, shoulders, ribs, hips, knees and ankles, as well as brachial plexus injury, venous pooling and diminished lung capacity.

21.11.2.1 Checklist for Surgery Requiring Access to Thoracic/Lumbar Spine in the Lateral Position

Table: Radiolucent modular operating table system

Positioning aids: Sheet as underlay, towel as stretch cover, gel head cushion with surgical cap, white disposable head cushion, two-arm positioning devices with gel pads for arms, Ulmer wheel, abdominal fixation belt, two body warming blankets, surgical cotton sheet as top cover, backrest, one three-sectioned support, two two-sectioned supports, three gel pads, disposable tunnel cushion.

Important: Attach upper arm at 90° to specially padded anaesthesia screen, sheets in the flank, legs parallel and padded with cushions and gel mats. Provide for pressure ulcer prophylaxis, particularly in the region of the trochanters, malleoli, calcanei and head of the fibula. Do not flex arms beyond 90° and do not position below the thorax (risk of plexus damage). Ensure the head is in orthograde position (risk of impaired blood perfusion). Ensure male genitals, in particular, are not restricted.

21.11.3 Supine Position

21.11.3.1 Checklist for Surgery to the Cervical Spine in the Supine Position
(Fig. 21.5a, b)

Table: Radiolucent modular operating table system

Positioning aids: Gel pads, half-roll, footrest, head ring, gauze dressings, Fixomull tape, brown Leukoplast tape, sheet for arm fixation, arm extender, backrest. Place a towel roll under the cervical spine or scapula. Extension of the arms ensures intraoperative fluoroscopy of the cervical spine is possible without superimposition of the scapulae. Provide pressure ulcer prophylaxis, particularly in the region of the heels, the elbows, the buttocks

21.11.4 Checklist for Surgical Procedures Requiring Access to the Lower Lumbar Spine in the da Vinci Position
(Fig. 21.6)

Table: Radiolucent modular operating table system

Positioning aids: Sheet as underlay, towel as stretch cover, gel head cushion with surgical cap, white disposable head cushion, two-arm positioning devices with gel pads for arms, Ulmer wheel, abdominal fixation belt, body warming blanket, surgical cotton sheet as top cover.

Important: Provide for pressure ulcer prophylaxis, particularly in the region of the buttocks and heels. Position gel cushions under both legs. Do not flex arms beyond 90° and do not position below the level of the thorax (risk of plexus damage). Ensure head and cervical vertebrae are in orthograde position.

References

1. Batson OV. The function of vertebral veins and their role in the spread of metastases. Ann Surg. 1940;112:139–49.
2. Norgore M. Clinical anatomy of the vertebral veins. Surgery. 1945;17:606.
3. McCulloch JA, Young PH. Microsurgery for lumbar disc hernia-tion. In: McCulloch JA, Young PH, editors. Essentials of spinal microsurgery. Philadelphia: Lippincott; 1998. p. 329–82.
4. Lipton S. Anesthesia in the surgery of retropulsed vertebral discs. Anaesthesia. 1950;5:208–12.
5. Tarlov IM. The knee chest position for lower spinal operations. J Bone Joint Surg Am. 1967;49:1193–4.
6. Wayne SJ. The tuck position for lumbar disc surgery. J Bone Joint Surg Am. 1967;49:1195–8.
7. Ray CD. New kneeling attachment and cushioned face rest for spi-nal surgery. Neurosurgery. 1987;20:266–9.
8. Stephens GC, Yoo JU, Wilbur G. Comparison of lumbar sagit-tal alignment produced by different operative positions. Spine. 1996;21:1802–6.
9. Hastings DE. A simple frame for operations on the lumbar spine. Can J Surg. 1969;12:251.
10. Relton JE, Hall JE. An operation frame for spinal fusion. A new apparatus designed to reduce haemorrhage during operation. J Bone Joint Surg Br. 1967;49:327–32.
11. NICE. Clinical-practice-guideline, the management of inadver-tent perioperative hypothermia in adults. National Collaborating Centre for Nursing and Supportive Care commissioned by National Institute for Health and Clinical Excellence (NICE). 2007. http://guidance.nice.org.uk/CG65. Accessed 23 Jan 2015.
12. Torossian A, Bräuer A, Höcker J, et al. Clinical practice guideline: preventing inadvertent perioperative hypothermia. Dtsch Arztebl Int. 2015;112:166–72.

Suggested Reading

Ali AA, Breslin DS, Hardman HD, Martin G. Unusual presentation and complication of the prone position for spinal surgery. J Clin Anesth. 2003;15:471–3.
Botsman O, Hyrkas J, Hirvensalo E, Kallio E. Blood loss, operating time, and positioning of the patient in lumbar disc surgery. Spine. 1990;15:360–3.
Callahan RA, Brown MD. Positioning techniques in spinal surgery. Clin Orthop. 1981;154:22–6.
Campbell K. Pressure points in the operating room. J Enterostomal Ther. 1989;16:119–24.
Chu YC, Tsai SK, Chan KH, et al. Lateral medullary syndrome after prone position for general surgery. Anesth Analg. 2002; 95:1451–3.
DiStefano VJ, Klein KS, Nixon JE, Andrews ET. Intra-operative analy-sis of the effects of position and body habitus on surgery of the low back. A preliminary report. Clin Orthop. 1974;99:51–6.
Ecker A. Kneeling position for operations on the lumbar spine. Surgery. 1949;25:112.
Ford LT. Position for lumbar disc surgery. Clin Orthop. 1977;123:104.
Guanciale AF, Dinsay JM, Watkins RG. Lumbar lordosis in spinal fusion. A comparison of intraoperative results of patient position-ing on two different operative table frames. Spine. 1996;21:964–9.
Keim HA, Weinstein JD. Acute renal failure. A complication of spine fusion in the tuck position. J Bone Joint Surg Am. 1970;52A:1248–51.

Knight DJW, Mahajan RP. Patient positioning in anesthesia. Contin Educ Anesth Crit Care Pain. 2004;4(5):160–3.

Krettek C, Aschemann D. Positioning techniques in surgical application. Heidelberg: Springer; 2006.

McNulty SE, Weiss J, Azad SS, et al. The effect of the prone position on venous pressure and blood loss during lumbar laminectomy. J Clin Anesth. 1992;4:220–5.

Ogbue MN, Jefferson P, Ball DR. Perioperative peripheral nerve injury. Anaesthesia. 2001;56:393–4.

Park CK. The effect of patient positioning on intraabdominal pressure and blood loss in spinal surgery. Anesth Analg. 2000;91:552–7.

Papantonio C, Wallop JM, Kolodner KB. Sacral ulcers following cardiac surgery: incidence and risks. Adv Skin Wound Care. 1994;7:24–36.

Pearce DJ. The role of posture in laminectomy. Proc R Soc Med. 1957;50:109.

Phillips NF. Berry & Kohn's operating room technique. 10th ed. St. Louis, MO: Mosby; 2004.

Prielipp RC, Morell RC, Buttworth J. Ulnar nerve injury and perioperative arm positioning. Anesthesiol Clin North Am. 2002;20:351–65.

Schonauer C, Bochetti A, Barbagallo G, et al. Positioning on surgical table. Eur Spine J. 2004;13(Suppl 1):S50–5.

Servant C, Purkiss S. Positioning patients for surgery. Cambridge: Cambridge University Press; 2002.

Sessler DI. Complications and treatment of mild hypothermia. Anesthesiology. 2001;95:531–43.

St-Arnaud D, Paquin M. Safe positioning for neurosurgical patients. AORN J. 2008;87(6):1156–72.

Sutterlin C, Rechtine GR. Using Heffington frame in elective lumbar spinal surgery. Orthop Rev. 1988;17:597–600.

Tao-Chen L, Lin-Cheng Y, Han-Jung C. Effect of patient position and hypotensive anesthesia on inferior vena cava pressure. Spine. 1998;23:941–7.

Part II

Anterior Upper Cervical Spine

Overview of Surgical Techniques and Implants for the Anterior Upper Cervical Spine

22

Meic H. Schmidt

22.1 Introduction and Core Messages

The upper cervical spine represents a unique biomechanical and anatomic region that requires specialized surgical techniques and implants. Most commonly, the upper cervical spine is affected by trauma (odontoid fractures and nonunions), occipital-cervical dislocations, or degenerative processes, particularly rheumatoid arthritis, which results in atlantoaxial instability. Trauma indications include Jefferson fractures with instability and disruption of the transverse ligament, odontoid fractures that are mobile in flexion and extension, and C1–2 dislocations. In rheumatoid degenerative instability of the C1–2 joints, the indications are also inclusive of decompression of the spinal cord and then subsequent stabilization. The four most common surgical techniques for the region are anterior odontoid screw fixation, transoral resection of the odontoid process, posterior C1–2 fixation, and anterior transarticular screw fixation [1–4].

22.2 Approaches

Approaches and implants for the anterior upper cervical spine are complex, corresponding to the unusual biomechanical and anatomic arrangement of that part of the spine. Some of them are not recommended as a stand-alone technique. Frequently, for example, a transoral resection of the odontoid is performed in conjunction with a posterior cervical fusion. Anterior approaches to the upper cervical spine are frequently based on modifications of the standard approach for anterior cervical discectomy and fusion, which is extended toward the head (cephalad).

22.2.1 Transoral Approach

There are two common transoral approaches for the treatment of rheumatoid arthritis or fracture/instability. The transoral resection is more commonly performed in rheumatoid disease for decompression of the spinal cord. This is frequently done through the mouth if the patient is able to open the mouth widely enough (Fig. 22.1). It requires a specialized retractor system, as described in Chap. 17. We do not usually place instrumentation using this approach.

22.2.2 Extraoral Ventral Retropharyngeal Approach

On rare occasions, a similar approach can be used for the placement of anterior transarticular screws (see Chap. 16). This can be done when there is C1–2 instability or an odontoid fracture (Fig. 22.2). The retropharyngeal approach is used, and then bilateral transarticular screws are passed from an anterior approach using a K-wire system. This can be done in combination with an odontoid screw. Typically, this procedure can also be done with K-wires and cannulated screws, but the K-wires must be carefully monitored so they do not migrate after insertion of the screws.

M. H. Schmidt (✉)
Department of Neurosurgery, University of New Mexico, Albuquerque, NM, USA
e-mail: MHSchmidt@salud.unm.edu

© Springer-Verlag GmbH Germany 2023
U. Vieweg, F. Grochulla (eds.), *Manual of Spine Surgery*, https://doi.org/10.1007/978-3-662-64062-3_22

Fig. 22.1 Photograph showing transoral exposure using the Spetzler–Sonntag retractor

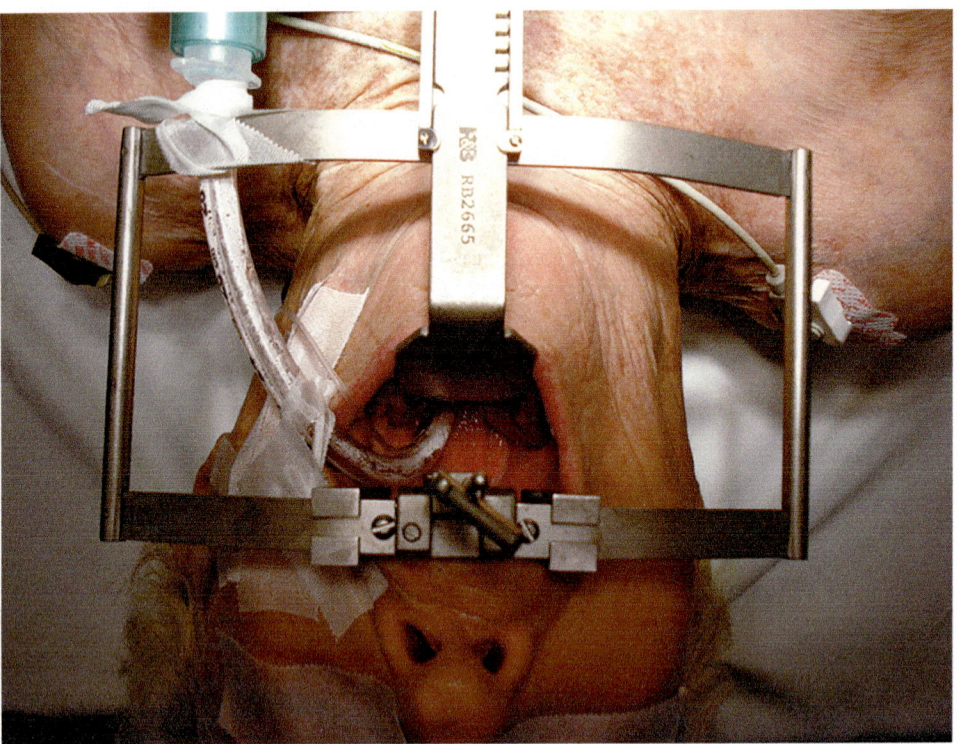

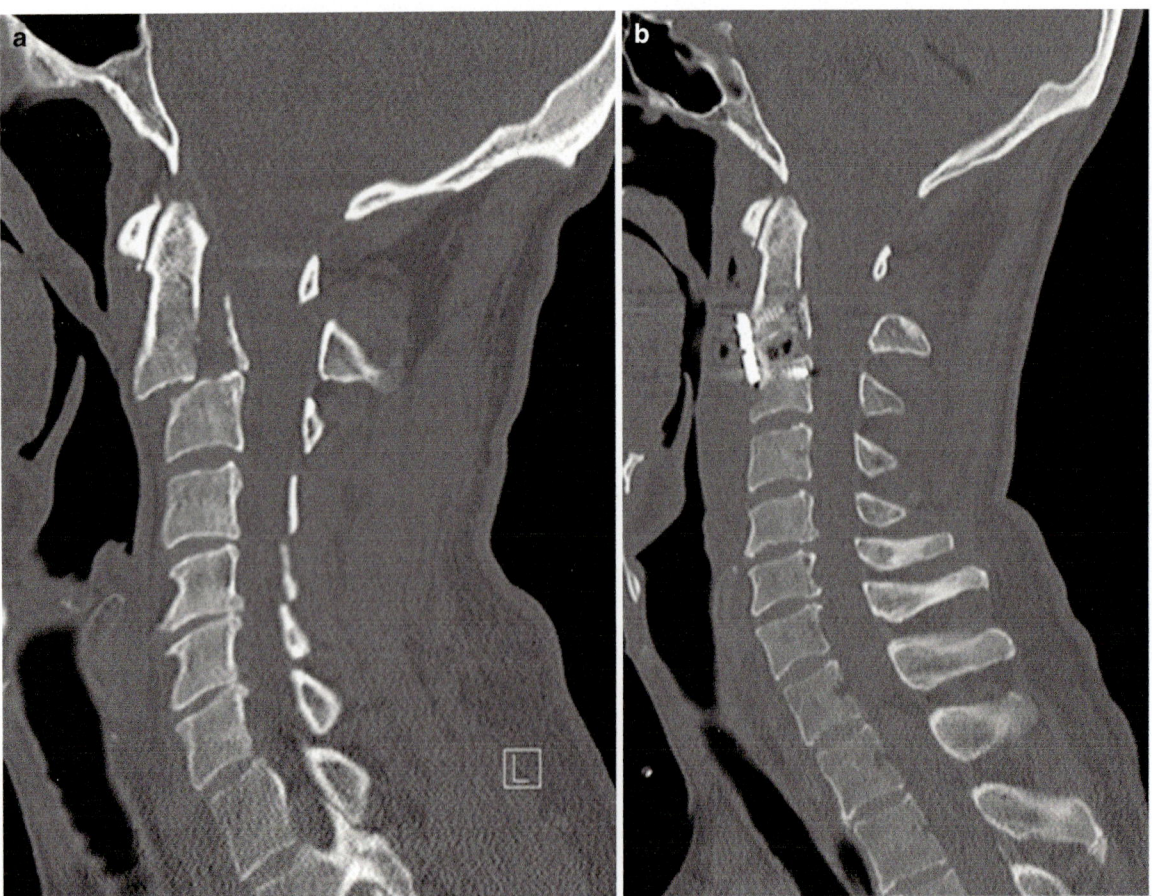

Fig. 22.2 Computed tomography scans showing C2/3 fracture dislocation (**a**) and C2/3 anterior cervical discectomy and fusion (**b**) using a retropharyngeal submandibular approach

22.3 Implants

22.3.1 Screws

The screws used for fixation in anterior approaches to the upper cervical spine are varied and depend on the approach used. With odontoid screw fixation, we use noncannulated screws, although others advise against their use. For the retropharyngeal approach, bilateral transarticular screws are typically used, sometimes in combination with an odontoid screw. Cannulated screws can be used. Anterior transarticular screws should be lag screws since this will "lag" together the C1/2 joint for fusion.

22.3.2 Plating

Anterior plating has been described but is rarely used. The predominant indication is traumatic instability after C1 fracture or resection of the odontoid. The Harms plating system has been described by Ruf et al. [1].

References

1. Ruf M, Melcher R, Harms J. Transoral reduction and osteosynthesis C1 as a function-preserving option in the treatment of unstable Jefferson fractures. Spine. 2004;29:823–7.
2. Russo A, Albanese E, Quiroga M, Ulm AJ. Submandibular approach to the C2–3 disc level: microsurgical anatomy with clinical application. J Neurosurg Spine. 2009;10:380–9.
3. Schmelzle R, Harms J. Craniocervical junction–diseases, diagnostic application of imaging procedures, surgical techniques. Fortschr Kiefer Gesichtschir. 1987;32:206–8.
4. Vender JR, Harrison SJ, McDonnell DE. Fusion and instrumentation at C1–3 via the high anterior cervical approach. J Neurosurg. 2000;92:24–9.

Odontoid Screw Fixation

23

Meic H. Schmidt

23.1 Introduction and Core Messages

Anterior odontoid screw fixation is ideal for fixation of unstable odontoid fractures and is superior to posterior C1–2 arthrodesis as it preserves C1–2 rotational movement and obviates the need for autograft bone harvest. This method has become increasingly popular since the time it was introduced by Bohler [1], and it is now widely used to treat unstable type II and shallow type III odontoid fractures [2–9]. The goals of odontoid screw fixation are immediate stabilization of type II odontoid fractures or shallow type III odontoid fractures with no need for external orthosis.

23.2 Indications

- Type II odontoid fractures
- Shallow type III odontoid fractures that have failed non-operative treatment
- Elderly patients who have failed halo fixation and external orthosis
- Patients that do not want to use halo fixation or external orthosis

23.3 Contraindications

- Severe associated C1 and C2 fractures
- Occipital cervical instability associated with type II odontoid fractures
- Fractures that are older than 18 months
- Patients that have excessive cervical kyphosis
- Patients with a large chest (barrel chest)
- Anterior oblique fracture (see Fig. 23.1a)

23.4 Technical Prerequisites

It is essential that the patient can be intubated fiberoptically by an experienced anesthesiologist. Neuromonitoring, including somatosensory evoked potentials (SSEPs) and motor evoked potentials (MEPs), can be performed.

Awake nasotracheal or fiberoptic intubation is used if there is instability in extension. Traditional laryngoscopic intubation is safe if the fracture reduces in extension. We highly recommend using two fluoroscopy machines for bilateral views simultaneously of the anterior-posterior (AP) upper cervical spine and the lateral upper cervical spine. Because we use the Aesculap anterior odontoid screw fixation system, which allows for intraoperative reduction of the odontoid fracture, we do not require complete preoperative reduction of the fracture.

23.5 Planning, Preparation, and Positioning

We routinely include the upper sternum and the neck in the sterile preparation. The patient is placed in the supine position with head immobilized with 10 lb of traction via a halter device. Alternatively, Gardner–Wells tongs can be used or halo traction can be used if the patient has already been in the

M. H. Schmidt (✉)
Department of Neurosurgery, University of New Mexico, Albuquerque, NM, USA
e-mail: MHSchmidt@salud.unm.edu

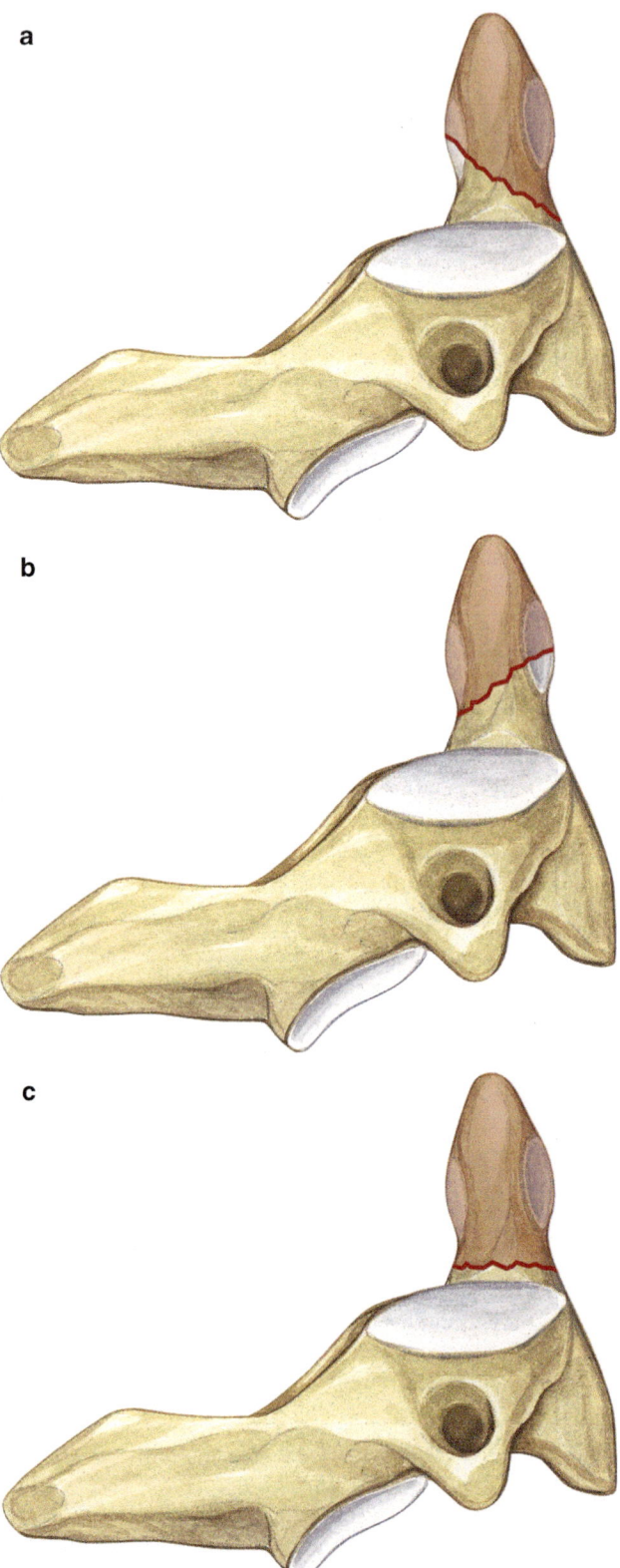

a

b

c

Fig. 23.1 Classification based on the direction of the slope of the fracture: anterior oblique (**a**), posterior oblique (**b**), and horizontal (**c**)

halo. We always place a shoulder roll between the shoulder blades to maximally extend the neck. To get a good AP view of the odontoid process, a radiolucent mouth gag is frequently used (a wine bottle cork can be notched into the teeth).

23.6 Operating Technique

23.6.1 Approach

- Lateral fluoroscopy is used to ensure the proper trajectory; we place a K-wire along the neck of the patient to ensure that the sternum does not interfere with the screw placement.
- Once this is done, we infiltrate the skin with epinephrine and perform a standard Cloward approach to the anterior spine (see Fig. 23.2).
- At the C5 level, we place a small unilateral midcervical incision in the skin crease. Then the platysma muscle is divided horizontally, and the plane between the pharynx and esophagus medially and the carotid sheath laterally is developed.
- We use blunt finger dissection to expose the cervical spine.
- The longus colli muscle is then incised and bilaterally elevated, and sharp-tooth cervical retractor blades are inserted firmly under these muscles and attached to a special retractor blade.
- Firm fixation is important because a fair amount of tension is placed on the retractor during the drilling and screw placement. After this retractor is placed, we use a Kittner dissector to sweep up the anterior cervical spine to approximately the level of C1.
- Once this dissection is completed, we place a superior angled retractor blade (see Fig. 23.2). This blade should reach up approximately to C1. A choice of six different blades is available.
- This retractor blade is then connected via a special retractor system to the lateral retractor blades. Once the retractor is in place, a working tunnel is created for the drilling and placement of the odontoid screws.

23.6.2 Instrumentation

- Using a sharp K-wire, we find the entry site at the inferior anterior edge of C2 on the lateral and AP fluoroscopy (see Fig. 23.3a). The entry point location is chosen based on whether one or two screws will be placed: If only one screw is placed, the entry point should be at the anterior

Fig. 23.2 The C5 skin incision and the position of the soft tissue retractors (with permission of Aesculap AG, Tuttlingen, Germany)

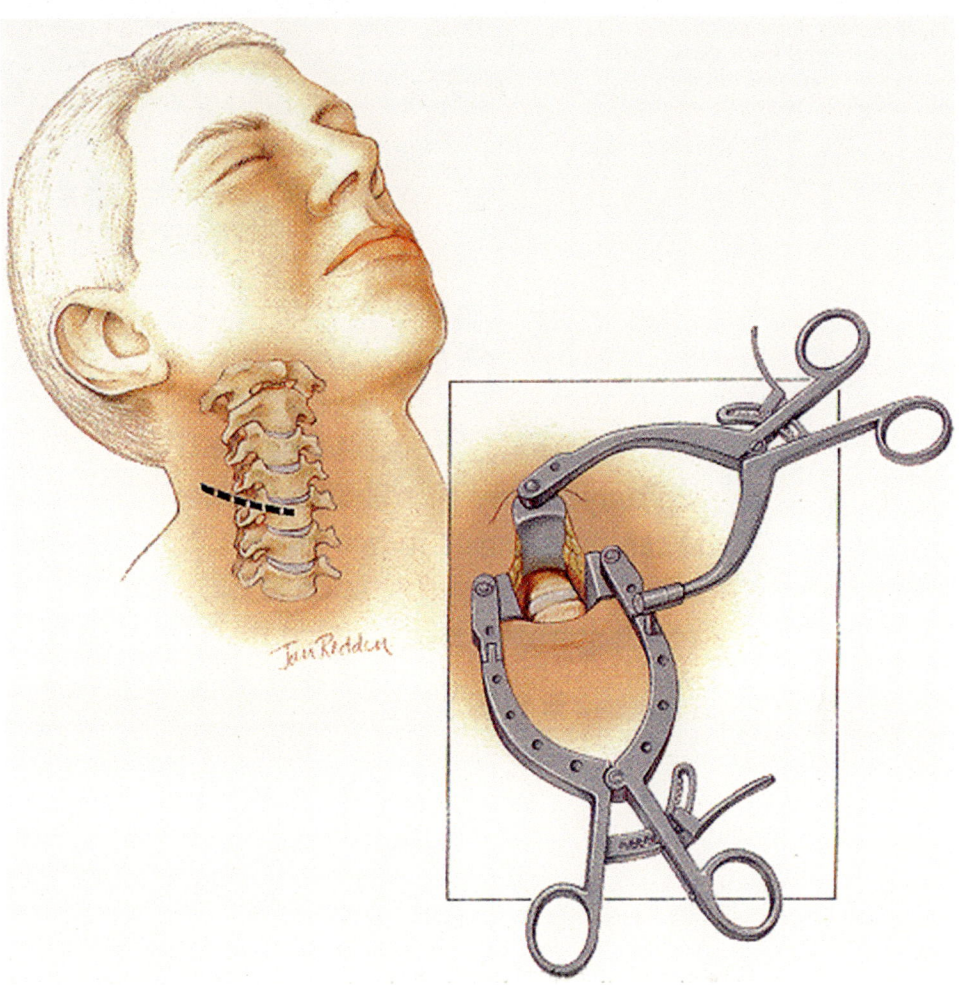

inferior edge of C2 at the midline. We place the entry point slightly laterally about 2–3 mm off the midline if two screws are to be placed.

- The K-wire is then manipulated under biplanar fluoroscopy and impacted approximately 5 mm into the C2 vertebral body (see Fig. 23.3a).
- Once the K-wire is impacted, we use a hollow cord drill that is passed over the K-wire, and a shallow groove is cut into the anterior face of C3 and the C2–3 annulus (Fig. 23.3).
- We then put together the inner and outer drill guides and pass them over the K-wire. The outer drill guide has spikes (see Fig. 23.4), which are carefully maneuvered over the C3 vertebral body under fluoroscopy.
- At this point, the K-wire frequently needs to be shortened with a wire cutter since it protrudes over the inner tube guide. It is important to leave at least 1 cm of the K-wire protruding beyond the inner tube guide in order to be able to remove it.

- The plastic impact sleeve is then fitted over the guide wire assembly, and a mallet is used to impact the spikes into the C3 vertebral body (see Fig. 23.5).
- The inner tube guide is then advanced until it contacts the inferior edge of C2. The surgeon at this point can manipulate the handle and adjust the cervical spine to the appropriate trajectory (see Fig. 23.6).
- The K-wire then can be removed without loss of alignment and positional stability. By lifting and depressing the guide tube assembly that is impacted into C3, the alignment between C1 and C2 can be carefully manipulated. If the odontoid process is retrolisthesed, the guide tube assembly can be depressed to get the optimal angle for drilling. This is monitored under fluoroscopy.
- Next, the drill is inserted through the drill guide and through the C2 odontoid process under AP and lateral fluoroscopy. The drill guide can be adjusted before the fracture site is crossed by depressing or elevating the C2–3 complex (see Fig. 23.7).

Fig. 23.3 After dissection of the retropharyngeal space, the K-wire is placed (**a**) and the entry site at C2/3 is drilled (**b**, **c**, **d**) (with permission of Aesculap AG, Tuttlingen, Germany)

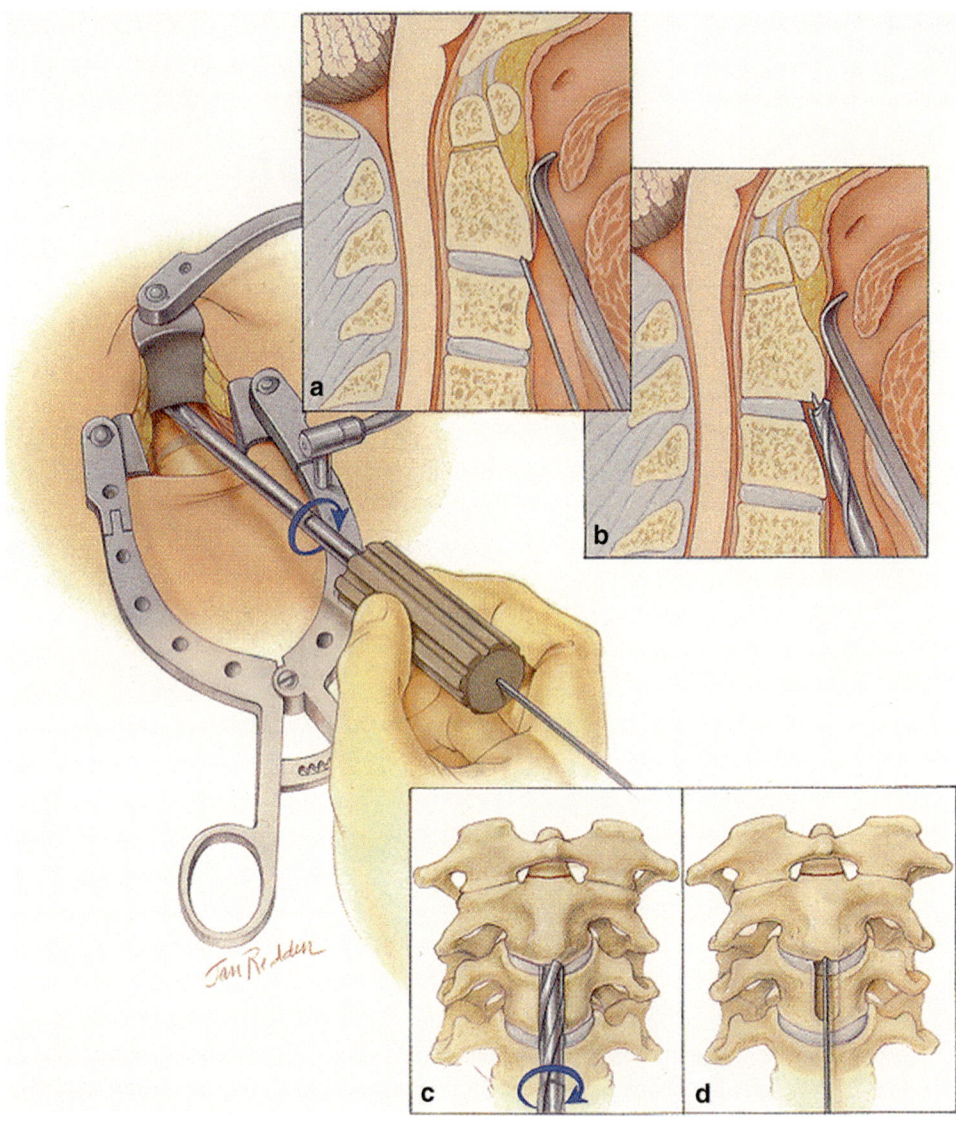

Fig. 23.4 Inner and outer drill guide assembly (with permission of Aesculap AG, Tuttlingen, Germany)

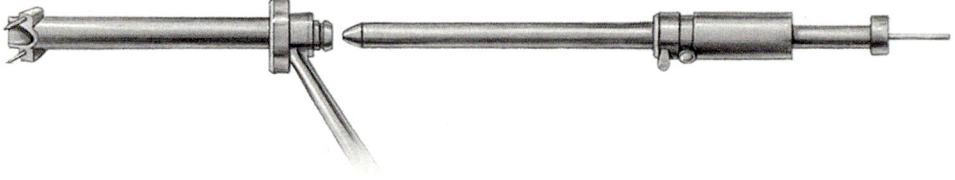

Fig. 23.5 Advancing the inner drill guide in the previously created C2/3 groove (with permission of Aesculap AG, Tuttlingen, Germany)

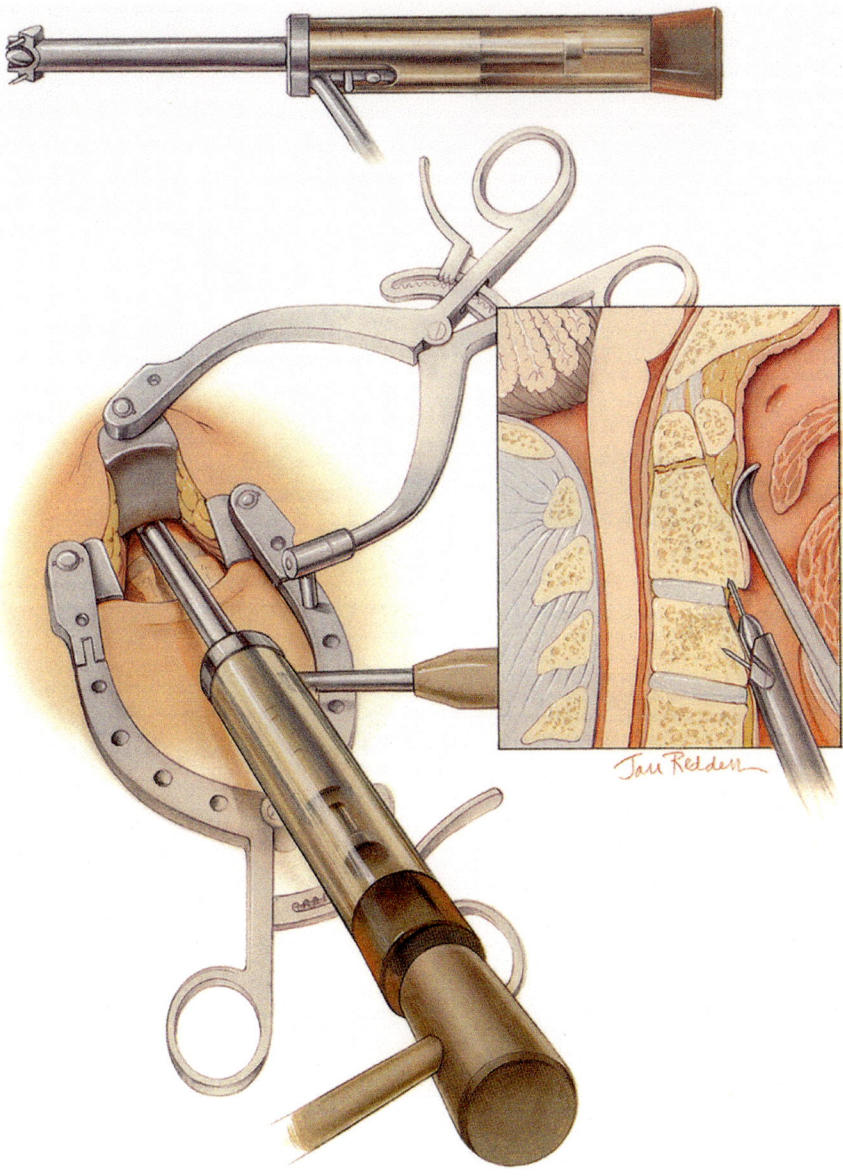

Fig. 23.6 Securing of the
teeth of the guide tube to C3
with impactor (with
permission of Aesculap AG,
Tuttlingen, Germany)

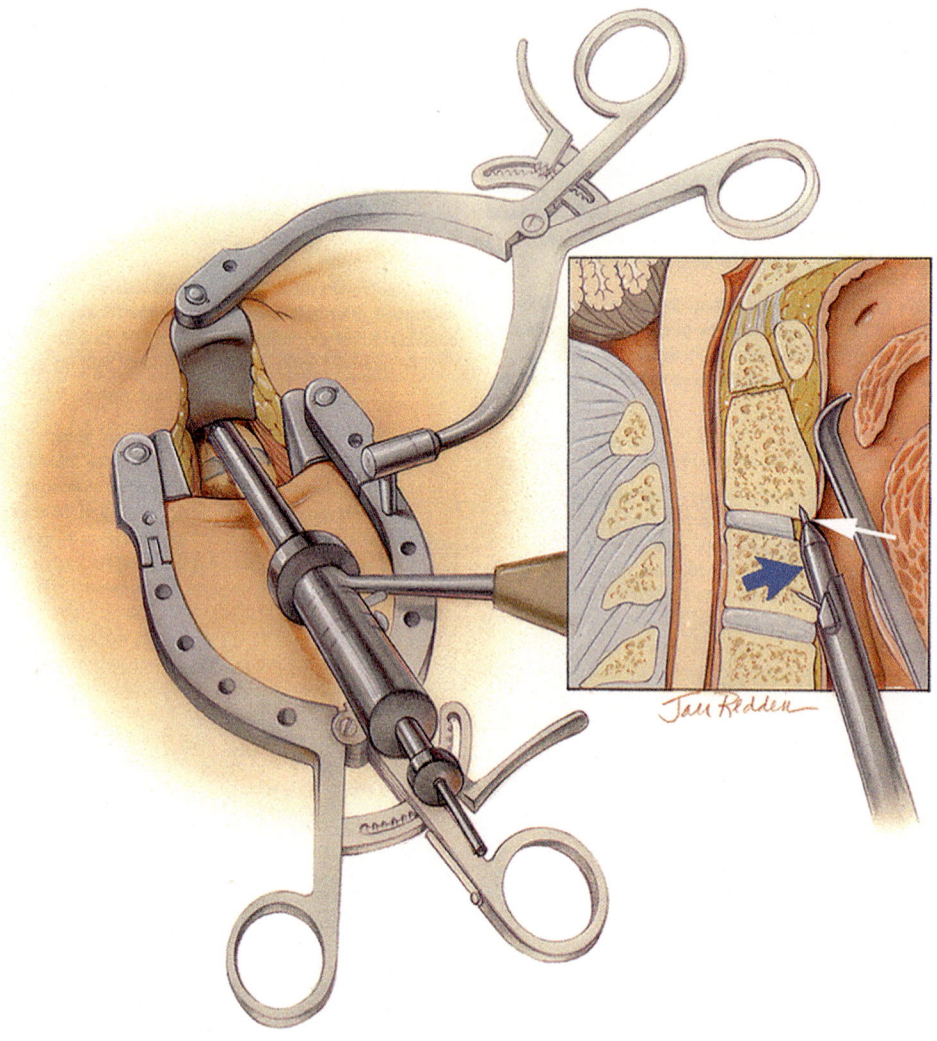

Fig. 23.7 The guide tube is
secured into the C3 vertebral
body to drill through C2 into
the apex of the odontoid tip
(with permission of Aesculap
AG, Tuttlingen, Germany)

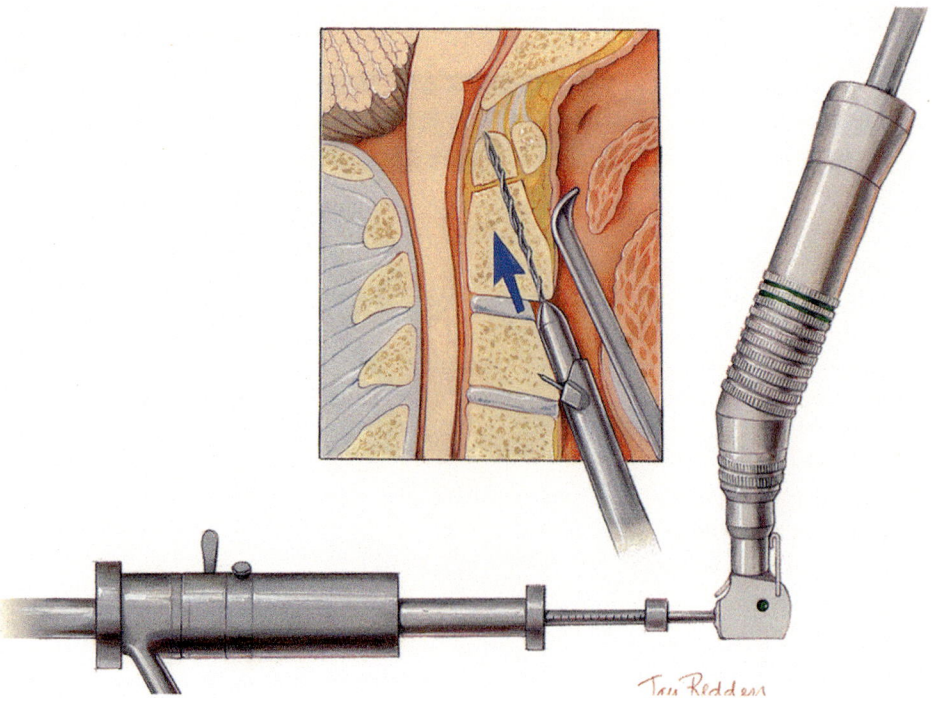

Fig. 23.8 After the drill is withdrawn, the hole is tapped, and the length of the screw is determined (with permission of Aesculap AG, Tuttlingen, Germany)

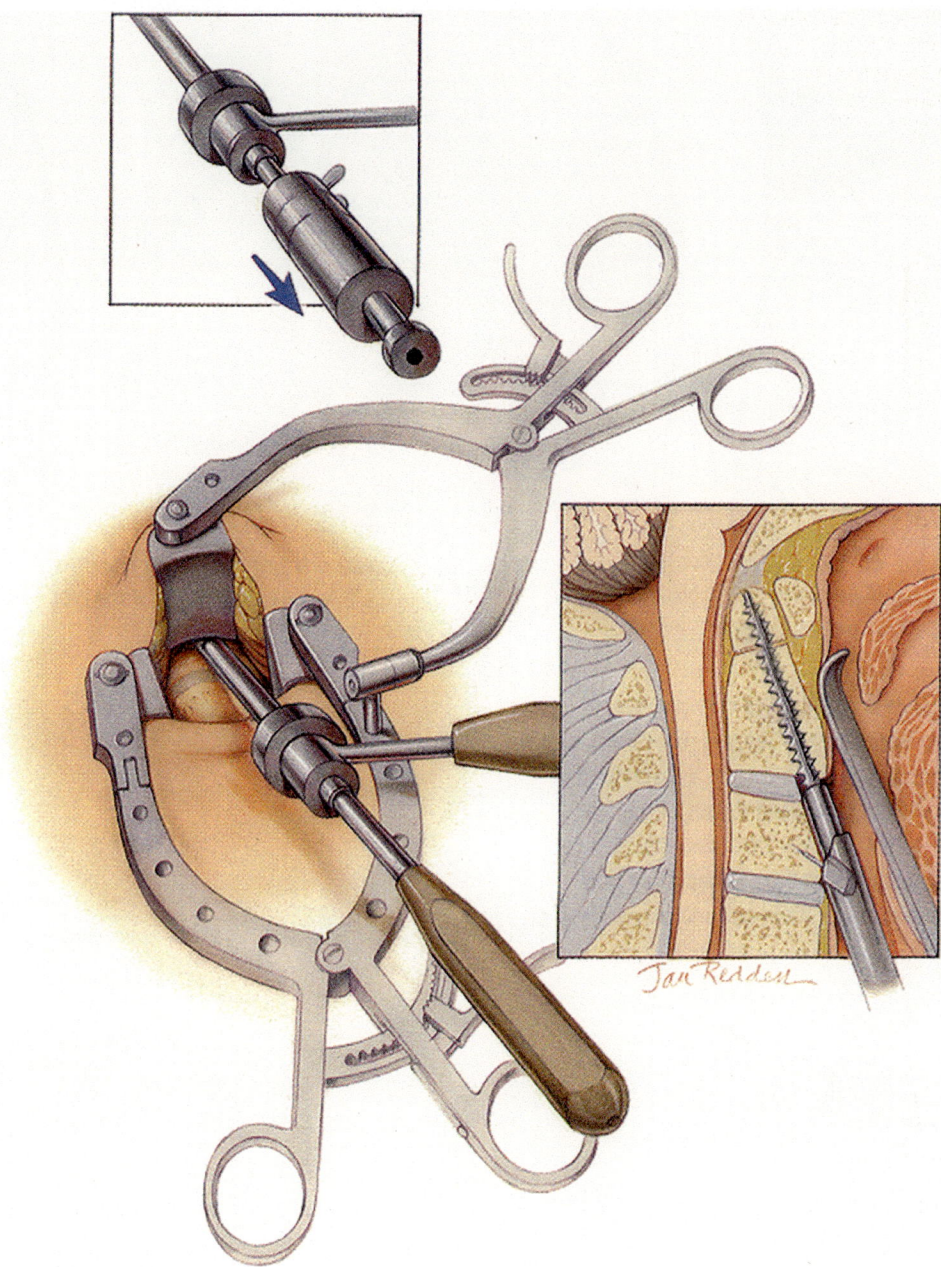

- Once the desired alignment has been achieved, the drill can be advanced through the tip of the odontoid process. In osteoporotic bone, in particular, it is important that the drill is placed bicortically through the apical cortex, which will prevent back out of the screw.
- The appropriate screw length is determined from the calibrated marks at the proximal end of the drill. A partially threaded screw is initially selected. Then, the drill is withdrawn, and a tap is inserted. In general, we tap the entire drill path bicortically through the tip of the odontoid process. The length of the screw can then be confirmed with the tap (see Fig. 23.8).

- After the tap is removed, we place the titanium screw under bilateral fluoroscopy until the distal cortex of the odontoid is fully engaged and sometimes draws back slightly to pull together the bone fragments. The "lag effect" assists with closing the fracture gap and the healing process (see Fig. 23.9).
- If a second screw is to be placed, the same process is repeated (see Fig. 23.10).
- Then, the retractors are removed, and the muscle is lightly approximated with 3.0 absorbable stitches, and the skin is closed. We generally do not place drains. The immediate stability can be confirmed by extending and flexing the neck under lateral fluoroscopy.

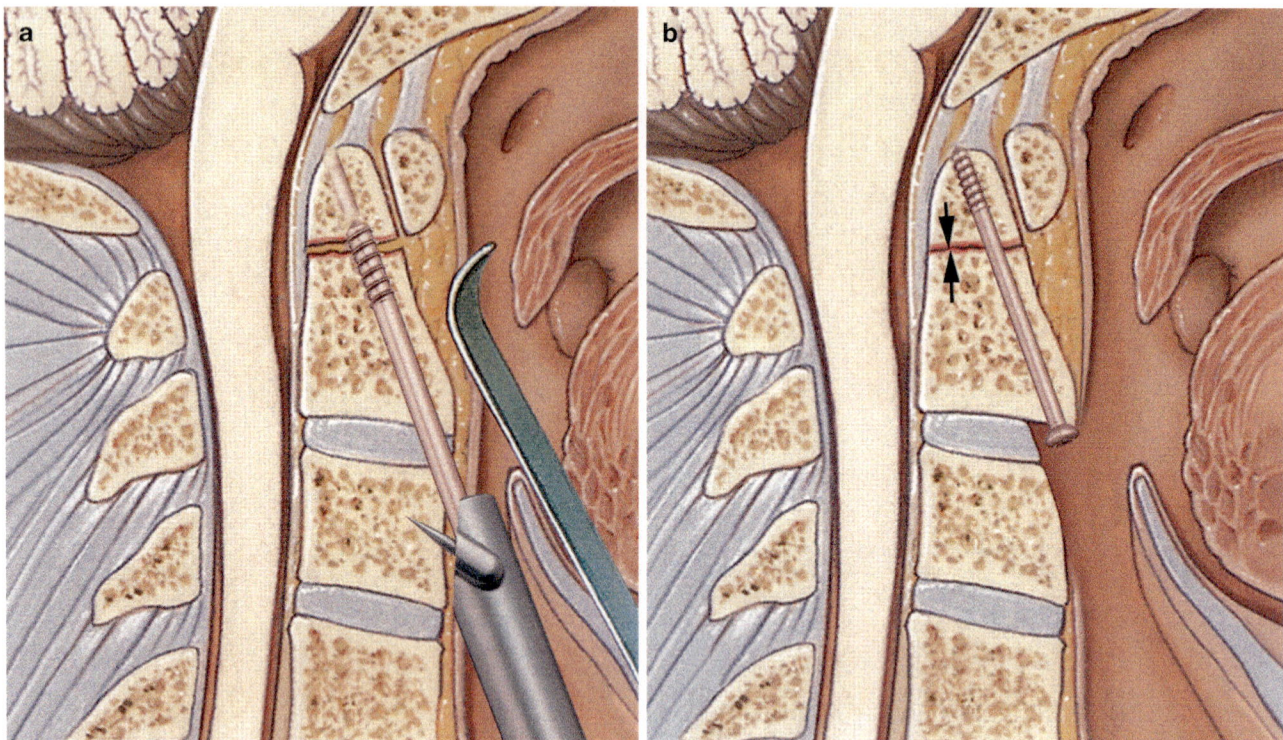

Fig. 23.9 Illustration of screw insertion (**a**) and the lag effect (arrows, **b**) (with permission of Aesculap AG, Tuttlingen, Germany)

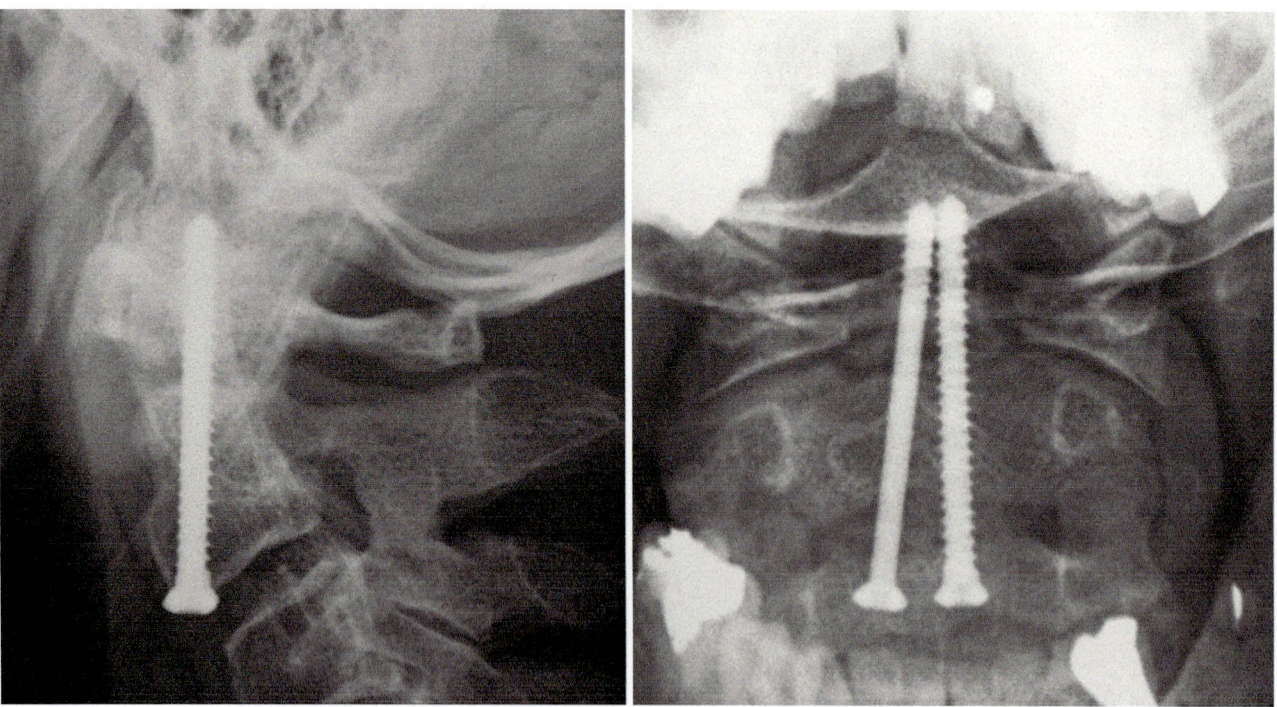

Fig. 23.10 Postoperative X-rays of odontoid screws (with permission of Klimo et al. [8])

References

1. Bohler J. Anterior stabilization for acute fractures and non-unions of the dens. J Bone Joint Surg Am. 1982;64:18–27.
2. Aebi M, Etter C, Coscia M. Fractures of the odontoid process. Treatment with anterior screw fixation. Spine. 1989;14:1065–70.
3. Apfelbaum RI. Anterior screw fixation for odontoid fractures. In: Rengachary SS, Wilkins RH, editors. Neurosurgery operative atlas, vol. 2. 3rd ed. Park Ridge: American Association of Neurological Surgeons; 1992. p. 189–99.
4. Apfelbaum RI, Lonser RR, Veres R, Casey A. Direct anterior screw fixation for recent and remote odontoid fractures. J Neurosurg. 2000;93:227–36.
5. Dunn ME, Seljeskog EL. Experience in the management of odontoid process injuries: an analysis of 128 cases. Neurosurgery. 1986;18:306–10.
6. Etter C, Coscia M, Jaberg H, et al. Direct anterior fixation of dens fractures with a cannulated screw system. Spine. 1991;16:S25–32.
7. Jenkins JD, Coric D, Branch CL Jr. A clinical comparison of one- and two-screw odontoid fixation. J Neurosurg. 1998;89:366–70.
8. Klimo P, Rao G, Apfelbaum RI. Microsurgical treatment of odontoid fractures. In: Mayer HM, editor. Minimally invasive spinal surgery. New York: Springer; 2005.
9. Montesano PX, Anderson PA, Schlehr F, et al. Odontoid fractures treated by anterior odontoid screw fixation. Spine. 1991;16:S33–7.

Anterior Transarticular Screw Fixation C1/C2

24

Uwe Vieweg and Meic H. Schmidt

24.1 Introduction and Core Messages

Anterior transarticular screw fixation is a useful minimally invasive technique for achieving C1–2 stabilization. This chapter describes the anterior transarticular screw fixation of the atlantoaxial joints using an anterior (Smith–Robinson) approach to the cervical spine. Cannulated or noncannulated screws can be inserted with a lateral angulation of 20° relative to the sagittal plane and a posterior angulation of 30° relative to the coronal plane. The advantages of this method are immediate stability, the elimination of external orthosis, and cost-effectiveness. This form of anterior transarticular screw fixation is as stable and rigid as posterior transarticular screw fixation [1–4].

24.2 Indications [5–8]

- Atlantoaxial instabilities (acute and chronic)
- C1–2 instability in cases where a posterior approach is impossible
- Failure of previous posterior treatment
- C1 type II odontoid combination fracture [5]

24.3 Contraindications

- Fracture of the C1–2 joint complex
- Vertebral artery with atypical course
- Some cases where neck is very short or thick
- Some cases with high barrel-shaped thorax

24.4 Equipment

Two C-arms for simultaneous anteroposterior and lateral fluoroscopy are essential for this technique. The settings and other equipment, and the operative approach, are the same as those for osteosynthesis using expansion screws (e.g., positioning device, rechargeable drill, appropriate screws for small fragments, Synthes odontoid screw system).

24.5 Planning, Preparation, and Positioning

The planning of the operation requires a CT to ensure that the C1–2 joint complex is intact (look out for rotational malalignment). The patient is put in a supine position, and the head is stabilized using a Mayfield headholder. Two C-arms are necessary to identify the anatomical structures of the upper cervical spine in the anteroposterior and lateral

U. Vieweg (✉)
Department of Conservative and Surgical Spine Therapy with Interdisciplinary Spinal Deformities Centre and Rummelsberg Sectional Center, Hospital Rummelsberg, Schwarzenbruck, Germany
e-mail: uwe.vieweg@sana.de

M. H. Schmidt
Department of Neurosurgery, University of New Mexico, Albuquerque, NM, USA
e-mail: MHSchmidt@salud.unm.edu

© Springer-Verlag GmbH Germany 2023
U. Vieweg, F. Grochulla (eds.), *Manual of Spine Surgery*, https://doi.org/10.1007/978-3-662-64062-3_24

Fig. 24.1 (**a**) Patient positioned on operating table. (**b**) Note the placement of two C-arm fluoroscopic units for anteroposterior (transoral) and lateral fluoroscopic control

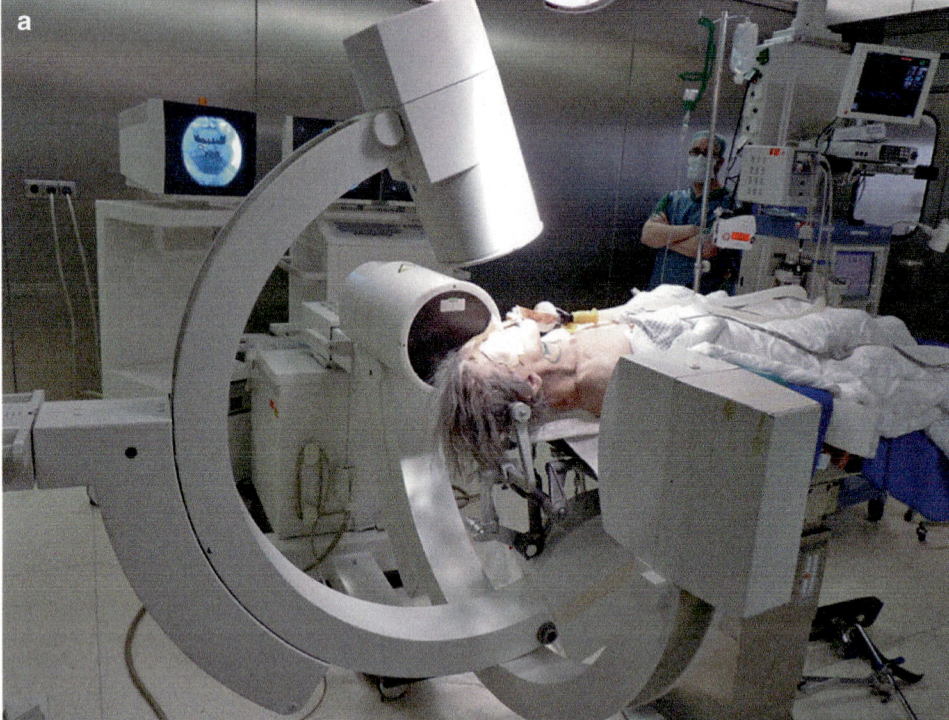

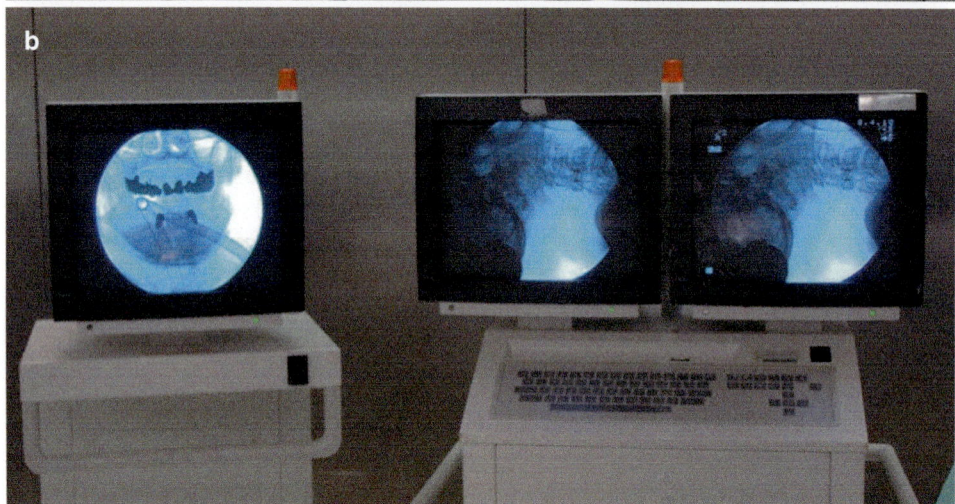

Fig. 24.1 (**a**) Patient positioned on operating table. (**b**) Note the placement of two C-arm fluoroscopic units for anteroposterior (transoral) and lateral fluoroscopic control

projections (see Fig. 24.1a, b). The site of the incision (usually at the C4/C5 level) is determined by placing a K-wire along the side of the neck in the intended direction of the screw and viewing it with the image intensifier (see Fig. 24.2).

24.6 Surgical Technique

24.6.1 Approach

- A transverse skin incision is recommended as, in most cases, only one segment is involved (for C3/C4, two fin-

gerbreadths caudal to the mandible at the level of the lingual bone; for C4/C5, at the level of the Adam's apple).
- Using a routine anterior approach to the cervical spine at the C4–5 level, the anterior side of the C2 vertebral body is exposed.
- The platysma is cut, and the superficial nuchal fascia is exposed. This is then cut longitudinally at the anterior edge of the sternocleidomastoid muscle.
- The sternocleidomastoid muscle is then moved to the side, exposing the two longus colli muscles beneath.
- Blunt dissection is carried out in the prevertebral facial plane using a side sweeping motion with a small gauze pad. Exposure of the upper half of C3 and the lower half

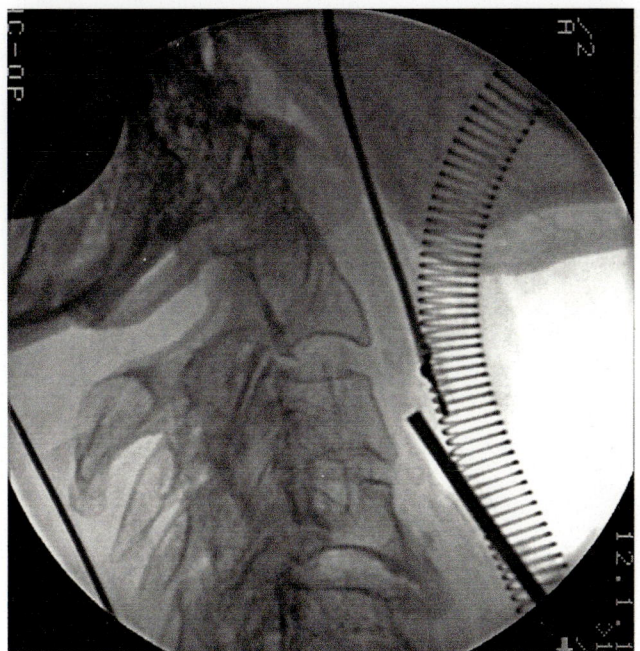

Fig. 24.2 K-wire along the side of the neck in the intended direction of the screws and viewed on the image intensifier

of C2 is usually sufficient. Preparation can often be carried out with the fingers.

24.6.2 Instrumentation

- The insertion point for the screws is at the midpoint of the C2 vertebral body in the medial third of the C1–2 articulation, just below the sulcus on the anterior side [9].
- After drilling and tapping, 3.5- or 4-mm small fragment screws are placed across the joint in the C1 massa lateralis, diverging about 20° and inclined upward about 30° (standard lag screw technique).
- It is absolutely essential that tissue protectors are used when drilling and tapping.
- Note: The use of cannulated screws and predrilling with a K-wire makes instrumentation much easier. The cannulated screw technique can be used for this (see Fig. 24.3).
- A threaded K-wire of 1.2-mm diameter and 20-cm length is advanced into the body of C2 in a posterior and superior direction at an angle of 20° to the coronal plane and 30° to the sagittal plane (see Fig. 24.3a, b).
- The length of the K-wire in the bone is measured with the ruler, indicating the length of screw required.
- The screw length is 20–25 mm. When odontoid screws are used, only the 28-mm screws may be readily avail-

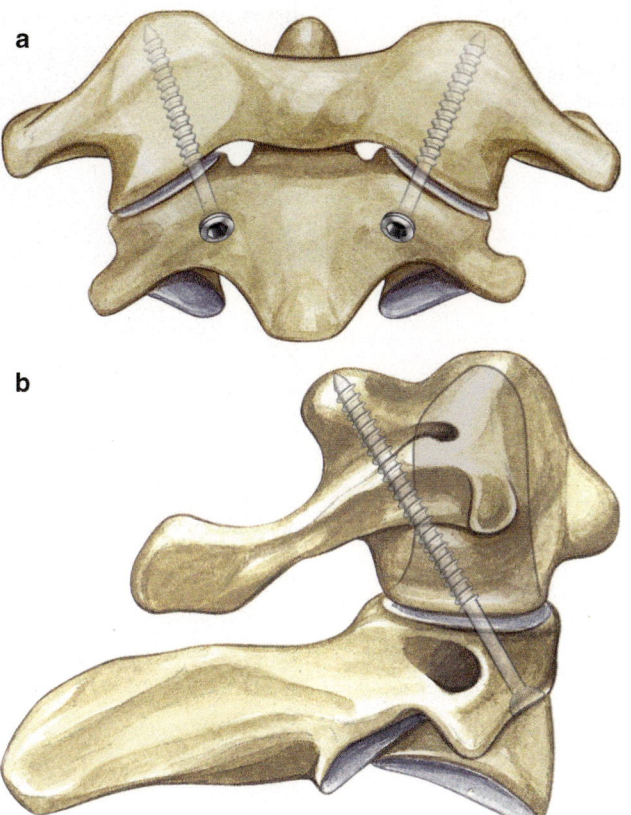

Fig. 24.3 Orientation of anterior transarticular screws relative to C1–2. (**a**) anteroposterior view (20°). (**b**) lateral view (30°)

able. It is possible to place these screws safely (see Fig. 24.4a–f).
- 3.5-mm cannulated fully threaded and short-thread screws can be used.
- Cannulated screws are inserted after predrilling of the subchondral bone of the joint surface of the lateral mass of C2 and C1.
- The screws are inserted using a cannulated screwdriver. Note: Observe the insertion of the cannulated screws on the lateral image intensifier to ensure that the K-wire does not advance in an anterior direction.
- The ventral portions of the C1–2 joint are decorticated, and spongiosa is applied (arthrodesis).

24.7   Tips and Tricks

- Do not go too far in a cranial direction and cross into the occipitoatlantal joint. If the screw trajectory is too lateral, there is a risk of injuring the vertebral artery.
- Odontoid and bilateral C1–2 transarticular screw fixation through a small anterior skin incision is an alternative

Fig. 24.4 Different CT images of the transarticular screws at C1–2 and the odontoid screw of an 82-year-old woman show an odontoid type II and C1 arc fracture. (**a**) Screws in the base of C2, (**b**) in the middle of the corpus C2, (**c**) the tip of the screws in the odontoid process and in the joint C1/C2, (**d**) lateral view of the screw in the right joint C1/C2, (**e**) odontoid screw, and (**f**) lateral view of the screw in the right joint C1/C2

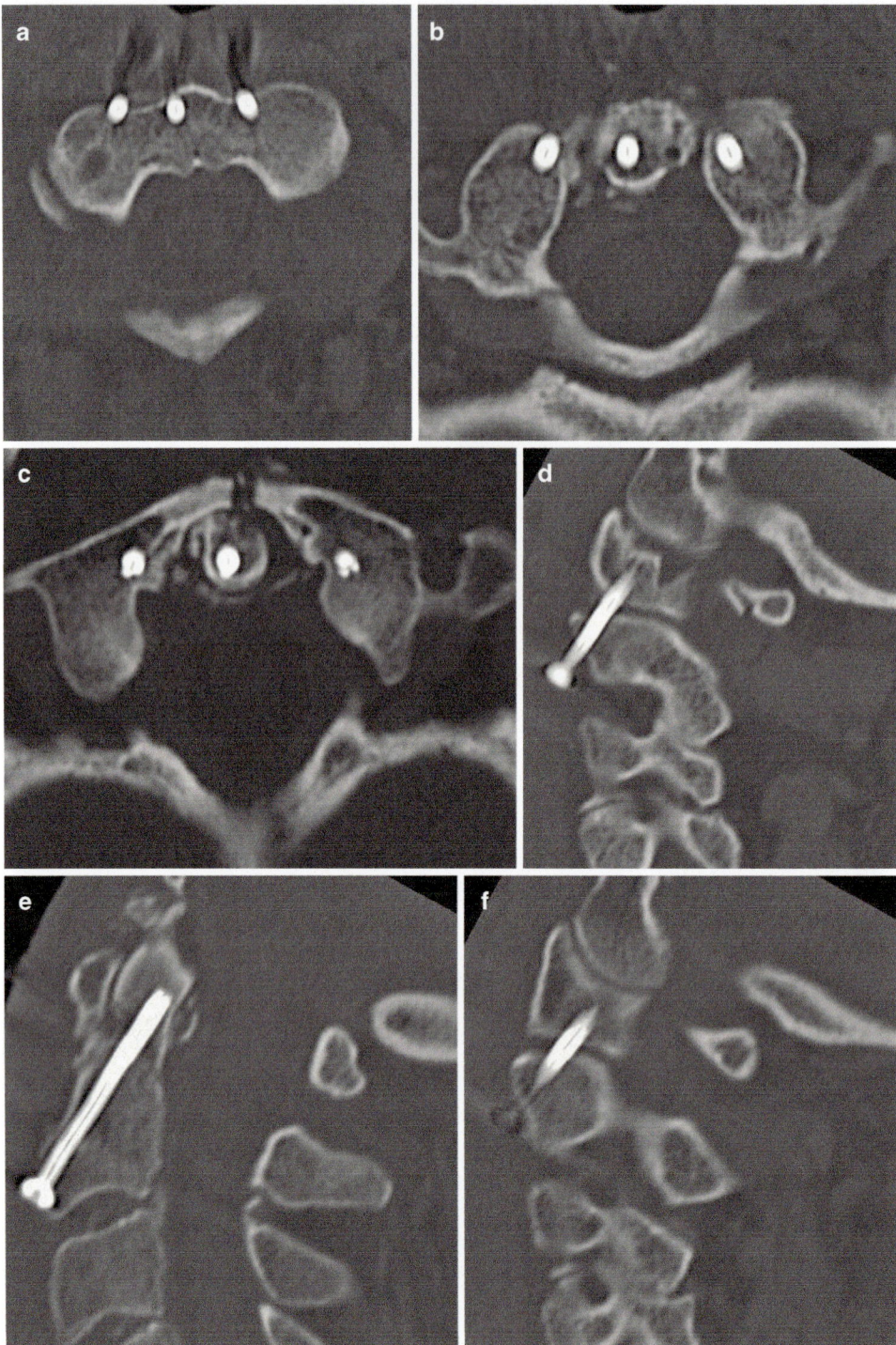

option for patients with odontoid fracture, worsened clinical state, and poor bone quality.
- This procedure is helpful in polytraumatized or elderly patients where surgery needs to be limited, but stability of the C1/C2 complex is absolutely essential.

References

1. Koller H, Kammermeier V, Ulbricht D, Assuncao A, Karolus S, van den Berg B, Holz U. Anterior retropharyngeal fixation C1–2 for stabilization of atlantoaxial instabilities: study of feasibility, technical description and preliminary results. Eur Spine J. 2006;15:1326–38.
2. Lu J, Ebrahim NA, Yonk H, et al. Anatomic considerations of anterior transarticular screw fixation for atlantoaxial instability. Point of view. Spine. 1998;23:1229–36.
3. Pepin JW, Boune RB, Hawkins RJ. Odontoid fractures with special references to the elderly patients. Clin Orthop Relat Res. 1985;193:178–83.
4. Reindl R, Sen M, Aebi M. Anterior instrumentation for traumatic C1-C2 instability. Spine. 2003;28:E329–33.
5. Dean Q, Jiefu S, Jie W, Yunxing S. Minimally invasive technique of triple anterior screw fixation for an acute combination atlas axis fracture: case report and literature review. Spinal Cord. 2009;48(2):174–7.
6. Kim SM, Lim TJ, Paterno J, Hwang TJ, et al. Biomechanical comparison of anterior and posterior stabilization methods in atlantoaxial instability. J Neurosurg. 2004;100(3 Suppl): 277–83.
7. Six E, Kelly DL. Technique for C1, C2 and C3 fixation in cases of odontoid fractures. Neurosurgery. 1981;8:374–7.
8. Vaccaro AR, Lehman AP, Ahlgren BD, Garfin SR. Anterior C1-C2 screw fixation and bony fusion through an anterior retropharyngeal approach. Orthopedics. 1999;22:1165–70.
9. Sen MK, Steffen T, Beckman L, et al. Atlantoaxial fusion using anterior transarticular screw fixation of C1-C2: technical innovation and biomechanical study. Eur Spine J. 2005;14: 512–8.

Transoral Resection of the Odontoid Process

25

Meic H. Schmidt and Uwe Vieweg

25.1 Introduction and Core Messages

The transoral approach to anteriorly placed lesions at the craniocervical junction is not new [1] but is still infrequently used by neurosurgeons for tumors in this region [2]. The anterior inferior aspect of the craniocervical junction constitutes the upper posterior wall of the oral cavity. The open oral cavity can therefore be used to access this region without disturbing the medulla.

25.2 Indications

- Spinal column tumor with neural compression
- Extradural metastatic tumor
- Irreducible subluxations
- Os odontoideum
- Rheumatoid pannus

25.3 Contraindications

- Inability to open the mouth widely for the transoral approach, that is, severe arthritis of the temporomandibular joints (TMJ)
- Intradural pathologies

M. H. Schmidt (✉)
Department of Neurosurgery, University of New Mexico, Albuquerque, NM, USA
e-mail: MHSchmidt@salud.unm.edu

U. Vieweg
Department of Conservative and Surgical Spine Therapy with Interdisciplinary Spinal Deformities Centre and Rummelsberg Sectional Center, Hospital Rummelsberg, Schwarzenbruck, Germany
e-mail: uwe.vieweg@sana.de

25.4 Technical Prerequisites

Fluoroscope, retractor system, long forceps, dissectors, and burrs are technical prerequisites. In general, any resection of the odontoid process results in instability. It is therefore most often performed in conjunction with posterior C1–2 fusion. Alternatively, the use of various screw systems and plating systems for anterior plating has been described [3].

25.5 Planning, Preparation, and Positioning

The transoral exposure of the clivus, atlas, and ventral aspect of C2 is commonly performed in our practice. After induction of general anesthesia, the patient is placed with the neck extended in the supine position. For the transoral approach, it is important to ensure that the patient can open his or her mouth sufficiently. This can frequently be a problem in patients with arthritic temporomandibular joints, which are common in rheumatoid patients. In such cases, the procedure can be modified to include transmandibular splitting, but this is not common. Regular intubation is performed, and we use the Spetzler–Sonntag retraction system to allow exposure of the oral cavity (Fig. 25.1). It is important to protect the teeth during the placement of this retractor. It is also important to protect the tongue since significant tongue swelling can occur if retraction is performed against the teeth. Some authors advocate nasal intubation, but we have found this unnecessary. Once the retractors are placed, the posterior pharynx is sufficiently exposed, and the C1 tubercle is palpated.

25.6 Operating Technique

25.6.1 Approach

- The surgical site is infiltrated with lidocaine and epinephrine, and the midline is incised with a monopolar cautery,

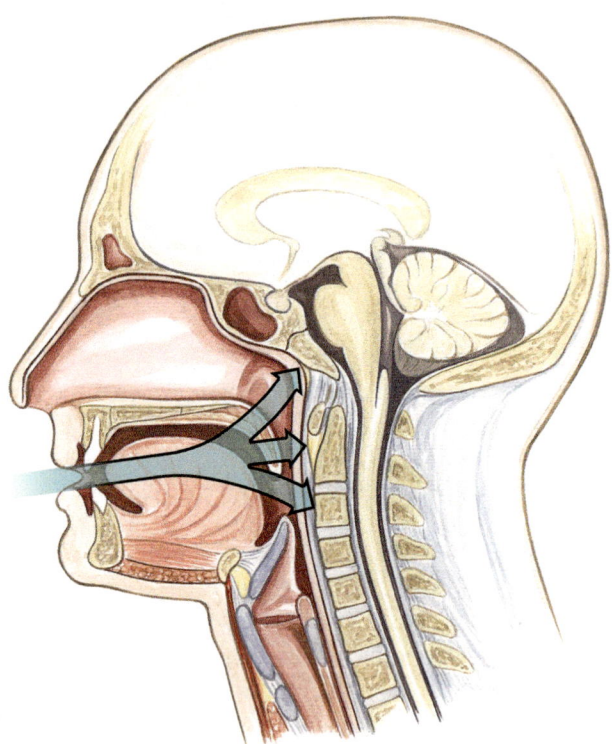

Fig. 25.1 Diagram of the upper cervical resections that can be performed cranially and caudally from a transoral approach

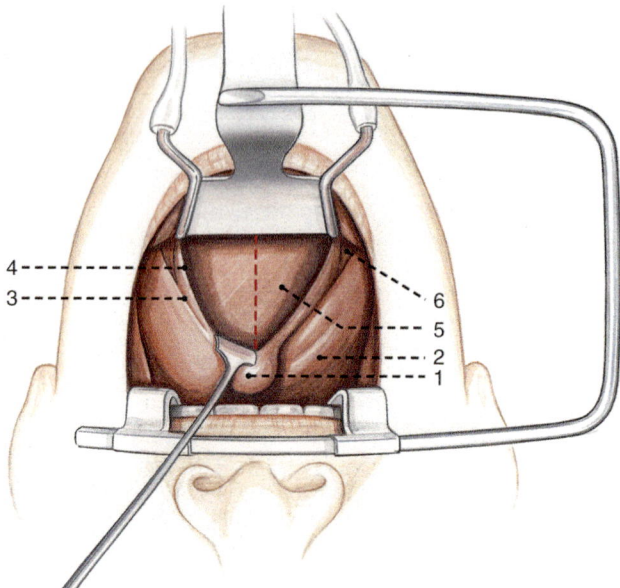

Fig. 25.2 Retraction of the soft palate with subsequent longitudinal incision of the dorsal wall of the pharynx (*1* Uvula, *2* palatum molle, *3* arcus palatoglossus, *4* arcus palatopharyngeus, *5* dorsal wall of pharynx with mucosa, *6* tonsilla palatina)

with the incision extending approximately 2–3 cm from the anterior arch of C1 to the bottom of C2.

- With this dissection, the bone is exposed, and the pharyngeal tissues are retracted laterally. This is greatly facilitated by placement of the retractor plate (see Figs. 25.2 and 25.3).
- Once the retractors are placed, we use the Midas Rex drill or remove the anterior aspect of the arch of C1.
- We then proceed with drilling of the C2 dens. It is important initially to preserve the outer shell of the C2 dens to prevent the soft tissues from falling into the surgical site.
- Once the C2 dens are eggshell thin, we remove the remaining tissues. This allows access for removal of the pannus in rheumatoid patients and decompression of the upper cervical canal.

25.6.2 Instrumentation (Additional)

- The transoral exposure of the posterior pharynx has been described by Schmelzle and Harms [4] for treatment of unstable Jefferson fractures.
- Reduction is achieved by placing the patient in traction. C1 and C2 are then exposed anteriorly (Fig. 25.4).
- Osteosynthesis is performed with a compression plate or a screw/rod system.

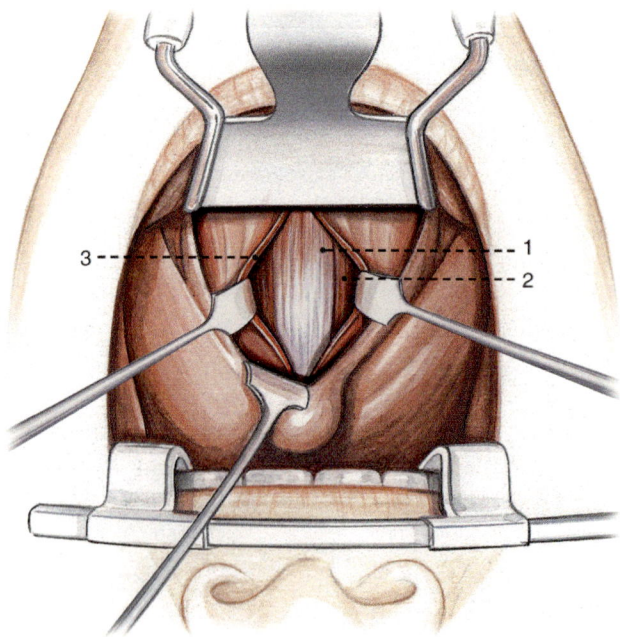

Fig. 25.3 After incision has been made in dorsal wall of pharynx (*1* longus colli muscle, *2* longus capitis muscle, *3* superior constrictor pharyngis muscle)

- Polyaxial screws are placed into both C1 lateral masses and then connected with a rod. This allows for preservation of the C1–2 motion segment in cases with Jefferson fractures [5].

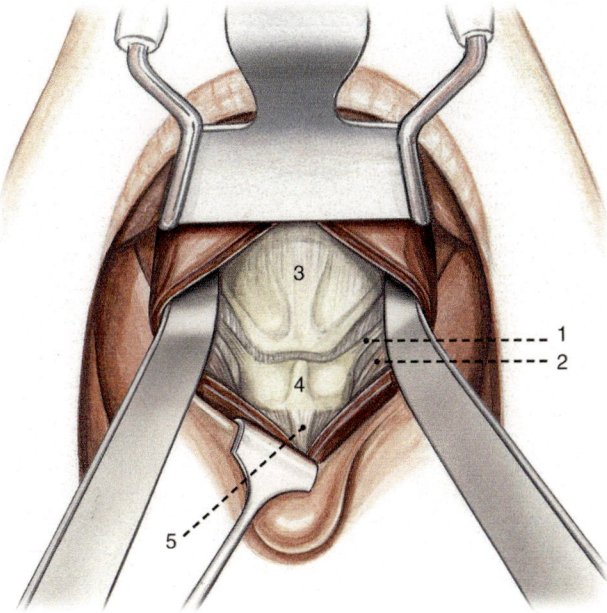

Fig. 25.4 Atlas and axis (*1* longus colli muscle, *2* longus capitis muscle, *3* corpus axis, *4* tuberculum anterius atlantis, *5* membrana atlanto-occipitalis anterior)

25.7   Tips and Tricks

- Reconstruction of the dens using a C2 prosthesis, as described by Jeszenszky et al. [6].
- Additional dorsal instrumentation and fusion of C1–C3.
- Primary dorsal instrumentation with decompression may also be considered for patients with rheumatoid arthritis.

References

1. Hall JE, Dennis F, Murray J. Exposure of the upper cervical spine for spinal decompression by mandible and tongue-splitting approach. J Bone Joint Surg Am. 1977;59A:121.
2. Russo A, Albanese E, Quiroga M, et al. Submandibular approach to the C2–3 disc level: microsurgical anatomy with clinical application. J Neurosurg Spine. 2009;10:380–9.
3. Vender JR, Harrison SJ, McDonnell DE. Fusion and instrumentation at C1–3 via the high anterior cervical approach. J Neurosurg. 2000;92:24–9.
4. Schmelzle R, Harms J. Craniocervical junction-diseases, diagnostic application of imaging procedures, surgical techniques. Fortschr Kiefer Gesichtschir. 1987;32:206–8.
5. Ruf M, Melcher R, Harms J. Transoral reduction and osteosynthesis C1 as a function-preserving option in the treatment of unstable Jefferson fractures. Spine. 2004;29:823–7.
6. Jeszenszky D, Harms J, Hadasch R, et al. C2 prosthesis allowing optimal stabilisation after C2 resection following destructive lesions. Eur Spine J. 1999;8(Suppl 1):S40.

Cervical Tong Extension and the Halo Fixator

26

Uwe Vieweg, Pia Borgas, and Kiril Mladenov

26.1 Introduction and Core Messages

The cervical tong (*Crutchfield, Gardner-Wells, Vinke*) has two slats, which pin the bony skull, in order to perform an extension procedure such as a luxation of the upper cervical spine, or in preparation for scoliosis operations. Skull tongs such as cone calipers are used in more severe cervical injuries. A halo ring may be indicated as an alternative to cervical tongs. Both instruments are inserted into the skull such that weighted traction can be applied to the cervical spine. A halo-ring with a vest forms a *halo fixator*. This can be used to immobilize the cervical spine after fractures and instabilities (injuries, infections), but also for spinal extension treatment before surgically correcting spinal deformations. In these situations, the halo-ring can either be used in combination with a halo-cast or a halo-vest. Extension techniques including the *halo-gravitation-extension or halo-pelvic-apparatus* are especially useful for the correction of spinal deformations. Furthermore, the halo fixator is largely used for pre-surgical extension treatments in patients with paralytic scoliosis, as well as temporary retention in patients who have undergone complex spine deformity operations after ventral release or mobilized osteotomies.

U. Vieweg (✉)
Department of Conservative and Surgical Spine Therapy with Interdisciplinary Spinal Deformities Centre and Rummelsberg Sectional Center, Hospital Rummelsberg, Schwarzenbruck, Germany
e-mail: uwe.vieweg@sana.de

P. Borgas
Faculty of Medical Sciences, University College London, London, UK

K. Mladenov
Department of Pediatric Orthopedic Surgery, AKK Altonaer Children's Hospital, Hamburg, Germany

26.2 Indications and Contraindications of Cervical Tong and Halo Fixator

The *cervical tong* has two slats, which pin the bony skull, in order to perform an extension, such as a luxation of the upper cervical spine, or in preparation for scoliosis surgery (see Fig. 26.1). Skull tongs such as cone calipers are used in more severe cervical injuries. Alfred S. Taylor first used such traction devices and skull-based traction in 1929 for cervical fractures and spinal injuries [1]. Introduced in 1973 by J. Gardner, the Gardner–Welss Tong (GWT) has become a popular method of spinal traction [2]. Different apparatus have been utilized for skeletal traction, including Crutchfield's caliber, Cone's caliber, Bluckburn's caliber, and halo traction [2, 3]. For traumatic lesions of the cervical spinal cord, the cervical tong allows for a dosed, temporary extension while the patient is on bed rest, with the possibility to reposition the spine. However, complete healing is not possible. During longer term bed rest, patients are at risk of cardiorespiratory, cerebrovascular, or thromboembolic complications. Complex mal-alignments cannot be restored using the cervical tong. It is also not possible to mobilize the patient into a standing position. Perry and Nickel therefore described the *halo fixator* in 1959 [4]. A halo system is a construction of a ring, pins, a superstructure and a vest (see Figs. 26.3 and 26.7). The halo ring is fixed to the skull with pins and is the anchor point for the superstructure at the head. The skull pins are fastened tight enough such that the halo ring is stabilized, as they are the main fixation points for the ring to the head. The vest is connected to the ring by the superstructure, which forms a rigid construction to immobilize the neck. The vest extends to the waist and is designed to fit comfortably and tightly around the body to maintain the initial alignment of the spine [5, 6]. The first application of the device was for patients for whom poliomyelitis had led to paralysis or the head and neck musculature, with consequent loss of head control. In the first version of the halo fixator, the ring was combined with a plaster cast. Through the application of modern synthetic materials and carbon rods, an MRI examination with the device is now possible. The device can be used to compress, distract, and

U. Vieweg, F. Grochulla (eds.), *Manual of Spine Surgery*, https://doi.org/10.1007/978-3-662-64062-3_26

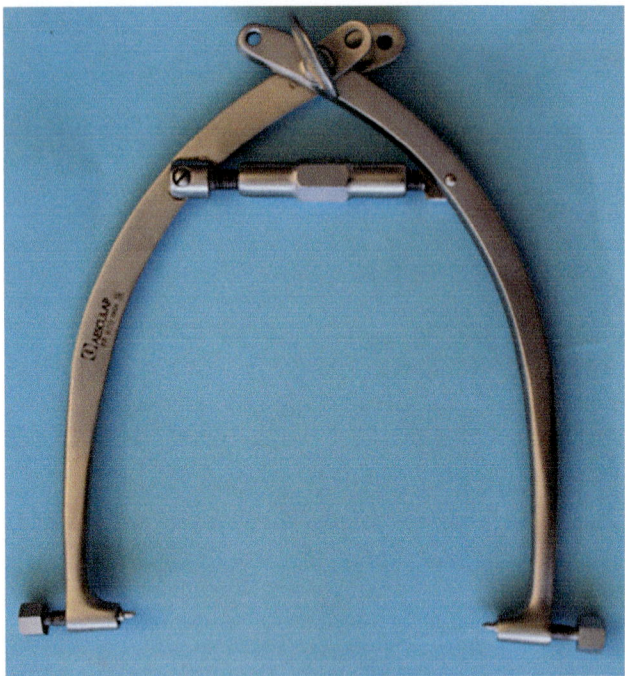

Fig. 26.1 Cervical traction tong (Aesculap AG, Tuttlingen, Germany) for extension of the neck vertebral, large size, pins adjustable hence not initial drilling

move the spine. The external halo fixator therefore offers an improvement to the cervical tong [5–8]. The disadvantage of the halo fixator however is that patients are restricted at home. Assistance with bodily hygienic care, as well as dietary intake is required, and the halo vest also posits an enormous psychiatric burden for patients. To protect the lining of the halo vest from moisture, the upper body may only be cleaned using a wet washcloth. One focus of application however remains the temporary immobilization and extension during a two-sided approach, after an upstream release or a mobilizing osteotomy, as part of complex corrective spinal interventions. However, the introduction of modern spinal osteosynthesis procedures has made the application of the halo fixator uncommon. Before rigid internal fixation methods were introduced and became more commonly used, the halo fixator was used as the first-line treatment of choice to stabilize the cervical spine for many cervical injuries [5].

The indications and contraindications for halo vest, halo-, and cervical tong extensions are largely identical. The indications are [3, 5, 6, 9–12]

- Injuries of the cervical spine,
- Temporary immobilization for patients with tumors and infections,
- Halo extension before or between operative spinal correction procedures,
- Pre-surgical extension of paralytic scoliosis, and
- Temporary extension after ventral release.

The contraindications are [7–9, 12–14]:

- Cranial fractures and intracranial injuries,
- Soft tissue infections of the skull,
- Children <3 years,
- Thorax injuries, and
- Paraplegia with respiratory muscle impairments.

Halo use in elderly patients remains controversial as recent evidence demonstrated extremely high mortality rates in patients 79 years and older [7, 8].

26.3 Cervical Tong Extension

26.3.1 Technical Prerequisites

Several different tongs are in common use. They always consist of a stainless steel or graphite body with two sharp-tipped titanium pins; one attached at each end. Their material make-up makes them compatible with magnetic resonance imaging (MRI). The pins are attached on each side of the skull to its outer table. The commonly used cervical tongs include the Crutchfield (small size, medium, large), Gardner–Wells, and Vinke tongs [1, 9, 15, 16]. The Vinke tongs are placed on the parietal bones, near the widest transverse diameter of the skull. The Gardner–Wells tongs are inserted slightly above the patient's ears. Alternative types include the Bremer Universal and Trippi–Wells tongs.

26.3.2 Technique

- Place the patient in the bed. Shave the patient's hair above the ear region.
- Infiltrate the skin with a local anesthetic.
- Avoid the temporal artery.
- Make a small incision superior to the ear in line with the auditory meatus (see Fig. 26.2a).
- The clamp is adapted to the cranial circumference of the patient with this set screw. After the pins have been firmly anchored in the cranial bone, the clamp is turned on with a wrench.
- Screw in the pin until it perforates the outer skull table.
- Tie the tong to a rope and attach weights (see Fig. 26.2b, c).

26.3.3 Direction of Traction and Calculated Weight

- Continuous traction is provided by weights applied to the external cervical fixation device via a rope and pulley system.

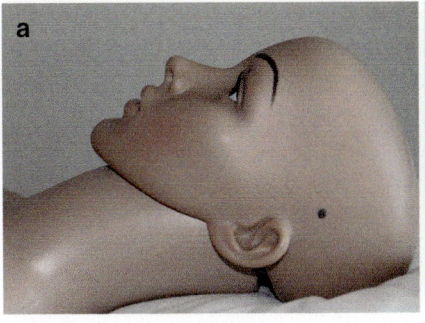
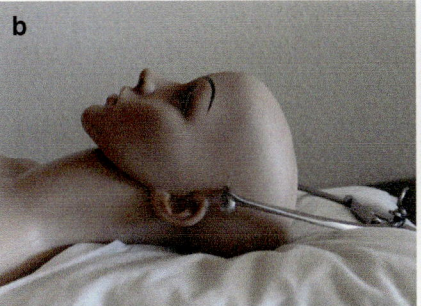
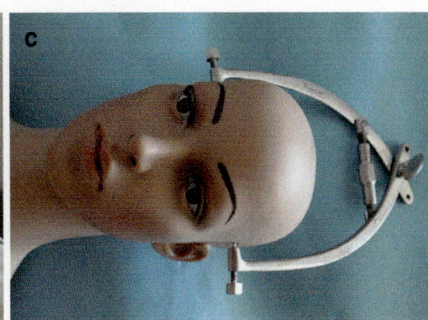

Fig. 26.2 (**a–c**) The fixation point for the pins is approximately 2 cm above the porus acusticus externus (**a**) before installation of the cervical tong; (**b** and **c**) after installation of the cervical tong

- Calculate the force required: *2.5 kg for the head and 1/2 kg per vertebra.*
- Adjust the height of the pulley, with the bed in anti-Trendelenburg position. Then apply the weights.
- Start with 6 kg and increase by 1 kg every 6 h until a maximum weight of 15 kg has been reached.
- Add the weights gradually while proceeding with radiographic imaging to determine reduction.
- The direction of extension must be in line with the auditory meatus.

26.3.4 Complications of Cervical Tong Extension

Possible complications of a cervical traction include bleeding of the temporal artery, pressure sores on the skull (this is preventable by avoiding a downward vector to the rope), skin sepsis or sepsis due to a subdural abscess, declining neurological status, and a squint due to fall out of the sixth cranial nerve [9, 10, 15, 16]. Saleh et al. [3] reported in a systematic literature review a 37.5% incidence rate of minor complications with the usage of a Gardner–Wells tongs which includes pin loosening, asymptomatical pin positioning, and superficial infections. Various cases reported more serious complications including perforation of the skull brain, brain abscesses, and neurovascular damage.

26.4 Halo Fixator

26.4.1 Technical Prerequisites

A halo fixator (see Figs. 26.3 and 26.7) may be required in adults or children. Different companies provide halo fixators (e.g., Bremer ACE Halo System; Johnson and Johnson Halo ring with vest; DAONSA, ReSolve Halo Vest; OSSUR ORTHOTICS, etc.). Some of these have special skull pins, which utilize a unique cutting head to significantly reduce bone destruction. Importantly, both halo vest and ring have to be

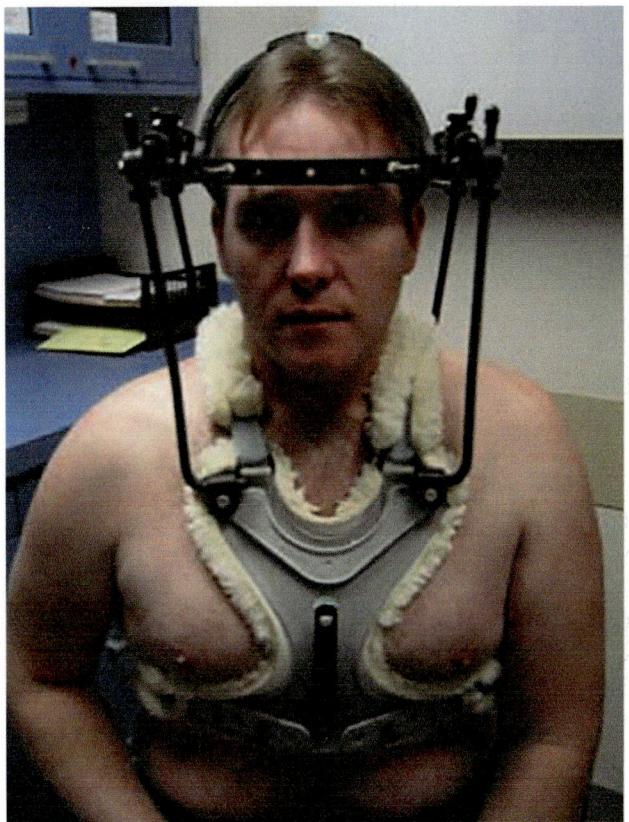

Fig. 26.3 A patient with a halo vest

sized prior to the procedure. The optimal ring size is 1–2 cm greater than the circumference of the patient's head [17]. Different variables influence the stability and comfort of the construct, as well as the complication rate. These variables include the pin location and the design of the pin, ring, and vest [2, 5, 13, 18]. The interaction site between pin and bone is the most likely and common location at which the halo fixator may fail. Ideally, the pin should be positioned 0.5 cm proximal to the eyebrow. Pins that were instead positioned 1 and 1.5 cm proximal were 10% and 30% less stable, respectively [18]. Thus, the fixation strength and pin–bone relationship are determined by the angle at which the pin contacts the bone [3, 5, 18]. Very important is the "safe zone" for placement of halo-fixator pins. Anterior pins are placed anterolaterally, approximately 1 cm above the orbital ring below the equator (area of widest circumferences) of the skull (see Figs. 26.4, 26.5 and 26.6).

26.4.2 Technique

- Halo traction is a two-stage procedure; first, attach the halo ring to the skull, subsequently apply the body cast and suspension construction to the ring (see Figs. 26.4, 26.5 and 26.6).
- In conscious patients, the halo ring can be placed under local anesthesia. Closed reductions, especially, should only be performed in conscious patients.
- Gloves should be worn and antiseptic swabs or a disinfectant used to clean the pin insertion areas. The skin and periosteal is then infiltrated with a local anesthetic.
- Stabilizing plates hold the ring in place. The optimal position of the ring is such that its lower margin lies just above the ears and approximately 0.5 cm above the eyebrows. It should be positioned inferior to the skull's equator (see Figs. 26.4, 26.5 and 26.6).
- When applying the ring, the patient should be sitting or in a supine position.
- While inserting the screws into the skull, the patient's eyelids should remain closed.

- Insert the anterior pins in the shallow groove on the forehead between the supraorbital ridges and frontal protuberances [17]. Note that four screws are required for adults, while six to eight are necessary for children.
- Screw the threaded skull pins into the skull's lamina externa with defined torque but without perforating the lamina interna.

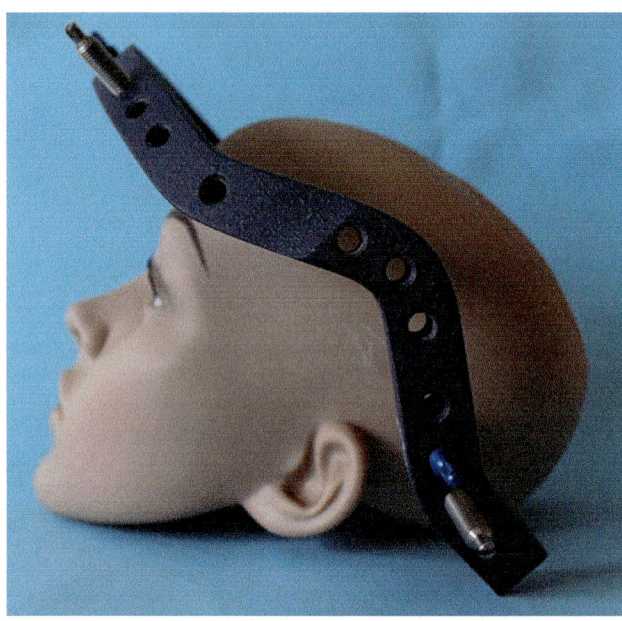

Fig. 26.5 With use of tongs, orient V over ears to fit around base of tong otherwise invert V to allow access to ears

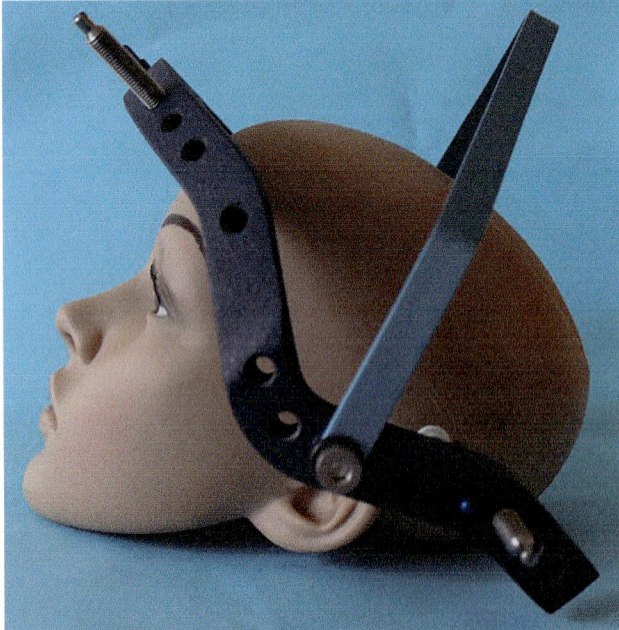

Fig. 26.4 The appropriate halo ring is placed with temporary positioning stabilization pins. The ring should allow 1–2 cm clearance from the skull. Care should be taken to prevent contact between the halo ring and the ears

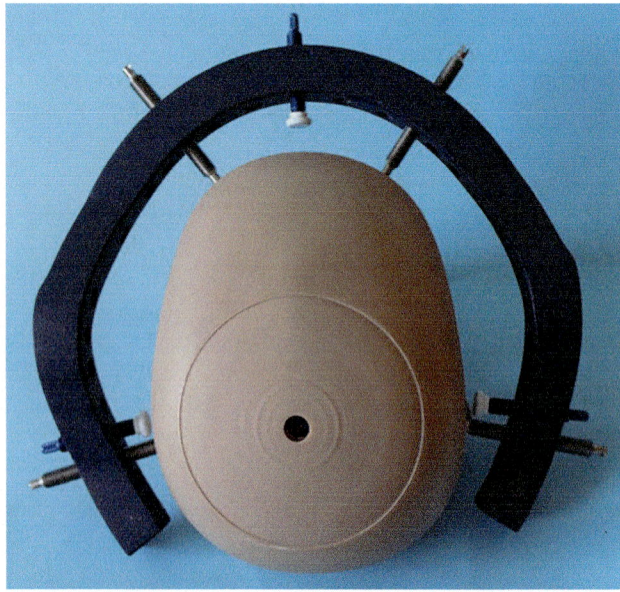

Fig. 26.6 Anterior screws are inserted 1 cm superior to the lateral 1/3 of the eyebrows. Initially, the permanent screws are tightened by hand, followed by the use of a torque driver. Pins opposite each other are tightened simultaneously

- Tighten the permanent screws by hand and subsequently tighten them further using a torque screwdriver. Tighten the diagonally opposing screws successively and simultaneously; this avoids pins from drifting and ensures greater stability.
- Remove the positioning pins and apply the lock nuts. These should be finger-tightened.
- Lastly, attach the halo ring to the vest or body cast, or apply an extension device (see Figs. 26.7 and 26.8) [17].

26.4.3 Post-Operative Care

The following are part of the post-operative care
- Daily cleaning of screw sites.
- Regular clinical observation of the patient's neurological status.
- A slow increase in distraction at the adjustable brace parts.
- A lateral radiograph of the cervical spine after application of the halo fixator, as well as during the treatment process.
- Modifying items of clothing to accommodate the brace; a larger clothing size may be required such that the neck opening is large enough to fit over the brace.
- Re-torqueing screws after 24 h, 3–4 days and then weekly until the halo is removed. This is because screws will loosen with time.

26.4.4 Removal of the Halo System

Patients must typically wear their halo for 12 weeks depending on the treatment. Upon removal of the halo system, patients are required to wear a collar for a period of weeks. Removal of the system is accompanied by an adjustment and balancing period, similar to when the halo was first applied. Since the neck has been held inactive for the treatment duration, patients may experience aching of the neck, back, and shoulders.

26.4.5 Complications of Halo Fixator

Complications are minor and include pin loosening, localized infections, periorbital oedema, superficial pressure sores, and unsightly scars. Major complications may include pin penetration, osteomyelitis, subdural abscesses, nerve palsies, fracture overdistraction, and persistent instability. However, complications can be well avoided by carefully placing the pins during the procedure, as well as participat-

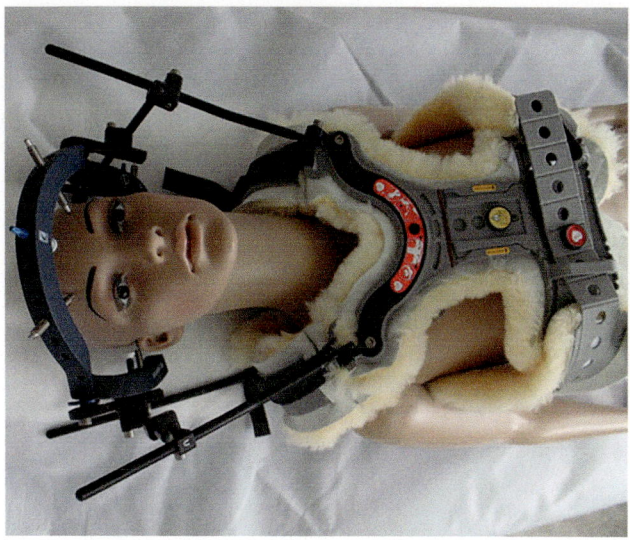

Fig. 26.7 The complete Halo fixator

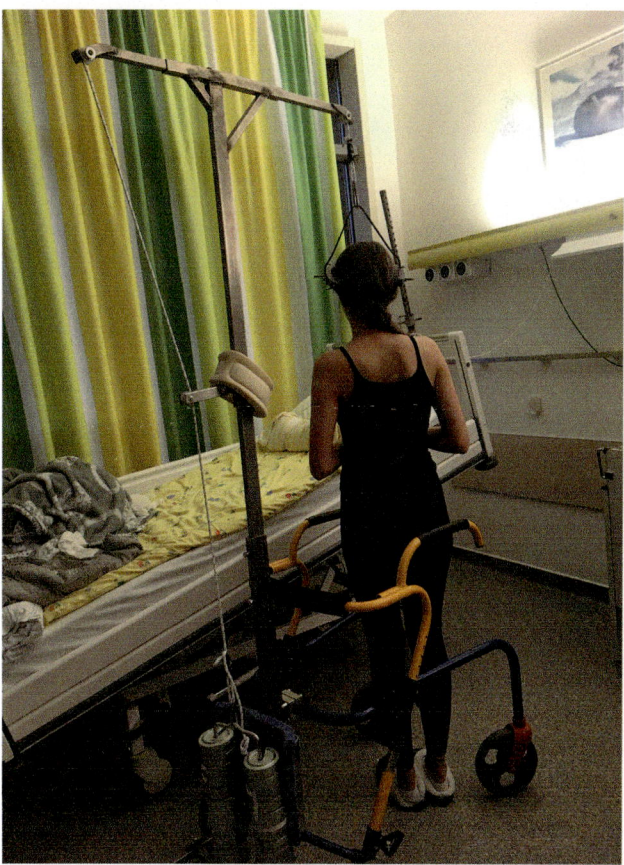

Fig. 26.8 Halo extension for the postoperative correction of a thoracolumbar scoliosis in standing position

ing in thorough post-operative care at the pin sites. In elderly patients, respiratory distress and other more life-threatening complications have been reported at a more concerning rate [5, 13, 19, 20].

References

1. Krag MH, Beynnon BD. A new halo-vest: rationale, design and biomechanical comparison to standard halo-vest designs. Spine. 1988;13:228–35.
2. Gardner WJ. The principle of spring-loading points for cervical traction: technical note. J Neurosurg. 1973;39:543–4.
3. Saleh H, Yohe N, Razi A, et al. Efficacy and complications of the use of Gardner-Wells tongs: a systematic review. J Spine Surg. 2018;4:123–9.
4. Perry J, Nickel VL. Total cervical-spine fusion for neck paralysis. J Bone Joint Surg Am. 1959;41:37–60.
5. Bono CM. The halo fixateur. J Am Acad Orthop Surg. 2007;15:728–37.
6. Grundy DJ. Skull traction and its complications. Injury. 1983;15:173–7.
7. Lopes A, Andrade A, Silva I, et al. Brain abscess after halo fixation for cervical spine. World Neurosurg. 2017;104:1047.e7–11.
8. Majercik S, Tashijan RZ, Biffl WL, et al. Halo vest immobilization in the elderly: a death sentence? J Trauma. 2005;59:350–6.
9. Glaser JA, Whitehill R, Stamp WG, Jane JA. Complications associated with the halo-vest. A review of 245 cases. J Neurosurg. 1986;65:762–9.
10. Loeser JD. History of skeletal traction in the treatment of cervical spine injuries. J Neurosurg. 1970;33:54–9.
11. Püschel K, Lignitz E, Saukko P, et al. Iatrogenic complications of extension treatment of injuries of the cervical vertebrae using Crutchfield tongs. Unfallchirurg. 1986;89:42–6. [In German].
12. Schulze W, Esenwein SA, Müller EJ, et al. Complications in the use of the halo fixator. Zentralbl Neurochir. 2001;62:2–9. [In German].
13. Anderson PA, Budorick TE, Easton KB, et al. Failure of halo vest to prevent in vivo motion with injured cervical spines. Spine. 1991;16:501–5.
14. Blauth M, Lange UF, Knop C, Bastian L. Spinal fractures in the elderly and their treatment. Orthopade. 2000;29:302–17. [In German].
15. Barsoum WK, Mayerson J, Bell GR. Cranial nerve palsy as a complication of operative traction. Spine. 1999;24:585–6.
16. Fraunhoffer M. Transverse syndrome following extension of a dislocation of the cervical spine with a Crutchfield bracket. Aktuelle Traumatol. 1986;16:164–6. [In German].
17. Schmolke S, Gosse F. The halo-fixateur. Oper Orthop Traumatol. 2008;20:3–12. [In German].
18. Ballock RT, Lee TQ, Triggs KJ, et al. The effect of pin location on the rigidity of the halo pin bone interface. Neurosurgery. 1990;26:238–41.
19. Garfin SR, Botte MJ, Waters RL, Nickel VL. Complications in the use of the halo fixation device. J Bone Joint Surg Am. 1989;68:320–5.
20. Hähnel H, Zippel H. Experiences with the external fixation of the cervical spine with the Halo-Yoke-System. Z Orthop. 1986;124:299–308. [In German].

Suggested Reading

Copley LA, Pepe MD, Tan V, et al. A comparison of various angles of halo pin insertion in an immature skull model. Spine. 1999;24:1777–80.

Hayes VM, Silber JS, Siddiqi FM, et al. Complications of halo fixation of the cervical spine. Am J Orthop (Belle Mead NJ). 2005;34:271–6.

Nickel VL, et al. The halo. A spinal skeletal traction fixation device. J Bone Joint Surg Am. 1969;50:1400–9.

Papagelopoulos PJ, et al. Halo pin intracranial penetration and epidural abscess in a patient with a previous cranioplasty: case report and review of the literature. Spine. 2001;26:463–7.

Prothmann KH, et al. An interesting case: inflammatory cerebral complications after Crutchfield-extension. Zentralbl Chir. 1989;114:1025–30. [In German].

Rinella A, Lenke L, Whitaker C, et al. Perioperative halo-gravity traction in the treatment of severe scoliosis and kyphosis. Spine. 2001;30:475–82.

Strohm PC, Muller CHA, Kostler W, et al. Halo fixator vest—indications and complications. Zentralbl Chir. 2007;132:54–9. [In German].

Vieweg U, Schultheiss R. A review of halo vest treatment of upper cervical spine injuries. Arch Orthop Trauma Surg. 2001;121:50–5.

Voor MJ, Khalily C. Halo pin loosening: a biomechanical comparison of experimental and conventional designs. J Biomech. 1998;31:397–400.

Weigel K, Wilms H. Cranial complications in extension therapy of cervical fractures. Riechert's modification of extension therapy. Chirurg. 1978;49:374–6. [In German].

Part III

Anterior Cervical Spine

Overview of Surgical Techniques and Implants

27

Tobias Pitzen, Jörg Drumm, Gregor Ostrowski, and Michael Ruf

27.1 Introduction and Core Message

This is a short overview on different techniques and implants for anterior decompression and fixation for the cervical spine. Degenerative disc diseases, ossifications of the posterior longitudinal ligament, vertebral body tumours, spondylodiscitis, and vertebral body compression fractures are amongst the most frequent cervical spine pathologies a spine surgeon has to deal with. All these are located within the anterior aspect of the cervical spine—which are the vertebral bodies and the discs. Thus, anterior cervical spine techniques as anterior decompression, fixation, and anterior possibilities of realignment are amongst the most popular and necessary ones within the armamentarium of a spine surgeon. Within this chapter, we will give a very short overview on different techniques for anterior decompression, fixation, and realignment within the cervical spine. Moreover, different anterior implants for dynamic and permanent osseous fixation, distributed by different companies are presented.

27.2 Approaches

The standard approach for anterior cervical spine C3–C7/T1 procedure is an antero-lateral approach as described by Cloward. Description here is slightly modified according to the authors experience and spreaders used. Take care, that the incision usually crosses the midline by 1 cm and reaches the medial edge of the sternocleidomastoid muscle. The incision should be placed above the centre of the lesion. An oblique incision is preferred by the authors, by careful subcutaneous/subfascial spreading even three or more segments can be reached. Once the superficial layer of the fascia has been split, the approach is medial to the sternocleidomastoid muscle, cranial or caudal to the omohyoid muscle and medial to the carotid artery to the anterior aspect of the spine that is reached between the left and right longus colli muscle. Self-holding sharp retractors are placed under the longus colli muscles, blunt retractors are used to spread the wound in cranio-caudal direction. A longitudinal incision is used, if the cervicothoracic junction has to be exposed. Now, the incision starts at the medial aspect of the caudal part of the sternocleidomastoid muscle and reaches the manubrium at its midline and is elongated 4–5 cm to its caudal aspect. Using blunt dissection, the soft tissue at the backside of the manubrium is detached and the manubrium is split using a chisel or saw. If unfamiliar, ask a thoracic surgeon for help. To the authors' opinion and experience, percutaneous and endoscopic approaches do not have any importance for anterior cervical spine surgery.

27.2.1 Tips and Tricks

1. Preferred side of the approach—there has been a long debate about this aspect. However, just two aspects dictate the side of the approach. (1) If there is a RLN palsy, choose the side of the palsy for approach. (2) If surgery is due to a tumour with extravertebral soft tissue mass, chose this side for approach.
2. To prevent RLN palsy, ask the anaesthetist to reduce cuff pressure after final placing of your retractors. This will reduce both dysphagia and incidence of RLN palsy.
3. If the patient had a surgical procedure at the anterior aspect of the spine before, check for RLN palsy. This is usually performed in the best way by laryngoscopy. Hoarseness must not be clinically evident!

T. Pitzen (✉)
Center for Spine Surgery, Orthopedics, and Traumatology, SRH Klinikum Karlsbad-Langensteinbach, Karlsbad, Germany
e-mail: tobias.pitzen@wkg.srh.de

J. Drumm · G. Ostrowski · M. Ruf
Center for Spine Surgery, SRH Klinikum Karlsbad-Langensteinbach, Karlsbad, Germany

© Springer-Verlag GmbH Germany 2023
U. Vieweg, F. Grochulla (eds.), *Manual of Spine Surgery*, https://doi.org/10.1007/978-3-662-64062-3_27

27.3 Techniques for Decompression

27.3.1 Uncoforaminotomy

This is a technique that may be used for anterior lateral decompression within the cervical spine for the indication of soft disc prolapse or spondylosis that compress a root. The main advantage is that the main parts of the disc are spared, range of motion is probably not affected significantly, no implants are necessary. However, the technique is not very easy to learn and take care of the vertebral artery that is pretty close to your high speed drill.

27.3.2 Discectomy

The technique of cervical spine discectomy is the basic one for anterior cervical spine decompression. No matter, if a one or more level discectomy or a one or more level vertebral body resection, you usually start by performing a cervical spine discectomy via anterior approach. Following anterior approach and placing of the retractor and spreading system, the anterior longitudinal ligament must be incised and removed with the disc by means of curettes and rongeurs. The authors prefer to remove the lateral aspects of the disc towards the uncus using a 4 mm Kerrison (Take care: the vertebral artery is very close here!) and to remove the anterior rim of the superior vertebra using a size 4 Kerrison. The bone chips taken this way are used to fill a cage. A cylindrical burr may be used to perform a rectangular shape of the disc space; a round burr is used to remove posterior osteophytes in the presence of an intact posterior ligament (Fig. 27.1). Alternatively, these spurs may be removed after resection of the posterior longitudinal ligament. Again, these bone chips may or even should be taken to fill a cervical spine fusion cage. When the disc is removed, you may try to recline the head and thus the c-spine by changing the position of the patient's neck and head on the head–neck rest. This is an important step for anterior realignment.

27.3.2.1 Tips and Tricks

1. The dura should be exposed, where its encroachment is less pronounced. This may reduce the risk of thecal sac perforation and chord contusion. However, in the presence of a free disc fragment (sequester), remove this first! Usually, the dura is apparent after this manoeuver.
2. In case of far lateral osteophyte, compressing the root, an uncoforaminotomy may be necessary. To do this, check the course of the vessel before surgery starts. Start surgery as usual, decompress the root. Place a cottonoid

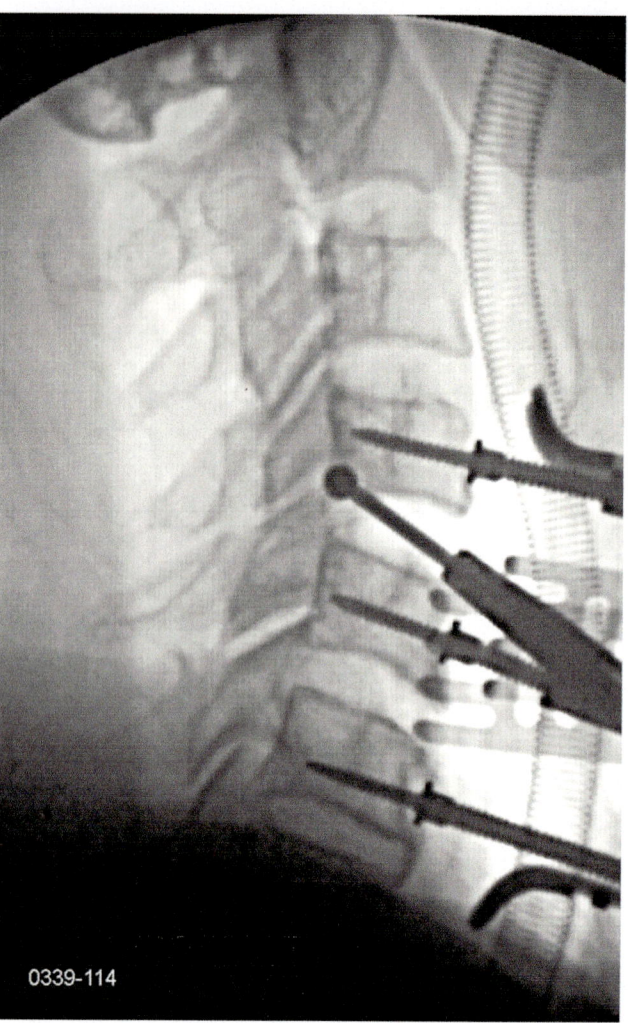

0339-114

Fig. 27.1 Lateral x-ray intraoperatively. A round burr is used to remove posterior osteophtyes

upon the root, then remove the anterior wall of the transverse foramen. Localize the vessel, place a penfield N 2 medial to the vessel to protect it. Then remove the uncus using a small chisel, take the fragment out. The cottonoid will protect the root during this manoeuver. Figure 27.2 is an example of a coronal CAT scan reconstruction following a left-sided uncoforaminotomy combined with cage insertion and anterior plating.

27.4 Vertebral Body Resection

Before a vertebral body resection is performed, all discs adjacent to the vertebral body should be removed as described above. The thecal sac should be exposed within

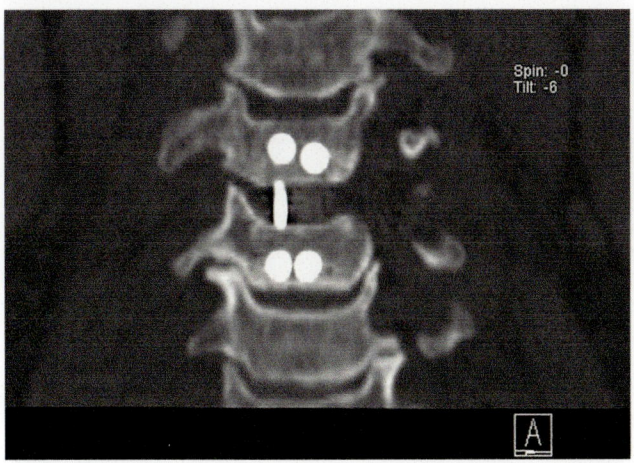

Fig. 27.2 Coronal CAT scan reconstruction following a left-sided uncoforaminotomy combined with cage insertion and anterior plating

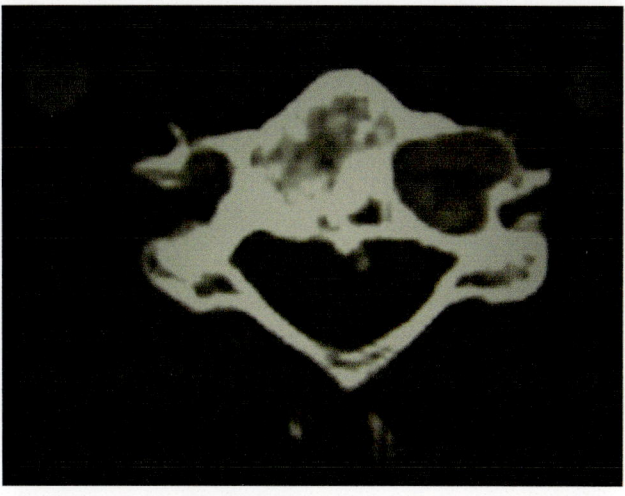

Fig. 27.3 Transverse CAT scan through a vertebral body with a VA looped into the vertebral body

the segment where spinal encroachment is least. Vertebral body resection starts using big size rongeurs. Again, the bone is taken to fill a cage. 8 mm of the vertebral body at each side of the midline are removed for median resection of a vertebral body—which is sufficient for placing a cage for vertebral body replacement. Use sharp drills to remove the posterior cortical shell down to the soft parts of the posterior longitudinal ligament. Resection of this may be performed finally using a size 2 Kerrison; the cuts are performed at the most lateral parts of the ligament. Finally, the ligament may be removed en bloc.

27.4.1 Tips and Tricks

1. Bone from the vertebral body resection—except in tumour and spondylitis cases—is ideal to fill into a VBR cage. Do so, do not use iliac crest in such cases.
2. Severe bleedings from venous vessels during VBR procedures are best controlled using a 5–6 mm diameter diamond burr on a high speed drill. Do not irrigate (!) until it gets dusty and dry. Bleeding has stopped usually, then ask for irrigation. This is better than the use of bone wax, which will contaminate your local bone graft.
3. Arterial bleeding from the midline (!) indicates that you are close to the thecal sac, upon the cortical shell or PLL. Take even more care now!

4. In some cases, the VA may be looped into the vertebral body. Figure 27.3 shows such a rare case. Be sure, before VBR, that this is not the case!

27.5 Spondylectomy

The term *Spondylectomy* is derived from the greek words "*Spondylos*—vertebra" and "*tomi*—cut" and therefore means a complete removal of the vertebra. This is usually indicated in case of primary bone tumours or single metastasis. Usually, spondylectomy first requires a complete removal of the posterior structures. Via anterior approach, the discs are excised and lateral circumferential dissection is performed until the vertebra can be removed "en bloc". Due to the relationship of both VA to the cervical spine, a classic en bloc removal as known from the thoracic or lumbar spine is not possible at the cervical level. If, however, radical removal is necessary between C1 and C6, it must be planned using VA occlusion tests, VA unilateral resection, or bypass procedures. Ask radiologists, vascular surgeons, and even more experienced spine surgeons for help. At the level of C7/T1, the VA are usually outside the spine (Fig. 27.4). Thus, a spondylectomy may be performed here in a two stage procedure: first remove the posterior parts, then the vertebral body en bloc. Figure 27.5 is an example of this. Figure 27.6 shows the sagittal MRI of the lesion before surgery, Fig. 27.7 the lateral x-ray after surgery.

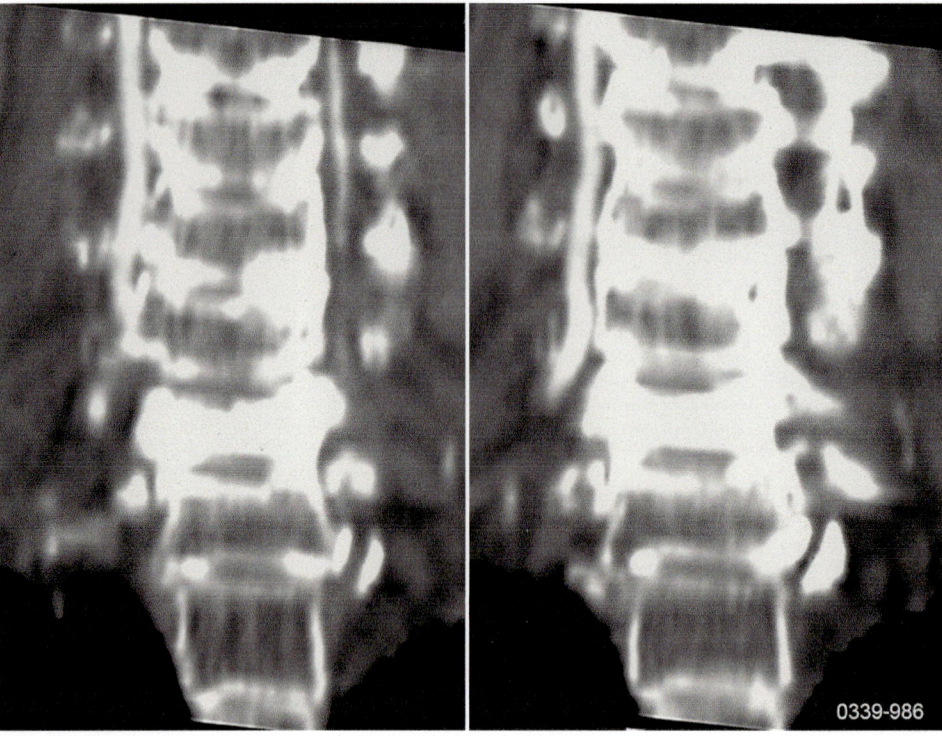

Fig. 27.4 Coronal CAT scan reconstruction of a patient with a C7 metastasis of a tonsillar carcinoma. At the level of C7, the VA are usually outside the spine

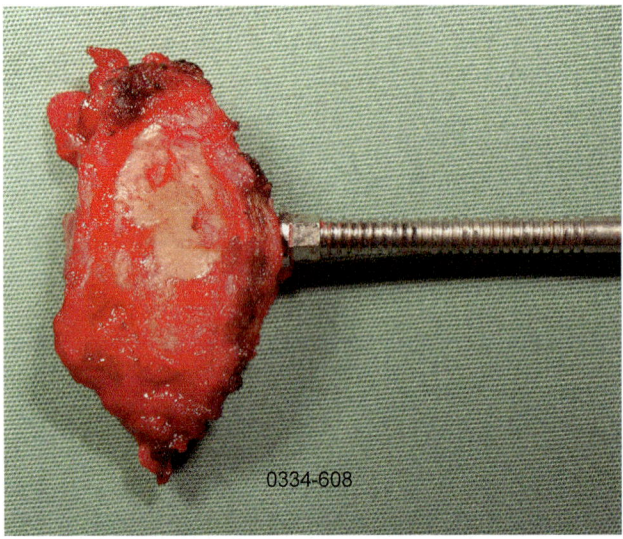

Fig. 27.5 Vertebral body C7—case from Fig. 27.4—removed en bloc

27.6 Techniques for Interbody Fixation

27.6.1 Cages

Cages are amongst the most successful implants within spine surgery and especially within cervical spine surgery within the last years. Obviously, these implants helped to solve and eliminate the problem of graft site morbidity, which was mainly not only a problem of long lasting donor site pain. Cages usually consist of titanium, PEEK, or car-bon fibre composite or the later ones with titanium spray covering to promote bony ingrowth. They usually have one or more perforations to allow bony ingrowth for long term stability and teeth/fins or similar for secure fixation after insertion until bony ingrowth is completed. It is believed that cages made from titanium have a greater tendency for settling, but the main disadvantage of these is that bony fusion is difficult to judge via x-ray or CAT scan and visu-alisation of soft tissue (tumour cases) is difficult if not impossible via MRI. Cages can be used to replace one single or more discs or to replace one or even more vertebral bod-ies. The function of cages may be described as follows: (1) Disc replacement, (2) Restoration of normal disc height, (3) Induction of bony fusion, (4). Stabilisation of the segment. This function is even more pronounced in cages, combined with anterior screws to be fixed within the vertebral bodies. There is a huge variety of cages available; Table 27.1 gives a short overview on cervical cages for disc replacement. Although the authors do not recommend (too expensive, too technical), they would like to mention cages for vertebral body replacement that include mechanisms to distract. There are some cages available with inclined endplates, thus giving the possibility to create some lordosis to the surgeon.

27.6.2 Disc Prostheses

Disc prostheses have been introduced into surgical treatment of the degenerative disc disease of the lumbar spine as early

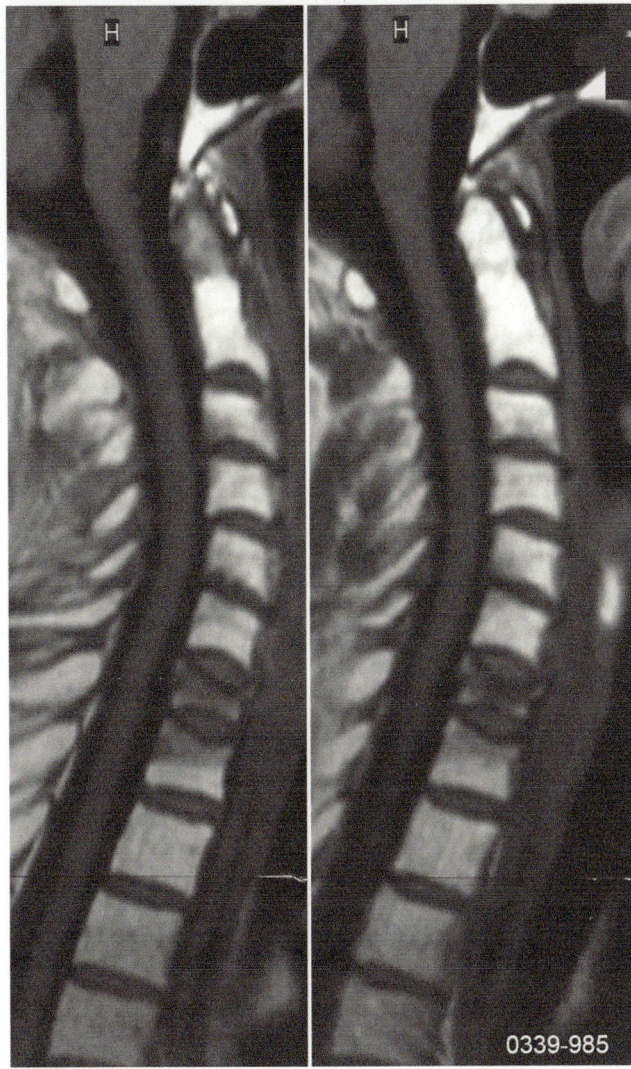

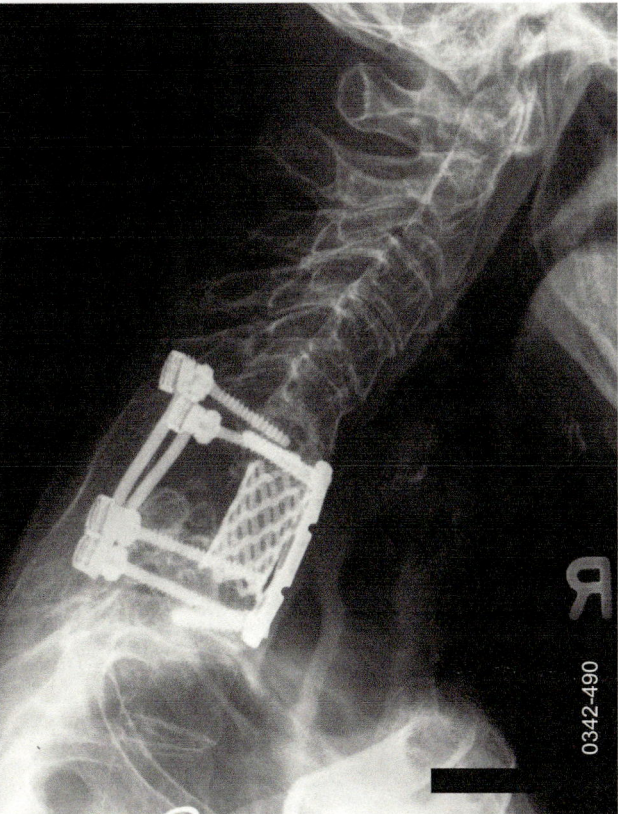

Fig. 27.7 Lateral x-ray after surgery, case from Figs. 27.4, 27.5, and 27.6

Fig. 27.6 Sagittal MRI of the lesion—case from Figs. 27.4 and 27.5—before surgery

as in 1960s, but disappeared from the market due to major problems until they had a second peak in the early 2000. Within the cervical spine, they became more popular when Hilibrand in 1999 reported that more than 25.6% of all patients having received an ACDF will receive an adjacent level disease within 10 years. Today, these values are known to be probably overestimated, but meanwhile cervical disc prostheses became a popular—and efficient—tool to deal with the problem of degenerative disc disease within the cervical spine. Initially, the clinical results are good and there has been some evidence that segmental motility may be preserved at least for a certain time. If, however, disc prosthesis will reduce the problem of ALD or if this is a natural history is still unclear. There are more and more data that genetics are the key point for ALD. Moreover, we face another problem in cervical spine disc replacement using prosthesis, that is heterotopic ossification. The problem of revision surgery,

however, is not as pronounced as it is (no big vessels) within the lumbar spine.

Twenty years after initial insertions of cTDR, it must be noted that there is currently no evidence that these implants produce a better outcome than ACDF or significantly reduce ALD.

Table 27.2 gives an overview of current implants designed and distributed by several companies.

27.6.3 Anterior Cervical Plating

Anterior cervical plating has been introduced into routine cervical spine surgery by Caspar in the 1980s to reduce graft-related complications. In fact, there is some evidence that anterior cervical plating may reduce complications such as graft compression fracture, graft dislocation, or pseudarthrosis healing. Every anterior cervical plate will add stability to a cervical spine segment in flexion—extension, axial rotation and lateral bending. However, complications such as screw loosening or even plate loosening as a consequence of screw loosening occurred in the presence of this plate. Thus, more recently, plating concepts in which the screws are connected to the plate—thus secured against screw back-out—

Table 27.1 Cages for cervical disc replacement distributed by different companies

	Solis Cage (Stryker)	Cervios (Synthes)		
PEEK				
Titanium		Syncage-C (Synthes)	Affinity (Medtronic)	
Other			Cornerstone (Medtronic)	Bengal (Depuy)

Table 27.2 Cervical disc prosthesis distributed by different companies

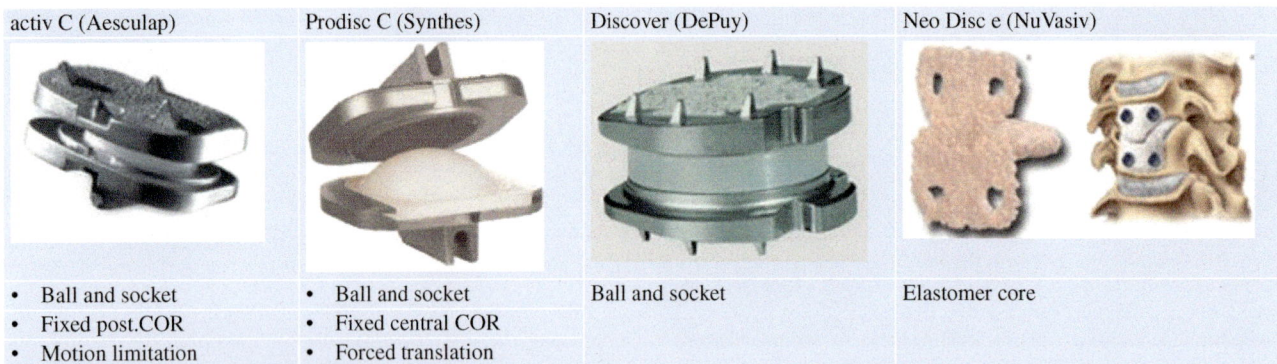

activ C (Aesculap)	Prodisc C (Synthes)	Discover (DePuy)	Neo Disc e (NuVasiv)
• Ball and socket • Fixed post.COR • Motion limitation	• Ball and socket • Fixed central COR • Forced translation	Ball and socket	Elastomer core

have been developed. Amongst these, rigid plate designs and dynamic plate designs will be discussed a little more in detail here: Rigid Plates do not allow any screw motility within the plate. Thus, they are believed to give more stability, especially in trauma cases. There is, however, some evidence that this is not the case. Loading of the interbody cage or graft is less pronounced when compared to dynamic plates. Dynamic plates allow some screw motility within the plate, with the consequence of graft or cage loading, thus resulting in higher speed of fusion and lower incidence of implant complications. Semiconstrained or semirigid or semidynamic plates are located—concerning the implant mechanics—some-where in between the mechanism of these two poles. There seems to be some evidence that dynamic plates reduce the rate of implant complications and have a tendency to a more rapid fusion when compared to rigid plates. On the other hand, rigid plates reduce the loss of height and lordosis after surgery when compared to dynamic ones. Clinical results are comparable or equal. Usually, plates are prebend to give some lordosis to the segments treated. In some models, the bending may be reduced or increased to adapt to the individual lordosis.

Table 27.3 gives a short overview on different implants, supplied by different companies.

Table 27.3 Different implants for anterior cervical plates distributed by different companies

	Aesculap	Synthes	Medtronic	DePuy
Dynamic	ABC	Vectra T	Premier	Swift
Semi-constrained	Caspar	CSLP variable angle	Venture/Zephir	Eagle Slim Loc Uniplate
Constrained		CSLP	Atlantis (Fixed Construct)	
Hybrid		Vectra / ACCS	Atlantis (Hybrid Construct)	Skyline

Suggested Reading

Apfelbaum RI, Kriskovich MD, Haller JR. On the incidence, cause, and prevention of recurrent laryngeal nerve palsies during anterior cervical spine surgery. Spine. 2000;25(22):2906–12.

Baily R, Badgley C. Stabilization of the cervical spine by anterior fusion. J Bone Joint Surg Am. 1960;42:565–94.

Bohler J, Gaudernak T. Anterior plate stabilization for fracture dislocations of the lower cervical spine. J Trauma. 1980;20:203–5.

Bose B. Anterior cervical fusion using Caspar plating: analysis of results and review of the literature. Surg Neurol. 1998;49:25–31.

Caspar W, Barbier DD, Klara PM. Anterior cervical fusion and Caspar plate stabilization for cervical trauma. Neurosurgery. 1989;25:491–502.

Caspar W, Geisler FH, Pitzen T, et al. Anterior cervical plate stabilization in one- and two-level degenerative disease: overtreatment or benefit? J Spinal Disord. 1998;11:1–11.

Chen IH. Biomechanical evaluation of subcortical versus bicortical screw purchase in anterior cervical plating. Acta Neurochir. 1996;138:167–73.

Cloward RB. The anterior approach for removal of ruptured cervical discs. J Neurosurg. 1958;15:602–17.

Connolly PJ, Esses SI, Kostuik JP. Anterior cervical fusion: outcome analysis of patients fused with and without anterior cervical plates. J Spinal Disord. 1996;9:202–6.

Emery SE, Bohlman HH, Bolesta MJ, et al. Anterior cervical decompression and arthrodesis for the treatment of cervical spondylotic myelopathy. Two to seventeen-year follow-up. J Bone Joint Surg Am. 1998;80:941–51.

Griffith SL, Zogbi SW, Guyer RD, et al. Biomechanical comparison of anterior instrumentation for the cervical spine. J Spinal Disord. 1995;8:429–38.

Grubb MR, Currier BL, Shih JS, et al. Biomechanical evaluation of anterior cervical spine stabilization. Spine. 1998;23:886–92.

Kaiser MG, Haid RW Jr, Subach BR, et al. Anterior cervical plating enhances arthrodesis following discectomy and fusion with cortical allograft. Neurosurgery. 2002;50(2):229–36.

Katsuura A, Hukuda S, Imanaka T, et al. Anterior cervical plate used in degenerative disease can maintain cervical lordosis. J Spinal Disord. 1996;9:470–6.

Lowery GL, McDonough RF. The significance of hardware failure in anterior cervical plate fixation. Patients with 2- to 7-year follow-up. Spine. 1998;23:181–7.

Morscher E, Sutter F, Jenny H, et al. Die vordere Verplattung der Halswirbelsaule mit dem Hohlschrauben-Plattensystem aus Titanium. Chirurg. 1996;57:702–7.

Panjabi MM, Isomi T, Wang JL. Loosening at the screw-vertebra junction in multilevel anterior cervical plate constructs. Spine. 1999;24:2383–8.

Paramore CG, Dickman CA, Sonntag VK. Radiographic and clinical follow-up review of Caspar plates in 49 patients. J Neurosurg. 1996;84:957–61.

Pitzen TR, Chrobok J, Stulik J, et al. Implant complications, fusion, loss of lordosis, and outcome after anterior cervical plating with dynamic or rigid plates: two-year results of a multi-centric, randomized, controlled study. Spine. 2009;34(7):641–6.

Pitzen T, Drumm J, Berthold C, et al. Degenerative cervical spine diseases: fusion vs. total disc replacement: what can be done when? Orthopade. 2018;47(6):467–73.

Rechtine GR, Cahill DW, Gruerenberg M, et al. The synthes cervical spine locking plate and screw system in anterior cervical fusion. Tech Orthop. 1994;9:86–91.

Smith GW, Robinson RA. The treatment of certain cervical spine disorders by anterior removal of the intervertebral disc and interbody fusion. J Bone Joint Surg Am. 1958;40:607–24.

Spivak JM, Chen D, Kummer FJ. The effect of locking fixation screws on the stability of anterior cervical plating. Spine. 1999;24:334–8.

Stulik J, Pitzen TR, Chrobok J, Ruffing S, et al. Fusion and failure following anterior cervical plating with dynamic or rigid plates: 6-months results of a multi-centric, prospective, randomized, controlled study. Eur Spine J. 2007;16(10):1689–94.

Swank ML, Lowery GL, Bhat AL, et al. Anterior cervical allograft arthrodesis and instrumentation: multilevel interbody grafting or strut graft reconstruction. Eur Spine J. 1997;6:138–43.

Wang JC, McDonough PW, Endow K, et al. The effect of cervical plating on single-level anterior cervical discectomy and fusion. J Spinal Disord. 1999;12:467–71.

Wang JC, McDonough PW, Endow KK, et al. Increased fusion rates with cervical plating for two-level anterior cervical discectomy and fusion. Spine. 2000;25:41–5.

Wang JC, McDonough PW, Kanim LE, et al. Increased fusion rates with cervical plating for three-level anterior cervical discectomy and fusion. Spine. 2001;26:643–7.

Zechmeister I, Winkler R, Mad P. Artificial total disc replacement versus fusion for the cervical spine: a systematic review. Eur Spine J. 2011;20(2):177–84.

Anterior Cervical Discectomy and Fusion

28

Frank Grochulla

28.1 Introduction and Core Messages

Anterior cervical discectomy and fusion (ACDF) is a widely used technique and has become the gold standard for the treatment of cervical radiculopathy. The surgical principles of the surgical treatment are the decompression of neurostructures, the restoration of the cervical lordosis, and the stabilization. The surgical outcome is mainly dependent on the decompression effect. Fusion rates are dependent on the number of levels treated. Actually, there is no evidence for the superiority of cage fusions compared to fusions with autologous bone graft from the iliac crest, except that of iliac crest donor site pain. In the 1950s, the first reports of anterior approaches to cervical disc pathology appeared. The two most common methods for ACDF were described by Robinson and Smith in 1955 [1] and by Cloward in 1958 [2]. Robinson and Smith did not decompress the neural structures and believed that osteophytes and herniated discs would be reabsorbed during immobilizing the segment.

28.2 Indications

- Single or multiple level soft disc herniation
- Single or multiple level spondylosis
- Ossification of the posterior longitudinal ligament (OPLL)
- Trauma (vertebral body fractures, subluxations, luxations)
- Tumors (vertebral body tumors or metastases)
- Infectious diseases

28.3 Contraindications

- Predominant posterior compression of the neural structures
- Isolated traumatic disruption of the posterior elements

28.4 Technical Prerequisites

The technical prerequisites are the microscope, different microsurgical instruments, retractor systems for ventral approach to the cervical spine (e.g., Caspar retractor system), high-speed drill, and the intraoperative fluoroscopy.

28.5 Planning, Preparation, and Positioning

ACDF is usually performed under general anesthesia with optimum muscle relaxation.

The patient is positioned supine on the operating table. A rolled towel or sandbag is placed under the cervicothoracic junction between the shoulders for head and neck extension. Head traction device incases with instability. Shoulder countertraction may be necessary, particularly in patients with short necks and for approaches to the lower cervical spine and the cervicothoracic junction. A right-sided approach is generally recommended because it is easier for the right-handed surgeon. Some authors recommend a left-side approach to reduce the risk of injury to the recurrent laryngeal nerve. However, a review of 328 cases [3] showed no association between the side of the approach and the incidence of recurrent laryngeal nerve symptoms. The location of the skin incision is estimated with a lateral fluoroscopic image.

F. Grochulla (✉)
Metropol Medical Center, Clinic for Orthopedics, Trauma Surgery and Spinal Surgery, Nuremberg, Germany
e-mail: frank.grochulla@mmc-nuernberg.de

© Springer-Verlag GmbH Germany 2023
U. Vieweg, F. Grochulla (eds.), *Manual of Spine Surgery*, https://doi.org/10.1007/978-3-662-64062-3_28

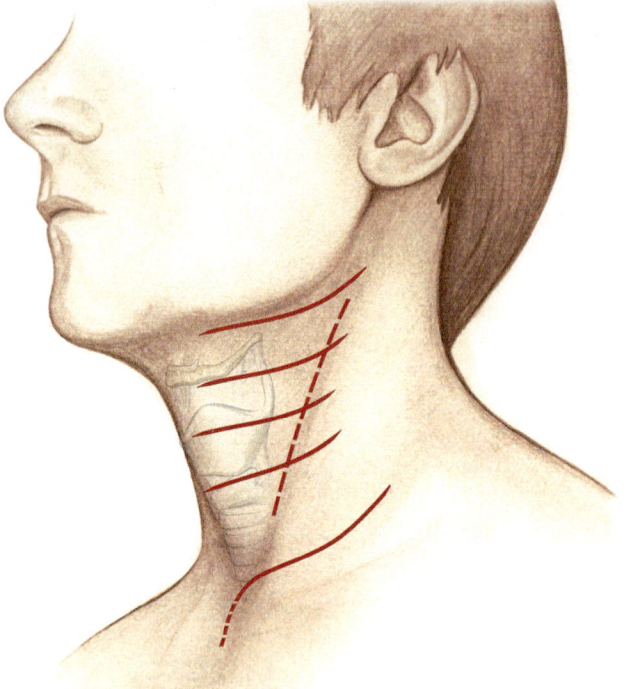

Fig. 28.1 Skin incision

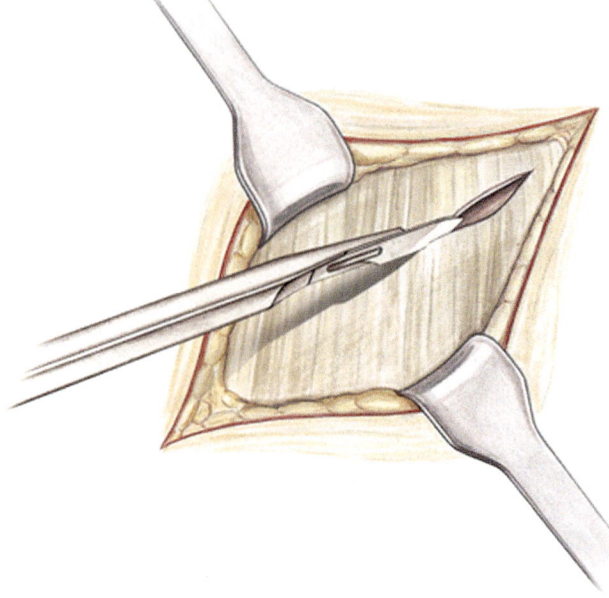

Fig. 28.2 Incision of the platysma muscle

28.6 Surgical Technique

28.6.1 Approach

- The skin incision (3–4 cm) is usually slightly oblique along Langer's lines; this provides the best possible cosmetic result (Fig. 28.1). A skin incision along the medial border of the sternocleidomastoid muscle may be used for multilevel disease.
- Dissection is carried sharply through the subcutaneous tissue. The platysma muscle may be sharply divided transverse or split longitudinally (Fig. 28.2).
- After subplatysmal dissection, the superficial fascia overlying the medial border of the sternocleidomastoid muscle is sharply divided.
- The following deep dissection between sternocleidomastoid muscle and carotid sheath laterally and trachea, esophagus, and strap muscles of the neck medially is performed careful with blunt finger dissection. In patients without previous ventral cervical surgery, blunt dissection is easily and safely accomplished. In patients with previous ventral cervical surgery, sharp dissection may be necessary. In this case, it is important to confirm that the sharp dissection remains dorsal to the esophagus and the hypopharynx. A placed nasogastric tube may be helpful to confirm the location of esophagus and hypopharynx by palpation.
- After entering the prevertebral space, the correct intervertebral disc is marked by fluoroscopy.
- The longus colli muscles are elevated from the vertebral bodies (Fig. 28.3) and discs bilaterally, and self-retaining

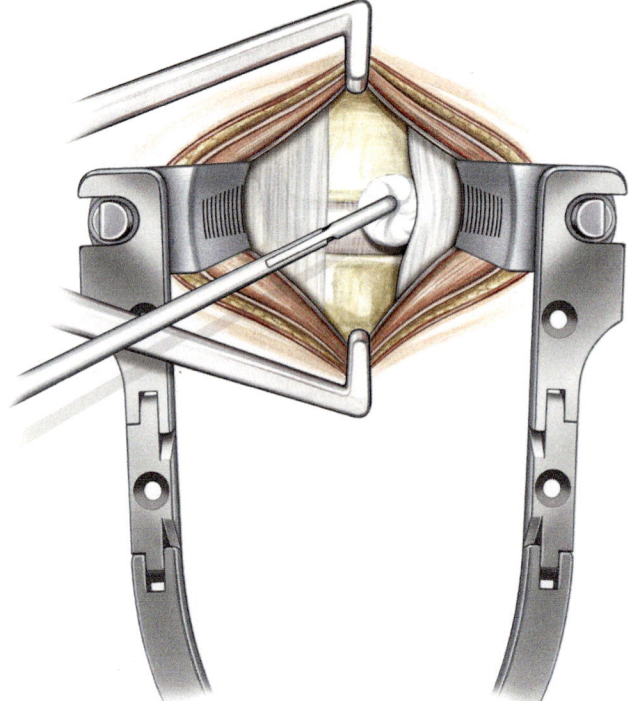

Fig. 28.3 The longus colli muscles are elevated from the vertebral bodies

retractors are placed under the longus colli muscle (Fig. 28.4).
- A drill guide is used to position the drill hole for the first distraction screw in the middle third of the inferior vertebral body (Fig. 28.5a). The drilling direction is orientated approximately parallel to the index disc space.

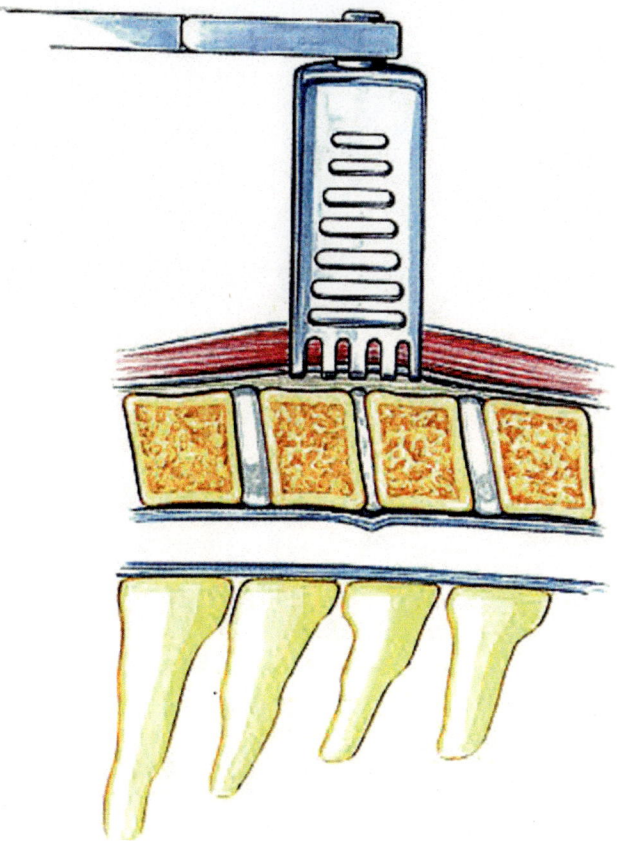

Fig. 28.4 Self-retaining retractors are placed under the longus colli muscle (with permission Aesculap AG, Tuttlingen, Germany)

28.6.2 Discectomy and Fusion

- The distraction screw is inserted through the drill guide with the screwdriver. The screw should not penetrate the posterior cortex of the vertebral body.
- After drilling the hole, the second distraction screw is placed into the middle third of the superior vertebral body parallel to the first screw (Fig. 28.5b).
- The distractor is pushed onto the distraction screws as far as possible up to the screw base plates.
- After distraction, an operating microscope with powerful illumination should be used to improve the magnification and lighting.
- Discectomy: following the incision of the anterior annulus (Fig. 28.6a), the disc is completely removed from the cranial and caudal end plates and in between the medial borders of the uncinate processes (Fig. 28.6b). Adequate posterior disc removal is accomplished when the white, vertically organized fibers of the posterior longitudinal ligament are well visualized.
- In the case of extruded and sequestered disc fragments (Fig. 28.6c), perforations of the posterior longitudinal ligament (OPLL) can be identified under microscopical view. It is important to open the OPLL to explore all sequestered epidural disc fragments. In most cases, it is not necessary to remove all portions of the OPLL, unless fragments have migrated bilaterally and extensively [4].

- If spondylosis/osteophytes are present, it is necessary to recreate an interspace height with parallel preparation of the end plates with cylindrical or coronial burrs and to remove posterior osteophytes with drills and Kerrison rongeurs.
- The complete resection of osteophytes is checked with a blunt hook under fluoroscopic control (Fig. 28.7).

28.6.3 Preparation of Bone Graft Side: Bone Graft Harvesting and Impacting of the Bone

- The bone graft site is prepared with curettes and burrs, as far as possible plane parallel.
- The height and a.p. depth of the intervertebral space are measured with a gauge (Fig. 28.8).
- Graft harvesting: the most commonly used area to harvest tricortical grafts for ACDF is the anterior iliac crest.
- A skin incision and muscular detachment with monopolar is performed over the anterior iliac crest.
- A tricortical bone graft with parallel cut edges is prepared (oscillating saw with appropriate size for the graft) (Fig. 28.9a). A graft cutter is set to the measured depth of the intervertebral space, and the correctly sized bone graft is then cut from the iliac crest (Fig. 28.9b).
- The bone graft is drilled and then screwed onto the graft holder (Fig. 28.10).
- The graft is impacted with slight press fit under image intensifier guidance.

28.6.4 Cages

- The use of structural autografts for ACDF is related to a relatively high rate of morbidity at the donor site in the range of 10–25%.
- As an alternative, a variety of interbody cages are now available for use in the cervical spine. The materials used are carbon fiber, polyether ether ketone (PEEK), titanium, or bioabsorbable implants. The cages can be classified into screw-in, box-type, and cylindrical design categories.
- Interbody cages should provide the immediate load-bearing capacity while allowing bony fusion.

28.6.5 Plating

- Indications and techniques for the use of anterior cervical plates are described in detail in Chap. 21

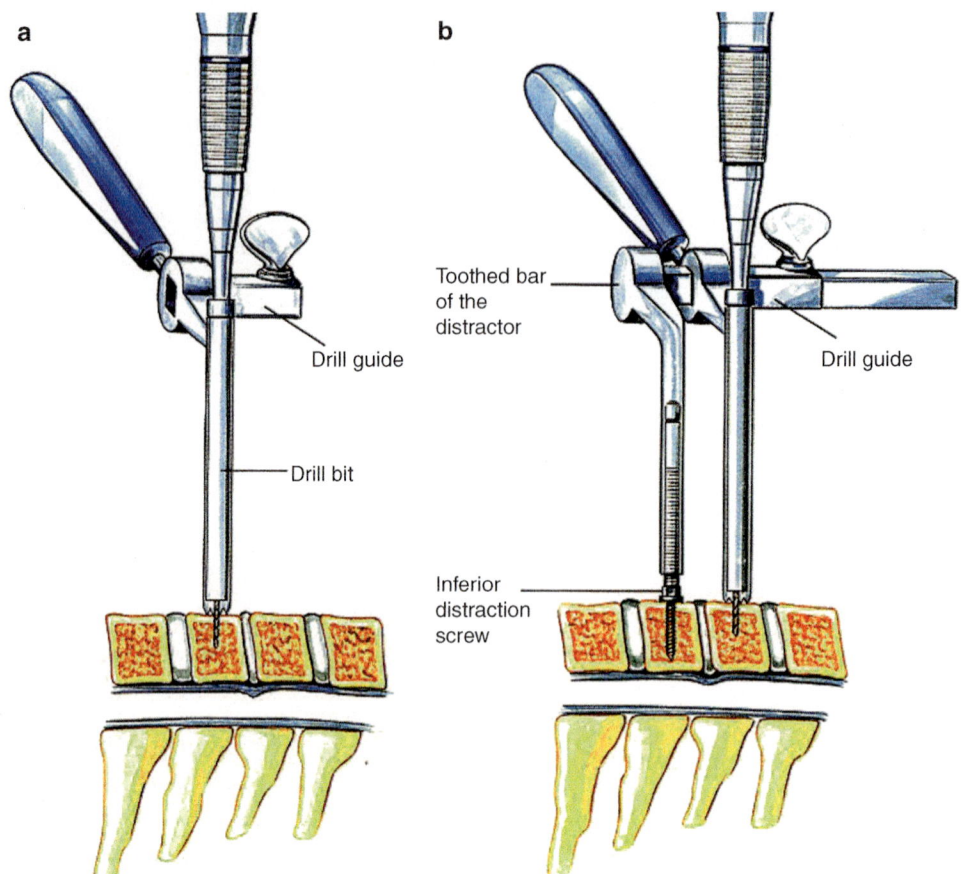

Fig. 28.5 (**a**) Positioning the first drill hole in the inferior vertebra with the drill guide. (**b**) Sitting the second (superior) distraction screw (with permission Aesculap AG, Tuttlingen, Germany)

28.7 Postoperative Care

Patients can be mobilized on the day of surgery approximately 4–6 h after surgery.

Soft drain for 24 h. In the case of ACDF, a soft collar is applied for 6–8 weeks postoperatively.

28.8 Tips and Tricks

- Monitoring of the endotracheal cuff pressure and its release after retractor placement can decrease the rate of recurrent laryngeal nerve temporary paralysis [5].
- Excessively, longus colli dissection can cause Horner's syndrome. The incidence varies from 0.2% to 2% [6, 7]. Therefore, longus colli dissection should be limited to 4 mm of the muscle.

- Each of the surgical steps must be monitored and performed individually using an image intensifier.
- Adequate visualization is essential for performing the decompression procedure safely. A microscope with powerful illumination should be used to improve the magnification and lighting.
- Width of decompression of the spinal canal: for an adequate decompression, an approximately 15-mm bony dissection centered over the midline is necessary. If nerve root decompression is part of the surgical procedure, a wider discectomy/decompression on one or both sides may be necessary.
- Manipulation of the nerve root is particularly problematic with the C5 nerve root, which appears to be more vulnerable to injury. Therefore, extreme care should be taken during performing discectomies in the level C4/5. C5 palsy is more common in posterior approaches.

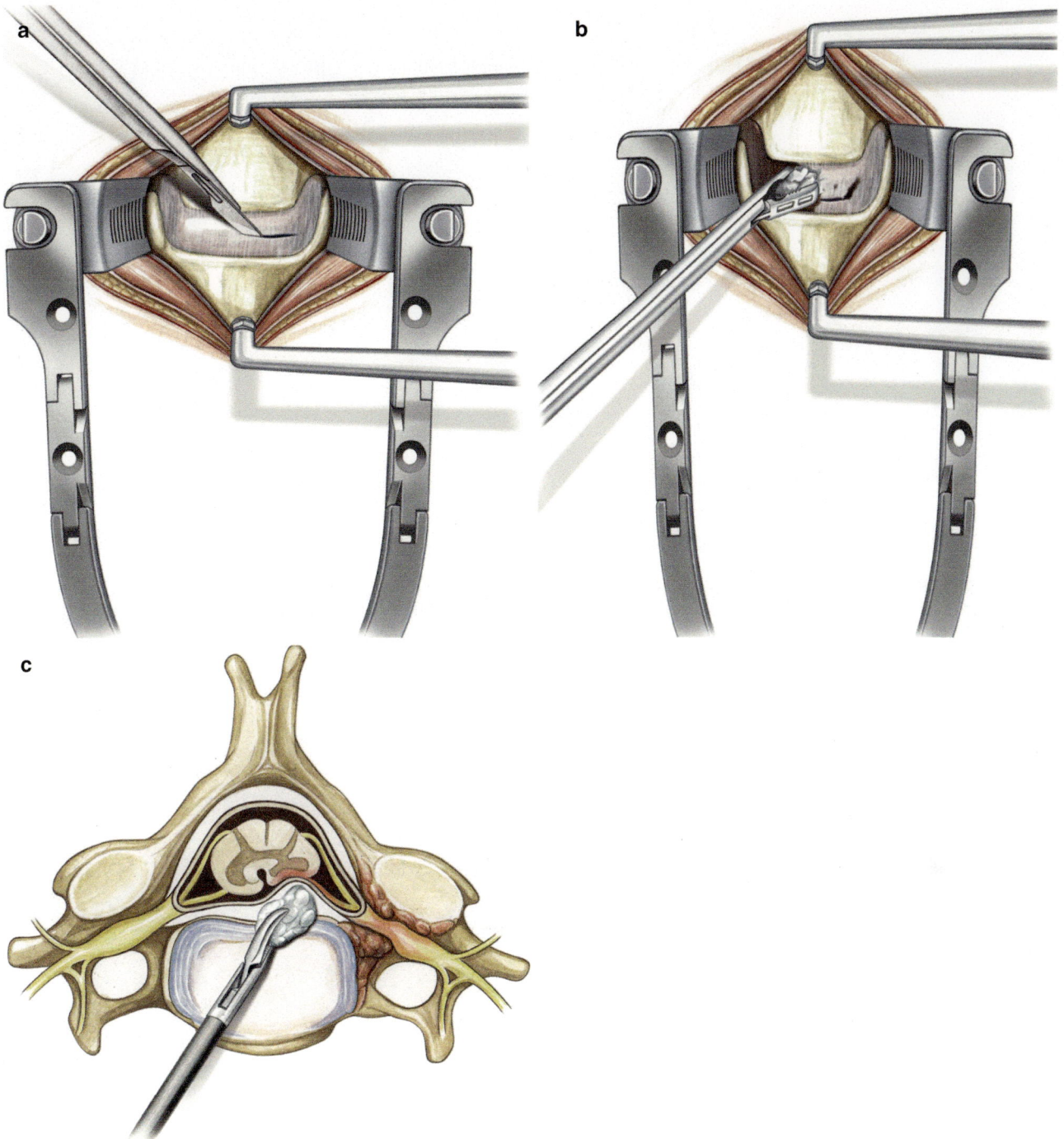

Fig. 28.6 (**a**) Incision of the anterior annulus. (**b**) The disc is completely removed. (**c**) Removal of sequestrates disc fragments

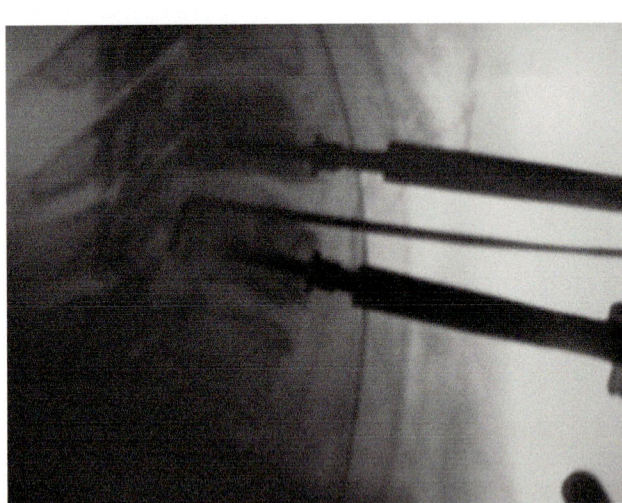

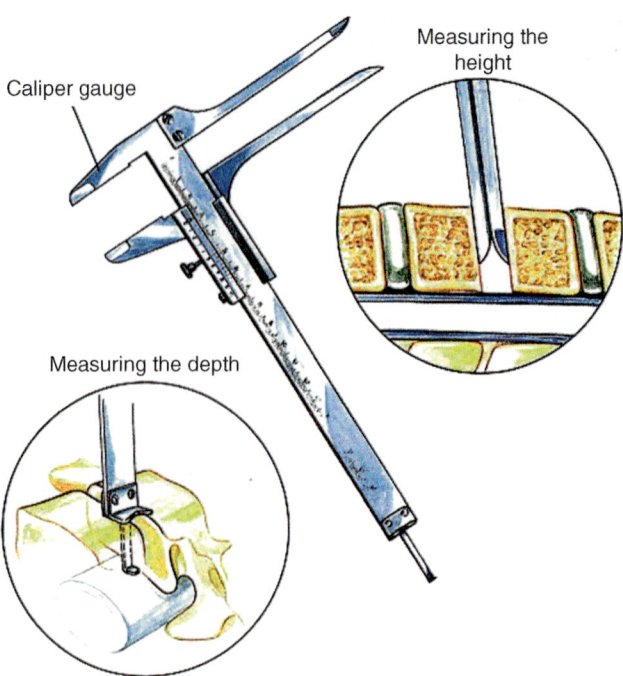

Fig. 28.7 Complete resection/decompression is checked with a blunt hook under fluoroscopic control

Fig. 28.8 Measuring the height and the depth of the intervertebral space (with permission of Aesculap AG, Tuttlingen, Germany)

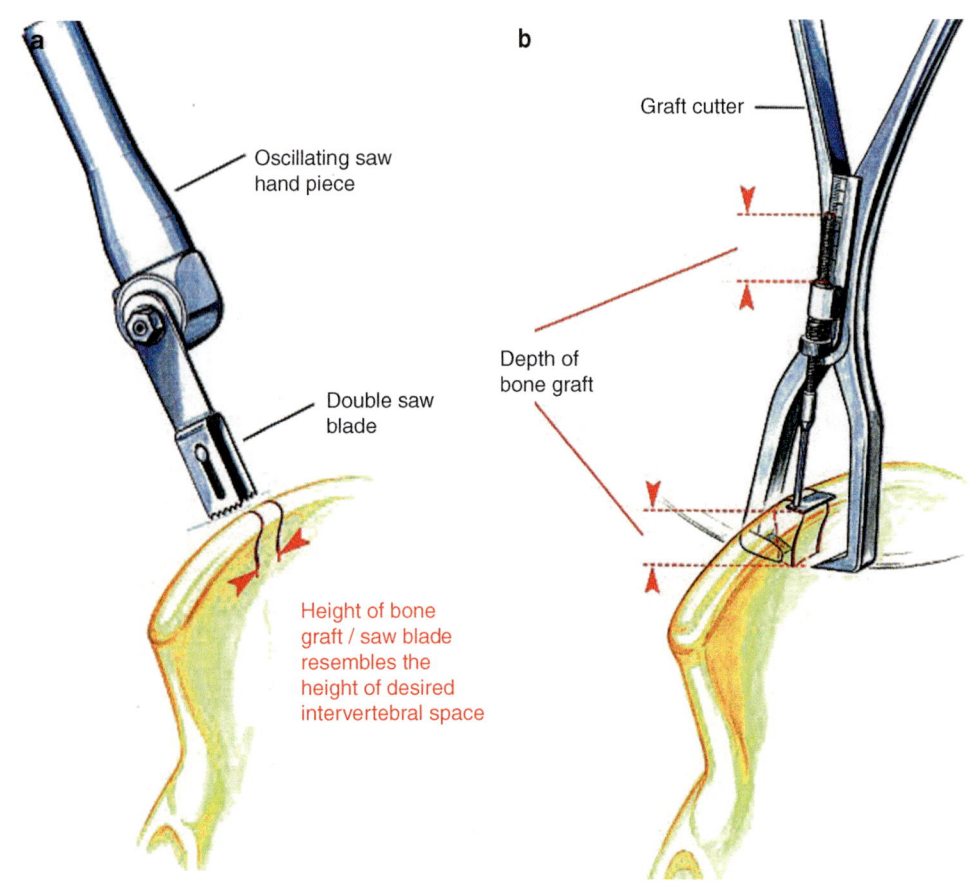

Fig. 28.9 (**a**) Bone graft harvesting from the iliac crest with oscillating saw. (**b**) Graft cutter (with permission Aesculap AG, Tuttlingen, Germany)

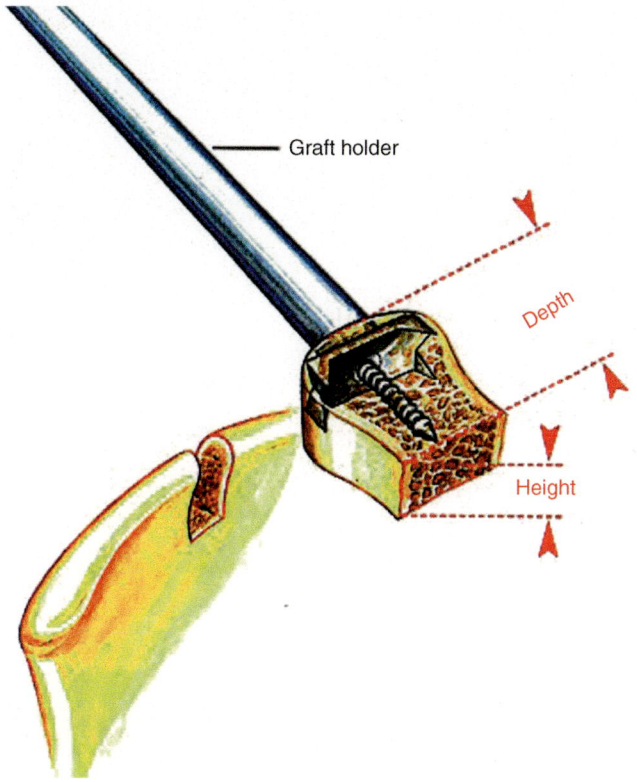

Fig. 28.10 The bone graft is drilled and screwed onto the graft holder
(with permission Aesculap AG, Tuttlingen, Germany)

References

1. Robinson RA, Smith GW. Anterolateral cervical disc removal and interbody fusion for cervical disc syndrome (abstract). Bull John Hopkins Hosp. 1955;96:223–4.
2. Cloward RB. The anterior approach for removal of ruptured discs. J Neurosurg. 1958;15:602–14.
3. Beutler WJ, Sweeney CA, Conolly PJ. Recurrent laryngeal nerve injury with anterior cervical spine surgery risk with laterally of surgical approach. Spine. 2001;26:1337–42.
4. McCulloch JA, Young PH, editors. Essentials of spinal microsurgery. Philadelphia: Raven Lippincott; 1998.
5. Apfelbaum RI, Kriskovich MD, Haller JR. On the incidence, cause, and prevention of recurrent laryngeal nerve palsies during anterior cervical spine surgery. Spine. 2000;25:2906–12.
6. Bertalanffy H, Eggert HR. Complications of anterior cervical discectomy without fusion in 450 consecutive patients. Acta Neurochir. 1989;99:41–50.
7. DePalma A, Rothmann R, Lewinnek G, et al. Anterior interbody fusion for severe cervical disc degeneration. Surg Gynecol Obstet. 1972;134:755–8.

Uncoforaminotomy

Kirsten Schmieder

29.1 Introduction and Core Message

In carefully selected cases and in experienced hands, this surgical method provides good clinical results and preserves motion in the affected segment [1, 2]. Uncoforaminotomy is a minimally invasive surgical technique. The approach uses the uncovertebral joint to create direct access to the neuroforamen. Within the bony canal, there is a close proximity between the bony borders and the nerve root. In cases of an additional hard or soft disc disease, a significant narrowing or obstruction is present. Via a ventral route on the side of the symptoms, the offending lesion is removed resulting in a decompression of the nerve root in its neuroforaminal segment. Since the disc itself is left in place, motion of the segment can be preserved [3, 4].

29.2 Indications

- Unilateral disc herniation
- Unilateral osseous foraminal stenosis
- Unilevel hard or soft disc disease
- Bisegmental foraminal obstruction
- Failed conservative treatment
- Neurological deficit correlating with the radiological finding

29.3 Contraindications

- Cervical myelopathy
- Multilevel hard or soft disc pathology
- Ossification of the posterior ligament
- Bilateral foraminal obstruction
- Segmental instability
- Kyphotic malalignment of the cervical spine

29.4 Technical Prerequisites

Fluoroscopy, operation microscope, adequate instrumentation for ventral discectomy (punches, forceps, ball piler), and drill (rosen und diamant, preferable high-speed drilling system).

- Caspar retractor system or similar retractor for ventral approach to the cervical spine
- No additional implantation system required

K. Schmieder (✉)
Department of Neurosurgery, University Hospital Knappschaftskrankenhaus Bochum, Bochum, Germany
e-mail: kirsten.schmieder@kk-bochum.de

© Springer-Verlag GmbH Germany 2023
U. Vieweg, F. Grochulla (eds.), *Manual of Spine Surgery*, https://doi.org/10.1007/978-3-662-64062-3_29

Fig. 29.1 Anterior approach to the cervical spine on the side of the offending lesion and the symptomatology

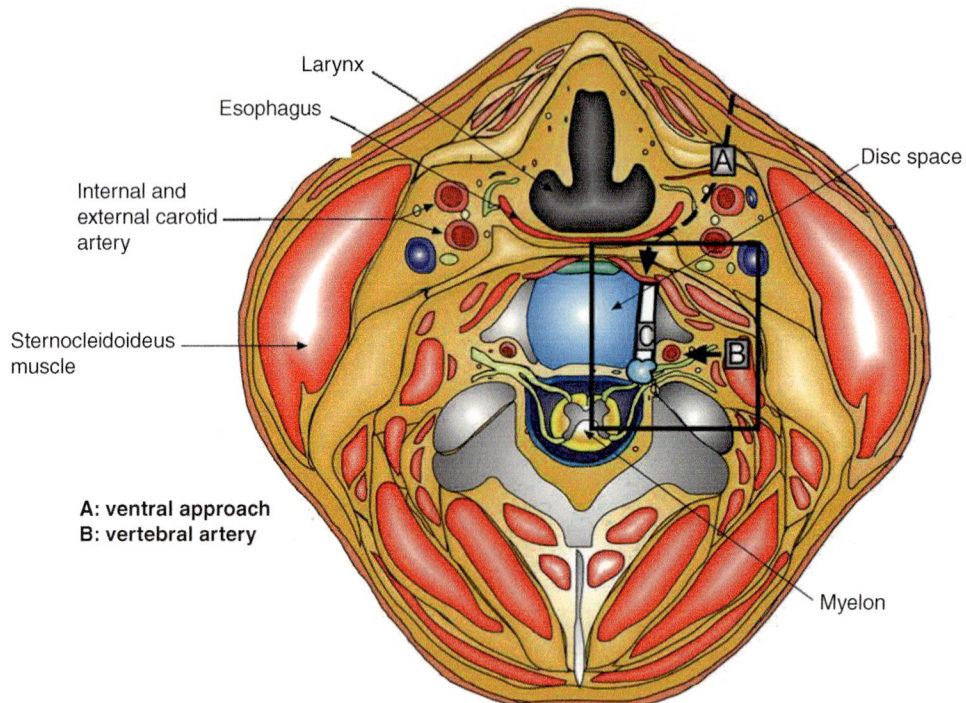

Larynx

Esophagus

Internal and external carotid artery

Sternocleidoideus muscle

Disc space

A: ventral approach
B: vertebral artery

Myelon

29.5 Planning, Preparation, and Positioning

Prior to surgery, MRI or CT scans are reviewed to see where exactly within the neuroforamen the offending process is located. Vertebral artery on the side of the approach has to be localized. Knowledge of normal anatomy of the uncovertebral joint and the surrounding structures is essential. The patient is placed on its back, and the head is on a horseshoe-like positioning device. The fluoroscopy is draped sterile.

29.6 Surgical Technique

29.6.1 Approach

An anterior approach to the cervical spine is performed on the side of the patient's complaints (Fig. 29.1). The skin incision is placed in relation to the affected segment on the anterior border of the sternocleidomastoid muscle about 3 cm long (same incision used for ACDF). At the ventral surface of the cervical spine, the self-retaining retractor is inserted and placed above the longus colli muscle (Figs. 29.2 and 29.3). No Caspar pins are placed in the adjacent vertebral bodies. After lateralization of the longus colli muscle at the level of the disc, the lateral border of the adjacent vertebral bodies is identified and the uncovertebral joint is localized (Fig. 29.4).

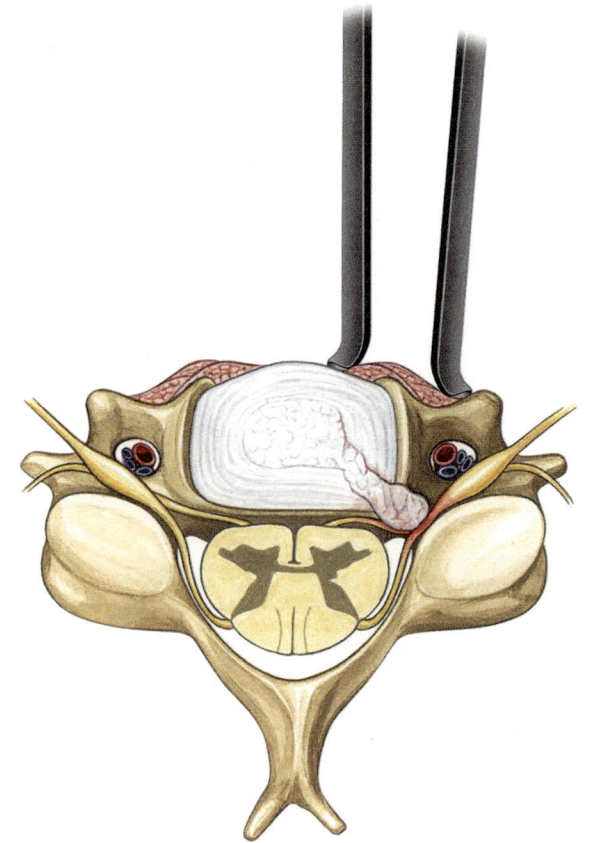

Fig. 29.2 Insertion of the retractor system

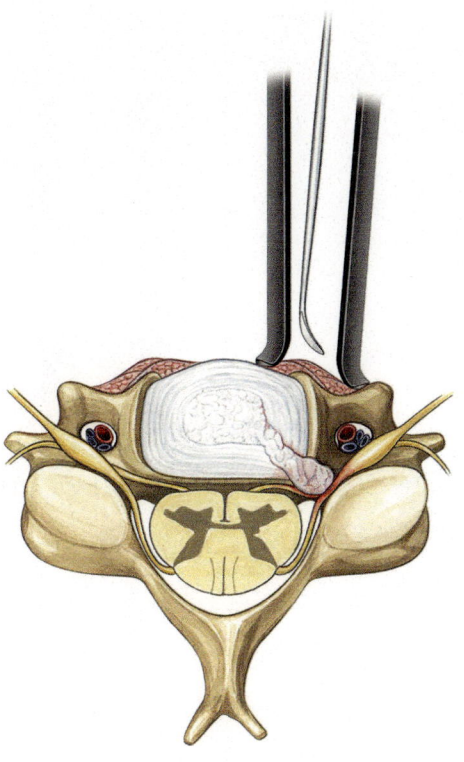

Fig. 29.3 Lateral mobilization of the longus colli muscle with a dissector

29.6.2 Microsurgical Decompression

- Drill an upper uncoforaminotomy down to the neuroforamen (Fig. 29.5) [5, 6].
- Prevent a too lateral drilling (vertebral artery!) [7, 8].
- Control the direction and depth with fluoroscopy [9].
- Beware that at level C6/7, the vertebral artery enters the cervical spine from lateral.
- Identify the neuroforamen after reaching the posterior border of the vertebral body (Fig. 29.6).
- Remove the longitudinal ligament above the nerve root.
- Remove offending disc material or osseous spurs.
- Identify the nerve root.
- Make sure that the lateral osseous portion of the neuroforamen is removed.
- Using a small dissector or nerve hook, the medial part of the foramen is checked (Fig. 29.7).
- Using a small punch, remaining parts of the longitudinal ligament are removed if necessary (Fig. 29.8a, b).
- Control the localization of the removed disc material with the morphology on the preoperative images.
- Follow the course of the nerve root into the neuroforamen (Figs. 29.9 and 29.10).

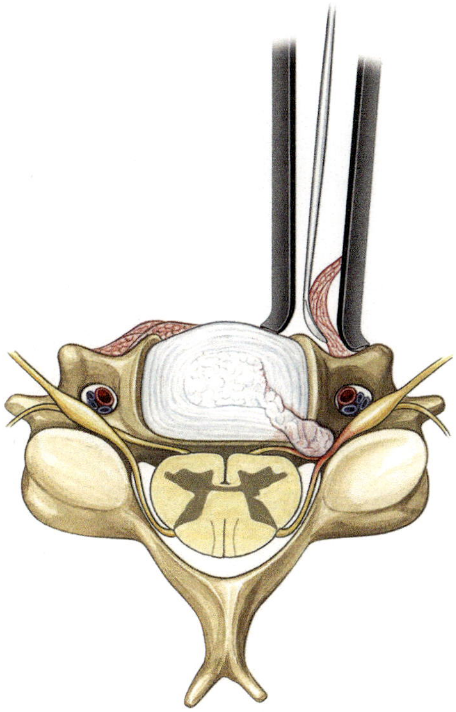

Fig. 29.4 Identification of the lateral border of the vertebral body and the uncus

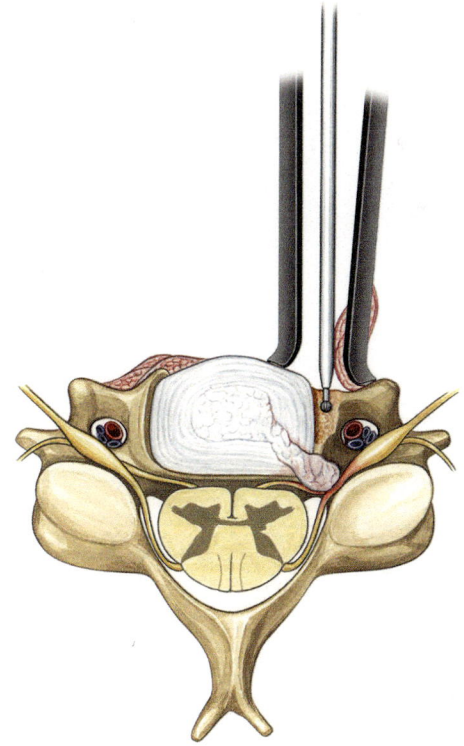

Fig. 29.5 Upper uncoforaminotomy with a high speed drill (cave: vertebral artery!)

a

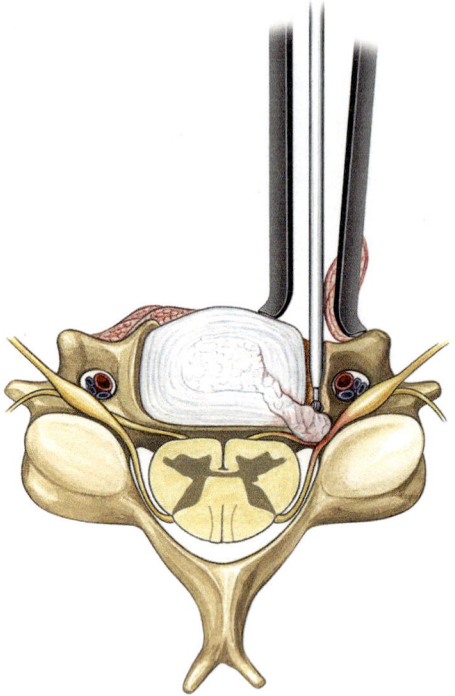

Fig. 29.6 Identification of the posterior border of the vertebral body and the neuroforamen

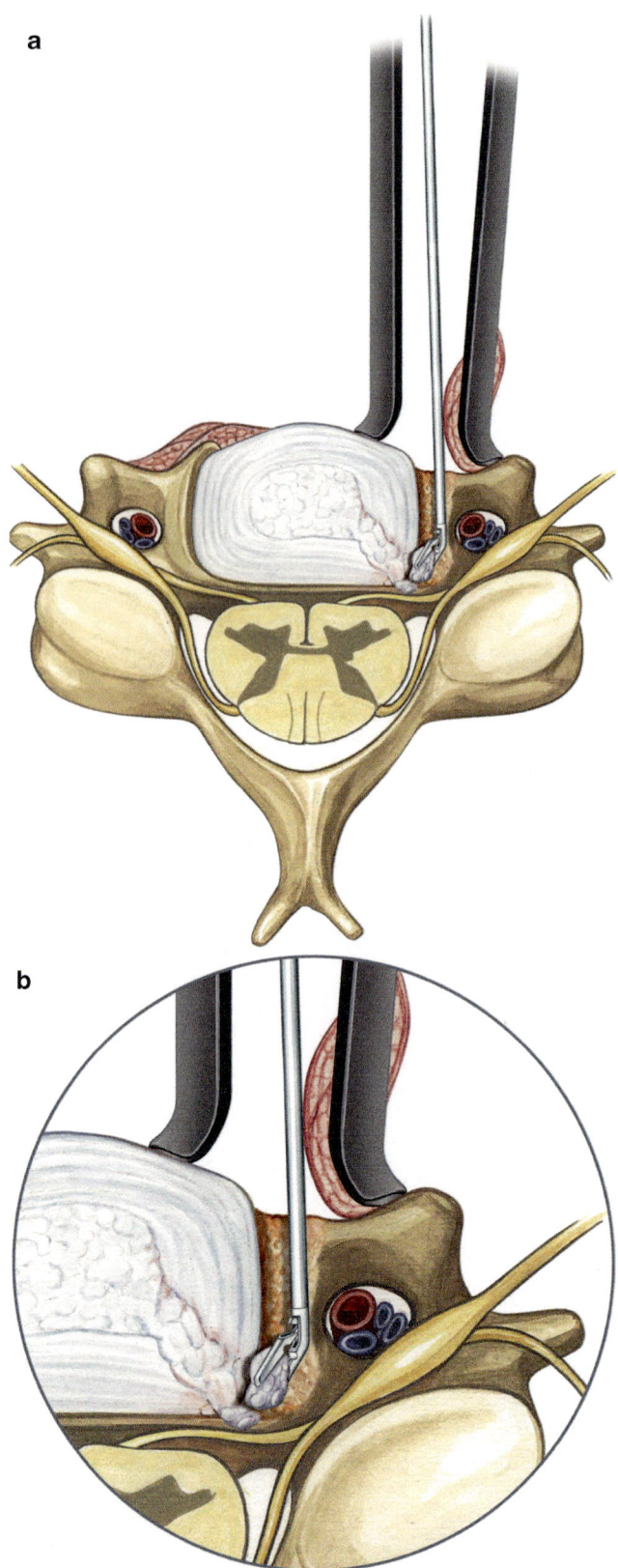

b

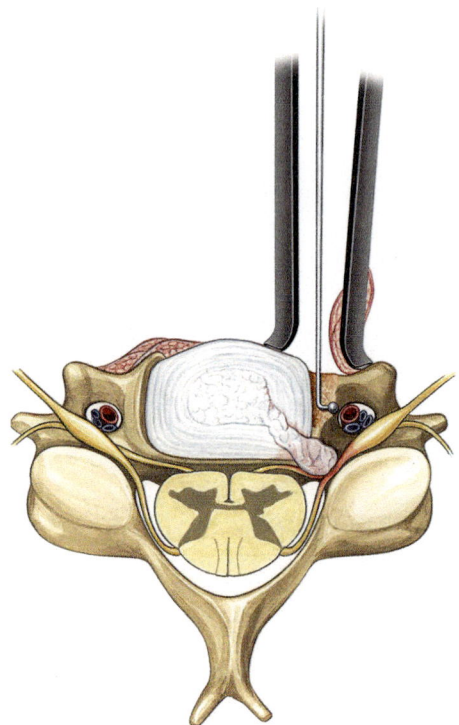

Fig. 29.7 Mobilization of the disc material with a nerve hook

Fig. 29.8 (**a, b**) Removal of the disc material with a small punch

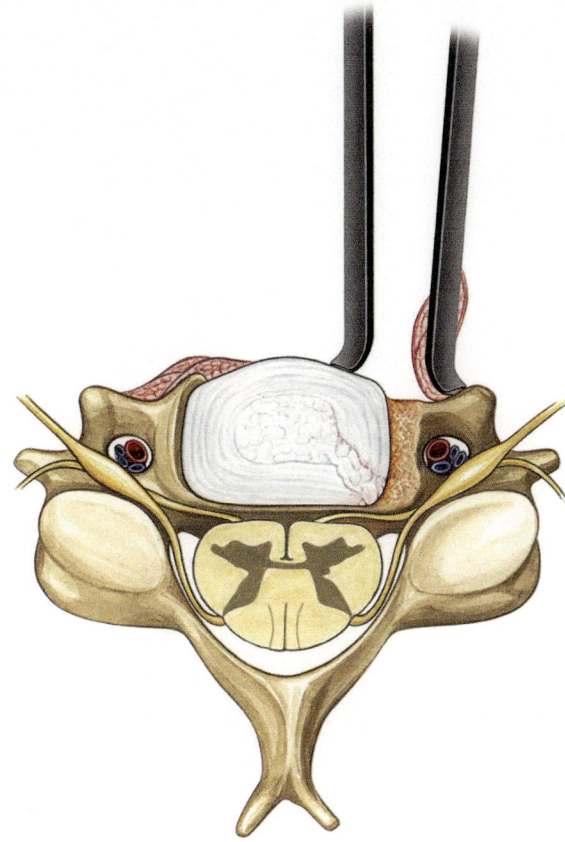

Fig. 29.9 Inspection of the nerve root in its intraforaminal part

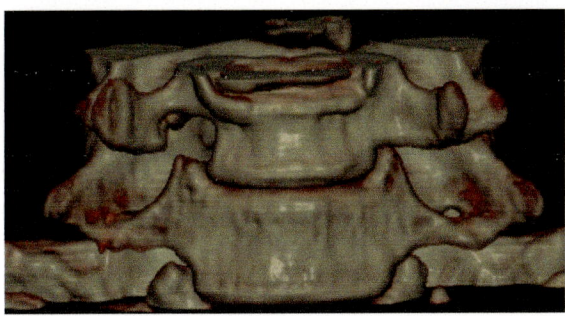

Fig. 29.10 Postoperative CT scan of the uncoforaminotomy

29.7 Tips and Tricks

- In the event of a venous bleeding from the epidural intraforaminal plexus, use a small collagen sponge and a cotton to apply gentle pressure and wait for some time. It will stop bleeding, and the removal of the material is possible. In some cases, a small piece of collagen sponge has to be left in place.
- If the insight into the neuroforamen is not sufficient, an enlargement of the uncoforaminotomy may be necessary. If so, drill away the adjacent part of the vertebral body offending the direct view into the neuroforamen.

References

1. Pechlivanis I, Brenke C, Scholz M, Engelhardt M, Harders A, Schmieder K. Treatment of degenerative cervical disc disease with uncoforaminotomy – intermediate clinical outcome. Minim Invasive Neurosurg. 2008;51:211–7.
2. Schmieder K, Kettner A, Brenke C, Harders A, Pechlivanis I, Wilke HJ. In vitro flexibility of the cervical spine after ventral uncoforaminotomy. Laboratory investigation. J Neurosurg Spine. 2007;7:537–41.
3. Jho HD. Microsurgical anterior cervical foraminotomy for radiculopathy: a new approach to cervical disc herniation. J Neurosurg. 1996;84:155–60.
4. Jho HD. Editorial: failed anterior cervical foraminotomy. J Neurosurg Spine. 2003;98:121–5.
5. Hayashi K, Yabuki T. Origin of the uncus and of Luschka's joint in the cervical spine. J Bone Joint Surg. 1985;67:788–91.
6. Orofino C, Sherman MS, Schlechter D. Luschka's joint – a degenerative phenomenon. J Bone Joint Surg. 1960;42:853–8.
7. Benazzo F, Alvarez AA, Nalli D, et al. Pathogenesis of uncus deformation and vertebral artery compression: histologic investigations of the uncus and dynamic angiography of the vertebral artery in the cadaveric spine. J Spinal Disord. 1994;7:111–9.
8. Ebraheim NA, Lu J, Haman SP, et al. Anatomic basis of anterior surgery on the cervical spine: relationships between uncus-artery-root complex and vertebral artery injury. Surg Radiol Anat. 1998;20:389–92.
9. Hirsch C, Schajowicz F, Galante J. Structural changes in the cervical spine – a study on autopsy specimens in different age groups. Acta Orthop Scand. 1967;109(Suppl):34–41.

Anterior Cervical Plating

30

Tobias Pitzen, Jörg Drumm, Gregor Ostrowski, and Michael Ruf

30.1 Introduction and Core Messages

Anterior cervical decompression and fusion using an autologous bone graft has been developed in the mid- and late 1950s of the last century by different groups (see Chap. 29). Using this technique for fixation of traumatic instability of the cervical spine, it was shown that the treated segment was prone to displacement [1]. To avoid graft complications such as graft dislocation or graft settling and to avoid the necessity of an external orthesis—i.e., a halo body jacket—anterior cervical plating was first used by Hermann [2], who published his experiences in 1975. Several other authors already had reported their results [2–4] when Caspar in 1989 [5] presented a standardized technique using a unique system of instruments for positioning, approach, decompression, fusion, and stabilization, as well suitable implants (bicortical screws and plates). Since then, the plate has been redesigned several times and monocortical screws as well as thicker revision screws have been developed and several other plate designs (dynamic, rigid, and others working between dynamic and rigid) have been developed. Two important questions arise connected to these design options of cervical plates:

1. *Is there a need for bicortical fixation?*

   Looking at the results of two biomechanical studies [6, 7], there is to the authors knowledge probably no need to fix a cervical plate with bicortical screws. These studies did not see any difference for three-dimensional segmental stability, screw pullout or insertional screw torque when bicortical screws versus monocortical screws were used. However, the screws should be chosen as long as possible their length should be around 80% of the depth of the vertebra and free spinning screws must be avoided, Fig. 30.1, also see Sect. 30.5.

2. *What type of plate: dynamic, rigid, or semi-dynamic or semi-rigid?*

   Current biomechanical concepts of anterior cervical spine plates are no longer completely unconstrained due to a possible screw pullout, resulting in loss of stability and/ or soft tissue compression. Dynamic plates, for example, allow screws to settle in cranio-caudal direction [8]. This design feature results in loading of the graft or cage during the ongoing fusion process. A more rapid fusion may be expected [9, 10]. Against pullout, however, the screws are secured by a special connection between the head of the screw and the plate, so that the screws should not be backed out. Rigid plate designs are characterized by a tight fixation between the head of the screws and the plate. They do not allow motion in any direction between the screws and the plate. Thus, this type of plate is often preferred, if highly unstable situations are diagnosed and brought to surgery. There is, however, no mechanical proof for this [11]. A clinical study—looking at speed of fusion, implant complication rate, loss of segmental lordosis, and segmental height—showed that a dynamic plate is more favorable with respect to speed of fusion and rate of implant-associated complications; a rigid plate is favorable when looking at loss of lordosis and height. There have been no sig-

T. Pitzen (✉)
Center for Spine Surgery, Orthopedics, and Traumatology, SRH Klinikum Karlsbad-Langensteinbach, Karlsbad, Germany
e-mail: tobias.pitzen@srh.de

J. Drumm · G. Ostrowski · M. Ruf
Center for Spine Surgery, SRH Klinikum Karlsbad-Langensteinbach, Karlsbad, Germany

© Springer-Verlag GmbH Germany 2023
U. Vieweg, F. Grochulla (eds.), *Manual of Spine Surgery*, https://doi.org/10.1007/978-3-662-64062-3_30

nificant differences in clinical aspects [9, 10]. It is difficult to transfer these results to other plates of other companies and even more if so called semi-rigid or semi-constrained designs—designs, placed within the dynamic ones and constrained (rigid) ones with respect to their mechanical properties—should be judged.

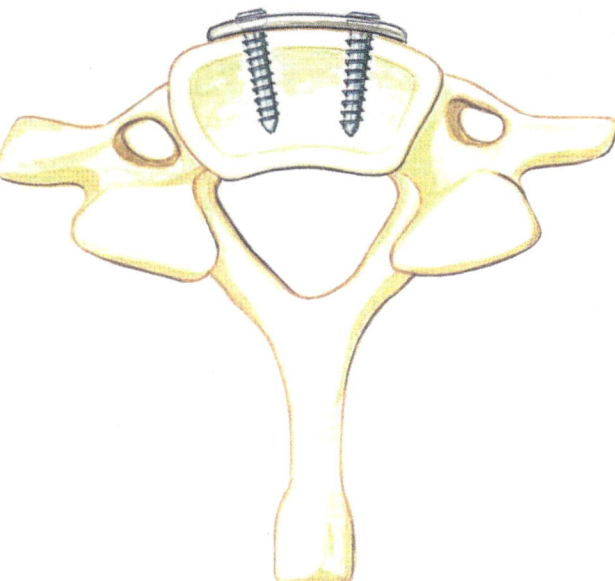

Fig. 30.1 Schematic drawing of the monocortical screws in place, axial view

30.2 Indications

In any pathology of the anterior aspect within the subaxial cervical spine treated by anterior decompression, bone graft (or cage) insertion an anterior plate, fixed by screws within the vertebral body may be used as an additional stabilization to increase initial stability, avoid graft/cage dislocation and accelerate the time to fusion. In particular, the main indications for this procedure include [5, 12–14]:

- Degenerative disease of the cervical spine (with the clinical signs of radiculopathy and/or myelopathy). The use of an anterior plate following monosegmental discectomy and fusion is usually not necessary, however recommended by the authors.
- Trauma. Note, that anterior plating is also sufficient in cases of less severe posterior instability [15]
- Tumor
- Rheumatoid instability
- Spondylodiscitis
- Failed surgery of the cervical spine

30.3 Contraindications

- Hypersensitivity to any of the implant materials

30.4 Technical Prerequisites

- Adjustable head neck-rest according to Caspar (Braun Aesculap, Tuttlingen, Germany), head fixed using a clamp according to Mayfield or Gardner–Wells, shoulders pulled down by tape,
- C-Arm,
- Preferred plate to be used, including set of screws and instruments

30.5 Surgical Technique

- Anterior cervical discectomy and graft/cage insertion is finished
- Resect remaining anterior osteophytes (create normal anatomic conditions)
- Length of the plate is determined using lateral fluoroscopy (it should not touch the adjacent discs and should be bend to the patient's individual lordosis, if possible. Please note: this is not possible with every type of plate!)
- Fix the plate temporarily by spikes in the upper and lower vertebral bodies exactly in the midline.
- Drill two burr holes into each vertebral body, insert the screws in a convergent angle. The screws should be as long as possible. However, perforation of the posterior cortical shell is not necessary (Figs. 30.1, 30.2, and 30.4). Again, there is no proof that bicortical screw fixation is necessary to ensure tight fixation [6, 7].
- Check the final situation by fluoroscopy. Figures 30.2 and 30.3 give an example of a perfectly placed 4-segmental ABC plate (Aesculap, Tuttlingen, Germany) in anterior- posterior (AP) as well as lateral projection, Figs. 30.4 and 30.5 depict the same projections for a vertebral body replacement procedure.

Figs. 30.2 and 30.3 Lateral and AP projection of a cervical spine x-ray, showing a 4 segmental plate in perfect position following 4 segmental ACDF with bone-filled cage

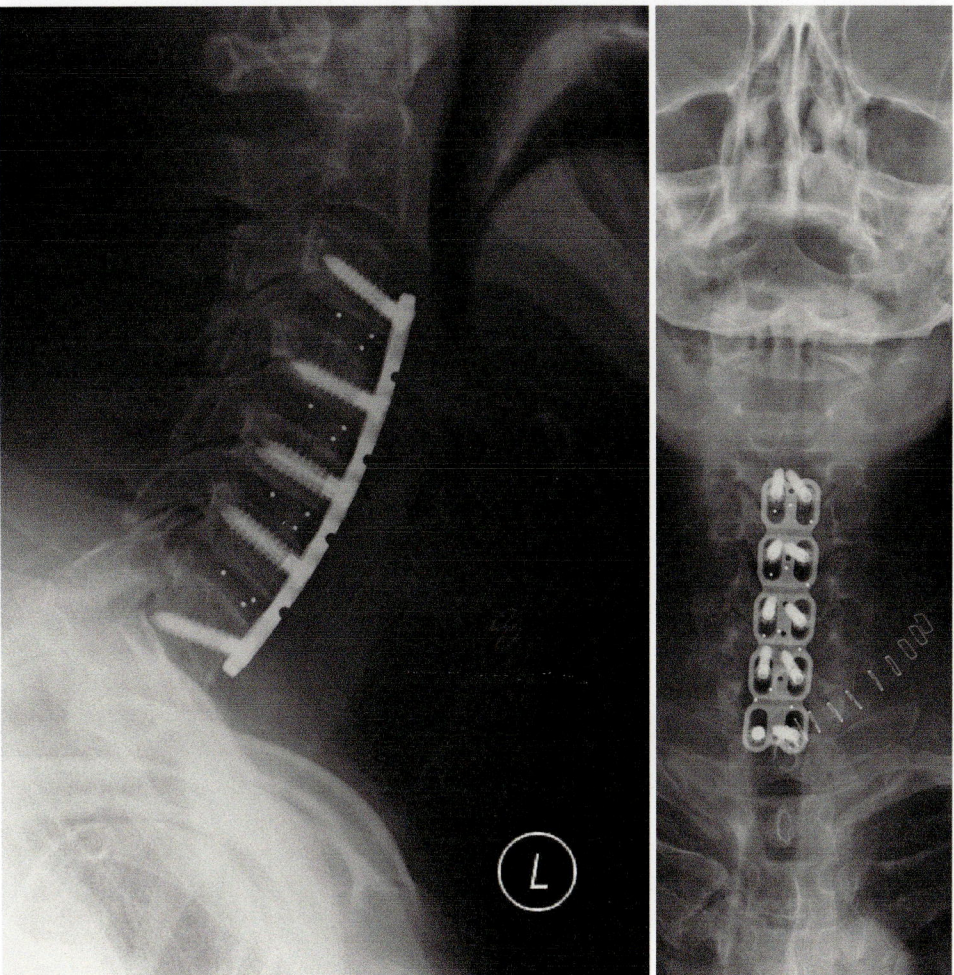

30.6   Tips and Tricks

- Note that any plate is designed to be fixed within the midline (Figs. 30.3 and 30.5). Fixing the plate in the midline prevents screw malpositioning toward the roots, which may happen if the plate is fixed lateral to the midline (Fig. 30.6). Therefore, it is beneficial to mark the midline at the initial steps of the surgery, before the longus colli muscle is detached. If this is not possible, there are two other options: give yourself an orientation where the midline is, by checking the zygapophyseal joints on both sides or take an x-ray in AP projection (not possible if you use Caspar's head neck rest as described above). However, using the technique described above, correct positioning of the plate is easy.

- If dynamic plates are used, it is of special importance, to use plates as short as possible (see Figs. 30.2 and 30.4): these plates allow the graft/cage to settle some millimeters into the adjacent vertebral body, thus resulting in a shortening of the anterior aspect. As a result, the plate may touch the adjacent discs, thus maybe producing some kind of adjacent level pathology. Thus, "think short" if using dynamic plates.
- The plate should be temporarily fixed with two or more spikes. Take care that these spikes are not placed within the holes of the distraction screws, this will NOT work.
- Although there is no evidence that filling the cervical spine cage is necessary for earlier fusion, it is easy to apply bone into the perforation of the cage used. To do so, grasp the bone from the adjacent anterior rims of the disc

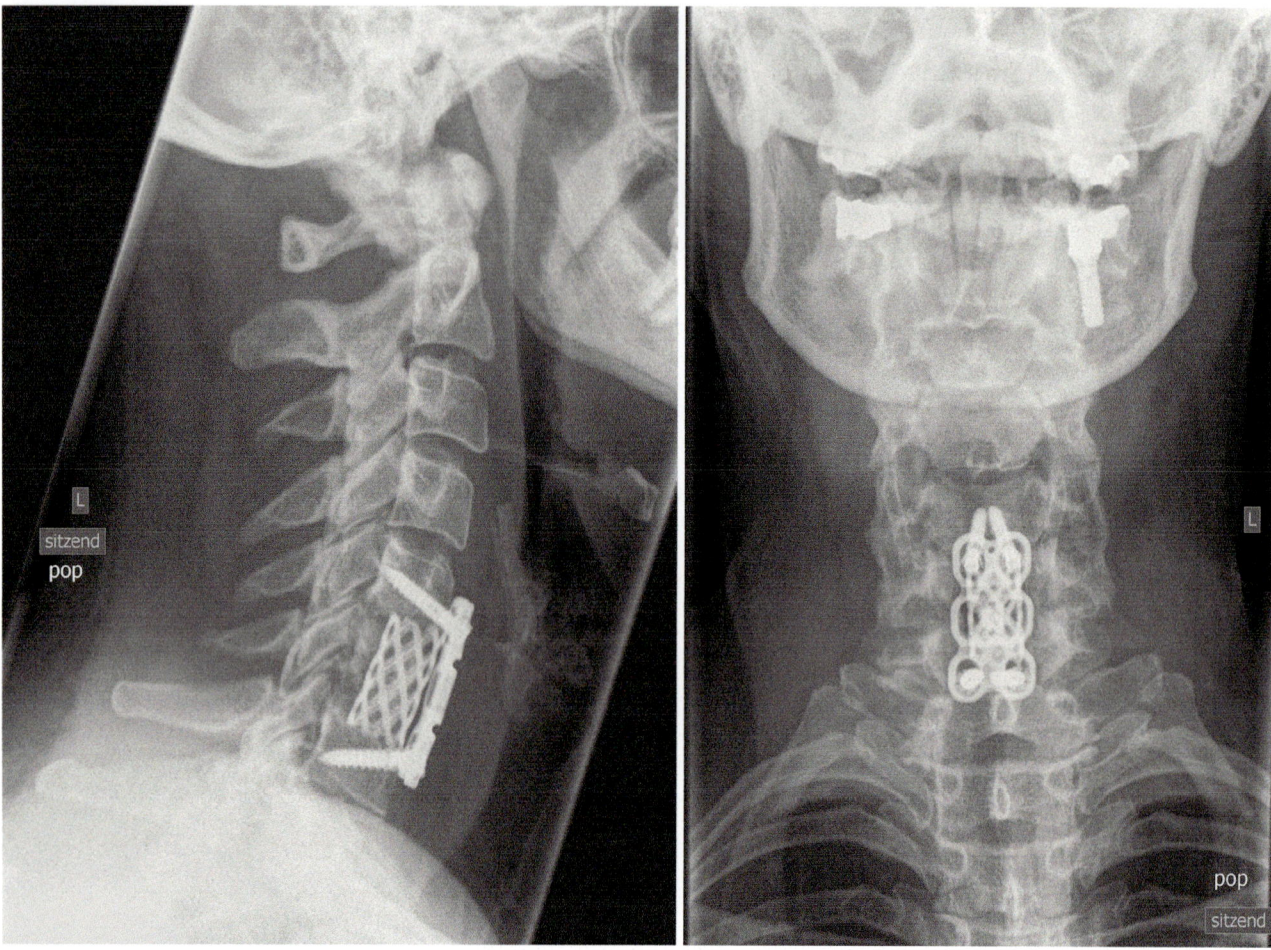

Figs. 30.4 and 30.5 Lateral and AP projection of a cervical spine x-ray. Vertebral body replacement C6, insertion of a Harms cage filled with autologous bone graft and an anterior dynamic plate. Please note the length of the plate (think short!) and the length of the screws: not bicortical, but approximately 80% of the vertebral body depth

removed. This technique has been described and evaluated by the authors [16].

- The importance of lateral fluoroscopy cannot be overemphasized, check the direction as well as the position of the screw. Again: To our knowledge, there is no proof that engaging the screws into the posterior cortical shell does increase the initial postoperative stability or pullout force or screw torque [6, 7]. Note, however, that the screws should be as long as possible. Therefore, the author prefers to orient the screws toward the adjacent discs if possible (Fig. 30.2).

- Insertional screw torque is important to obtain tight implant fixation [17]. Therefore, if the screw can just be inserted with very low torque, or the screw is even free spinning, do not hesitate to use a thicker screw (revision or rescue screw) or to enlarge the burr hole, to fill the burr hole with bone cement (methylmetacylate cement) and to insert the screw again. After hardening of the cement, the screw is finally tightened with usually very high torque [18]. The authors never saw any implant loosening using this technique. You also may use a rescue screw with thicker core and outer diameter.

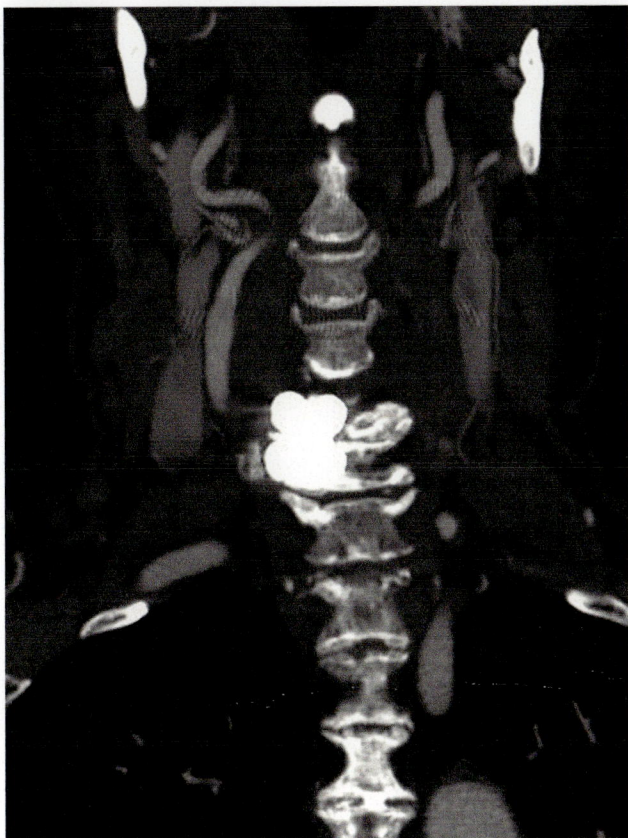

Fig. 30.6 Coronal CAT scan reconstruction: Plate fixed outside the midline, potentially harmful to roots and vertebral artery

References

1. Van Petegham PK, Schweigel JF. The fractured cervical spine rendered unstable by anterior cervical fusion. J Trauma. 1979;19:110–4.
2. Hermann HD. Metal plate fixation after anterior fusion of unstable fracture dislocationof the cervical spine. Acta Neurochir. 1975;32:101–11.
3. Böhler J, Gaudernack T. Anterior plate stabilization for fracture-dislocations of the lower cervical spine. J Trauma. 1980;20:203–5.
4. Orozco DR, Llovet TR. Osteosintesis en las lesiones traumaticas y degeneratives de la columna vertebral. Revista Traumatol Chirurg Rehabil. 1972;1:45–52.
5. Caspar W, Barbier D, Klara PM. Anterior cervical fusion and Caspar plate stabilization for cervical trauma. Neurosurgery. 1989;25:491–502.
6. Pitzen T, Wilke HJ, Caspar W, Steudel WI, Claes L. Evaluation of a new monocortical screw for anterior cervical fusion and plating by a combined biomechanical and clinical study. Eur Spine J. 1999;8:382–7.
7. Pitzen T, Barbier D, Tintinger F, Steudel WI, Strowitzki M. Screw fixation to the posterior cortical shell does not influence peak torque and pullout in anterior cervical plating. Eur Spine J. 2002;11:494–9.
8. Brodke DS, Gollogly S, Alexander Mohr R, Nguyen BK, Dailey AT, Bachus AK. Dynamic cervical plates: biomechanical evaluation of load sharing and stiffness. Spine. 2001;26:1324–9.
9. Pitzen TR, Chrobok J, Stulik J, Ruffing S, Drumm J, Sova L, Kucera R, Vyskocil T, Steudel WI. Implant complications, fusion, loss of lordosis, and outcome after anterior cervical plating with dynamic or rigid plates: two-year results of a multi-centric, randomized, controlled study. Spine. 2009;34(7):641–6.
10. Stulik J, Pitzen TR, Chrobok J, Ruffing S, Drumm J, Sova L, Kucera R, Vyskocil T, Steudel WI. Fusion and failure following anterior cervical plating with dynamic or rigid plates: 6-months results of a multi-centric, prospective, randomized, controlled study. Eur Spine J. 2007;16(10):1689–94.
11. Dvorak MF, Pitzen T, Zhu Q, Gordon JD, Fisher CG, Oxland TR. Anterior cervical plate fixation: a biomechanical study to evaluate the effects of plate design, endplate preparation, and bone mineral density. Spine. 2005;30(3):294–301.
12. Caspar W, Geisler F, Pitzen T, et al. Anterior cervical plate stabilization in one – and two – level degenerative disease: overtreatment or benefit? J Spinal Disord. 1998;11:1–11.
13. Caspar W, Pitzen T, Papavero L, Geisler FH, Johnson TA. Anterior cervical plating for the treatment of neoplasms in the cervical spine. J Neurosurg. 1999;1:27–34.
14. Caspar W, Pitzen T. Anterior cervical fusion and trapezoidal plate stabilization for re – do surgery. Surg Neurol. 1999;52:345–52.
15. Pitzen T, Lane C, Goertzen D, Dvorak M, Fisher C, Barbier D, Steudel WI, Oxland TR. Anterior cervical plate fixation: biomechanical effectiveness as a function of posterior element injury. J Neurosurg. 2003;99:84–90.
16. Pitzen T, Kiefer R, et al. Filling a cervical spine cage with local autograft: change of bone density and assessment of bony fusion. Zentralbl Neurochir. 2006;67:8–13.
17. Ryken TC, Clausen JD, Traynelis VC, Goel VK. Biomechanical analysis of bone mineral density, insertion technique, screw torque, and holding strength of anterior cervical plate screws. J Neurosurg. 1995;83:324–9.
18. Pitzen TR, Drumm J, Bruchmann B, Barbier DD, Steudel WI. Effectiveness of cemented rescue screws for anterior cervical plate fixation. J Neurosurg Spine. 2006;4(1):60–3.

Cage Implantation in the Cervical Spine

31

Uwe Vieweg

31.1 Introduction and Core Messages

Anterior cervical discectomy is the most common surgical procedure used to treat damaged cervical discs. Its goal is to relieve pressure on the nerve roots or on the spinal cord by removing the ruptured disc. In the operation, the soft tissues of the neck are separated, and the disc is removed. In order to maintain the normal height of the disc space, the surgeon may choose to fill the space with a bone graft or cage. This chapter describes the implantation of a fusion cage [1–3].

31.2 Indications [1–9]

- Degenerative disease of the cervical spine with clinical signs (radiculopathy, myelopathy) as described in Chap. 19.
- Single or multilevel soft disc herniation.
- Disc ligament injuries with additional plating.

31.3 Contraindications

- Predominant posterior compression of the neural structures.

31.4 Technical Prerequisites

Fluoroscopy, operating microscope, adequate instrumentation for ventral discectomy (punches, forceps), high-speed drill (rose and diamond), Caspar retractor system (see

U. Vieweg (✉)
Department of Conservative and Surgical Spine Therapy with Interdisciplinary Spinal Deformities Centre and Rummelsberg Sectional Center, Hospital Rummelsberg, Schwarzenbruck, Germany
e-mail: uwe.vieweg@sana.de

Fig. 31.8) or similar retractor for ventral approach to the cervical spine. A ring retractor system (Synthes Synframe) is an alternative. Different interbody fusion cages can be used (see Fig. 31.12a–f).

31.5 Planning, Preparation, and Positioning

The patient is positioned supine on the operating table, and the head is supported on a Mayfield horseshoe headrest. General anesthetic giving optimal muscle relaxation is administered. The neck is placed in a neutral position with the aid of fluoroscopy. Note: shoulder roll placed between scapulae to increase neck extension in this patient whose fracture reduced in extension (see Fig. 31.1). The arms are tucked to the side. Wrist restraints with long extensions or shoulder tape can be useful to enhance X-ray visualization (see Fig. 31.2a–c). The location of the incision is estimated

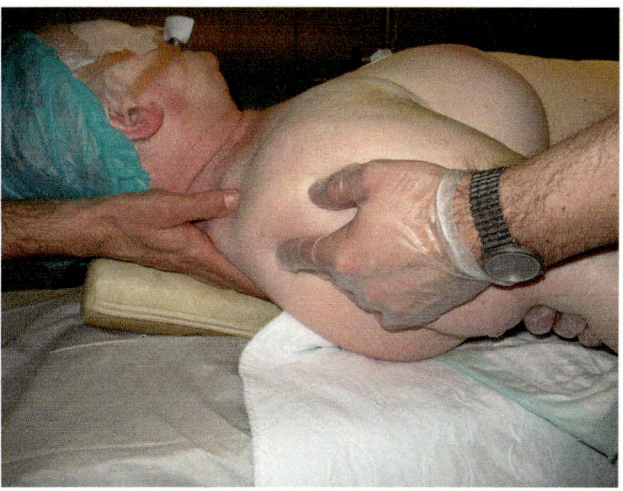

Fig. 31.1 Positioning of the patient with a roll placed between the shoulder blades. Padding is placed under the shoulders

U. Vieweg, F. Grochulla (eds.), *Manual of Spine Surgery*, https://doi.org/10.1007/978-3-662-64062-3_31

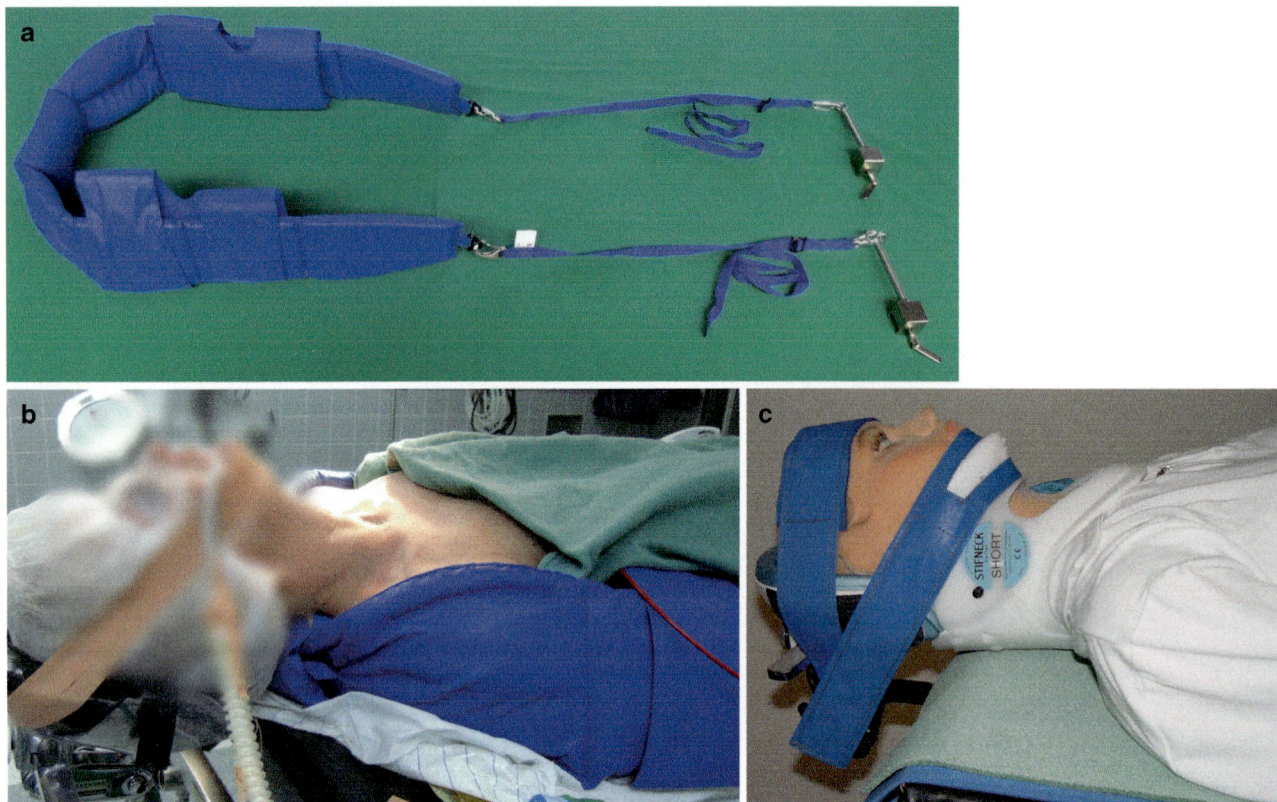

Fig. 31.2 (**a–c**) Special shoulder-, arm-, head-fixation systems

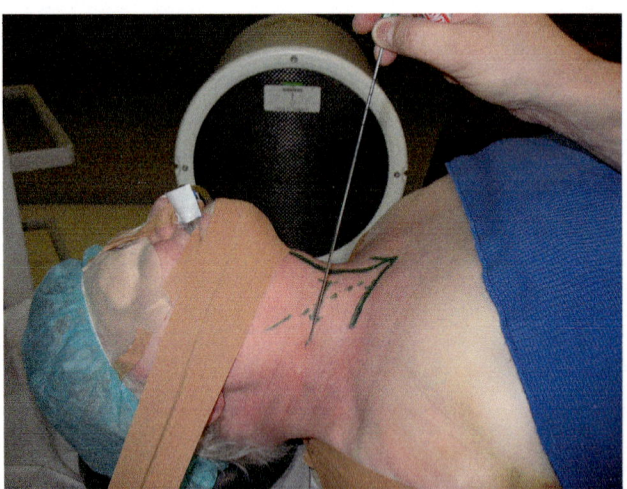

Fig. 31.3 Marking of the skin incision with the aid of the C-arm

using the lateral fluoroscopic image (see Fig. 31.3). Localization of the skin incision to the level of pathology via external landmarks (see Fig. 31.4): hard palate–arch of atlas, lower border of mandible–C2/3, hyoid–C3, thyroid cartilage–C4/5, cricoid cartilage–C6 and carotid tubercle (anterior transverse process)–C6.

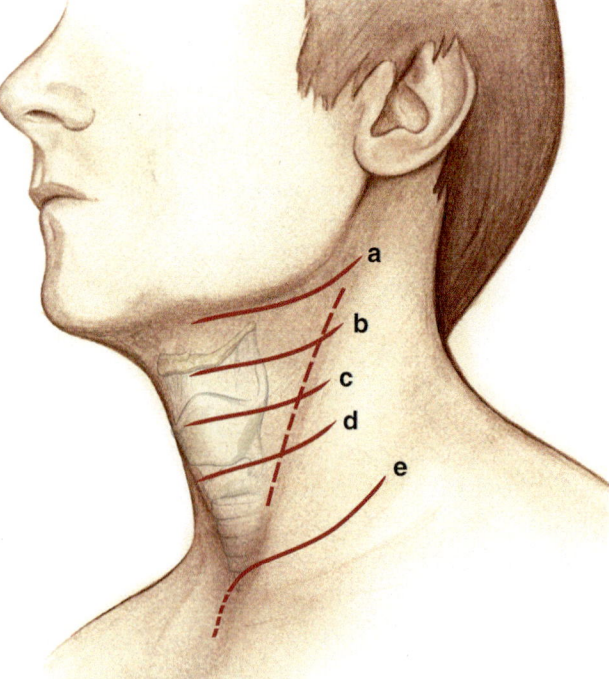

Fig. 31.4 (**a**) Skin incision in relation to the anatomical level. External landmarks are hard palate–arch of atlas, (**b**) lower border of mandible–C2/3, (**c**) hyoid–C3, thyroid cartilage–C4/5, (**d**) cricoid cartilage–C6, (**e**) carotid tubercle (anterior transverse process)–C6

31.6 Surgical Technique [1–3, 6, 8]

31.6.1 Approach

- The Cloward standard approach to the anterior cervical spine [2] is recommended (see Fig. 31.6).
- A transverse skin incision should be made on the left or right side for access. The author prefers access from the right. (see Fig. 31.4 demonstrated the incisions on the left side.) The recurrent laryngeal nerve may be traumatized during the deepest layer of the approach. Many surgeons prefer a left side approach because the nerve takes a more predictable course on this side, descending into the thorax with the carotid sheath, curving around the aortic arch and ascending between the trachea and esophagus to supply the larynx. On the other hand, a right-side approach may be easier for a right-handed surgeon. Yet, the recurrent laryngeal nerve descends with the carotid sheath and curves around the subclavian artery to ascend into the neck at a higher level than on the left.
- The incision should be medial to the anterior border of the sternomastoid muscle and should extend to the midline. For cosmetic reasons, we recommend a diagonal incision along the Langer's line. Alternatively, a longitudinal incision can be made along the anterior edge of the sternocleidomastoid muscle.
- The skin is undermined in a cranial and caudal direction.
- Immediately following the incision, the platysmas muscle is identified and incised (see Fig. 31.5). Directly beneath the skin lies the platysma, which may be divided longitudinally (in line with the fibres) with the tip of the index fingers.

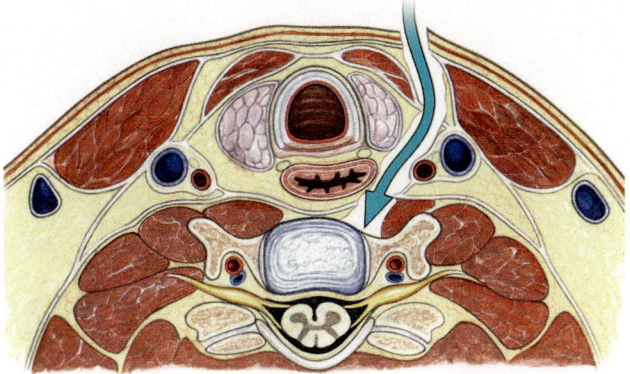

Fig. 31.6 Axial schematics of the Smith–Robinson approach (standard anterolateral approach) to the middle anterior cervical spine, trachea, strap muscle, longus coli muscle, pretracheal fascia, prevertebral fascia, superficial fascia

Alternatively, the platysma may be divided, without functional consequences, in line with a transverse incision.

- The deep cervical fascia is next identified as an investing layer that splits around the sternocleidomastoid. It is superficial to all of structures of the neck except the platysma and external jugular vein. The sternocleidomastoid may now be gently laterally retracted (see Fig. 31.5).
- Blunt dissection using scissors reveals the carotid sheath (carotid artery, internal jugular vein, vagus nerve).
- When the omohyoid muscle has been found, it should be passed either cranially (C2–5) or caudally (C5–T2) or should be severed.
- The trachea and esophagus are moved toward the middle, and the carotid artery and jugular vein are moved to the side. Both are then protected with metal retractors which can occasionally cause a sore throat or hoarseness for a short time after surgery.
- The attachments of the longus colli muscle are separated on both sides by means of alternating use of scissors, bipolar forceps, and swab (see Fig. 31.7).
- The relevant disc is localized using intraoperative fluoroscopy.
- Once the correct level has been identified, the longus colli muscles are moved away from the lateral edge of the anterior cervical vertebra so that retractors will be able to engage the tissue (see Fig. 31.8).
- Ventral spondylophytes are removed with a high-speed drill or Luer.
- After exposure of the anterior aspects of the spine and detachment of the medial insertion of the longus colli muscles on both sides, the soft tissue is retracted using the Caspar cervical retractor. Retractor valves are inserted under the belly of each muscle (see Fig. 31.8). The cervical ring of the Synframe retractor system can also be used as an alternative.

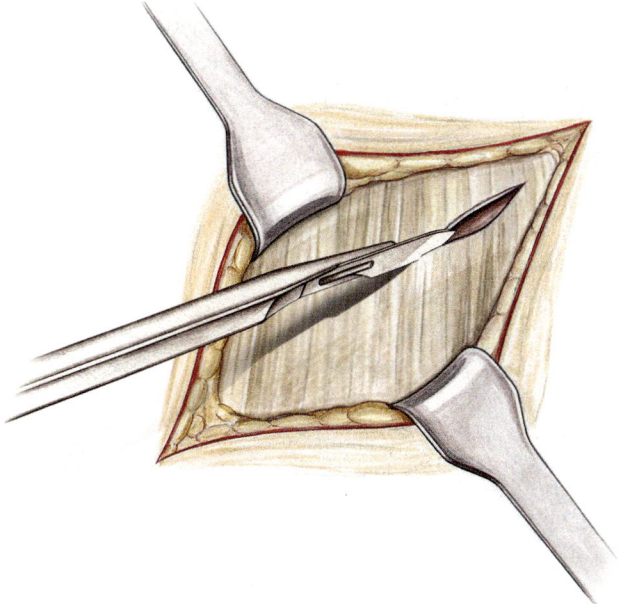

Fig. 31.5 Identification and incision of the platysmas muscle

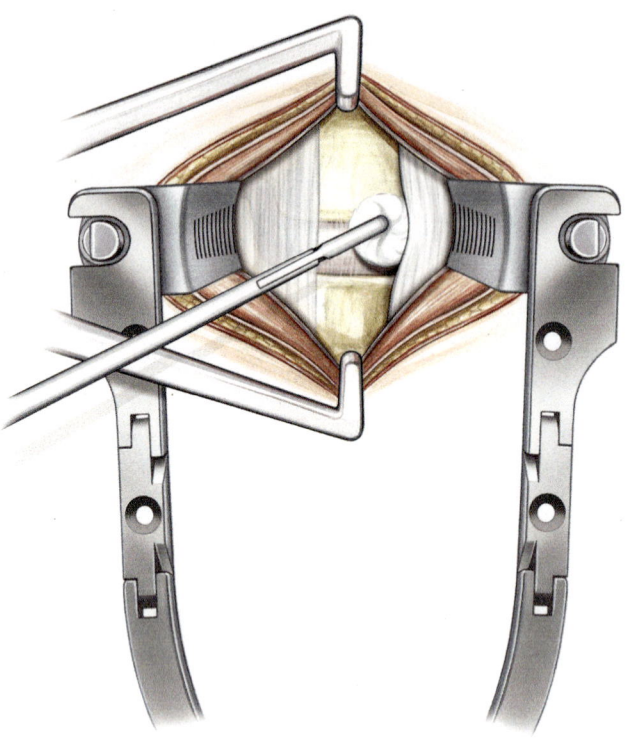

Fig. 31.7 Pushing the two longus colli muscles aside with small swabs

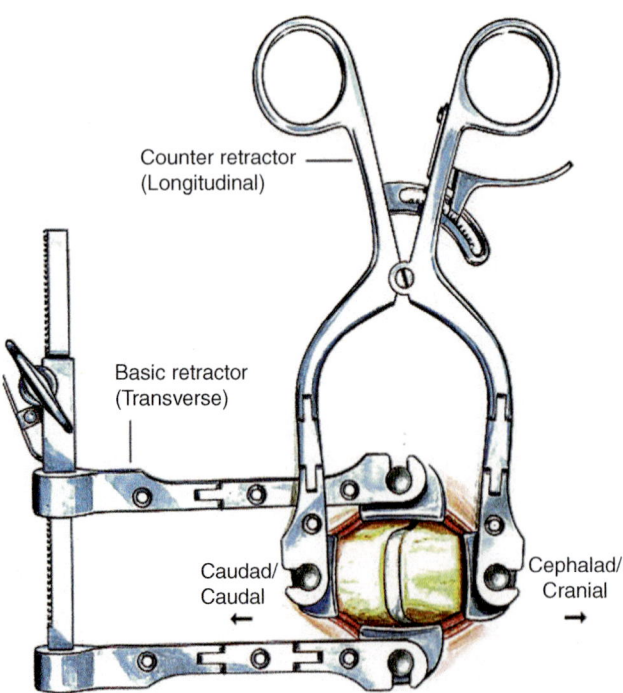

Counter retractor (Longitudinal)

Basic retractor (Transverse)

Caudad/Caudal

Cephalad/Cranial

Fig. 31.8 Caspar cervical retractor system in position. (With permission of Aesculap AG, Tuttlingen, Germany)

31.6.2 Discectomy and Decompression

- The midline between the two longus colli muscles is marked using a small diamond burr.
- The Caspar distraction screws are positioned. Note: they should be placed centrally in the midline of the vertebral body.
- A drill guide is used to position the drill hole for the first distraction screw in the middle of the inferior vertebral body. The drilling depth of the drill is fixed at 8 mm to exclude the possibility of inadvertent penetration into the spinal canal. The drilling direction is usually approximately parallel to the adjacent vertebral end plates. The screw should not penetrate the posterior cortex (see Chap. 19). Screws with self-cutting threads should be used. The correct choice of thread length is determined by the anteroposterior diameter of the vertebral body. The screw should not penetrate the posterior cortex.
- The distraction screw is inserted through the drill guide using the screwdriver. Care must be taken to screw in the distraction screw right up to its base plate in order to embed it firmly in the vertebral body. This prevents screw pullout during the distraction process.
- After removing the moveable distractor arm, the drill guide is fitted onto the toothed distractor bar, and this assembly is positioned over the distraction screw which is already in place.
- After drilling in the center of the vertebral body, the second (superior) distraction screw is screwed in, and the drill guide assembly is removed. The drill guide is subsequently taken off the distractor bar and replaced by the moveable distractor arm.
- The disc is then excised near the anterior longitudinal ligament and detached using a sharp spoon and curette (Fig. 31.9).
- The disc should be completely removed from the cranial and caudal end plates and laterally from the uncovertebral joints, with Kerrison rongeurs and straight curettes (see Fig. 31.10a, b).
- Discectomy is completed under mild distraction, and decompression of the neural structures is then performed. The posterior longitudinal ligament is normally retrieved and detached as far as is necessary to remove osteophytes using the longitudinal ligament dissector.
- The dorsal spondylosis is ablated with a high-speed burr and punch, and the posterior longitudinal ligament is removed. Note: when the high-speed diamond burr is used to remove the dorsal edge or dorsal osteophytes, care should always be taken to ensure that the end plates remain undamaged.

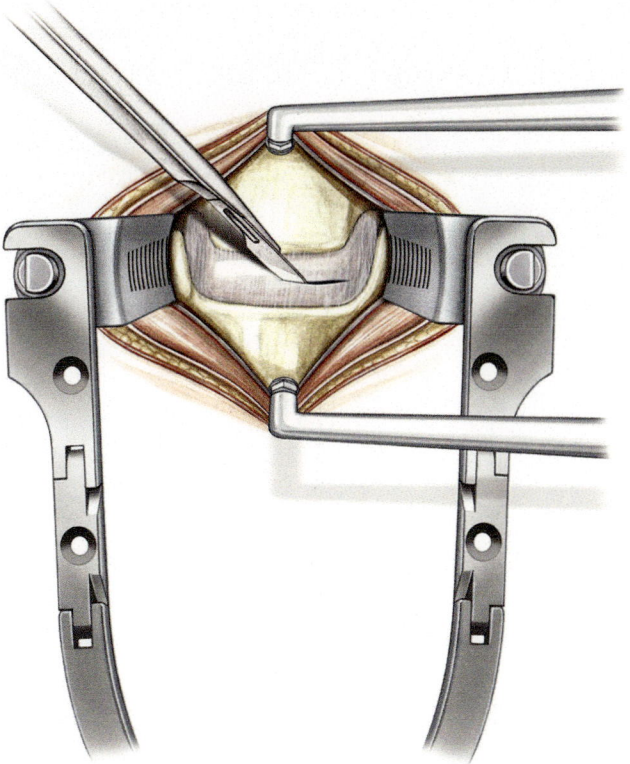

Fig. 31.9 Cutting into the disc with a microscapel

- After the disc has been removed, the posterior longitudinal ligament is also removed revealing the anterior aspect of the dura.

31.6.3 Cage Implantation

- Once the neural structures have been fully decompressed, the appropriate implant size can be determined with the aid of the trial implants (see Fig. 31.11a).
- Using the insertion instrument set, the cage is introduced into the intervertebral space (see Fig. 31.11b). The implant should usually lie centrally about 1–2 mm in front of the rear edge.
- By relaxing the Caspar retractor, the ligaments are reactivated so that the implant is held securely in the intervertebral space (see Fig. 31.11c). The cage must be firmly held and not easy to move!

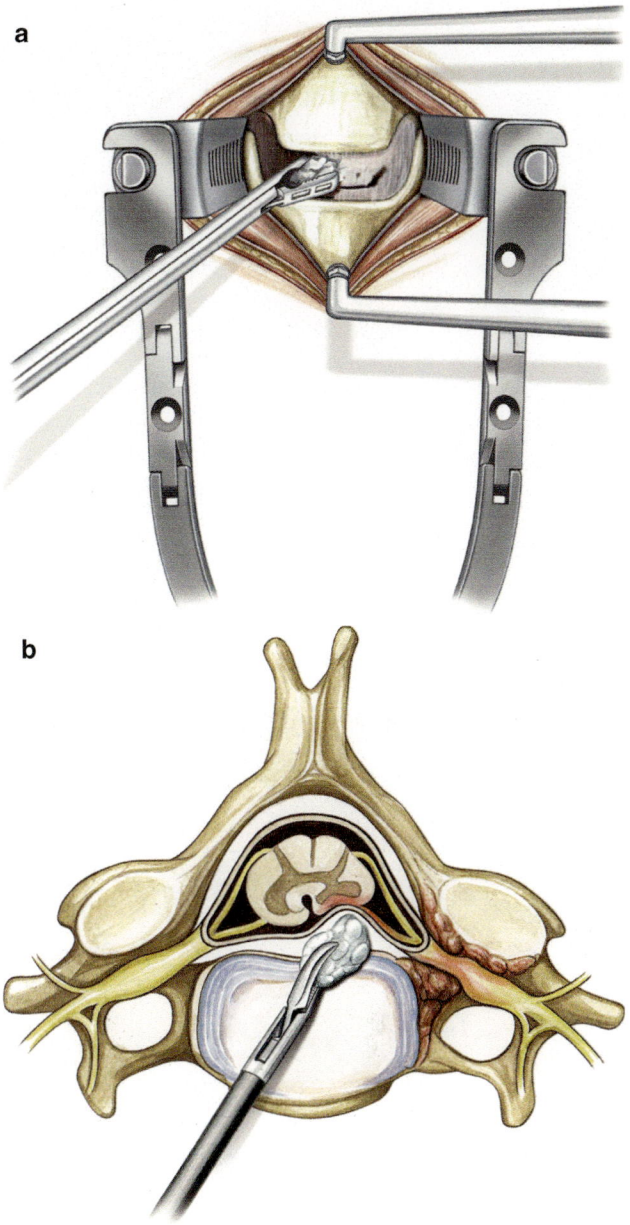

Fig. 31.10 (**a, b**) Removal of the disc with rongeurs

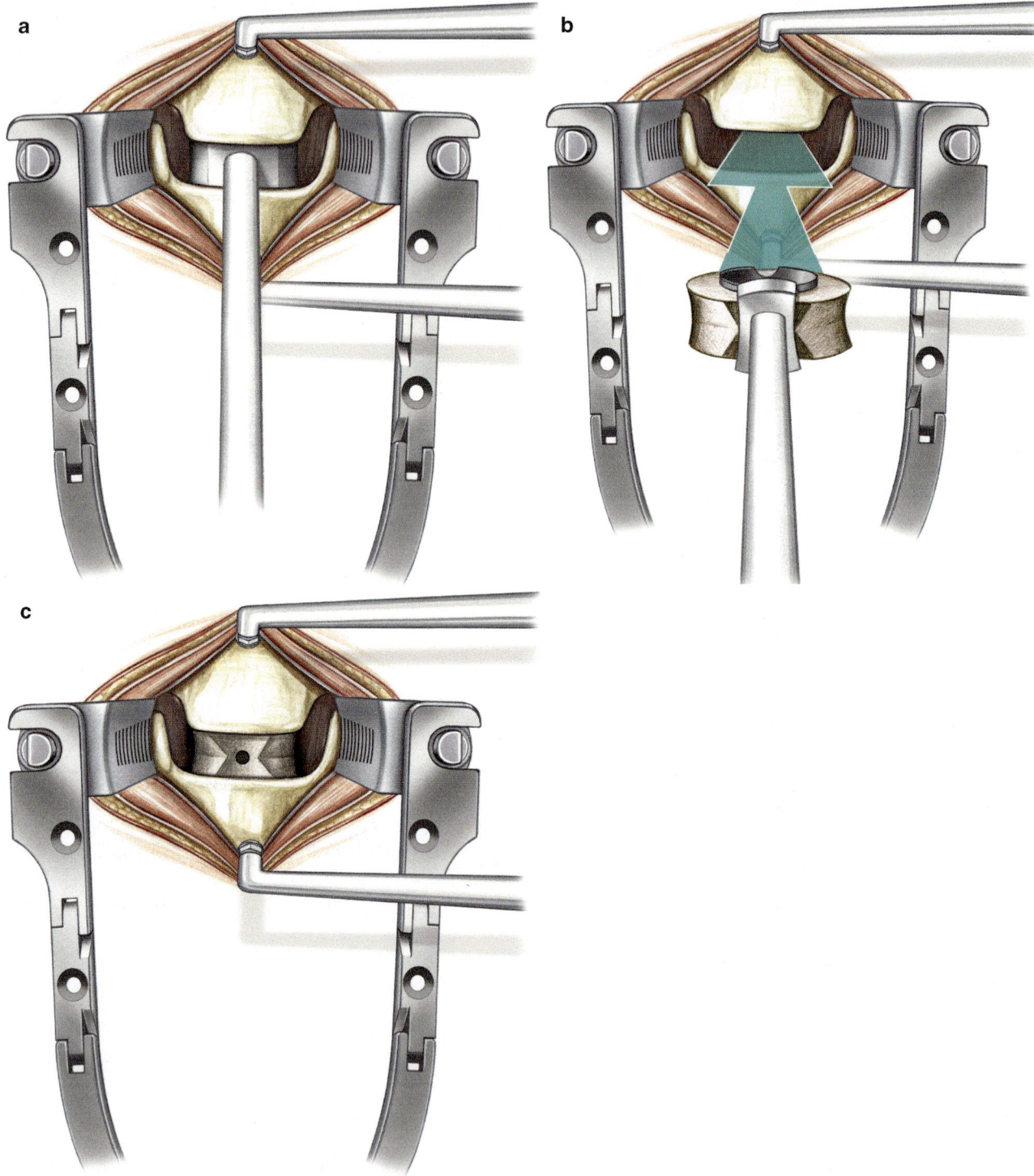

Fig. 31.11 (**a**) Determining implant size. (**b**) Cage implantation. (**c**) Cage in situ

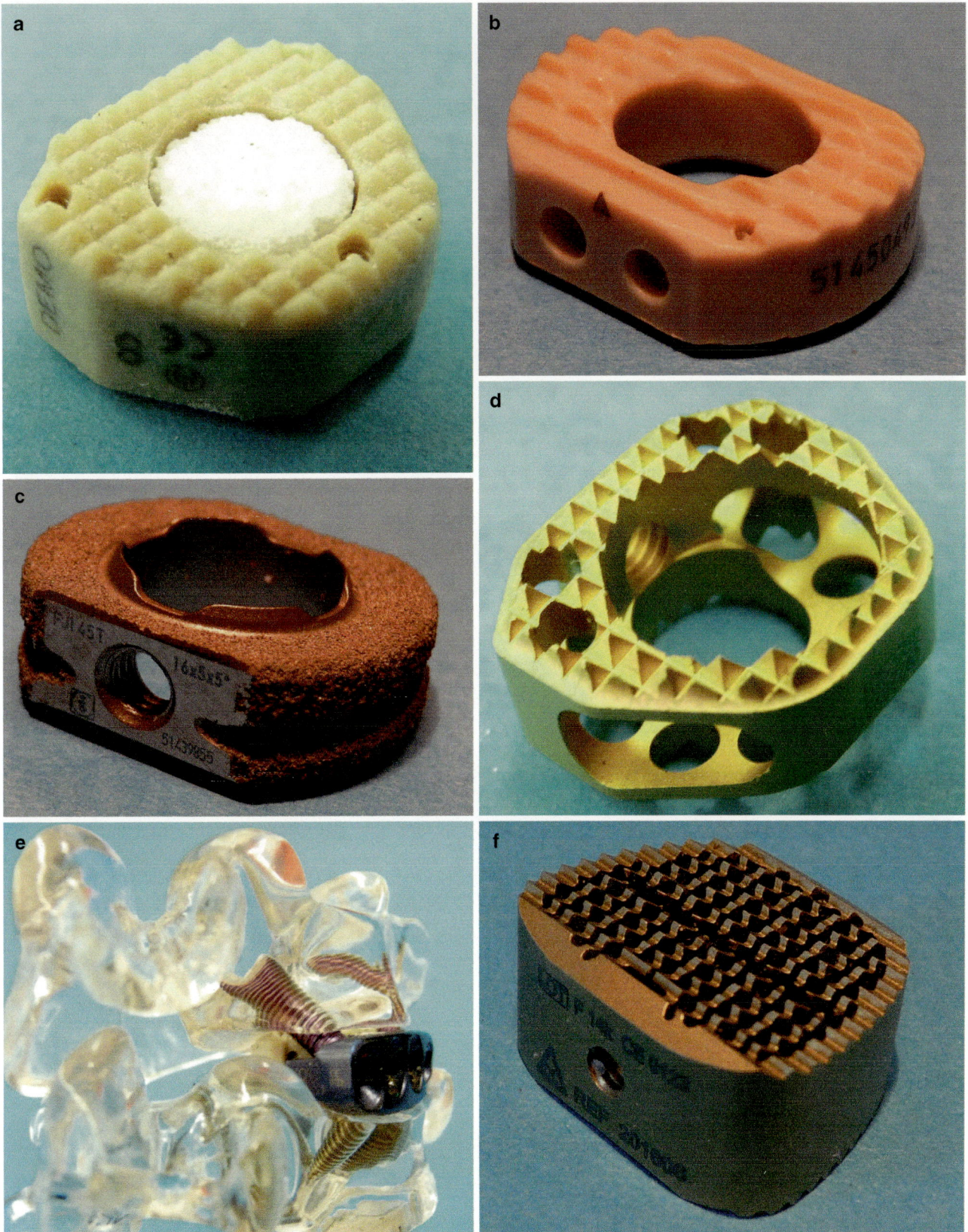

Fig. 31.12 Different interbody fusion cages. (**a**) Syncage with Chronos (Synthes). (**b**) C-Space PEEK (Aesculap). (**c**) C-Space Titan Plasmapore-coated (Aesculap). (**d**) Cervios Titan cage (Synthes). (**e**) Zero-P cage with integrated plate (Synthes). (**f**) Hydro Deltacor

References

1. Bailey RW, Badgley CE. Stabilization of the cervical spine by anterior fusion. J Bone Joint Surg Am. 1960;42:565–94.
2. Bartels RH, Donk RD, Feuth T. Subsidence of stand-alone cervical carbon fiber cages. Neurosurgery. 2006;58(3):502–8.
3. Cloward RB. The anterior approach for removal of ruptured discs. J Neurosurg. 1958;15:602–17.
4. Bednar DA, Al-Tunaib AW. Failure of reconstitution of open-section, posterior iliac-wing bone graft donor sites after lumbar spinal fusion. Observations with implications for the etiology of donor site pain. Eur Spine J. 2005;14(1):95–8.
5. Chen Y, Lu G, Wang B, et al. A comparison of anterior cervical discectomy and fusion (ACDF) using self-locking stand-alone polyetheretherketone (PEEK) cage with ACDF using cage and plate in the treatment of three-level cervical degenerative spondylopathy: a retrospective study with 2-year follow-up. Eur Spine J. 2016;25(7):2255–62.
6. Faldini C, Chehrassan M, Miscione MT, et al. Single-level anterior cervical discectomy and interbody fusion using PEEK anatomical cervical cage and allograft bone. J Orthop Traumatol. 2011;12(4):201–5.
7. Kao TH, Wu CH, Chou YC, et al. Risk factors for subsidence in anterior cervical fusion with stand-alone polyetheretherketone (PEEK) cages: a review of 82 cases and 182 levels. Arch Orthop Trauma Surg. 2014;134(10):1343–51.
8. Moon HJ, Kim JH. The effects of anterior cervical discectomy and fusion with stand-alone cages at two contiguous levels on cervical alignment and outcomes. Acta Neurochir. 2011;153(3):559–65.
9. Sasso RC, Smucker JD, Hacker R, et al. Clinical outcomes of BRYAN cervical disc arthroplasty: a prospective, randomized, controlled, multicenter trial with 24-month follow-up. J Spinal Disord Tech. 2007;20(7):481–91.

Implantation of a Cervical Disc Prosthesis

Uwe Vieweg

32.1 Introduction and Core Messages

Anterior cervical decompression and interbody fusion with an internal fixation device (ACDF, or anterior cervical decompression and fusion) has, for some time, been the classic treatment for cervical spondylosis, but this technique could result in accelerated degeneration of the adjacent level. It was hypothesised that this degeneration could be prevented or at least decelerated by replacing the diseased disc with a prosthesis, and thus preserving motion. Over the last decades, numerous disc prostheses designs have been developed and have been approved for specific indications. The evidence available to-date indicates that they help to prevent or slowdown degeneration of the adjacent disc and segment [1, 2]. Disc replacement can restore the physiological curvature and range of motion of the cervical vertebrae to a greater extent than other forms of treatment [3–5]. Implantation of a cervical disc prosthesis consists of two fundamental steps. The first is decompression of the neural structures, for which a conventional approach via the left or right blood vessel compartment is usually taken. The second step involves thorough preparation of the site followed by secure, central placement of the implant in the prepared space.

32.2 Indications

Clear

Clinically proofed and accepted
- Soft disc prolapse.
- Symptomatic cervical discopathy with neck and/or arm pain with or without neurological-deficit concordant with MRI of disc pathology.

Questionable

- Preoperative segmental kyphosis or "straight neck."
- Narrow, hard disc.
- Acute myelopathy with MRI signal changes.
- Osteophytic and sclerotic changes of the vertebral bodies.
- Anterior or posterior longitudinal ligament ossifications.

U. Vieweg (✉)
Department of Conservative and Surgical Spine Therapy with Interdisciplinary Spinal Deformities Centre and Rummelsberg Sectional Center, Hospital Rummelsberg, Schwarzenbruck, Germany
e-mail: uwe.vieweg@sana.de

U. Vieweg, F. Grochulla (eds.), *Manual of Spine Surgery*, https://doi.org/10.1007/978-3-662-64062-3_32

32.3 Contraindications

- Spinal deformities following trauma and laminectomy.
- Spondylarthrosis, facet joint degeneration.
- Chronic degenerative spinal stenosis.
- Segmental instability (more than 3 mm of translation).
- Segmental immobility (segmental mobility less than 2° in flexion and extension).
- Chronic myelopathy.
- Osteoporosis.
- Metal (CoCrMo) allergy.
- Pregnancy, rheumatoid arthritis, systemic illness.
- Deformation of the end plates.

32.4 Technical Requirement

- Head fixed using a clamp according to Mayfield or Gardner–Wells.
- C-arm.
- Microscope.
- High-speed drill.

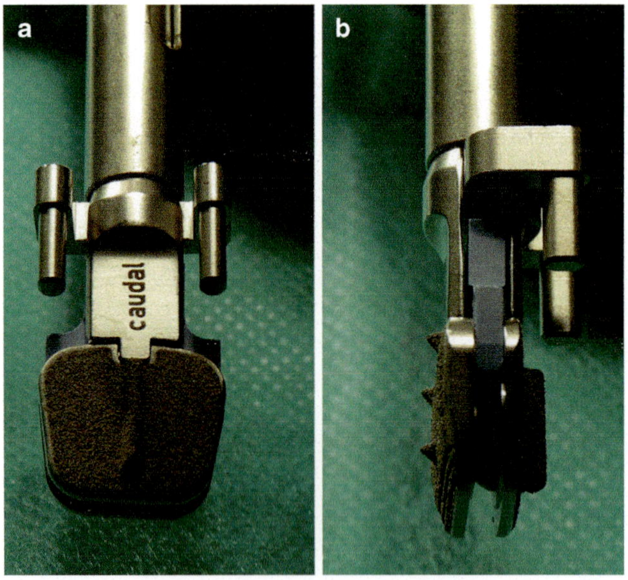

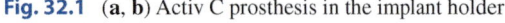

Fig. 32.1 (**a, b**) Activ C prosthesis in the implant holder

The primary goal of cervical arthroplasty is to remove the pathologically herniated disc while maintaining disc height and preserving motion. This chapter describes the implantation of the activ C prosthesis. The activ C intervertebral disc prosthesis is used to replace intervertebral discs in the cervical spine. The activ C intervertebral disc prosthesis consists of two components: superior prosthesis plate with spikes for anchoring in the vertebral body and inferior prosthesis plate with integrated polyethylene inlay and central anchoring fin for fixation in the vertebral body. The prosthesis plates and the polyethylene inlay together form a ball-and-socket joint. The polyethylene inlay is anchored to form-fit in the inferior prosthesis plate (see Fig. 32.1).

The activ C intervertebral disc prosthesis is available in six different sizes (XS, S, M, L, XL, and XXL) and up to three different heights (5, 6, and 7 mm). Activ C intervertebral disc prostheses are supplied fully pre-assembled.

Many designs have been advocated as replacements for cervical discs. They consist of either articulating or non-articulating components constructed from various materials (see Table 32.1 and Fig. 32.2).

32.5 Planning, Preparation, and Positioning

- Patient's neck is placed in a neutral position, not in hyperlordosis which is routinely used for anterior fusion techniques (see Fig. 32.3b).
- If necessary, the operating position is adjusted according to a preoperative X-ray of the patient standing in a neutral position.
- Positions of the head, the cervical spine, and the patient are fixed.
- Radiographic visibility of the relevant segments (lateral and anteroposterior (AP) views) is ensured.

Note: Positioning of the patient's neck in hyperlordosis can result in inappropriate positioning of the prosthesis. During the operation, the alignment of the prosthesis and the spinal segment can wrongly appear as 'correct'. As soon as

Table 32.1 Different artificial disc prosthesis with different design details [3, 4, 6–12]

Device	Prestige	Activ C	Bryan	ProDisc C	Cervicore	Porous coated motion
Company	Medtronic	Aesculap	Medtronic	Synthes	Stryker	
Articulating materials	Metal-metal	Metal-polyethylene	Metal-polyethylene	Metal-polyethylene	Metal-metal	Metal-polyethylene
Theoretical centre of rotation location	Superior vertebra	Directly below the inferior plate	Within implant	Inferior vertebra	Superior and inferior vertebra	Inferior vertebra
Initial fixation	Screws	Combination of spikes and keel	Milled bone	Keels	Screws and spikes	Ridges

Fig. 32.2 Classification of different designs for cervical arthroplasty by the Cervical Spine Study Group on "artificial cervical nomenclature" [13]

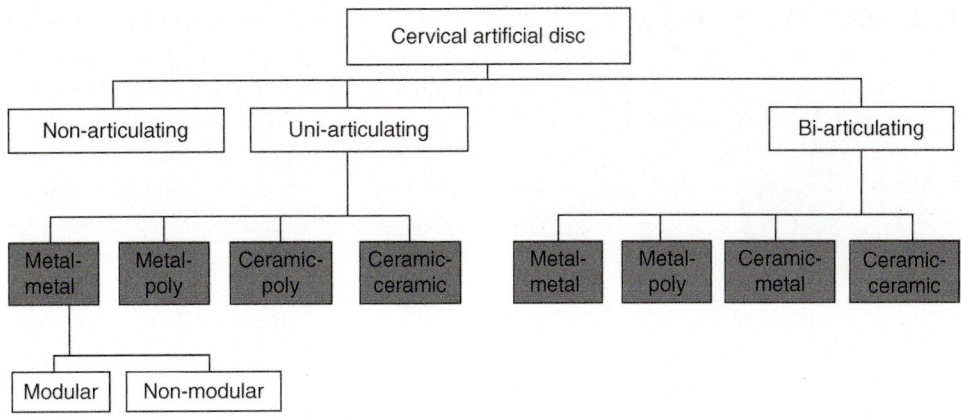

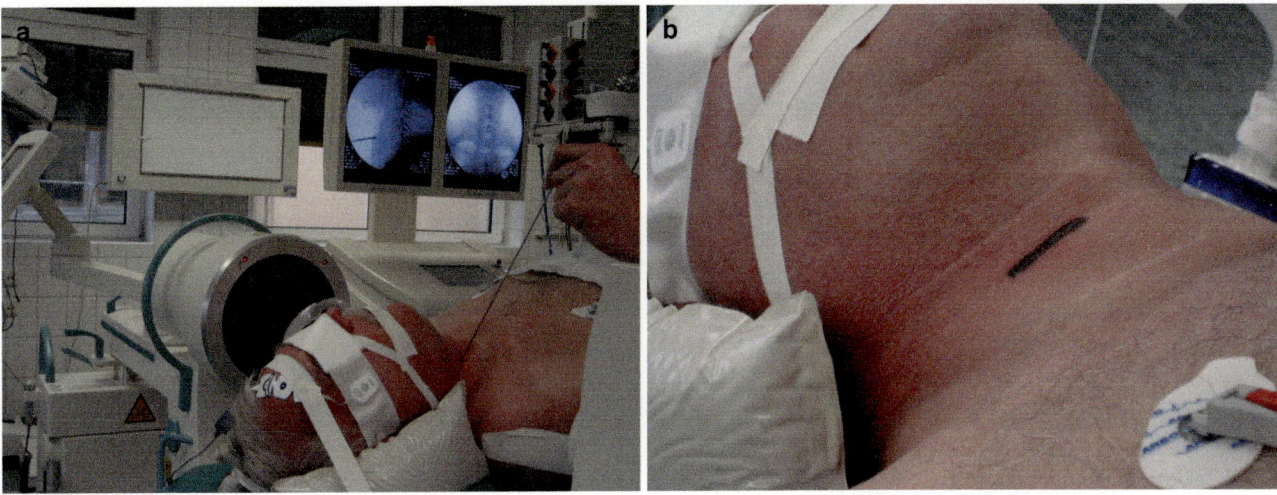

Fig. 32.3 Skin incision (**b**) and planning of the skin incision. A horizontal "'cosmetic'" skin incision targeted with fluoroscopy (**a**)

the spine returns to a neutral position in post-operative daily life, the segment and the prosthesis can fall into a kyphotic position.

32.6   Surgical Technique

32.6.1   Approach

- A standard anterolateral approach allows a precise view of all anterior parts of the cervical spine that are affected during a discectomy and the implantation of a disc prosthesis.
- Subaxial cervical spine can be approached from the right or left side depending on surgeon's preference.

- Most surgeons approach the upper part from the right and the lower part (C5/6 and C6/7) from the left side because of the anatomical positions of the recurrent nerves.
- A horizontal 'cosmetic' skin incision, targeted using fluoroscopy, is currently preferred (see Fig. 32.3b).
- The medial sheet is sharply cut, and the anterior spine is accessed by approaching between the neuromuscular bundle (v. jugularis, a. carotis, vagus nerve) and the visceral organs (trachea and oesophagus).
- Cutting of the pre-vertebral lamina allows sharp dissection of the walls of the medial longus colli muscle. This step is important in order to anchor the wound distractor firmly and safely (regarding oesophagus) beneath the muscle bundles. Alternatively, a Synframe (Synthes) or Caspar retractor (Aesculap) (see Fig. 32.4) can be used.

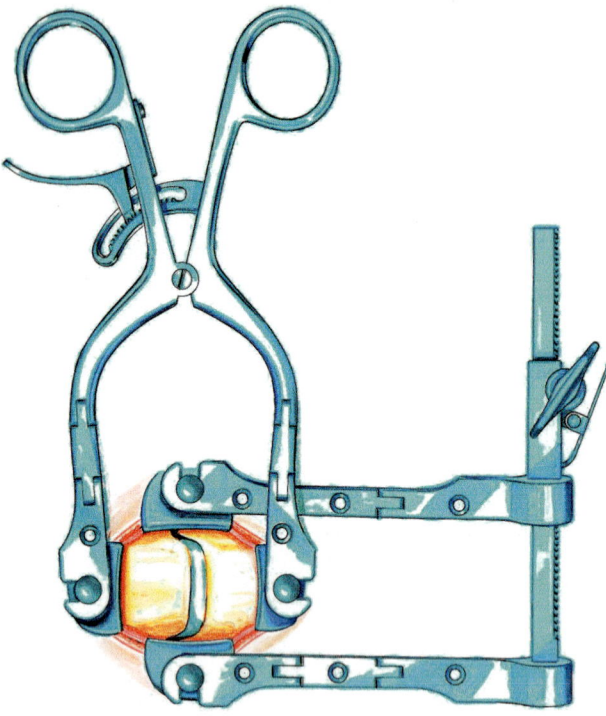

Fig. 32.4 Caspar retractor. The PEEK material provides enough biomechanical stability and, which features of radiolucency excellent visibility in both lateral and AP fluoroscopic view (With permission of Aesculap AG, Tuttlingen, Germany)

32.6.2 Instrumentation

- Midline marking.
  The midline of the vertebral body in the sagittal plane is usually determined from the following anatomic landmarks: position of the longus colli muscles, axis of symmetry of the anterior vertebral surface, and midline between the processi uncinati (see Fig. 32.4). The midline is most reliably determined in AP X-rays from the position of the spinous processes and the midline between the uncinate processes. The midline must be permanently marked with a bone chisel or high-speed drill or by inserting midline pins/Caspar. After verification of the midline position, the pins can be removed and replaced with the Caspar screws, using the same bone hole screws (see Fig. 32.5a, b). *Note*: A final check of the midline should be made after placing the trial implant in the disc space.
- Preparation of the disc space.
  Discectomy is performed using standard procedures. The cartilaginous end plate has to be removed completely but care should be taken to avoid any damage to the integrity of the bony end plates. Decompression of neural elements has to be precise and complete (microsurgical technique). In lateral soft disc prolapse, the posterior longitudinal ligament can be preserved as a tension band on the asymptomatic side and in the midline. Burrs, cutters, reamers, or drills can be used for foraminal decompression or cutting off the posterior osteophytes. Bone preparation should be

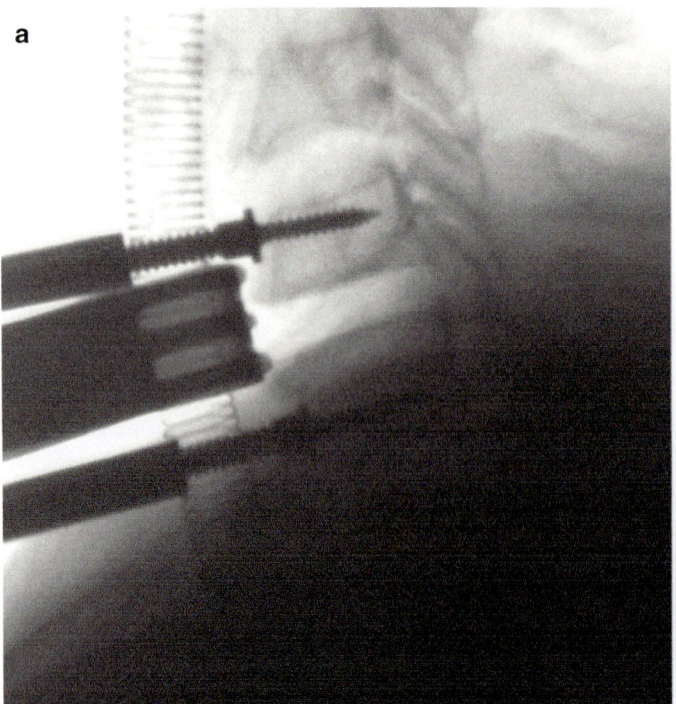
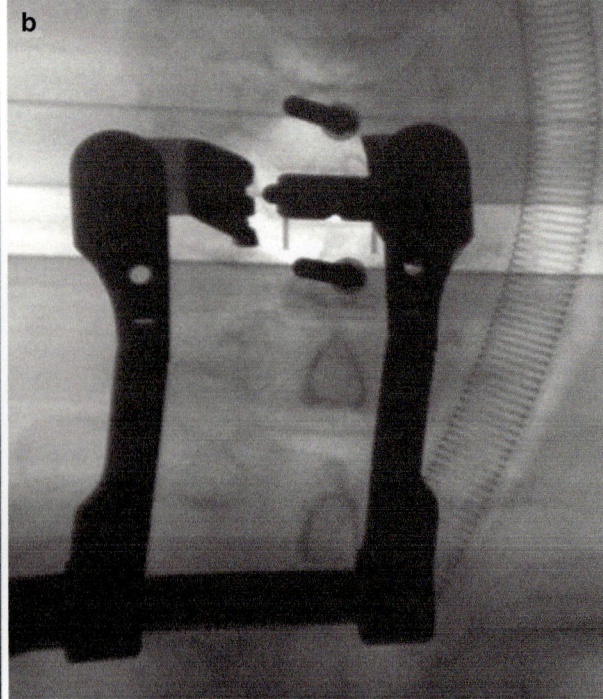

Fig. 32.5 Position of the midline marking pins or Caspar screws (**a**—lateral; **b**—AP view)

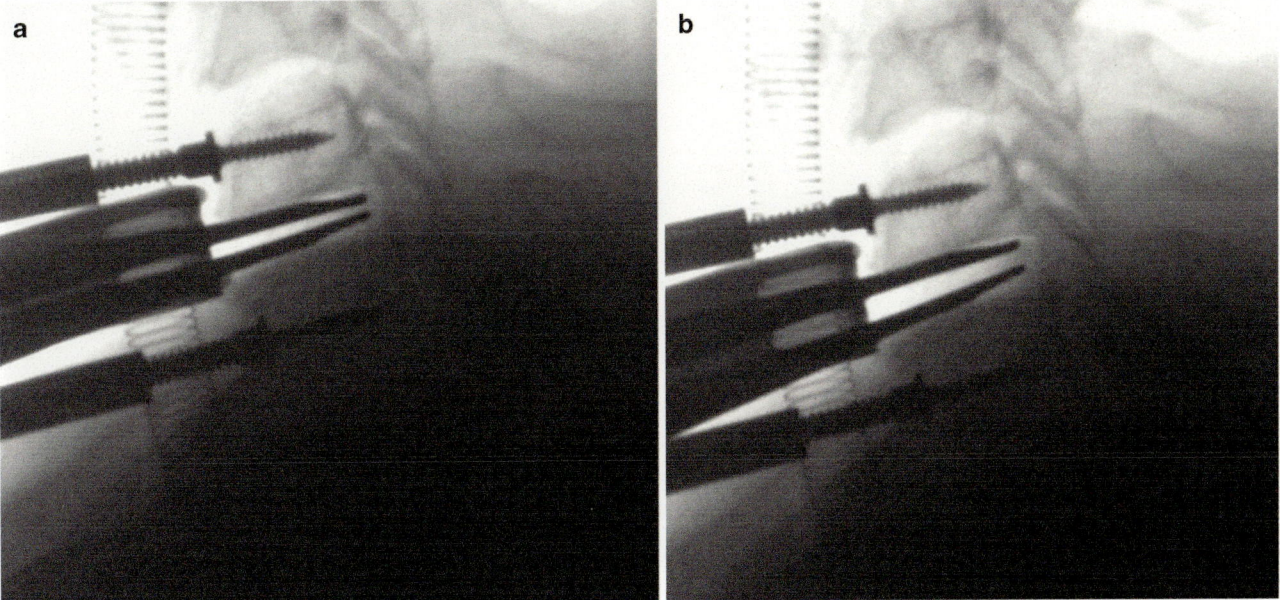

Fig. 32.6 Distraction forceps are used for distracting the treated segment. (**a**) Without and (**b**) With distraction

kept minimal in order to avoid creating too much bone powder as this can serve as a focal point for later ossification. Preparation of the posterior uncus should be limited to one-third of the total structure to avoid instability of the segment.

• Distraction with Caspar retractor or distraction forceps.
  Once the midline has been determined and the disc compartment prepared (partial discectomy), the Caspar screws for the distractor are inserted.
  Note: For fusion procedures, the Caspar screws are usually applied centrally in lateral alignment, and the distraction force is transmitted via their shafts. In activ C implantation, however, the Caspar distractor serves as a distraction holding device. The self-locking mechanism assures its stability and keeps the vertebral end plates parallel. Maximal distraction force is created by means of distraction forceps, and the interbody distance enlargement is passively followed by moving the distractor longitudinally.
  Distraction forceps are used for distracting the treated segment. The forceps are applied to the posterior part of the intervertebral space under fluoroscopic control. Distraction is increased gradually in parallel fashion. Step-by-step distraction allows relaxation of the ligaments (see Fig. 32.6a, b). The height of the space in the treated segment should be compared with adjacent segments to avoid over-distraction. Careful observation of joint fissure enlargement can be helpful. The forceps are equipped with a locking mechanism to hold the distance.

• Trial implant (see Fig. 32.7a, b).
  Inserting the trial implant–verifying the size of the required disc implant.

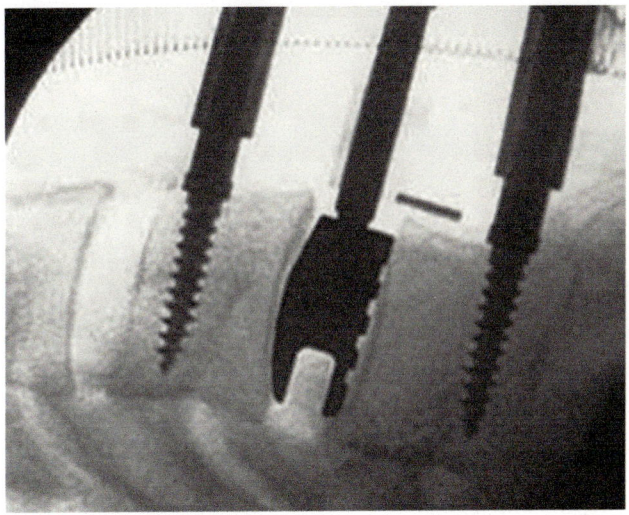

Fig. 32.7 Under X-ray control, tap the trial implant into the disc compartment until the safety stop touches the anterior side of the vertebral body

The safety stop position is adjusted in the AP direction with the adjusting wheel. The safety stop is moved forward by turning the adjusting wheel counterclockwise and backwards by turning the adjusting wheel clockwise. Initially, the safety stop is moved forward as far as possible. The trial implant is then tapped into the disc compartment until the safety stop touches the vertebral body from anterior. The size (depth and height) of the trial implant is inspected under X-ray control. If necessary, adjusting wheel is turned clockwise to move the safety

Fig. 32.8 (**a, b**) Preparation of the keel groove. The figures show burr holes (No. 1 and 2) in lateral X-ray view. The latter runs immediately next to the trial implant. Both burr holes end 1.5 mm in front of the posterior edge of the trial implant

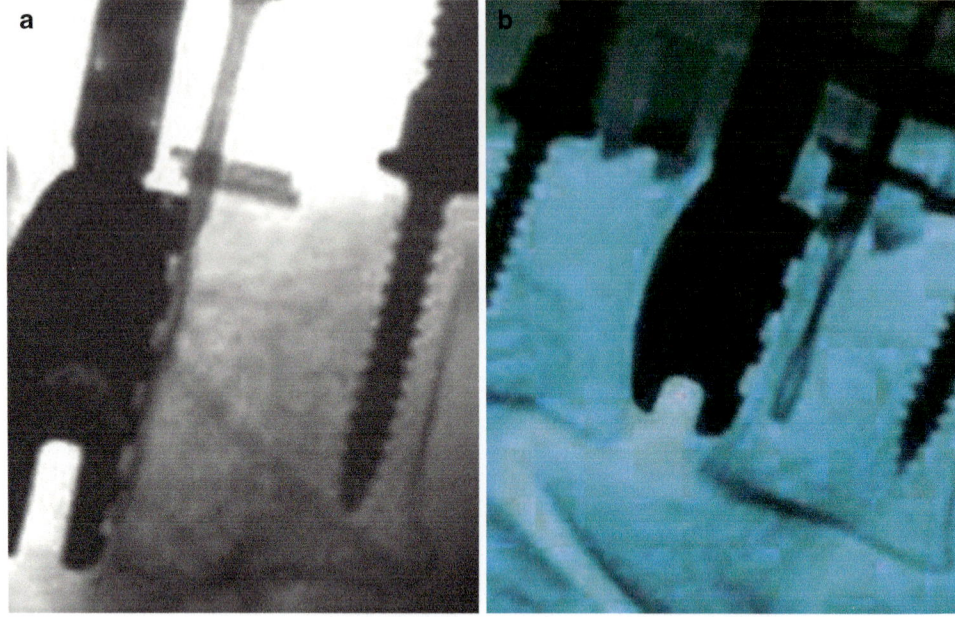

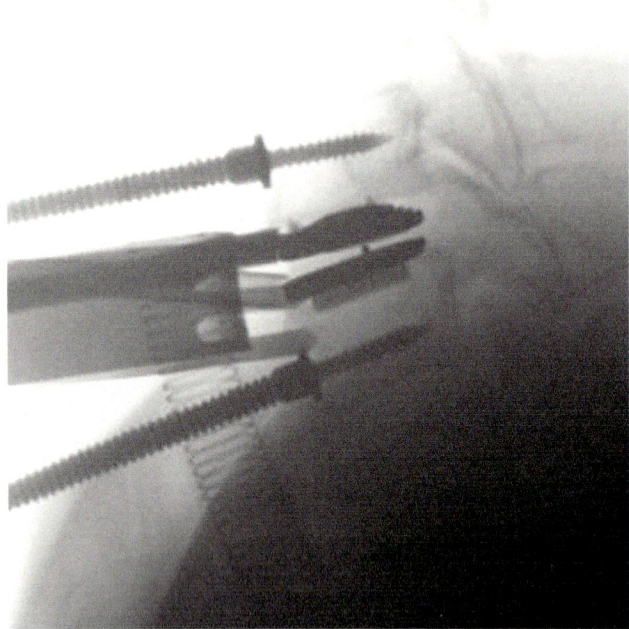

Fig. 32.9 Implantation of the prosthesis. The prosthesis is carefully inserted in the disc compartment by guiding the keel into the prepared keel groove

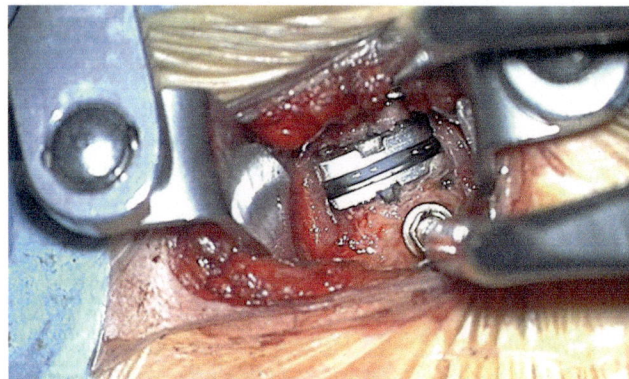

Fig. 32.10 Prosthesis in situ

stop back and push the trial implant in a posterior direction. Once the final position has been reached, the distraction is released to see the actual angulation of the segment. The distractor can be removed completely for a better view. The trial holder is unlocked and removed. *Note*: The trial implant is introduced in the distracted position. Over-

distraction must be avoided. The trial implant should not be introduced too far posterior. *The midline and sagittal midplane must be respected.* Once the keel groove has been reamed, the position of the prosthesis is fixed and can no longer be changed.

- Preparation of the keel bed, keel groove, and reaming (see Fig. 32.8a, b).
- Implantation of the artificial disc (see Figs. 32.9 and 32.10).
    - Corresponding to the trial implant used.
    - Apply slight distraction with the Caspar distractor.
    - Attach the appropriate prosthesis to the insertion instrument.
    - Introduce the artificial disc under lateral fluoroscopic control.

– Detach the insertion instrument.
– Check the final position in AP and lateral view.
– Correct the position if necessary.
– Release distraction.
– Check the position of the artificial disc.

32.7   Tips and Tricks

- The surgeon naturally has a duty to explain the potential complications of disc prosthesis.
  The operation can lead to infection, occasionally even sepsis and meningitis; secondary bleeding with or without respiratory problems; injury of the oesophagus, trachea, carotid artery, and jugular vein; injury of the recurrent nerve, spinal cord, and nerve roots; and cerebrospinal fluid fistula. Dislocation and migration of the implant must also be considered. With regard to the cervical spine itself, the possible complications are a loss of lordosis and increase in kyphosis, narrowing of the disc space, fracture of the end plates, and heterotopic ossification (HO).
- When explaining the operation, it is important to describe alternative methods such as fusion techniques, dorsal decompression, and conservative treatment (physiotherapy, manual therapy osteopathy, and pain treatment).
- The dorsal edges of the bones should be sealed with bone wax.
- Choosing the appropriate prosthesis size and insertion position should prevent subsidence or extrusion of the prosthesis.

References

1. Chang UK, Kim DH, Lee MC, et al. Changes in adjacent level disc pressure and facet joint force after cervical arthroplasty compared with cervical discectomy and fusion. J Neurosurg Spine. 2007;7:33–9.
2. Sekhon LH. Cervical arthroplasty in the management of spondylotic myelopathy: 18-month results. Neurosurg Focus. 2004;15:E8.
3. Anderson PA, Rouleau JP. Intervertebral disc arthroplasty. Spine. 2004;29:2779–86.
4. Anderson PA, Sasso RC, Rouleau JP, et al. The Bryan cervical disc: wear properties and early clinical results. Spine J. 2004;4:303S–9S.
5. DiAngelo DJ, Puttlitz CM. Biomechanical aspects associated with cervical disk arthroplasty. In: Kim DH, Cammisa FP, Fessler RG, editors. Dynamic reconstruction of the spine. New York/Stuttgart: Thieme; 2006.
6. Boden SD, Balderston RA, Heller JG, et al. An AOA critical issue. Disc replacements: this time will we really cure low-back and neck pain? J Bone Joint Surg Am. 2004;86:411–22.
7. Kim SW, Shin JH, Arbatin JJ, et al. Effects of a cervical disc prosthesis on maintaining sagittal alignment of the functional spinal unit and overall sagittal balance of the cervical spine. Spine. 2008;17:20–9.
8. Lafuente J, Casey AT, Perzold A, et al. The Bryan cervical disc prosthesis as an alternative to arthrodesis in the treatment of cervical spondylosis. J Bone Joint Surg Br. 2005;87:508–12.
9. Leung C, Casey AT, Goffin J, et al. Clinical significance of heterotopic ossification in cervical disc replacement: a prospective multicenter clinical trial. Neurosurgery. 2005;57:759–63.
10. Lin EL, Wang JC. Total disk arthroplasty. J Am Acad Orthop Surg. 2006;14:704–14.
11. Mummaneni PV, Haid RW. The future in the care of the cervical spine: interbody fusion and arthroplasty. J Neurosurg Spine. 2004;1:155–9.
12. Nabhan A, Ahlhelm F, Shariat K, et al. The Pro-Disc C prosthesis: clinical and radiological experience 1 year after surgery. Spine. 2007;32:1935–41.
13. Jaramllo-de La Torre J, Grauer JN, Yue JJ. Update on cervical disc arthroplasty: where are we and where are we going? Curr Rev Musculoskelet Med. 2008;1:124–30.

Percutaneous Anterior Endoscopic Cervical Decompression

Stefan Hellinger

33

33.1 Introduction and Core Messages

As a bridge between open [1] and percutaneous therapy [2], endoscopy of the cervical spine started to be used at the beginning of the 1990s, following good experiences on the lumbar spine [3–5]. The principle of microsurgery is combined with the minimally invasive principles by bringing the optical level to the forefront of pathology. Access morbidity has been significantly reduced by the percutaneous access technique. Furthermore, a large proportion of the intervertebral disc, in particular most of the fibrous ring, is preserved. The pathology is only removed selectively in the area of the nucleus pulposus and on the dorsal fibrous ring. This preserves the remaining biomechanical function of the degenerated intervertebral disc. By means of tried and tested minimally invasive methods under vision, such as the use of a laser to ablate and shrink tissue, the risk of complications has been further reduced, at the same time enhancing efficiency. The advancement of the endoscopic technique with increased miniaturization of the telescope and working options led to restriction of use (e.g., LASE system). Our objective was to create an adequate working space in front of the telescope while preserving the minimally invasive approach. This was achieved by the use of dilation sheaths, which force the base plate and upper plate apart in the manner of a Caspar retractor and permit a working field of 5 mm or 6 mm. Here, visualization is sufficient to expose the ventral epidural space. A swiveling maneuver of the endoscope enables the dorsal section of the intervertebral disc to be visualized from one uncovertebral joint to the other. Removal of disc material is limited to the pathologic part, in a similar way to arthroscopic meniscus surgery. Equally, the surgeon has to become accustomed to the fact that limited viewing fields are lined up rather than in joint arthroscopy. An irrigation system is used to rinse the ablated disc material out of the viewing field and to achieve partial hemostasis.

33.2 Indications and Contraindications

Indications are
Clinically proofed and accepted
- Soft disc prolapse.
- Symptomatic cervical discopathy with neck and/or arm pain with or without neurological deficit concordant with MRI of disc pathology questionable
- Preoperative segmental kyphosis or "straight neck."
- Narrow, hard disc.
- Acute myelopathy with MRI signal changes.
- Osteophytic and sclerotic changes of the vertebral bodies.
  Contraindications are
- Serious cervical spinal stenosis.
- Migrated free disc sequestration.
- Pronounced spondylosis with large osteophytes.
- Collapsed disc space with or without instability.
- Calcifications of the posterior spinal ligament.

S. Hellinger (✉)
OOCC München MVZ, Munich, Germany
e-mail: info@ooccm.de

© Springer-Verlag GmbH Germany 2023
U. Vieweg, F. Grochulla (eds.), *Manual of Spine Surgery*, https://doi.org/10.1007/978-3-662-64062-3_33

As further instruments for endoscopic intervertebral disc surgery are developed, the scope of application can undoubtedly be extended up to endoscopic fusion technology [6].

33.3   Technical Requirement

- Endoscopic System for anterior cervical endoscopic decompression with endoscope and fitting rongeurs, burrs, and endokerrisons (Storz, Wolf, Joimax, Spinendos).
- Videosystem.
- Radiofrequency (e.g., Elliquence) or laser for coagulation.
- Flouroscope.

For the endoscopic decompression, we use an enhanced percutaneous endoscopic cervical discectomy (PECD) set. The main component is a 4 mm diameter endoscope with a fiberoptic telescope and a 1.9 mm working channel. Other systems come in different sizes. This enables the camera to be attached to the optical cable, which reduces the weight and improves the balance of the endoscope during use. Suitable instruments for the working channel are available. A laser or radiofrequency unit can be used, as can a variety of working sleeves, particularly dilation sleeves. The intervention is generally performed under general anesthesia. An operation under local anesthesia and analgosedation in the case of risk patients is also possible. The patient is positioned in the same way as for conventional anterior cervical

discectomy on the back with a caudalization of the shoulders. It is advisable to maintain a state of readiness for an open surgical procedure, and to keep an operating microscope available. The level of the intervertebral disc that is to be operated on is marked using the C-arm. Then an approximately 5 mm skin incision is made at this level on the right side, medially to the sternocleidomastoid muscle, and the platysma is exposed without cutting. Following lateralization of the carotid artery and the jugular vein, and medialization of the larynx, trachea, esophagus and thyroid gland by applying pressure with the index finger and middle finger, the anterior surface of the cervical spine can be touched. Under fluoroscopy, an 16 or 18G spinal needle is then inserted into the intervertebral disc, preferably in the midline, via the skin incision (Fig. 33.1). The position of the needle is checked in at least two planes with the C-arm. The direction of the needle is toward the extrusion verified on MRI. Then a guidewire and various obturators can be placed on the intervertebral disc via the needle (Fig. 33.2). A 5 mm or 6 mm working sleeve, depending on the height of the disc and the system, is inserted into the anterior fibrous ring via the last obturator. The working sleeve can now be advanced further into the disk space. The procedure is facilitated by using a trephine and a shaver. Under endoscopic vision (Figs. 33.3 and 33.4), the intervertebral disc can be curetted in a channel as far as the posterior fibrous ring. The pathological region of the posterior fibrous ring, previously identified by imaging, determines the angle of entry into the

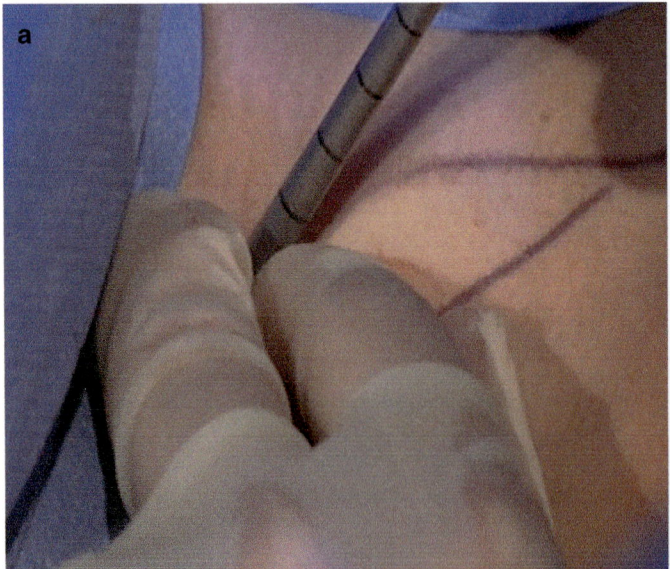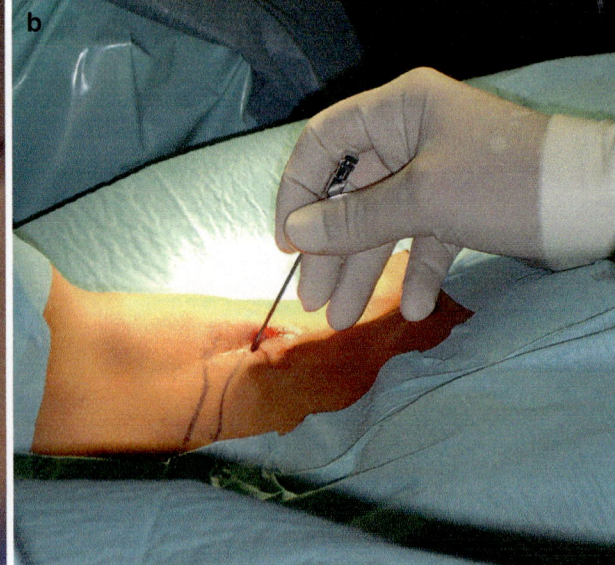

Fig. 33.1 (**a**) Intraoperative photograph shows lateralization of the carotid artery and the jugular vein, and medialization of the larynx, trachea, esophagus and thyroid gland by applying pressure with the index

finger and middle finger, this allows the anterior surface of the cervical spine to be touched. Under fluoroscopy, a dilator is then inserted into the intervertebral disc. (**b**) Needle placement

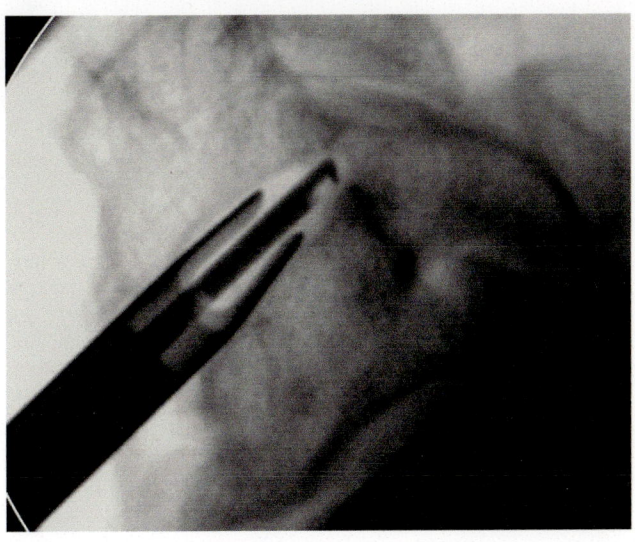

Fig. 33.2 Intraoperative flouroscopy demonstrates the working canula placed in the intervertebral disc with an instrument

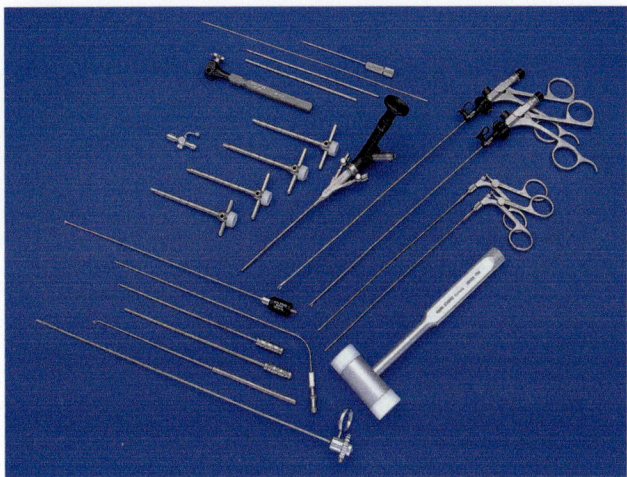

Fig. 33.4 For the endoscopic decompression we use an enhanced PECD set from Storz. The main component is a 4 mm diameter endoscope with a fiberoptic telescope and a 1.9 mm working channel

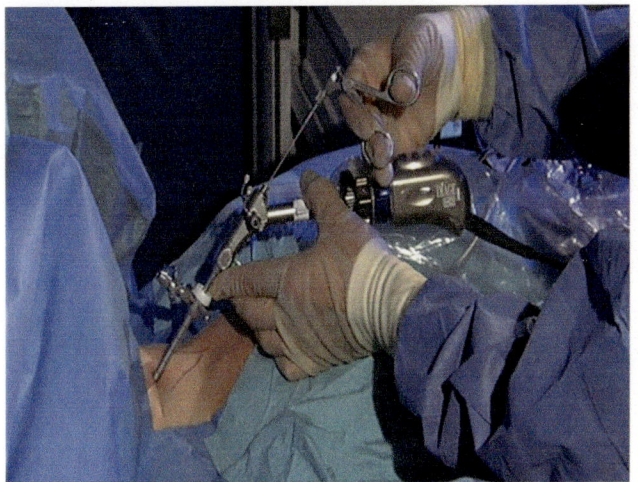

Fig. 33.3 The placement of the cervical endoscope for discectomy and decompression

intervertebral disc. This section of the disc is located and ablated together with the prolapsed disc tissue. When so doing, the working area can, if necessary, be extended as far as the uncovertebral joints by swiveling the endoscope. If required, the excision forceps or a microkerrison can be used to carefully open the posterior spinal ligament and expose the epidural space. Similarly, relatively small osteophytes can be ablated under fluoroscopic vision using the ring curette or kerrison. Furthermore, intervertebral disc material that is still floating freely can be ablated and stabilized by laser or radiofrequency. A final check is carried out with the palpation hook.

33.4 Complications

The complication rate of percutaneous cervical decompression is extremely small, as is the case with non-endoscopic percutaneous procedures. In our patients, there have been no complications to date. Various complications have been discussed in the literature. In a multicenter study, 1750 cervical endoscopic interventions on the cervical spine, employing different techniques, have been recorded around the world. In four cases, discitis occurred, in one case there was a permanent sensory deficit, and in 5 cases nerve lesions with motor damage was found. This corresponds to an average incidence of complications in 0.6% of cases. Other, rare events to be found in publications are vessel injuries with hematoma, in one case a carotid injury, damage to autonomic nerves with Horner syndrome, and two cases with recurrent laryngeal nerve lesion out of 1200 interventions [7]. Inadequate decompression when using the endoscopic technique is reflected in the incidence of secondary operations. The multicenter study quotes 28 relevant cases, which represents 1.6%.

33.5 Tips and Tricks

- It is obligatory to explain potential risks of complications up to carotid or dural injuries and an eventual necessary change to open surgery.
- The limits of the endoscopic anterior techniques have to be clarified in front of the patient and the alternatives such as fusion techniques, dorsal decompression, and conservative treatment must be specified.

- In the beginning of the surgery, it is helpful to start with a small incision to gain mobility and to make a blunt dissection to the anterior spine with a mosquito clamp.
- The use of a shaver can fasten the transdiscal approach to the anterior ligament.

References

1. Hankinson HL, Wilson CB. Use of the operating microscope in anterior cervical discectomy without fusion. J Neurosurg. 1975;43(4):452–6.
2. Hellinger J. Technical aspects of the percutaneous cervical and lumbar laser-disc-decompression and nucleotomy. Neurol Res. 1999;21(1):99–102.
3. Lee SH, Lee SJ, Park KH, et al. Comparison of percutaneous manual and endoscopic laser diskectomy with chemonucleolysis and automated nucleotomy. Orthopade. 1996;25(1):49–55. in German
4. Chiu JC, Negron F, Clifford T, et al. Micro decompressive percutaneous endoscopy: spinal discectomy with new laser thermodiskoplasty for non-extruded herniated nucleus pulposus. Surg Technol Int. 1999;8:343–51.
5. Fontanella A. Endoscopic microsurgery in herniated cervical discs. Neurol Res. 1999;21(1):31–8.
6. Hellinger S. The fullendoscopic anterior cervical fusion: a new horizon for selective percutaneous endoscopic cervical decompression. Acta Neurochir Suppl (Wien). 2011;108:203–7.
7. Chiu J. Clifford T Cervical endoscopic discectomy with laser thermodiskoplasty. In: Savitz MH, Chiu JC, Yeung AT, editors. The Practice of Minimally Invasive Spinal Technique. Richmond: AAMISMS Education; 2000. p. 141–8.

Overview of Surgical Techniques and Implants

34

Stefan Schären

34.1 Introduction and Core Messages

A posterior approach to the cervical spine is indicated in posteriorly situated lesions or as a supplement to anterior surgery. Great advancements in posterior instrumentation have been made over the last decades. Today, modern versatile rod-screw systems allow easy and stable fixation from the occiput to the upper thoracic spine. If surgery is indicated, the choice of the approach depends on etiology and location of the pathology and the functional spinal stability considering the options for appropriate decompression and stabilization. Posterior decompressive approaches are suited for cases of posteriorly situated lesions compressing the spinal cord and/or the exiting nerve roots. As an advantage, the posterior approach is relatively simple not being compromised by neural or vascular structures and can easily be extended if necessary. Also, the posterior bony elements are usually very strong, providing excellent purchase for implants even in the osteoporotic spine. Nevertheless, intact anterior column is an important prerequisite for a stable long-term result. In cases of anterior column defect or kyphotic deformity, anterior or combined approaches are indicated. Thanks to the continuous evolution of spinal instrumentation technology over the last decades, versatile and powerful implants are available that meet the specific demands of the cervical spine, adding immediate stability and increasing the fusion rate. The strength of the constructs allows minimal, if any, external bracing. In addition, the latest generation of implants is designed to be compatible with MRI and allows to rapidly assess adequate decompression of neural structures or progression of pathological lesions being treated. Due to the specific characteristics and the techniques of stabilization for the craniocervical junction, the atlantoaxial articulations, and the subaxial cervical spine will be discussed separately. In reality, pathologies rarely respect artificial boundaries but cross the various regions. Frequently, techniques must be combined. The modern modular implants which have been developed in the past decade are adapted to meet these specific anatomical characteristics.

34.2 Approach and Positioning

The patient is placed in prone position with cushion under his chest. Alternatively, a vacuum mattress or a spine frame may be used. The head is fixed in slightly flexed position on a padded U-shaped headrest. Alternatively, a Mayfield clamp can be used. A laterally placed image intensifier should be installed in fixed position. As with occipitocervical fusion, the neutral position of the head must be verified under image intensifier and compared to preoperative standard lateral radiograph. Reduction and traction (always under image intensifier) are possible if necessary (fracture dislocation, rheumatoid arthritis). The shoulders are pulled down with adhesive straps. Shaving of the back of the head and of the neck is required (patient must be informed prior to surgery!). A standard midline approach is performed, and the posterior elements of the spine of the levels to be addressed are exposed.

34.3 Occipitocervical Fusion

The craniocervical junction comprising occiput, atlas, and axis represents a complex transition zone from the cranium to the cervical spine. Its characteristic anatomy differs fundamentally from the subaxial spine. More than 50% of the flexion/extension and rotation of the head and neck occur in

S. Schären (✉)
Department of Orthopaedic Surgery/Spine, University Hospital, Basel, Switzerland
e-mail: sschaeren@uhbs.ch

© Springer-Verlag GmbH Germany 2023
U. Vieweg, F. Grochulla (eds.), *Manual of Spine Surgery*, https://doi.org/10.1007/978-3-662-64062-3_34

241

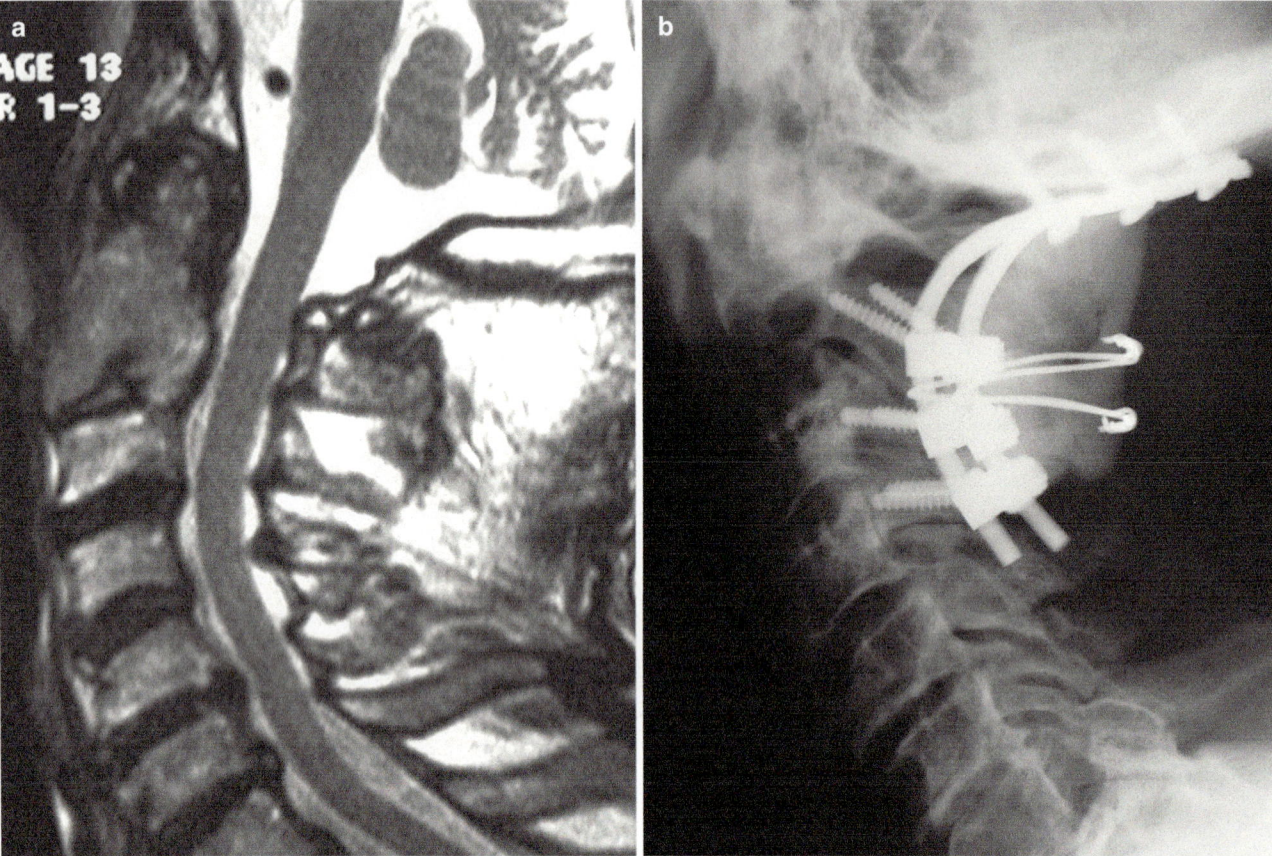

Fig. 34.1 (**a**, **b**) T2-weighted sagittal MRI of an 81-year-old patient with invalidating neck pain shows infiltration of corpus and dens axis by plasmocytoma (1A). Occipitocervical (C0–C4) stabilization with

Cervifix® (Synthes, Oberdorf, Switzerland) was performed. In view of the malignant underlying disease of the lesion, the construct was augmented with PMMA (1B)

this area. As a result, high biomechanical forces and strong lever arms are acting and challenging the attempt of surgical stabilization. In order to neutralize these biomechanical forces, instrumentation constructs must therefore have adequate dimensions and sufficient rigidity. At the same time, the systems must offer great flexibility to be easily adapted to the multiple anatomical variations and leave enough room for grafting, allowing for bony fusion to take place. The first occipitocervical fusion was reported in 1927 by Foerster [1], who inserted a fibular graft between the occiput and C7 to stabilize a progressive atlantoaxial dislocation after an odontoid fracture. Since then, multiple methods of fusion in this area have been developed: simple onlay bone grafts with halo immobilization; wire, pin, or hook constructs; rigid metallic loops or rectangles fixed to the bone with wires or screws. Today, modular rod-screw systems have become the standard for occipitocervical stabilization in adults [2–4]. The systems can be fixed either by lateral mass screws or transpedicular screws to the subaxial spine and be attached to the suboccipital bone by plates. They are easy to contour and provide rigid internal fixation allowing immediate mobilization with no or minimal external support, while the fusion is taking place. High fusion rates are reported [2, 5]. In several biomechanical studies, superior stability of the

rod-screw systems could be demonstrated [4, 6]. Most stable are constructs including C2 reducing the number of segments to be included in the fusion [7]. For good and safe anchoring to the suboccipital bone, it is essential to study preoperatively the thickness of the bone and the position of the dural sinuses on CT scans. In an anatomical study, the thickness was found to be 8 mm and more extending from the occipital protuberance bilaterally for 23 mm [8]. In pediatric patients, internal fixation techniques have been applied more hesitantly partly because fusion without internal fixation is achieved more easily and partly because the implants did not suit the smaller anatomy. Today, smaller implants are available, and there is a tendency toward internal fixation also in children [9]. Only anatomic constraints in children less than 1 year old usually still require fusion with onlay techniques (Fig. 34.1).

34.4 Atlantoaxial Fusion

Techniques for isolated C1–2 fusion have gradually evolved over the last several decades since Gallie described the placement of a notched bone graft between the posterior arch of the atlas and the spinous process of C2 secured by sublaminar

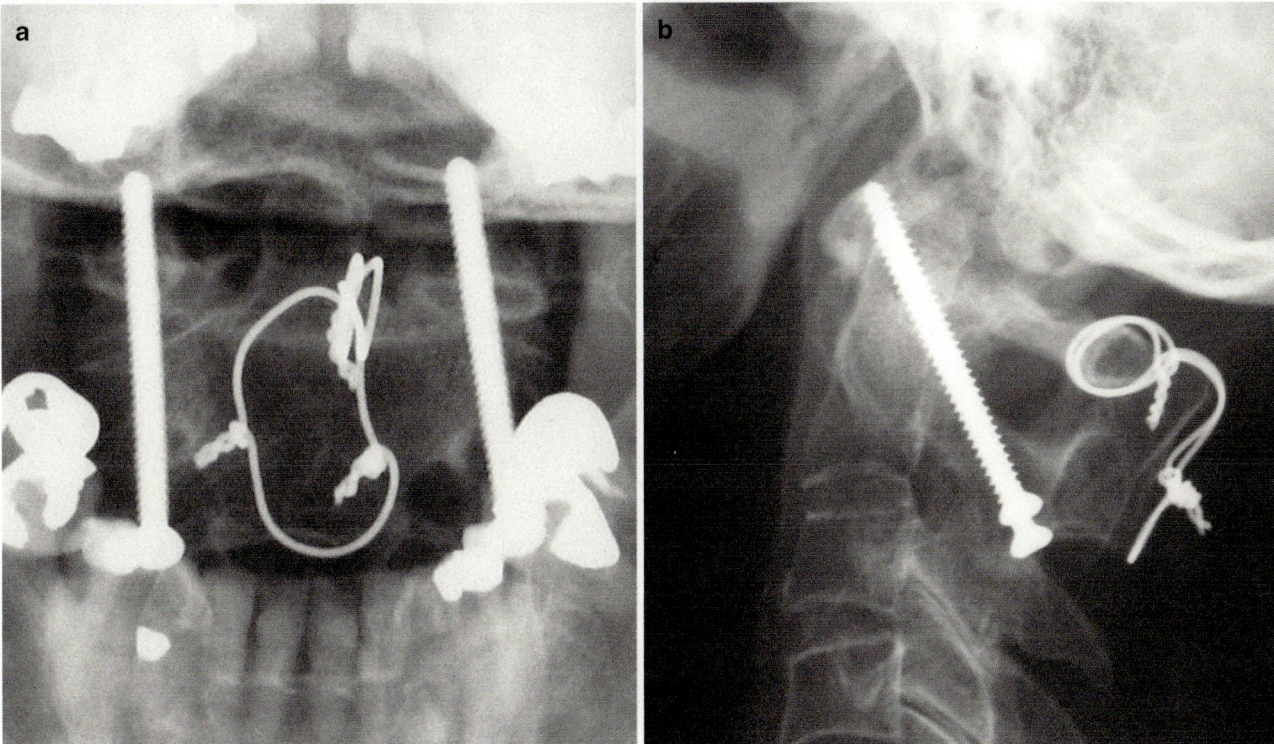

Fig. 34.2 (**a, b**) A 73-year-old female patient with painful atlantoaxial osteoarthritis. Transarticular screw fixation C1–C2 was performed showing solid fusion and stable implants at 24 months postoperatively

wires in 1939 [10]. The single midline fixation point provided only limited rotational stability requiring rigid postoperative immobilization, preferably a halo. Modifications by Brooks and Sonntag aimed to increase the rotational stability [11, 12]. The introduction of transarticular screws fixing the lateral masses of C1 and C2 by Magerl presented a major breakthrough in posterior atlantoaxial fixation [13]. The transarticular screws provide immediate stabilization. Mostly, a Gallie-type interspinous bone graft with or without wires is added providing a very stable three-point fixation. In case of incomplete or fractured posterior arch of the atlas, the atlantoaxial joints can be opened and packed with bone graft. Preoperatively, the diameter of the isthmus of C2 must be determined on CT reconstructions for safe passage of the screws without injury to the vertebral artery. If no safe screw can be inserted, unilateral C1–2 facet screw fixation with interspinous bone graft wiring was reported to still provide excellent stability leading to high fusion rates [14]. Drilling and insertion of the screws are performed under lateral fluoroscopic control. A specific aiming device and computer assistance can further increase safety of the technically demanding procedure [15, 16]. Olerud modified the Magerl technique in 2001, adding a clamp for C1 posterior arch fixation obviating the need for posterior wiring [17].

The only true contraindication for transarticular screws remains fixed/irreducible subluxation of C1–2. Trying to

overcome this shortcoming, Harms and Melcher described a novel technique of atlantoaxial stabilization in 2001 using polyaxial head screws inserted in the lateral mass of C1 and the pedicle of C2 [18]. The screws are bilaterally connected by rods. Fluoroscopically guided reduction of the atlantoaxial articulation can be performed if necessary, and a cancellous onlay bone graft can be used for fusion. In contrast to the transarticular screws, the lateral atlantoaxial joints are not affected, allowing removing the implants if only temporary fixation is required. Biomechanically, several studies demonstrated superior almost identical rigid internal fixation for the Magerl and the Harms technique [19]. Regarding safety, C2 pedicle screw placement was reported to have nearly the same anatomic risk of vertebral artery injury as transarticular screw placement (Fig. 34.2) [20].

34.5 The Subaxial Cervical Spine

Originally, various wiring techniques and laminar clamps systems have been used to stabilize the subaxial spine. Both methods provided only limited stability especially in rotation and translation, necessitating prolonged external fixation. Nevertheless, the incidence of nonunion and loss of correction was high. Sublaminar wires and laminar hooks also carried the risk of neurovascular injury. Lateral

Fig. 34.3 (**a–c**) Transdiscal fracture C5/6 in a 61-year-old patient with ankylosing spondylitis (3A). Considering the highly unstable injury in ankylosing spondylitis, posterior stabilization of C3/T2 using a polyaxial screw and rod system (Synapse, Synthes, Oberdorf, Switzerland) and fusion of C5/6 using iliac crest autograft were performed

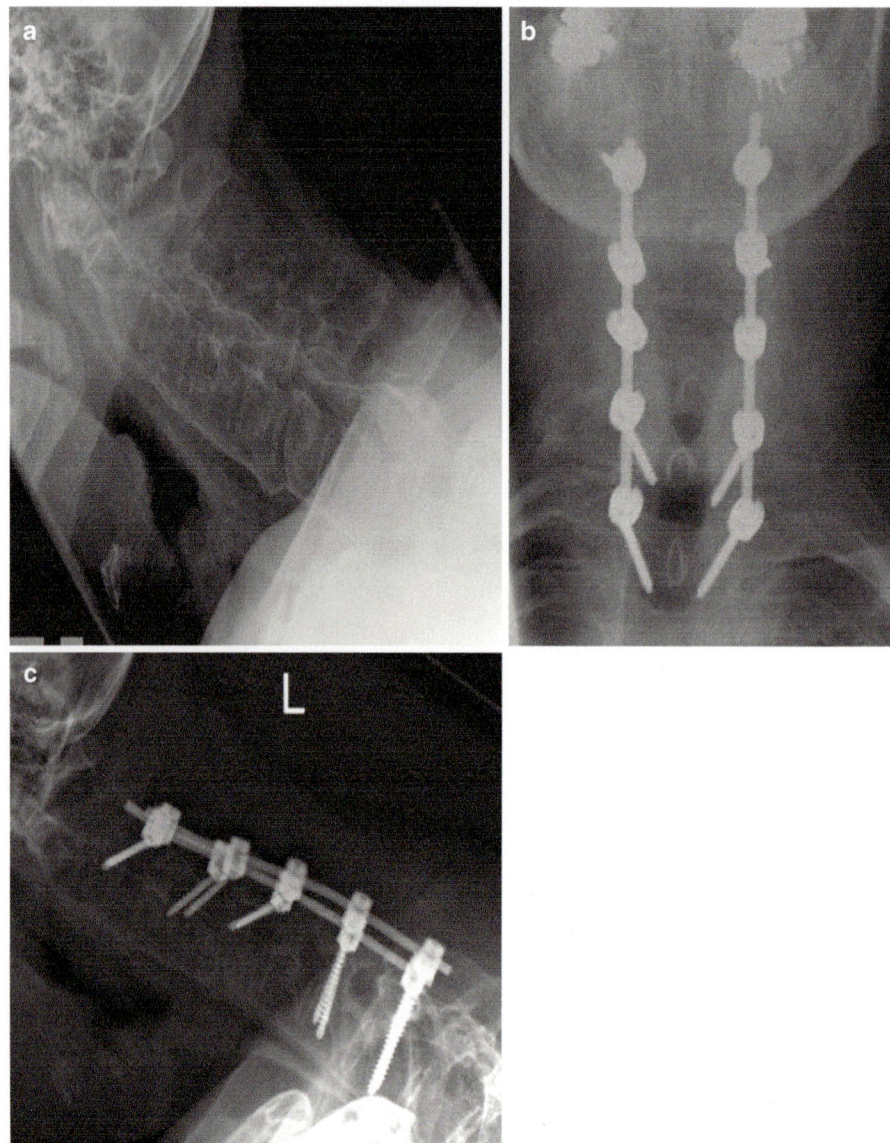

mass plate systems first described by Roy-Camille were biomechanically superior to laminar wire or clamp fixation [21]. In addition, unlike posterior laminar wiring or clamping, lateral mass plates did not require the presence of the posterior elements, which are often removed to facilitate decompression. However, the plates still were associated with a number of disadvantages like the given position of the screw holes, the limited insertion angle, and the insufficient angular stability between screw and plate. Subsequently, various versatile screw-rod systems have been developed which have become the standard for posterior stabilization [22, 23]. Its modular design allows easy contouring and offers almost unlimited flexibility regarding orientation and location of the screws. If necessary, the stabilization can easily be extended to the occiput and/or the thoracic spine. The screw-rod systems are anchored with lateral mass screws inserted according to the technique of Magerl or An [22, 24]. In recent years, pedicle screws for the cervical spine have been established as an alternative [2, 23]. Safety and accuracy of the technically demanding pedicle screws could be improved using computer navigation [16]. Biomechanically, the modern angle-stable screw-rod systems particularly with transpedicular fixation provide the most rigid stability reducing the risk of implant failure until fusion takes place and allowing instrumentation of fewer segments (Fig. 34.3).

References

1. Foerster O. Die Leitungsbahnen des Schmerzgefühls und die chirurgische Behandlung der Schmerzzustände. Berlin: Urban & Schwarzenburg; 1927.

2. Abumi K, Takada T, Shono Y, et al. Posterior occipitocervical reconstruction using cervical pedicle screws and plate-rod systems. Spine. 1999;24:1425–34.

3. Jeanneret B. Posterior rod system of the cervical spine: a new implant allowing optimal screw insertion. Eur Spine J. 1996;5:350–6.

4. Richter M, Wilke HJ, Kluger P, et al. Biomechanical evaluation of a new modular rod-screw implant system for posterior instrumentation of the occipito-cervical spine: in-vitro comparison with two established implant systems. Eur Spine J. 2000;9:417–25.

5. Schaeren S, Jeanneret B. Occipitocervical instrumentation. Tech Orthop. 2002;18:87–95.

6. Oda I, Abumi K, Sell LC, et al. Biomechanical evaluation of five different occipito-atlanto-axial fixation techniques. Spine. 1999;24:2377–82.

7. Finn MA, Fassett DR, Mccall TD, Clark R, et al. The cervical end of an occipitocervical fusion: a biomechanical evaluation of 3 constructs. Laboratory investigation. J Neurosurg Spine. 2008;9:296–300.

8. Ebraheim NA, Lu J, Biyani A, et al. An anatomic study of the thickness of the occipital bone. Implications for occipitocervical instrumentation. Spine. 1996;21:1725–30.

9. Anderson RC, Ragel BT, Mocco J, et al. Selection of a rigid internal fixation construct for stabilization at the craniovertebral junction in pediatric patients. J Neurosurg. 2007;107(1 Suppl):36–42.

10. Gallie WE. Fractures and dislocations of the cervical spine. Am J Surg. 1939;46:495–9.

11. Brooks AL, Jenkins EB. Atlanto-axial arthrodesis by the wedge compression method. J Bone Joint Surg Am. 1978;60:279–84.

12. Sonntag VKH, Dickman CA. Craniocervical stabilization. Clin Neurosurg. 1993;40:243–72.

13. Magerl F, Seemann PS. Stable posterior fusion of the atlas and axis by transarticular screw fixation. In: Kehr P, Weidner A, editors. Cervical spine, vol. 1. Vienna: Springer; 1987.

14. Grob D, Bremerich FH, Dvorak J, et al. Transarticular screw fixation for osteoarthritis of the atlanto axial segment. Eur Spine J. 2006;15:283–91.

15. Gebhard JS, Schimmer RC, Jeanneret B. Safety and accuracy of transarticular screw fixation C1-C2 using an aiming device. An anatomic study Spine. 1998;23:2185–9.

16. Richter M, Mattes T, Cakir B. Computer-assisted posterior instrumentation of the cervical and cervico-thoracic spine. Eur Spine J. 2004;13:50–9.

17. Olerud S, Olerud C. The C1 claw device: a new instrument for C1-C2 fusion. Eur Spine J. 2001;10:345–7.

18. Harms J, Melcher RP. Posterior C1-C2 fusion with polyaxial screw and rod fixation. Spine. 2001;26:2467–71.

19. Richter M, Schmidt R, Claes L, et al. Posterior atlantoaxial fixation: biomechanical in vitro comparison of six different techniques. Spine. 2002;27:1724–32.

20. Yoshida M, Neo M, Fujibayashi S, Nakamura T. Comparison of the anatomical risk for vertebral artery injury associated with the C2-pedicle screw and atlantoaxial transarticular screw. Spine. 2006;31:E513–7.

21. Roy-Camille R, Saillant G, Judet T, et al. Traumatismes recents Des Cinq Dernieres Vertebres Cervicales Chez L'Adulte (Avec et sans complication neurologique). Sem Hop. 1983;59:1479–88.

22. Jeanneret B, Schaeren S. Posterior stabilization of the cervical and upper thoracic spine with the CerviFix®. Oper Orthop Traumatol. 2004;16:89–116.

23. Richter M. Posterior instrumentation of the cervical spine using the neon occipito-cervical system part 2: cervical and cervicothoracic instrumentation. Oper Orthop Traumatol. 2005;17:579–600.

24. An HS, Gordin R, Renner K. Anatomic considerations for plate-screw fixation of the cervical spine. Spine. 1991;16:S548–51.

Foraminotomy

35

Frank Grochulla

35.1 Introduction and Core Messages

Posterior foraminotomy at the cervical spine is a minimal invasive microsurgical technique for the posterior decompression of nerve roots affected by lateral soft disc herniations or spondylotic formations in the foramen. The nerve root should be decompressed without affecting the stability of the cervical spine. Furthermore, this procedure is a motion preservation technique.

35.2 Indications

- Lateral/foraminal soft disc herniation with nerve root compression and associated radicular symptoms.
- Osteophytic foraminal nerve root compression with radicular symptoms.

35.3 Contraindications

- Pathology near the midline, myeloradiculopathy.
- Instability of the motion segment.

35.4 Technical Prerequisites

High-speed burr, microscope, fluoroscopy, microsurgical instruments, Mayfield frame.

35.5 Positioning

- Patient is placed in a prone position (Fig. 35.1).
- Three-point pin fixation device such as Mayfield tongs to secure the head (Fig. 35.2).
- *Note*: The neck should be slightly flexed and kept in horizontal plane. Extreme flexion should be avoided as it may produce spinal cord ischemia.
- The table is placed in a head-up position (20–30°).
- Cushions or rolled blankets are applied under the chest and the pelvis to avoid abdominal compression (with secondary elevation of venous pressure of the epidural venous plexus).
- The patient is positioned in a prone position with rigid pin fixation to the skull.
- The cervical spine and head are in a neutral position or slightly flexed.
- X-ray is performed to determine the target level and to plan exactly the minimal invasive approach.

35.6 Surgical Technique [1–6]

- "Classic" paramedian 2 cm skin incision across the target level and incision of the fascia.
- Subperiostal dissection of the muscular and ligamentous tissues along the laminae of interest.
- The facet joint is exposed with the lateral mass above and below the target level.
- A tubular retractor system with black-coated surfaces (to avoid glare under microscopical view) is applied (Fig. 35.3).
- An alternative to the classic approach is the minimally invasive paramedian approach with 1.5-cm skin incision (under microscope or endoscope assistance).
- X-ray at this time is essential to confirm the correct level.
- Using a high-speed burr under the microscope, the foraminotomy is started at the junction between the lateral

F. Grochulla (✉)
Metropol Medical Center, Clinic for Orthopedics, Trauma Surgery and Spinal Surgery, Nuremberg, Germany
e-mail: frank.grochulla@mmc-nuernberg.de

© Springer-Verlag GmbH Germany 2023
U. Vieweg, F. Grochulla (eds.), *Manual of Spine Surgery*, https://doi.org/10.1007/978-3-662-64062-3_35

247

Fig. 35.1 Positioning in the prone position

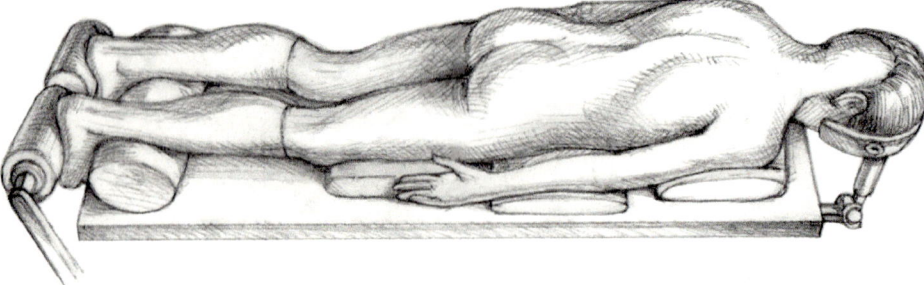

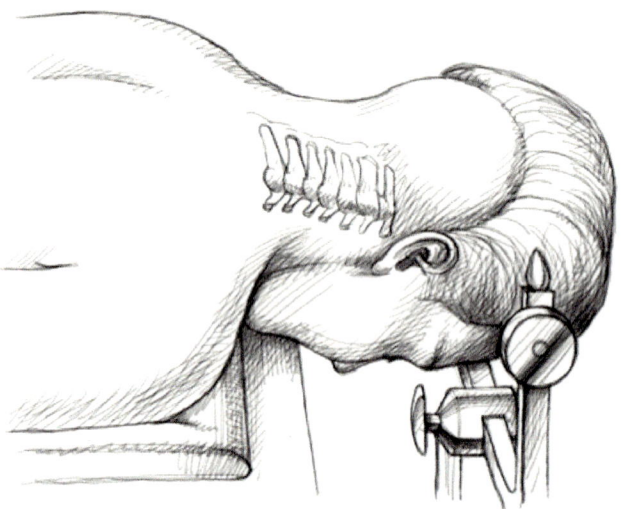

Fig. 35.2 Optional pin fixation of the head

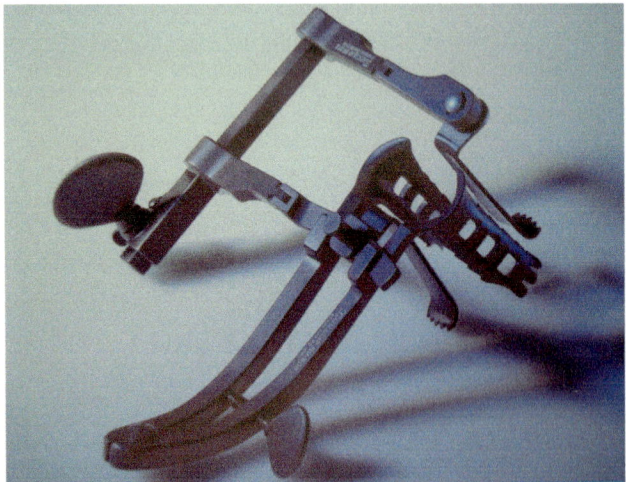

Fig. 35.3 Caspar tubular retractor system

- The size of the keyhole foraminotomy is approximately 8–10 mm in diameter.
- Careful blunt dissection and resection of the ligamentum flavum will expose at first the lateral portion of the dura as an anatomical landmark. Epidural venous bleeding from the perineural plexus or from the epidural plexus in the lateral spinal canal is a frequent problem at this time. A series of careful coagulations of the epidural tissues followed by cuttings with microscissors will avoid major epidural venous bleedings. If persistent venous bleeding occurs after coagulation, the use of hemostatic agents (e.g., Floseal, Fa. Baxter) is helpful to achieve absolute hemostasis.
- The nerve root, the axilla of the nerve root, and the lateral part of the dura are exposed.
- Soft disc sequestrations are often located in the axilla of the nerve root. When the compressed root has been exposed, a short blunt nerve hook is placed in the axilla, and the nerve root is retracted superiorly. It is important to be certain that the entire nerve root is retracted (separate dural sleeves of the motor and sensory roots may occur!). In the case of separated dural sleeves, the smaller motor nerve root is located anterior and caudal to the larger sensory root.
- After retraction, a blade is used to open the posterior longitudinal ligament, and disc herniation is then removed with small forceps. An adequate decompression is achieved, when the nerve root expands with CSF pulsations (Fig. 35.5).
- After removal of disc fragments, there is often additional space so that the foramen can be better explored and enlarged.
- Hemostasis and thorough irrigation of the wound.
- Wound closure: the paravertebral muscles, nuchal ligament, subcutaneous tissues, and skin are sutured.

35.7 Postoperative Care

- Soft collar for 2–4 weeks.
- Anti-inflammatory medication and muscle relaxant.
- Progressive neck exercise program.

aspect of the interlaminar space and the medial border of the facet joint (Fig. 35.4a, b). One-third of the upper and lower laminae are drilled away, and laterally one-third but never more than one half of the facet joint is removed. The bone where the superior articular facet of the inferior vertebra meets the pedicle is also removed to gain access to the nerve root axilla.

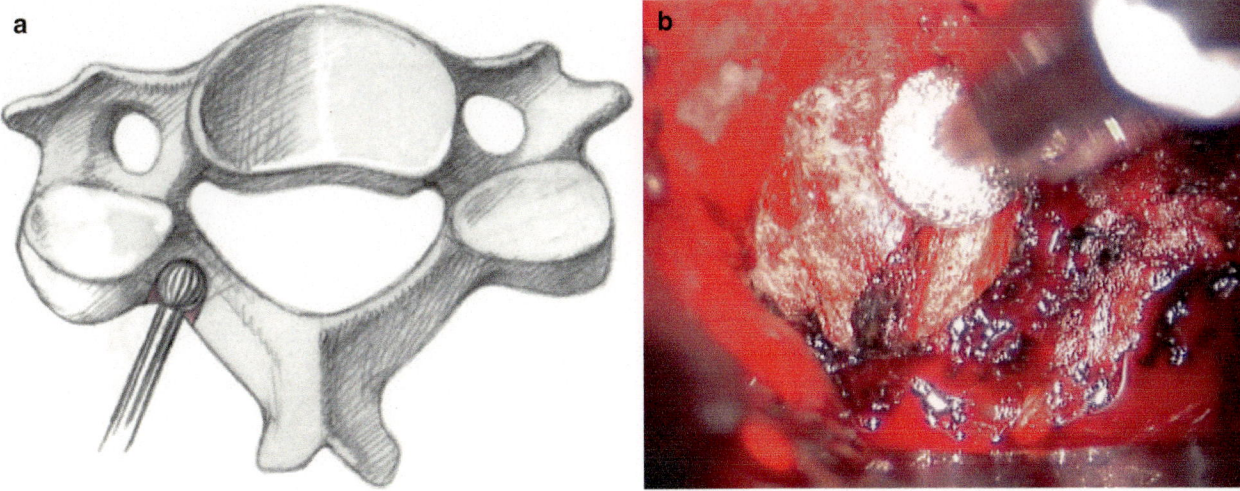

Fig. 35.4 (**a**) The foraminotomy is started at the junction between the lateral aspect of the interlaminar space and the medial border of the facet joint. (**b**) High-speed burr under microsurgical view

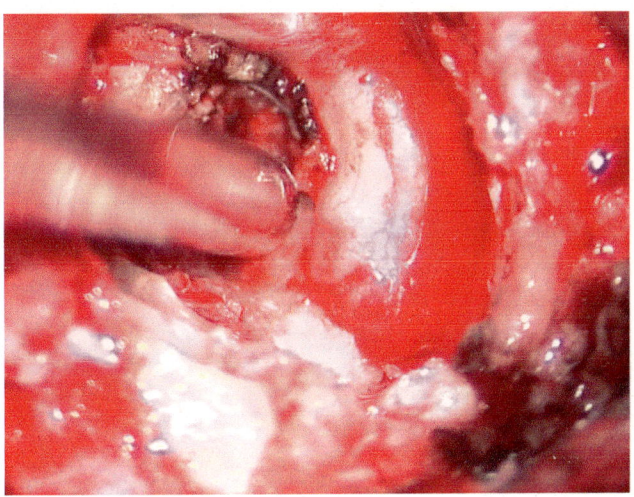

Fig. 35.5 Nerve root C8 after decompression

35.8   Complications and Pitfalls

Spinal cord and/or nerve root injury, CSF leakage, postoperative compressive hematoma, laceration of the vertebral artery, inadequate removal of the disc herniation or spondylotic bars with persistent radicular symptoms, deep paraspinous, or epidural wound infection.

35.9   Tips and Tricks

- Correct and careful positioning is important to reduce bleeding.
- The lateral facet capsule should be spared.
- When bleeding from the epidural venous plexus is encountered, it can be managed by the use of hemostatic agents such as Floseal (Baxter).

References

1. Burke TG, Caputy A. Microendoscopic posterior cervical foraminotomy: a cadaveric model and clinical application for cervical radiculopathy. J Neurosurg. 2000;93:126–9.
2. Chen BH, Natarajan RN, An HS, Andersson GB. Comparison of biomechanical response to surgical procedures used for cervical radiculopathy: posterior keyhole foraminotomy versus anterior foraminotomy and discectomy versus anterior discectomy with fusion. J Spinal Disord. 2001;14:17–20.
3. Clark CR. The cervical spine. 4th ed. Philadelphia, PA: Lippincott Williams & Wilkins; 2005. p. 1031–42.
4. Collias JC, Roberts MP. Posterior surgical approaches for cervical disk herniation and spondylotic myelopathy. In: Schmidek HH, Sweet WH, editors. Operative neurosurgical techniques: indications, methods and results. 4th ed. Philadelphia, PA: WB Saunders; 2000. p. 2016–27.
5. Fessler RG, Khoo LT. Minimally invasive cervical microendoscopic foraminotomy: an initial clinical experience. Neurosurgery. 2002;51:S37–45.
6. Gala VC, O'Toole JE, Voyadzis JM, et al. Posterior minimally invasive approaches for the cervical spine. Orthop Clin North Am. 2007;38:339–49.

Laminoplasty

Frank Grochulla

36.1 Introduction and Core Messages

The aims of the laminoplasty are to expand the spinal canal, to secure spinal stability, and to preserve the protective function of the spine [1]. Preservation of mobility is also a goal of this procedure for multiple-level involvement. Cervical laminoplasty was developed in the early 1970s for the treatment of cervical myelopathy due to multilevel spondylosis or multilevel ossification of the posterior longitudinal ligament. Since then, a variety of laminoplasty techniques have been described (Figs. 36.1, 36.2, and 36.3). In this chapter, the laminoplasty with the hardware-augmented open-door technique is described [2].

36.2 Indications

- Patients with cervical spinal canal stenosis (AP spinal canal diameter < 13 mm) due to developmental multilevel spondylotic and ossification of the posterior longitudinal ligament origin, with straight or lordotic cervical alignment.

36.3 Contraindications

- Cervical spine instability.
- Severe cervical kyphosis.

36.4 Technical Prerequisites

High-speed burr, microscope, X-ray, microsurgical instruments, Mayfield frame, special laminoplasty systems (e.g., New Bridge Laminoplasty System (Blackstone Medical)).

36.5 Planning, Preparation, and Positioning

- Patient is placed in a prone position (Fig. 36.4).
- Three-point pin fixation device such as Mayfield tongs to secure the head.
- The neck should be slightly flexed and kept in a horizontal plane. Extreme flexion should be avoided as it may produce spinal cord ischemia.
- The table is placed in a head-up position (20–30°).
- Cushions or rolled blankets are applied under the chest and the pelvis to avoid abdominal compression (with secondary elevation of venous pressure of the epidural venous plexus).

F. Grochulla (✉)
Metropol Medical Center, Clinic for Orthopedics, Trauma Surgery and Spinal Surgery, Nuremberg, Germany
e-mail: frank.grochulla@mmc-nuernberg.de

© Springer-Verlag GmbH Germany 2023
U. Vieweg, F. Grochulla (eds.), *Manual of Spine Surgery*, https://doi.org/10.1007/978-3-662-64062-3_36

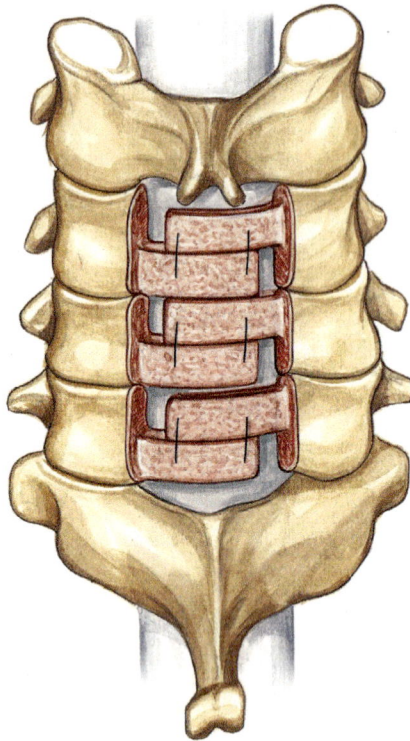

Fig. 36.1 Z-laminoplasty

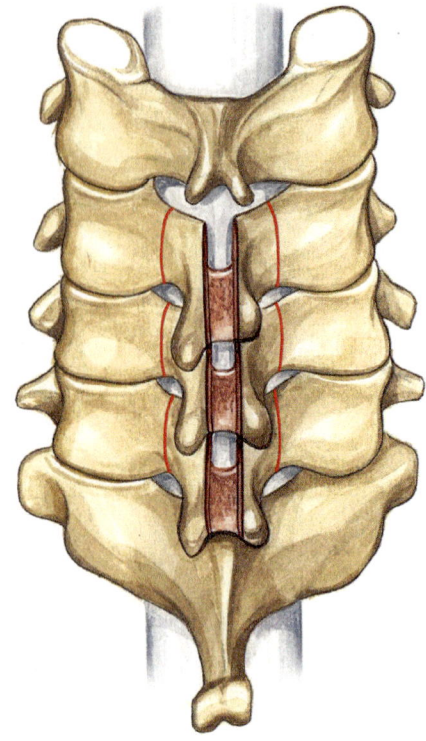

Fig. 36.3 Kurokawa laminoplasty

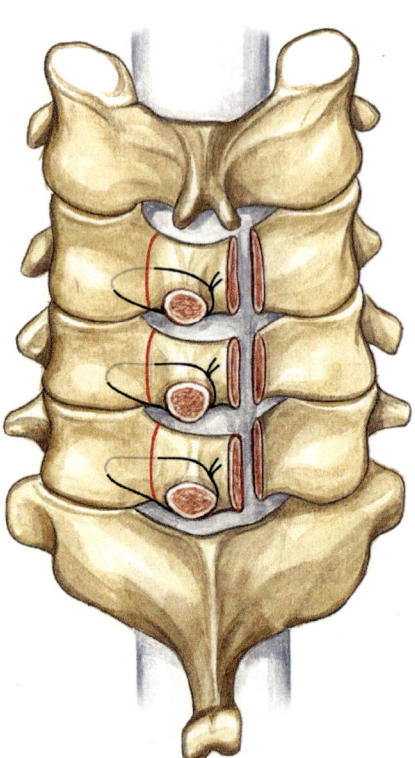

Fig. 36.2 Open-door laminoplasty

36.6   Surgical Technique

- Midline skin incision across the target region. For a C3–C7 laminoplasty, a 10–12-cm incision from the spinous processes C2 to C7/T1 may be adequate.
- Midline fascia incision to the level of the ligamentum nuchae.
- Dissection along the margin of this deep fascia to avoid bleeding. In the conventional posterior median approach, major blood vessels are not encountered.
- Careful dissection of the paraspinous muscles in a subperiosteal plane with Cobb, curved periosteal elevator, and cautery. Exposure until the lateral portion of the facet joint capsules is identified.
- Care should be taken not to violate the attachment of the semispinalis cervicis muscles at the inferior tip of the C2 spinous process (important for the maintenance of cervical lordosis).
- The open-side gutter is made first with a steel burr at the junction of the laminae and the facet joints. Perforation and resection of the ventral cortex with a diamond burr and/or a thin-bladed Kerrison rongeur.

Fig. 36.4 (**a–c**) Positioning of the patient

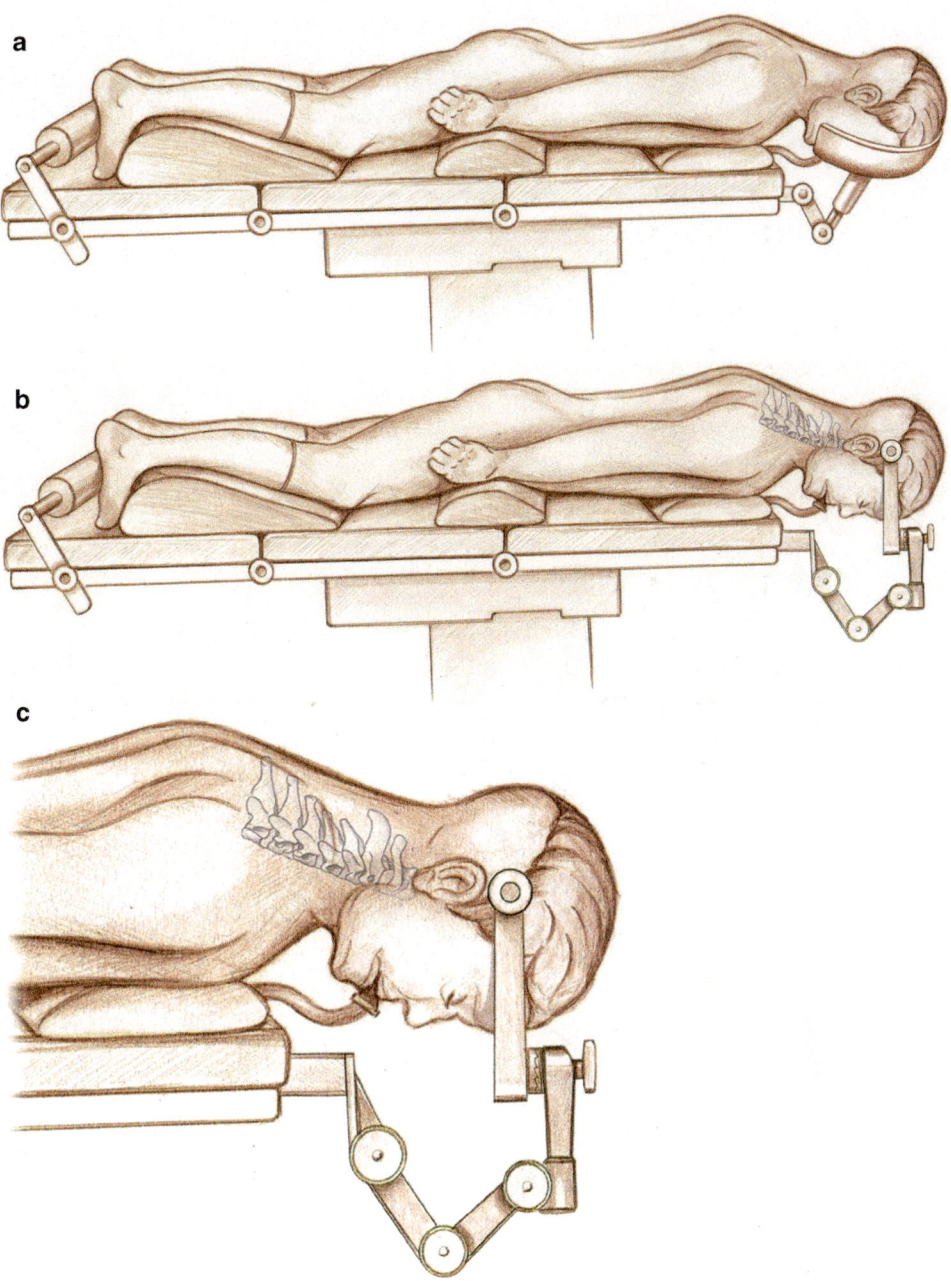

a

b

c

- Resection of the ligamentum flavum at the upper and lower end of the laminar door, usually at C2/3 and C7/Th1 with a thin-bladed Kerrison rongeur.
- The hinge-side gutter is made with a high-speed steel burr (Figs. 36.5 and 36.6). A thin rim of bone – a part of the ventral cortex – is left.
- Opening procedure (Fig. 36.7): The tip of one side of the laminar elevator is placed under the ventral surface of the lamina at the open side, and the lamina is lifted slightly to expand the gap. The spinous process can be held in the expanded position by an assistant. Then the next lamina is lifted in the same manner. During the opening procedure, the remaining soft tissues and adhesions in the open side should be excised with microdissectors and scissors to avoid tension.
- With the lamina in expanded position, the appropriate miniplate size can be determined by inserting the trial implants into the laminar gap (Fig. 36.8).
- A single- or double-bend miniplate is selected by placing the plates on the laminar expansion (Fig. 36.9).
- A variety of screws (self-tapping and self-drilling) are available to secure the miniplate.

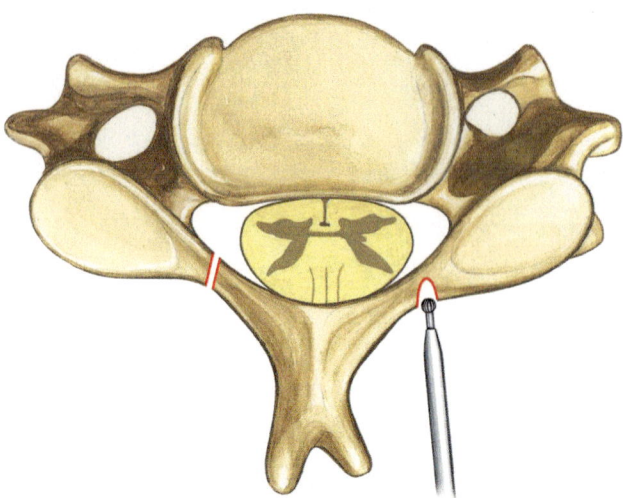

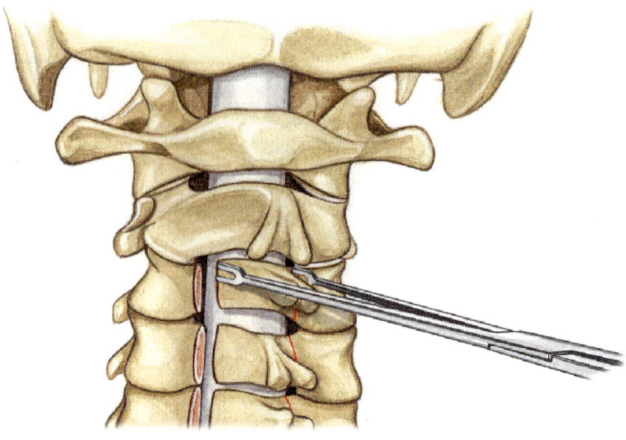

Fig. 36.7 Posterolateral view showing the elevation of the lamina

Fig. 36.5 With a thin cut the lamina is separated on the side with predominant symptoms. On the opposite side, a hinge is created in the lamina (Springer)

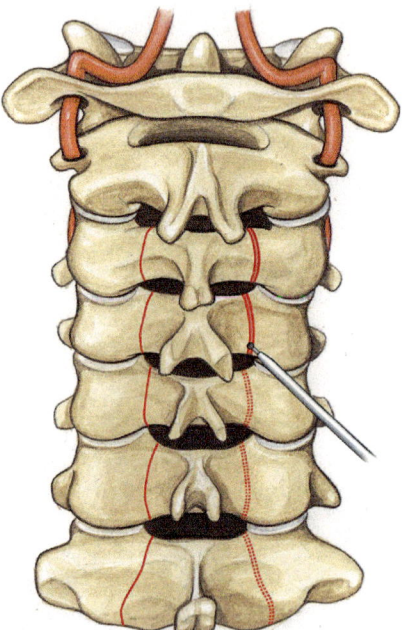

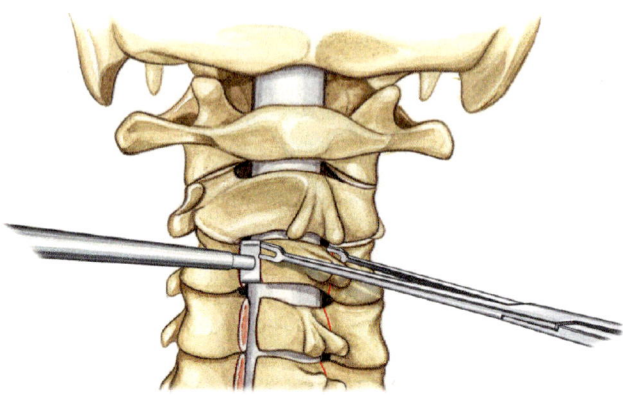

Fig. 36.8 Determination of the appropriate size and shape of the allograft with a trail spacer

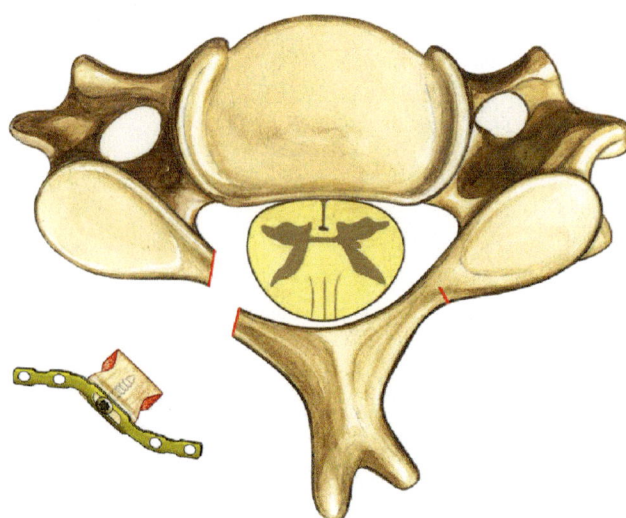

Fig. 36.6 Posterior view of the vertebral levels showing the laminar cuts and the hinges

- The first screw of proper size should be placed immediately lateral to the gap. Self-tapping screws require drilling prior to insertion.
- Two screws on each side of the gap should be placed (Fig. 36.10).
- Insertion of the remaining miniplates (Fig. 36.11).
- A drainage tube is placed subfascial/epidural.
- The paravertebral muscles, nuchal ligament, subcutaneous tissues, and skin are sutured.

Fig. 36.9 Introducing of the construct with the miniplate and a bone piece or spacer

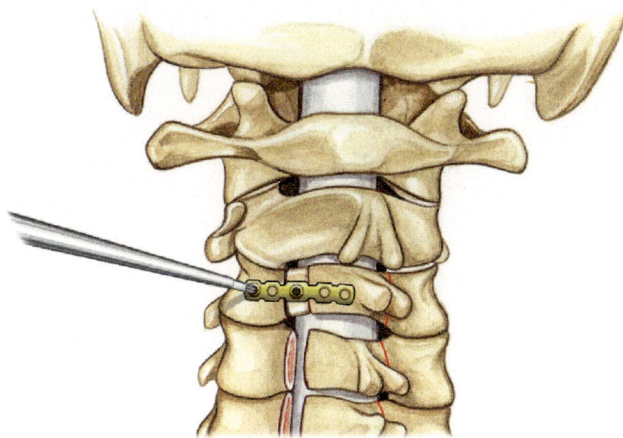

Fig. 36.10 Fixation of the miniplate with self-tapping screws on the right side

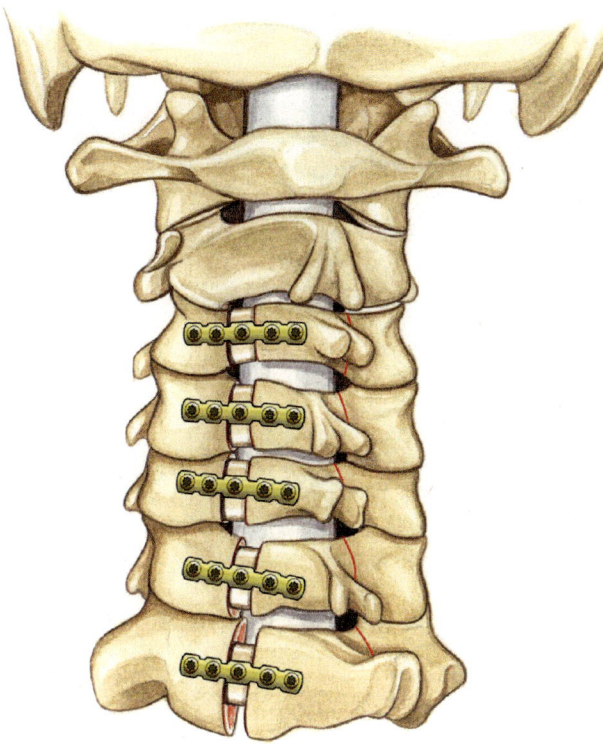

Fig. 36.11 Illustration after open-door laminoplasty of the cervical spine using a spacer plate system

36.7 Postoperative Care

- The patients are allowed to mobilize 4–6 h postoperatively.
- Soft cervical collar for 3–4 weeks.
- Instructions for general neck movement after 3–4 weeks, mild progressive neck exercise program.

36.8 Tips and Tricks

- Correct and careful positioning is important to reduce bleeding.
- When bleeding from the epidural venous plexus is encountered, it can be managed by the use of hemostatic agents such as Floseal (Baxter).
- Care should be taken during repair of the nuchal ligament for maintained good alignment postoperatively.

References

1. Ratliff JK, Cooper PR. Cervical laminoplasty: a critical review. J Neurosurg. 2003;98(Spine 3):230–8.
2. Hirabayashi K, Watanabe K, Wakano K, et al. Expansive open-door laminoplasty for cervical spinal stenotic myelopathy. Spine. 1983;8:693–9.

Occipital Cervical Stabilization with Rod-Screw Systems

37

Grégoire P. Chatain, Meic H. Schmidt, and Michael A. Finn

37.1 Introduction and Core Messages

Modern screw-based occipitocervical constructs enable immediate stabilization of the craniocervical junction [1–5]. Various screw trajectories allow for concomitant decompression and the creation of biomechanically stable constructs in a broad array of conditions. Bony fusion is successful in >95% of cases without requiring the use of rigid external immobilization. The goals of segmental instrumented occipitocervical fusion are stabilization of the craniocervical junction, reduction of deformity, minimization of segments immobilized, and bony fusion of instrumented segments.

37.2 Indications

- Traumatic instability.
- Rheumatoid disease/inflammatory arthropathies.
- Degenerative disease.
- Infection.
- Congenital malformations.
- Neoplasia.

37.3 Contraindications

- Aberrant vertebral artery anatomy may preclude the use of some screw constructs.

37.4 Technical Prerequisites

Fluoroscopy, positioning device (e.g., padded rolls), rigid head holder (e.g., Mayfield), and adequate implants and instruments are mandatory for the procedure.

In addition, neural monitoring consisting of somatosensory-evoked potentials and motor-evoked potentials is used in cases of significant instability or cervicomedullary compression. We additionally plan our screw trajectories on a three-dimensional workstation (StealthStation, Medtronic, Inc., Minneapolis, MN) preoperatively. We are now using the O-arm (Medtronic, Inc.) in lieu of fluoroscopy for intraoperative navigation and confirmation of the adequacy of hardware placement in cases with difficult anatomy. This system, however, makes the immediate confirmation of alignment upon positioning in the highly unstable spine difficult, and fluoroscopy is still used in these circumstances.

37.5 Planning, Preparation, and Positioning

Prior to surgery, a plan is created that is specific for the patient's anatomy and the goals of the procedure. Particular attention is given to the anatomy of the vertebral arteries as they course through the pars of the atlas. Three-dimensional multiplanar reconstructed images are helpful in planning screw trajectories across this area (Fig. 37.1). Anatomy permitting, transarticular screws are the preferred option as they provide excellent fixation and are the lowest cost construct. If another construct variant, including C1 lateral mass screws, C2 pars or pedicle screws, or C2 laminar screws, is planned, the placement is also planned in advance. The use of laminar

G. P. Chatain · M. A. Finn (✉)
Department of Neurosurgery, School of Medicine, University of Colorado, Aurora, CO, USA
e-mail: gregoire.chatain@cuanschutz.edu

M. H. Schmidt
Department of Neurosurgery, University of New Mexico, Albuquerque, NM, USA

© Springer-Verlag GmbH Germany 2023
U. Vieweg, F. Grochulla (eds.), *Manual of Spine Surgery*, https://doi.org/10.1007/978-3-662-64062-3_37

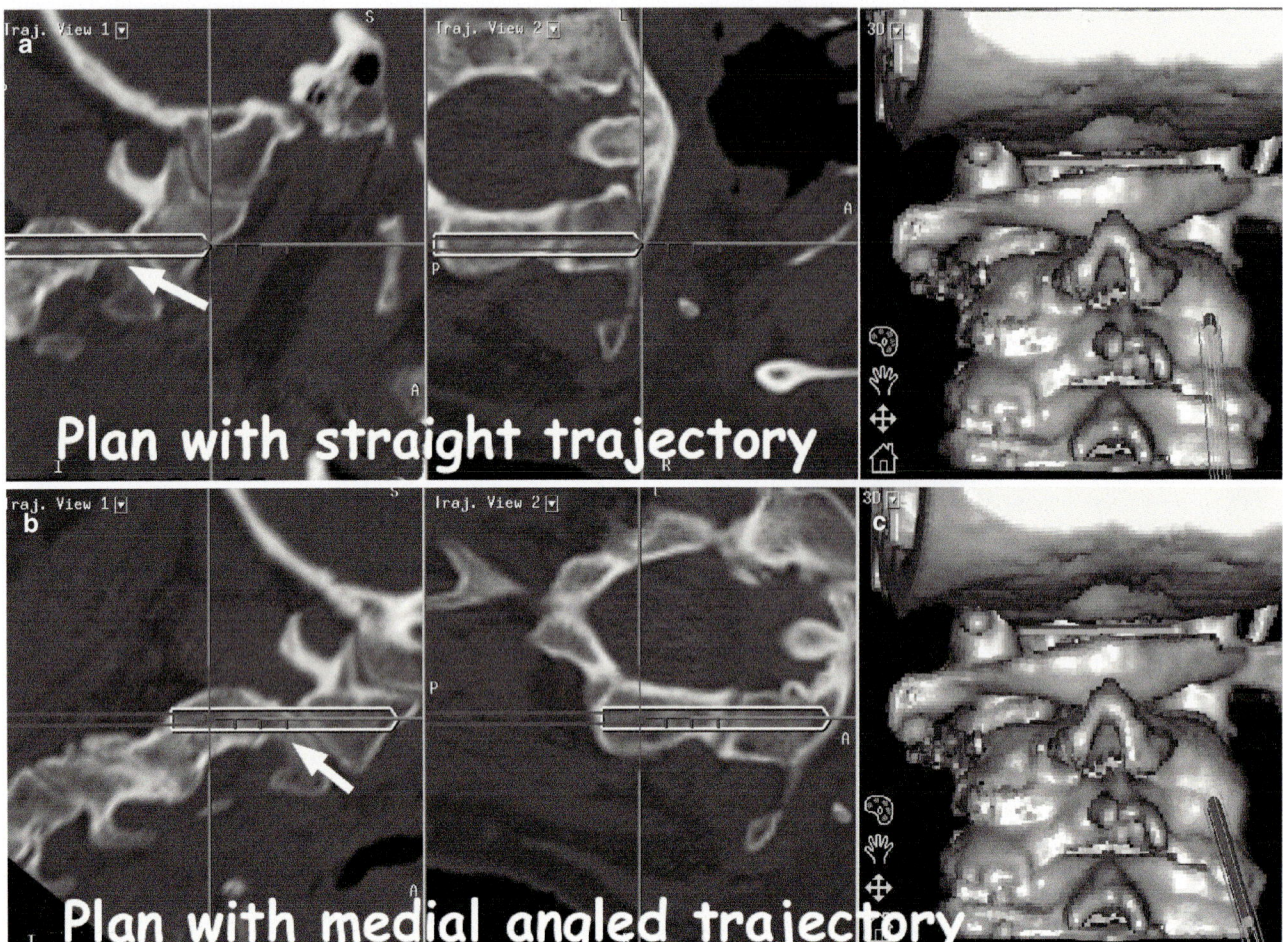

Fig. 37.1 Multiplanar three-dimensional reconstructions on the Stealth Workstation. (**a**) A straight screw trajectory results in violation of the vertebral canal. (**b**) A slight medial trajectory enables placement of transarticular screw entirely within bone. (**c**) Three-dimensional sur-face anatomy shows trajectory and allows for easy identification of starting position relative to bony landmarks. (With permission of Finn and Apfelbaum [2])

screws is reserved as an option of last resort as laminar screws reduce the area over C2 for graft placement and bony fusion and have been shown to be biomechanically inferior to other options in occipitocervical constructs. In cases of significant instability, awake fiberoptic intubation is performed. Baseline evoked potentials are obtained, the patient's head is fixed in a cranial fixator, and the patient is rolled into the supine position onto padded rolls. The patient's head is kept in a neutral position and locked into place. Immediate postpositioning lateral fluoroscopic imaging is performed to ensure adequacy of alignment, and postpositioning evoked potentials are obtained. Loss of potentials mandates a return to supine position and the performance of a wake-up test. It is critical that the patient be placed in a gaze-neutral or slight downward position as fusion of the craniocervical junction in an upward position can lead to gait problems, and fixation in a downward position can contribute to dysphagia. The patient is prepped and draped from just above the inion to the upper thoracic spine to allow for the placement of guide tubes if transarticular screws are used.

37.6 Surgical Technique

37.6.1 Approach

- A midline incision is created from the level of the inion to the spinous process of C3.
- The avascular midline raphe is developed to expose the dorsal bony elements, which are dissected in a subperiosteal fashion. The occiput is exposed from the inion to the foramen magnum and laterally to the medial edge of the mastoids.
- The atlas is exposed laterally to its articulation with the axis if placement of lateral mass screws is planned. Bleeding from the epidural venous plexus may be encountered at this time and is controlled with bipolar electrocautery and powder Gelfoam (Pfizer, New York, NY) and thrombin. If Songer cables are to be used to secure the bone graft, the soft tissues are circumferentially dissected off the arch of atlas with curettes.

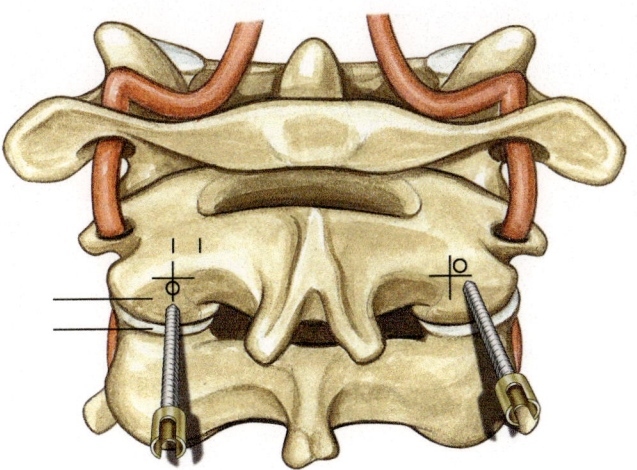

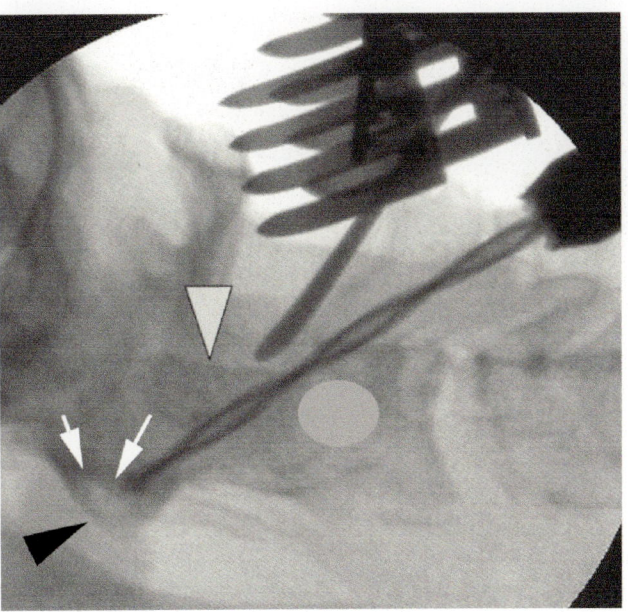

Fig. 37.2 The typical entry points for transarticular/pars screws (*left*) and pedicle screw (*right*) in C2 are illustrated with crosshairs indicating the midline. Transarticular/pars screws enter 2–3 mm cephalad to C2–3 lateral mass articulation and 2–3 mm medial to the canal. They are typically angulated at 40° in the sagittal plane and 0–10° medially in the axial plane. C2 pedicle screws enter in the upper outer quadrant of the C2 pars and are angulated approximately 20° medially and superiorly

- The axis is exposed laterally to the pars and the facet articulation of C2–3, with care taken not to disrupt the joint.
- Exposure of the subaxial spine is undertaken if an extended construct is planned. The interspinous and supraspinous ligaments between C2 and C3 are preserved.

37.6.2 Instrumentation

- Atlantoaxial screw fixation is undertaken first. The use of C3 screws may preclude placement of transarticular and C2 pars screws.

37.6.2.1 Transarticular Screw Fixation

- The entry point is identified (Fig. 37.2), and the medial edge of the pars is developed with curettes to identify the lateral boundary of the spinal canal. The typical entry point is 2–3 mm medial to this edge and 2–3 mm superior to the C2–3 joint. The entry site can vary depending on patient-specific anatomy.
- The entry site for the percutaneous drill guide is identified using fluoroscopy and a radiopaque marker (e.g., drill bit) placed alongside the patient in the trajectory of the screw. The typical entry site is at the level of the high thoracic spine. Here, a small (~1.5 cm) incision is created, and a subcutaneous/intramuscular tunnel is created to the screw entry site.

Fig. 37.3 The drill trajectory for TAS placement is demonstrated. The drill is aimed toward the upper part of the anterior arch of C1 (*black arrowhead*) to its final exit site through the anterior cortex of the lateral mass of C1 (*white arrows*). Resistance is felt as the drill passes through the C1–2 joint (*white arrowhead*) and again as the drill passes through C1 anteriorly. The Penfield dissector is placed on the pars and used as a marker to correlated intraoperative observations with fluoroscopic imaging. The *shaded circle* represents the area of the vertebral canal. (With permission of Gluf et al. [4])

- Once the percutaneous drill guide has been placed, the inner drill guide is removed, and a starting awl is placed through the drill guide to create a starter hole at the entry site. The screw tract is then created by using a power drill with fluoroscopic guidance (Fig. 37.3). An instrument (e.g., a Penfield 4 dissector) can be placed on the dorsum of the pars as a radiographic marker for the dorsum of the pars. The drill should be aimed to exit on the upper half of the C1 lateral mass.
- More recently, intraoperative navigation has been described for safe and accurate placement of K-wire preventing damage to vital structures whilst drilling [6].
- The tract is tapped, and a 4.0 mm polyaxial screw is placed.

37.6.2.2 C1 Lateral Mass Screws

- The C2 nerve root is retracted caudally, and the entry point on the C1 lateral mass is identified. The typical entry point is on the middle prominence of the lateral mass. The posterior arch may need to be drilled to access this point.
- The C2 nerve can be taken in cases of crowded anatomy. Ligating the nerve proximal to the ganglion reduces the incidence of bothersome post-operative dysesthesia [7].

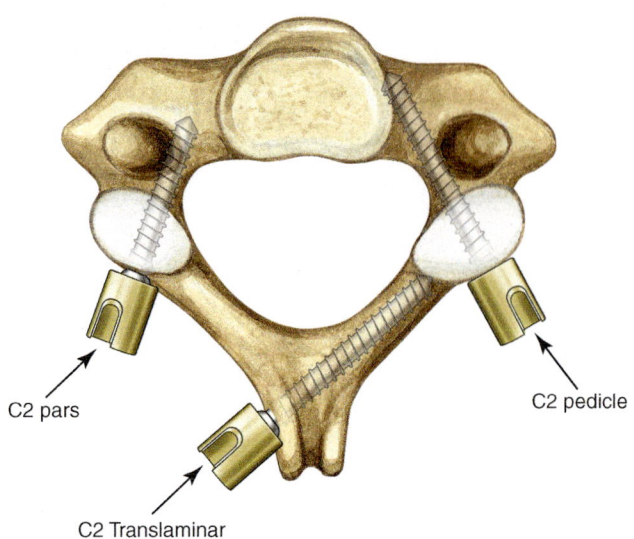

Fig. 37.4 Varying trajectories for C2 pars, pedicle, and laminar screws

- The tract is started with a high-speed burr. A high-speed drill with a protective drill guide is then used to create the pilot hole. The trajectory is slightly medial in the axial plane and parallel to the arch of C1 in the sagittal plane and directed toward the anterior tubercle with fluoroscopy.
- The tract is tapped, and a partially threaded polyaxial screw is placed, which may reduce the incidence of occipital neuralgia.

37.6.2.3 C2 Pars Screws

- The entry point, trajectory, and setup are identical to those used in transarticular screw fixation (Fig. 37.4). The length of the screw is determined on preoperative image reconstructions.

37.6.2.4 C2 Pedicle Screws

- The typical entry point is identified in the upper outer quadrant of the C2 lateral mass and marked with a high-speed drill (Fig. 37.2). Preoperative image reconstructions help determine the exact entry point, trajectory, and screw length.
- The screw tract is created with a high-speed drill at a typical trajectory of approximately 20° medial and 20° cephalad.

37.6.2.5 C2 Laminar Screws

- The typical entry point is identified and marked at the junction of the spinous process and lamina, with a cephalad entry on one side and a caudal entry on the opposing side (Fig. 37.5). The entry point should be in line with the slope of the contralateral lamina.

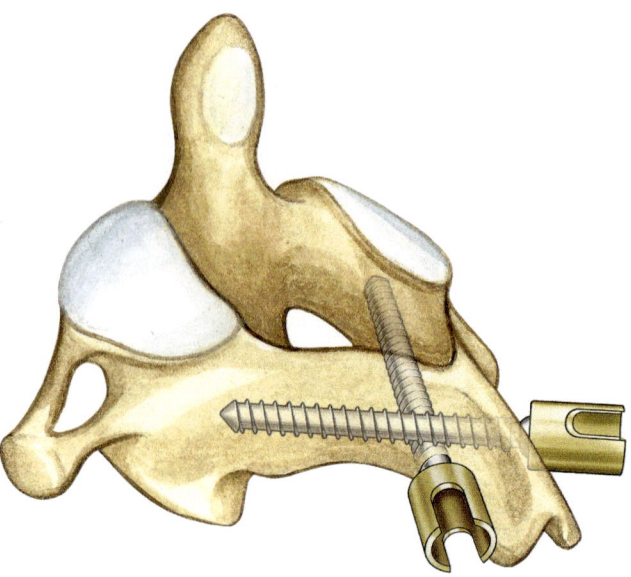

Fig. 37.5 Illustration demonstrating trajectories of crossed laminar screws

- The screw tract is drilled and tapped, and the screw is placed. Up-going curettes can be used to confirm absence of anterior screw breakout.
- The contralateral screw is placed just caudal to the first screw.

37.6.2.6 Occipital Plate

- Many occipital plate variants are commercially available [5] (Fig. 37.6). Key attributes to consider include ease of use, bulk, and location of screw placement. The bone is the thickest in the midline and thins out rapidly laterally (Fig. 37.7). Screws placed in the midline therefore provide the greatest resistance to pullout.
- Bony ridges on the subocciput are smoothed out with the high-speed burr to provide for a flush plate fit. The upper screw in the plate is placed first. For midline screws, a pilot hole is created with a power drill to a depth of 6 mm. The drill stop is increased in 2 mm increments until the deep cortex is penetrated. For lateral screws, bony thickness is measured on preoperative computed tomography scan, and prospective tracts are created in the same manner.
- The entire depth of the pilot tract is tapped, and 4.5 mm blunt-tipped screws are placed. The first screw is completely tightened after placement of the second screw.
- 3.5 mm rods are shaped to fit the screw heads and the plate. Hinged rods and right-angle connectors can be used to aid in connecting elements. Adequacy of head position is confirmed prior to final tightening of the construct.

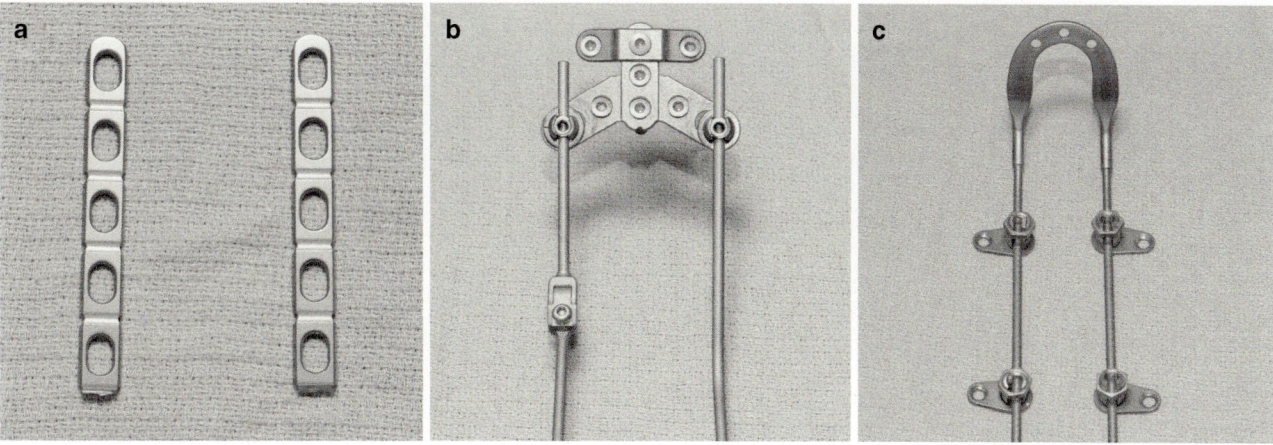

Fig. 37.6 Variations of screw-based occipitocervical instrumentation constructs. Those shown in (**b** and **c**) allow for the placement of a midline screw. (With permission of Finn et al. [3])

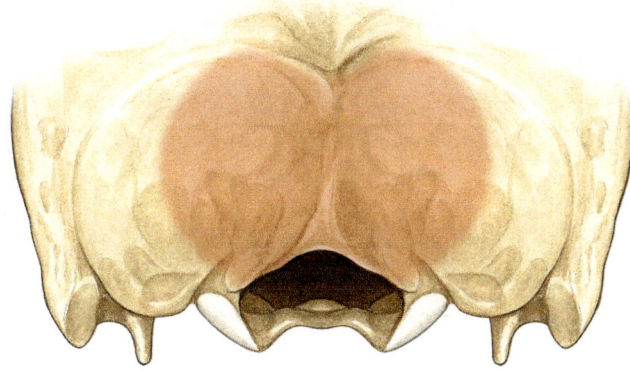

Fig. 37.7 Illustration demonstrating the optimal locations for placement of occipital screws, with *whiter areas* representing areas of thicker bone

- An alternative to occipital plating is the occipital bolt technique. It is achieved by drilling paramedian burr holes and placing bolts in the suboccipital bone from an "outside-in" or "inside-out" fashion. This technique has the advantage of bolstering robust lateral fixation point when compared to other lateral fixation systems.
- Tricortical iliac crest allograft is preferred in most patients and has been shown to have good fusion results. The graft is shaped to fit flush against the posterior bony elements. A V-shaped notch is cut into the bottom to accommodate the spinous process of C2. The fusion bed is decorticated, and Songer cables are used to secure the graft. A screw is placed in the cephalad end of the graft to secure it to the occiput.
- If the C2 nerve roots are ligated, the C1-2 joints can be decorticated and packed with bone to provide another surface for fusion.

- As bone morphogenetic protein (BMP) has been shown to improve fusion rates in the lumbar spine, its judicious and parsimonious use in high-risk patient may be a reasonable surgical option. Its utilization remains an off-label in this application, however, and when used, its application must be kept away from neural elements.
- Postoperative orthoses are typically not used in non-trauma patients with good bone quality and good screw purchase.

37.6.2.7   Occipital Condyle Screw
- Occipital condyle screws can offer an additional fixation point in the occipital bone which may be particularly helpful in patients who have had posterior fossa surgery.
- After the occiput and posterior elements of upper cervical spine are exposed using approach described above, the occipital condyle exposure can proceed. The soft tissue of the condylar fossa is dissected away from the atlantoocipital joint using a combination of blunt and sharp dissection whilst being mindful of the vertebral artery course. Once the foramen magnum is identified, its posterior rim can be followed laterally to find the condyles.
- The posterior emissary vein should be recognized and coagulated using bipolar cautery.
- Although entry site can vary depending on patient-specific anatomy, typical entry point for condyle screw is shown in Fig. 37.8.
- A starting hole is made with a high-speed burr or awl through the condyle cortical surface. With the aid of either fluoroscopic guidance or intraoperative navigation, the remainder of the tract is created with a drill. The screw trajectory is then tapped. Although screw size can vary

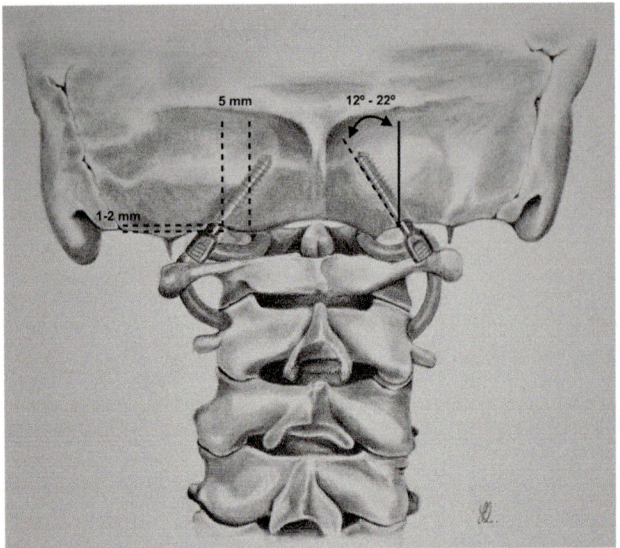 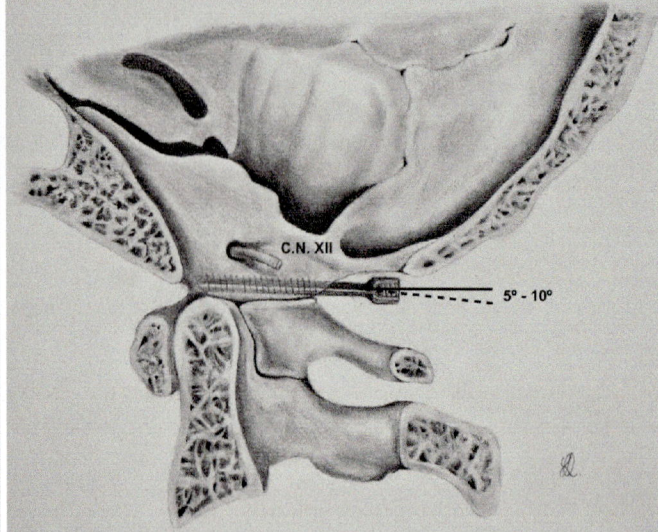

Figs. 37.8 and 37.9 The typical entry points for condyle screw are illustrated. Condyle screws enter 5 mm lateral to foramen magnum and 1–2 mm superior to the atlantooccipital joint (Fig. 37.8). They are typi-cally angulated at 5–10° in the sagittal plane (Fig. 37.9) and 12–22° medially in the axial plane. (With permission of artist Clarisse Lavech)

based on patient's anatomy, a 20 mm screw is usually placed.
- The condylar screws can then be connected to adjacent instrumentation with rods in the standard fashion.

37.6.2.8 C0–C1 Transarticular Screw
- Occipital-C1 transarticular screw offers an option in the rare setting of Occ-C1 instability or as a means to strengthen Occ-C1 fixation when using longer constructs.
- Biomechanically, stability at the junction is robust during lateral bending and rotation but found to be inferior in flexion extension [8].
- Although large individual variation exists mandating consideration of patient-specific anatomy with advanced imaging, ideal screw trajectory based on anatomical study [9, 10].
- Entry points are prepared with a high-speed drill or awl. The screw tract is created by using a drill under fluoroscopic guidance or intraoperative navigation and is subsequently tapped with 3.5 mm tap; 28–34 mm screws are typically utilized.
- Detailed understanding of the patient's anatomy is imperative as the occipital condyle is surrounded by critical neurovascular structures including brainstem medially, hypoglossal nerve superiorly, vertebral artery posterolat-erally, sigmoid sinus superolaterally, and internal carotid anteriorly.

37.7 Tips and Tricks

- Careful examination of patient-specific anatomy is critical to planning screw combinations and trajectory.
- Preoperative planning on a three-dimensional workstation can be invaluable in planning screw trajectories in difficult cases.
- Occasionally, patients are placed in a halo vest preoperatively and allowed to walk to ensure adequacy of head position. If adequate, the patient is positioned in the halo vest, which is removed only after the halo ring is secured to the operative bed. This technique ensures the patient's final head position will be adequate for ambulation and deglutition.

References

1. Du JY, Aichmair A, Kueper J, et al. Biomechanical analysis of screw constructs for atlantoaxial fixation in cadavers: a systematic review and meta-analysis. J Neurosurg Spine Feb. 2015;22(2):151–61.
2. Finn MA, Bishop FS, Dailey AT. Surgical treatment of occipitocervical instability. Neurosurgery. 2008;63(5):961–8.

3. Gluf WM, Schmidt MH, Apfelbaum RI. Atlantoaxial transarticular screw fixation: a review of surgical indications, fusion rate, complications, and lessons learned in 191 adult patients. J Neurosurg Spine. 2005;2:155–63.

4. Winegard CD, Lawrence JP, Friel BC, et al. A systematic review of occipital cervical fusion: techniques and outcomes. J Neurosurg Spine. 2010;13(1):5–16.

5. Lee KM, Yeom JS, Lee JO, et al. Optimal trajectory for the atlanto-occipital transarticular screw. Spine. 2010;35(16):1562–70.

6. Eliott RE, Kang MM, Smith ML, et al. C2 nerve sectioning in posterior atlantoaxial instrumented fusions: a structure review of the literature. World Neurosurg Dec. 2012;78(6):697–708.

7. Finn MA, Apfelbaum RI. Atlantoaxial transarticular screw fixation: update on technique and outcomes in 269 patients. Neurosurgery. 2010;66(3 Suppl):184–92.

8. Hara T, Iwamuro H, Ohara Y, et al. Efficacy of atlantoaxial Transarticular screw fixation using navigation-guided drill: technical note. World Neurosurg Feb. 2020;134:378–82.

9. Gonzalez LF, Crawford NR, Chamberlain RH. Craniovertebral junction fixation with transarticular screws: biomechanical analysis of a novel technique. J Neurosurg Spine. 2003;98:202–9.

10. Yan W, Zhang C, Zhou X, et al. Safe angle scope for posterior atlanto-occipital transarticular screw fixation. Neurosurgery. 2009;65:499–504.

Michael Winking

38.1 Introduction and Core Messages

Several techniques are known for treatment of an atlanto-axial instability. Posterior transarticular screw fixation first published by Grob and Magerl (1987) is the most rigid way to achieve this aim [1–3]. The C1–C2 joint functions primarily in rotation and secondarily in flexion and extension. Therefore, in stabilization of this segment, it is mandatory that flexion-extension, lateral bending, and axial rotation are restricted. The direction of the screws in the transarticular screw technique reduces motion in all degrees of freedom, which results directly in high segmental stability. Additionally, this technique prevents a slippage of the segment. However, only the interlaminar bone graft between C1 and C2 will achieve the final stability through bony fusion [1–11].

38.2 Indications

Instability of C1–2 due to:
- Rheumatoid arthritis.
- Odontoid fractures.
- Os odontoideum.
- Arthrosis of C1–2.

38.3 Contraindications

- Aberrant course of the vertebral artery between C1 and C2.
- Physical size of the C2 isthmus is too small.

M. Winking (✉)
ZW-O Spine Center, Klinikum Osnabrück, Osnabrück, Germany
e-mail: info@zw-o.de

- Irreducible deformity of the C1–2 junction.
- Prominent kyphosis of the cervico-thoracic junction.
- Destruction of the lateral mass of C1.

38.4 Technical Prerequisites

Preoperative 3D-CT for planning of the virtual screw pathway, navigation system (optional), fluoroscopy, Mayfield clamp, cannulated screws (optional), and titanium wiring cable.

38.5 Planning, Preparation, and Positioning

To avoid any intraoperative surprise, detailed preoperative planning using CT is mandatory. Several questions have to be answered before starting the surgery:
- What is the distance between the estimated pathway of the screws and the vertebral artery?
- Does the vertebral artery have an aberrant course?
- Is the diameter of the C2 interartical portion big enough for a 3.5 mm screw?
- Is there a risk of drill deviation due to osteochondrosis of the joints?
- The best way to answer these questions is via a preoperative 3D-CT scan for virtual assessment of the navigation of the screws (Fig. 38.1).

Additionally, flexion/extension X-rays will identify the amount of mobility in the C1–2 segment and the chance of reducing a dislocation of the joints (Fig. 38.2). The correct drilling direction can be limited by a prominent kyphosis in the cervico-thoracic junction. Preoperatively, the estimated drilling trajectory should be checked. The MRI is more a supplemental imaging to identify the pathology as well as the spinal cord and the course of the vertebral arteries (Fig. 38.3). For surgical plannings, its information is not sufficiently enough. When the patient is still lying in supine position, the Mayfield clamp is fixed. Take care the patient has not had previous cranial surgery

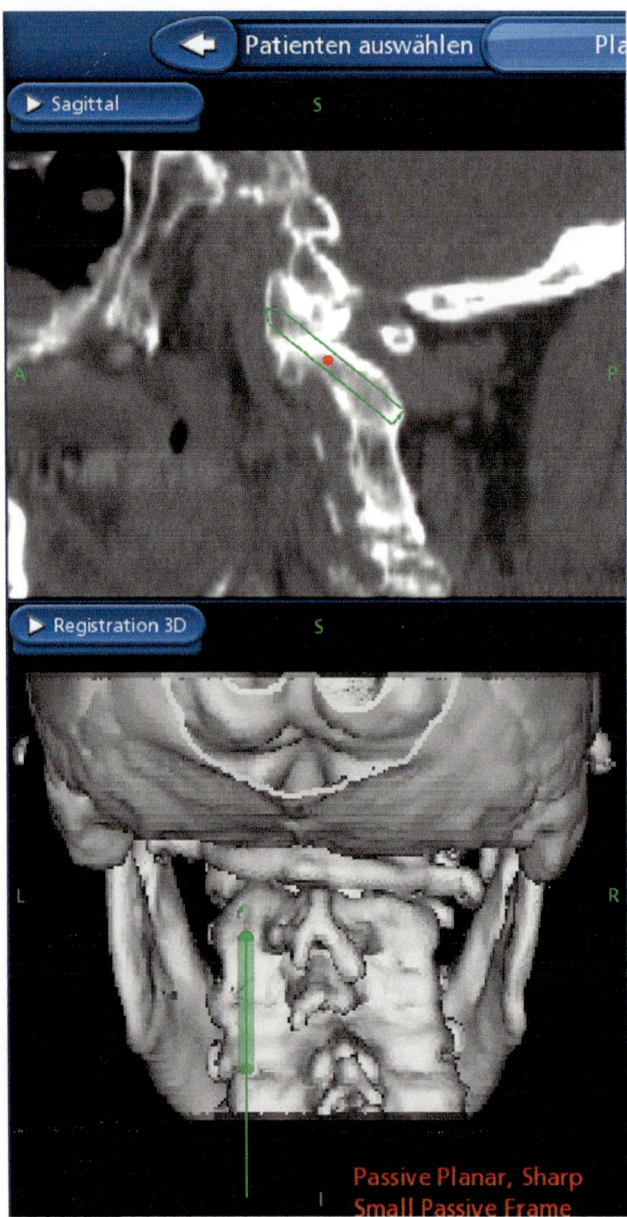

Fig. 38.1 Sagittal CT scan (3D reconstruction) with trajectory for the screws

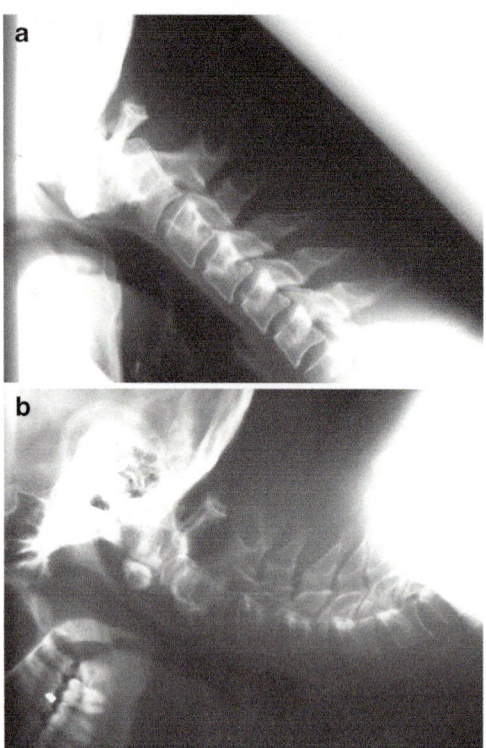

Fig. 38.2 Preoperative flexion and extension X-ray in a patient with atlanto-axial instability due to rheumatoid arthritis

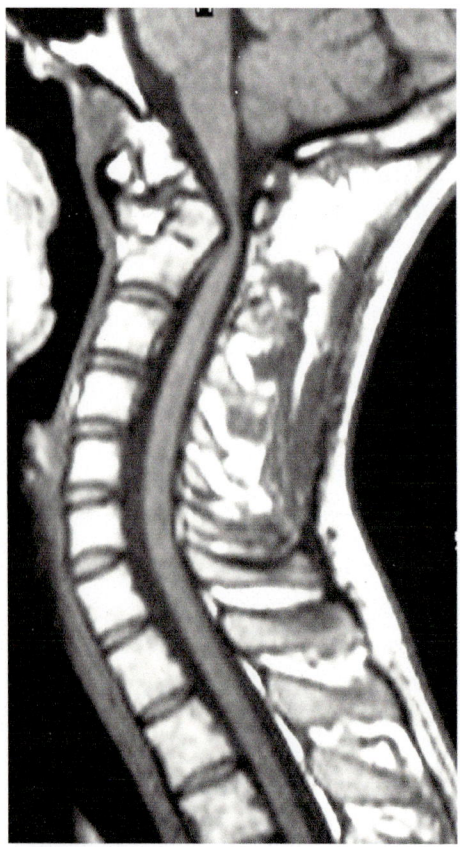

Fig. 38.3 Lateral MRI showing the spinal cord compression

(an X-ray of the cranium before surgery is necessary). Now the patient is turned over on the operating table into prone position.

Definitive fixation of the Mayfield clamp to the operating table is done after AP and lateral fluoroscopy. The upper cervical spine should be positioned in exact derotation and a slight extension. A potential atlanto-axial deviation should be adjusted. Check the estimated drilling trajectory. A prominent kyphosis of the cervico-thoracic junction can limit the access. Pull back the cervical spine slightly to adjust the trajectory. The shoulders should be positioned alongside the body fixed with a slight pull in caudal direction (Fig. 38.4). This will reduce intraoperative bleeding because the intramuscular veins are compressed. Make sure that the intravenous catheters work

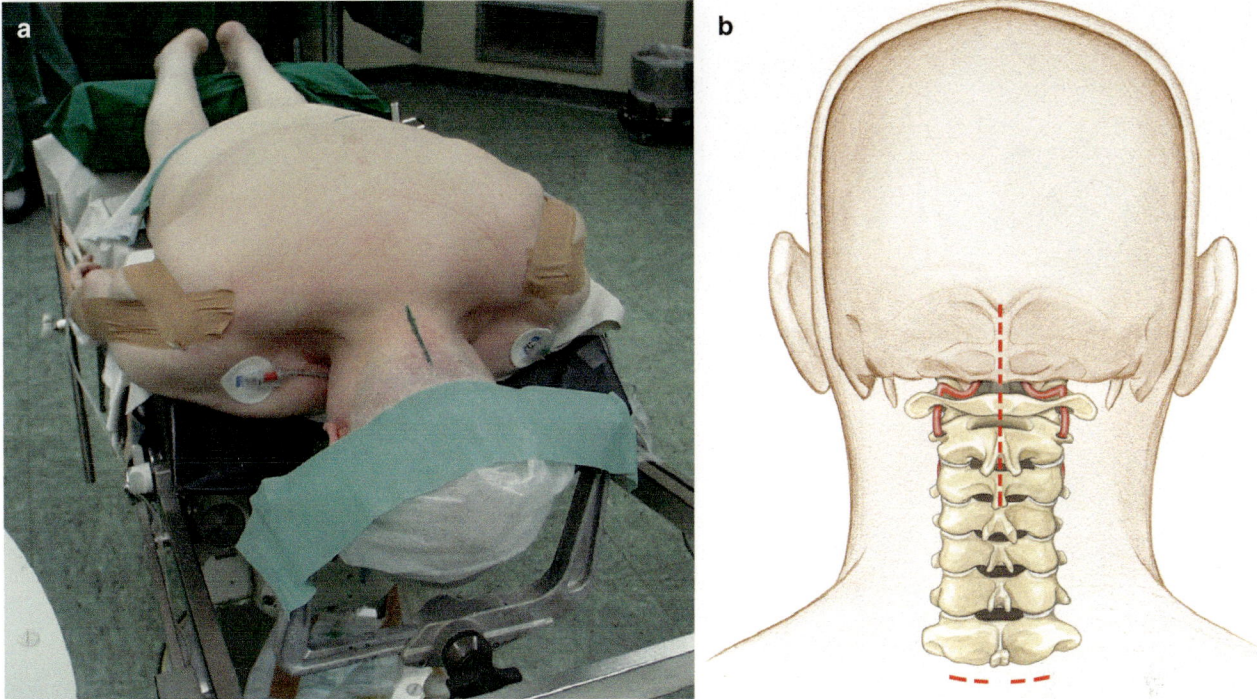

Fig. 38.4 (**a**) The patient is positioned while monitoring vertebral position under lateral fluoroscopy. (**b**) Illustration of the midline skin incision and the additional skin incisions lateral to C7

well. During surgery, the treatment of any anesthesiological emergency can be complicated by the prone position of the patient and the sharp fixation of the head.

38.6   Surgical Technique

38.6.1 Approach

- A midline incision from the occiput to C7 is performed (Fig. 38.4a, b).
- Cut the subcutaneous tissue until you identify the nuchal ligament.
- Stay accurately in the midline to reduce venous bleeding.
- Identify the spinous processes from C2 to C4.
- By electrocautery, remove the splenius and semispinalis muscle from the spinous processes (Fig. 38.5).
- Remove the muscles bilaterally from C3 and C4 by blunt preparation.
- Leave the capsules from C2/3 and C3/4 protected. Identify the C2/3 facet.
- Dissect bilaterally the lower part of the obliquus capitis inferior muscle to identify the arch of C2.
- Remove the rectus capitis minor muscle insertions from the dorsal arch of C1. With blunt preparation, the lamina of C1 is dissected, stopping short of the sulcus of the vertebral artery (Fig. 38.5).
- Remove the atlanto-axial membrane. The preparation should be done with a sharp dissector subperiosteally.

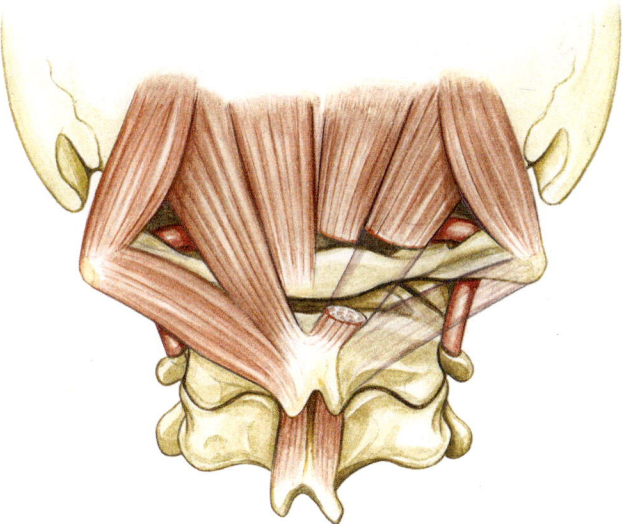

Fig. 38.5 Anatomical situation after resection of *M. rectus* capitis posterior and *M. obliquus* capitis inferior

Now the lamina of C1 can be identified for later wiring. Identify the joint of C1. During this step, the periradicular venous plexus can be damaged. The bleeding can be controlled by bipolar coagulation, better by compression with hemostatic substances.

- Identify the inner cortical border of the isthmus of C2 with a nerve hook, which will guide the later drilling direction.

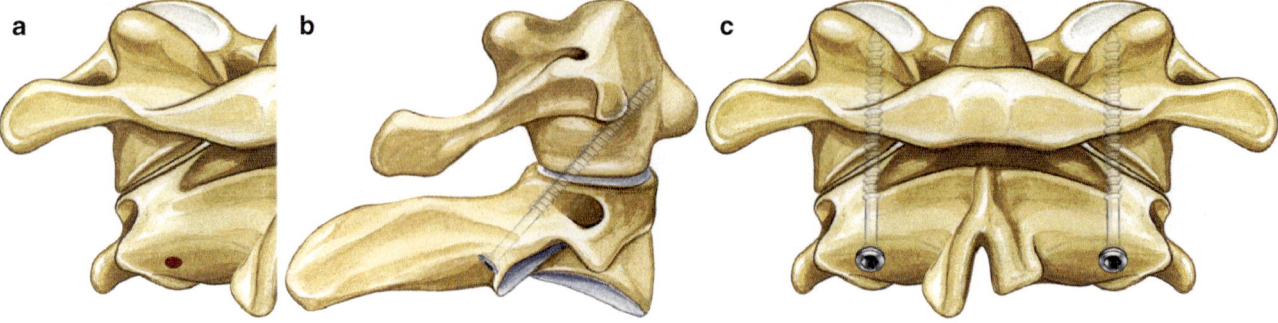

Fig. 38.6 (**a–c**) Drill placement, starting point, and drilling direction for transarticular screwing

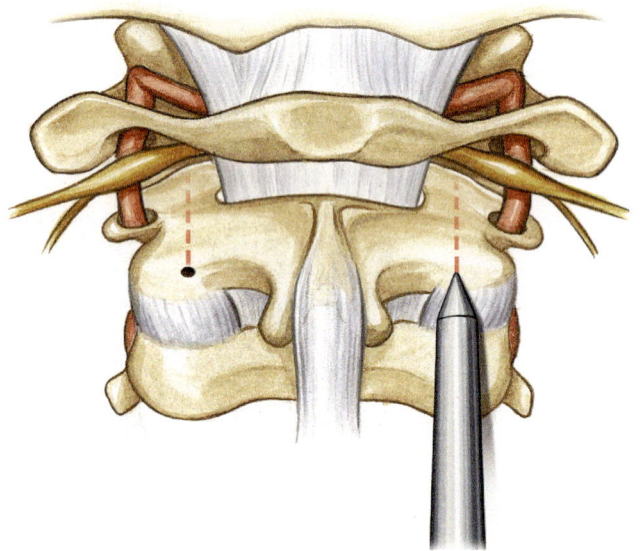

Fig. 38.7 Details of the surgical anatomy. The desired screw placement is just lateral to the edge of the spinal canal. It will traverse the isthmus of C2 and the C1–C2 articulation

38.6.2 Instrumentation

- The starting point for screw placement is typically 2–3 mm cephalad to the lower border of the C2 facet and 2–3 mm lateral to the medial cortical border of the C2 isthmus (Fig. 38.6a).
- The entry point is opened with an awl (Fig. 38.7).
- Using lateral fluoroscopy, a guide wire is drilled toward the superior aspect of the anterior C1 ring (Fig. 38.6b).
- Sometimes percutaneous skin incisions (beneath C7) are necessary to ensure the right angulation toward C1 (Fig. 38.8). The drilling direction is orientated slightly medially, parallel to the inner wall of the isthmus of C2. During drilling, the direction is controlled with a nerve hook attached to the isthmus.
- In cases of an osteochondrotic C1 joint, the guide wire may drift from its planned direction as it passes the joint space. Drilling with reduced pressure under continuous

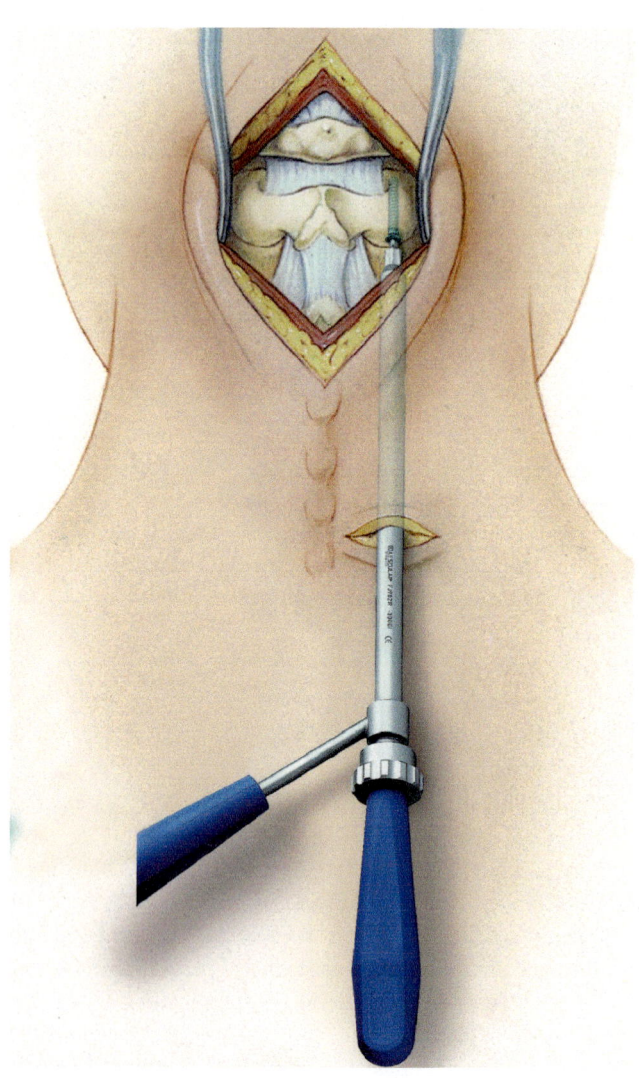

Fig. 38.8 Introducing of the transarticular screw in the AP view. (With permission of Aesculap AG, Tuttlingen, Germany)

fluoroscopy will help keep the right trajectory. After positioning, a guide wire is used as a track for the cannulated 3.5 mm drill. Use fluoroscopic guidance to ensure that the guide wire is not moved forward during drilling.

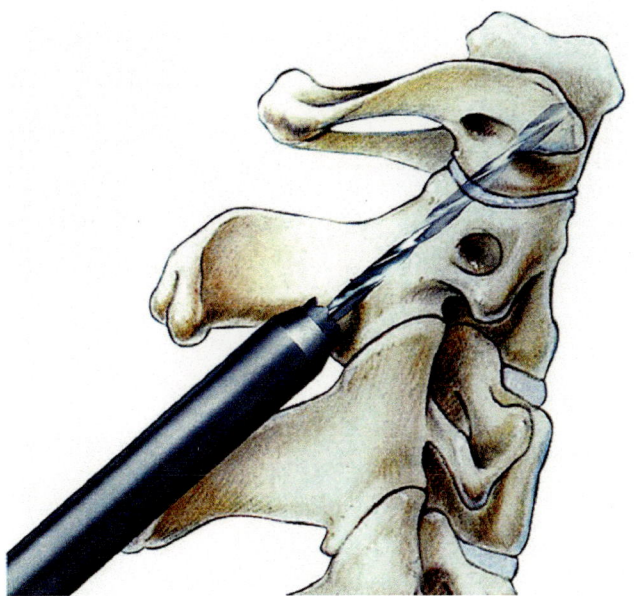

Fig. 38.10 Drilling. (With permission of Aesculap AG, Tuttlingen, Germany)

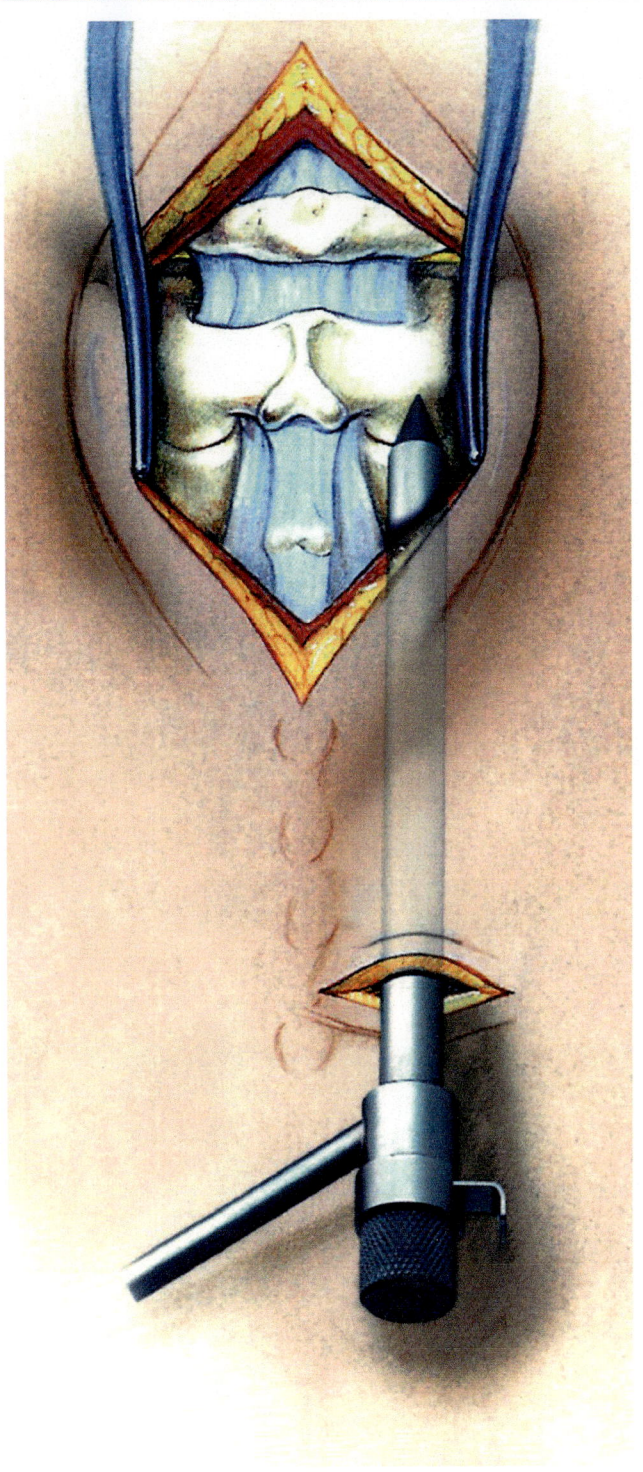

Fig. 38.9 Placement of the guide tube (with obturator) through a stab wound into the field

- After threading, screws with a length between 38 and 50 mm are inserted.
- AP and lateral fluoroscopy will assess the screw direction.
- In case of a persistent dislocation between C1 and 2 joint, C1 can be pulled back using a towel clamp which is fixed

at the C1 lamina (Fig. 38.9). Alternatively, you can push C2 spinous process. Under lateral view fluoroscopy, you see the adjustment. Using a guide wire for first drilling the cannulated instruments and screws gives the advantage that the drilling channel can be recovered at the temporarily fixed C1–2 joint. After having inserted both screws, the spinous process of C2 should be gripped with a towel clamp and pulled back to check the C1–2 stability (Figs. 38.8, 38.10, 38.11, and 38.12).

38.6.3 Bone Graft

- For fusion and long-term stability, an additional bone graft is necessary.
- Best stability will be achieved by a tricortical bone graft from the iliac crest.
- To prepare the implantation bed, the surface of the C1 and C2 lamina is decorticated. Proceed with caution with the thin C1 lamina, which may be fractured by a brisk debridement.
- The cable loop passes beneath the dorsal arch of the atlas in midline from caudally to cranially. A notch, which is cut into the lamina near the spinous process of C2, will hold the loop. The bone graft is clamped between both laminae. The two free ends of the cable are pulled slightly and crimped over the bone block. Additional spongious bone chips can be used to cover the remaining decorticated areas (Fig. 38.13).
- For closure, the detached deep cervical muscles are fixed to the spinous process of C2. The wound is closed in multilayer fashion.

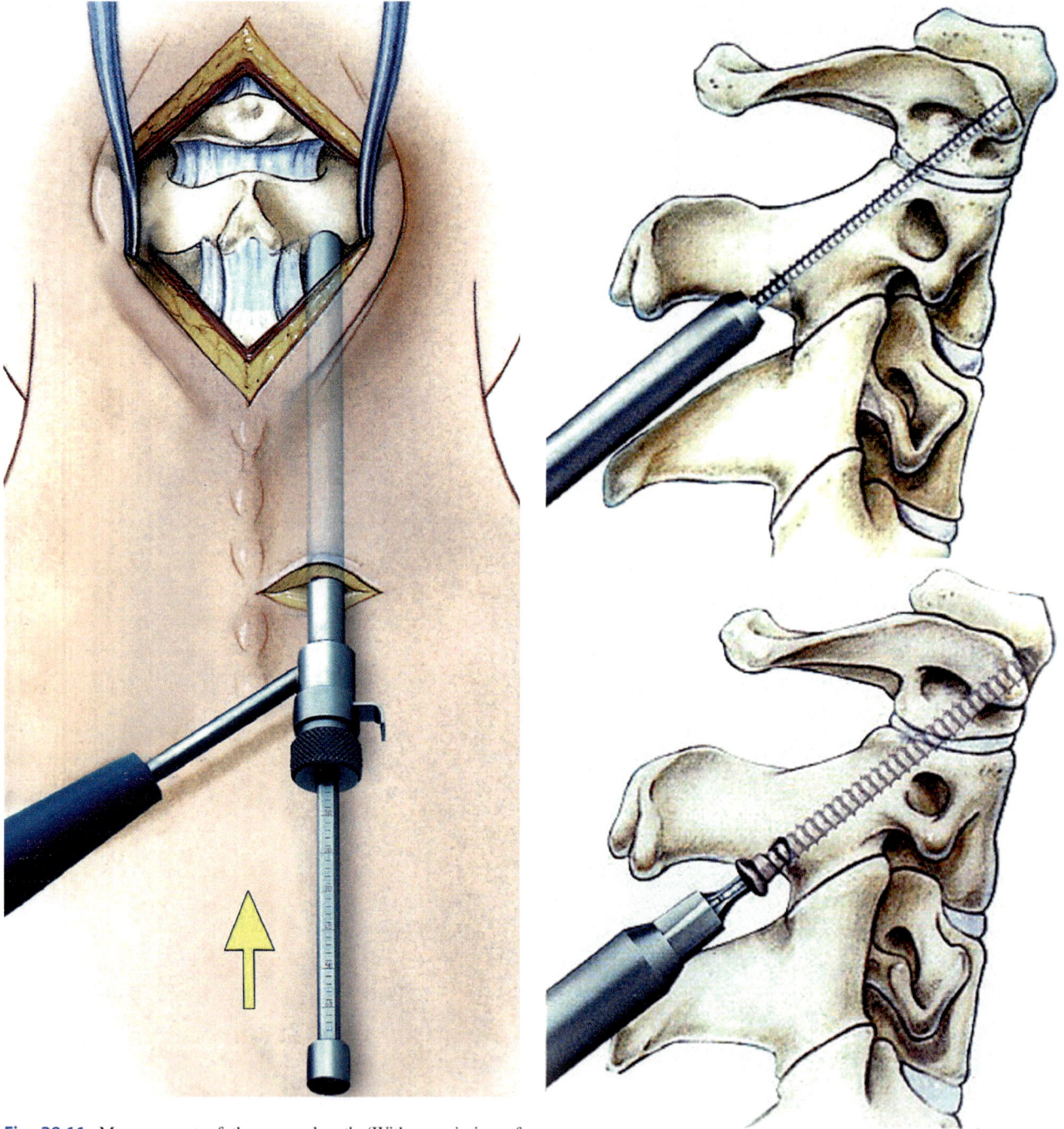

Fig. 38.11 Measurement of the screw length (With permission of Aesculap AG, Tuttlingen, Germany)

Fig. 38.12 Taping and introducing of the transarticular screw in the lateral view (With permission of Aesculap AG, Tuttlingen, Germany)

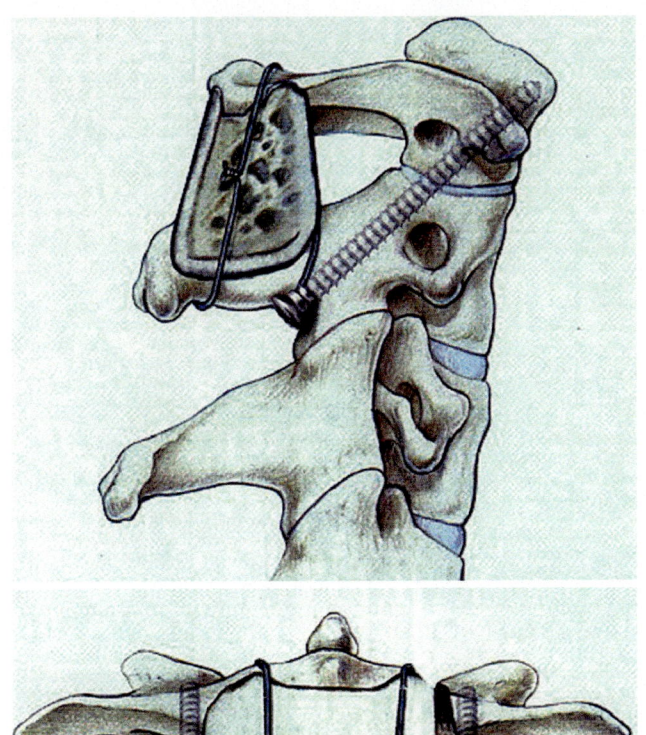

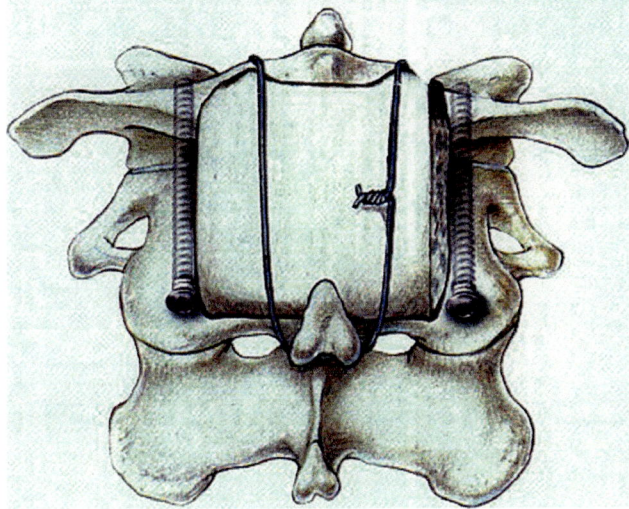

Fig. 38.13 Illustration after transarticular fixation and wiring C1/C2 with an additional bone graft between the arch of C1 and C2. (With permission of Aesculap AG, Tuttlingen, Germany)

38.7 Postoperative Treatment

A cervical (Philadelphia) collar is applied for 6 weeks. For follow-up, radiographs are taken immediately after surgery, after 6 days and 6–8 weeks, respectively (Fig. 38.14a, b). Especially in rheumatoid arthritis, a long-term follow-up is necessary to detect a later subaxial instability. Isometric exercises are started once it has been established that there is no screw loosening.

38.8 Tips and Tricks

The complication feared most of all is an injury of the vertebral artery. The symptom is severe bleeding (pulse synchronous) out of the borehole. In these cases, transarticular screwing should be avoided on this side. Bleeding can be stopped only by closing the hole with hemostatic agents. In cases of heavy arterial bleeding, a shorter screw which does not enter the canal of the vertebral artery may be the only way to stop the bleeding. Unilateral screwing with bone graft apposition will give sufficient stability in these cases. A postoperative angiography is recommended. In rare cases of split atlas, bone apposition is limited. In those cases, bone graft must be attached to the C1–2 facet. By using modern computer-assisted navigation or a screw-guided template system, the risk of malposition of the screws can be reduced [12, 13].

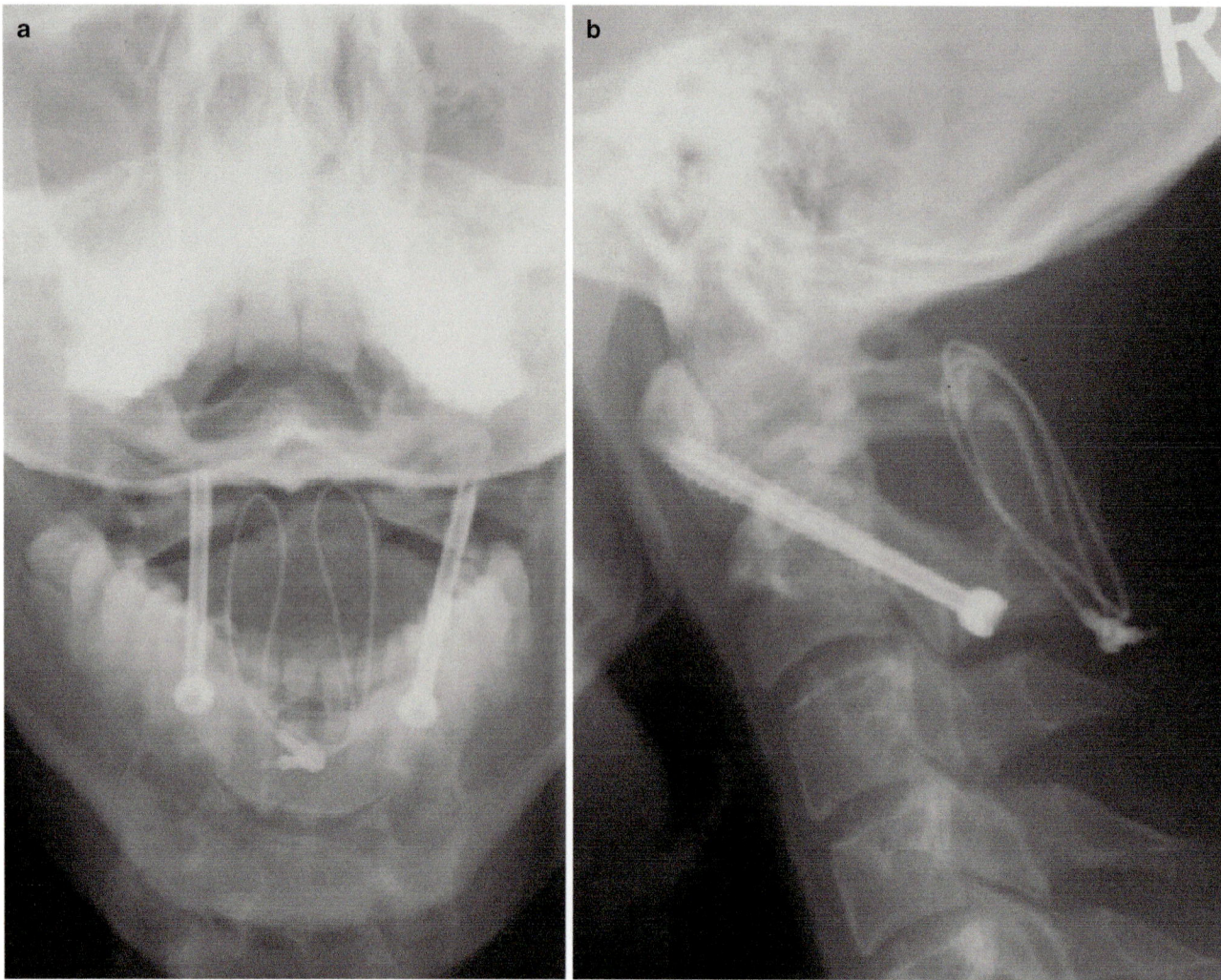

Fig. 38.14 (**a** and **b**) Postoperative X-ray after C1–C2 transarticular screwing in a patient with os odontoideum

References

1. Grob D, Crisco JJ, Panjabi MM, et al. Biomechanical evaluation of four different posterior atlantoaxial fixation techniques. Spine. 1992;17:480–90.
2. Grob D, Jeanneret B, Aebi M, Markwalder T. Atlanto-axial fusion with transarticular screw fixation. J Bone Joint Surg Br. 1991;73B:972–6.
3. Grob D, Magerl F. Operative Stabilisierung bei Frakturen von C1 und C2. Orthopade. 1987;16:46–54.
4. Brooks AL, Jenkins EB. Atlanto-axial arthrodesis by the wedge compression method. J Bone Joint Surg Am. 1978;60:279–83.
5. Dickman CA, Sonntag VKH, Papadopoulos S, et al. The interspinous method of posterior atlantoaxial arthrodesis. J Neurosurg. 1991;74:190–8.
6. Gallie WE. Fractures and dislocations of the cervical spine. Am J Surg. 1939;46:495–9.
7. Jeanneret B, Magerl F. Primary posterior fusion C1 in odontoid fractures: indications, technique, and results of transarticular screw fixation. J Spinal Disord. 1992;5:464–75.
8. Magerl F, Seeman PS. Stable posterior fusion of the atlas and axis by transarticular screw fixation. In: Kehr P, Weidner A, editors. Cervical spine. Berlin: Springer; 1987.
9. Mandel IM, Kambach BJ, Petersilge CA, et al. Morphologic considerations of C2 isthmus dimensions for the placement of transarticular screws. Spine. 2000;25:1542–7.
10. Marcotte P, Dickman CA, Sonntag VKH, et al. Posterior atlantoaxial facet screw fixation. J Neurosurg. 1993;79:234–7.
11. Weidner A, Wähler M, Chiu ST, et al. Modification of C1-C2 transarticular screw fixation by image-guided surgery. Spine. 2000;25:409–14.
12. Kaneyama S, Sugawara T, Sumi M, et al. A novel screw guiding method with a screw guide template system for posterior C-2 fixation: clinical article. J Neurosurg Spine. 2014;21:231–8.
13. Uehara M, Takahashi J, Hirabayashi H, et al. Computer-assisted C1-C2 transarticular screw fixation "Magerl technique" for atlantoaxial instability. Asian Spine J. 2012;6:168–77.

C1–C2 (Harms) Technique

39

Christian Schultz

39.1 Introduction and Core Messages

There is a broad range of options for stabilization of the atlantoaxial complex. To achieve stability, often fusion was used between the laminar arches C1/C2. The persisting motion was the reason for the high failure rates for this kind of single posterior fusion. To increase the fusion rate, Magerl introduced the transarticular screw fixation C1/C2 in 1987 [1]. The Harms technique of stabilizing C1–C2 using fixation of the C1 lateral mass and the C2 pedicle with polyaxial screws and rods is a further option when utilizing the posterior approach. Advantages are reduction of C1/C2, protection of the C1/C2 joint, and possibility of screw removal after healing to regain C1/C2 range of motion. Moreover, the Harms technique reduces the risk of vertebral artery lesion in comparison to the transarticular screw fixation because the screw angulation is easier in patients with kyphotic spine compared to the transarticular screw fixation according to Magerl.

39.2 Indications

- C1/C2 instability caused by trauma, tumor, and inflammatory conditions.
- Nonfusion of odontoid fractures.
- Revision after failed odontoid screw fixation.
- Unstable Jefferson fractures.

- Disruption or laxity of the transverse ligament caused by trauma, local disease processes, or local effects of systemic diseases.
- Nonfusion, instability after alternative fixation techniques.

39.3 Contraindications

- Anatomical variation of the vertebral artery.

39.4 Technical Prerequisites

Utilization of C-arm for intraoperatively lateral and AP fluoroscopy control, the use of navigation could be useful. Endotracheal anesthesia, positioning device (e.g., Mayfield head clamp), and adequate implants and instruments (the distal part of the screw should not be threaded to preserve the C2 nerve). The S4 Cervical System (Aesculap) is one suitable implant for the C1/C2 Harms technique. Other suitable implants are, for example, the Oasys System (Stryker) or the Quartex Stabilization System (Globus Medical).

39.5 Planning, Preparation, and Positioning

Preoperative CT scan is performed to estimate the pathology, the run of the vertebral artery, and to examine anatomical variation. Furthermore, information about the pedicle anatomy is obtained to choose suitable implant sizes. The patient is placed in the prone position, head and neck are secured with the desired sagittal alignment, and positioning is done while monitoring vertebral position under lateral fluoroscopy. Preoperative closed reduction may be done by positioning if possible. After final supporting of the head in a pin head holder, again preoperative alignment is confirmed by using a lateral fluoroscopy.

C. Schultz (✉)
Augsburg, Germany
e-mail: schultz.christian@gmx.de

39.6 Surgical Technique

39.6.1 Approach

- Surgical approach with a midline incision from the occiput to the spinal process C3 and further preparation similar to the C1/C2 transarticular screw fixation.
- Preparation in lateral direction and exposure of the posterior elements of C1/C2. Dissection of the lamina of C2 and the C2 pars interarticularis to remove soft tissue and to identify the landmarks for the C2 pedicle screw insertion.
- To dissect the entry point in the C1 lateral mass, the greater occipital nerve (dorsal ramus of C2) has to be retracted in a caudal direction.

39.6.2 Instrumentation (Using the S4 Cervical System)

Insertion of the C1 Lateral Mass Screw

- The landmarks for the C1 lateral mass screw are below the posterior lamina of C1, above the C1/C2 joint in the center of the posterior lateral mass (see Fig. 39.1) [2].
- The use of a guiding tube is recommended to ensure a safe procedure without endangering the greater occipital nerve, as well as the vertebral artery which both lie very close to the screw entry point.
- The cortical bone is opened by using a bone awl through the guiding tube (see Fig. 39.2).
- The hole is drilled with the 2.9-mm-diameter drill for 4.0-mm-diameter screws under fluoroscopy control. The appropriate trajectory is 10–20° ascending direction, parallel to the plane of the C1 posterior arch in the lateral view and 10° toward the midline in the axial plane. Drilling must be bicortical; the drill has a scale for length measurement and the possibility of a safety stop (see Fig. 39.3).
- Although the screws are self-tapping, cortical tapping is recommended (see Fig. 39.4) [3].
- Bicortical screw insertion under fluoroscopy control (see Fig. 39.5), to preserve the C2 nerve and the dorsal ramus, the distal part of the screw is not threaded (smooth shank screw) (see Fig. 39.6).

Insertion of the C2 Pedicle Screw

- The landmarks for the C2 pedicle screws are the medial and cranial part of the pars interarticularis in the middle between the upper and lower articular surfaces of C2. This technique was first described by Judet in 1962 [3].
- After opening, the cortical bone drilling is performed with the 2.4-mm-diameter drill for 3.5-mm-diameter screws (if favored angle screw is preferred, 2.9-mm drill

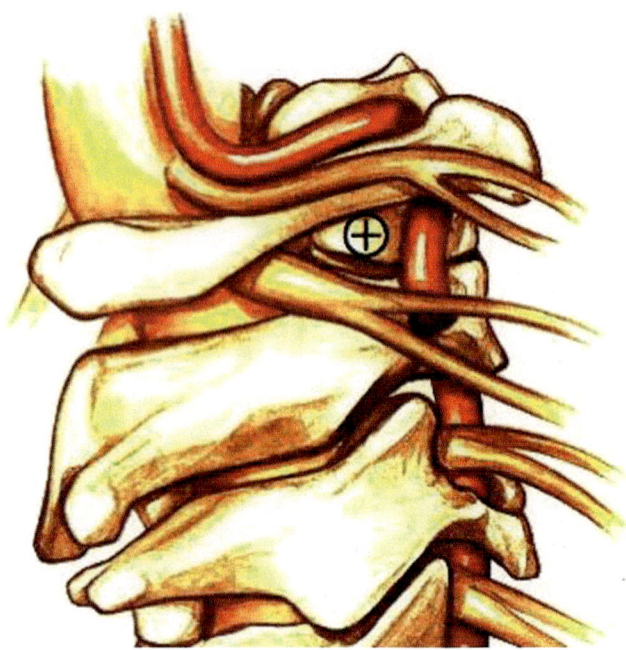

Fig. 39.1 Landmarks for the C1 screw insertion (With permission of Aesculap AG, Tuttlingen, Germany)

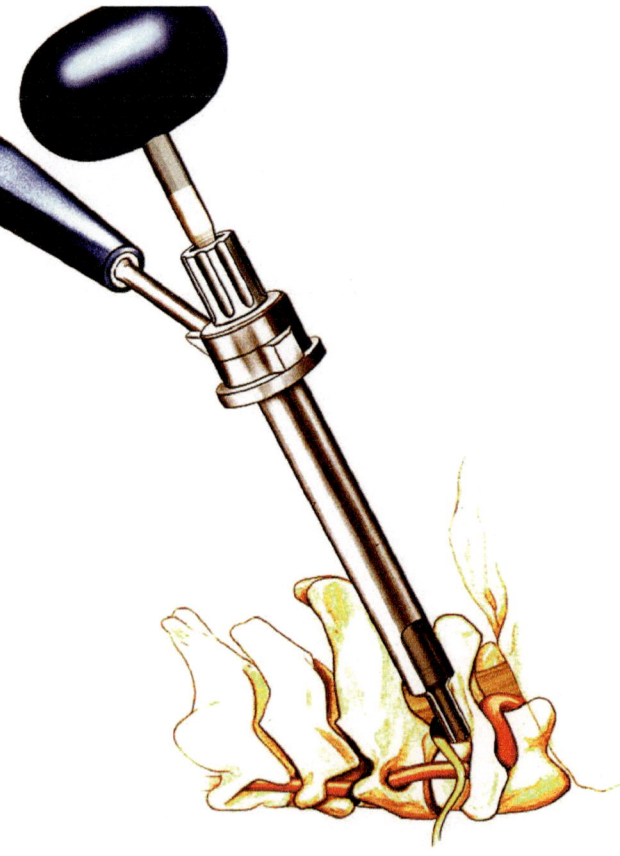

Fig. 39.2 Opening the cortical bone by using a bone awl through the guiding tube (With permission of Aesculap AG, Tuttlingen, Germany)

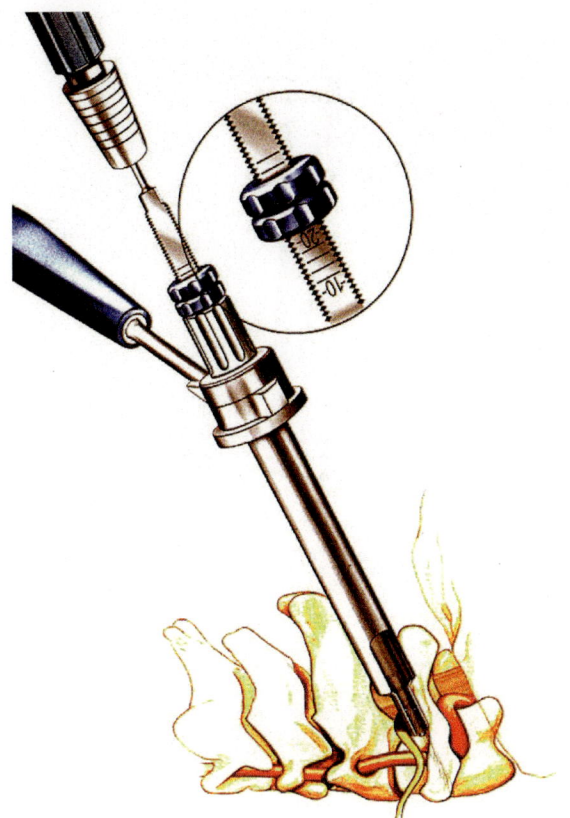

Fig. 39.3 Drilling the bicortical hole (With permission of Aesculap AG, Tuttlingen, Germany)

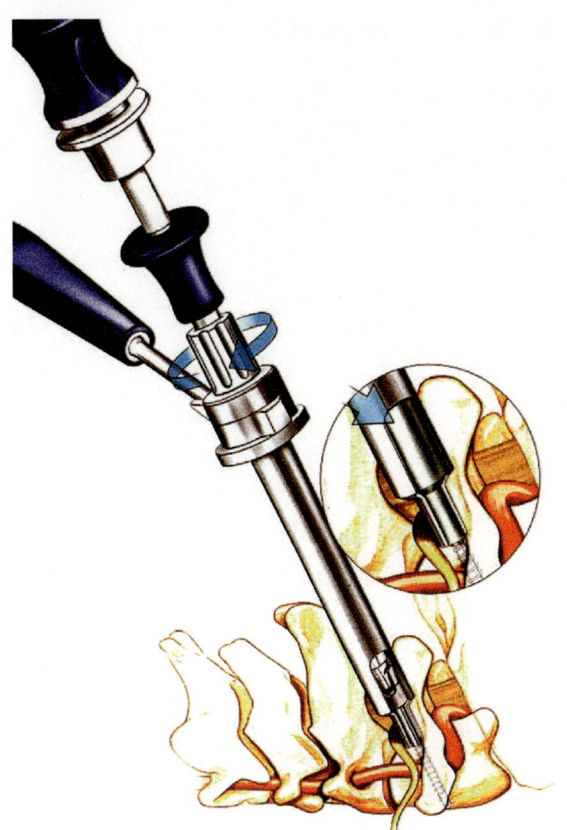

Fig. 39.5 Screw insertion (With permission of Aesculap AG, Tuttlingen, Germany)

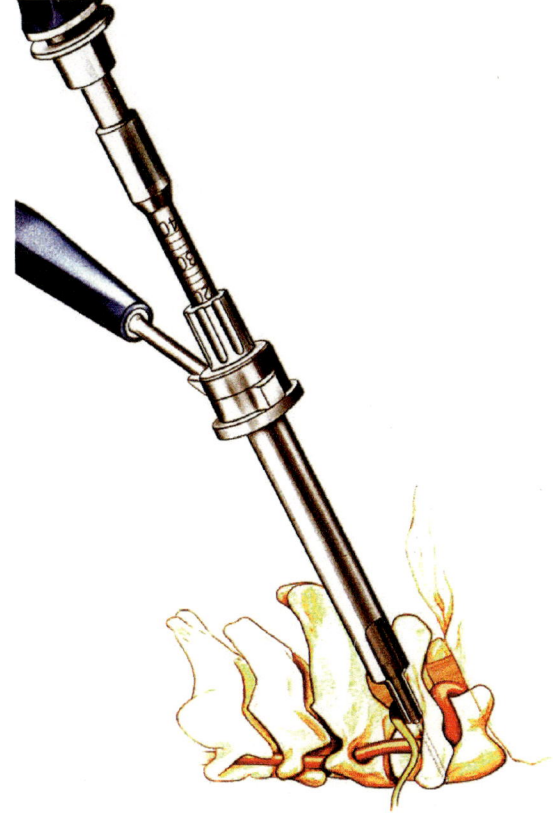

Fig. 39.4 Cortical tapping (With permission of Aesculap AG, Tuttlingen, Germany)

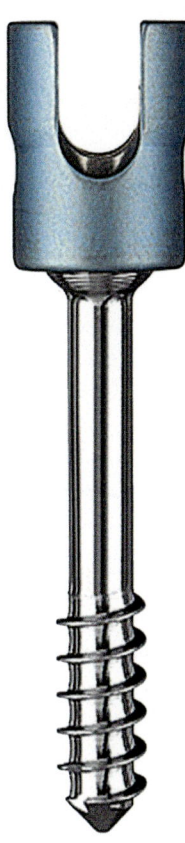

Fig. 39.6 Smooth shank screw (With permission of Aesculap AG, Tuttlingen, Germany)

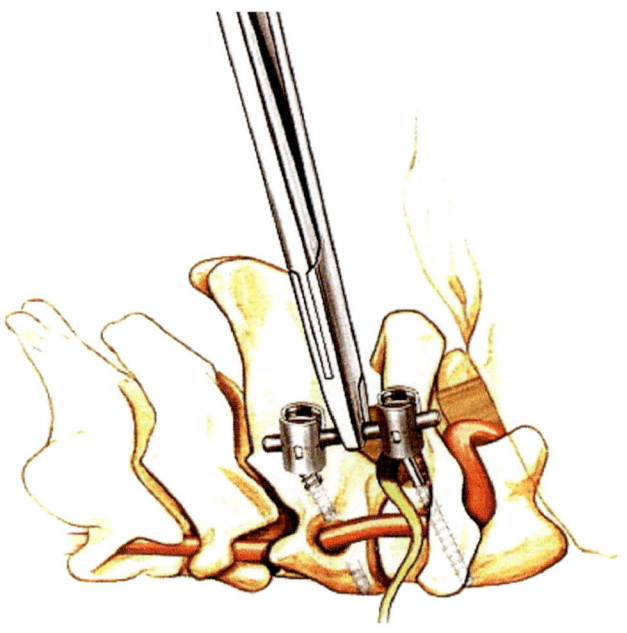

Fig. 39.7 Rod insertion (With permission of Aesculap AG, Tuttlingen, Germany)

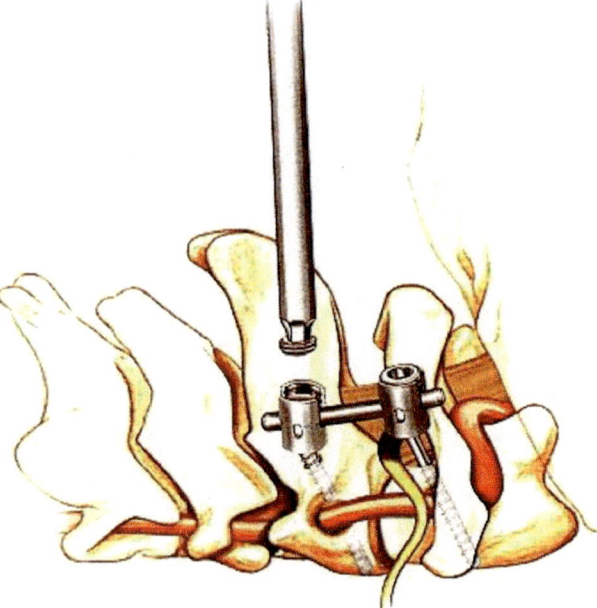

Fig. 39.8 Set screw insertion (With permission of Aesculap AG, Tuttlingen, Germany)

is used for 4.0-mm-diameter screw) under fluoroscopy control. The drill trajectory is 20–30° cranially under lateral fluoroscopy control and 20–25° in a convergent direction in the axial plane.
- Bicortical insertion of a polyaxial screw with suitable length.
- If necessary, reduce C1/C2 in the desired position by adjusting the screws or by manipulation of the head.

Rod Insertion
- Insertion of the rod and with the rod in place the set screws can be inserted to tighten the construct and fix the rod with the polyaxial screws (see Figs. 39.7, 39.8, and 39.9).
- To achieve fusion between the laminar arches, bone grafting can be considered.

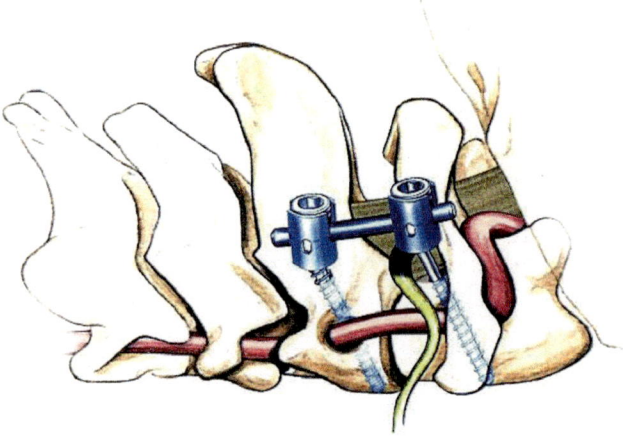

Fig. 39.9 Final construct (With permission of Aesculap AG, Tuttlingen, Germany)

insertion of the screw and compression with the screw head controls bleeding.

39.7 Postoperative Care

Soft collar for a period of 6–8 weeks.

39.8 Tips and Tricks

Opening the cortical bone and drilling frequently causes bleeding of the venous plexus; bleeding control by bipolar electrocautery may risk a nerve injury, as an alternative quick

References

1. Harms J, Melcher RP. Posterior C1-C2 fusion with polyaxial screw and rod fixation. Spine. 2001;26:2467–71.
2. Stulik J, Vyskocil T, Sebesta P, et al. Harms technique of C1-C2 fixation with polyaxial screws and rods. Acta Chir Orthop Traumatol Cechoslov. 2005;72:22–7.
3. Magerl F, Seeman PS. Stable posterior fusion of the atlas and axis by transarticular screw fixation. In: Kehr P, Weidner A, editors. Cervical spine. Wien: Springer; 1987. p. 322–7.

Rod-Screw Stabilization of the Posterior Cervical Spine

Uwe Vieweg

40.1 Introduction and Core Messages

Posterior rod-screw systems have a history of successful clinical use. The posterior rod-screw technique, with the screw positioned in the lateral mass or transpedicularly, provides a stable tension band system. For fixation to the occiput, an occiput plate has been designed. The complete system includes top-loading screws, rods, offset connectors, cross connectors, clamps, laminar hooks, and occiput screws and plates.

40.2 Indications

- Upper and lower cervical spine instabilities (rheumatoid arthritis, anomalies, traumatic instabilities, infections, tumours, deformities).
- Anterior fusions requiring additional posterior stabilization.
- Instability associated with deficiency of the posterior elements from laminectomy or fractures.

40.3 Contraindications

- Significant damage to the vertebral bodies.

40.4 Technical Prerequisites

Fluoroscopy, positioning device (e.g. padded rolls), rigid head holder (e.g. Mayfield), and adequate implants (polyaxial rod-screw systems) and instruments are essential for the procedure.

40.5 Planning, Preparation, and Positioning

A CT for preoperative planning is recommended (anatomical variation, confirm pedicle orientation, planning of implant size, etc.). The patient is placed on the operating table in the prone position and secured with the desired sagittal alignment. Accurate positioning is especially important when fixing the occiput to the cervical and thoracic spine. Confirm proper alignment using an image intensifier or radiograph prior to draping. The neck and shoulder are prepped and draped in the usual manner. The sitting position is an alternative.

40.6 Surgical Technique

40.6.1 Approach

- A posterior midline incision is performed.
- The incision is taken down through the subcutaneous tissue and facia with electrocautery.
- If fusion is to include the occiput, exposure should be extended to the external occipital protuberance.
- All soft tissue is removed from the posterior bone structures, and the lateral mass is identified. The medial border of the lateral mass is the valley at the junction of the lamina and lateral mass. The lateral boundary is the far edge of the lateral mass. The superior and inferior borders are the respective cranial and caudal facet joints.

U. Vieweg (✉)
Department of Conservative and Surgical Spine Therapy with Interdisciplinary Spinal Deformities Centre and Rummelsberg Sectional Center, Hospital Rummelsberg, Schwarzenbruck, Germany
e-mail: uwe.vieweg@sana.de

© Springer-Verlag GmbH Germany 2023
U. Vieweg, F. Grochulla (eds.), *Manual of Spine Surgery*, https://doi.org/10.1007/978-3-662-64062-3_40

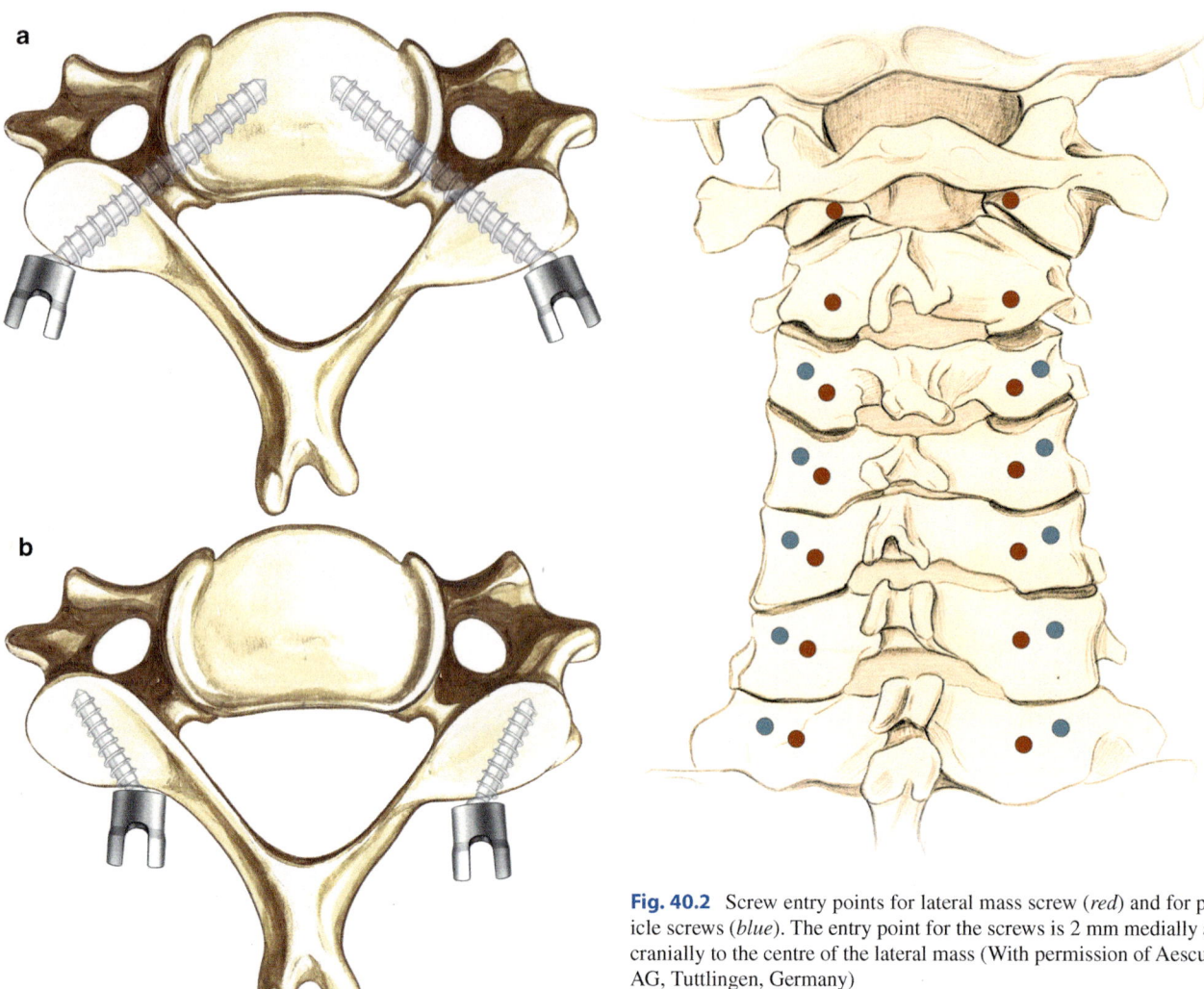

Fig. 40.2 Screw entry points for lateral mass screw (*red*) and for pedicle screws (*blue*). The entry point for the screws is 2 mm medially and cranially to the centre of the lateral mass (With permission of Aesculap AG, Tuttlingen, Germany)

Fig. 40.1 Pedicle screw (**a**) and lateral mass screw (**b**) (With permission of Aesculap AG, Tuttlingen, Germany)

40.6.2 Instrumentation [1–3]

Rod-Screw Stabilization without Occiput

- In general, the screws can be placed in two different ways—either (a) transpedicular, with pedicle screws inserted from lateral to medial through the pedicle or (b) lateral mass, with lateral mass screws inserted from medial to upper lateral (see Fig. 40.1a, b). Though there are dangers associated with the insertion of cervical pedicle screws, their use is advantageous in some clinical conditions when increased load bearing is necessary [4].

- Depending on the anatomy, different entry points for the screws may have to be chosen. The entry point for the lateral mass screws is more medial than the entry point for the pedicle screws. The entry point for the lateral mass screw lies 2 mm medially and cranially to the centre of the lateral mass (see Fig. 40.2).

- The lateral mass screws are placed as described by Magerl [5] (see Fig. 40.3). Note: in order to achieve the correct drilling direction, partial resection of the spinous process, which is in the way, may be helpful.

- The screw trajectory is about 20–25° outwards (lateral to the spinous process) and 30–40° cranially. The cranial angulation attempts to parallel the facet joint. *Note*: the inclination of the surface can be determined by inserting a fine dissector into the joint.

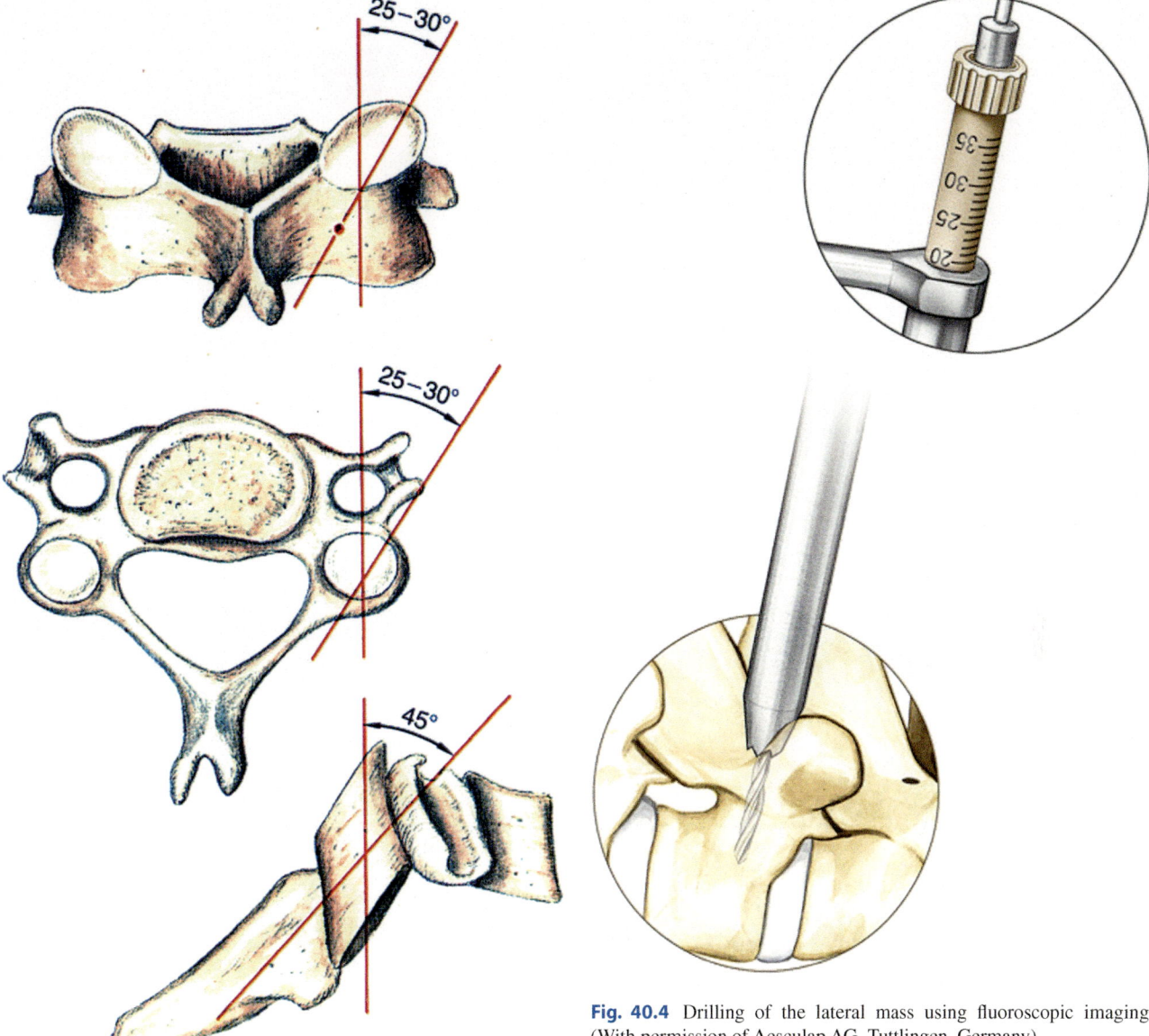

Fig. 40.4 Drilling of the lateral mass using fluoroscopic imaging (With permission of Aesculap AG, Tuttlingen, Germany)

Fig. 40.3 Positioning of the lateral mass screws as described by Magerl. The screw orientation is about 20–25° outwards (lateral to the spinous process) and 30–40° cranially. The cranial angulation attempts to parallel the facet joint (With permission of Aesculap AG, Tuttlingen, Germany)

- An awl may be used to open the cortex. Alternatively, a 1–2 mm drill hole can be made using a small decortication burr.
- The lateral mass is drilled with an adjustable drill guide using fluoroscopic imaging. Note: the drill guide is initially set at 12 mm. The depth of the hole is checked with a depth sounder (see Figs. 40.4 and 40.5). The length of the adjustable drill guide is increased in 1 to 2 mm increments until the drill penetrates the far cortex.
- With the pedicles or lateral mass prepared and the proper screw length determined, the appropriate screws are inserted into the predrilled holes bilaterally, using the self-holding polyaxial screwdriver (see Figs. 40.6 and 40.7).
- Once the screw is inserted, the position of the polyaxial head is optimized for rod insertion using a screw body manipulator.

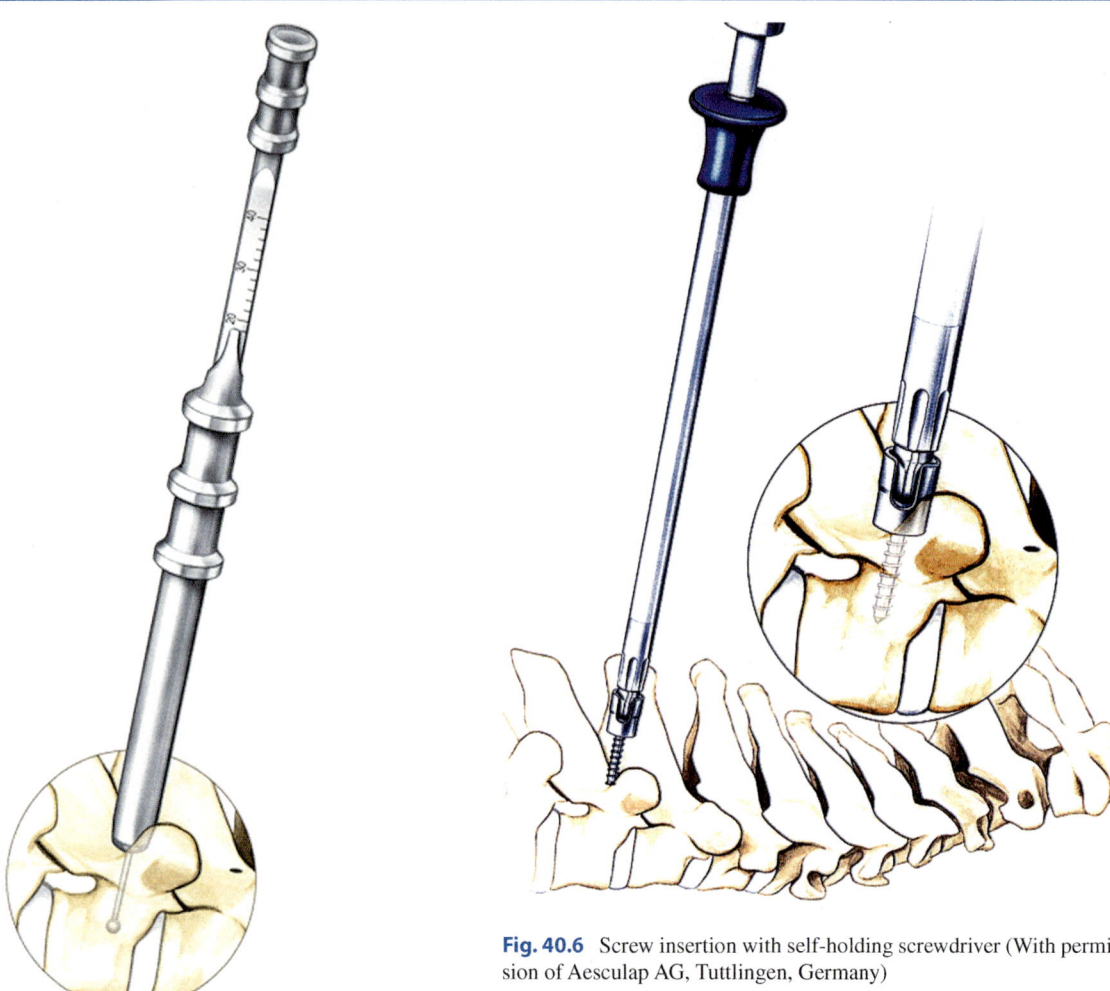

Fig. 40.6 Screw insertion with self-holding screwdriver (With permission of Aesculap AG, Tuttlingen, Germany)

Fig. 40.5 The hole is checked for penetration with a depth gauge (With permission of Aesculap AG, Tuttlingen, Germany)

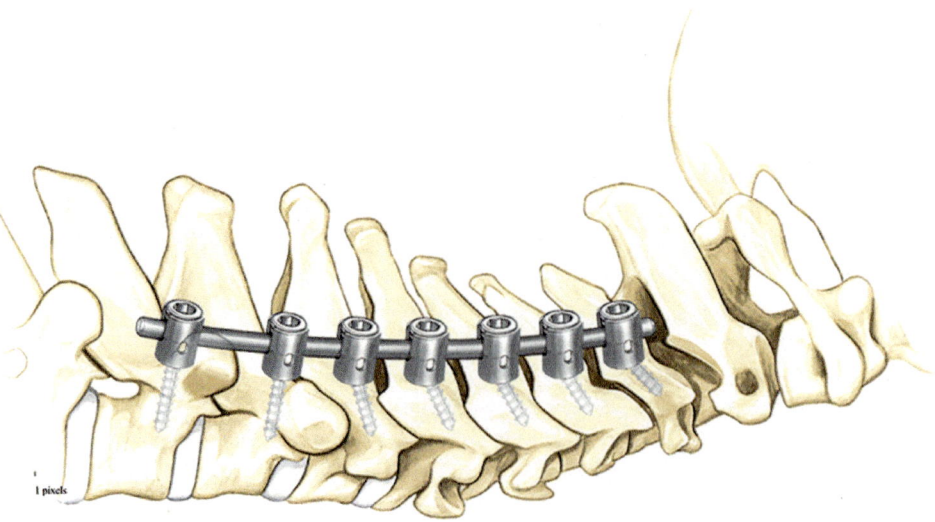

Fig. 40.7 Complete rod-screw construct C3-Th2 (With permission of Aesculap AG, Tuttlingen, Germany)

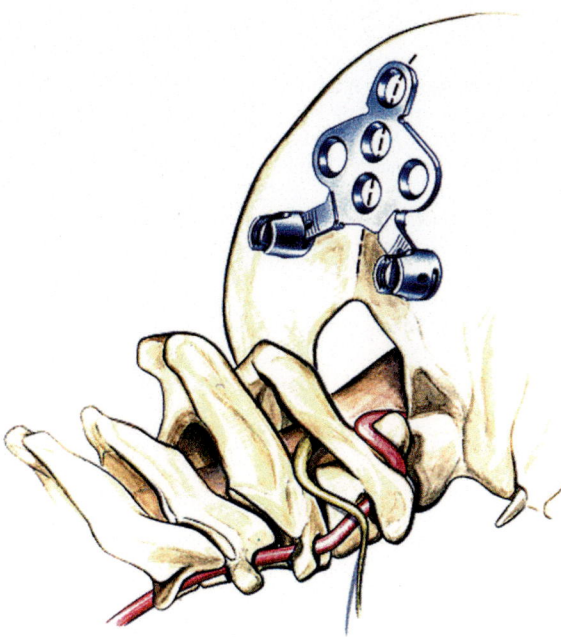

Fig. 40.8 Positioning of the occipital plate (With permission of Aesculap AG, Tuttlingen, Germany)

- After the insertion of the screws, and prior to insertion of the rods, the lordotic alignment of the cervical spine should be verified via intraoperative lateral fluoroscopy. A trial rod template can be used to aid in rod contouring or trimming to the required length.
- Insertion of the set screw in the polyaxial body is started by turning the instrument counterclockwise until a click is heard or felt. The set screws are hand tightened with the set screw starter and then finally tightened to the predefined optimum torque with a torque-limiting screwdriver and the countertorque handle.
- Cancellous bone graft is applied over the decorticated laminae and articular masses.

Rod-Screw Stabilization with Occiput

- The occiput plate should be placed medial to the external occipital protuberance and the foramen magnum. The greatest stability of the plate is achieved by midline fixation at the inion where the bone thickness is highest (see Fig. 40.8).
- A drill guide can be used to hold the plate onto the occiput. Note: even if the drill depth was measured before

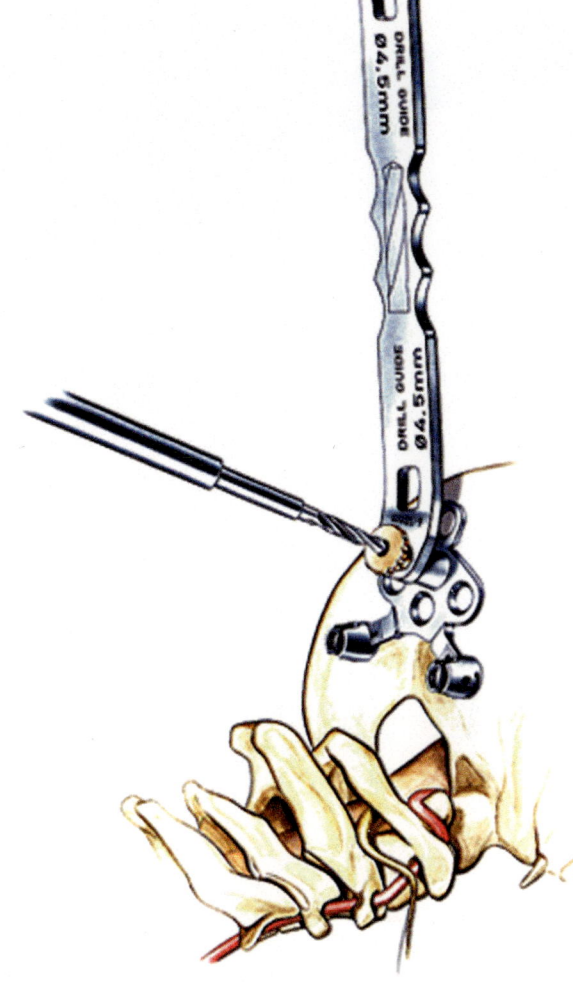

Fig. 40.9 Drilling of the occipital bone (With permission of Aesculap AG, Tuttlingen, Germany)

surgery, proceed with care to prevent damage to the dura (see Fig. 40.9).
- By using the tap guide and the tap, the drilled hole is further prepared for insertion of the occipital screws.
- The occipital screws are inserted, and the plate is fixed on the occipital bone. The occipital screws can be inserted in the appropriate holes using a screwdriver (see Fig. 40.10).
- To connect the occipital plate to the cervical spine, a prebent rod is inserted into the rod receptacles and fixed with set screws.
- Finally, the set screws have to be locked using a torque wrench and countertorque handle (see Fig. 40.11).

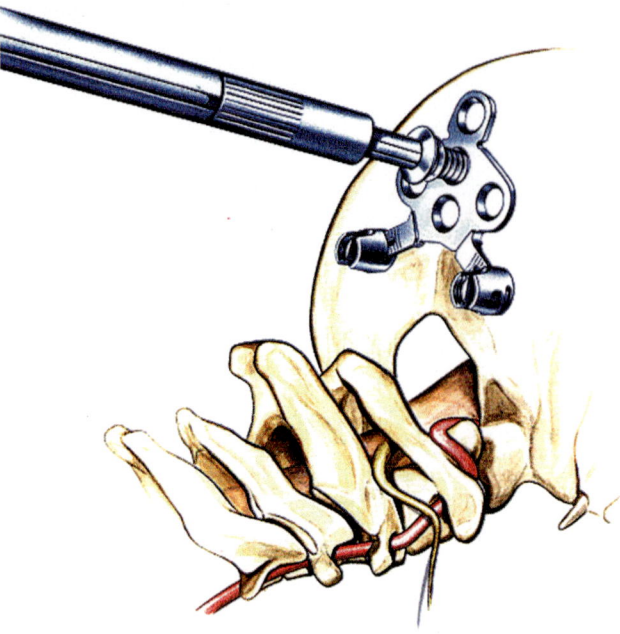

Fig. 40.10 Screw insertion in the occipital bone (With permission of Aesculap AG, Tuttlingen, Germany)

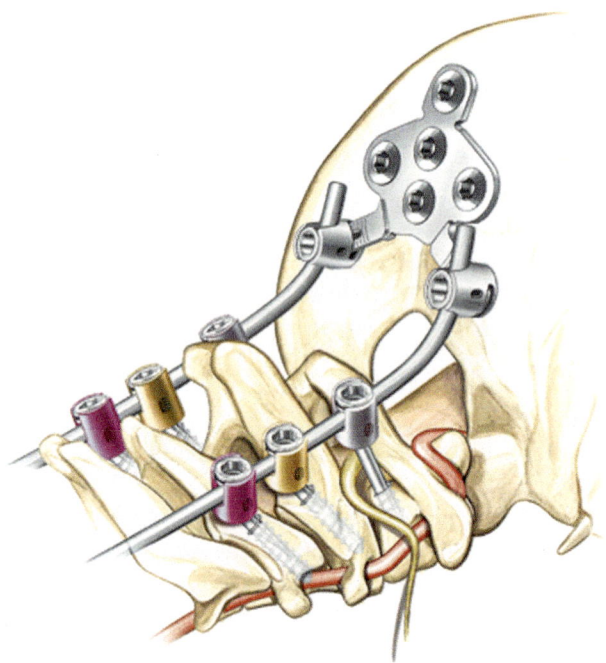

Fig. 40.11 Complete construct (With permission of Aesculap AG, Tuttlingen, Germany)

References

1. Aebi M, Thalgott JS, Webb JK. Chapter 6: posterior techniques lower cervical spine. In: AO ASIF principles in spine surgery. Berlin/Heidelberg: Springer; 1998. p. 54–76.
2. Dickman CA, Sonntag VKH, Marcotte P. Techniques of screw fixation for the upper cervical spine. BNI Q. 1992;8:9–26.
3. Dickman CA, Douglas R, Sonntag VKH. Occipitocervical fusion: posterior stabilization of the craniovertebral junction and upper cervical spine. BNI Q. 1990;6:2–14.
4. Dunlap BJ, Karaikovic EE, Park HS, et al. Load sharing properties of cervical pedicle screw-rod constructs versus lateral mass screw-rod constructs. Eur Spine J. 2010;19(5):803–8. Epub 2010 Feb 2
5. Magerl F, Grob D. Dorsal fusion of the cervical spine with the hook plate. In: Kehr P, Weidner A, editors. Cervical spine. 2nd ed. Berlin: Springer; 1987.

Part V

Anterior Thoracic Spine

Overview of Surgical Techniques and Implants

41

Christian Schultz

41.1 Introduction and Core Message

The chapter gives an overview to the different approaches (extended anterior cervical approach, periscapular approach and cervical thoracic approach with osteotomy of the manubrium to the upper thoracic spine; posterolateral transthoracic approaches to the mid-level and lower thoracic spine), different approach techniques (open/mini-open approach, microendoscopic approach) and different implants (plate-screw systems, rod-screw systems, vertebral body replacements) for the anterior thoracic spine.

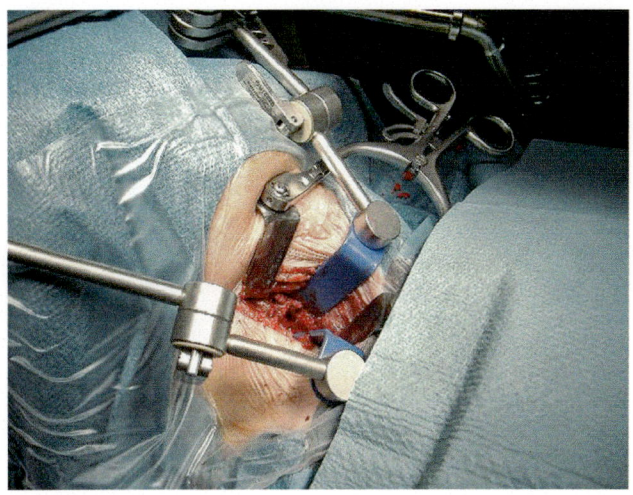

Fig. 41.1 Anterior approach to the cervicothoracic junction

41.2 Approaches

41.2.1 Open/Mini-Open Anterior Approach to the Cervicothoracic Junction (T1–T2)

- Caudally extension of the standard anterior lower cervical approach to dissect between the trachea and the esophagus medially and the innominate vessels inferolaterally.
- Exposure of the anterior wall of the vertebral bodies and the intervening discs (see Fig. 41.1).
- Identification of internal jugular vein, common carotid artery, the recurrent laryngeal nerve and the thoracic duct.

  With this approach, it is usually possible to attain the vertebral bodies T1 and T2; in some individual cases, one can reach the T3/T4 level. For more caudal access, there is a need for median sternal bone resection [1].

41.2.2 Open/Mini-Open Anterior Approach to the Upper Thoracic Spine (Level T3–T4)

- Common cervicosternal approach with an osteotomy of the clavicle and an individual-sized sternotomy depending on the extent of the pathology.
- In case of sternotomy, the brachiocephalic vein has to be ligated.

  Because of the ligation and section of the left brachiocephalic vein, the risk of injury of the thoracic duct increases. The superior intercostal vessels should be preserved.

  Alternative to decrease the morbidity:
- Exposure of the level T1 to T4 between the right brachiocephalic vein and the brachiocephalic artery.

  The level T4–T5 can be exposed between the superior vena cava and the ascending aorta using a transmanubrium approach without ligation and section of the left brachiocephalic vein.

C. Schultz (✉)
Augsburg, Germany
e-mail: schultz.christian@gmx.de

41.2.3 Lateral Approach to the Upper Thoracic Spine

- Skin incision at the inferior scapula.
- Dissection of the latissimus dorsi and the serratus muscle to fold away the scapula.
- Intercostal opening or resection of the ribs depending on the extend of pathology.

This approach can lead to significant morbidity because of the extensile muscle dissection [2].

41.2.4 Open/Mini-Open Approaches to the Mid-Level Anterior Thoracic Spine (Level T5–T9)

Standard anterior approach until the level T9 is by a right posterolateral thoracotomy:

- Positioning on the left side (vacuum bed), abduction of the right arm 120°.
- Skin incision depending on the level and extend of pathology.
- Dissection of the latissimus dorsi muscle if necessary and as distal as possible.
- Dissection of the serratus muscle also as distal as possible to avoid lesions of the long thoracic nerve and the lateral thoracic artery.
- Intercostal approach to the spine, in rare cases rib resection.

On the T4 level, the azygos arch ends in the superior vena cava. The azygos arch crosses the vagus nerve running on the surface of the esophagus. The anterior intercostal veins from the higher vertebral bodies end in the vertex of the azygos arch crossing the vertebral bodies perpendicularly (Fig. 41.2). The sympathetic trunk and ganglia continue to be nearby the rib heads [3].

41.2.5 Open/Mini-Open Approaches to the Lower Anterior Thoracic Spine (Level T10–T12)

Standard anterior approach to the lower levels is the left lateral thoracotomy:

- Skin incision on the tenth rib.
- Dissection of the latissimus dorsi muscle and intercostal thoracotomy (Fig. 41.3).

This approach leads into the costodiaphragmatic recess, and with an additional diaphragm split, it is possible to reach the level L2 [4].

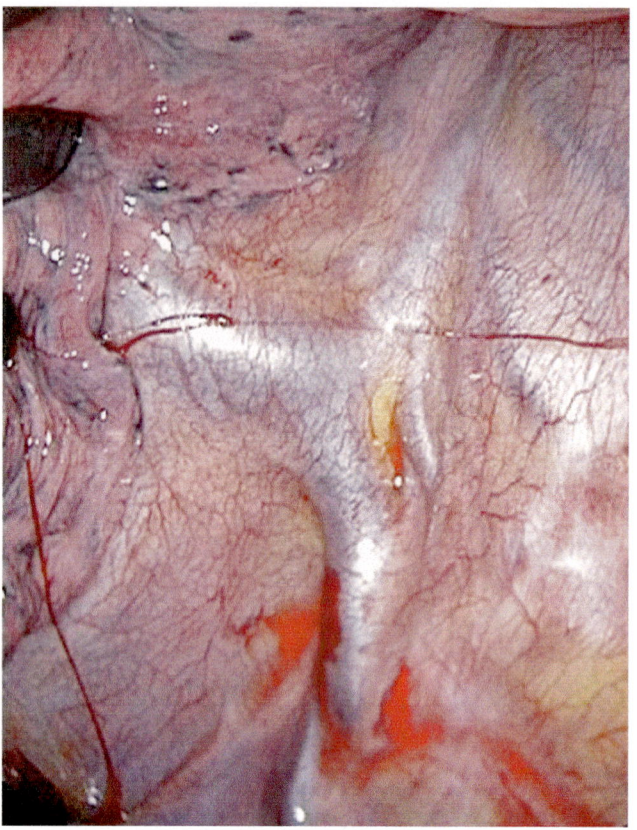

Fig. 41.2 View at the azygos vein at the level T5

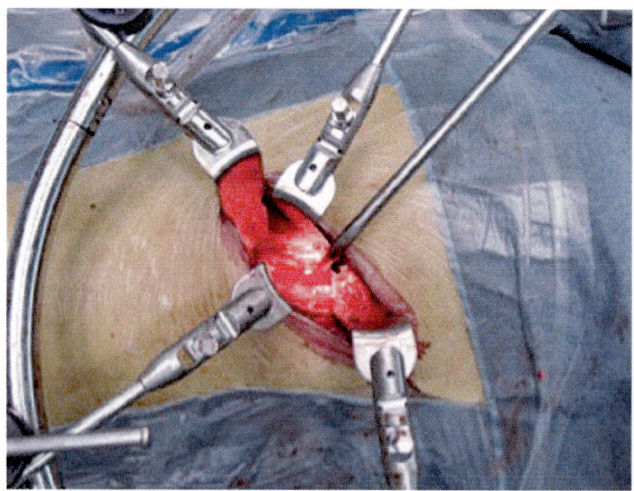

Fig. 41.3 Open approach to the lower anterior thoracic spine with the SynFrame Retractor System (DePuySynthes)

Fig. 41.4 Trocar positioning for the endoscopic approach to the level T6 from the *right side*

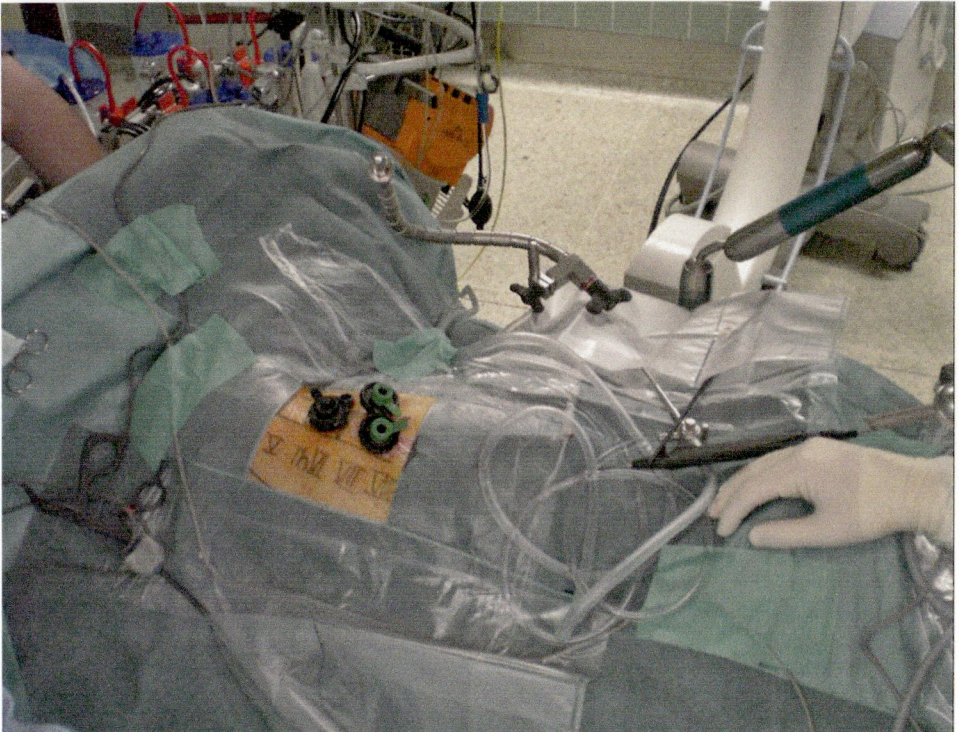

41.2.6 Endoscopic Approaches Upper Anterior Thoracic Spine (Level T2–T4)

Demanding nearly transaxillary approach for experienced surgeons:
- Positioning on the left side, arm lifted upwards.
- Four portals with the working portal above the pathology, the camera portal caudal in the same line, suction and irrigation portal anterocranial, and the retractor portal caudal.

The thoracodorsal and axillary vessels, the long thoracic nerve and the brachial plexus could be compromised. For these thoracic levels, the open approach still is the standard approach [5].

41.2.7 Endoscopic Approaches Mid-Level Anterior Thoracic Spine (Level T5–T8)

Because of the position of the great vessels and the heart approach from the right side:
- Lateral position on the left side.
- Portal position as stated above (Fig. 41.4).

The side of approach depends on the position of the aorta; therefore, a preoperatively CT or MRI is desirable.

41.2.8 Endoscopic Approaches Lower Level Anterior Thoracic Spine (Level T9–T12)

Because of the liver, the lower levels have to be approached from the left side:
- The working portal is also located above the pathology, the camera portal is located two intercostal spaces cranial to the working portal and suction and retractor portal are each located anterior.

41.3 Implants

41.3.1 Rod-Screw and Plate-Screw Systems

These implants for stabilisation of the anterior spine are usually used combined with bone graft or additional implants like vertebral body replacements (VBR). The new implants provide an angle-stable constrained construct with four-point stability like the TRUSS Thoracolumbar Plate (Globus Medical) or the MACS TL System (with permission of Aesculap, Tuttlingen, Germany) (Fig. 41.5) with:
- Low profile, smoothed edges and a safe screw insertion due to the monocortical screw design.
- A design for open and endoscopic procedures with.
- Cannulated instruments and implants to simplify the endoscopic application with k-wire-guided instrumentation.

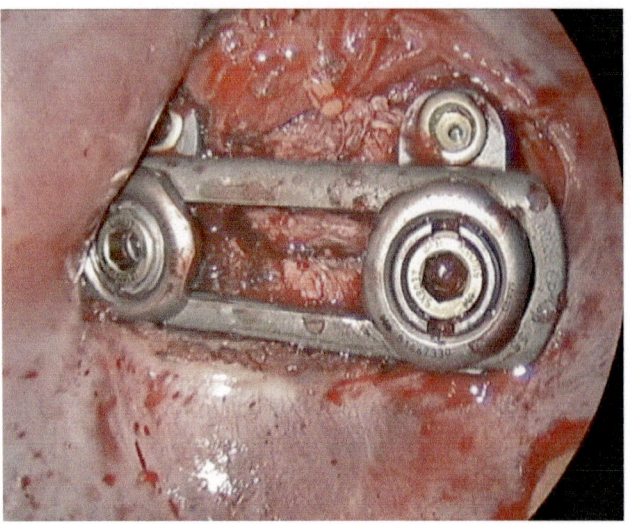

Fig. 41.5 MACS TL Implant (with permission of Aesculap, Tuttlingen, Germany) with iliac crest bone graft T12

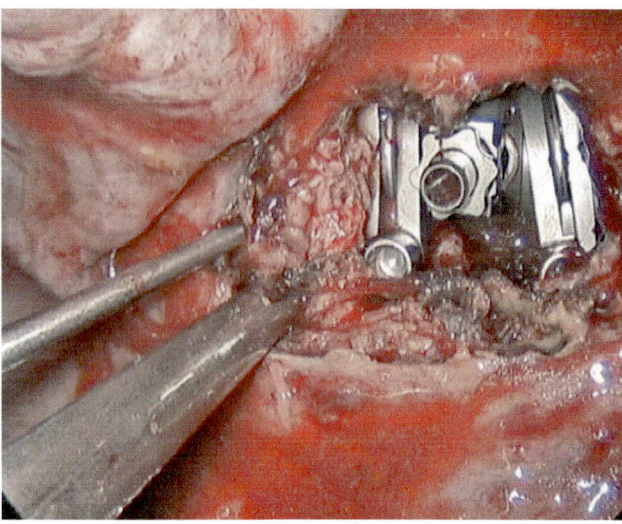

Fig. 41.6 Hydrolift VBR (with permission of Aesculap AG, Tuttlingen, Germany) T10

41.3.2 Vertebral Body Replacement (VBR)

For special indications, like multilevel corporectomy in tumour cases, there are still non-expandable cages available like the titanium mesh cage SynMesh (DePuySynthes). They are designed to fill with bone to achieve healing and resulting in stability. Alternatives are the Trabecular Metal VBR's (Zimmer Biomet). Amongst other things, the endoscopic approaches and the request for primary stability have the use of expandable titanium cages for vertebral body replacement well established. Commonly, today's devices are mechanically expandable like the Obelisc (Ulrich) and the XRL Vertebral Body Replacement (DePuySynthes).

There are further designs like the Fortify I (Globus Medical) with integrated titanium plates and screws for additional stabilization between vertebral body and spacer.

Advantages of these devices:

- Small size of the compressed VBR.
- Adjustment of the height of the VBR to the length of the cavity.
- High primary stability.

Because of the manually application until the VBR fits tightly into the resection area, there is usually no reliable feedback of the applied forces. Especially in case of reduced bone quality an overextension could lead to an impression of the end plates. The Hydrolift (Aesculap) is an example for a VBR (Fig. 41.6) with special features to avoid these complications:

- Hydraulic manometer-controlled distraction.
- Continuously adjustable endcaps to improve force transmission at the bone–cage interface.

References

1. Xiao ZM, Li ZX, De Feng G, et al. Surgical management for upper thoracic spine tumors by a transmanubrium approach and a new space. Eur Spine J. 2007;16:439–44.
2. Anderson TMMK, Jl M. Approaches to anterior spinal operations: anterior thoracic approaches. Ann Thorac Surg. 1993;55:1447–52.
3. Cauchoix J, Binet JP. Anterior surgical approaches to the spine. Ann R Coll Surg Engl. 1957;21(4):234–43.
4. Ikard Robert W. Methods and complications of anterior exposure of the thoracic and lumbar spine. Arch Surg. 2006;141:1025–34.
5. Cheung KMC, Al Ghazi S. Approach-related complications of open versus thoracoscopic anterior exposures of the thoracic spine. J Orthop Surg. 2008;16:343–7.

Anterolateral Endoscopic Stabilization

42

Oliver Gonschorek

42.1 Introduction and Core Messages

The use of minimally invasive techniques in thoracoscopically assisted procedures allows the reconstruction of the anterior column after vertebral fractures of the thoracolumbar region with reduced approach morbidity. Further indications are secondary reconstruction after malalignment and non-union and resection of tumour and metastasis. After resection of the destroyed discs and vertebra, vertebral body replacement together with an angle-stable double-rod instrumentation results in a biomechanical stable anterior column. The aims of this procedure are: reconstruction and stabilization of the anterior column, decompression of the spinal canal, resection of destroyed discs, restoration of the sagittal alignment, early functional treatment, and reduced comorbidity by using the minimally invasive approach.

42.2 Indications [1, 2]

42.2.1 General

- Unstable fractures between T3 and L3.
- Fractures A1.2, A1.3 and A2 with kyphosis >15° [3].
- Burst fractures A3 (main indication) [3].
- Tumour and metastasis.
- Secondary operations, that is, after malalignment and non-union.

O. Gonschorek (✉)
Department of Spine Surgery, BGU Trauma Center Murnau, Murnau, Germany
e-mail: oliver.gonschorek@bgu-murnau.de

42.2.2 Monosegmental Anterior Spondylodesis

- Incomplete burst fracture A3.1 and A1.2 fractures.
- Good bone quality (young patient, no osteoporosis).
- One destroyed disc.

42.2.3 Bisegmental Anterior Spondylodesis

- Burst (split) fractures A3.2/A3.3, Pincer fracture A2.3 [3].
- Two destroyed discs.

42.3 Contraindications

- Limited general condition.
- Restricted cardiopulmonary function.
- Severe thoracic trauma.
- Acute post-traumatic lung failure.

42.4 Technical Prerequisites

Fluoroscopy, carbon table, vacuum mattress, thoracoscopy unit (see Fig. 42.1), special thoracoscopical instruments (Fig. 42.2), monosegmental cages (i.e. Tantalum, Zimmer Spine, monosegmental procedure), expandable cages (i.e. Hydrolift, Aesculap, bisegmental procedure), angle-stable double-rod system (MACS, Aesculap). For monosegmental spondylodesis, bone grafts may be used. Due to the harvest morbidity, we prefer to use a non-expandable cage, that is, Tantalum (Fig. 42.3). Small expandable cages may be used as well. However, in most cases, they are too big. For bisegmental spondylodesis, expandable cages are advantageous (Fig. 42.4). Beside the mentioned Hydrolift (Aesculap), there are many other products (VLift, Stryker; Obelisk, Ulrich; Xtenz, Königsee). For lateral stabilization, an

© Springer-Verlag GmbH Germany 2023
U. Vieweg, F. Grochulla (eds.), *Manual of Spine Surgery*, https://doi.org/10.1007/978-3-662-64062-3_42

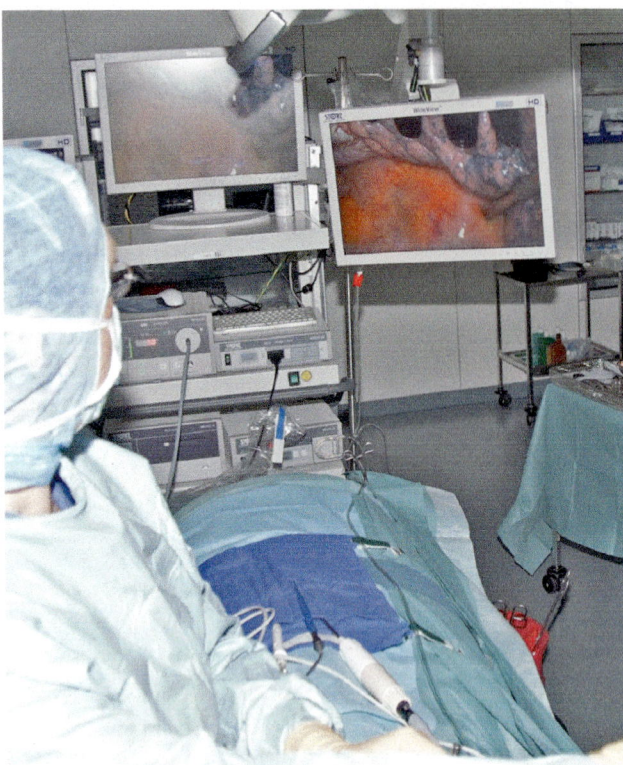

Fig. 42.1 The thoracoscopy unit with three HD screens allows all participants an excellent view

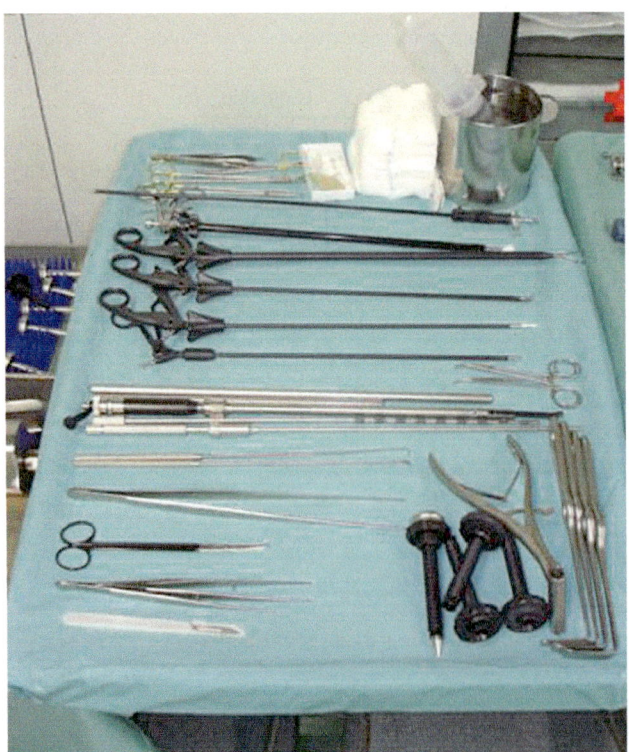

Fig. 42.2 Special instruments are necessary to operate under endoscopical control

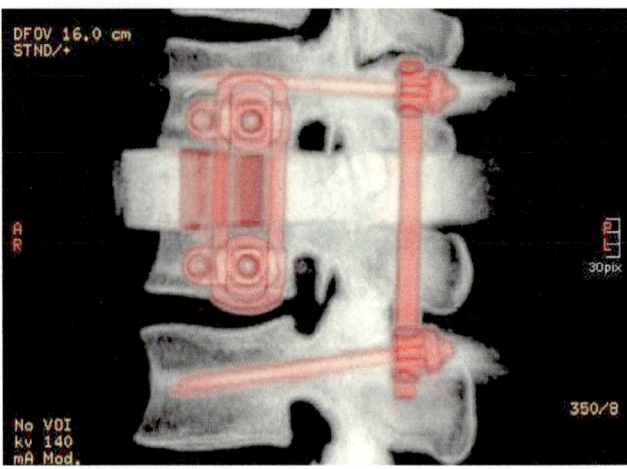

Fig. 42.3 Monosegmental spondylodesis with Tantalum cage and MACS shown as 3D-CT scan

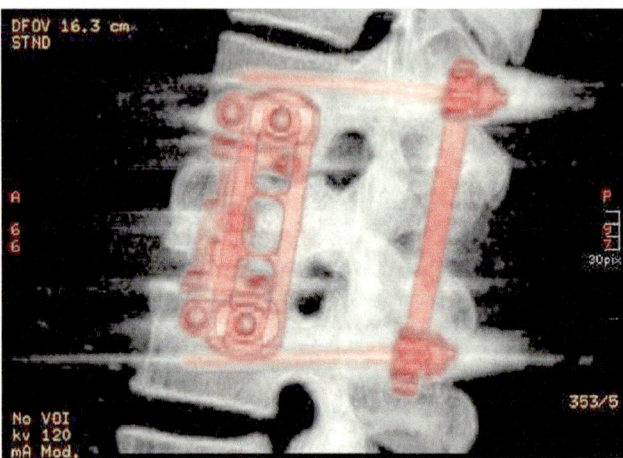

Fig. 42.4 Bisegmental spondylodesis with Hydrolift and MACS shown as 3D-CT scan

angle-stable system should be used. Alternatives to the MACS system are Xia anterior (Stryker) and Telefix or Arcofix (Synthes), respectively [4, 5].

42.5 Planning, Preparation and Positioning

The CT scan is used to measure the sizes of all implants to be used during the anterior spondylodesis. During the operation, measurements are re-evaluated using intraoperative special measuring devices and fluoroscope. Navigation may be useful. Stable lateral positioning on the right side of the patient on a carbon table is performed using a vacuum mattress. Free tilt of the C-arm must be checked. Entrance points for the working and optical channels and the target area are marked on the skin using the fluoroscope (see Fig. 42.5).

Fig. 42.5 Patient in lateral position on a vacuum mattress; approaches are marked under fluoroscopic control

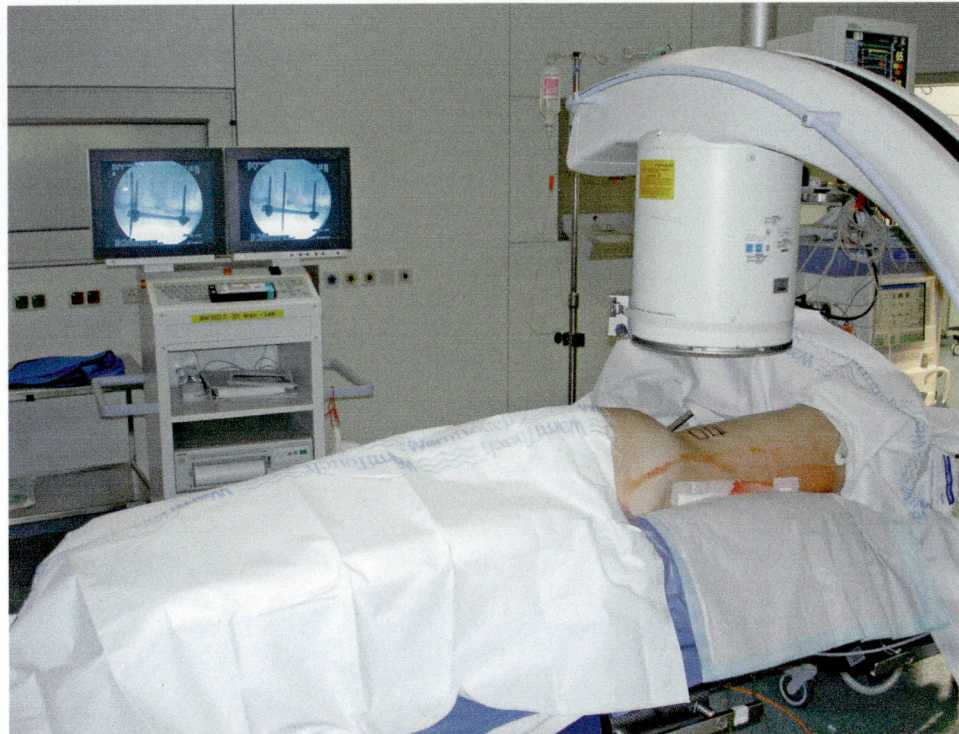

42.6 Surgical Technique

42.6.1 Approach

- Four trocars are placed after the one-lung ventilation has started, the first one using a mini-open procedure to avoid lung lesions (see Fig. 42.6).
- From this point, all operative steps are under thoracoscopic control.
- Lung retractor and suction instrument are inserted using the anterior portals; the working channel is caudal posterior.
- To reach L1–3, a diaphragm split is necessary [6].

42.6.2 Instrumentation

- A K-wire is placed in the vertebra superior to the fractured one using the K-wire impactor under fluoroscopic control. The correct position is close to the ground plate ~1 cm from the posterior border (see Fig. 42.7).
- The entry hole is prepared using a cannulated punch (see Fig. 42.8).
- The posterior polyaxial screw, the polyaxial plate and the centralizer have to be preassembled and then placed over the K-wire (see Fig. 42.9).
- To avoid the risks by pushing forward the K-wire, it has to be removed after the initial turns.
- The polyaxial plate is then screwed down but not tightened. The precise alignment may be controlled by fluoroscope.

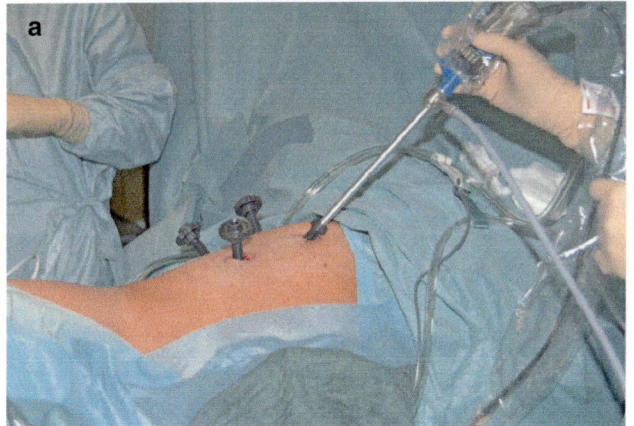

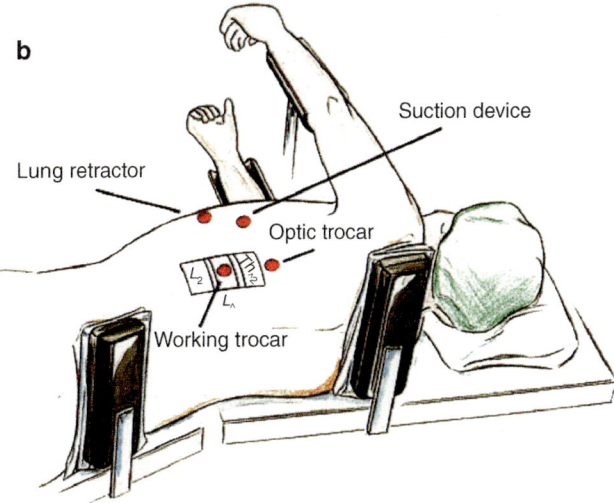

Fig. 42.6 (**a**) Situs with the portals for endoscopic operation technique. (**b**) Illustration of the portal placements. (With permission of Aesculap AG, Tuttlingen, Germany)

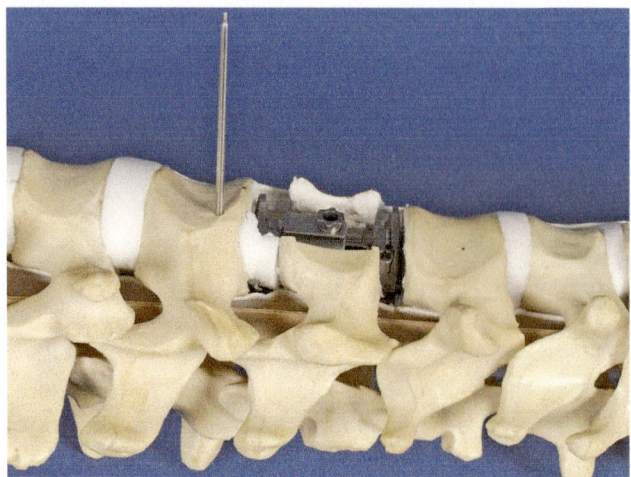

Fig. 42.7 K-wire placed close to the end plate of the vertebra

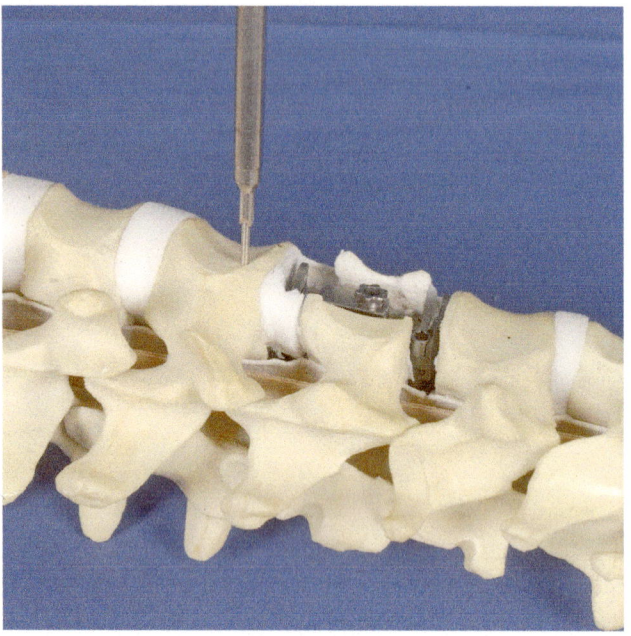

Fig. 42.8 Entry hole prepared by punch

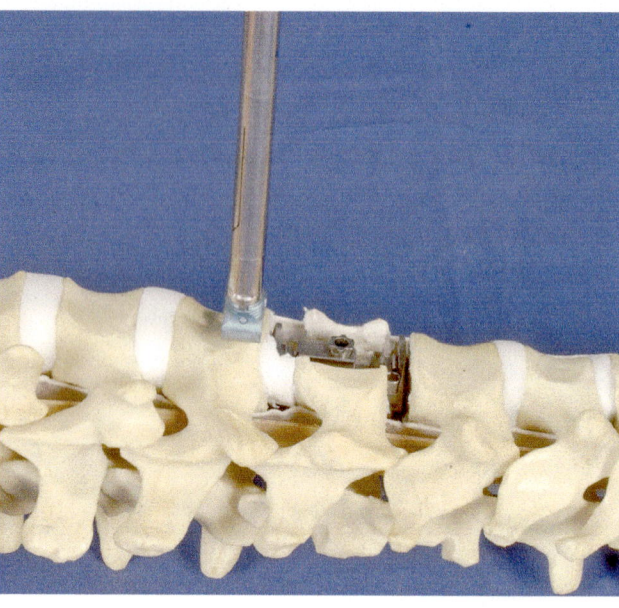

Fig. 42.9 The polyaxial screw together with the polyaxial plate is placed over the K-wire

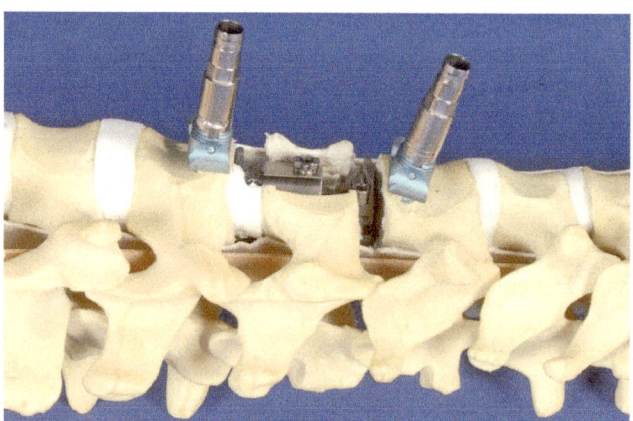

Fig. 42.10 Both polyaxial plates and screws together with the centralizer in place

- Same procedure has to be performed with the second screw (see Fig. 42.10).

42.6.3 Monosegmental Procedures

- The second screw has to be placed close to the ground plate of the fractured vertebra.
- The ruptured intervertebral disc and the fractured parts of the vertebra are resected.
- The cancellous bone of the remaining vertebra is compressed by using the probes of the cage.
- The Tantalum cage is then inserted in a 'press-fit technique'.

42.6.4 Bisegmental Procedures

- The second screw has to be placed close to the end plate of the adjacent vertebra.
- Both discs are resected and partial corpectomy is performed.
- The expandable cage is inserted and expanded.
- Cancellous bone graft (from the resected vertebra) is attached laterally.
- The double-rod system configured as a frame plate is laid onto the clamping elements (see Fig. 42.11) and fixed by nuts, using a torque of 15 Nm (see Fig. 42.12).
- A guide sleeve is inserted to place the anterior screw after opening the cortex using a punch (see Fig. 42.13).

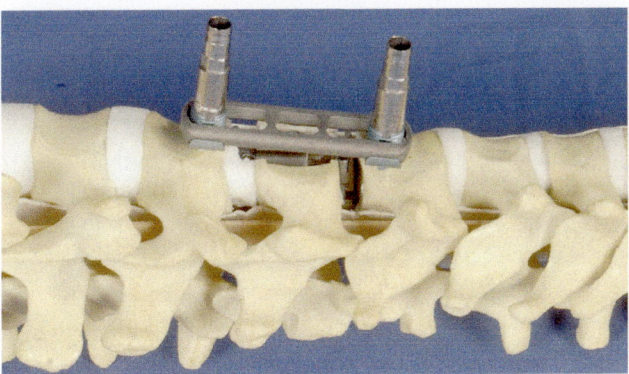

Fig. 42.11 Insertion of the frame plate

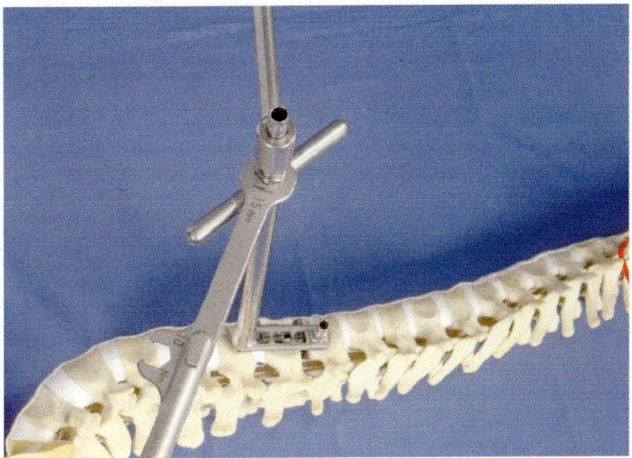

Fig. 42.12 The frame plate is fixed to the clamping elements firmly using a torque wrench

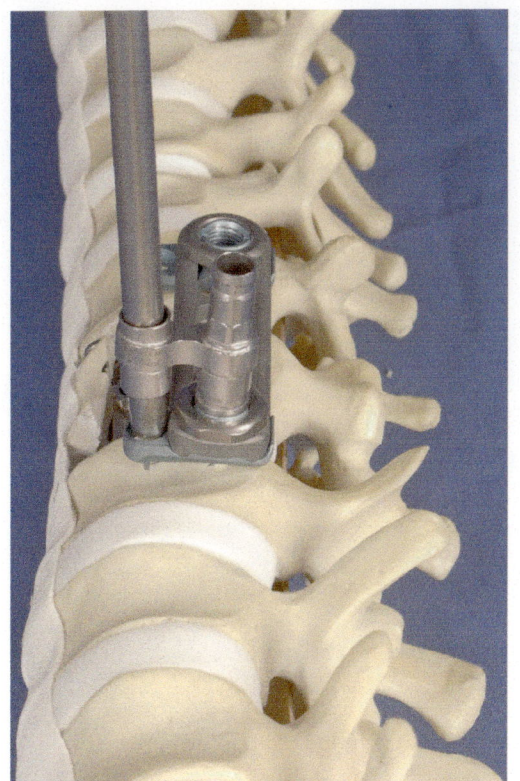

Fig. 42.13 Entry hole for the anterior screw is prepared by punch

- The anterior screws are inserted through the guide sleeve (see Fig. 42.14).
- The guiding sleeve is then removed and the polyaxial mechanism is locked by inserting a locking screw (see Figs. 42.15 and 42.16).
- If a diaphragma split has been performed, the gap in the diaphragma is closed using adaptive sutures.
- A chest tube is placed with its end in the costodiaphragmatic recess, and all instruments and trocars are removed, the portals closed.
- The posterior screws are tightened down to press the plate firmly to the vertebra (see Fig. 42.17).

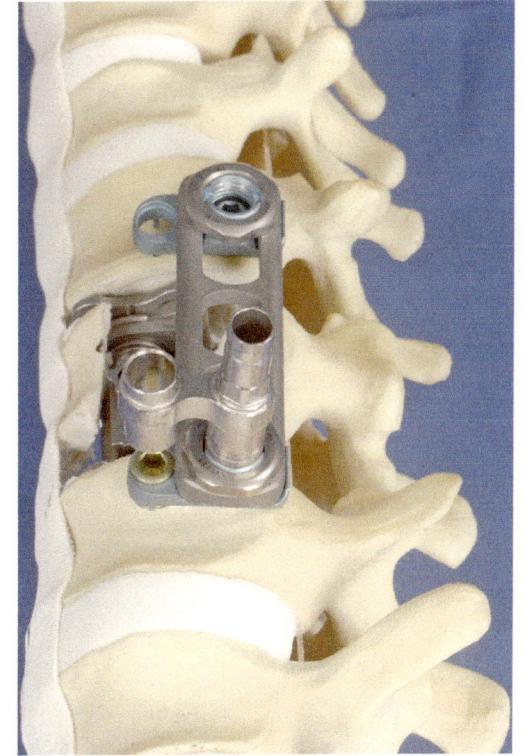

Fig. 42.14 Anterior screw in place

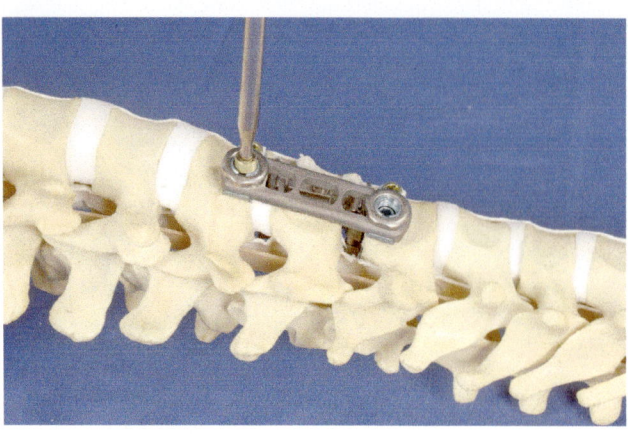

Fig. 42.15 Locking of the polyaxial mechanism

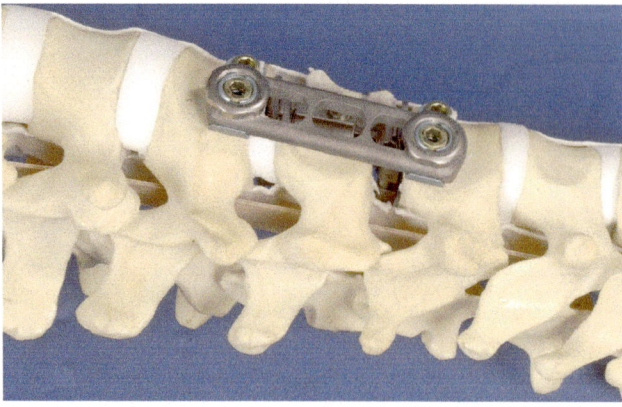

Fig. 42.16 Final construction of the MACS in a bisegmental anterior spondylodesis (with hydrolift as expandable cage)

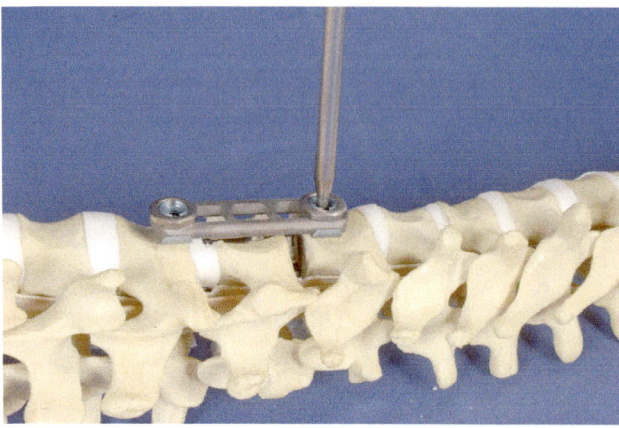

Fig. 42.17 The frame plate is tightened to the vertebra

42.7   Tips and Tricks

- Screwdrivers should be inserted perpendicular to the screws. This is facilitated by 'switching over the rib' using one working portal.
- Posterior screws together with the polyaxial plate – once correctly placed – may serve as a 'navigation frame' during the resection of the fractured vertebra. Thereby, orientation on the thoracoscopic view is facilitated.
- The K-wires and screws should be placed close to the end plates. So it is very unlikely to set lesions to the segmental vessels.

References

1. Beisse R, Potulski M, Beger J, et al. Entwicklung und klinischer Einsatz einer thorakoskopisch implantierbaren Rahmenplatte zur Behandlung thorakolumbaler Frakturen und Instabilitäten. Orthopade. 2002;31:413–22.
2. Gonschorek O, Bühren V. Verletzungen der thorakolumbalen Wirbelsäule. Orthop Unfall Up2date. 2006;1:195–222.
3. Magerl F, Harms J, Gertzbein SD, et al. A comprehensive classification of thoracic and lumbar injuries. Eur Spine J. 1990;3:184–201.
4. Josten C, Katscher S, Gonschorek O. Therapiekonzepte bei Frakturen des thorakolumbalen Überganges und der Lendenwirbelsäule. Orthopade. 2005;34:1021–32.
5. Raju S, Balabhadra V, Kim DH. Thoracoscopic decompression and fixation (MACS-TL). In: Kim DH, Fessler RG, Regan JJ, editors. Endoscopic spine surgery and instrumentation. New York: Thieme; 2005.
6. Kim DH, Jahng TA, Balabhadra RS, et al. Thoracoscopic transdiaphragmatic approach to thoracolumbar junction fractures. Spine. 2004;4:317–28.

Vertebral Body Replacement

43

Jürgen Nothwang

43.1 Introduction and Core Messages

The anterior support in thoracolumbar spine fractures and in some special cases of tumour diseases is one of the most important steps for reconstructing the shape of the vertebral column to preserve satisfying long-term results. A lot of biomechanical and clinical investigations confirm the necessity of anterior reconstruction in bisegmental posterior stabilizations to avoid posterior implant failure. Potential of healing of a bisegmental corticocancellous graft is limited. With vertebral body replacements (VBR), the loss of correction after removal of the posterior stabilization device is small. VBRs with expandable components (Fig. 43.1) allow an adapted anterior defect bridging and open the possibility of anterior reduction.

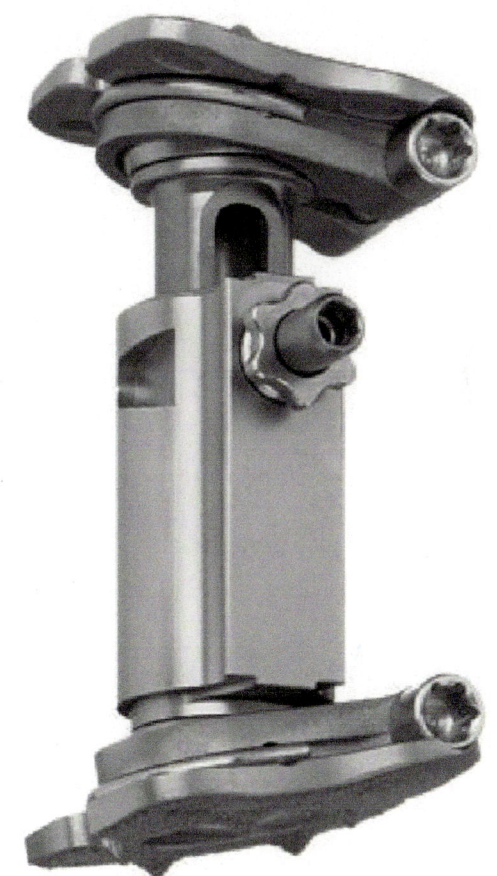

Fig. 43.1 Expandable vertebral body replacement system Hydrolift (Aesculap) (With permission Aesculap AG Tuttlingen, Germany)

43.2 Indications

Indication of vertebral body replacement is depending on the entity of the lesion, bone quality, and general condition of the patient. A careful analysis of the pathology protects further complications. We have to remind that even in endoscopic techniques, the perioperative risk [1–3] is respectable.

J. Nothwang (✉)
Rems-Murr-Klinik Schorndorf, Department for Trauma Surgery and Orthopedics, Schorndorf, Germany
e-mail: juergen.nothwang@freenet.de; jnothwang@khrmk.de

- Fractures of thoracolumbar spine (Type A2.3, A3.2., A3.3., Type B and C1 fracture in combination of bisegmental fractures of the vertebral body, Type C2.2 and C3 fractures with severe destruction of the vertebral body).
- Total corporectomy/spondylectomy in primary tumour treatment,
- Metastases of vertebral body in epithelial tumours with mild prognosis: corporal destruction >40% (lumbar spine) and 60% (thoracic spine) [4].
- Persistent instability after total vertebral collapse due to osteoporosis,
- Post infectious, post-traumatic or kyphotic deformities in degenerated diseases (Fig. 43.2).

43.3 Contraindications

- Reduced general conditions of the patient: pulmonary and cardiac risk factors (ASA risk score ≥ IV, NYHA score IV).
- Pre-existing lung diseases with mayor reduction of vital capacity, pleural diseases as pleural rind, adhesions of the lung, and residuals after lung contusion may disable a thoracic transpleural approach and one-lung ventilation in endoscopic approach.
- Disturbance of haemostasis.
- Extensive osteoporosis with severe pre-existing deformities.
- Bad prognosis in tumour diseases and reduced general conditions of the patient.
- Malformation of the thorax and its cavity, and.
- Previous surgery with the same approach (relative).

43.4 Technical Prerequisites

Fluoroscopy, radiolucent operating table, retraction device, rip raspatory, rip resector, light source, long instruments, thoracotomy set, lung retractor, electric scissor and hook for preparation of the pleura parietalis, osteotomes, hook probes, sharp and blunt rongeurs, Kerrisson rongeur, curettes, clip applicator and if disposable, shaver for disc preparation. *Not only for endoscopic preparation ultrasound dissector is helpful and enables an operation technique with reduced blood loss.*

For endoscopic techniques, there is further need for three chip camera, 30° angled rigid scope, light source, monitors, video-recorder and printer, irrigation/suction unit, fan retractor.

In endoscopic technique, double tube for one-lung ventilation intraoperatively is mandatory. Further advantages might be offered by three-dimensional thoracoscopy [5].

43.5 Basic Clinical and Biomechanical Messages

- Reduced load-bearing capacity of the anterior column (i.e. burst fractures, extended vertebral body defects) is the mayor risk for loss of correction and implant failure [6–8].
- Several biomechanical investigations have demonstrated the breakage of the posterior implant under cyclic load [9, 10].
- In vitro biomechanical investigations showed that the maximum load was lower in the strut grafted spines, when compared with those with pedicle fixation only [11]. It is also of concern that the potential of healing of a bisegmental corticocancellous graft is limited. Pseudarthrosis and even fractures of the grafts are described [12].
- To minimize principle loss of correction, a metallic titanium or peek expandable (Fig. 43.1) vertebral body replacement can offer higher guarantee [13–15].
- Collapse of the VBR implant into the vertebral body remains a point of concern [7, 16]. Several clinical and in vivo measurements confirm force reduction in the first two months after operation due to subsidence of the implant [17].
- Currently, little is known about the amount of loads which is created by VBRs and which stresses the end plates under daily life movements [16, 17]. Additional axial loads in upright position in interaction with individual factors due to bone mineral density further modify the resistance capabilities. In rotatory instabilities, VBR + anterolateral plate+ posterior screw-rod-system offers the highest stability in biomechanical testings compared to the normal spine [18]. The contribution of the muscle corset to spinal stability is still well known, its effects in spinal instability not yet [19].
- In poor bone quality, the subsidence of VBR into the endplate may cause an increased loss of correction [15]. Our clinical experience that a near endplate anterior vertebroplasty in adjacent level can provide good results is found in literature [20].
- The question of near endplate vascularisation, which is interrupted by cementing, is not answered in the end.

Fig. 43.2 (**a** and **b**)
Posttraumatic and
degenerative deformity:
preoperative X-rays. (**c** and **d**)
Postoperative X-rays after
ventrodorsal reconstruction

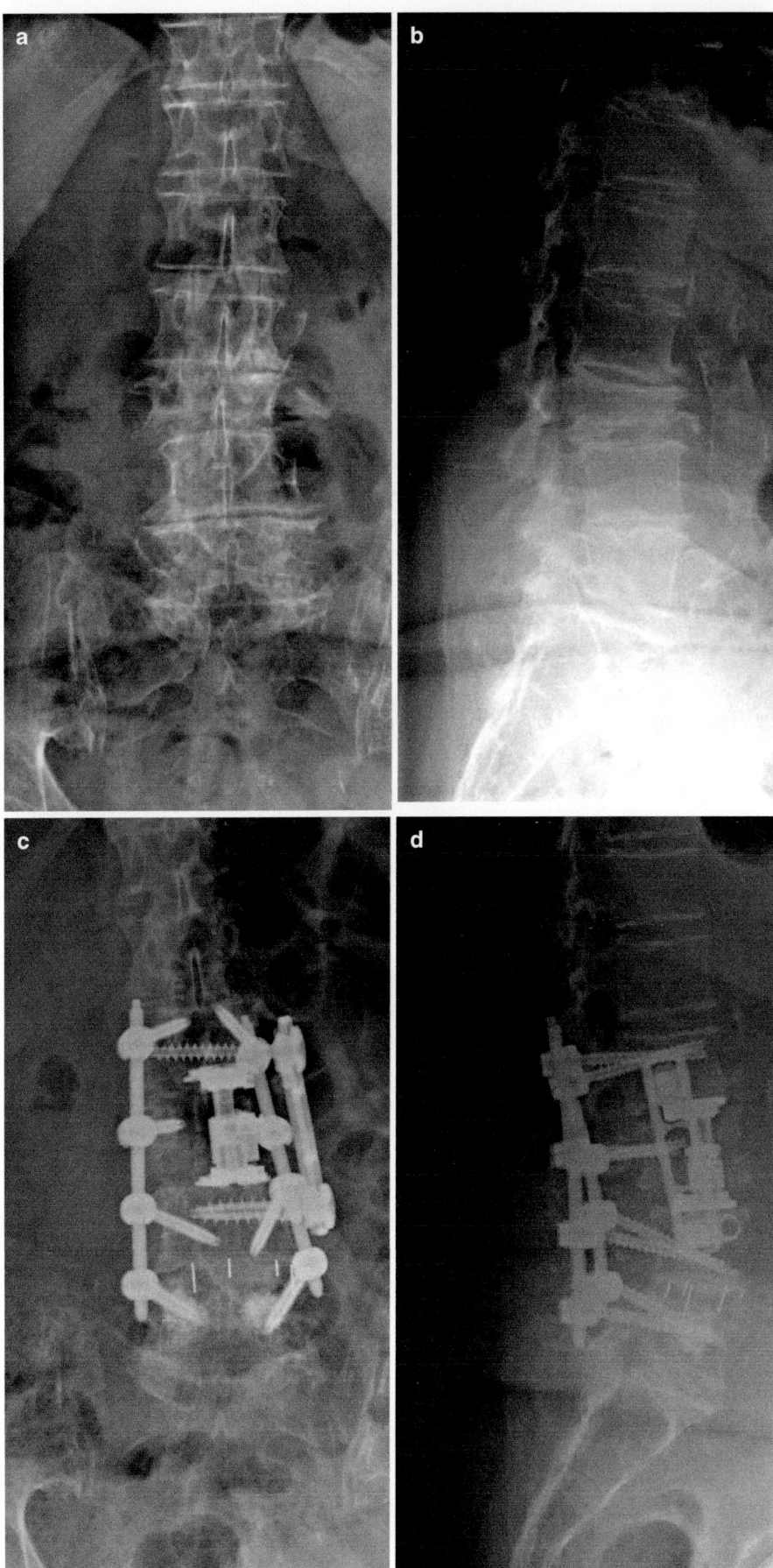

43.6 Planning, Preparation and Positioning

- Analysis of the preoperative x-rays and CT scans to evaluate the region of lesion and special conditions of the vessels (King-King phenomenon, atypical veins). In some special cases, Angio CT or MRI may provide further information of blood supply and FSU.
  Attention is demanded to the number of lumbar vertebrae and stump rips to identify the correct segment level.
- Measurement of FSU height is recommendable, especially cranial T9. In small patients, the predetermined space is smaller than the smallest expandable VBR, and the strategy of treatment has to be modified. (*In endoscopic approaches, the patient should be informed of switching to open procedure techniques if endoscopic approach has to be quit by technical reasons or complications.*)
- Preoperative preparation of the patient should include shaving of the operative field and catheter of urinary bladder. (In our experience, in transthoracic operations further preparations as intestinal preparation by laxatives are dispensable, even if a split of diaphragm is necessary).
- Right-side positioning is chosen in all lesions of T9 and lower, left-side positioning above T9. (This decision is due to the course of the vessels, which by trend prefer a Dexter course lower than T9 and a sinistral one in the upper regions).
- A straight lateral position should be favoured. With fluoroscopy, the posterior wall has to form a singular line and the end plates should be hit perpendicular to the radiologic beam.
- In the lower lumbar, spine positioning of the patient depends on the pelvic rim. In some cases, a backward tilting of the table is necessary to provide access to the target area.
- The patient has to be fixed in pillars with anterior and posterior support. To avoid decubital problems to the legs, we use a special bedding pillow, so-called 'tunnel' and gel blankets to protect bony prominences.
- Before starting the operation under fluoroscopic control, the incisions are marked. Especially in endoscopic approach, the definition of the portals is one of the most important steps.
- In minimal open and endoscopic approaches, the incision of the working channel should be exactly in projection to the target area. The length of the skin incision depends on the presumed size of the vertebral body replacement (Fig. 43.3).
- In endoscopic technique, which we prefer in thoracic spine surgery and at thoracolumbar junction, the portal for the endoscope should be marked two segments above

the working channel, the incisions of the fan retractor and the suction form of a trapezoid.

43.7 Surgical Technique

43.7.1 Approach

- We always start the operation with the working channel (Fig. 43.3)
  (It has the largest size, and the success of one-lung ventilation can be controlled visually without danger of lung damage even in case of adhesions.)
  In thoracolumbar junction, attention should be given to the course of the diaphragmal line, especially in cases of raised dome position.
- In case of pleural adhesions, due to former inflammations, mobilize pleura visceralis through the working channel. Develop an anterior portal, then change position to the abdominal side of the patient and continue pleural mobilization to reach the lateral vertebral surface from anterior portal under guidance of endoscope, which then is positioned through the working channel.
- If elasticity of the chest is obviously limited, we recommend a limited resection of the rip in projection to the target segment to reduce stress and risk of intraoperative rip fracture. If required, the bone of the rip can be saved for grafting.
  Usually in the upper thoracic spine, the resection of the rip is necessary due to the horizontal and narrow course of the rips.
- In terms of the further steps in endoscopic approach, see the specific chapter.
- If diaphragma's split is necessary, we expose the line of insertion with the fan retractor and then incise it with the help of an electric hook or scissor. After having opened the diaphragma in the line of insertion, a split of the diaphragma follows and the fan retractor can be placed into the diaphragma's gap. With the same instruments, the parietal pleura is incised in a T-shape and mobilized anteriorly and posteriorly.
- The segmental vessels of the target vertebral body are mobilized, closed with clips and dissected.
- The adjacent discs are identified and cut with a long-armed scalpel.
- With a raspatory, the disc is separated from the endplates and finally removed with Kerrison rongeurs.
- If decompression of the spinal canal is necessary, the lower border of the pedicle is identified and the base of the pedicle is then resected in a cranial direction with the help of a Kerrison rongeur and punches.

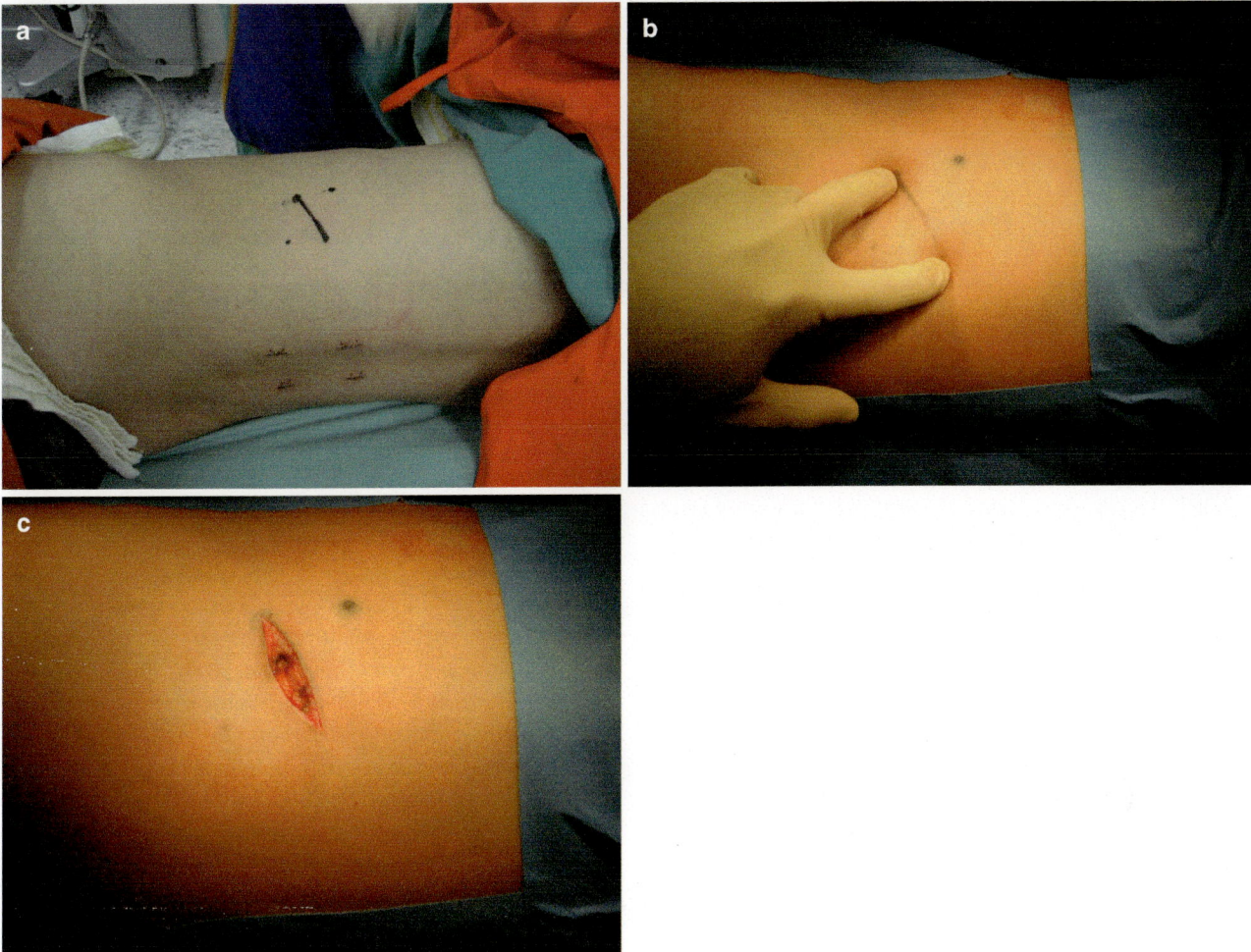

Fig. 43.3 (**a**) Positioning of the patient for minimal invasive lumbotomy an incision line exactly in projection to the target area. (**b**) Slight skin extension for a smaller approach. (**c**) Size of incision for minimal invasive lumbotomy for a VBR

- Having finished the resection, the clearance of the spinal canal can be performed.
- The bed for the vertebral body replacement has to be prepared and modelized by chisels. Angulated chisels are available to shape the corners precisely (Fig. 43.4a).
- The end plate and the suitable length of the vertebral replacement can be appreciated by test implants (Fig. 43.5a, b).
- Choose a size close to the measured length to create high stiffness of the spacer and avoid weakening of the implant by long expansion's distance.
- The ex situ angle of the end plate can be gently fixed along with the safety screw for distraction.
- With a holding device, the VBR is inserted (Fig. 43.6).
- Under fluoroscopic control the VBR is placed in a midline position in both planes.

- The safety screw is opened and the spacer can be expanded
- and hydraulically controlled (Fig. 43.7).
- The compression forces should not pass 30 atm.
- The screws for end-plate fixation are opened to allow optimal adaption to the end plates of the next segments.
- If ideal positioning is achieved, all screws have to be tightened by torque wrench.
- With the preparation of the spacer's bed, usually plenty enough cancellous bone graft can be harvested, used for lateral spondylodesis and covering of the VBR.
- In osteoporosis, vertebroplasty of the adjacent vertebral bodies is recommendable to avoid subsidence of the implant. The cement augmentation should be applied close to the endplates (Fig. 43.8).
- In tumorous diseases, cement augmentation should be considered to enlarge local stability (so-called compound spondylodesis).

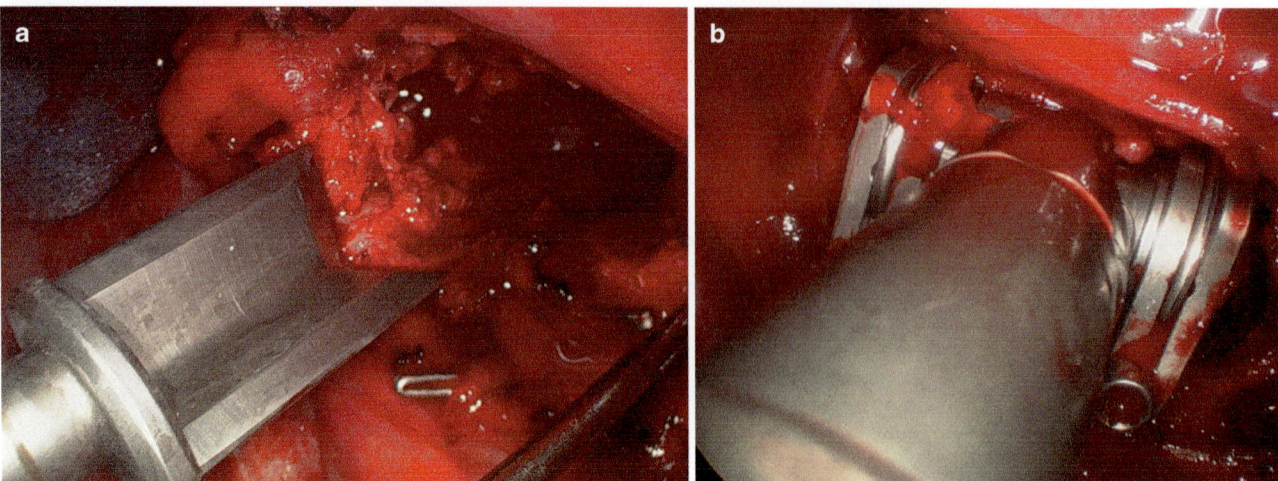

Fig. 43.4 (**a** and **b**) Endoscopic preparation of the bed of VBR by angulated chisels and insertion of the VBR

43.8   Tips and Tricks

- A strict lateral positioning of the patient is extremely important to avoid malposition of the VBR. *Respecting the correct position means eliminating any risk of spinal canal compromising.*
- If the collapse of the lung hasn't been succeeded totally, it is possible to push the lung back by an abdominal cloth.
- To reduce the frequency of fluoroscopic control, we mark the midline of the adjacent vertebral bodies in the lateral view by k-wires before starting the vertebral body resection. In our experience, further fluoroscopy is not required until the definite implantation of the VBR.
- Having clipped the segmental vessels, due to the anatomically more stable situation, we always start the osteotomy anteriorly with a 2 cm chisel, parallel to the anterior vertebral border. In a second step, the posterior osteotomy follows. This avoids a 'swinging' of the vertebral body with a higher safeness during osteotomy.
- Always respect the curvated shape of the anterior border of vertebral body to minimize risk of vascular damage.
- In case of anterior kyphectomy, good results can be achieved, if the anterior longitudinal ligament is completely cut in the level of the discs (Zielke-adapted procedure [21]).

- Use the largest implant which can be inserted in the prepared cavity without additional forces.
- If reduction is desired, the angle of the VBR endplates must be definitely fixed in the favoured position before introduction of the spacer. For this procedure, special templates are provided by the companies.
- In the lower lumbar spine, it is sometimes difficult to reach the posterior locking screw riskless, especially after anterior spinal decompression. In these cases, it is helpful to measure the necessary angle in the CT-scan and prefix the locking screw definitely before insertion of the VBR.
- The aim of the vertebral replacement is to achieve high contact zones between the VBR endplates and the endplates of the adjacent vertebral bodies. The larger the contact zone, the lesser the risk of implant penetration.
- Infiltration of intercostal space where the thoracic drainage is inserted reduces postoperative pain. If harvesting bone graft from the anterior or posterior iliac crest is required, we recommend periostal denerving by electric knife and finally infiltration with Ropivacain®.

At the end of a transpleural reconstruction, we applicate 250 ml Ropivacain per infusion into the pleura. In our experience, this significantly reduces the patients demand for central effective analgesics.

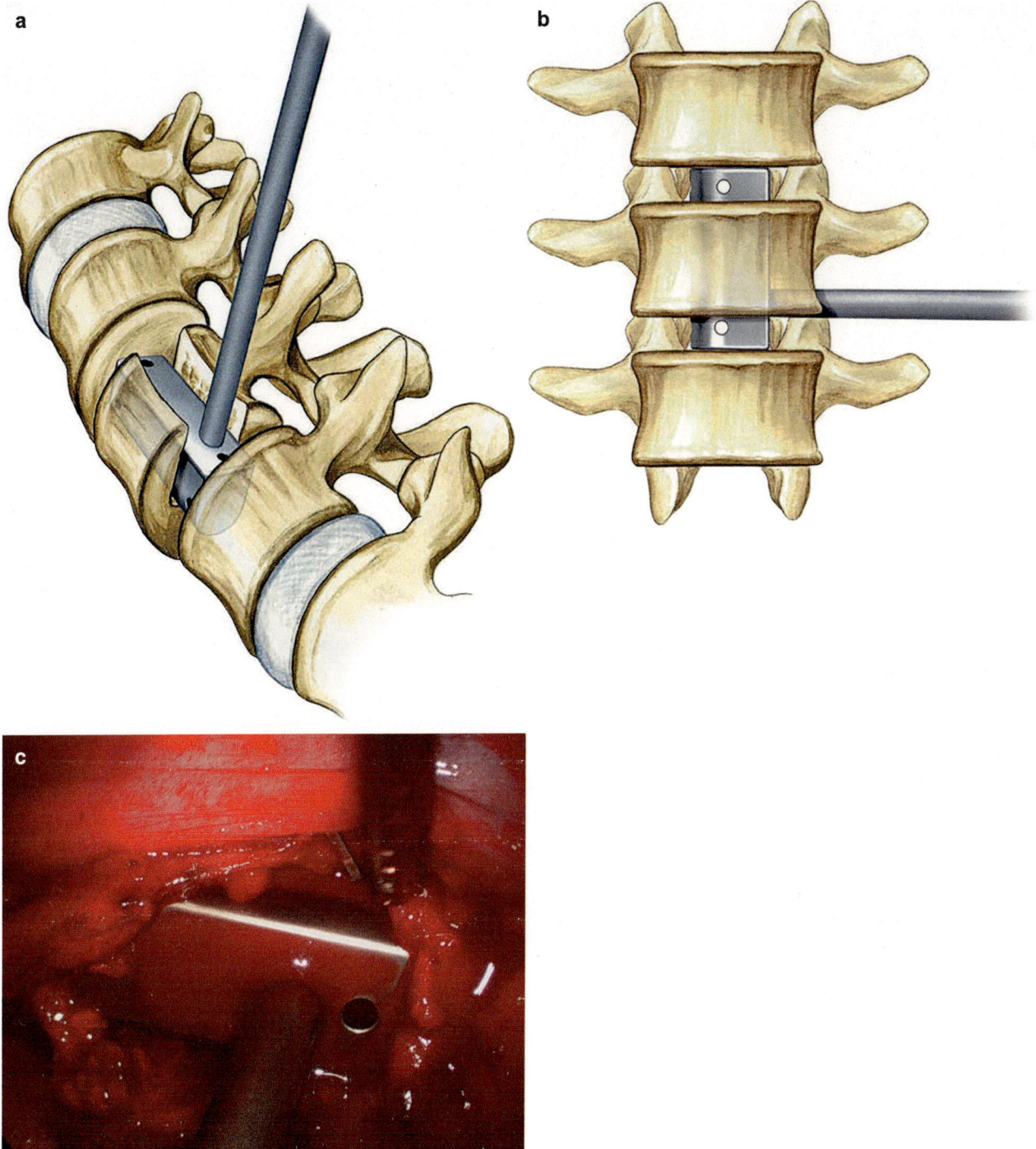

Fig. 43.5 (**a**, **b**) Measurement device for the ident length of the implant. (**c**) Endoscopic intraoperative view of the measurement device in the prepared implant bed (With permission Aesculap AG, Tuttlingen, Germany)

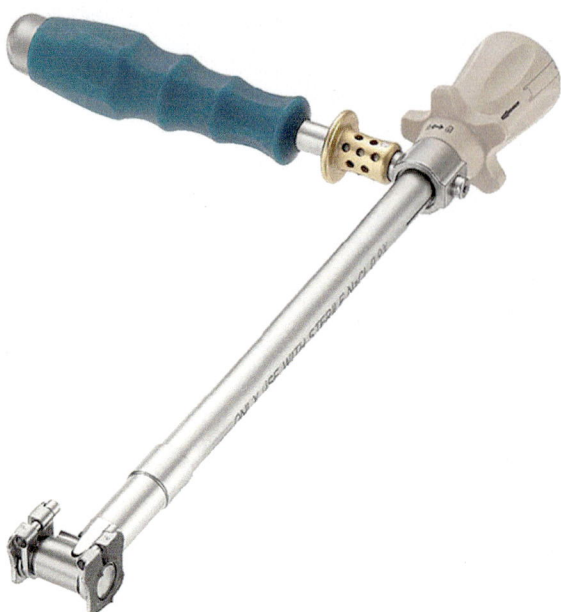

Fig. 43.6 Holding instrument for the vertebral body replacement (VBR) device. (With permission Aesculap AG, Tuttlingen, Germany)

Fig. 43.7 (**a**) Positioning of the VBR and expansion under pressure control (With permission Aesculap AG, Tuttlingen, Germany) (**b**) intraoperative situation with the holding instrument

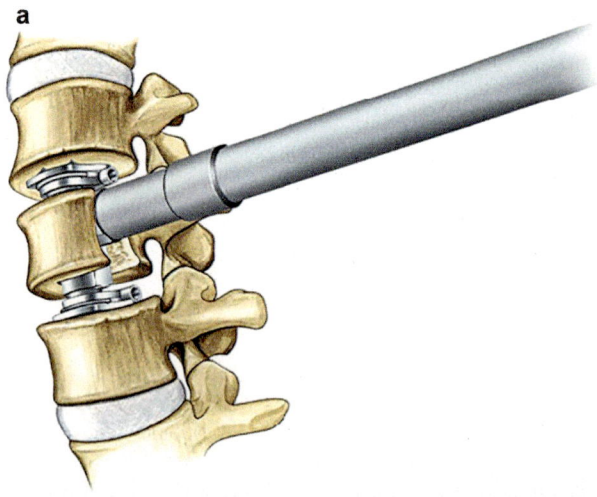

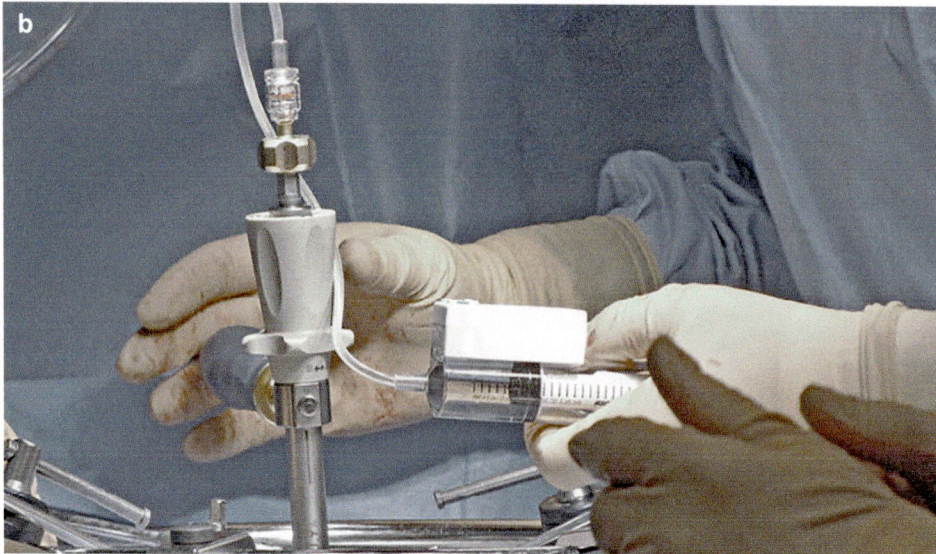

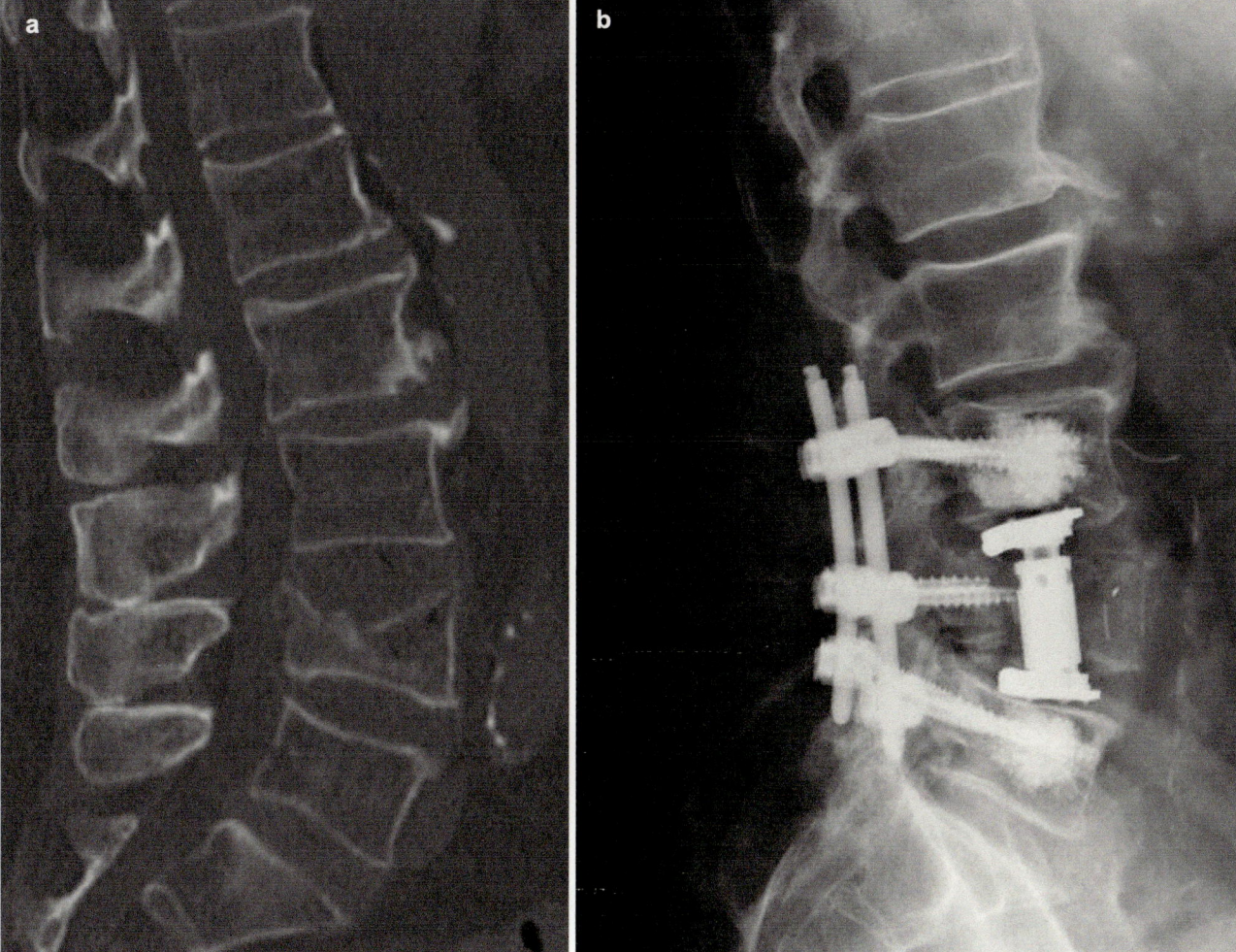

Fig. 43.8 (**a**) Pre- and (**b**) postoperative X-ray of pathologic fracture of L4 with augmentation of the adjacent levels with PMMA- cement and posterior augmented pedicle screw

References

1. Beisse R. Complications of endoscopic surgery of the spine. Trauma Berufskrankh. 2005;7(Suppl 2):321–6.
2. Lee C-H, Wu M-H, Li Y-Y, Cheng C-C, Lee C-Y, Huang T-J. Video-assisted thoracoscopic surgery and minimal access spinal surgery compared in anterior thoracic or thoracolumbar junctional spinal reconstruction: a case-control study and review of the literature. BioMed Res Int. 2016;2016:6808507. https://doi.org/10.1155/2016/6808507.
3. Matschke S, Wagner C, Davids D, et al. Complications in endoscopic anterior thoracolumbar spinal reconstructive surgery. Eur J Trauma. 2006;23(3):215–26.
4. Taneichi H, Kaneda K, Takeda N, Abumi K, Satoh S. Risk factors and probability of vertebral body collapse in metastases of the thoracic and lumbar spine. Spine. 1997;22(3):239–45.
5. Smits AJ, Deunk J, and. Bloemers F.W. Three-dimensional thoracoscopic surgery for spine fractures: a technical report with first results and experiences. Global Spine J. 2018:1–6.
6. McLain RF, Sparling D, Benson DR. Early failure of short segment pedicle instrumentation for thoraco-lumbar fractures. A preliminary report. J Bone Joint Surg Am. 1993;75:162–9.
7. Sasso RC, Cottler HB. Posterior instrumentation and fusion for unstable fractures and fracture dislocations of the thoracic and lumbar spine. Spine. 1993;18:450–560.
8. Reinhold M, Schmölz W, Canto F, Krappinger D, Blauth M, Knop C. An improved vertebral body replacement for the thoracolumbar spine. A biomechanical in vitro test on human lumbar vertebral bodies. Unfallchirurg. 2007;110(4):327–33.
9. Cripton PA, Jain GM, Wittenberg RH, et al. Load sharing characteristics of stabilized lumbar spine segment. Spine. 2000;25(1):170–9.
10. Cunningham BW, Sefter JC, Shono Y. Static and cyclic biomechanical analysis of pedicle screw spinal constructs. Spine. 1993;18(12):1677–88.
11. Maiman DJ, Pintar F, Yoganandan N, Reinhartz J. Effects of anterior vertebral grafting on the traumatized lumbar spine after pedicle screw-plate fixation. Spine. 1993;18:2423–30.
12. Knop C, Blauth M, Bühren V, et al. Operative treatment of thoracolumbar fractures – results of a prospective multicenter study by the

working group "spine" of the German Society of Trauma Surgery Part 3 follow-up. Unfallchirurg. 2001;104:583–600.

13. Kreinest M, Schmahl D, Grützner PA, Matschke S. Radiological results and clinical patient outcome after implantation of a hydraulic expandable vertebral body replacement following traumatic vertebral fractures in the thoracic and lumbar spine: a 3-year follow-up. Spine. 2017;42(8):482–9.

14. Nothwang J, Ulrich C. The reconstruction of the anterior column of thoracolumbar spine fractures. Osteosynthese Int. 2000;8:1–6.

15. Vieweg U, Solch O, Kalff R. Titandistraktionselement als Wirbelkörperersatz bei instabilen Berstungsfrakturen der Brust- und Lendenwirbelsäule - Eine retrospektive Studie bei 30 Patienten. Zentralbl Neurochir. 2003;64:58–64.

16. Rohlmann A, Dreischarf M, Zander T, Graichen F, Strube P, Schmidt H, Bergmann G. Monitoring the load on a telemeterised replacement for a period of up to 65 months. Eur Spine J. 2013;22:2575–81.

17. Rohlmann A, Graichen F, Bender A, et al. Loads on a telemeterized vertebral body replacement measured in three patients within the first postoperative month. Clin Biomech. 2008;23(2):147–58.

18. Ulmar B, Erhard S, Unger S, Weise K, Schmoelz W. Biomechanical analysis of a new expandable vertebral body replacement combined with a new polyaxial antero-lateral plate and/or pedicle Screw and rods. Eur Spine J. 2012;21:546–53.

19. Maciaszek J. Muscle training for the stability of the spine. Trend Sport Sci. 2017;2(24):59–65.

20. Geiger F, Kafchitsas K, Rauschmann M. Anterior vertebroplasy of adjacent levels after vertebral body replacement. Eur Spine J. 2011;20:1385–92.

21. Richter A, Quante M, Macherei A, Halm H. Modified primary stable ventral derotation spondylodesis with Halm-Zielke instrumentation for the treatment of idiopathic scoliosis. Operative Orthopädie Traumatolol. 2010;22:164–76.

Anterior Correction of Scoliosis

Cornelius Wimmer

44.1 Introduction and Core Messages

In 1969, Dwyer developed instrumentation for spinal correction and fixation through an anterior approach [1]. The Dwyer device is a cable attached to vertebral bodies with large screws. The discs are removed and compression is applied on the convex side of the curve. This is powerful system with a lot of complications such as pseudarthrosis, cable fractures and loss of correction. Postoperative bracing was necessary (Fig. 44.1). In 1976, Zielke [2] developed a modification of Dwyer system using a rod of 3,2 mm instead of the cable. The application of the Zielke derotation technique using the solid flexible rod allows controlled production of lordosis and lessens kyphosis (Fig. 44.2). There was a high rod breakage rate. Over the years, double-rod systems with powerful correction and postoperative mobilization without braces have been developed and are currently the state of the art [3–9].

44.2 Indication

Indication is idiopathic scoliosis in the thoracic or thoracolumbar or lumbar spine (Lenke 1 and 5 [10, 11]). The cranial end fusion level should not be higher than T4, and the caudal end level should be utmost L4. The curve should be flexible with a coronal Cobb measurement of at least 45° and should not exceed 90°. Bending films are necessary to ensure the flexibility of the fractional curve. Treatment is only possible for a single major curve.

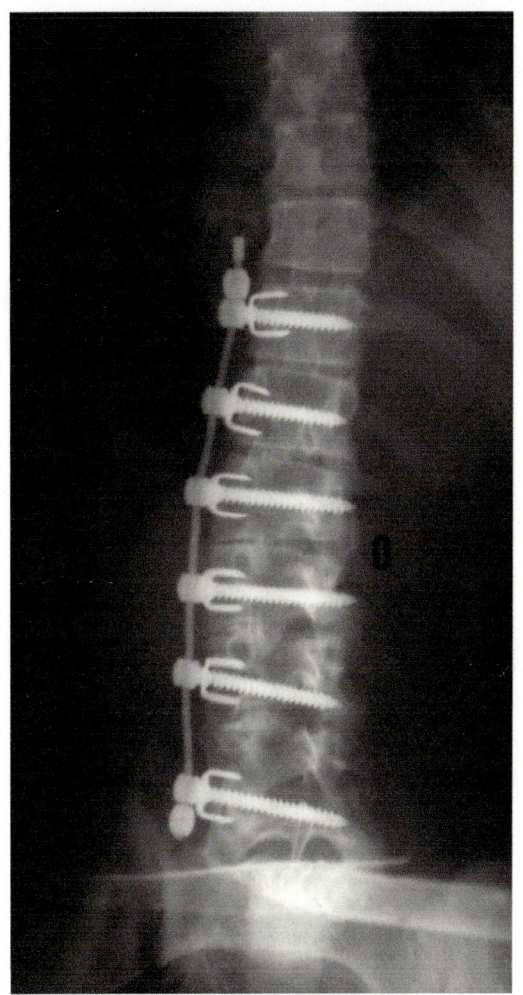

Fig. 44.1 Postoperative x-ray after Dwyer instrumentation

44.3 Contraindication

Absolut contraindication is an osteoporosis, infection, allergic reaction to the metal of the implant, structured kyphosis in the major curve, minor curve that does not correct to 25° on

C. Wimmer (✉)
Department of Spine Surgery, Trauma Center, Trostberg, Germany
e-mail: ProfWimmer@t-online.de

© Springer-Verlag GmbH Germany 2023
U. Vieweg, F. Grochulla (eds.), *Manual of Spine Surgery*, https://doi.org/10.1007/978-3-662-64062-3_44

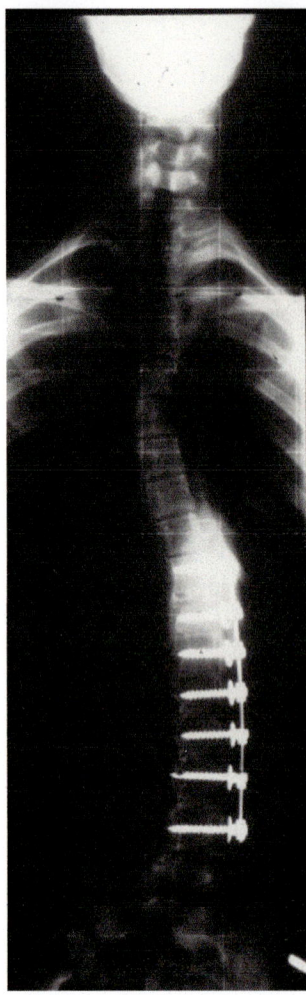

Fig. 44.2 Postoperative x-ray after VDS instrumentation

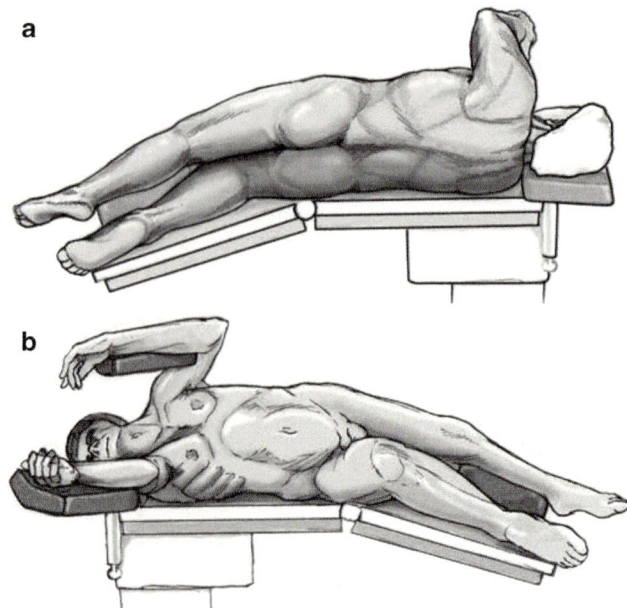

Fig. 44.3 (**a**, **b**) Positioning of the patient in lateral decubitus position with the convex side of the curve elevated

- Double lumen tube,
- Controlled hypotension,
- Neuromonitoring with MEPs,
- Fluoroscopy,
- Chest tube,
- Cell saver.

44.5.1 Approach [13–16]

If the curve to be instrumented is a thoracolumbar curve, lumbar or thoracic curve, a thoracolumbar, lumbar retroperitoneal or thoracic approach can be used.

44.5.1.1 Thoracic Approach

Once the patient is positioned (Fig. 44.4a), perform a curvilinear incision along the rib that is one level higher than the most proximal level to be instrumented (Fig. 44.4b). Perform the incision along the rib. Expose and excise the rib. Enter the chest and retract the lung (Fig. 44.4c, d). Identify the vertebral bodies and carefully dissect the muscle laterally of the vertebral disc spaces. Divide the prevertebral fascia in direction of the spine. Identify the segmental arteries over the waist of each vertebral body, isolate and ligate them (Fig. 44.4e). Expose the bone extraperiostally. The exposure from T7 to T11 is simple. A double thoracotomy is necessary for six or more levels. The second thoracotomy is best performed at T11.

bending film, sagittal malalignment with pathological kyphosis cranial or caudal of the instrumented segments [12].

44.4 Positioning of the Patient

Place the patient in the lateral decubitus position with the convex side of the curve elevated (Fig. 44.3a, b).

44.5 Technical Prerequisites

- X-ray of the whole spine in standing ap and lateral view,
- Bending films to detect flexibility of single major, double major or triple major curve,
- Measurement of the Cobb angles,
- CT scan of the part of the instrumentation,
- MRI to detect intraspinal pathology (tethered cord, diastematomyelie, Arnold Chiari Malformation),

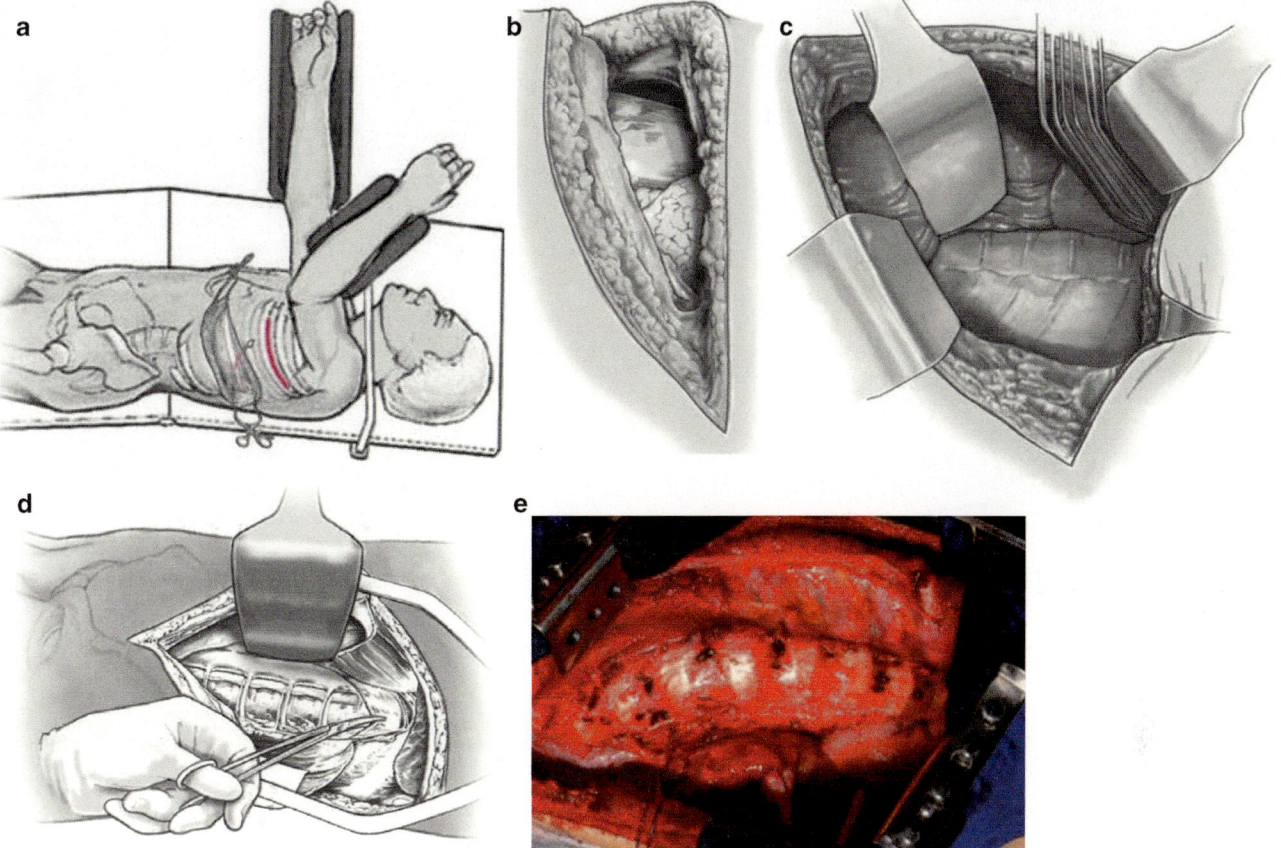

Fig. 44.4 (**a**) Skin incision for thoracolumbar approach. (**b**) Exposure after opening thorax. (**c**) Exposure of thorax with diaphragm. (**d**) Exposure of spine before ligation of segmental vessels. (**e**) Intraoperative view after ligation of segmental vessels

44.5.1.2 Thoracoabdominal Approach

Once the patient is positioned, perform a curvilinear incision along the rib that is one level higher than the most proximal level to be instrumented. Perform the incision along the rib and extend it distally along the anterolateral abdominal wall just lateral to the rectus abdominus muscle. Expose and excise the rib. Enter the chest and retract the lung. Identify the diaphragm as a separate structure:

Remove the diaphragm from the chest cavity and continue with retroperitoneal dissection distally. Enter the chest cavity transpleurally through the bed of the rib. Use the electrocautery to divide the diaphragm close to the chest wall. Leave a small tag of diaphragm for reattachment. Now expose the retroperitoneal space. Dissect the peritoneal cavity and split the oblique muscles and transvers muscles in line with the skin incision and exposure distally as far as necessary. Identify the vertebral bodies and carefully dissect the muscle psoas laterally to the vertebral disc spaces. Divide the prevertebral fascia in the direction of the spine. Identify the segmental arteries over the waist of each vertebral body, isolate and ligate them. Expose the bone extraperiostally.

44.5.1.3 Lumbar Extraperitoneal Approach

Place the patient in a lateral decubitus position with the convex side up (Fig. 44.5a). Perform a midflank incision from the midline anteriorly to midline posteriorly. Divide the abdominal oblique muscles in line with the incision, split the transversal muscle (Fig. 44.5b). Dissect the peritoneum anteriorly. Posterior dissection allows access to the spine. Repair any inadvertent entry into the peritoneum immediately because it may not be identifiable later. Locate the major vessels in the midline, divide the segmental arteries and veins and ligate them.

44.5.1.4 Disc Excision

The disc can be felt as soft, rounded protuberant area of the spine compared with the concave surface of the vertebral body. Divide the annulus sharply with a long handled scalpel and remove it (Fig. 44.6). Remove the nucleus pulposus with rongeurs and curets. If necessary, remove the anterior or posterior longitudinal ligaments. Remove the cartilaginous endplates using a ring curet or osteotome. Obtain hemostasis with Gelfoam. Significant correction of the curve occurs dura

b

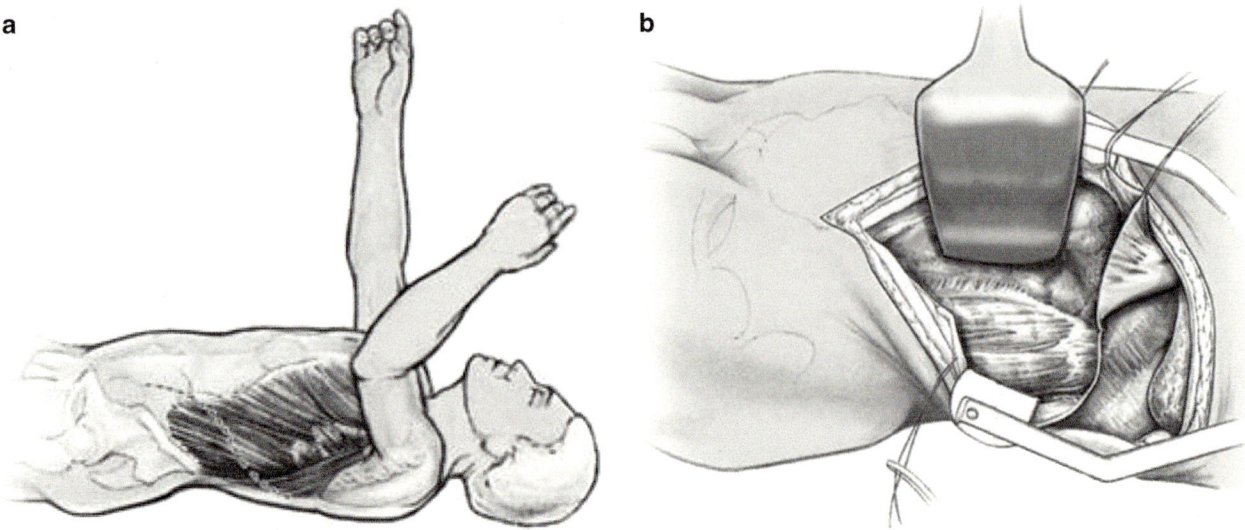

Fig. 44.5 (**a**) Skin incision for lumbar approach. (**b**) Exposure of spine in extra peritoneal approach

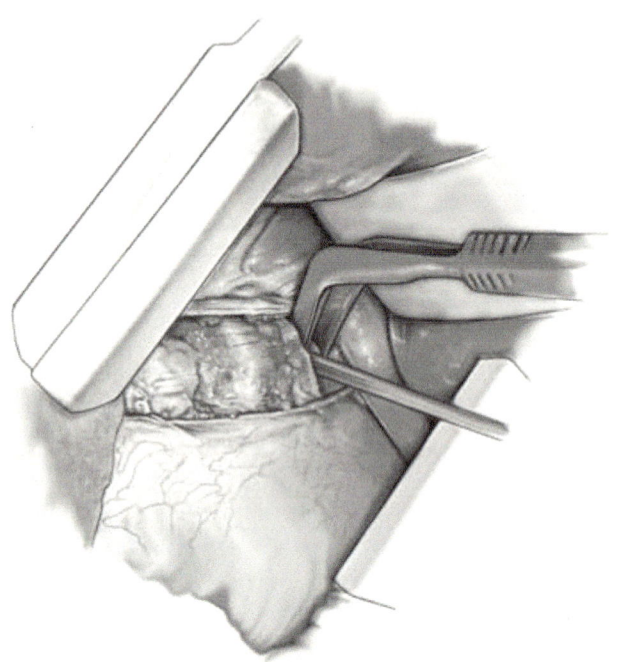

Fig. 44.6 Preparation of disc space

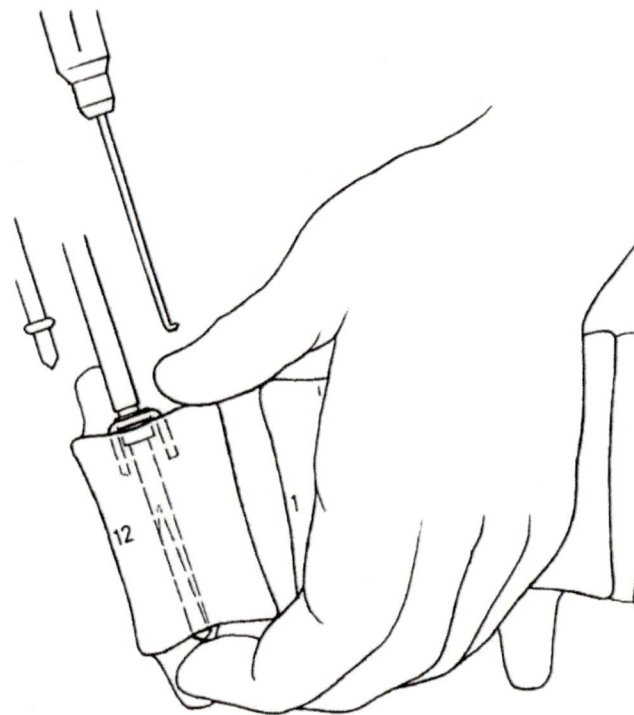

Fig. 44.7 Opening of cortex with a short sharp awl, followed by a long blunt awl, which is pushed through the contralateral cortex. Penetrating awl can be felt with the index finger

ing the discectomies, and it becomes more flexible and more easily correctable. Sometimes more flexibility is needed to make osteotomy of the rib cabs in thoracic spine.

44.5.1.5 Anterior Instrumentation

After exposure of the spine and removal of the disc, insert monoaxial bone screw (Expedium DePuy Synthes) into each vertebral body. The Expedium screws are available in 5 mm and 6 mm diameter. If possible, use a larger screw due to better pull-out strength.

Anatomy dictates whether you can use a single or double rod construct. Instrument the apical vertebra first. Insert a staple and use an awl to create a hole in the side of the vertebral body through the hole of the staple. Direct the hole parallel to the endplates and slightly in a posterior to anterior direction (Fig. 44.7). Impact the awl in the hole. This is the starting hole of the vertebral body screw. It is not necessary to

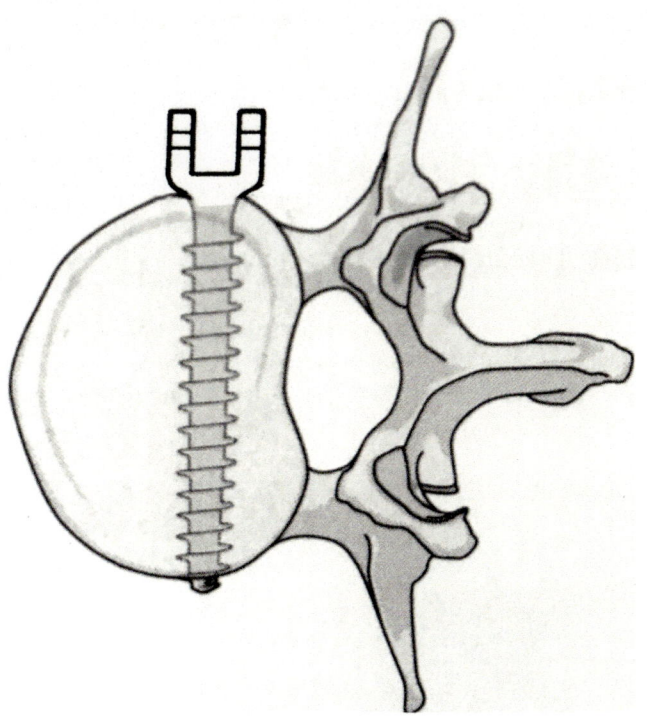

Fig. 44.8 Insertion of bone screw parallel to endplate and in slightly posterior anterior direction

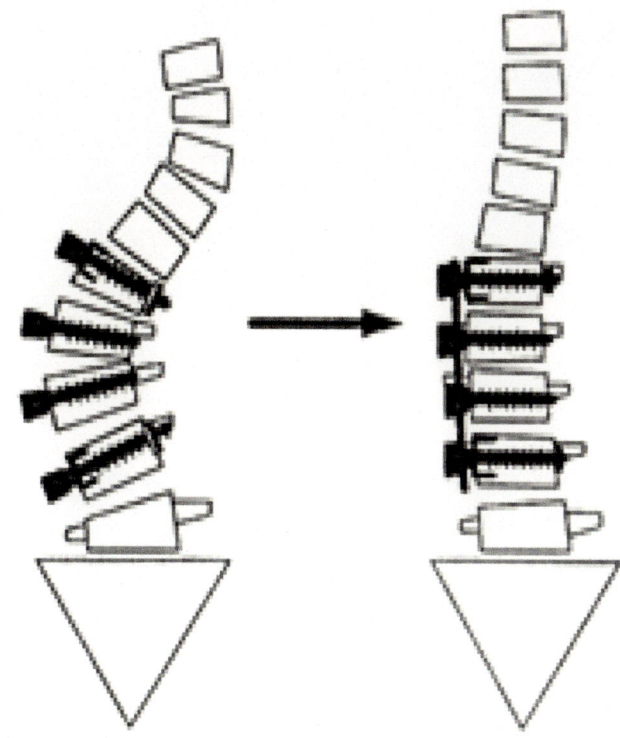

Fig. 44.9 Principles of the anterior correction with compression in a lumbar scoliosis

drill or tap a vertebral body. The screws are self-tapping. With the slotted screwdriver, insert a bone screw of appropriate length through the staple. Direct the screw parallel to the end-plate and to a point on the vertebral body on the other side palpable by the fingertip. Use a fingertip to guide the screw through the vertebral body. The screw should pass completely through the opposite cortex, and the finger should be able to feel one or two threads on the opposite cortex (Fig. 44.8). The screw length is based on the accurate measurement of the width of the vertebral body with a depth gauge. The screws should be placed in a relatively straight line, cephalad to cau-dal. Cut your rod to the length and contour it to maintain nor-mal lumbar lordosis or thoracic kyphosis. Place the rod into the head of the screws on the caudal end of your instrumenta-tion. Then seat it successively in each more proximal screw (Fig. 44.9). Tighten the insert screw enough to hold the rod in place but still allow rotation of the rod. Rotate the rod 90°; after rotation, the disc space opens up. Now place bone graft from the rib or from the bone bank in the anterior aspect of the disc space [14, 17–21]. This helps to prevent any kyphos-ing effect of the instrumentation. Fill the remainder of the disc space with smaller pieces of bone graft.

Obtain further correction of the curve by compressing towards the apical screw. This also helps to lock the bone graft into place. First, tighten the apical screw and then use a compressing device to compress the screws towards the apex

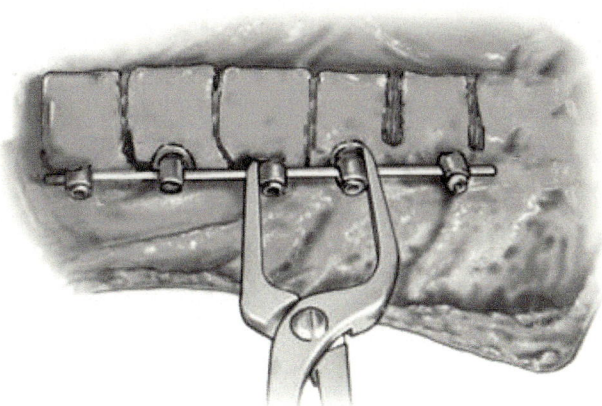

Fig. 44.10 Compression device in a segmental correction of the spine

both proximally and distally (Fig. 44.10). Tighten the insert screws completely to prevent any further rotation. Place remaining bone strips into the disc interspaces and along the area of the periosteal stripping (Figs. 44.11, 44.12a–d, and 44.13a, b).

Suture the pleura over the upper end of the rod. Insert a chest tube in case the thoracic cavity has been entered. Close the chest wall muscle layers in a routine manner.

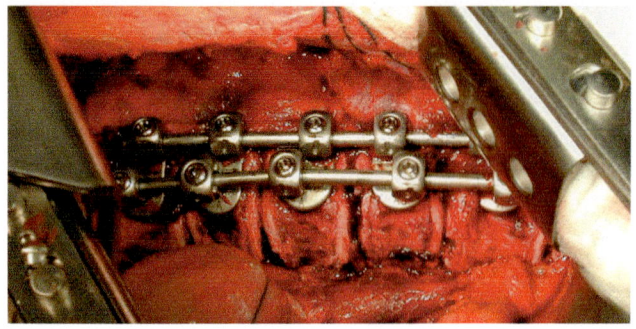

Fig. 44.11 Intraoperative view of corrected deformity with a double-rod construction of thoracolumbar scoliosis

44.6 After Treatment

The chest tube usually is left in place for 48–72 h. It is removed when the drainage decreases to less than 50 ml for two consecutive 8 h periods. The patient is to be kept on bed rest until the chest tube is removed. Afterwards the patient is allowed to stand up without brace given that the bone quality is good and the bone screw has a high fit, if not a TLSO should be used for three up to six months.

A Foley catheter is necessary to monitor urine output because urinary retention is common. An ileus is expected after anterior surgery which usually lasts 2 or 3 days.

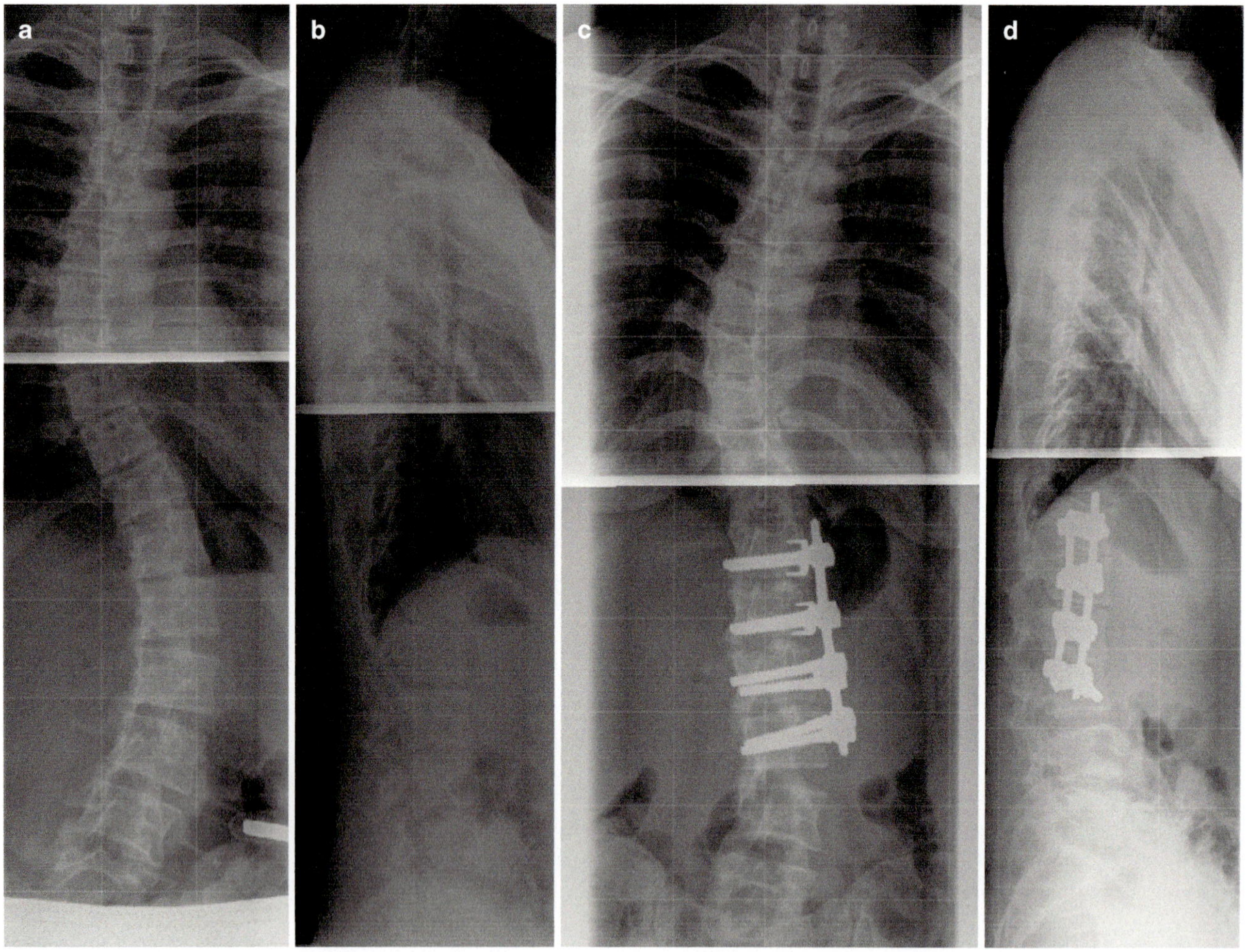

Fig. 44.12 (**a**) Preoperative x-ray in ap view of lumbar curve of 47° in an 18-year-old patient. (**b**) Preoperative x-ray in lateral view in an 18-year-old patient. (**c**) Postoperative x-ray in ap view of a lumbar curve after correction of 10° in an 18-year-old patient. (**d**) Postoperative x-ray in lateral view in an 18-year-old patient

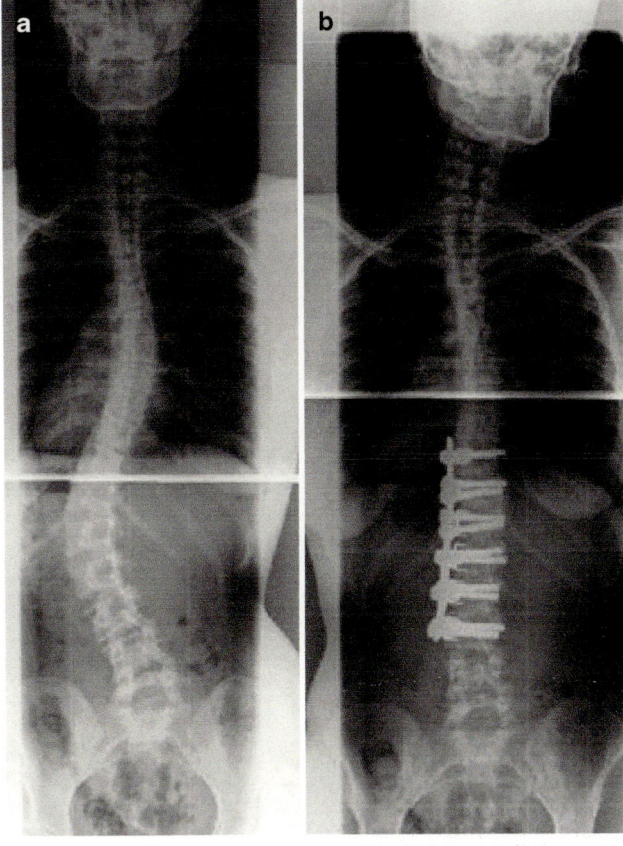

Fig. 44.13 (**a**) Preoperative x-ray in ap view of a thoracolumbar curve of 49° in a 15-year-old patient. (**b**) Postoperative x-ray in ap view of a thoracolumbar curve of 3° in a 15-year-old patient

References

1. Dwyer AF, Newton NC, Sherwood AA. An anterior approach to scoliosis. A preliminary report. Clin Orthop Relat Res. 1996;62:192–202.
2. Zielke K. Ventral derotation spondylodesis. Results of treatment of cases of idiopathic lumbar scoliosis (author's translation). Z Orthop Ihre Grenzgeb. 1982;120(3):320–9.
3. Bullmann V, Halm HF, Niemeyer T. Dual-rod correction and instrumentation of idiopathic scoliosis with the Halm-Zielke instrumentation. Spine. 2003;28:1306–13.
4. Burton DC, Asher MA, Lai SM. Patient-based outcomes analysis of patients with single torsion thoracolumbar-lumbar scoliosis treated with anterior or posterior instrumentation: an average 5- to 9-year follow-up study. Spine. 2002;7:2363–7.
5. Halm H, Liljenqvist U, Niemeyer T. Halm-Zielke instrumentation (Münster anterior double rod system) as an improvement over Zielke-VDS. Surgical method and preliminary results. Z Orthop Ihre Grenzgeb. 1997;135:403–11. In German
6. Halm HF, Liljenqvist U, Niemeyer T. Halm-Zielke instrumentation for primary stable anterior scoliosis surgery: operative technique and 2-year results in ten consecutive adolescent idiopathic scoliosis patients within a prospective clinical trial. Eur Spine J. 1998;7:429–34.
7. Hopf CG, Eysel P, Dubousset J. Operative treatment of scoliosis with Cotrel-Dubousset-Hopf instrumentation. New anterior spinal device. Spine. 1997;22:618–27.
8. Kaneda K, Shono Y, Satoh S. New anterior instrumentation for the man-agement of thoracolumbar and lumbar scoliosis. Application of the Kaneda two-rod system. Spine. 1996;21:1250–61.
9. Kaneda K, Shono Y, Satoh S. Anterior correction of thoracic scoliosis with Kaneda anterior spinal system. A preliminary report. Spine. 1997;22:1358–68.
10. Lenke LG, Betz RR, Haher TR. Multisurgeon assessment of surgical decision-making in adolescent idiopathic scoliosis: curve classification, operative approach, and fusion levels. Spine. 2001;26:2347–53.
11. Lenke LG, Betz RR, Harms J. Adolescent idiopathic scoliosis: a new classi-fication to determine extent of spinal arthrodesis. J Bone Joint Surg Am. 2001;83:1169–81.
12. Richter A, Quante M, Macherei A, Halm H. Die modifizierte primärstabile ventral Derotationsspondylodese mit dem Halm Zielke Instrumentarium (HZI) zur Behandlung der idiopathischen Skoliose. OOT. 2010;2:164–76.
13. Canale ST. Campbell`s operative orthopaedics; 2003. p. 1818–25.
14. Saraph VJ, Krismer M, Wimmer C. Operative treatment of scoliosis with Kaneda anterior spine system. Spine. 2005;30:1616–20.
15. Turi M, Johnston CE, Richards BS. Anterior correction of idiopathic scoliosis using TSRH instrumentation. Spine. 1993;18:417–22.
16. Vavruch L, Brink RC, Malmqvist M, et al. H surgical outcomes of anterior versus posterior fusion in Lenke type 1 adolescent idiopathic scoliosis. Spine. 2019;2019:14.
17. Rajpal S, Resnick DK. Rod cantilever techniques. Neurosurgery. 2008;63:157–62.
18. Betz RR, Harms J, Clements DH III. Comparison of anterior and posterior instrumentation for correction of adolescent thoracic idiopathic scoliosis. Spine. 1999;24:225–39.
19. Cotrel Y, Dubousset J, Guillaumat M. New universal instrumentation in spinal surgery. Clin Orthop Relat Res. 1988;227:10–23.
20. Giehl JP, Zielke K, Hack HP. Die ventrale Derotationsspondylodese nach Zielke. Orthopedic. 1989;18:101–17.
21. Kim YJ, Lenke LG, Bridwell KH. Prospective pulmonary function compari-son of anterior spinal fusion in adolescent idiopathic scoliosis: thoracotomy versus thoracoabdominal approach. Spine. 2008;33:1055–60.

Dynamic Scoliosis Correction: A Motion-Preserving Surgical Technique for Scoliosis

45

Per Trobisch

45.1 Introduction and Core Messages

The standard treatment for idiopathic scoliosis exceeding more than 40° at skeletal maturity is spinal fusion. However, motion-preserving surgical techniques are emerging. A decade ago, Randy Betz and colleagues published a series of papers sharing their experience with Vertebral Body Stapling (VBS) [1–3]. Although, short-term results were very promising, only few selected patients were considered good candidates. These were skeletally very immature patients with Risser stage 2 or less, as well as patients with moderate curves that do not exceed 35° in the thoracic spine or 40° in the lumbar spine [3, 4]. Implant strength was considered being responsible for failures, and in 2011, Nitinol staples that were used for VBS were replaced with stronger implants—a specific anterior screw-cord construct (Fig. 45.1). In accordance to VBS, the new technique has been popularized as Vertebral Body Tethering (VBT) [4, 5]. Since 2011, approximately 2.000 patients have received this surgical treatment worldwide. While the indication window was kept very narrow in the first few years, it is not continuously widening. Today, even more rigid and severe curves that exceed 60° and do not bend down to less than 30° or patients that are closer to skeletal maturity (Risser 3 and 4) can be operated. In some cases, disk releases may be required to facilitate curve correction. Disk releases can be considered as de-tethering technique. Therefore, some surgeons in the United States prefer the term Anterior Scoliosis Correction (ASC) over VBT. In Germany, anterior scoliosis correction can easily be confused with the very popular Ventral Derotation Spondylodesis. Therefore, we have used the term Dynamic Scoliosis Correction (DSC) in Germany since its introduction. Motion-preserving surgery mainly uses two ways for curve correction following the Hueter–Volkmann principle—growth modulation and osseous remodeling. Growth plates that are compressed decrease growth, whereas distracted growth plates accelerate growth [4]. DSC therefore reverses the effect that scoliosis has on the natural history.

45.2 Indication

VBT is a growth modifying technique; therefore, it should be performed before skeletal maturity. The ideal candidate still has to be defined. In the early phases, VBT was mainly indicated for patients with significant remaining growth. Some surgeons recommended VBT only for patients with open triradiate cartilage. Patients with curve magnitudes between 40° and 60° who had good flexibility were considered to be most suitable. Additionally, structural lumbar curves represented a contraindication because of the unknown effect that VBT may have had on the sagittal profile, potentially reducing lumbar lordosis [4]. However, with increasing experience, as well as improved surgical techniques, including the introduction of disk releases and derotation techniques, surgeons are now widening their indication criteria and also changed the term VBT to ASC (in the US) or DSC (in Germany). Nowadays, even double major curves, as well as rigid curves and curves with more than 60° are still being indicated for surgery (Fig. 45.2). If the severity of a curve allows to be monitored, we recommend DSC at Risser stage 2 or 3 as long as the curve has not exceeded 60°. In these

P. Trobisch (✉)
Eifelklinik St. Brigida, Department of Spine Surgery, Simmerath, Germany
e-mail: per.trobisch@artemed.de

© Springer-Verlag GmbH Germany 2023
U. Vieweg, F. Grochulla (eds.), *Manual of Spine Surgery*, https://doi.org/10.1007/978-3-662-64062-3_45

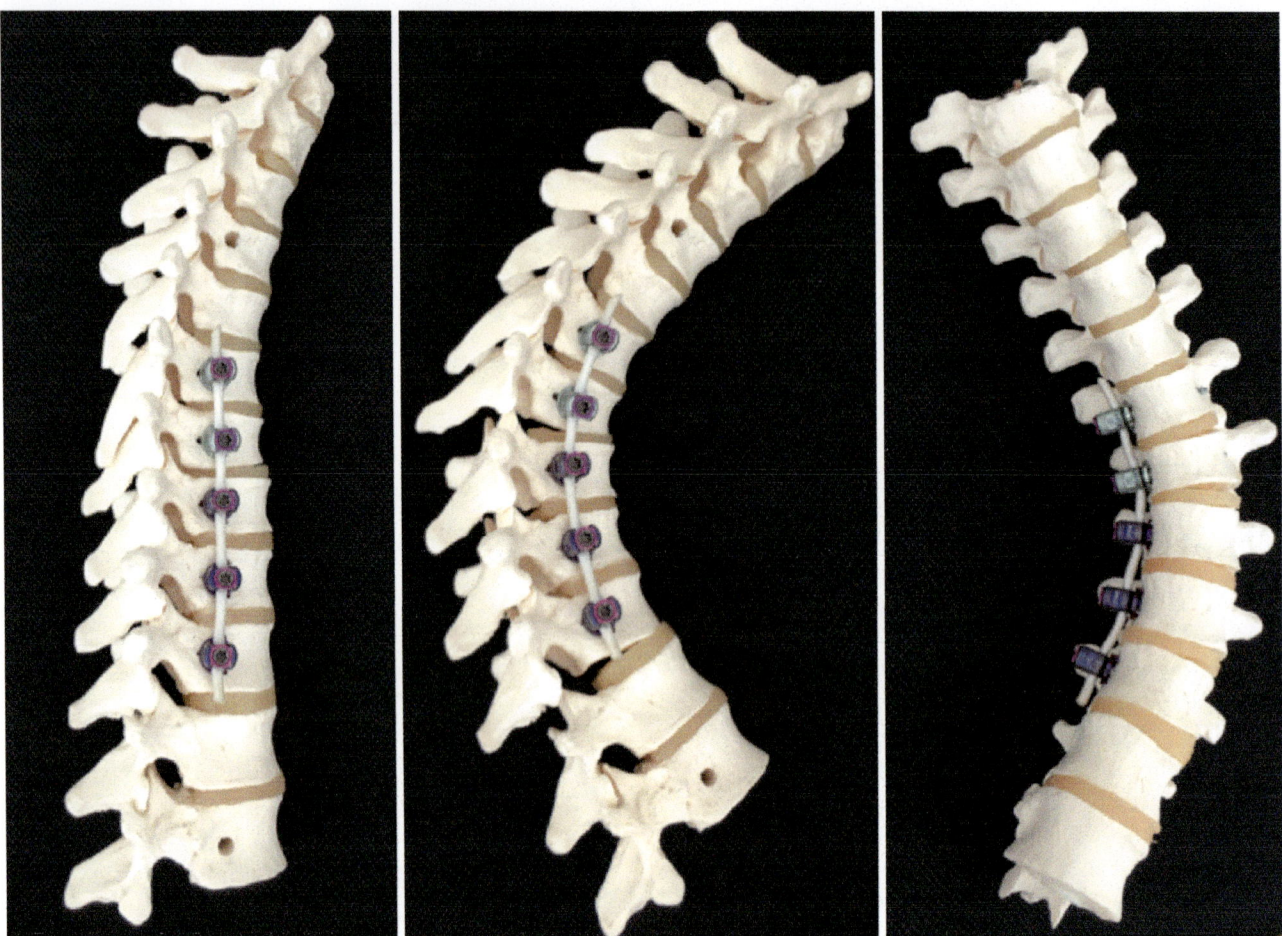

Fig. 45.1 Model of a thoracic spine that is "tethered" with an anterior screw-cord combination. Left: neutral position, Middle: flexed position, Right: right-bent position

cases, overcorrection can be eliminated as potential complication, disk releases are usually not yet required and correction of scoliosis to less than 30° at skeletal maturity is very likely. We also recommend DSC for lumbar curves (Lenke type 5) that exceed 40° or secondary curves that can be classified as Lenke lumbar-C modifier. In our opinion, these patients benefit even more from non-fusion surgery to prevent spinal fusion ending in the lumbar spine. With the compressive force being lateral, we have not seen a kyphosing effect in our patients (Fig. 45.3).

So far, we have not faced any absolute contraindications for DSC except maybe significant pulmonary restrictions. While patients with left-sided thoracic curves and right-sided lumbar curves have been considered as being contraindicated during our early phase, we have now found that surgical treatment is not much more complicated as the aorta usually falls anterior and the liver can be manually retracted (Fig. 45.4). At this point, we do not recommend DSC for congenital or neuromuscular scoliosis but consider these patients as potential candidates in the future.

45.3 Surgical Technique

45.3.1 Set-up and Positioning

Double-lumen intubation as well as intraoperative electrophysiologic neuromonitoring is recommended. Patients are positioned in a strict lateral position with the convex side facing up. We use soft bolsters under the axilla and the pelvis. The patient is fixed to table with tapes. Pre-operative X-rays are supposed to confirm correct lateral positioning and to provide an estimation of curve correction that is achieved with positioning.

45.3.2 Approach

We prefer a mini-open approach to the spine. Thoracic curves often require instrumentation from T5 to T12. For these cases, we use one 5 cm long mini-open approach above T11 and another one above T7. Usually three vertebrae can be

Fig. 45.2 Pre- and postoperative radiograph after single-stage double-sided DSC for a double major curve in a 13-year-old girl with Risser stage 0

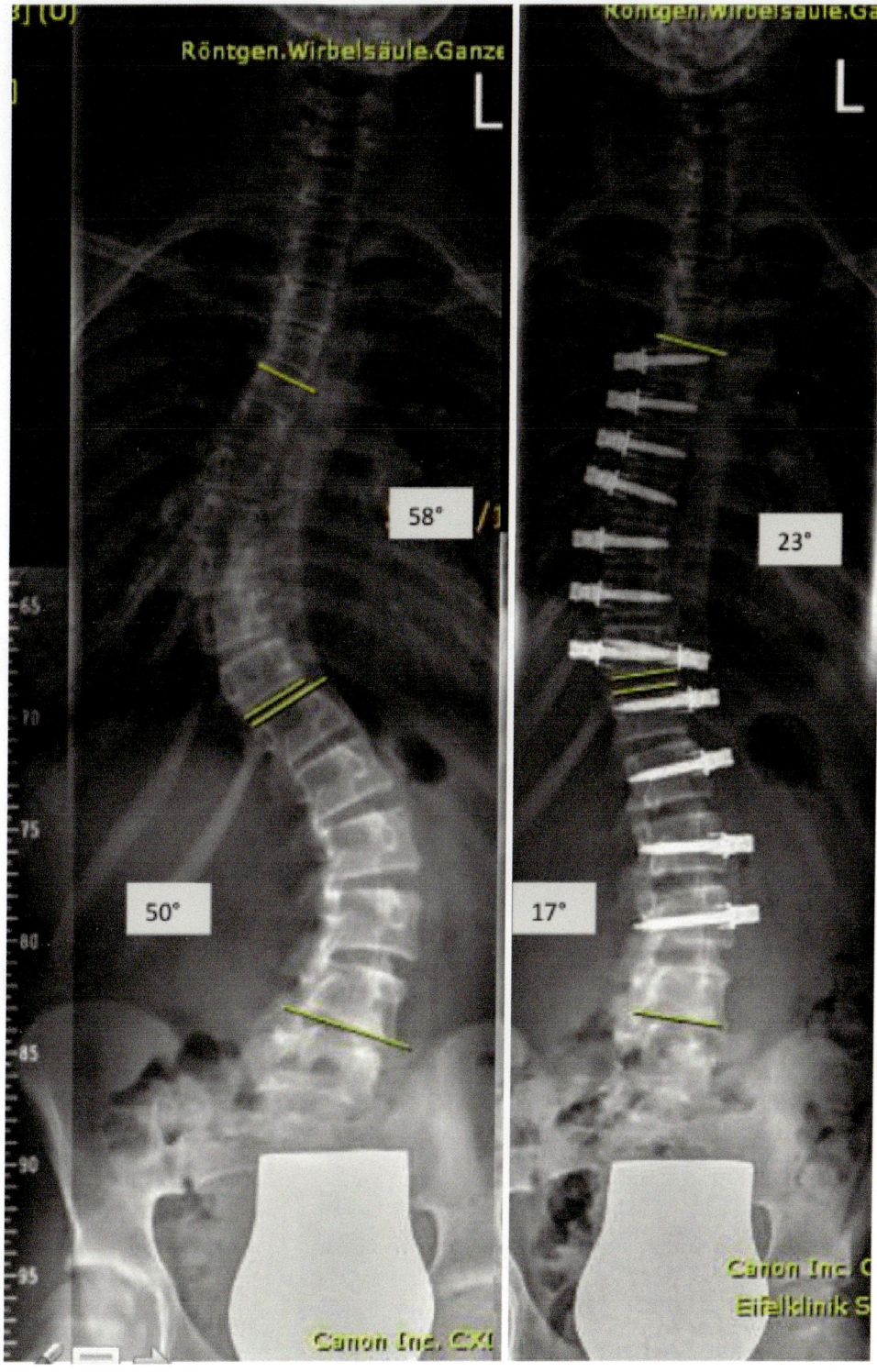

instrumented through one approach (e.g. T6-T12). Additionally, we use one to three thoracoscopic portals to improve visualization and retraction of the lung and the diaphragm, as well as instrumentation of T5 (Fig. 45.5). Lumbar curves often required instrumentation from T10 to L3. For these cases, we recommend a mini-open retroperitoneal approach for instrumentation of L2 to L3 (L4 when required). The psoas is temporarily retracted posterior. Transpsoas instrumentation is not recommended. Instrumentation of L1 and higher is performed through a mini-open intercostal approach, usually above T11 or T12. A diaphragm split will help with instrumentation of L1.

Fig. 45.3 Lateral radiograph pre- and 1 year post-operatively of a 13-year-old patient (Risser 3) with DSC from T10 to L3. Instrumentation into the lumbar spine has not shown to have a kyphosing effect

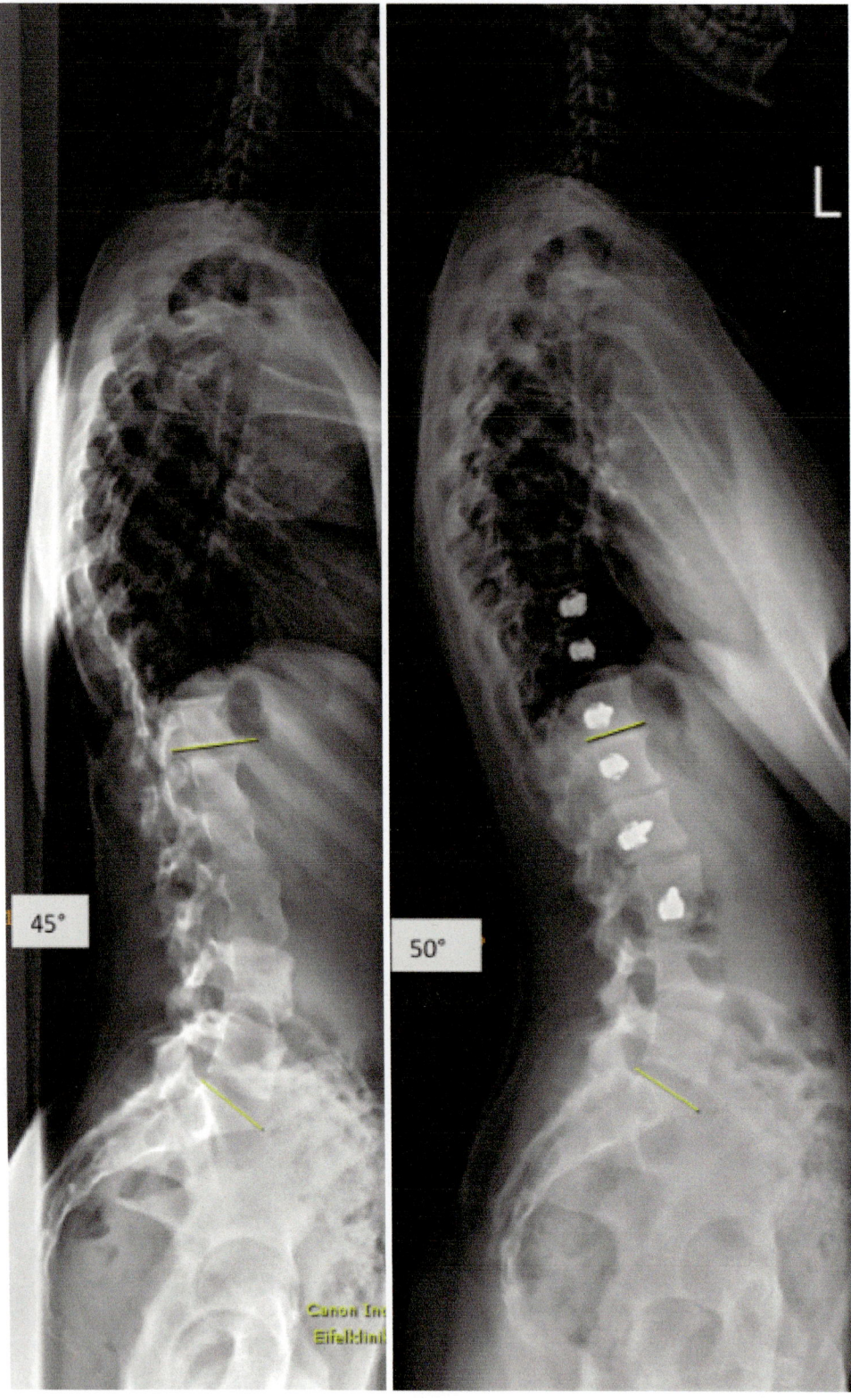

Fig. 45.4 Pre- and postoperative radiograph of a 12-year-old girl (Risser 0) after left-sided DSC from T7 to L1

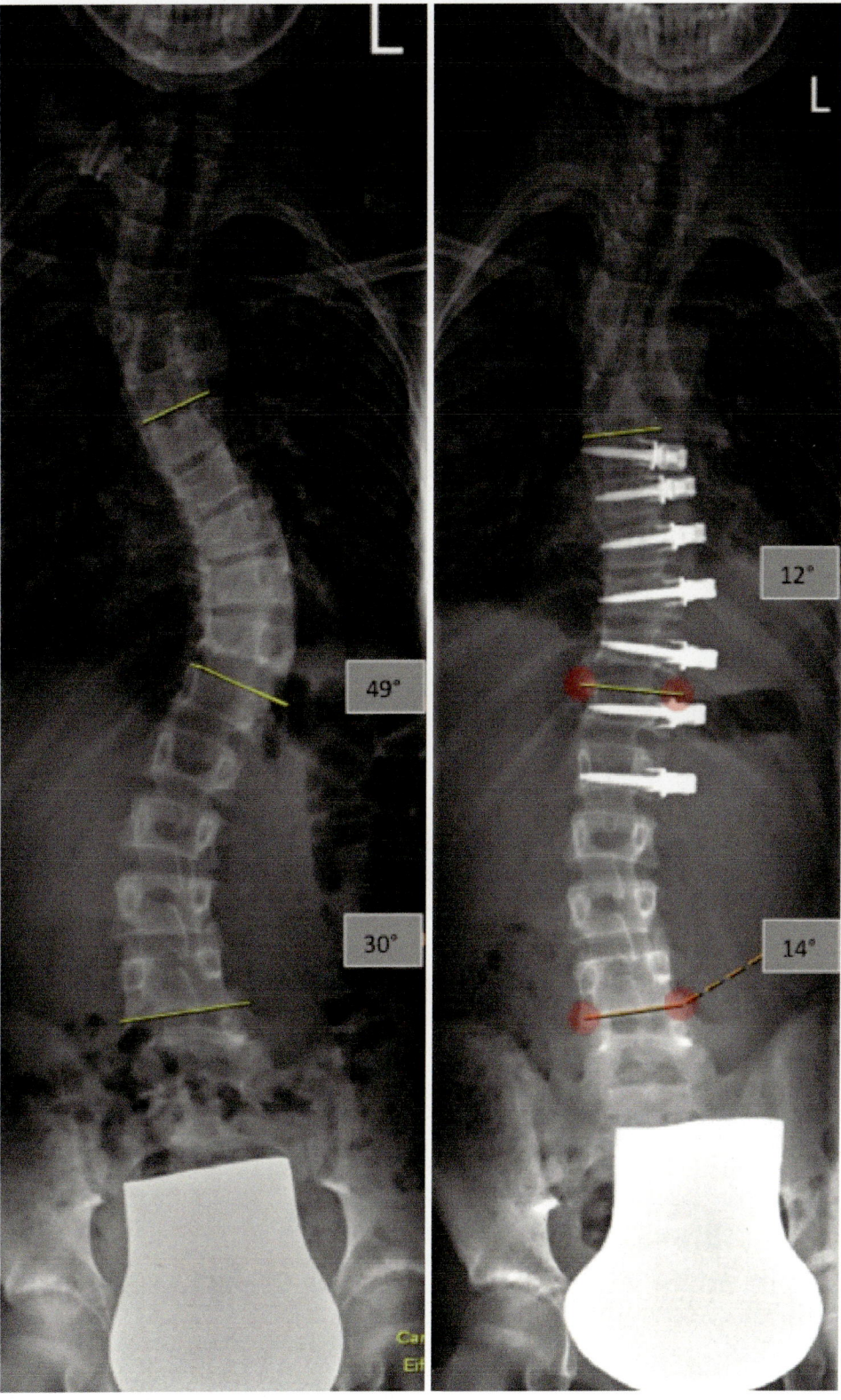

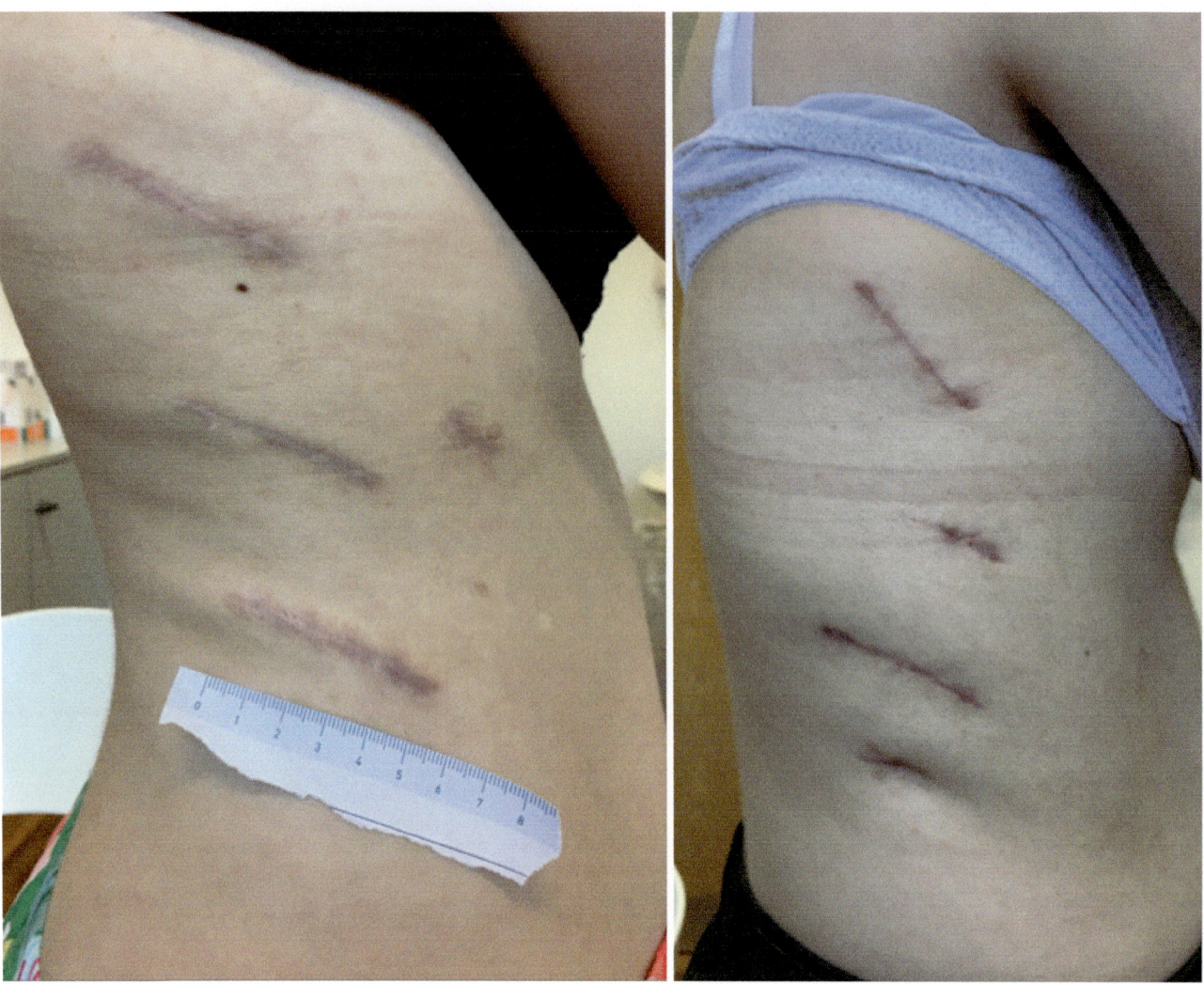

Fig. 45.5 Left: 6 months after instrumentation from T6 to L2 using three mini-open incisions of 5 cm length each plus one thoracoscopic portal; right: 6 weeks after instrumentation from T5 to T12 using two mini-open incisions plus two thoracoscopic portals

45.3.3 Instrumentation

A staple is required to decrease proximal screw windshielding. The screw canal is prepared with a probe under fluoroscopic guidance. Markers on the probe will define screw lengths. Meticulous screw length measurement is required in the mid thoracic spine due to the vicinity of the thoracic Aorta on the left that is not visualized during right-sided surgery. However, bicortical screw purchase is required (Fig. 45.6). Screw entry point is the center of a vertebral body except for apical levels where the entry point is more posterior with the screw aiming anterior. The cord is locked into the screw from cranial to caudal with segmental compression and derotation of the apical levels. The goal is to have a level disk between each screw. For very rigid curves, one or more disk releases may be required. A small window is cut into the lateral annulus from the anterior longitudinal ligament to the pedicle. The window is supposed to close after segmental compression. The cord is cut with a knife or a cord-cutter approximately 1 cm caudal of the lowest screw.

45.3.4 Instrumented Levels

The upper instrumented vertebra (UIV) equals the upper end vertebrae—usually T5 or T6 for thoracic curves and T10 or T11 for lumbar curves. The lower instrumented vertebra (LIV) equals the touching vertebra—the vertebra that is just touching the central sacral vertical line. LIV for thoracic curves usually is at T11 or T12 but can be as low as L2 in patients with severe trunk shift. LIV for lumbar curves usually is L3 and sometimes L4. For patients with bilateral curves that need to be instrumented, double-sided instrumentation of the transitional level is required (Fig. 45.2).

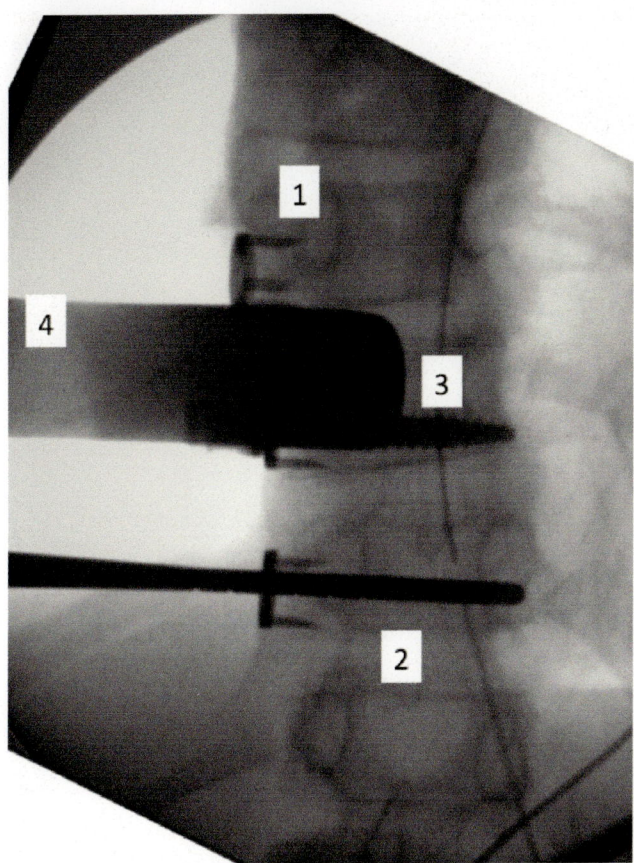

Fig. 45.6 Intraoperative radiograph: (1) Staple, (2) Staple with probe for canal preparation, (3) Staple and screw with bicortical purchase, (4) Retractor for lung and diaphragm protection

45.3.5 Postoperative Care

Patients are monitored in the intensive care unit as long as a chest tube is required. Chest tubes are removed when the output decreases to less than 200 cc in 24 h, which is achieved in most patients on the first or second postoperative day (POD). We recommend early mobilization; most patients walk on POD 1, with walking on stairs on POD 3 to 5. We initially use patient-controlled analgesia but switch to oral analgesics after 2 or 3 days. Patients are discharged between POD 4 and 7. We do not give restrictions for weight bearing or spinal motion.

References

1. Betz RR, Kim J, D'Andrea L. An innovative technique of vertebral body stapling for the treatment of patients with adolescent idiopathic scoliosis: a feasibility, safety, and utility study. Spine. 2003;28:255–65.
2. Betz RR, Ranade A, Samdani AF. Vertebral body stapling. A fusionless treatment option for a growing child with moderate idiopathic scoliosis. Spine. 2010;35:169–76.
3. Trobisch PD, Samdani A, Cahill P, Betz RR. Vertebral body stapling as an alternative in the treatment of idiopathic scoliosis. Oper Orthop Traumatol. 2011;23:227–31.
4. Jain V, Lykissas M, Trobisch P, et al. Surgical aspects of spinal growth modulation in scoliosis correction. Instr Course Lect. 2014;63:335–44.
5. Baroncini A, Trobisch P. Wachstumsmodelierende und nichtversteifende Skoliosechirurgie. Medizinisch-Orthopädische Technik. 2017;2:7–10.

Vertical Expandable Prosthetic Titanium Rib (VEPTR)

46

Cornelius Wimmer and Uwe Vieweg

46.1 Introduction and Core Messages

VEPTR stands for *Vertical Expandable Prosthetic Titanium Rib*. The purpose of implantation of a VEPTR is to correct deformities of the thorax and the spine in children. The VEPTR is a special form of the devices known as growing rods. In 1993, Campbell published an overview of the use of the VEPTR in the treatment of thoracic insufficiency syndrome (TIS). The device consists of a curved expandable prosthetic titanium rib with several holes in a row that allows it to be fixed at the desired length. In general, 6 months after initial implantation, intervention is necessary to extend the device. It is fixed in place between two ribs (*rib-to-rib*), a rib and the lumbar spine (*rib-to-lumbar lamina*) or between a rib and the ilium (*rib-to-ilium*). The correction of scoliosis is not achieved by means of direct effects on the individual vertebrae requiring correction but rather the device achieves the desired outcome by means of acting on the rib thorax [1]. In very young children, a VEPTR device can be used for growth-correcting treatment of congenital scoliosis [1–3]. Typically, there are three different forms of fixation. In cases of distortion of the thorax, thoracotomy on the concave side is used for osteotomy of rib synostosis and opening of the ribs with the help of a rib spreader. The device is then introduced as a rib-to-rib implant. In cases of thoracic lumbar distortion, a laminar hook is used to introduce the device as a rib-to-lumbar spine implant. In addition, it is also possible to fix the device to the pelvis.

46.2 Indications and Contraindications

46.2.1 Indications

Use of the device is indicated in [1, 4, 5]:

1. Primary thoracic insufficiency syndrome (TIS) due to a three-dimensional deformity of the thorax.
   - Thoracic congenital scoliosis with concave-fused ribs.
   - Progressive congenital scoliosis of the thorax with concave-fused ribs or flail chest as a result of missing ribs.
   - Progressive congenital neurogenic or idiopathic scoliosis of the thorax without rib anomalies.
   - Hypoplastic thorax syndrome.
   - Acquired posterolateral chest wall defects.
2. Secondary thoracic insufficiency due to lumbar kyphosis (non-gibbus).
3. Early onset scoliosis (EOS).

46.2.2 Contraindications

Contraindications are [1]:

- Absent diaphragmatic function.
- Completed bone growth.
- Severe kyphosis >70° per Cobb.
- Children over the age of 10 years.

C. Wimmer
Department of Spine Surgery, Trauma Center, Trostberg, Germany

Department of Orthopaedic Surgery, University of Innsbruck, Innsbruck, Austria
e-mail: ProfWimmer@t-online.de

U. Vieweg (✉)
Department of Conservative and Surgical Spine Therapy with Interdisciplinary Spinal Deformities Centre and Rummelsberg Sectional Center, Hospital Rummelsberg, Schwarzenbruck, Germany
e-mail: uwe.vieweg@sana.de

© Springer-Verlag GmbH Germany 2023
U. Vieweg, F. Grochulla (eds.), *Manual of Spine Surgery*, https://doi.org/10.1007/978-3-662-64062-3_46

- Children aged under 6 months.
- Known allergy to any of the materials of the implant.
- Infections at the site of surgery.
- Inadequate soft tissue for coverage of the VEPTR.
- Inadequate strength of bone for attachment of the VEPTR.
- Absence of proximal and distal ribs for attachment of the VEPTR.

46.3 Technical Prerequisites

46.3.1 Implant

VEPTR II device: vertical expandable prosthetic titanium rib II (see Fig. 46.1: rib-to-rib, Fig. 46.2 rib-to-lumbar spine).

46.3.2 Diagnosis

Required for diagnosis and surgical planning are x-rays of the entire spinal column, CT and MRT images of the spinal column, cardiological examination including an electrocardiogram and pulmonary function test.

46.3.3 Intraoperative Set-up

Required instruments are a C-arm, double lumen tube, a neuromonitoring system, a Bülau drain catheter, a sucker device with thin lead, a bipolar coagulator, special spreader and compression forceps for the introduction and expansion of the implant.

46.4 Technique

46.4.1 Patient Positioning

Place the patient in a lateral decubitus position similar to that required for a standard thoracotomy. To protect against brachial plexus injury, do not extend the shoulder more than 90°. If a hybrid construct is being implanted, it is also possible to place the patient in the prone position for better mobilisation of the intercostal muscles.

46.4.2 Implantation Procedure

- Make a J-shaped thoracotomy incision without disrupting the periosteum overlying the ribs.

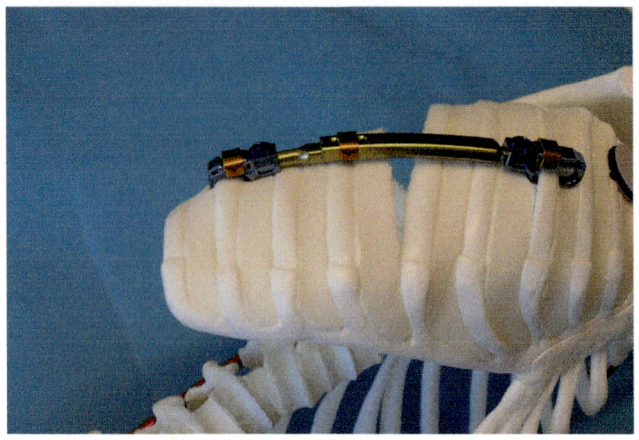

Fig. 46.1 Rib to rib. The VEPRT is attached to a superior rib and to an inferior rib: (1) Rib hook cap, (2) Closure for extension Bar, (3) Rib hook, (4) Proximal extension, and (5) Distal extension

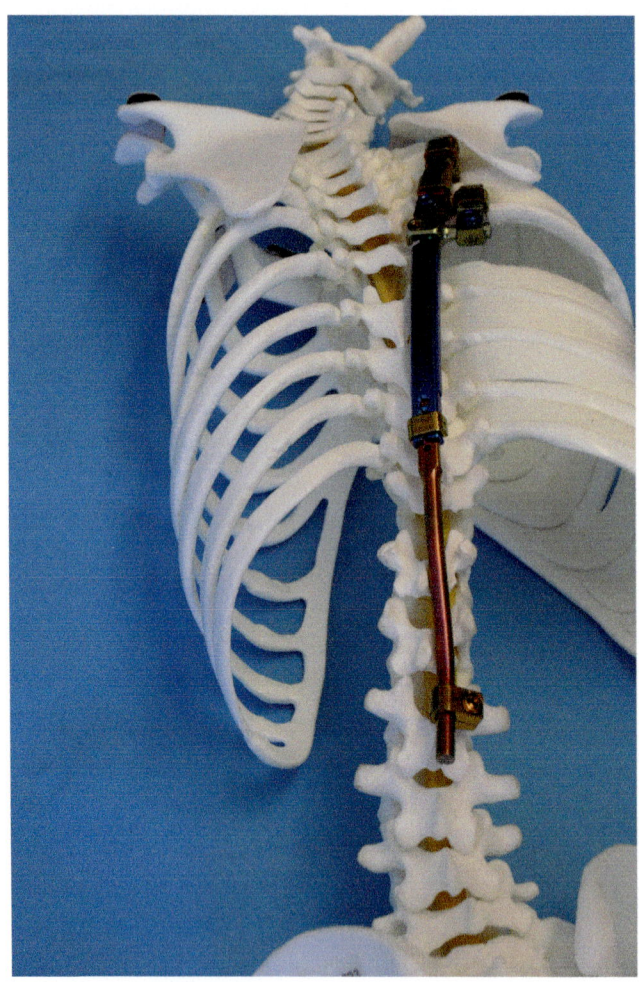

Fig. 46.2 Rib-to-lumbar lamina. The VEPRT is attached to a rib and the lumbar spine: (1) Rib hook cap, (2) Closure for extension, (3) Rib hook, (4) Proximal extension, and (5) Distal extension

- Retract the skin flaps. Continue the incision and elevate the paraspinal muscles medially only to the tips of the transverse processes. Gently elevate the scapula to expose the middle and posterior scalene muscle.

46.5 Rib-to-Rib (see Fig. 46.1)

- First insert the cranial implant. Identify the cranial rib that is to serve as the cranial attachment point. Mark the position and verify by means of radiographic imaging. *Note*: Because of the risk of brachial plexus impingement, do not choose the first rib as the superior point of attachment.
- Make a 1 cm incision into the intercostal muscles both above and below the position for the planned attachment to the cranial rib. Use a periosteal elevator to carefully elevate the periosteum of the rib next to the lung. Take care not to damage the soft tissue surrounding the rib so as to preserve rib vascularity and the neurovascular bundle. Use a trial rib hook to prepare the rib for the rib hook. *Note:* In the case of smaller patients, in whom a small rib hook is to be used employ the small trial rib hook for preparation.
- Select a rib hook in the size determined by the trial rib hook. Using the rib hook holder, position the underside of the rib hook in the space between periosteum and rib and turn the hook until it sits correctly.
- Select a rib hook cap appropriate to the anatomy of the patient.
- With the help of holding forceps, insert the rib hook cap into the intercostal space above the rib, rotate the cap distally until it slots into the rib hook. Ensure hook and cap are correctly aligned.
- Put a closure for the extension bar into the lock impactor. To lock the rib hook/rib cap combination together, precisely align the holes of the rib cap and rib hook. Use a hammer to firmly strike the impactor to fix the closure in place.
- Attach the 2 ft. for the rib distractor to the retractor. Using this assembly, distract the ribs as necessary. Alternatively, use a bone spreader to carefully distract the chest wall at the site of the opening wedge thoracostomy.
- If distraction proves difficult, additional resection of medially fused ribs may be necessary. Only resect visible bone directly next to the spine.
- Measure the distance between the expandable portion of the construct to determine the required proximal extension. **Note:** Measure the expandable portion over the dis-tracted thorax between the cranial rib and the thoraco-lumbar attachment point (rib-to-lamina/ilium) or between cranial and caudal rib (rib-to-rib).
- Cut and contour the rod to the size of the required proximal extension.
- Retain at least 11 mm of the straight rod to ensure that this section of the proximal extension will sit correctly in the rib hook. Use the measuring instrument to verify that the rod section is long enough to be seated securely in the rib hook. Any remaining rod can be cut and/or contoured to fit the anatomy of the patient. Select a distal extension that corresponds to the size of the proximal extension.
- Use the trial rod to determine the contour of the rod section of the distal extension. Do not bend the T-shaped end of the distal extension that connects with the proximal extension. Bend only the rod section of the distal extension using the rod bender. Alternatively, the bending irons and the rod benders can be used to contour the frontal section. Cut the rod section to the required length using the rod cutter. **Note:** If implanting a rib-to-rib construct, the rod sections of the proximal and distal extensions must have a length of at least 11 mm to ensure that they will sit correctly in the rib hook.
- Before introducing the distal extension, insert it in the proximal extension so that the caudal hole of the proximal extension is directly above the hole in the furthest caudal position of the distal extension.
- Using the offset impactor, put a closure for the extension bar in place in the hole. Gently tap the impactor with a hammer to seat the closure in place. Ensure the closure is correctly seated.

46.5.1 Rib-to-lamina or Ilium (see Fig. 46.2)

- Make a 4 cm paraspinal incision on the concave side of the curve of the lumbar interspace selected preoperatively.
- Use the lamina feeler to separate the ligamentum flavum unilaterally from the underside of the lamina to provide for good anchorage of the lamina hook on the bone; make sure the interspinal ligament remains intact. Resect the ligamentum flavum to provide passage for the hook. Select an appropriate lamina hook.
- Attach the hook pointing downwards with the adjustment screw in the most lateral position. Use the lamina hook holding forceps to position the hook in the required site on the lumbar lamina.

- If necessary, the hook can be additionally secured using heavy, non-absorbable suture thread wrapped around the posterior spinous process. Make a 4 cm longitudinal incision slightly laterally to the posterior superior iliac spine. Identify the posterior third and middle third of the iliac crest. Make a 1 cm transverse incision in the mid substance of the apophysis so that there are equal cartilage layers above and below the incision. Pass the periosteal elevator through the incision in the apophysis and widen it to form a tunnel and then pass the elevator along the medial cortical surface of the iliac crest until the tip of the elevator is just lateral to the sacroiliac joint. Select an appropriate ala-hook or S-rod. If using an S-rod, cut the rod to the appropriate length and contour as necessary. Use the small hexagonal screwdriver to attach an extension connector or a parallel connector to the ala-hook or S-rod.
- With the help of the rod holder, position the ala-hook or S-hook on the iliac crest medial to the wing of the ilium. Attaching to the lamina hook (rib-to-lumbar lamina)/ala-hook or S-rod (rib-to-ilium).
- From the proximal incision, create a tunnel through the paraspinal muscles to just above the caudal attachment point. Insert the end of the distal extension in the tip of a no. 20 thoracic catheter and carefully pass this proximal to distal to the caudal attachment point.
- If attaching to a lamina hook (rib-to-lumbar lamina construct), guide the distal extension into the lamina hook.
- If attaching to an ala-hook or S-hook (rib-to-ilium construct), insert the distal extension into the extension connector or parallel connector. Use the small hexagonal screwdriver to tighten the screws of the extension connector or parallel connector.

46.6   Postoperative Care

Patients with an implanted VEPTR device should not be braced. Patients may require additional wound protection to prevent inadvertent rubbing or bumping of the wound.

46.7   Complications

Unfortunately, the initial enthusiasm with which this technique of spine-sparing deformity correction was welcomed has progressively subsided with the increasing number of reports on complications, including the detection of extraspinal ossifications along the implants and across ribs [5] (Figs. 46.3, 46.4, and 46.5).

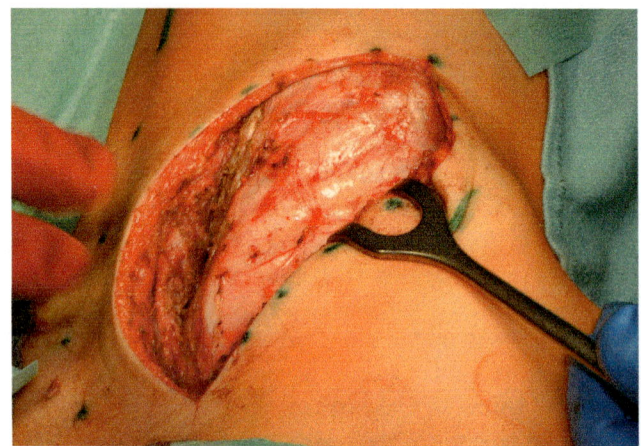

Fig. 46.3 Frontal radiograph of the spine of a 5-year-old boy with a progressive neuromuscular scoliosis

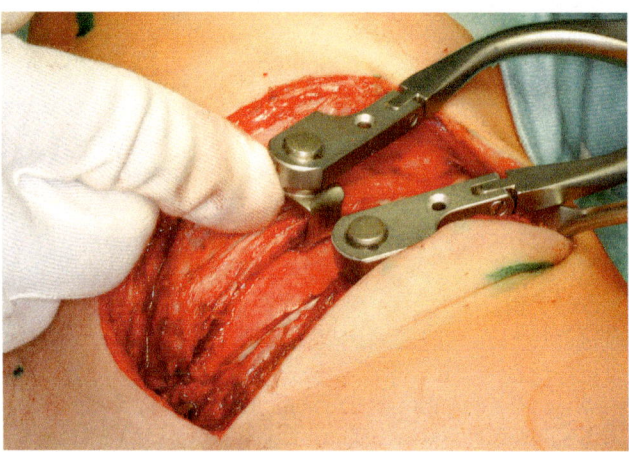

Fig. 46.4 Frontal radiograph 12 months after initial implantation of a rib-to lamina construct (VEPTR)

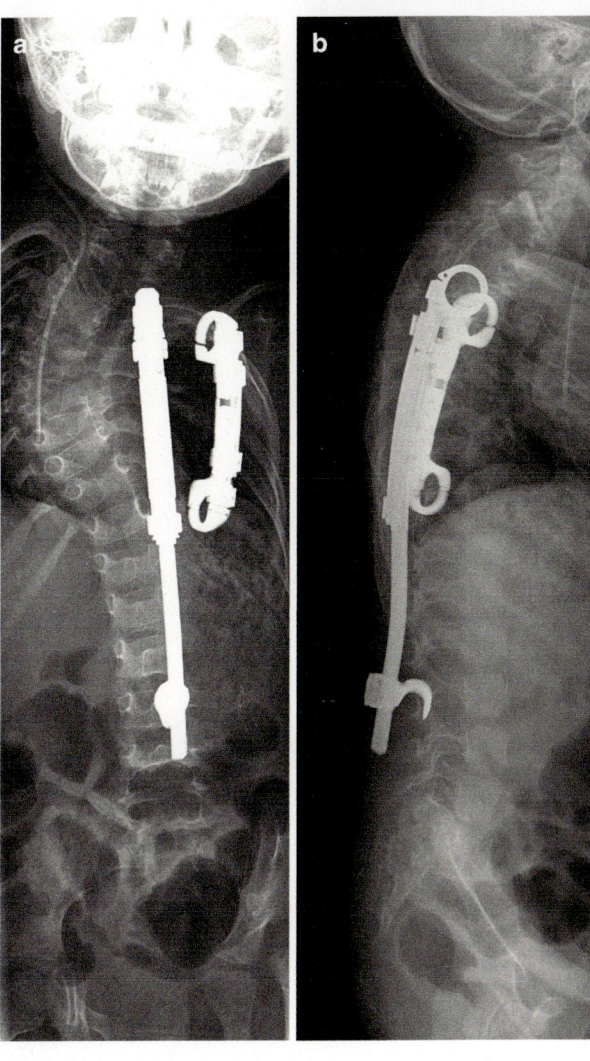

Fig. 46.5

References

1. Wimmer C, Wallnoefer P, Pfandlsteiner T. Operative treatment of scolioses with the VEPTR instrumentation. Oper Orthop Traumatol. 2010;22(2):123–36. in German
2. Campbell RM Jr, Smith MD, Mayes TC, et al. The characteristics of thoracic insufficiency syndrome associated with fused ribs and congenital scoliosis. J Bone Joint Surg A. 2003;85–A(3):399–408.
3. Campbell RM Jr. VEPTR: past experience and the future of VEPTR principles. Eur Spine J. 2013;22(Suppl 2):106–17.
4. Drebor RS, Katsarov A. Poland syndrome: use of vertical expandable prosthetic titanium rib system before walking age-a case report. Surg J. 2016;2:e91–5.
5. Studler D, Haßler C. Long term outcome of vertical expandable prosthetic titanium rib treatment in children with early onset scoliosis. Ann Transl Med. 2020;8(25):1–7.

Part VI

Posterior Thoracic Spine

Overview of Surgical Techniques and Implants

Paulo Tadeu Maia Cavali

47.1 Introduction and Core Messages

Currently, the instrumentation of thoracic spine is a rigid construction. There is no dynamic instrumentation system for the thoracic spine, except for early onset scoliosis, where growing systems can be applied. This means that achieving an arthrodesis is the goal of an ideal spine stabilization, and the use of implants does not substitute the procedure of bone grafting. Many factors are involved in selecting the type of system (screws, hooks, wires, plates, rods, etc.) and function (tension band, bridge fixation, buttressing, derotation, compression, etc.) to be employed. The surgeon has to always understand the following factors: surgeon familiarity with techniques, host bone quality, mechanism of injury, direction of instability, degree of instability, expected level of patient loading, graft bone quality, availability of implants, necessity of postoperative immobilization, and time of tissue healing. Harrington in the 1960s developed the first generation of spinal instrumentation using a hook-based distraction, Luque in the 1970s and 1980s developed the second generation of instrumentation, using a segment fixation technique with sublaminar wires, and Cotrel and Dubousset in the 1980s first brought up rigid segmental hook-based fixation which gave rise to all types of implants using screws and hooks with enormous biomechanical versatility [1]. The objectives of this chapter are to discuss the different implants and different techniques for the treatment of scoliosis, kyphosis, and fracture.

47.2 Implants

The implants employed in the posterior thoracic spine constructs are wires, hooks, and pedicle screw systems from different companies (see Fig. 47.1a, b).

47.2.1 Wiring Systems

Although the sublaminar wiring techniques are no longer common in the thoracic spine, a number of wire-rod techniques continue to be routinely employed. The Luque technique is the most common and employs sublaminar wires in each vertebra as additional anchors. These wires are then wrapped around rods of nonrigid segmental spine constructs. Indications commonly include the neuromuscular scoliosis (see Fig. 47.2a, b), scoliosis including a thoracic lordosis and some cases of osteoporotic spine, where they are used as a hybrid construct with pedicle screw. Wiring techniques do not provide axial stability, and they are a poor choice for stabilization of pathologic processes including anterior column insufficiency such as tumors and fractures. Another limitation of these techniques is the lacking rotation correction of scoliosis. In addition, these methods have a high risk of iatrogenic neurologic injury with the sublaminar wires passage being in the spinal canal and moving there during the fixation and reduction maneuvers. The contraindications to wiring system are patients with kyphosis or canal stenosis and those related to biomechanic insufficiencies.

47.2.2 Hooks

There are a variety of hooks with different characteristics. Basically, three types of hooks can be used: pedicle hooks, laminar hooks, and transverse process hooks (see Fig. 47.3). Pedicle hooks, resting on the lamina of the instrumented vertebrae and the superior articular process

P. T. M. Cavali (✉)
Department of Scoliosis os Hospital AACD-Sao Paulo,
Sao Paulo, Brazil
e-mail: paulo.escolioseaacd@uol.com.br

Fig. 47.1 (**a**) Sublaminar wires. The Luque instrumentation. (**b**) Types of pedicles screws and hooks. Implants of S4 System by Aesculap

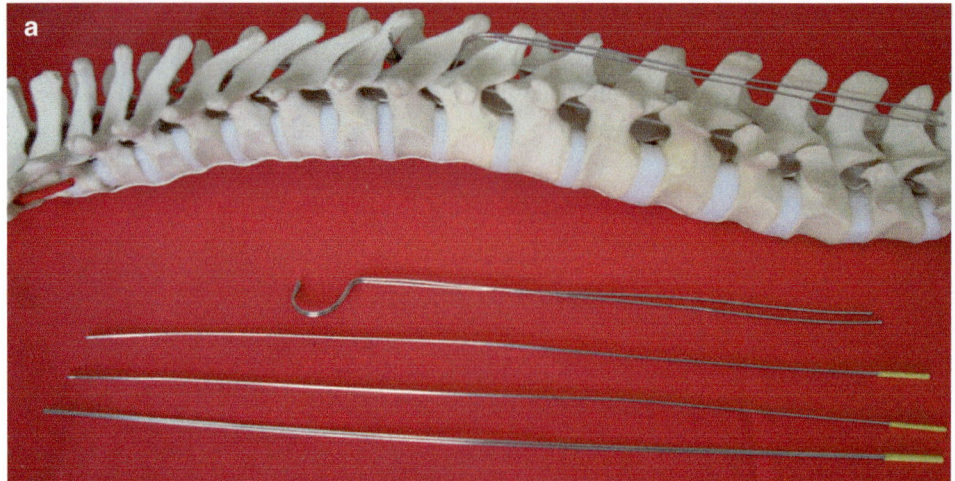

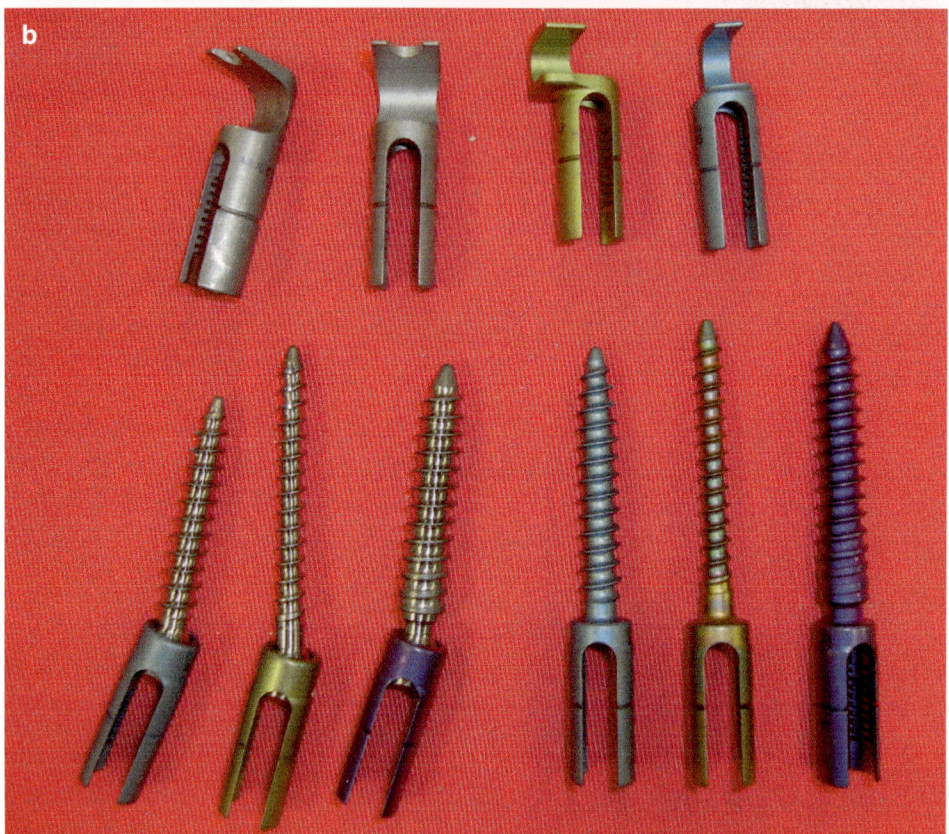

of next distal vertebrae, are the strongest hooks. They are always directed cephalad so that their "u" shaped tip embraces the pedicle and provides maximal stability concerning rotation and translation maneuvers. These implants can be placed from T1 to T10. Some of these hooks have additional features such as the possibility of being locked to the pedicle. Laminar hooks are available in a variety of designs. Variations in the blade width and style allow for an optimized hook–bone interface. These hooks may be placed in supralaminar or infralaminar positions dependent upon the required distraction or compression forces. Transverse process hooks have less risk of iatrogenic cord injury because they are out of the spinal canal. Usually, these implants are combined with a pedicle hook or a pedicle screw. This claw is the strongest hook construct, and it is very helpful in hyperkyphosis correction and can be added to transpedicular constructs to protect the screws from pullout.

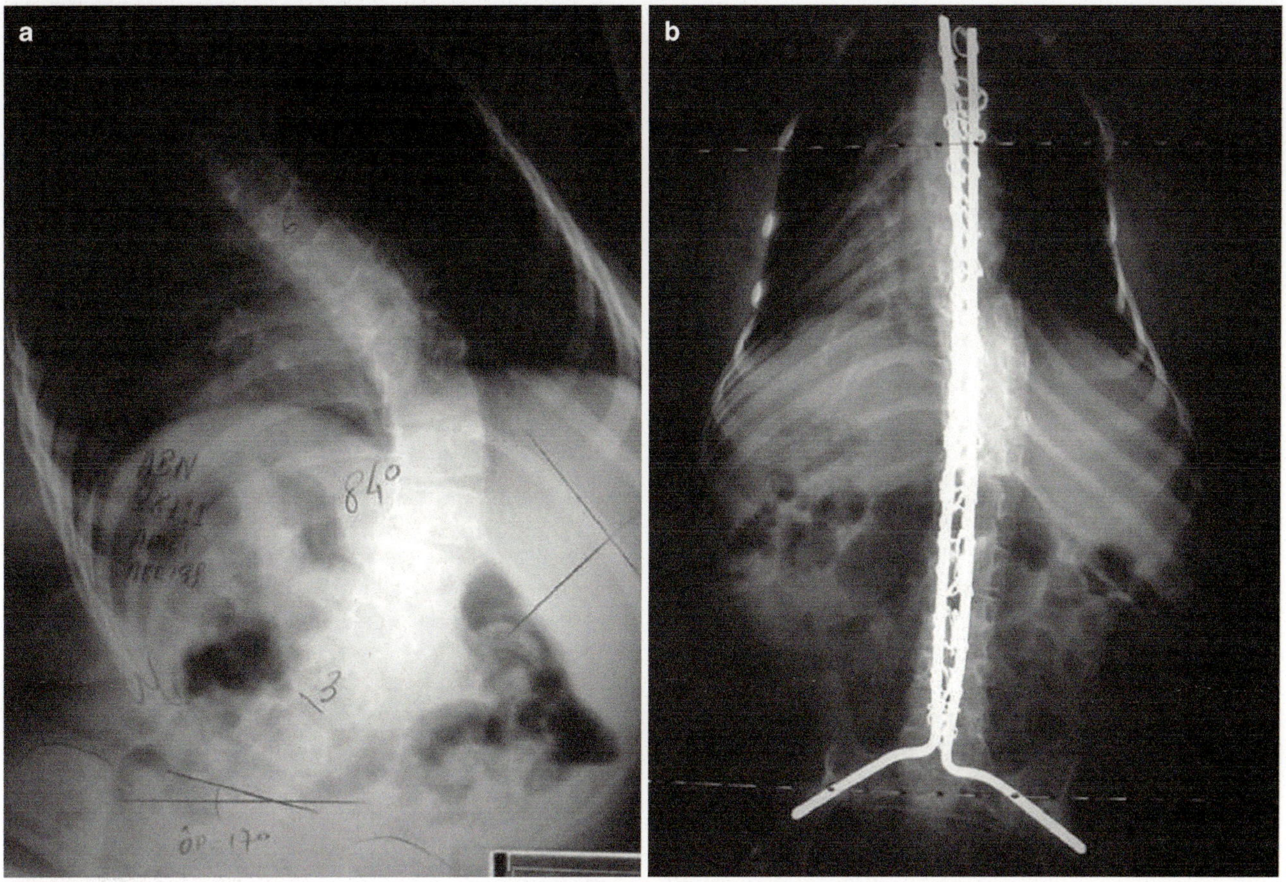

Fig. 47.2 (**a**) Preoperative image of neuromuscular scoliosis. (**b**) Surgical treatment of neuromuscular scoliosis with sublaminar wires technique

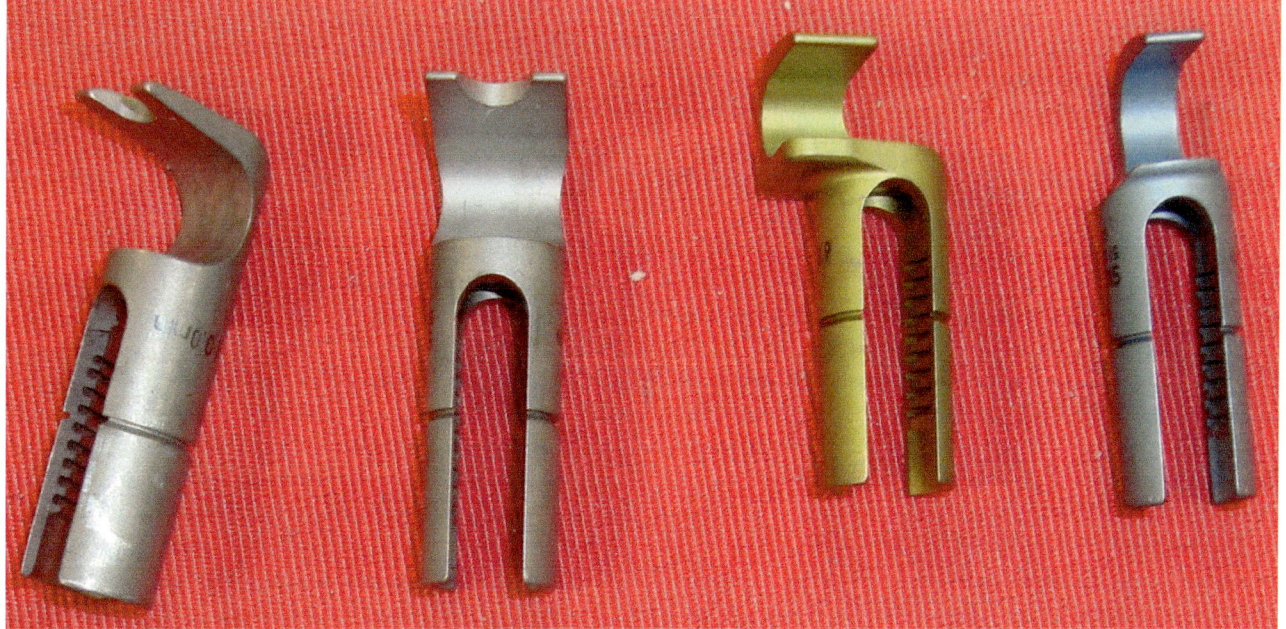

Fig. 47.3 Three types of hooks: pedicle, transverse process, and laminar hooks. Implants of S4 System by Aesculap

47.2.3 Pedicle Screw

The pedicle screw is the strongest implant because it is inserted into the vertebral body.

47.3 Special Surgical Techniques

47.3.1 Correction of Kyphosis [2–6]

The operative surgery for kyphosis is based on cantilever maneuvers and compression forces. Compression causes shortening of posterior column of the thoracic spine. Distraction is not allowed because of the high neurological risk. The standard construction for the treatment of a flexible thoracic kyphosis includes instrumentation reaching from T2 to L1. For the rigid kyphosis, prior to the posterior instrumentation, any kind of osteotomy (pedicle subtraction or Smith–Petersen) or anterior disc and ligaments release should be performed when necessary. Cranial implants are inserted using a claw on each side. The claw can be combined with a pedicle screw in T3 and a transverse process hook in T2 or a pedicle hook in T3 and transverse process hook in T2. In either construction, the superior laminar hook can be substituted by a transverse process hook. The important feature of the claw mechanism is the compression between the two superior vertebrae on either side to avoid a pullout of the cranial implants. The claw can also be used by leaving one vertebra in between (for example T2 and T4). If necessary, more than one claw construct per side can be done on the superior part of instrumentation. Pedicle screws or hooks are inserted as preoperatively planed. The preference at the caudal end is the use of pedicle screws. These can be supplemented with laminar hooks to resist the pullout force. Depending upon the curve rigidity, it may be necessary to insert pedicle screws in all vertebrae. Using the rod benders, 6 mm rods are precontoured to the desired sagittal plane kyphosis. The rods are then inserted into the upper pedicle screws or specialized pedicle hooks. With the rods applied in the correct sagittal plane, the claw constructs are locked. The rods are then reduced to the next caudal implants by applying uniform force on each rod with a rod pusher or rod holder. Compression is then applied to the implant in direction of the proximal claw construct. The nut can then be tightened to maintain the achieved correction before moving on to the next distal implants and repeating the procedure. At the end of the construct, two rod holders are applied to the rods, which are gently pushed down together onto the pedicle screws at T12 and L1. Once the rods are reduced onto these distal implants, the connectors and nuts are screwed on and compression is applied against the proximally adjacent fixed implant or a rod holder placed in between. Then the nuts are tightened. Finally, two cross-links are applied close to the ends of the instrumentation.

47.3.2 Correction of Scoliosis [1, 6, 7]

The most common pattern of idiopathic scoliosis is the right thoracic curve, and it is an ideal example to illustrate the principles of correction. The surgical treatment of scoliosis is based on many factors: age of patient, curve flexibility, Lenke classification (or other), frontal and sagittal balance, quality of bone, bone graft, patient clinical condition, structure of hospital, and availability of implants, as well as the surgeon's familiarity with the techniques among others. There are many ways to surgically reduce a scoliosis. It is utmost important to correctly apply the principles of correction. The follow technique using USS by Synthes is one option. The proximal and distal end vertebrae are identified on AP standing and lateral bending, fulcrum bending, or traction and lateral standing X-rays. The classic instrumentation of the right thoracic curve extends from T4 to L1. After posterior approach and intraoperative imaging to confirm the appropriate levels, the implants can be inserted, starting from the concave side and going to the convex side. The amount of implants (pedicle screws or hooks) depends upon the preoperative plan. The more implants are used and the more vertebrae are instrumented, if the potential of correction is greater. The foundation of the construct is established with pedicle screws placed in T12 and L1 caudally and in T4 and T5 cranially, on the concave side. On the convex side cranially, the implants are inserted as a claw construct, and it is applied between T4 and T5. Caudally, pedicle screws are inserted also at T12 and L1. The apical vertebra is usually T8 or T9 and is instrumented with pedicle screws, if possible on both sides. Additional instrumentation can usually be placed at alternating levels; however, additional implants must be used in larger and stiffer curves. A 6 mm rod template is placed in the desired sagittal plane on the concave side between the T4 and L1 screws. This template is used for the calculation of the final rod length while keeping in mind that the spine will automatically and passively elongate during the correction maneuvers. The rod template is then removed, and the appropriate size rod is contoured to the desired sagittal plane and cut to length. The rod can then be inserted into the T4 and L1 implants on the concave side, and collars and nuts are applied on both levels, but the nut is only tightened at L1 while maintaining the sagittal orientation of the rod. Using the complex reduction forceps (persuader), the intervening implants are brought to the rod using translation force. It is important not to apply force beyond that which the bone can withstand. In flexible curves, the apical implants are brought to the rod with the persuader. If the curve is stiff, do not primarily proceed to the reduction of apical implants and direct your attention to the convex side. The convex-contoured rod is now applied as a kind of lateral cantilever maneuver. The rod is inserted into the proximal claw inserted at T4 and T5. The claw is then compressed, and the nuts are tightened (T4 and T5) to ensure stability of the implants while the rod is maintained in a strict sagittal position. The convex rod is then pushed toward the midline using the rod holder to laterally engage the pedicle screws at T6, repeating the procedure at T8, T10, T12, and finally at L1. It is important not to tighten these nuts at this stage because this would prevent further correction on the concave side. At this moment, only the pedicle screw at L1 on concave side and the screws of the claw on the convex side have the nuts tightened to the rod, all the other implants connected to the rods have the nuts loose. The apical screws on the concave side will now have to be translated toward the concave rod using persuader forceps. After completing the coupling of implants to the rod on both sides of the spine in this way, the spine will have passively found its own length. The individually instrumented vertebrae are then sequentially derotated as they are secured to the rod starting from each end. This is achieved by placing a derotation force through the sticks attached to each of the implants, using the L handle and 6 mm socket wrench to tighten the nuts. It is important to hold the end vertebrae in their normal, neutral position prior to commencing this process in order to avoid transference of the torque force from instrumented to the uninstrumented spine. Cross-links are applied at the extremities of the instrumentation. Decortication of the posterior elements and osteotomy of the facet joints are important steps before the bone-grafting procedure.

47.3.3 Stabilization of Fractures

The principles of treatment of fractures of the thoracic spine are to correct the deficient part of the injured spine using appropriate forces, support, and stabilization methods. The use of any type of fracture classification will be helpful to choose the principles and proper implant system.

A good example for using these principles is the Universal Spine System—fracture module by Synthes. This system can be used in the middle and low thoracic spine. It is not recommended in the upper thoracic spine because the pedicles are too small and the instrumentation may be too prominent at these levels. In this system, the implants act as a tension band, a buttress, and a neutralization system. USS allows a lordosation, distraction, compression, as well as fixation, in a neutral position. Another important point is that the fulcrum of corrective forces can be adjusted by applying half rings. The important features of this system are: Schanz screws, clamps with separate fixation for rods, and Schanz screws and the half-ring clamps. The use of Schanz screw allows easy reduction of the vertebral body in the sagittal plane. The USS fracture clamps have separate fixations for rods and Schanz screws; it allows a range motion of + or − 18° in the sagittal plane of the Schanz screws. Also, it is possible to do compression or distraction independently of

the Schanz screw angle. The half-ring clamps can move the fulcrum of the corrective forces away from the posterior wall of the vertebral body. When all four Schanz screws have been inserted, the rods of the fracture module are applied to the Schanz screws using fracture clamps with the rods lying medially to the Schanz screws. The clamps are left loose.

47.3.3.1 Reduction and Fixation of Fractures with Intact Posterior Wall

The posterior ends of the Schanz screws are manually approximated until the desired correction of the kyphosis has been attained. The set screws on the clamps must remain loose so that the clamps can slide freely toward each other during the reduction maneuver. The center of rotation then lies at the posterior edge of the vertebral body. By creating the lordosis, the vertebral body will be distracted anteriorly, and the disc space and disc height can be restored by ligamentotaxis. Place the cannulated socket wrenches over the caudal Schanz screws and tilt them cranially to create lordosis in the spine. The posterior nuts are then locked. The same procedure is performed on the cranial Schanz screw in order to reestablish the correct sagittal plane. The appropriate posterior nuts are tightened to fix the angle between the Schanz screws and the rods. At this stage, it is necessary to distract the Schanz screws to reestablish the normal height of the injured disc and vertebra. A half-ring clamp is placed and locked in the center of each rod between the clamps. Distract the spreader forceps and check the procedure with the image intensifier. When the desired distraction is obtained, tighten the set screws and remove the rings.

47.3.3.2 Reduction and Fixation of Fractures with Fractured Posterior Wall

In this type of fractures, there is a danger that the posterior wall fragments might displace posterior into the spinal canal during the correction of the kyphosis by compressing the posterior ends of the Schanz screws. It is important to protect the posterior wall against compression. Distraction is used to reconstitute the height of the vertebral body and disc space.

Two half rings are placed on each of the 6 mm rods prior to reduction with the Schanz screws. A distance of 5 mm between the half rings and the clamp is allowed for every 10° of attempted kyphosis correction. When approximating the ends of the Schanz screws, the clamps will soon touch the half rings, and the center of rotation is transferred posterior to the level of the rods instead of the posterior wall. The lordosis is checked with a lateral image intensifier view. The posterior-opening nuts are tightened to secure the correction, and the set screws on the clamps are fixed. This procedure is repeated for the other Schanz screws. The half rings are then removed. Distraction is performed between the Schanz screws to obtain the height of the vertebral body.

After fracture reduction and stabilization, anterior surgery may be required for biomechanical purposes in case of significant vertebral body comminution, osteoporosis, or incomplete clearance of the spinal canal with persistent neurological deficit.

47.4 Tips and Tricks

- The pedicle screw is the most powerful implant because of its three-column insertion. An appropriate utilization of these implants, therefore, requires an understanding of their mechanical properties as well as the properties of alternative devices and models of constructions.
- If the placement of a pedicle screw is difficult, it is possible to open the spinal canal and, through direct visualization of pedicle, introduce the pedicle screw. If in doubt, instrumentation should be avoided, especially when optimal purchase and placement are in doubt.
- The principle of ligamentotaxis for posterior fragments reduction of fracture is valid only if the posterior longitudinal ligament is intact. When the posterior longitudinal ligament is disrupted, then indirect decompression of the spinal canal should not be done using this procedure. Images from a CT scan or an MRI can demonstrate the disruption of the posterior longitudinal ligament with the sign of a reverse cortical sign of the posterior wall fragment.
- The use of half rings can be avoided by using rod holders.
- The use of sticks or Schanz screw can be substituted by any kind of elongated screw to allow for cantilever force or other systems.

References

1. Winter RB, Lonstein JE. Congenital thoracic scoliosis with unilateral unsegmented bar and concave fused ribs. Spine. 2007;32:E841–4.
2. Cho KJ, Bridwell KH, Lenke LG, et al. Comparasion of smith-Petersen versus pedicle subtraction osteotomy for the correction of fixed sagittal imbalance. Spine. 2005;30:2030–7.
3. Gill JB, Levin A, Burd T, et al. Corrective osteotomies in spine surgery. J Bone Joint Surg Am. 2008;90:2509–20.
4. Heary RF, Bono CM. Pedicle subtraction astronomy in the treatment of chronic, posttraumatic kyphotic deformity. J Neurosurg Spine. 2006;5:1–8.
5. Macagno AE, O'Brien MF. Thoracic and thoracolumbar kyphosis in adults. Spine. 2006;19(Suppl):S161–70.
6. Mohan AL, Das K. History of surgery for the correction of spinal deformity. Neurosurg Focus. 2003;14(1):e1.
7. Aebi M, Arlet V, Webb JK. AOSPINE manual. Principle and techniques, vol. 1. New York: Thieme; 2007.

Stabilization of the Thoracic Spine with Internal Fixator

48

Robert Morrison and Uwe Vieweg

48.1 Introduction and Core Messages

The preparation of the pedicle within the thoracic spine requires precise preoperative planning. The anatomical structures marking the entry point, the pedicle orientation, and diameter must be known prior to the operation. Performing an adequate preoperative planning including CT scans is elemental for planning of the instrumentation and selection of the correct screw placement. The anatomy of the pedicle and the vertebra is quite different in different parts of the thoracic spine (e.g., special anatomy of Th1). In cases of very small pedicle diameters, especially within the middle thoracic spine, only a parapedicular screw placement may be possible. In cases of small pedicle diameter or poor intraoperative radiological picture quality (obese patient, etc.), navigational screw placement is recommended. Due to the lower axial load within the upper thoracic spine and the stabilization through the rib cage, an additional anterior stabilization is not as often necessary as in the lumbar spine.

48.2 Indications

- Fractures of the thoracic spine.
- Degenerative disorders.
- Deformities/scoliosis.
- Tumors or infections of the spine.

R. Morrison (✉)
Spine & Scoliosis Center, Asklepios Klinik Bad Abbach, Germany
e-mail: r.morrison@asklepios.com

U. Vieweg
Department of Conservative and Surgical Spine Therapy with Interdisciplinary Spinal Deformities Centre and Rummelsberg Sectional Center, Hospital Rummelsberg,
Schwarzenbruck, Germany
e-mail: uwe.vieweg@sana.de

48.3 Contraindications

- Osteopenia/osteoporosis (relative contraindication).
- Ongoing infection within the instrumented vertebra (relative contraindication).
- Poor medical condition of the patient (possibly absolute contraindication).
- Small pedicles make transpedicular stabilization impossible (relative contraindication).

48.4 Technical Prerequisites

Fluoroscopy, special cushions (e.g., Wilson Frame etc.), radiolucent operating table, possibly additional intraoperative electrophysiological monitoring (SSEP, MEP). Facultative, a spinal navigation system can be used.

48.5 Planning, Preparation, and Positioning

Preoperative measurement includes the pedicle diameter, and especially the transverse diameter. Within the thoracic spine, this should be done with a CT scan. If the transverse diameter is large enough to carry the screws, the preoperative planning can take place. The correct *entry point* can be found after identifying the necessary landmarks. These include the facet joint with its borders and the transverse process. Intraoperatively, the entry point is located in the lateral half of the oval area of the pedicle in the AP fluoroscopy. This also includes measuring the transverse diameter of the pedicles (Table 48.1). The *orientation of the pedicle* can be gauged in lateral radiographs or even more precise using CT scans. Sagittal reconstructions of the planning-CT for the cranial-caudal angle and coronary scans for the lateral deviation are advised (Fig. 48.1). These two values show a great variation within the thoracic spine [1, 2]. The *pedicle length* also shows great variations. The correct screw length cannot be gauged intraoperatively in lateral fluoroscopy, as the ante-

Table 48.1 Showing the average pedicle diameter, transverse angle corresponding to the midline, and the inclination angle of the pedicle orientation corresponding to the superior end plate

Vertebra	Gender	Transversal pedicle diameter (mm)	Transversal angle of the pedicle (°)	Inclination angle of the pedicle (°)
Th 1	M	8.8	39	23
	F	10.4	29	20
Th 2	M	6	35	23
	F	6.7	28	20
Th 3	M	4.1	22	22
	F	5.3	22	19
Th 4	M	3.9	29	23
	F	3.8	19	17
Th 5	M	4.6	24	25
	F	4	17	19
Th 6	M	3.6	26	27
	F	4	15	24
Th 7	M	4.5	25	24
	F	4.6	11	19
Th 8	M	5	29	20
	F	4.6	9	18
Th 9	M	5.3	21	18
	F	5.5	12	18
Th 10	M	5.6	20	18
	F	6	17	17
Th 11	M	8.3	22	20
	F	8.8	15	19
Th 12	M	8	15	20
	F	9.4	11	18

Adapted from Ebraheim et al. [1]

rior cortex has a convex shape. When deciding for a screw length, one must keep in mind that 60% of the pullout force is achieved in the pedicle and 15–20% additionally in the cancellous bone of the vertebral body [3]. So the screw should rather be chosen too short than too long.

48.5.1 Anatomical Specifications of the Thoracic Spine

- Small pedicle diameter (smallest in the midthoracic spine T3–T8) [4]. The screw diameter should be 75–80% of the transverse pedicle diameter.
- The medial cortex of the pedicles is much stronger than the lateral wall, making the lateral perforation much more common [5].
- Very small pedicle diameters make transpedicular screw placement impossible in such cases (Fig. 48.1c).
- Plain radiographs in two planes are often not enough to plan the instrumentation in the thoracic spine; in such cases, a CT scan is necessary.

48.6 Surgical Technique

48.6.1 Approach

- Open access via a midline incision. The incision should be two segments longer than the intended length of fusion. The subcutis is dissected to the fascia, and wound retractors are applied. The fascia is detached on both sides using a diathermy knife close to the bone. Great caution has to be taken, to leave the interspinous ligaments within the cranial segments intact to prevent a PJK (proximal junction kyphosis). The paraspinal structures are retracted with a raspatory. The muscles are retracted to expose the costal processes (Fig. 48.2).
- Alternatively, an additional laminotomy can be performed. This is used when a safe identification of the pedicles cannot be found during the operation (rare indication). In such cases, the lamina is resected to display the medial side of the pedicles. Then the screws can be placed as described above.

48.7 Instrumentation

48.7.1 Trajectory

- Entry point can be found at the intersection of the vertical line along the middle of the superior articular process and the horizontal line through the top of the transverse process. Distances to other landmarks can be misleading in the thoracic spine due to the great anatomical variability [1] (Fig. 48.2).
- The pedicle is opened with a pedicle awl, followed by consecutive deepening with a pedicle trocar. The length of the screw can be seen on the side of the trocar. To verify the intact pedicle walls, the walls of the canal are tested with a ball-tip pedicle probe.
- Within the thoracic spine, the screws will have a decreasing convergence toward the midline (20–25° in T1 to 5° in T4–12) (Table 48.1) (Fig. 48.3).
- To make room for the screwhead, it is advisable to resect part of the medial cortex of the transverse process (Red marking in Fig. 48.3).
- The screws should be placed parallel to the superior end plate if possible. Alternatively, a slanted introduction is also possible. Thereby, the tip of the screw is aimed toward the anterior edge of the inferior end plate (Choose higher entry point!) (Fig. 48.4).
- *Parapedicular screw placement* [6].

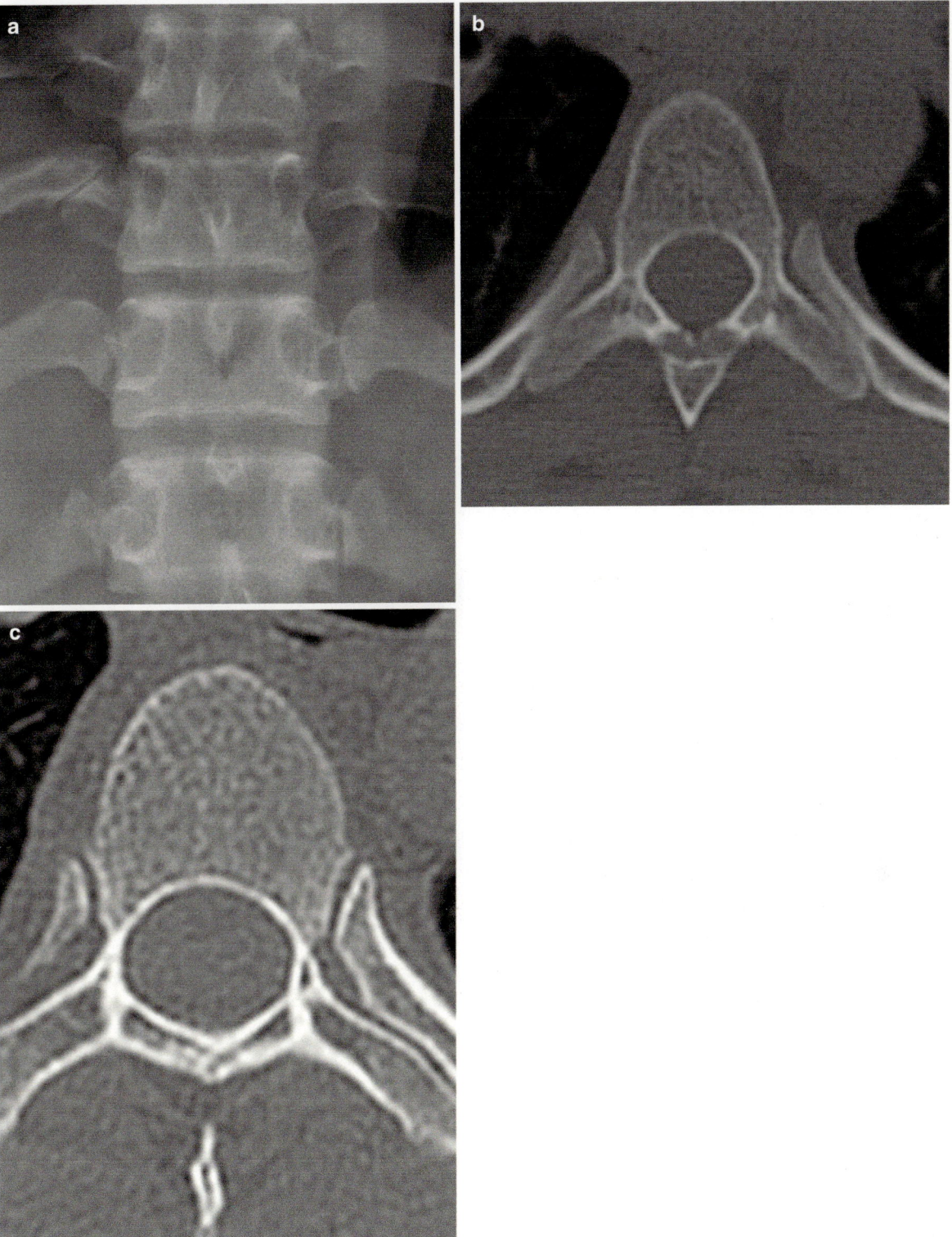

Fig. 48.1 (**a**) Plain radiograph of the thoracic spine in AP view and (**b**) corresponding CT scan in axial view showing the pedicle width and orientation (**c**) Example of very thin pedicles

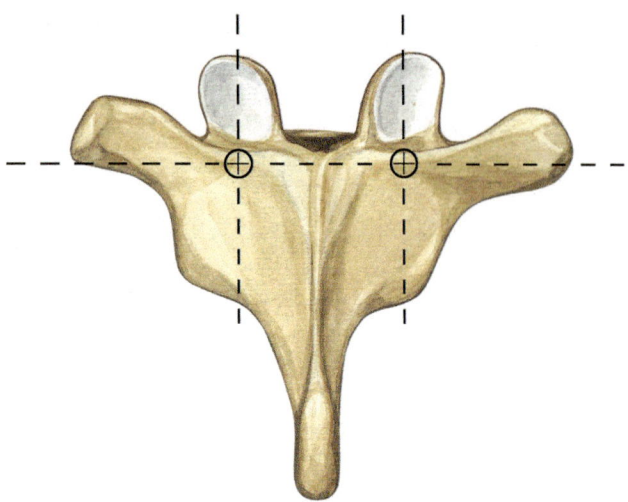

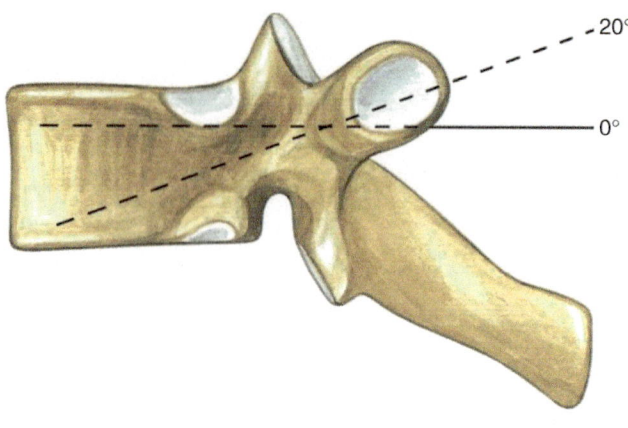

Fig. 48.4 Entry point of the transpedicular screw in the thoracic spine in a lateral view. Angulation depending upon the desired positioning

Fig. 48.2 Entry point of the transpedicular screw in the thoracic spine, when planning a screw placement parallel to the superior end plate

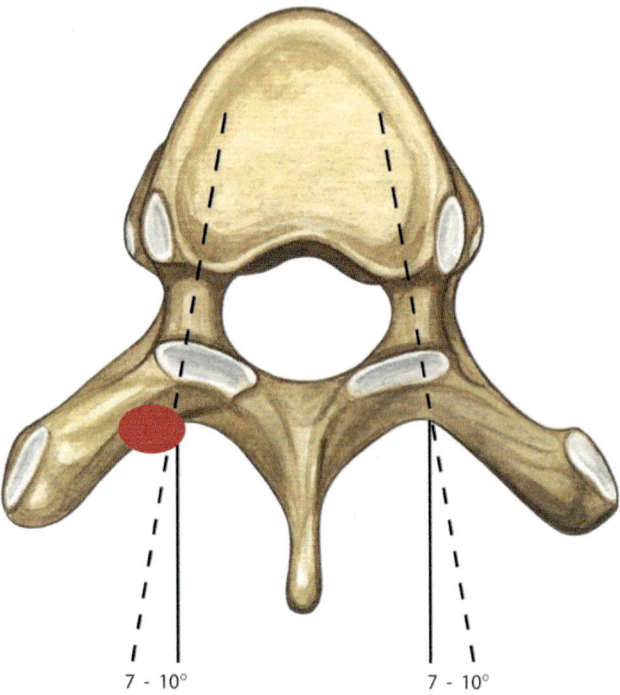

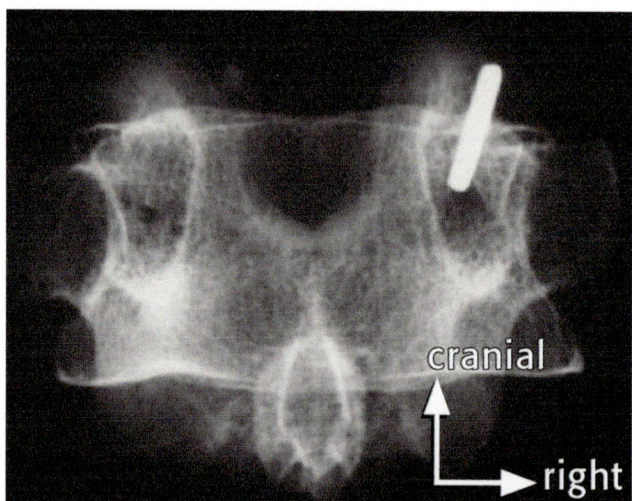

Fig. 48.5 Superior view of typical extrapedicular screw placement

Fig. 48.3 Entry point of the transpedicular screw in the thoracic spine, with an angulation of 7–10° toward the midline

In cases of narrow pedicles, a transpedicular trajectory would cause a burst fracture of the pedicles. In such cases, a more lateral entry point is chosen. The trajectory starts at the tip of the transverse process and enters the vertebral body via the costotransversal joints (Figs. 48.5). This technique involves a greater risk of penetration of the pleural cavity.

48.8   Tips and Tricks

- Start out by marking the entry points with K-wires or short pins using the fluoroscopy in the AP direction.
- The correct positioning and orientation can be verified by adjusting the fluoroscopy to where the K-wire is a "point," which lies clearly within the pedicle.
- The positioning of the patient is especially important when instrumenting the mid thoracic spine (T3–6), as the scapula interferes with the lateral fluoroscopy.
- Laying the arms next to the patient's body can help to lower the scapula. A clear lateral view has to be achieved prior to draping.

References

1. Ebraheim NA, Xu R, Ahmad M, et al. Projection of the thoracic pedicle and its morphometric analysis. Spine. 1997;22:233–8.
2. Vaccaro AR, Rizzolo SJ, Allardyce TJ, et al. Placement of pedicle screw in the thoracic spine. Part one: morphometric analysis of the thoracic vertebrae. J Bone Joint Surg Am. 1995;77:1193–9.
3. Weinstein JN, Rydevik BL, Rauschning WJN. Anatomic and technical considerations of pedicle screw fixation. Clin Orthop Relat Res. 1992;284:34–46.
4. Panjabi MM, Takata K, Goel V, et al. Thoracic human vertebrae. Quantitative three-dimensional anatomy Spine. 1991;16: 888–901.
5. Kothe R, O'Holleran JD, Liu W, et al. Internal architecture of the thoracic pedicle: an anatomic study. Spine. 1996;21:264–70.
6. Husted DS, Yue JJ, Fairchild TA, et al. An extrapedicular approach to the placement of screws in the thoracic spine: an anatomic and radiographic assessment. Spine. 2003;28:2324–30.

Transpedicular Stabilization with Freehand Technique on the Thoracic Spine

Paulo Tadeu Maia Cavali

49.1 Introduction and Core Messages

The use of pedicle screws has become popular during the past decade, first in applications involving the lumbar spine and subsequently in thoracic spine surgery. Pedicle screws also prevent the need to place instrumentation within the spinal canal-like sublaminar wiring or hooks, which create the risk of neurological injury. Transpedicular stabilization (TS) has been shown to resist flexion and extension loads, as well as torsional loads better than other devices. Especially in spinal deformity surgery, the use of TS provides better correction and maintenance than system with hooks and wires. Disadvantages of pedicular screws are related to the misplacement of pedicle screws which can lead to disastrous complications such as vascular or neural injuries. Accurate and safe placement of screw within the pedicle is a crucial step during the surgery. There are many proven techniques used to insert pedicle screws, including fluoroscopic or radiographic guidance, stereotactic guidance system based on computed tomography, direct visualization of pedicle with the use of a laminotomy, and the freehand technique (without intraoperative image guidance). The freehand techniques use established surface landmarks and direct palpation of internal pedicle and vertebral structure. The objective of this chapter is to describe the freehand technique for transpedicular stabilization in the thoracic spine.

49.2 Indications

- Deformities such as scoliosis and kyphosis.
- Trauma with fractures and/or dislocations.
- Tumors and other pathologic fractures.

49.3 Contraindications

- Intense osteoporosis.
- Small pedicle with diameter smaller than 4.0 mm.
- Inadequate anterior column support.

49.4 Technical Prerequisites

Fluoroscopy, positioning device (e.g., Wiltse frame), intraoperative neuromonitoring with somatosensory-evoked potentials (SSEP), transcranial electric motor-evoked potentials (TMEP), and electromyography (EMG) are some tech-

P. T. M. Cavali (✉)
Department of Scoliosis os Hospital AACD-Sao Paulo, Sao Paulo, Brazil
e-mail: paulo.escolioseaacd@uol.com.br

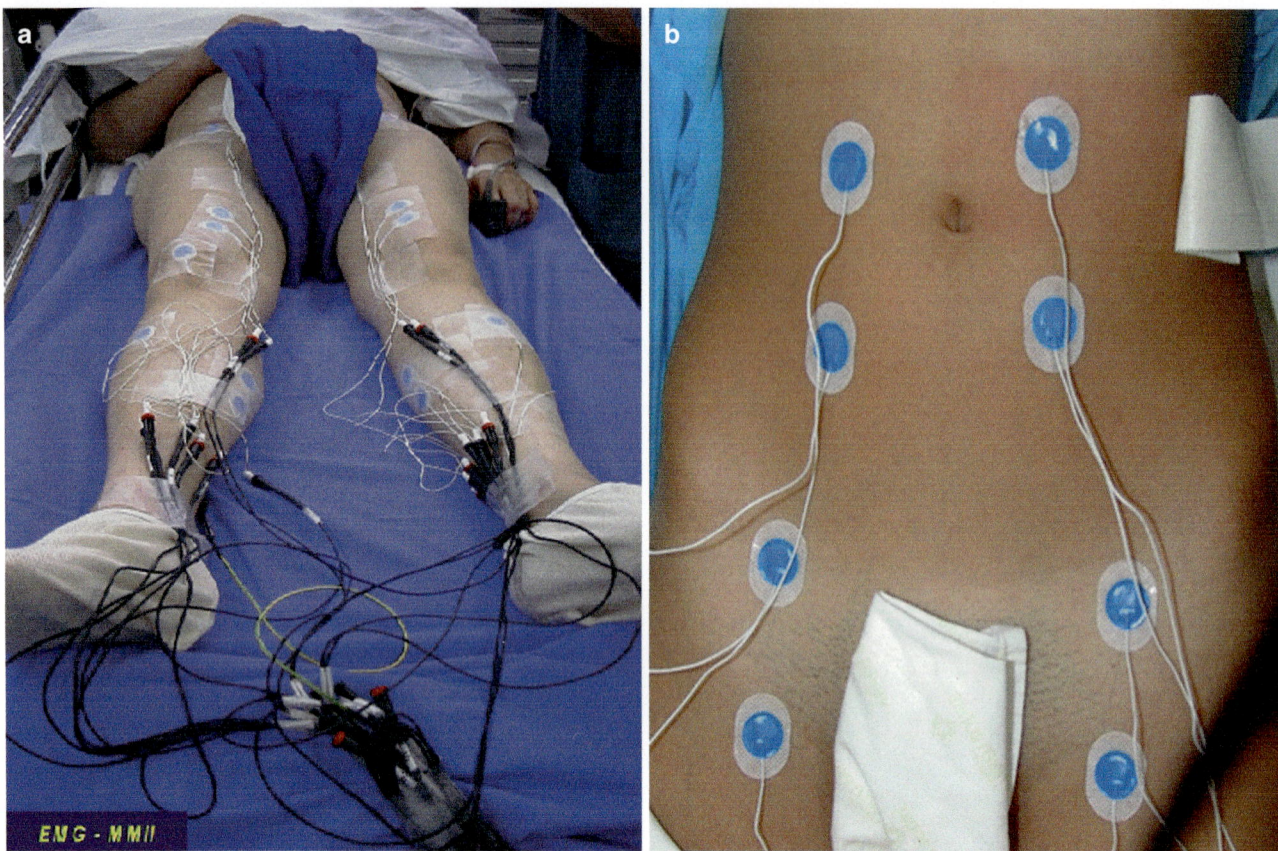

Fig. 49.1 Intraoperative monitoring with somatosensory-evoked potentials (SSEP) and transcranial electric motor-evoked potentials (TMEP). The thoracic nerve roots from T6–T12 are performed with EMG from rectus abdominus muscle

nical prerequisites. The SSEP and TMEP provide evaluation of cord function, and triggered EMG gives information about any contact of screw with neural structures as spinal cord or nerve roots (see Fig. 49.1). Adequate implants and instruments. There are many pedicle screw systems in the market. Most of them are able to stabilize the thoracic spine. In the thoracic spine, the area to set up the instrumentation is smaller than lumbar one; it means that the profile of head of screws, rods, and connectors must fit well for each patient to avoid prominence in the skin.

49.5 Planning, Preparation, and Positioning

Prior to surgery, the patient's X-ray is reviewed to assess pedicle diameter, length, and its orientation. Knowledge of normal pedicle morphometry is essential to proper placement of pedicle screw.

The lateral images with the patient in prone position on the operative table give orientation of screws for each verte-

bra in sagittal plane (see Fig. 49.2). For deformities surgeries, the level of spine instrumentation and the number and local of screws depend on many features such as classification, stiffness, and magnitude of curve. The patient is positioned prone on a radiolucent operative table. The abdomen and thorax are permitted to hang freely.

49.6 Operative Technique

49.6.1 Approach

- The midline posterior approach is the avenue for placement of thoracic instrumentation. It is performed with wide subperiosteal exposure of the posterior bony elements to the level of the transverse processes (see Fig. 49.3). This significantly more wide exposure beyond the facet and out into the transverse process is important to identify all anatomical landmarks.
- Transverse process and the base of superior facet are used as landmarks. With a 2 mm osteotome, approximately

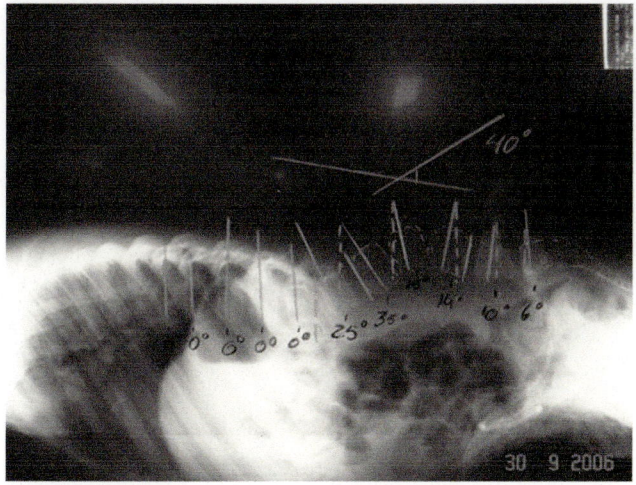

Fig. 49.2 Preoperative X-ray with the patient in prone position on the operative table. The measurement of the sagittal angle of all pedicles to be instrumented

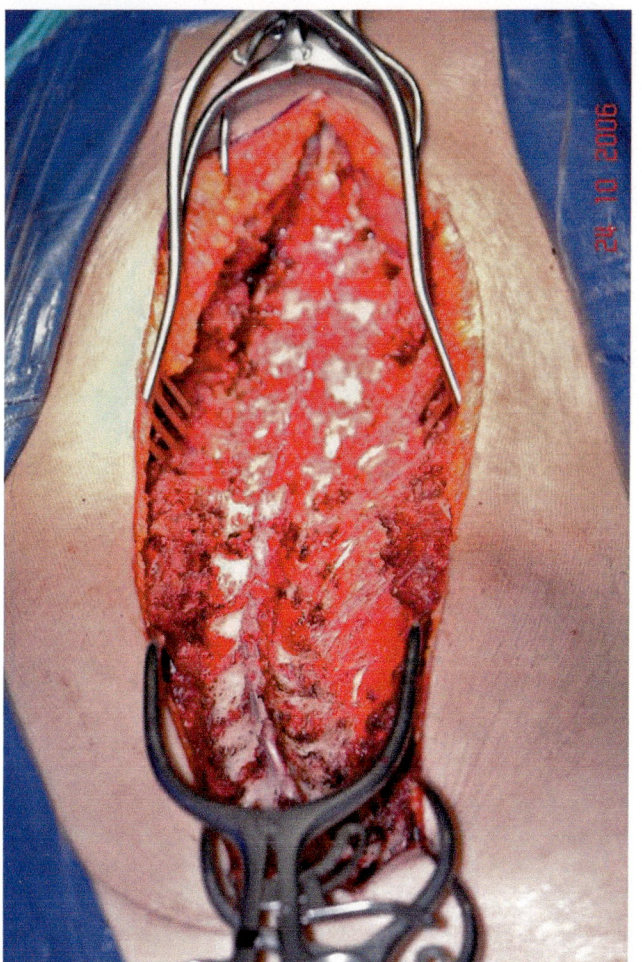

Fig. 49.3 The wide posterior exposure of the thoracic spine

5 mm of inferior articular process is removed so as to expose the base of the superior articular process.

49.6.2 Instrumentation [1–6]

- The starting point for each thoracic level is slightly variable and is based on the posterior element anatomy of the transverse process and the base of superior articular facet. The ideally entry point in the thoracic pedicle is at the junction of a horizontal line along the inferior border of facet joint and vertical line at the junction of the outer third and inner two-thirds of the facet joint. The starting point in the proximal region (T1–T3) is at the middle of transverse process; in the mid- and lower thoracic region, it is at superior third of transverse process, and in T12, the entry point is at middle and tip of transverse process (see Fig. 49.4).
- Before making the entry into the pedicle, initial neuromonitoring recordings with SSEP and TMEP are performed to establish the preinstrumentation neural status of the patient.
- The entry point is made rough with rouger or a 3.5 mm acorn-tipped burr to prevent slippage of awl, to visualize of cancellous bone, and to create space to lodge the head of pedicle screw.
- Then the further passage in the pedicle is made with appropriate amount of ventral pressure using the gearshift (2 mm blunt-tipped pedicle finder).
- The surgeon must be careful to the axial and sagittal position of vertebrae space to position the probe down the pedicle shaft appropriately. The information about the axial and sagittal angle is given by the images obtained preoperatively.
- In the thoracic spine without scoliosis and kyphosis, the pedicle finder should be angled 7–10 toward the midline and 10–20 caudally. When the spine is deformed or scoliotic, these angles are different and asymmetrical.
- The trajectory of pedicle screw is completed with the gearshift going down to the pedicle and reaching the cancellous bone near to anterior cortex of vertebra body. At this moment, new neuromonitoring recordings are performed with SSEP, TMEP, and EMG. The EMG is taken with direct stimulation of gearshift inserted into the pedicle trajectory. These data are used to investigate the integrity of pedicle trajectory (see Fig. 49.5).
- The surgeon sensitivity during the penetration of cancellous bone through the pedicle to vertebral body is an important step and depends on appropriate learning curve. Any sudden advancement of the pedicle finder suggests penetration into soft tissue, and thus a pedicle wall violation or vertebral body violation has occurred. Decision of screw diameter and length is based on preoperative assessment but confirmed intraoperatively.

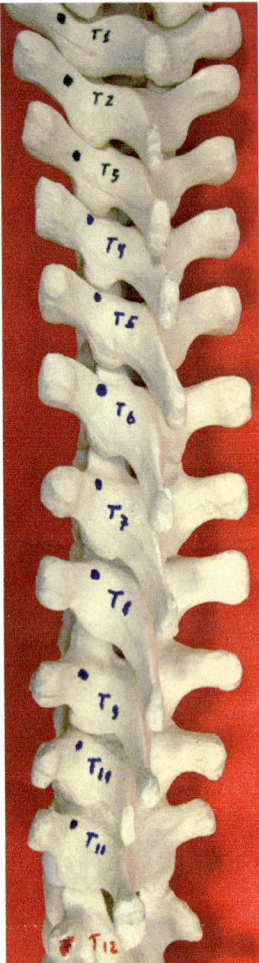

Fig. 49.4 The starting point for each thoracic pedicle

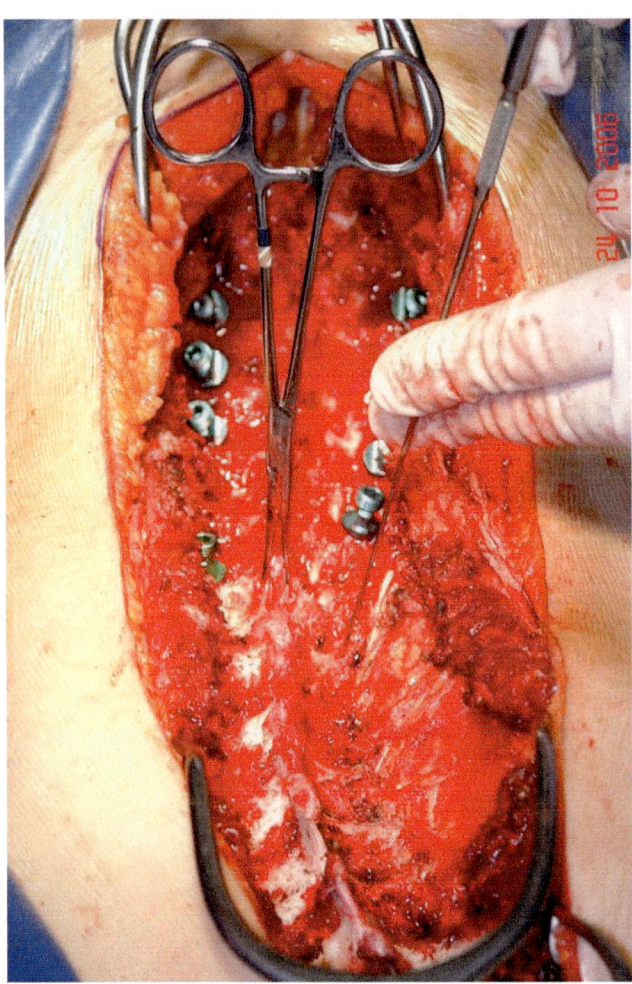

Fig. 49.6 Palpation of five walls of pedicle tract with flexible ball-tipped probe

- It is important to avoid penetration of the anterior cortex to prevent visceral and vascular injuries. Approximately 90% of strength of the screw comes from the pedicle and posterior half of the vertebral body.
- Once the trajectory of pedicle screw is completed and neuromonitoring data have not demonstrated any signal of wall violation, the pedicle finder (gearshift) is removed. The tract is visualized to make sure that only blood is coming out.
- Excessive bleeding from the pedicle hole may indicate epidural bleeding secondary to medial wall violation, and the presence of cerebrospinal fluid means more medial violation with dural lesion.
- At this point, if any of these situation occurs such as inappropriate neuromonitoring data or signs of violation of pedicle wall, there is an opportunity to redirect the pedicle finder into an appropriate position in the pedicle so that complete intraosseous borders can be obtained.
- Palpation of pedicle tract is the next step. With a flexible ball-tipped probe, the five walls are palpated (see Fig. 49.6).

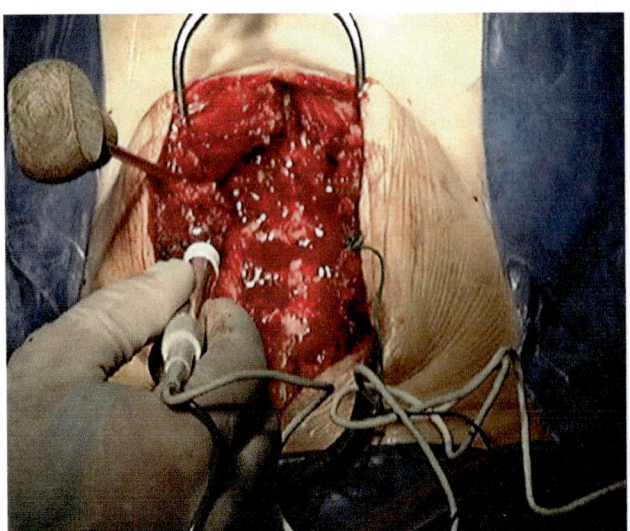

Fig. 49.5 The EMG with direct stimulation of gearshift immediately after complete perforation of pedicle trajectory

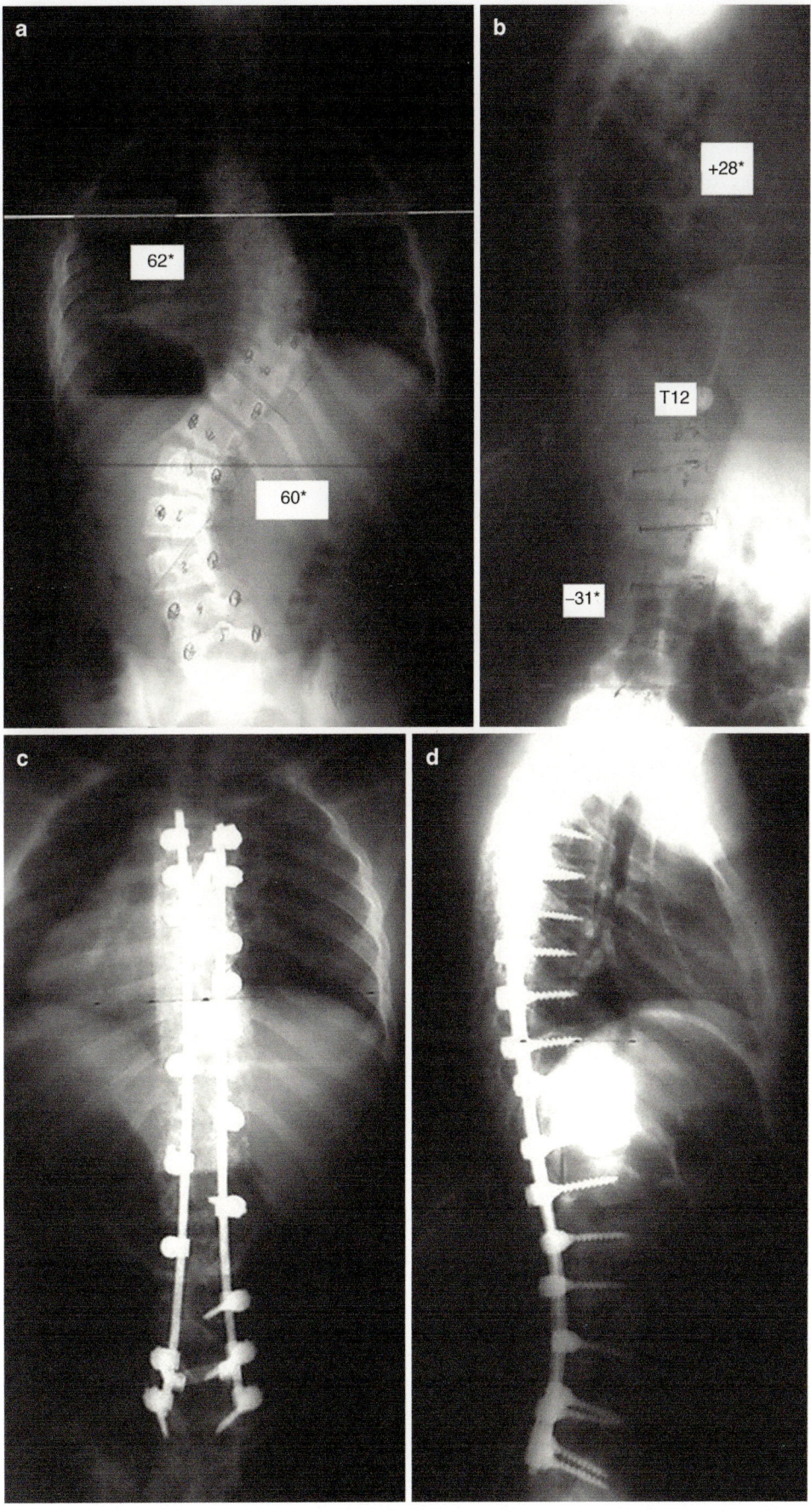

Fig. 49.7 Preoperative assessment of the patient (**a**, **b**) and intraoperative confirmation and documentation immediately after complete instrumentation (**c**, **d**)

- The integrity of five walls: medial, lateral, superior (cranial), inferior (caudal), and floor (anterior cortex) is essential to insert the screw. The most important walls are medial and inferior because of the presence of the spinal cord and nerve root, respectively. In the literature, the critical violation of any pedicle wall is defined as more than 2 mm, and the most common violated wall is the lateral followed by the medial one.
- The measurement of pedicle tract is performed with the same flexible ball-tipped probe after confirmation of integrity of the five walls. Then the tract is tapping, and an adequate screw in length and diameter is inserted into the pedicle.
- The next imperative step is the confirmation and documentation of intraosseous placement of all pedicle screw via images using fluoroscopy or radiography at the end of surgery (Fig. 49.7) and by neuromonitoring data performed after insertion of each screw during the surgery with SSEP, TMEP, and triggered EMG.
- With the screws inserted in appropriated position, the previously rods are placed according to the preoperative plan.

49.7   Tips and Tricks

- In order to prevent violation of the medial wall of pedicle, the half medial part of the superior facet and its caudal projection must be avoided (see Fig. 49.8).
- If the pedicle screw was misplaced and its reposition was not possible in the appropriate place, the screw can be inserted by the in-out-in technique (more lateral and more convergence technique).
- The insertion of pedicle screw in scoliotic spine can be difficult, especially on the concave side; then the orientation of the surface of superior facet can be helpful once the direction of pedicle screw has an angle

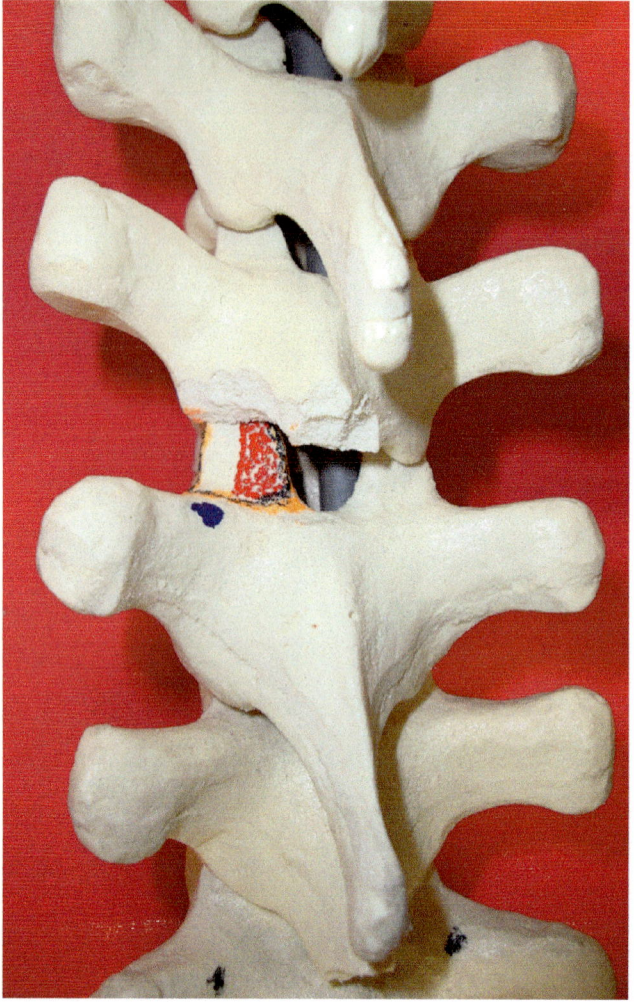

Fig. 49.8 The *red region* is the half medial part of the superior facet (must be avoided), and the *blue landmark* is the entry point of pedicle screw

slightly perpendicular to the surface of the superior facet. This is useful for axial and sagittal orientation (see Fig. 49.9).

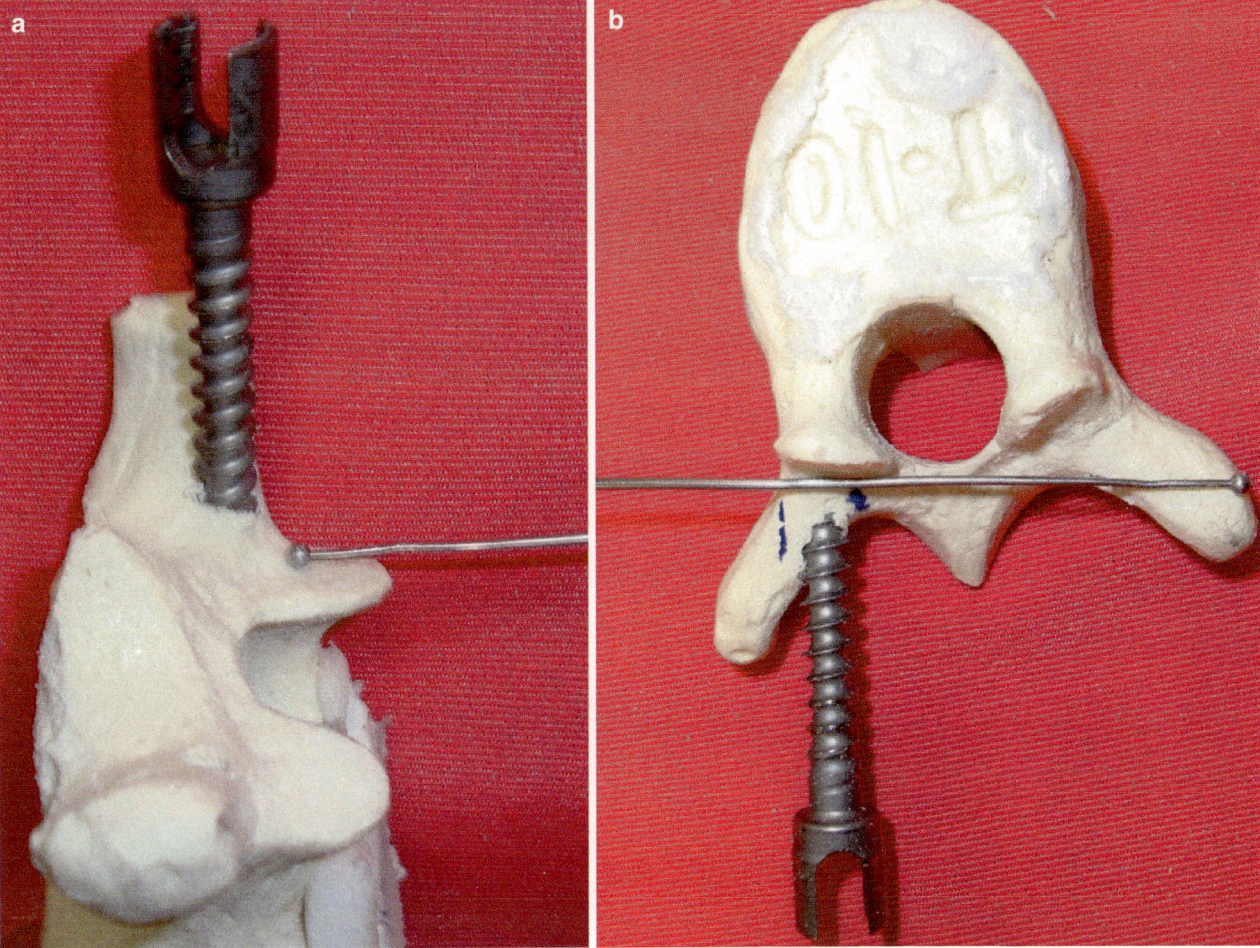

Fig. 49.9 The perpendicular relationship between axis of pedicle and surface of superior facet, even in sagittal plane (**a**) as in the axial plane (**b**)

References

1. Bergeson RK, Schwend RM, DeLucia T, et al. How accurately do novice surgeons place thoracic pedicle screws with the free hand technique? Spine. 2008;33(15):E501–7.
2. Chung KJ, Suh SW, Desai S, et al. Ideal entry point for the thoracic pedicle screw during the free hand technique. Int Orthop. 2008;32:657–62.
3. Kim YW, Lenke LG, Kim YJ, et al. Free-hand pedicle screw placement during revision spinal surgery. Spine. 2008;33:1141–8.
4. Modi HN, Suh SW, Fernandez H, et al. Accuracy and safety of pedicle screw placement in neuromuscular scoliosis with free-hand technique. Eur Spine J. 2008;17:1686–96.
5. Ofiram E, Polly DW, Gilbert JRTJ, et al. Is it safer to place pedicle screws in the lower thoracic spine than in the upper lumbar spine? Spine. 2007;32:9–54.
6. Schizas C, Theumann N, Kosmopoulos V. Inserting pedicle screws in the upper thoracic spine without the use of fluoroscopy or image guidance. Is it safe? Eur Spine J. 2007;16:625–9.

Posterior Correction of Adolescent Idiopathic Scoliosis (AIS)

Torsten Bräuer

50.1 Introduction and Core Message

Operative correction of AIS has evolved tremendously over the last decades trending in the favored use of posterior correction by means of all-pedicle-screw-constructs, stiffer rods, higher screw density, and last but not least intraoperative neuromonitoring (IONM) substantially supporting intraoperative distraction and de-rotation of the deformed spine rendering highly effective correction. A satisfactory correction of AIS is favored by the use of fixed angle screws (FAS) versus multiaxial screws (MAS), due to the fact of unsurpassed stability of FAS in comparison to all other pedicle screw designs. The use of FAS, whenever possible, may address more effectively correction of the deformity both in the coronal plane by transporting FAS on stiff rods in a controlled manner leading to a relatively elongation of the posterior spine, as well as in the sagittal plane by allowing to introduce superior forces on the screws with less deterioration of the screw stability in order to perform consequent spine de-rotation with a modified DVR procedure removing the AIS pathognomonic hunchback.

50.2 Indications

Adolescent Idiopathic Scoliosis (AIS) (see Fig. 50.1) is stated in current literature with an average prevalence of 0.47–5.2% and therefore has to be considered as a common disease interfering with patients attaining puberty. The female-to-male ratio can vary substantially from 1.5:1 to 3:1 and will grow with increasing age. Curves with higher Cobb angles will affect girls even more: female-to-male ratio gains in curves between 10° and 20° from 1.4:1 to curves above

40° up to 6:1. The threshold for operative treatment of AIS are COBB angles of 40°–50° in order to prevent rising COBB angles later in life of the patient, if not treated. AIS can occur as a single, double, or triple curve and may be located in the thoracic spine, the lumbar spine or both thoracic and lumbar spine. Natural history of untreated AIS is reported in recent literature to be back pain (even though not disabling), cosmetic concerns and suggests that AIS does not lead to severe long-term health consequences—in contrast to reports from the late twentieth century reporting severe back pain, pulmonary disablement, increased risk of early death, and social isolation (Figs. 50.2, 50.3, 50.4, 50.5, and 50.6).

50.3 Contraindications

The main contraindication to posterior scoliosis surgery would be medical instability and inability to survive surgery. Predominantly most of the AIS patients eligible for posterior correction and fixation find oneself in ASA I and II with no or little evidence for osteopenia/osteoporosis (Figs. 50.7, 50.8, 50.9, 50.10, 50.11, and 50.12).

50.4 Technical Prerequisites

FAS (fixed angle screws—enabling more consequent correction), MAS (multiaxial screws—primarily used by the author as most proximal implant averting proximal junctional kyphosis [PJK]) which substitutes FAS if preferred. The use of hooks instead of pedicle screws is possible, however in recent times, is less prevalent but provides on occasion to be used as a salvage procedure when applying pedicle screws is not achievable. Stiffer (CoCr stronger than Titanium Alloy) and thicker rods (stiffness increases to the fourth power of its diameter!), cross-connectors (not mandatory with a screw density tending to 2.0), bending bars which provide faster, smoother, more efficient, and harmonic contouring of the rods, avoiding (in comparison to the use of the French bender

T. Bräuer (✉)
Spine Section of the Orthopedic Department Norwegian University of Science and Technology (NTNU), Trondheim, Norway
e-mail: Torsten.Brauer@stolav.no; torsten.brauer@hotmail.com

© Springer-Verlag GmbH Germany 2023
U. Vieweg, F. Grochulla (eds.), *Manual of Spine Surgery*, https://doi.org/10.1007/978-3-662-64062-3_50

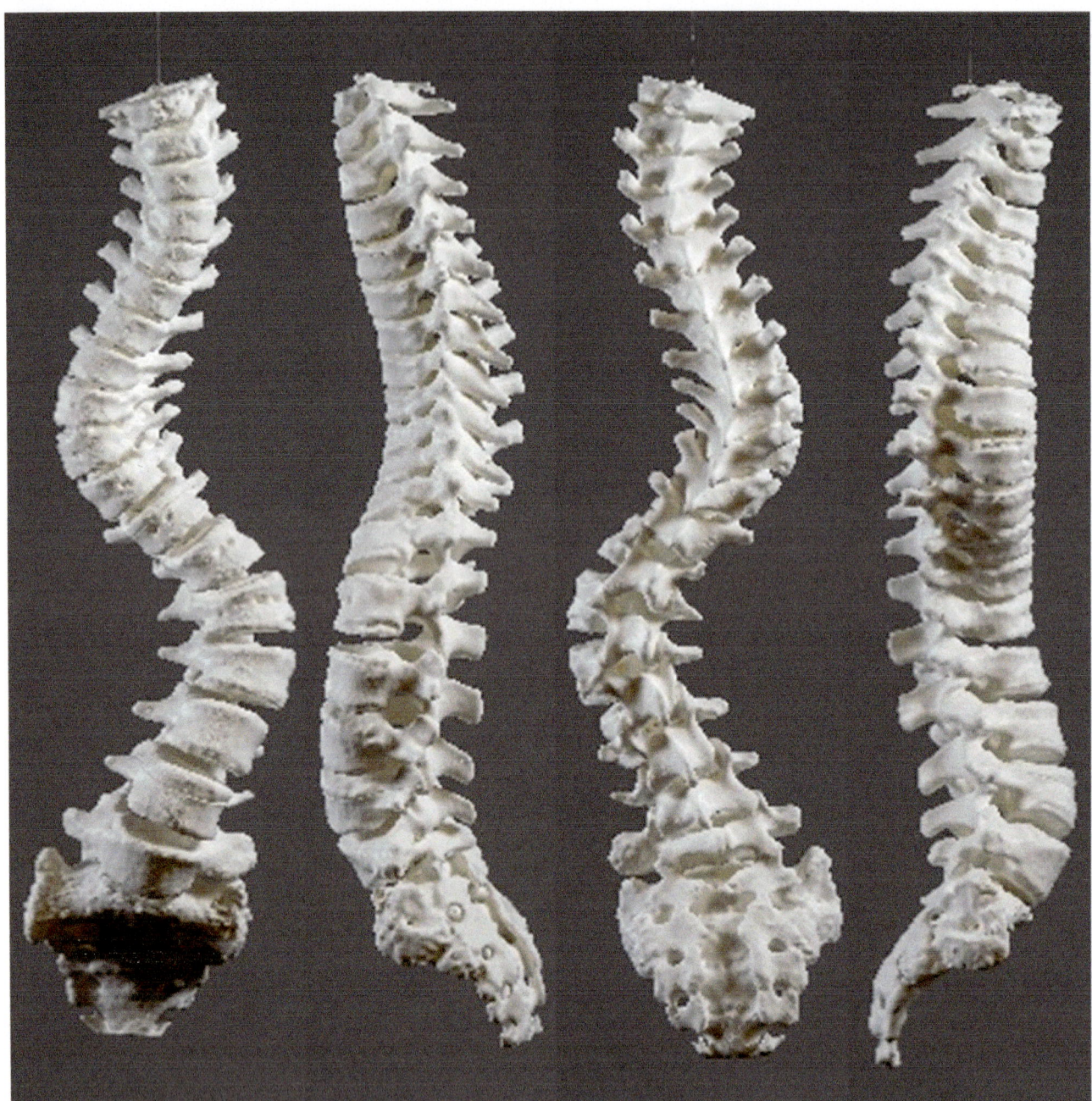

Fig. 50.1 3D-print in 4 aspects (from anterior-left-posterior-right) in the ratio 1 to 1 of the presented AIS case, which was obtained preoperatively on the basis of a low-dose CT

forceps) multiple break-points of the rods which may weaken the stability of the rod in the long run (CoCr less forgiving than Titanium alloy for interchanging bending). Likewise several rod reducers to accomplish on the level inserting of the rod to the screws protecting against undesirable "pull-out" of the FAS/MAS and by doing so eliminating the need for reduction tabs. The author encourages the bilateral use of distraction forceps to assist scheduled screw transport on the rods (explicit explanation of the technique follows in the course of this chapter), just as well the use of four counter

torques enabling to perform a modified straight forward Direct Vertebral Rotation (DVR). Besides coronal and in situ benders for exceeding contouring of the already screw-inserted rods for additional correction of the spinal deformity and a radiolucent table to ease X-ray control after completed setting of the screws, especially if there is the desire to use fluoroscopic assisted or intraoperatively navigated setting of the pedicle screws instead of freehand placement.

Last but not least, Intraoperative Neuromonitoring (IONM), which has become the gold standard providing

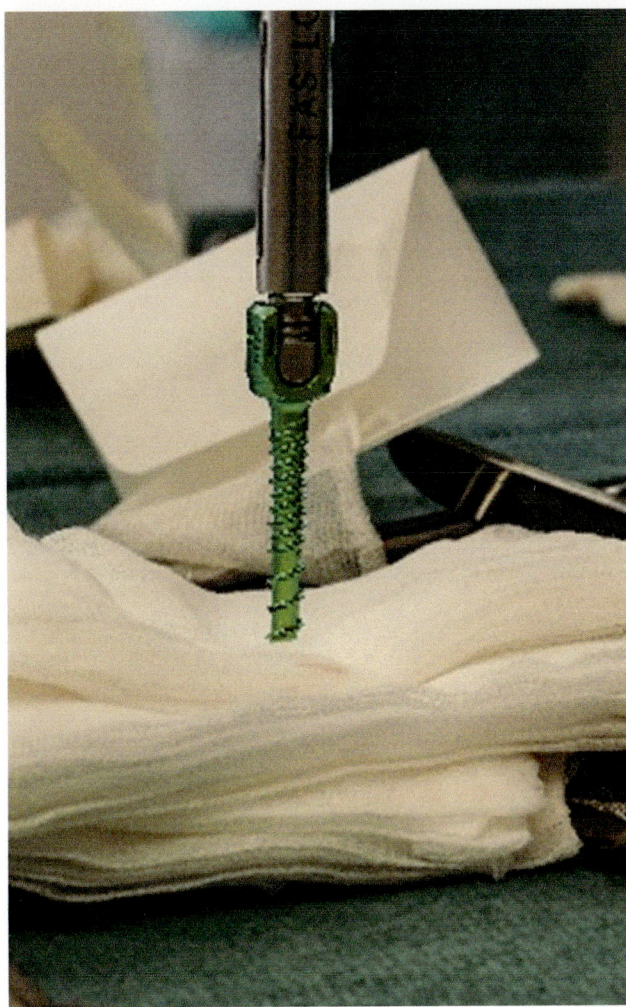

Fig. 50.2 Monoaxial pedicle screw (FAS)

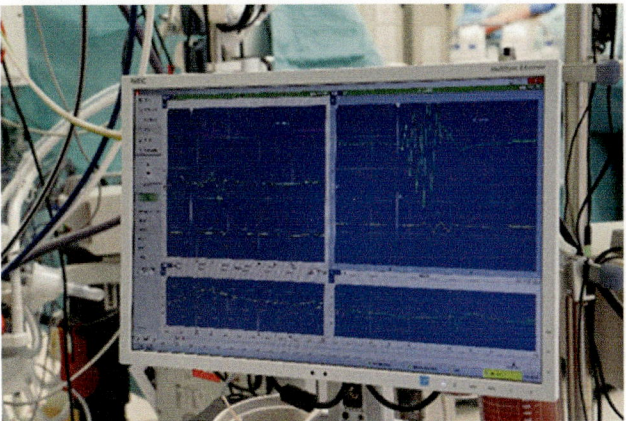

Fig. 50.4 32-Channel intraoperative neuromonitoring

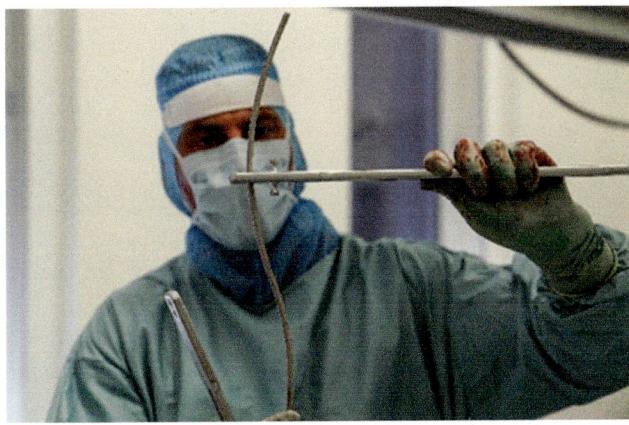

Fig. 50.3 Forming of the CoCr-rod using bending bars with less pressure point generation compared to the use of a French bender and the option of deforming the metallic microstructure more by tension than by pressure

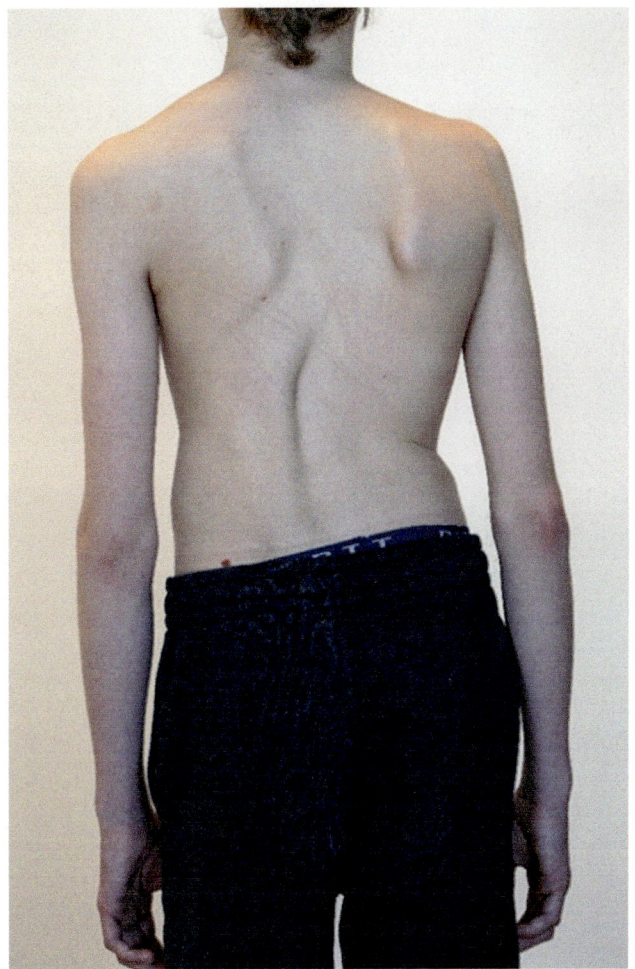

Fig. 50.5 Posterior aspect displaying shoulder imbalance, thoracic, and thoracolumbar hunchback

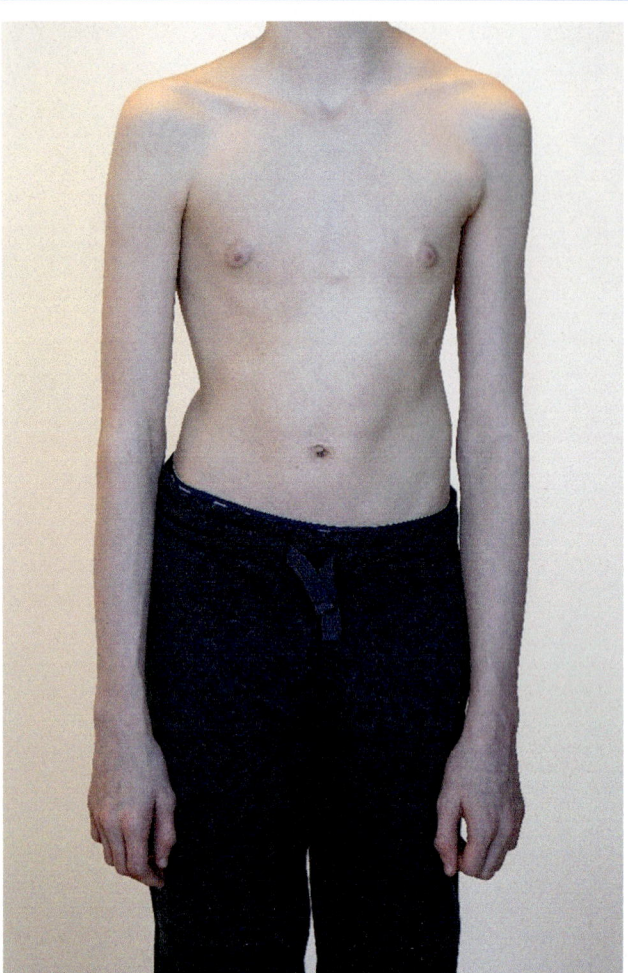

Fig. 50.6 Anterior aspect

both SSEPs (somatosensory-evoked potentials) and MEPs (motor-evoked potentials) and offering maximal security for the time being, has to be considered as compulsory to inhibit neurologic disaster to the best possible conditions.

50.5 Planning

The purpose of AIS correction is to achieve optimal deformity improvement by maintaining as much as possible mobile motion segments in the vertebral column. Preoperative evaluation focuses on details of curve location, magnitude, and flexibility. These parameters are used in combination with patient maturity factors (e.g., RISSER-sign, menarche) to determine optimal treatment decision, but definitive studies are not yet available that put in order specific surgical tactics. The goal is at all times to fuse as little of the spine as possible while effectively treating existing major curvature. At present, the Lenke classification system is regularly used

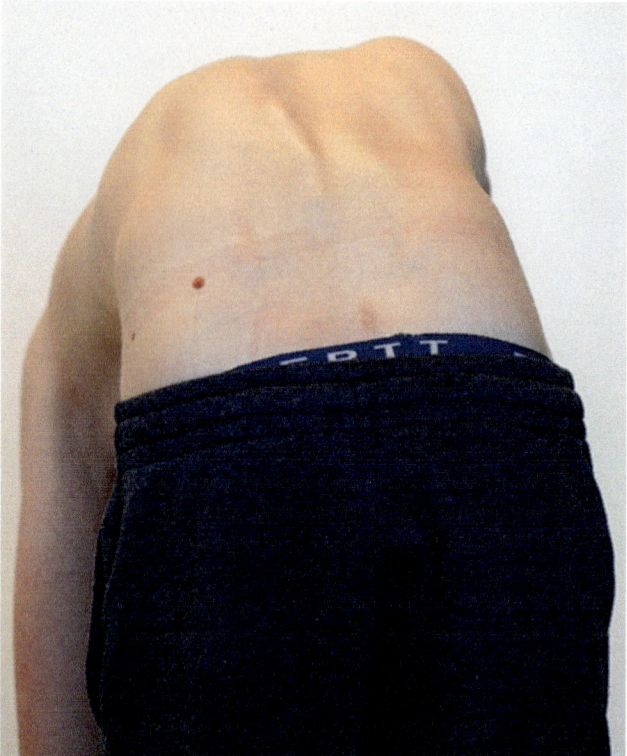

Fig. 50.7 Better visibility of both thoracic and thoracic lumbar gibbus when bending the patient forward

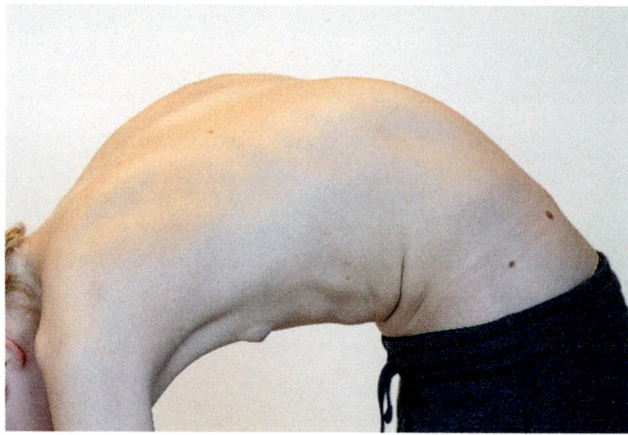

Fig. 50.8 Side view presenting the rotation in both the thoracic and thoracic lumbar spine appearing as double hunchback

to categorize adolescent idiopathic scoliosis. This system, first published in 2001, consists of the following three components:
- Curve type (1, 2, 3, 4, 5, or 6).
- Lumbar spine modifier (A, B, or C).
- Sagittal thoracic modifier (−, N, or +).

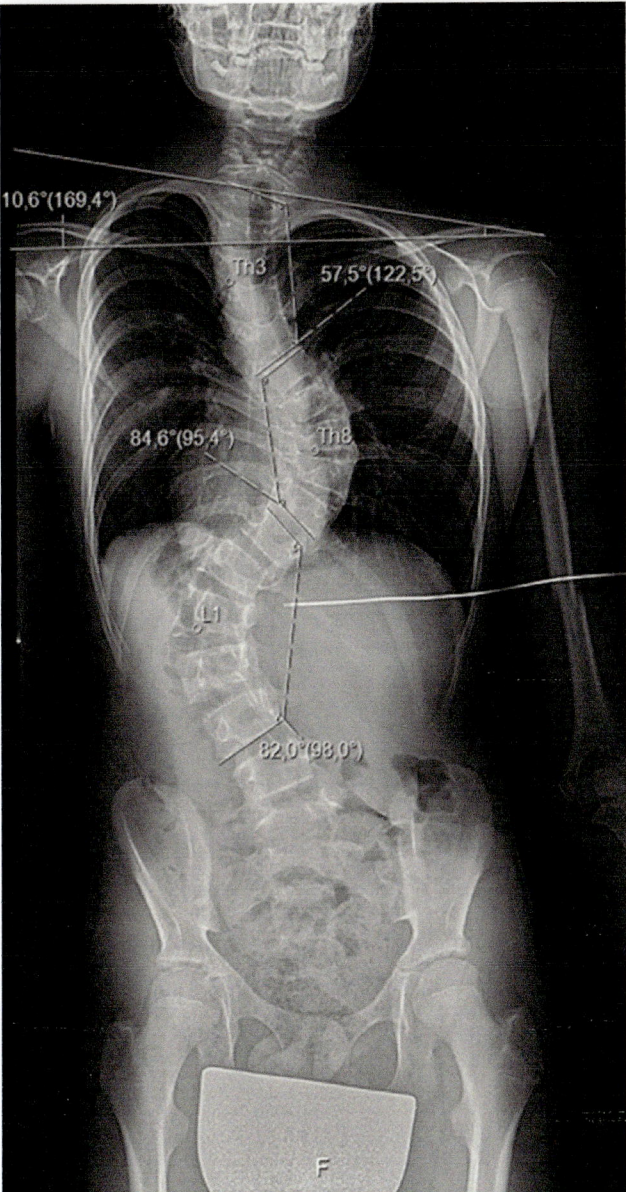

Fig. 50.9 X-ray coronal view Lenke type 4CN Triple Major

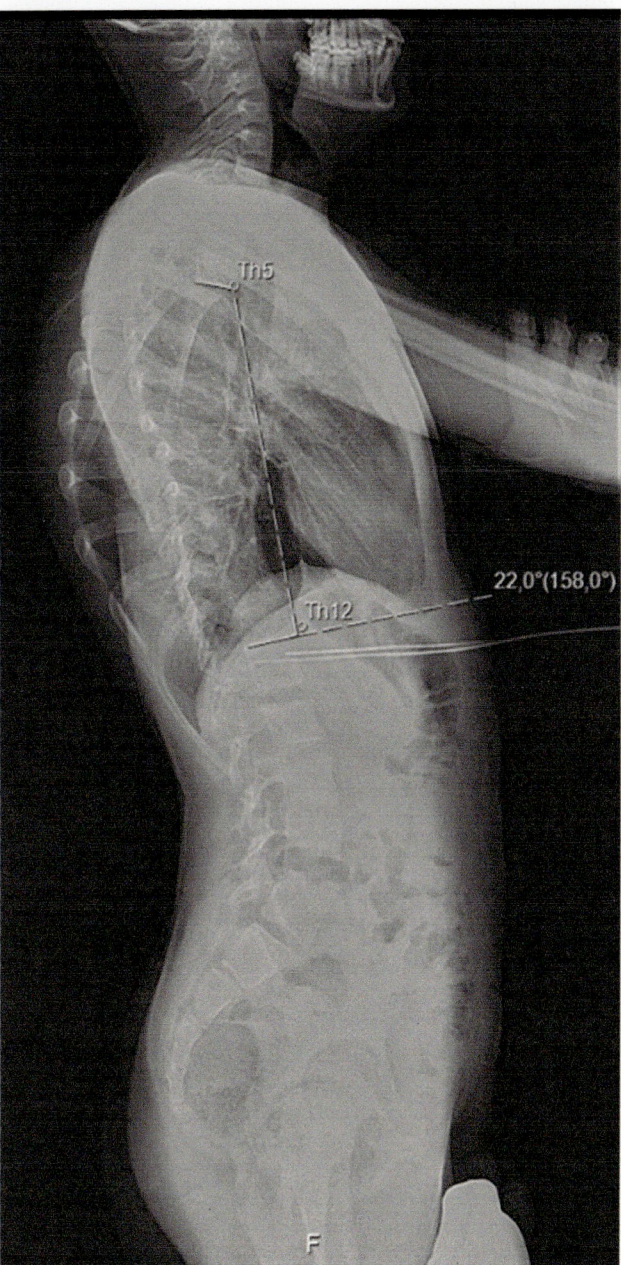

Fig. 50.10 X-ray sagittal view Lenke type 4CN Triple Major

On coronal and sagittal radiographs, the six types specified by Lenke et al. have specific characteristics that distinguish structural and nonstructural curves in the proximal thoracic (PT), main thoracic (MT), thoracolumbar (TL), and lumbar (L) regions. Regional curves are measured, the major curve is recognized, and a determination is made as to whether the minor curve is structural (i.e., curve does not bend out on bending pictures below 25°). The curve is then allocated to the relevant numeric type (1 through 6). The lumbar spine modifier is made on the relation of the center

sacral vertical line (CSVL) to the apex of the curve. If the CSVL passes between pedicles of apical lumbar vertebrae, the modifier A is assigned; if it touches a pedicle, the modifier B is assigned; and if it does not touch apical lumbar vertebrae, the modifier C is assigned. The sagittal thoracic modifier is based on the sagittal Cobb angle from T5 to T12. If the angle is less than 10° (hypokyphotic), the modifier is assigned; if it is 10–40° (normal), the modifier N is assigned;

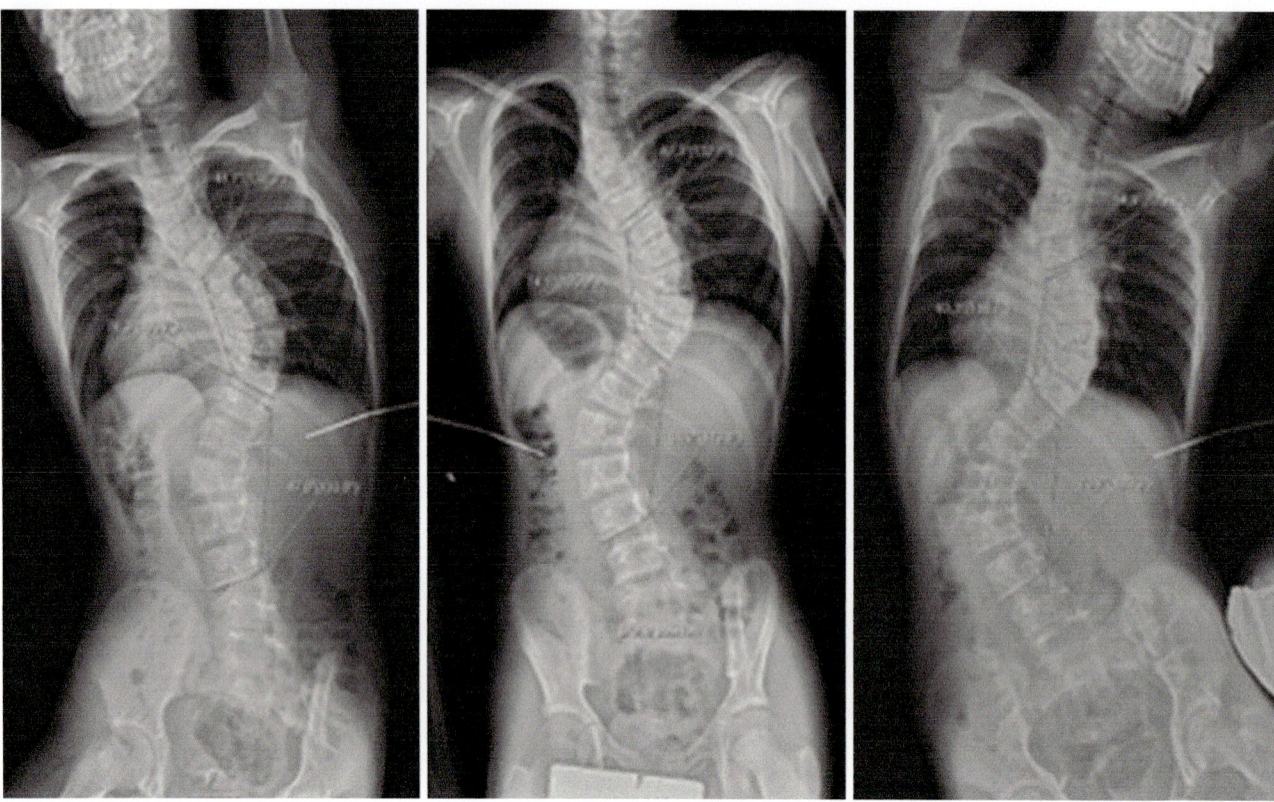

Fig. 50.11 *Left* and *right*: X-ray bending pictures confirming rigidity in all three curves/ the center: X-ray supine position depicting the real existing curvatures intraoperatively in a prone position

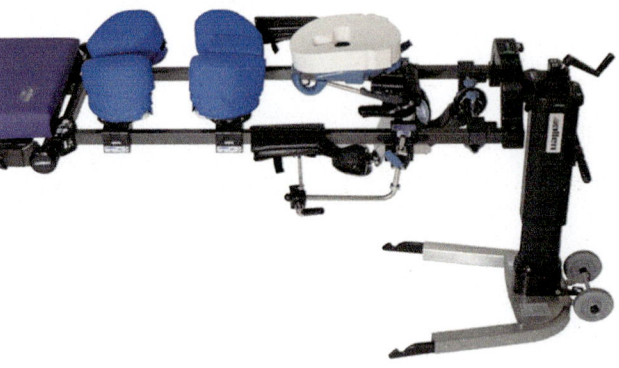

Fig. 50.12 ALLEN operating table

and if it exceeds 40° (hyperkyphotic), the modifier + is assigned. The Lenke classification can be of great help to plan the numbers of vertebrae to fuse (mostly COBB-to-COBB angle in structural curves to conserve motion in the non-structural curve/−s also described as "selective fusion"), however even with optimal pre-operatively planning, reality can show in some cases postoperatively—the need to extend the fixation in order for the patient to have proper balanced three-dimensionally.

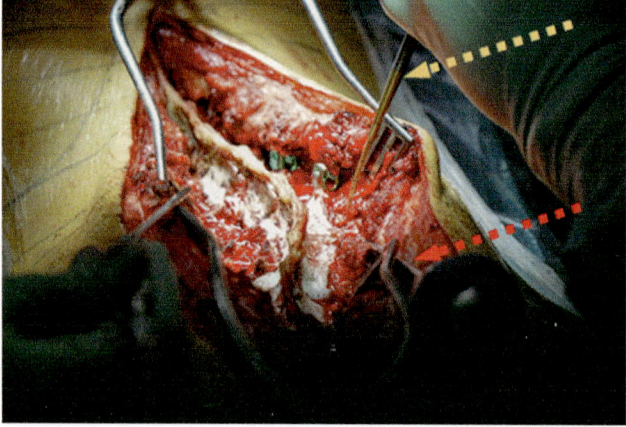

Fig. 50.13 *Yellow arrow:* gear shift positioned prior to penetration of the pedicle

50.6 Positioning

The patient is supported in a prone position on a radiolucent operating table (e.g., Jackson table or Allen table) (see Fig. 50.13). Positioning of the patient should assure least possible pressure upon the vena cava with the intention of minimalizing intraoperative loss of blood and preventing possible skin lesions due to extensive duration of the operative procedure.

50.7   Surgical Technique

Surgical technique benefits a great deal by better understanding the pathogenesis of AIS: when reaching puberty, the growth in the anterior wall of the corpus vertebrae in patients with AIS is "outrunning" the growth of the posterior wall resulting in a flat thoracic spine with an apical lordosis/hypokyphosis. The plumb line from C7 falls eventually behind/posteriorly to L5 with a concurrently introduction of an unnatural rotation in the main (structural) curve/−s which induces the growth of a hunchback. Nature's solution to deal with the anteriorly gain in anterior height of the vertebrae in order to prevent imbalance in the sagittal plane appears to give way by emerging a rotation as the minor biomechanical drawback in contrast to sagittal imbalance. The consistent analysis of the origin of AIS (and basically all deformities of the spine) may be a good help in correcting them: the derotation of the scoliotic spine removes the hump but at the same time brings back to light the original pathogenesis of AIS, which is the relative, anterior space requirement causing the rotation in the scoliotic spine, so that sagittal balance can be sustained. At the same time, anatomical derotation of the scoliotic spine produces an undesirable hypokyphosis. To avoid this, it is recommended to elongate the posterior structures of the spine starting from the apex of the primary curve, which can be achieved by transporting the pedicle screws on the rods using distraction forceps—closely controlled by intraoperative neuromonitoring.

50.7.1   Approach

A midline incision is performed with the customary subperiosteal exposure of the posterior bony elements. Scrupulous dissection will be beneficial concerning minimizing tissue damage, blood loss, and ultimately providing best possible fusion rate. Blunt dissection with gauze compresses instead of exceedingly usage of wound retractors may be supportive to complete optimal access and walking the thin line between hemostasis and preventable in situ rhabdomyolysis.

50.7.2   Instrumentation

The use of pedicle screws in correction of deformities also in the thoracic spine has become the gold standard in line for reported three column control of the vertebra, improved cor-

onal, sagittal and rotational correction, minimal loss of correction over time, lower pseud arthrosis rates, lower implant failures, and earlier return to activities. Several screw insertion techniques are described in the literature, for example, fluoroscopic assisted, Funnel technique, intraoperative navigation, electronic conductivity device, and freehand placement. The choice of the screw insertion technique is up to the personal preference of the surgeon. In the current selected operative case, the freehand technique was chosen which is also a topic of this book and is described in detail. In the following figure, the yellow arrow shows the gear shift before the penetration of the pedicle. At the given entry point for the pedicle screw, the cortical part of the lamina dorsalis has been removed beforehand in order to better haptically grasp the cancellous part of the pedicle. The gear shift illustrated here is pointed and bent. The tip points laterally in order to guarantee the integrity of the medial pedicle wall in the best possible way, which assures approx. 65% of the stability of the pedicle screw inserted later, while an intact lateral pedicle wall stands for approx. 35% of the stability of the pedicle screw. The gear shift is pushed approx. 10–15 mm into the pedicle with alternating rotations of the gear shift to the right and left. Experience shows that light, alternating rotations can facilitate safe and precise penetration, especially in the usually thin, narrow pedicels on the concave side of the scoliosis. After approximately 10–5 mm penetration of the pedicle with the gear shift, the tip of the gear shift is in the immediate vicinity where the pedicle merges into the vertebral body. It is recommended to pull the gear shift directly out of the pedicle at this point without any rotational movements. The gear shift is turned outside the pedicle with 180° and then inserted into the preformed pedicle screw channel with the tip pointing medially. Continue with the same pressure and rotation movements as before to the desired length of the pedicle screw channel. Although modern pedicle screw designs have self-tapping threads, it is preferable to use a pre-tap with a diameter 1 millimeter minor than that of the intended pedicle screw diameter to achieve a press-fit situation, and thus optimum stability of the pedicle screw (Figs. 50.14, 50.15, 50.16, 50.17, 50.18, 50.19, and 50.20).

The red arrow points to another gear shift that palpates the lateral boundary of the superior articular process and is then inserted from proximally to distally into the costo-transversal joint and then further pushed with nimble pressure approx. 10 mm. A slight movement of the gear shift from lateral to medial allows the haptic as well as optical representation of the lateral pedicle wall. Usually it is recommended to select the entry point for the pedicle screw approx. 2 mm medial from the lateral pedicle wall displayed with the gear shift. After thorough probing and integrity testing of the five walls that define the screw channel (floor-superior-inferior-lateral-medial), the pedicle screw is inserted (for FAS up to the resulting stop, i.e., when the floor of the screw head lies per-

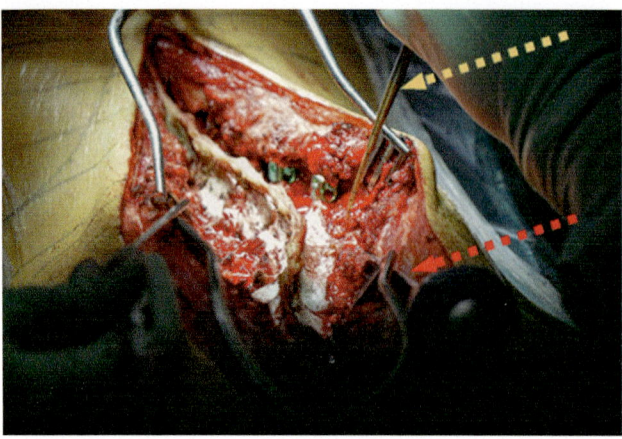

Fig. 50.14 *Yellow arrow:* gear shift positioned prior to penetration of the pedicle. *Red arrow:* indicating gear shift palpating the lateral boundary of the superior articular process unveiling the lateral border of the pedicle

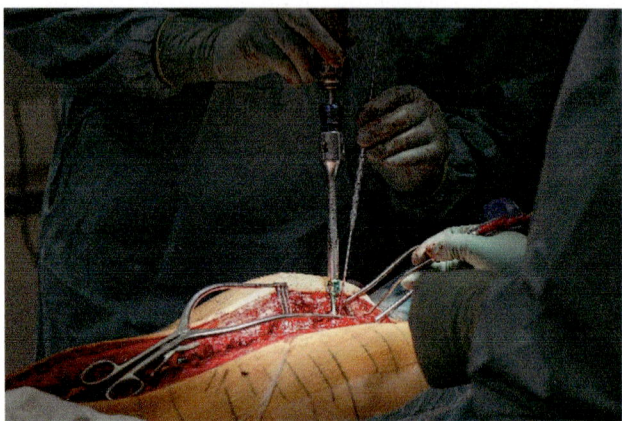

Fig. 50.15 After thoroughly palpating of the preformed pedicle screw channel with a probe follows the introduction of the pedicle screw

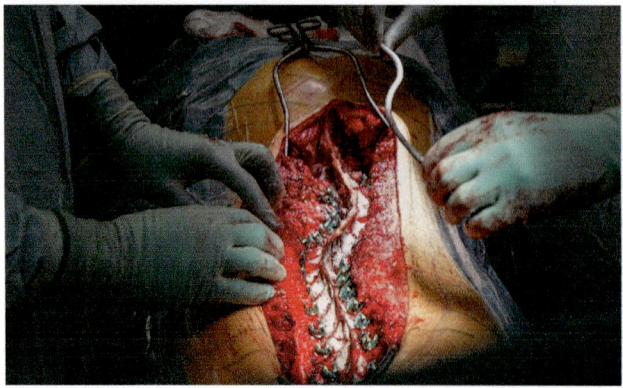

Fig. 50.16 The fittingly adjusted rod should compare to the given anatomy in the surgical site

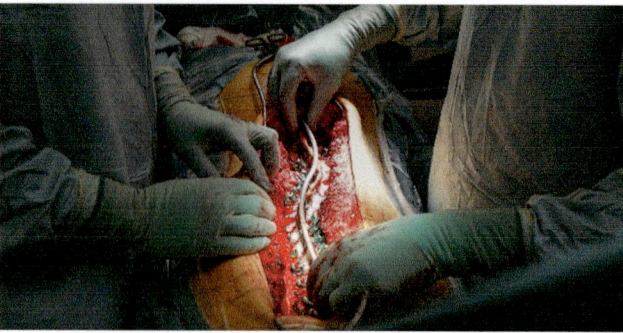

Fig. 50.17 Ideally, the appropriate rod can be placed on the spinal processes in the given surgical case indicating a proper fit

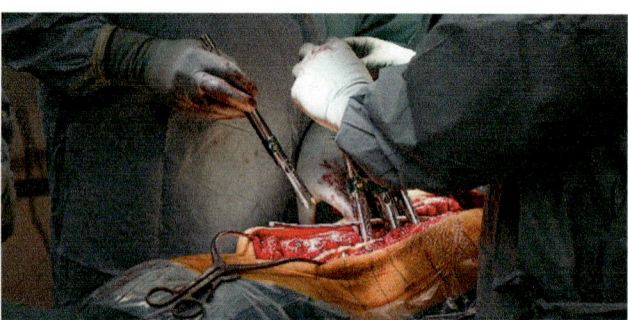

Fig. 50.18 Mount the rod reducer on the screw heads and insert the rod

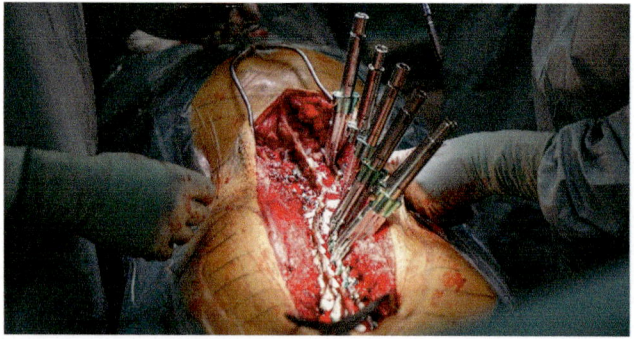

Fig. 50.19 With the help of rod reducers, the rod is consistently and without substantial force transfer brought into the screw heads and secured with the set screws

pendicular to the dorsal lamina and stops). When all planned pedicle screws are set, the rod is adjusted. For practical reasons, it may be helpful to adjust the rod at first for the side on which the concavity of the primary curve is found. The spinal processes are an additional aid in modifying the rod, as can be seen in the figure, the adjusted rod follows its course. Several rod reducers are placed on the screw heads to

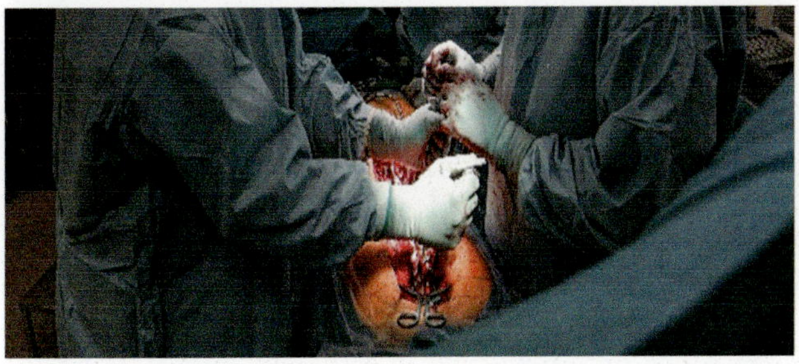

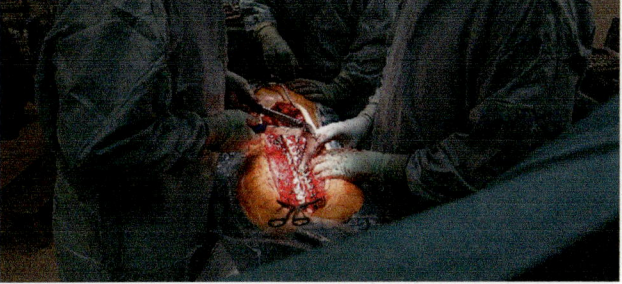

Fig. 50.20 90° rotation of the rod with the rod holder clamps from medial to lateral

Fig. 50.21 It follows both the definite profile adjustment of the rod and simultaneous an additional correction of the spinal deformity by using the coronal benders

minimize the load on the screws and their corresponding mobility segments. The rod is then inserted into the rod reducer. With the help of the rod reducers, the rod can be guided consistently and without significant effort into the heads of the pedicle screws. The rod holder forceps are used to rotate the rod by 90°. The rod is secured in the pedicle screw heads during rotation with set screws on top. The last plastic shape change of the rod is performed with the coronal benders to achieve further correction in the coronal plane. The other rod is applied in the same way on the contralateral side and fittingly adapted in its shape. The consecutive derotation takes place directly at the motion segment which is defined by two vertebrae with the vertebral disc between them. Four counter-torques are placed on each of the four attached pedicle screws in the motion segment. The extension of the relatively shortened posterior structures of the scoliotic spine is done bilaterally with distraction forceps between the proximal and distal pedicle screw pairs, while the set screws are loosely attached to the pedicle screw heads. After the distance between all four pedicle screws have been elongated on the rods to the matching height, the two counter torques on the convex side are carefully moved in the direction of the anterior spine, while the two counter torques on the concave side are guided in the direction of the spinal process at the same time. The inclination angle of all four pedicle screws in the motion segment in relation to the midline structures can be clearly seen from the long counter-torques. Ideally, with the same inclination angle, the pedicle screws are on the identical level in sagittal direction; in coronal level, the screws point with the tip toward the center of the anterior vertebral body. In this way, the achieved derotation can be visualized before the intraoperative X-ray control. Within the instrumented spine, all other motion segments are derotated in the same manner. The technique with four counter torques, compared with similar derotation techniques, may allow also a turning force within the intervertebral disc of the motion segment, which could optimize the derotation even more if desired. Once the three-dimensional correction has been completed, an X-ray inspection can be carried out (Figs. 50.21, 50.22, 50.23, 50.24, 50.25, 50.26, and 50.27).

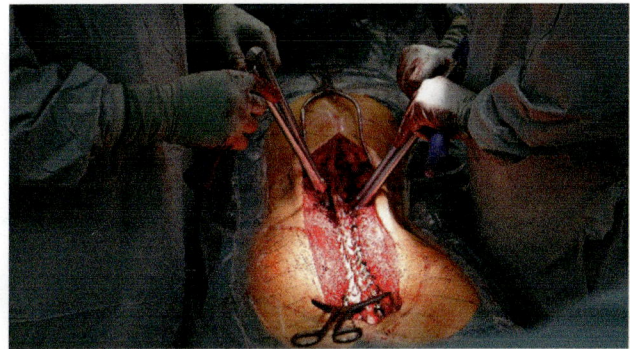

Fig. 50.22 Customized DVR technique with four counter torques mounted on four screw heads in the motion segment

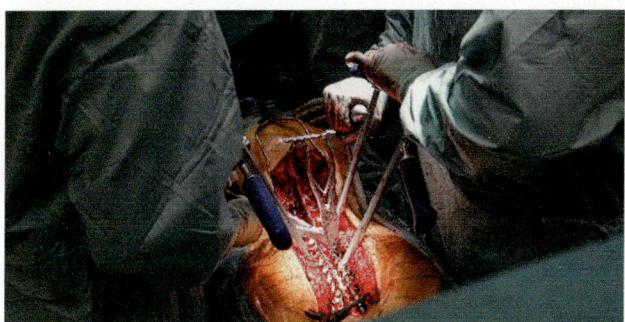

Fig. 50.23 Elongation of the motion segment by enlarging the distance of the screw heads on the rods performed with distraction forceps

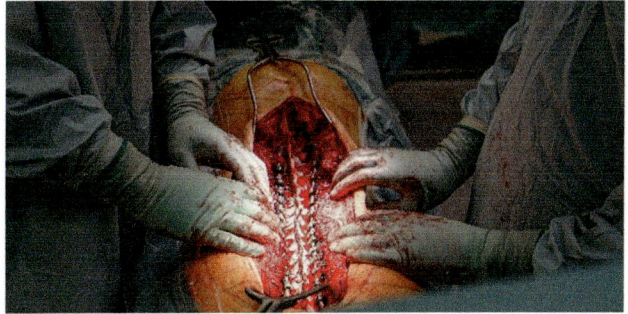

Fig. 50.24 Final check of the performed deformity correction (visual and with x-ray)

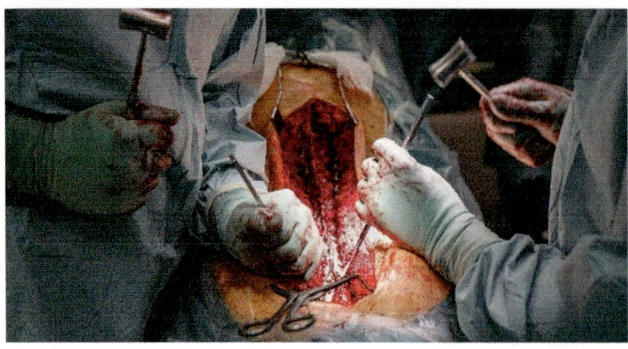

Fig. 50.25 Decortication and autologous bone transplantation inside the performed instrumentation

Operation is concluded by a consistent bilateral decortication of the lamina dorsalis within the instrumented spinal column in order to achieve optimal spondylodesis.

50.7.3 Postoperative Treatment

The postoperative therapy involves an effective pain treatment which in turn enables an early and optimal mobilization of the patient. The intrathecal morphine instillation carried out by the surgeon at the start of the operation and/or the introduction of two EDAs in the spinal canal after performed decortication of the instrumented spine can provide

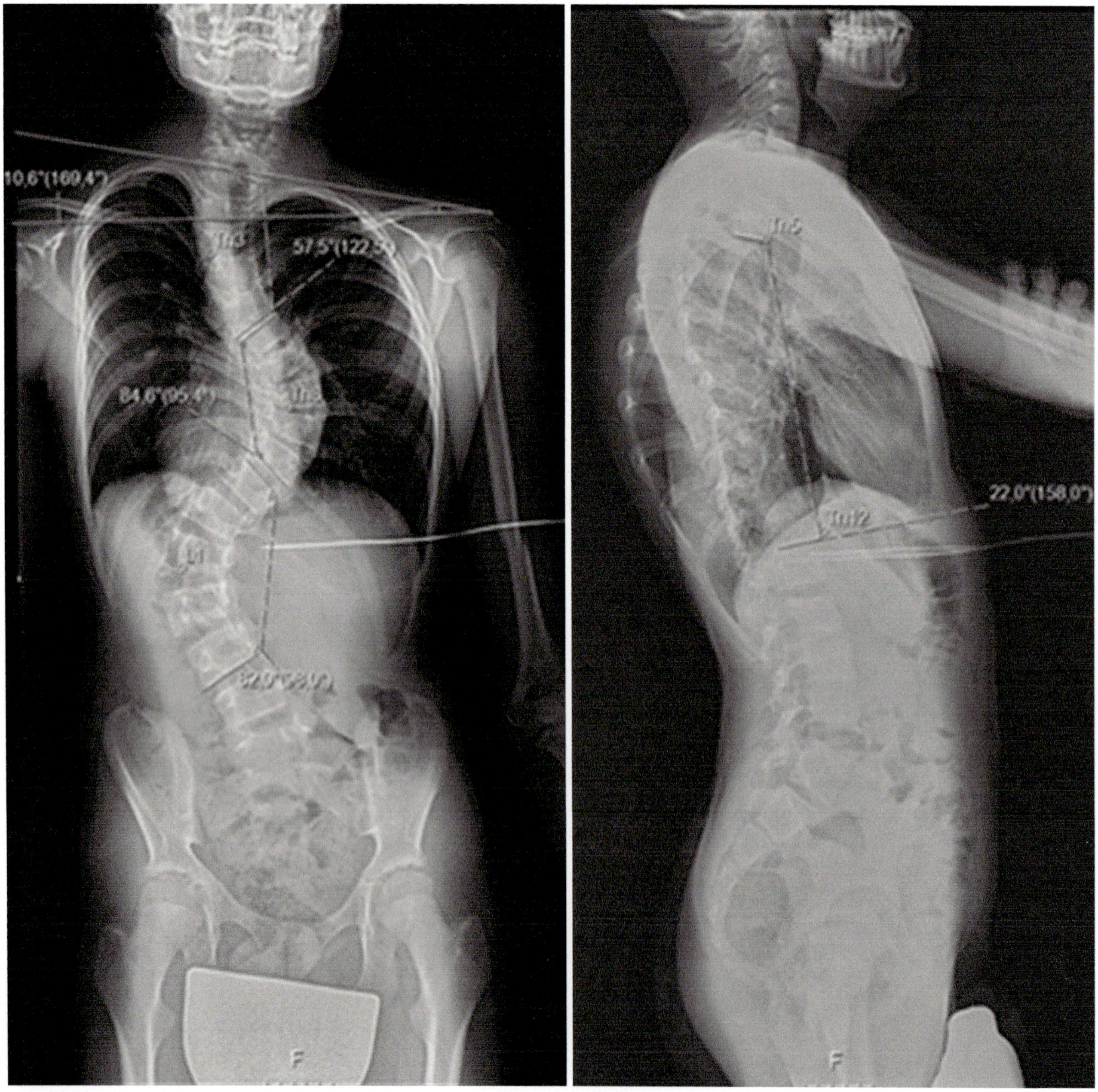

Fig. 50.26 Preop. X-rays showing LENKE type 4CN Triple Major

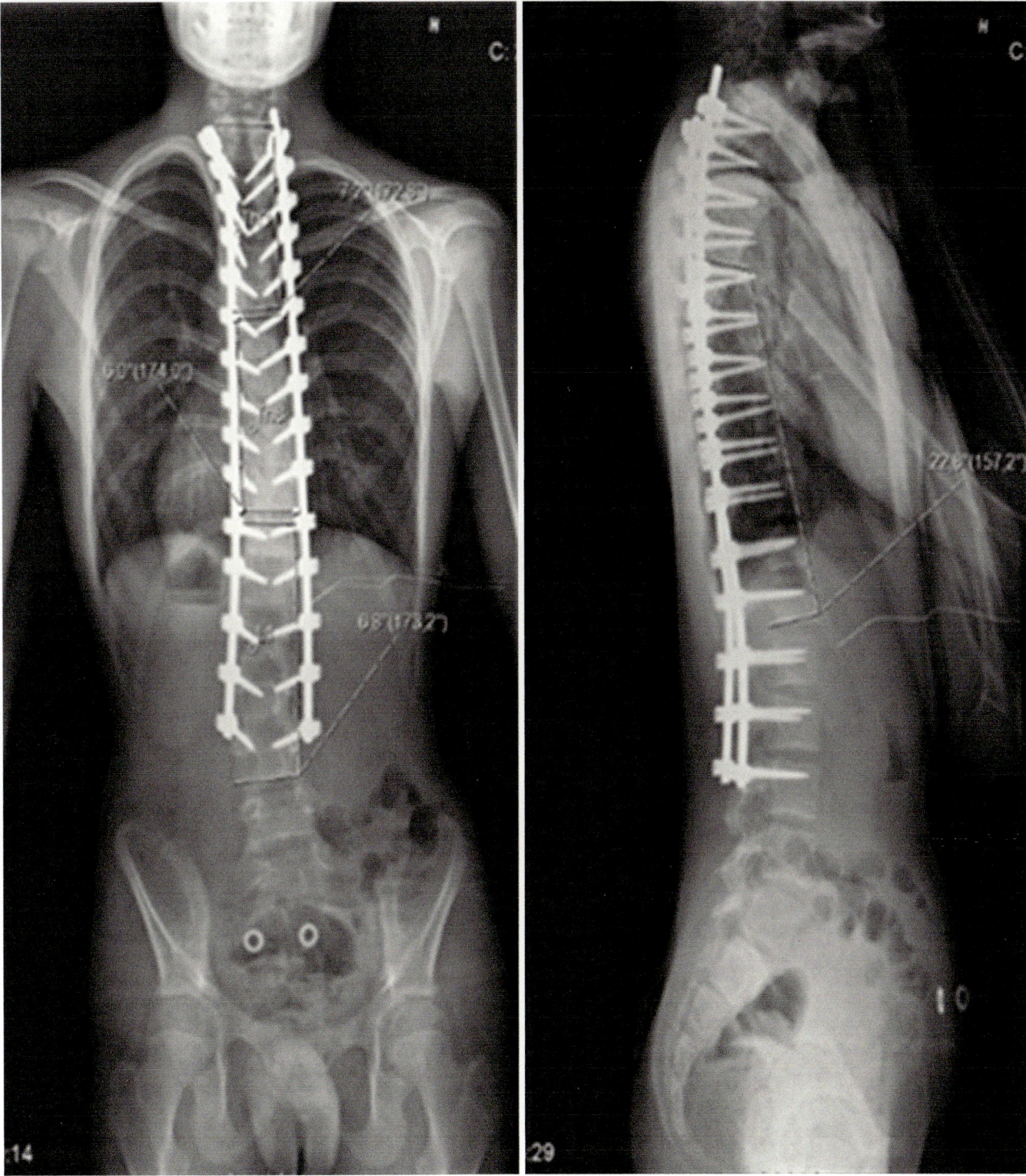

Fig. 50.27   2 year postop. X-ray

satisfactorily postoperative pain treatment accompanied by Paracetamol, morphine, and morphine-like drugs, as well as short-term use of NSAIDs. Total postoperative admission time is usually expected to be 4–7 days.

50.8 Tips and Tricks

- Operative 3D corrections of spinal deformities pose highly complex challenges to the surgeon. The acquisition of the necessary skills may require a correspondingly longer period of time and is undoubtedly made easier by a targeted training at institutions with a sufficiently high volume of deformity interventions to be performed.

- As is so often the case in surgical disciplines, a both well-designed and performed approach pays off in the correction of spinal deformities as well: the overview of the surgical site considerably facilitates more precise and easier placement of the pedicle screws, enables more atraumatic surgery by taking into account the anatomical structures, which in turn decreases significantly tissue damage— hence take down intraoperative blood loss— and benefits the patient in recovering faster.

- When placing the pedicle screw at the respective level, it may be recommended to consider the potential entry point of the pedicle screw on the contralateral side while simultaneously adjusting the intended direction of the pedicle screw channel on the ipsilateral side; ideally, the "virtual" pedicle screw channel on the contralateral side and the real one on the ipsilateral side should point toward each other. This procedure deems effective in preventing misplacement of the pedicle screw with either undesirable proximal penetration of the pedicle into the intervertebral disc or distal penetration which may compromise the nerve root.

- Considering the potential entry points of the pedicle screws before preparing the actual screw channel allows a smoother placement of the pedicle screws in line to each other. The subsequent insertion of the rod is then made considerably more convenient.

- Both of the above mentioned advices for placing the pedicle screws from S1 to Th1 may be of assistance to use polyaxial screws (MAS), as well as exclusively monoaxial screws (FAS) in extensive constructs.

- The mutually mixing of MAS and FAS in longer constructs should be carefully considered, as the significantly greater distance between the MAS-screw head (measured from the lamina dorsalis to the lower border of the inserted rod) compared to the FAS-screw head causes a hypomochlion (center of rotation of a joint) in the MAS-screw head which may give rise to the risk of pull-out moment in FAS.

- Self-image and self-understanding of the adolescent patients is—at a time when physical perfection is openly favored—far more negatively influenced by the observable hump than by the scoliosis/spinal curvature itself. The trade-off in the successful de-rotation of the hump can lead to a concurrent undesired intensification of the already preoperatively existing hypokyphosis. The extension of the spinal posterior structures with pedicle screw transport on rigid CoCr rods can counteract the formation of hypokyphosis but cannot completely protect against it. An optimal and patient satisfactory derotation of the hump has probably been achieved at the point where further derotation would fall short of the preoperative existing kyphosis, and thus threatening a stable sagittal balance of the spine.

References

1. Akbarnia Y. Thompson: the growing spine. Berlin Heidelberg: Springer-Verlag; 2011.
2. Danielsson AJ. Natural history of adolescent idiopathic scoliosis: a tool for guidance in decision of surgery of curves above 50°. J Child Orthop. 2013;7:37–41.
3. Dunn J, Henrikson NB, Morrison CC, et al. Screening for adolescent idiopathic scoliosis evidence report and systematic review for the US preventive services task force. JAMA. 2018;319(2):173–87.
4. Konieczny MR, Senyurt H, Krauspe R. Epidemiology of adolescent idiopathic scoliosis. J Child Orthop. 2013;7:3–9.
5. Weiss HR, Karavidas N, Moramarco M, Moramarco K. Long-term effects of untreated adolescent idiopathic scoliosis: a review of the literature. Asian Spine J. 2016;10(6):1163–9.
6. Wong HK, Tan KJ. The natural history of adolescent idiopathic scoliosis. Indian J Orthop. 2010;44(1):9–13.

Thoracic Vertebrectomy and Spinal Reconstruction Via Posterior or Combined Approaches

51

M. Ruf, J. Petrovics, G. Ostrowski, and T. Pitzen

51.1 Introduction and Core Message

Thoracic vertebrectomy and spinal reconstruction via posterior or combined approaches is a demanding technique for surgical treatment of spinal tumors that require a complete resection of the entire vertebra, including the posterior structures (lamina, facet joints, transverse processes, pedicles) as well as the anterior structures (vertebral body). This entire *en bloc vertebrectomy* or *spondylectomy* entails a complete disruption of the continuity of the spine with severe instability. Depending on the extension of the underlying pathology, the resection comprises one or more vertebrae, usually with resection of the adjacent ribs within their proximal part. This technique allows for resection of tumors in one piece including a healthy layer (marginal or wide resection). There is some evidence that local recurrence is reduced and long-term survival is more probable [1–3]. However, the technique creates a relevant instability necessitating a biomechanically sound reconstruction that is able to take loads and to withstand flexion/extension, lateral bending, and left-right axial rotation.

51.2 Indication

- Primary malignant tumors.
- Semimalignant tumors.
- Isolated spinal metastasis with long life expectancy.

M. Ruf (✉) · G. Ostrowski
Center for Spine Surgery, SRH Klinikum Karlsbad-Langensteinbach, Karlsbad, Germany
e-mail: michael.ruf@srh.de

J. Petrovics · T. Pitzen
Center for Spine Surgery, Orthopedics, and Traumatology, SRH Klinikum Karlsbad-Langensteinbach, Karlsbad, Germany

51.3 Contraindication

- Tumor infiltration of the spinal cord.
- Tumor infiltration in essential adjacent organs.
- Multiple metastasis (relative).
- Prognosis infausta.

51.4 Technical Prerequisites

Fluoroscopy, radiolucent operating table, thoracotomy resp. laparotomy equipment, intraoperative electrophysiological monitoring (SSEP/MEP), vertebral body replacement devices, adaptable to every size of defect (titanium mesh cages (Harms), expandable cages), posterior instrumentation with different diameters, transition rods if necessary at the cervicothoracic region.

51.5 Planning

Conventional radiographs, computed tomography, and MRI are essential to assess localization and extension of the tumor. Computed tomography of brain, thoracic chest, and abdominal cavity as well as bone scintigraphy are necessary to exclude further tumor and metastases, so widespread disease. Using all radiographic information, the border of the tumor is exactly identified. Every vertebra that is involved has to be included completely into the intended resection, also including affected ribs and surrounding soft tissue with a wide safety distance. As the vertebra contains the spinal cord, the area has to be defined where the bony ring can be opened with sufficient distance to the tumor (Fig. 51.1). Then an appropriate approach is chosen to remove the tumor in one piece (posterior or combined). In tumors with a pronounced perfusion, segmental arteries above and below the feeding artery, as well as the feeding artery itself, should be embolized preoperatively. Pre- and intraoperative neuromonitoring (SSEP, MEP) is strongly recommended.

© Springer-Verlag GmbH Germany 2023
U. Vieweg, F. Grochulla (eds.), *Manual of Spine Surgery*, https://doi.org/10.1007/978-3-662-64062-3_51

A score is proposed as a tool for surgical strategy for metastatic spine tumor, including grade of malignancy, visceral metastases, and bone metastases. Tomita et al. advised the surgical classification of spinal tumor (Figs. 51.2 and 51.3) based on the pattern of local vertebral tumor progression [4].

The Spinal Instability Neoplastic Score (SINS) was developed for assessing patients with spinal neoplasia. It identifies patients who may benefit from surgical consultation or intervention. It also acts as a prognostic tool for surgical decision making [5].

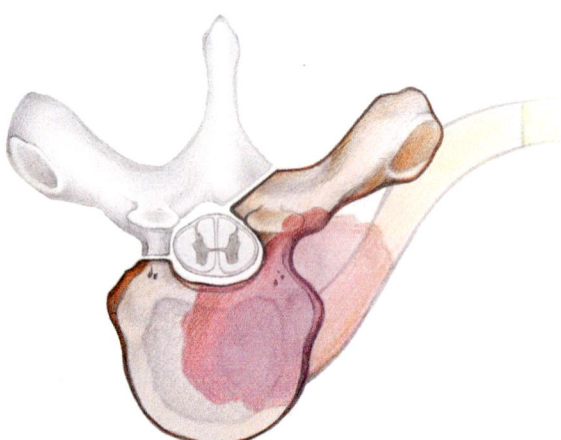

Fig. 51.1 Artist's view to illustrate preoperative planning of the opening of the spinal canal with sufficient distance to the tumor. The canal is opened at the position of the gaps, thus giving a safety margin around the tumor mass

51.6 Surgical Technique

Total en bloc vertebrectomy is the most aggressive surgical treatment for spinal tumors. It comprises a complete resection of the posterior structures and stabilization by a posterior approach, as well as the resection of the vertebral body via costotransversectomy or an additional anterior approach.

51.6.1 Posterior Approach

Tumor lesions that do not exceed to adjacent structures can be resected by a posterior approach with costotransversectomy [6]. This technique provides an adequate exposure of all three columns through a single posterior approach. It allows for en bloc corpectomy and sufficient stabilization with anterior support. The spinal cord can be observed during the whole resection maneuver. A clear disadvantage of the procedure is the limited visualization and control of the great vessels especially when the tumor exceeds the border of the vertebral body.

- Patient in prone position on radiolucent table under general anesthesia.
- Midline skin incision and subperiostal dissection of muscles far lateral to expose the proximal ribs. In case of tumor expansion to the posterior muscles, dissection leaves the muscles at the resectate.
- Placement of pedicle screws typically two levels below and above affected vertebra/vertebrae.

Fig. 51.2 Tomita's surgical classification of spinal tumors [4]

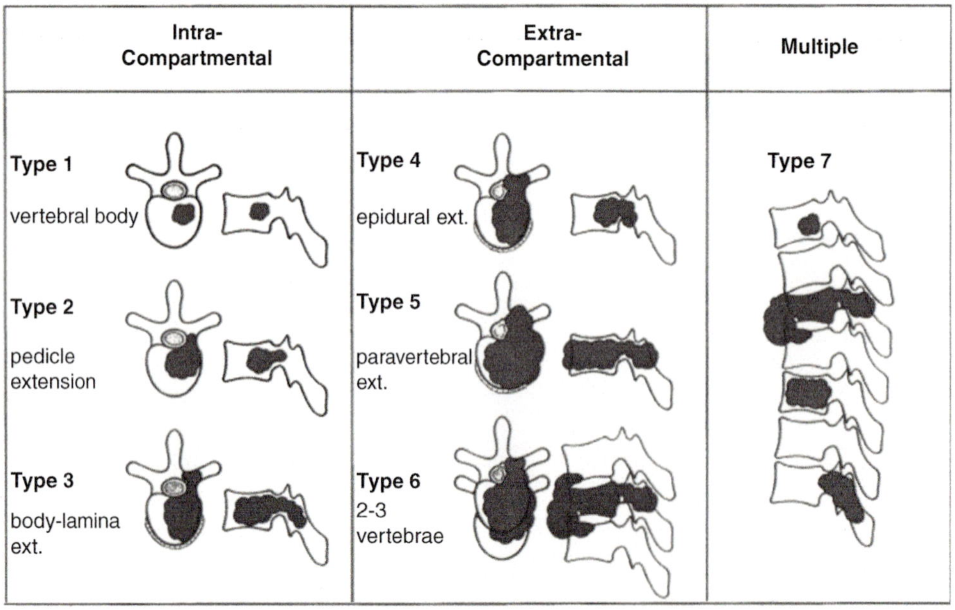

Intra-Compartmental	Extra-Compartmental	Multiple
Type 1 vertebral body	**Type 4** epidural ext.	**Type 7**
Type 2 pedicle extension	**Type 5** paravertebral ext.	
Type 3 body-lamina ext.	**Type 6** 2–3 vertebrae	

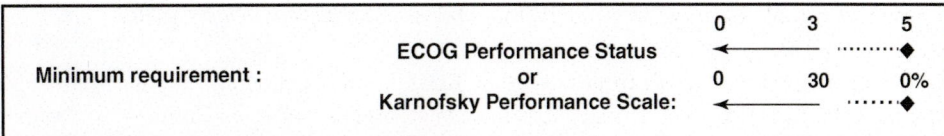

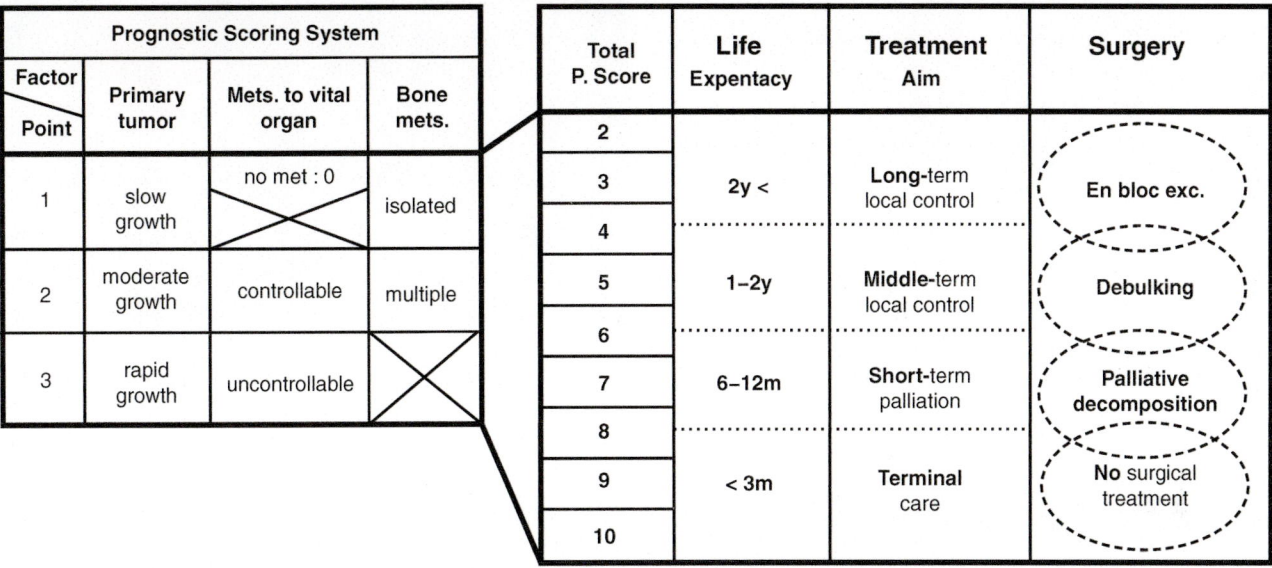

Fig. 51.3 Surgical strategy for spinal metastasis [4]

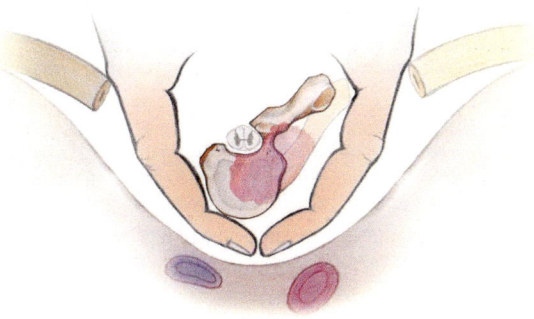

Fig. 51.4 Artist`s view for blunt dissection around the vertebral body

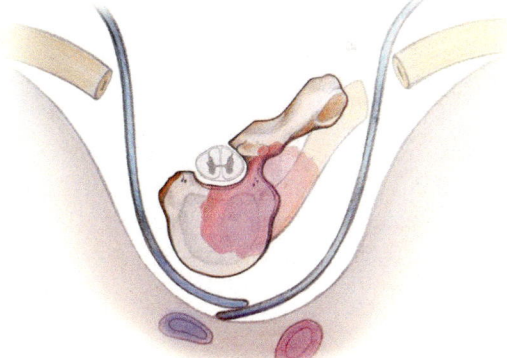

Fig. 51.5 Artist`s view of how the spatula protects the anterior structures

- The ribs on the affected level are transected lateral to the costotransverse joints with sufficient distance to an eventual tumor infiltration.
- The pleura is bluntly separated from the ribs and the vertebra. The aorta is carefully dissected from the anterior aspect of the vertebral body (Fig. 51.4). The segmental vessels are ligated if necessary.
- Blunt spatulae are inserted to protect the anterior lying vessels (Fig. 51.5).
- The lamina, facet joints, and pedicle are now cut and removed according to the preoperative planning (Fig. 51.1). The spinal cord and the nerve roots are visualized.

- The nerve roots at the affected level(s) are ligated and cut.
- The disks above and below the tumor-infiltrated vertebra/ae are incised and removed from both sides including the posterior longitudinal ligament. A temporary rod is inserted for stabilization alternatingly at the contralateral side.
- The spinal cord is carefully dissected from the posterior wall.
- When the resection of the vertebral body is intended by the posterior approach, it is now carefully rotated around the dural sac and removed en bloc (Fig. 51.6).

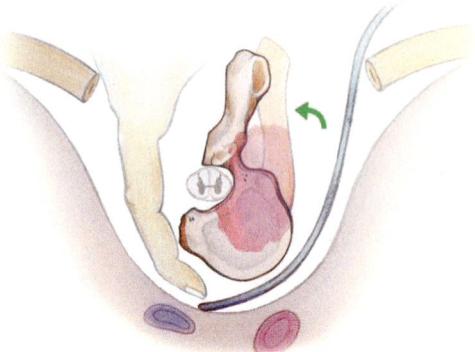

Fig. 51.6 Removal of the vertebral body including pedicle/transverse process en bloc

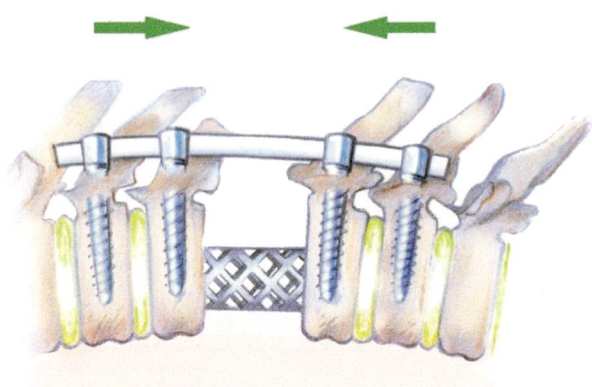

Fig. 51.7 Anterior support, posterior compression

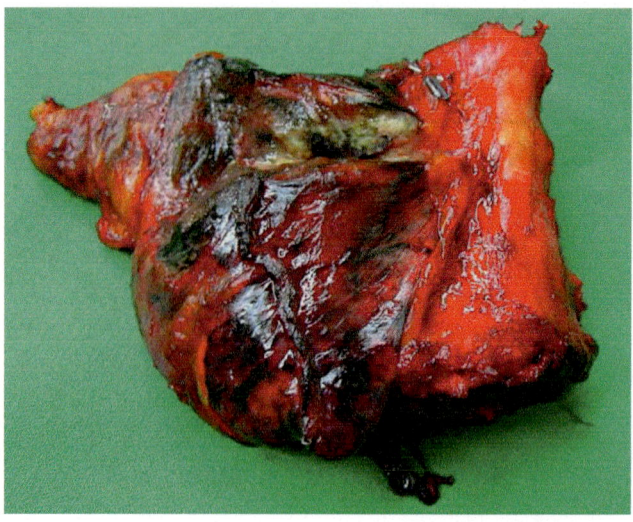

Fig. 51.8 Photograph of an en bloc specimen, including three vertebral bodies and the infiltrated upper lobe of the lung

- Debridement of the adjacent endplates. Reconstruction of the anterior column with an anterior support (Harms cage, filled with bone cement / expandable cage) (Fig. 51.7).
- Insertion of both rods, compression via the instrumentation (Case 1).

51.6.2 Anterior Approach

When the tumor exceeds the anterior border of the vertebral body with infiltration of the adjacent soft tissues (vessels, lung), an additional anterior approach is necessary. This approach allows for a widespread visualization of the anterior vessels (aorta, azygos vein, segmental vessels), pleura and lung, mediastinum. In case of infiltration of the lung or major vessels, a thoracic surgeon or cardiovascular surgeon should be consulted. It may be necessary to dissect the bronchus and the pulmonary vessels at the hilus

first to mobilize a pulmonary lobe, which allows leaving the lobe in one piece with the vertebral bodies (Fig. 51.8). Important arteries may be replaced by a vascular prosthesis (Fig. 51.9).

51.6.2.1 Thoracic Approach (T4–T9)

For thoracotomy in the midthoracic spine, the right-sided approach is preferred to avoid the aorta. However, a left-sided approach may be necessary when the tumor expands at the left side to dissect the segmental vessels and mobilize the aorta.

- Anesthesia with a double-lumen endotracheal tube for single lung ventilation is recommended. To decrease the risk of atelectasis, reinflate the lung every 30 min.
- The patient is placed in lateral decubitus position with the desired side up on the table with elevated arm.
- After dissection of the trapezius muscle and mobilization/dissection of the serratus anterior muscle, thoracotomy is performed usually 1–2 ribs above the involved segment. Osteotomy of the lower rib distally facilitates a sufficiently dimensioned approach.
- The margins of the tumor are localized under fluoroscopic control; the disks adjacent to the planned resectate are marked.
- The parietal pleura is usually left at the tumor. The segmental vessels at the tumor level are ligated close to the aorta, the aorta is carefully mobilized. The intervertebral disks are incised and removed (most parts of the disks, especially posterior annulus, posterior longitudinal

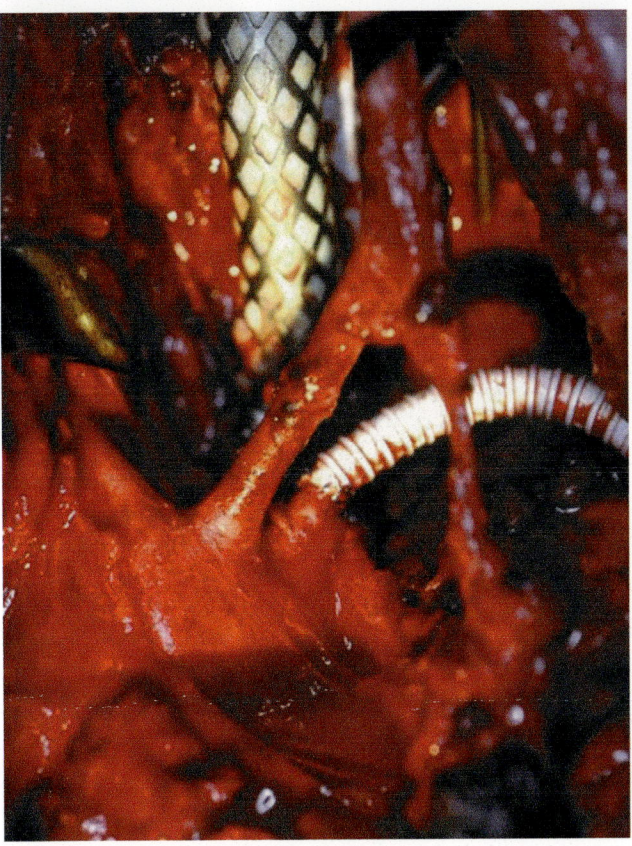

Fig. 51.9 Intraoperative situs after resection of a cervicothoracic tumor with infiltration of the subclavian artery; goretex substitute of the vessel

ligament, and annulus of the contralateral side should already be removed by the posterior approach).

• The tumor resectate is now mobile and can be carefully lifted from the spinal cord. It is removed in one piece.

• The adjacent endplates are debrided and an anterior column support is inserted. A meshgraft can be used to close the defect of the parietal pleura.

• A second posterior approach can be performed to apply compression forces at the posterior instrumentation, thus increasing the overall stability of the construct (Case 2).

51.6.2.2   Thoracolumbar Approach (T9–T12)

• In the thoracolumbar region, a left-sided approach is preferred.

• The planning and positioning in lateral decubitus position is similar to a midthoracic approach.

• If a phrenotomy is necessary, the peritoneal sac is mobilized starting at the costodiaphragmatic angle. The diaphragm is cut close to the costal insertion.

• Ligation of the segmental vessels, mobilization and removal of the tumor, as well as the stabilization is similar as described for the midthoracic area.

• If needed, the psoas muscle can be removed in one piece with the tumor.

51.6.2.3   Cervicothoracic Junction

• The patient is placed in a supine position.

• A common left-sided approach to the lower cervical spine is performed.

• Complete or partial osteotomy of the sternum after release of the soft tissue dorsal to the sternum.

• Dissection of the omohyoides, sternohyoideus, and sternothyroideus muscles.

• The inferior thyroid artery is ligated and transsected.

• If necessary, the brachiocephalic vein may be ligated and cut.

• A blunt dissection in front of the vertebral column is possible down to T4. Esophagus and trachea are retracted medially, thoracic duct and vessels laterally (Case 3).

51.7   Tips and Tricks

• A meticulous dissection and mobilization of the tumor by the posterior approach extremely facilitates the anterior part of the surgery. All connections to the surrounding structures that can be reached from posterior should be cut from posterior.

• When to use an additional anterior approach – it is not always easy to answer. Based on our experience, we suggest the following strategy: if mobilization of the big vessels is too difficult and the tumor mass is too big, use an additional anterior approach.

• The use of autologous bone or bone substitute in the primary tumor resection surgery is hindering the postoperative CT and MRI imaging in detecting early tumor recurrences. Bone may be added after a longer tumor-free interval to achieve a lifetime bony fusion.

• In case of resection of two or more vertebrae with pedicles, the nerve roots at the tumor side must be cut in the spinal canal to allow the removal of the vertebrae without traction at the spinal cord. The dura can be sutured after removal of the tumor.

• Compression of the facet joints of the adjacent vertebrae via the instrumentation increases the rotational stability. In short monovertebral fixations, a cross-link is able to resist rotational forces (Case 4).

• Take care to check SSEP and MEP in the patient before anesthesia is injected; so, you will not be surprised in case neuromonitoring is not possible due to any reason!

51.8 Clinical Cases

Case 1 Aneurysmatic Bone Cyst

A 27-year-old male with nonspecific, nontraumatic back pain at mid-thoracic level. After complete preoperative diagnostics (CT, MRI) (see Figs. 51.10a–c and 51.11) and additional angiographic embolization, an en bloc vertebrectomy T8 and 9 (see Figs. 51.12a, b and 51.13) via costotransverectomy, instrumentation with internal fixator system T6 to 11, and vertebral body replacement with a titanium mesh cage filled with bone cement were performed.

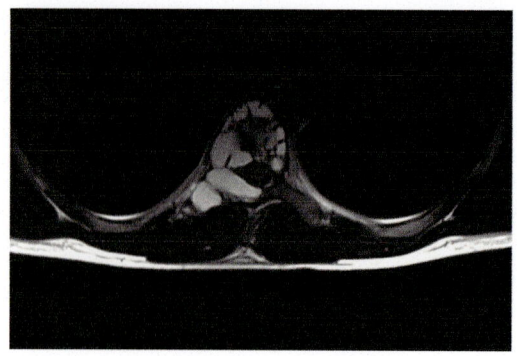

Fig. 51.11 Preoperative MRI scan, axial view, Case 1

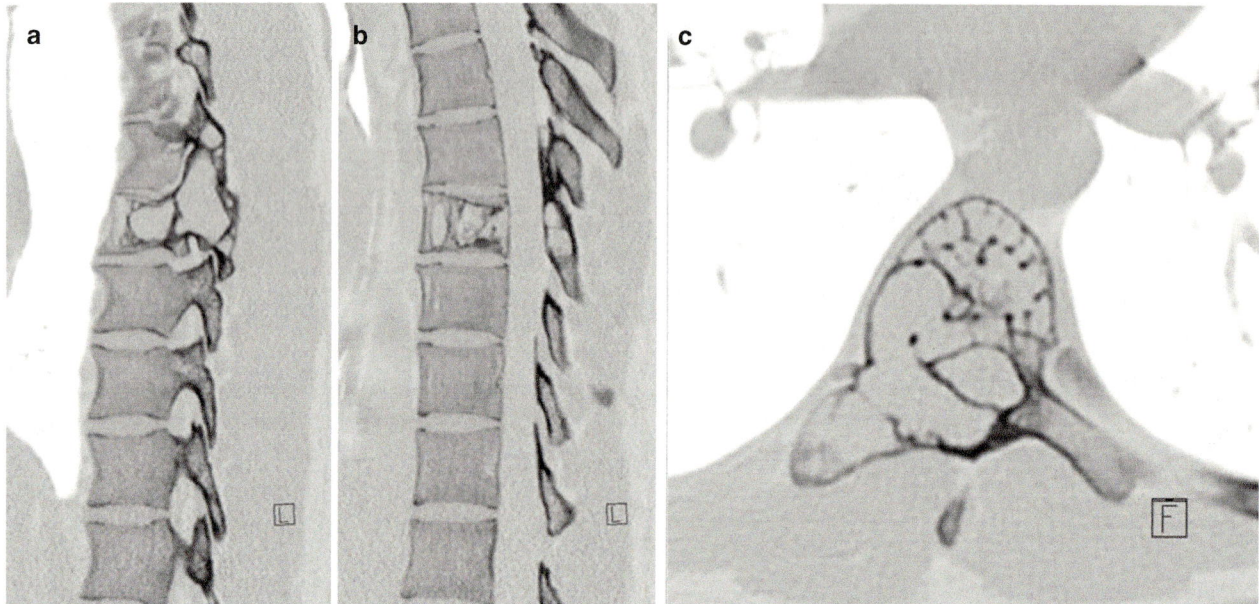

Fig. 51.10 Preoperative CT scans with sagittal (**a**, **b**) and axial views (**c**), Case 1

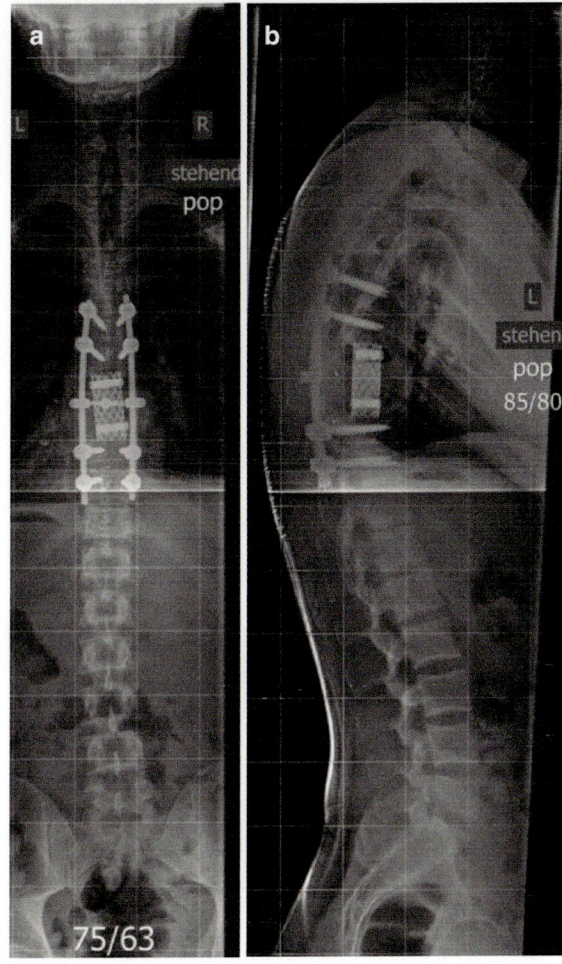

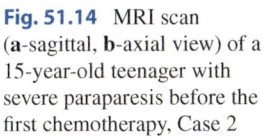

Fig. 51.12 Postoperative whole spine x-ray (**a**-AP, **b**-lateral view) after en bloc vertebrectomy T8 and 9 via costotransversectomy, instrumentation with internal fixator system, and vertebral body replacement with a titanium mesh cage filled with bone cement, Case 1

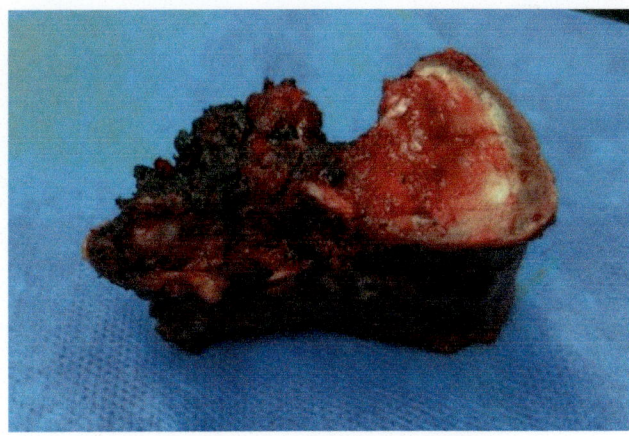

Fig. 51.13 Photograph of the en bloc specimen (aneurysmatic bone cyst), Case 1

Case 2 Ewing's Sarcoma

A 15-year-old teenager with severe paraparesis which was caused by a tumor in the level T8. Under emergency conditions, a laminectomy was performed to decompress the spinal cord (histology: Ewing's sarcoma). A chemotherapy according to Ewing protocol was performed (see Figs. 51.14a, b and 51.15a, b). The surgical therapy consisted of a posterior-anterior en bloc resection of T8 with the adjacent rib and posterior muscle, instrumentation T6 to 10, and vertebral body replacement with titanium mesh cage filled with bone cement (see Figs. 51.16, 51.17, and 51.18).

Fig. 51.14 MRI scan (**a**-sagittal, **b**-axial view) of a 15-year-old teenager with severe paraparesis before the first chemotherapy, Case 2

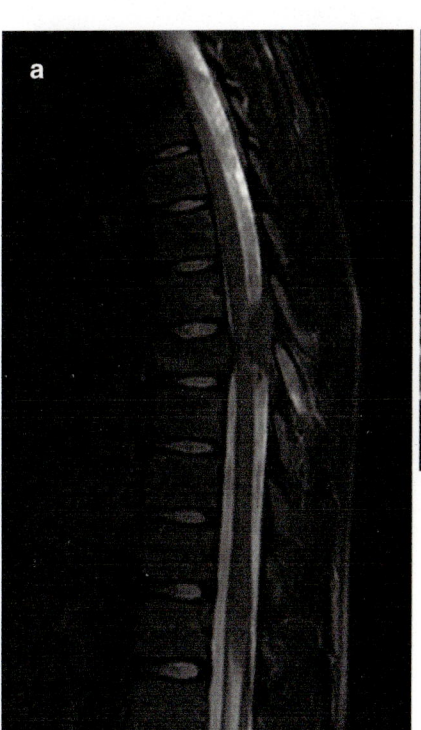

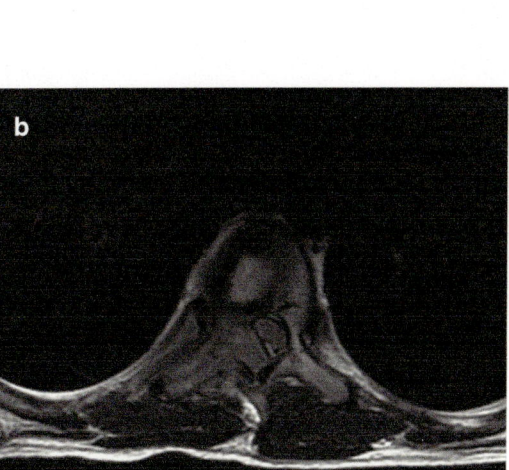

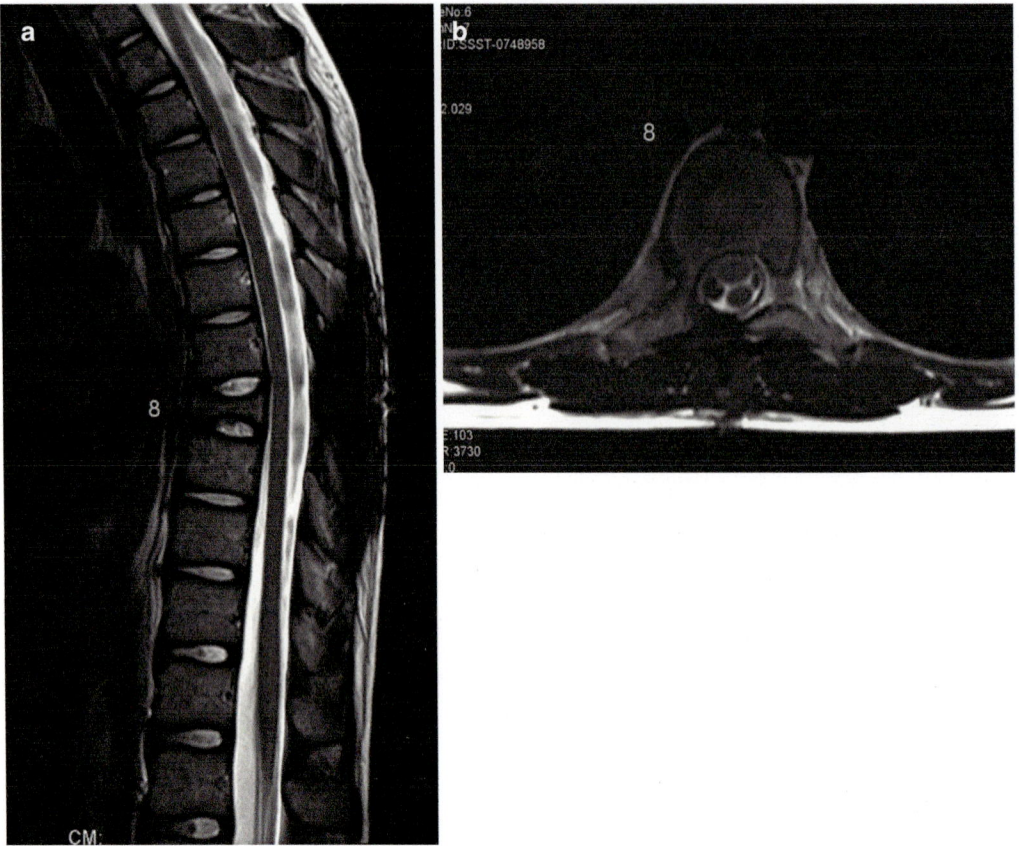

Fig. 51.15 MRI scan (**a**-sagittal, **b**-axial view) after the chemotherapy according to Ewing protocol, Case 2

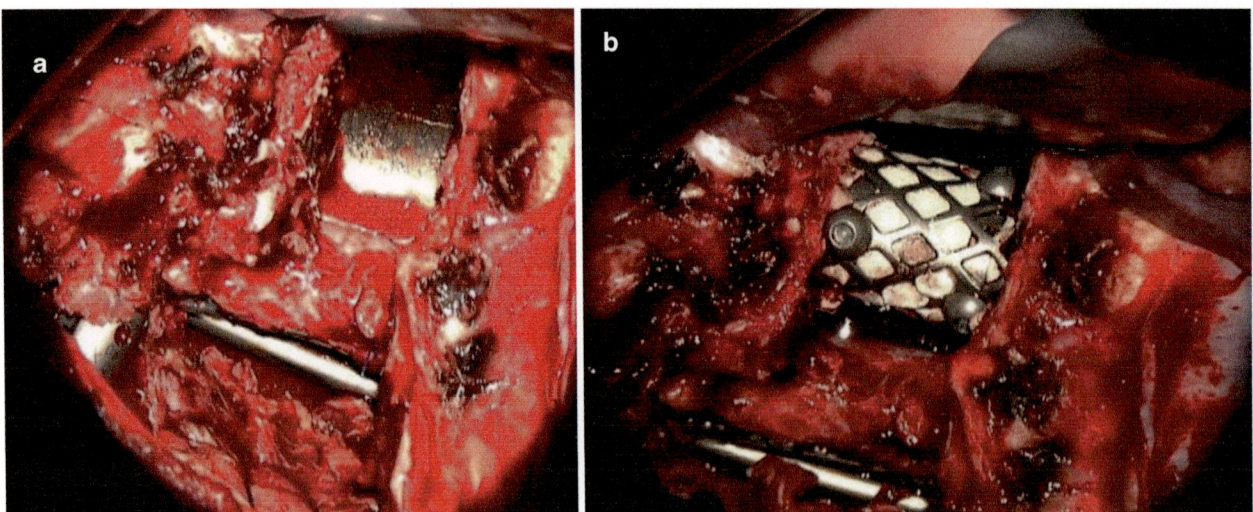

Fig. 51.16 Intraoperative view (right-sided thoracotomy), (**a**) defect following vertebrectomy (above) with a spatula in place, myelon with ligation of the nerve root (middle), posterior instrumentation, and (**b**) vertebral body replacement with titanium mesh cage filled with bone cement

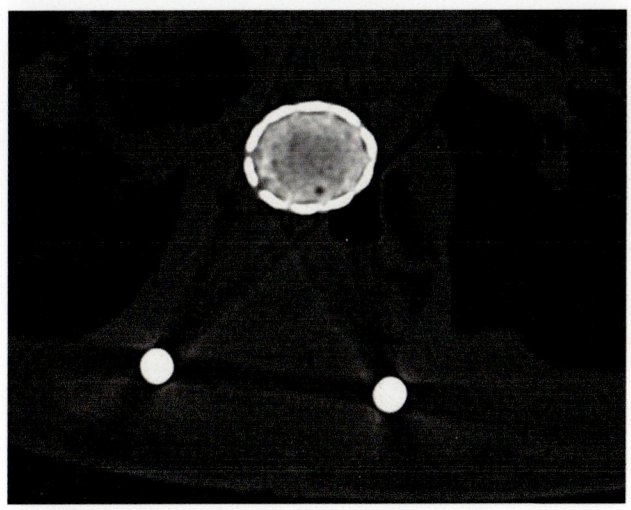

Fig. 51.17 Axial CT scan following the total en bloc vertebrectomy, Case 2

Case 3 Giant Cell Bone Tumor

A 29-year-old male with a destructive giant cell bone tumor T1, T2, and T3; status post vertebroplasty, laminectomy, and instrumentation C7 to T3 elsewhere (see Fig. 51.19a–d). A two-stage surgery was performed with (1) posterior pedicle screw instrumentation C5 to T6 with laminectomy T1–3 and tumor mobilization via costotransversectomy and (2) anterior vertebrectomy T1, T2, and T3 and vertebral body replacement with titanium mesh cage filled with bone cement via sternotomy (see Figs. 51.20a, b and 51.21).

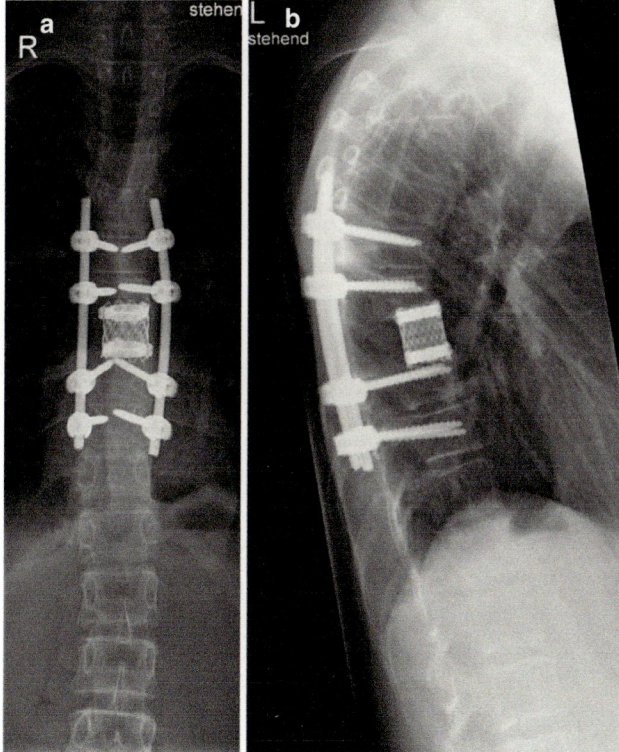

Fig. 51.18 Postoperative AP (**a**) and lateral X-ray scan (**b**) after posterior-anterior en bloc resection of T8, instrumentation T6 to 10, and vertebral body replacement with titanium mesh cage filled with bone cement, Case 2

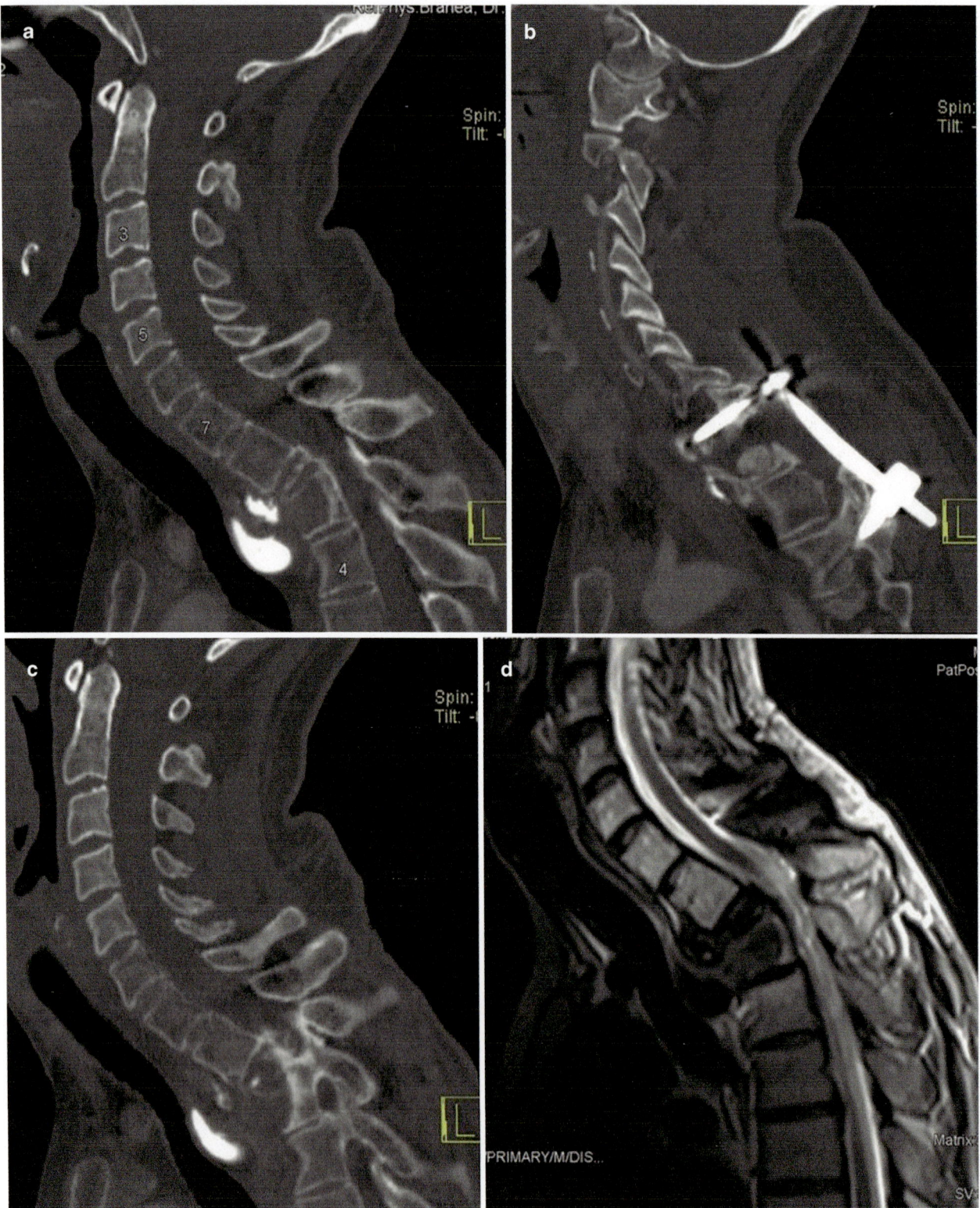

Fig. 51.19 Preoperative CAT (**a–c**) and MRI (**d**) scans after vertebroplasty, laminectomy, and instrumentation C7 to T3 elsewhere, Case 3 (histology: destructive giant cell bone tumor)

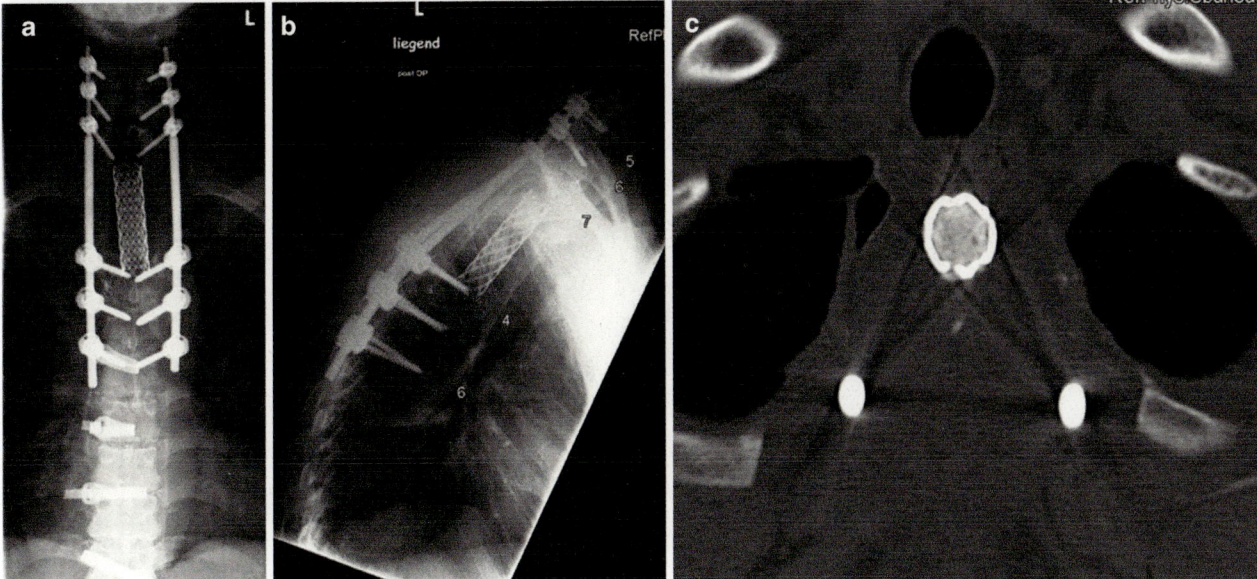

Fig. 51.20 Postoperative X-rays in the AP (**a**) and lateral (**b**) view and CAT scan (**c**), Case 3

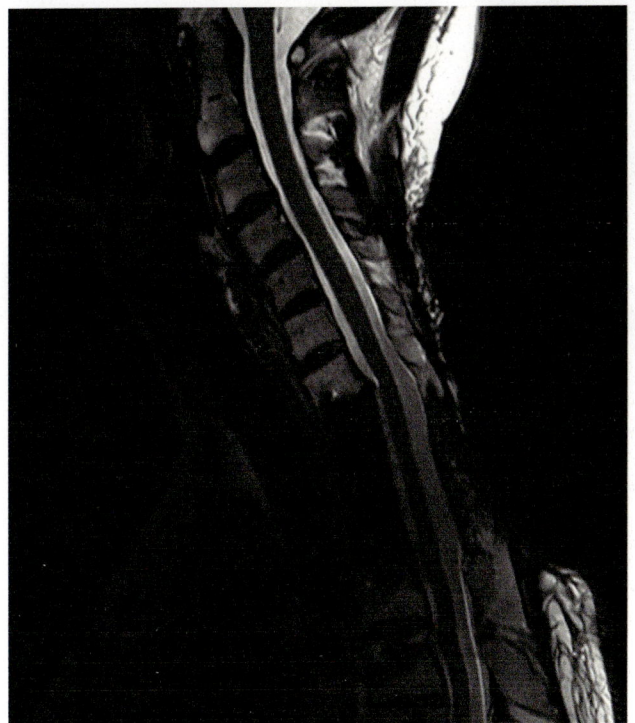

Fig. 51.21 MRI scan at 5-year follow-up with no evidence of tumor recurrence, Case 3

Case 4 Osteoblastoma

An 8-year-old boy with an osteoblastoma L3, status post curettage and filling with calcium sulfate (see Fig. 51.22a, b) elsewhere in a hospital. A posterior-anterior-posterior en bloc resection of L3 with instrumentation and fusion L2 to L4 was performed (see Figs. 51.23 and 51.24a, b).

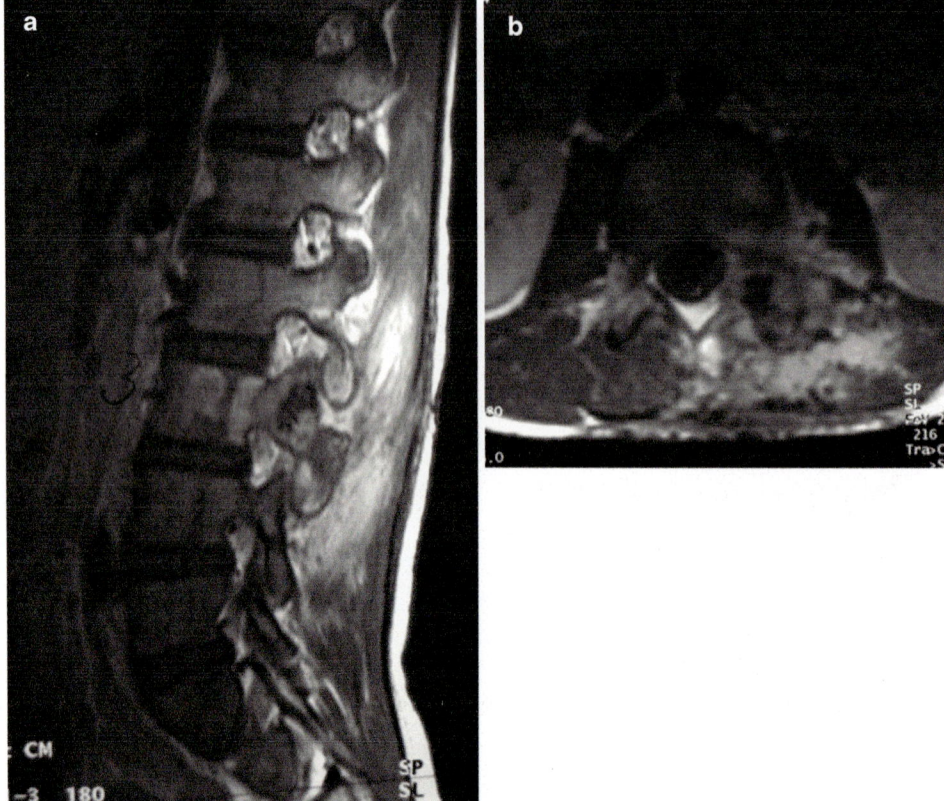

Fig. 51.22 Preoperative MRI in sagittal (**a**) and axial (**b**) view of an 8-year-old boy (histology: osteoblastoma) after curettage and filling with calcium sulfate, Case 4

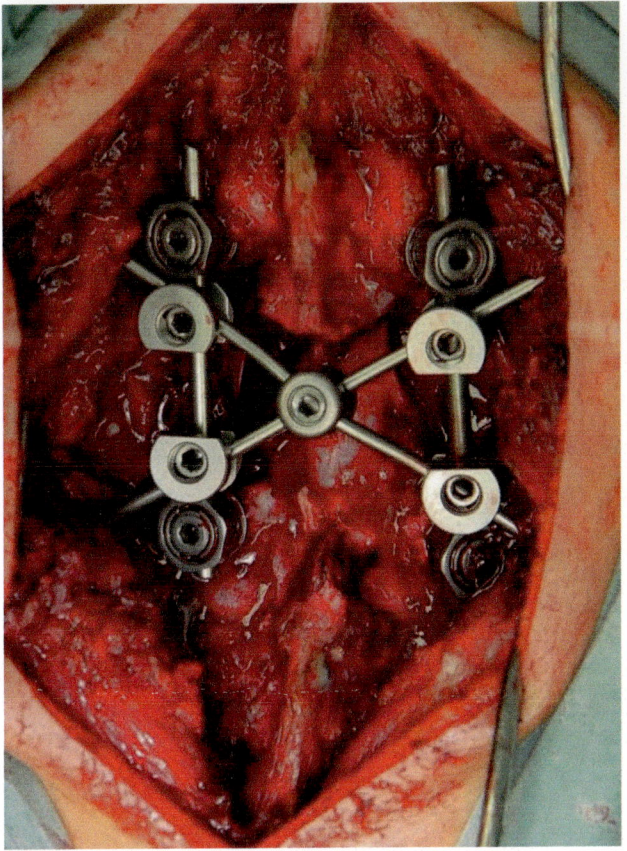

Fig. 51.23 Intraoperative view, short instrumentation L2 to L4, cross-link connector to compensate shear and rotational forces

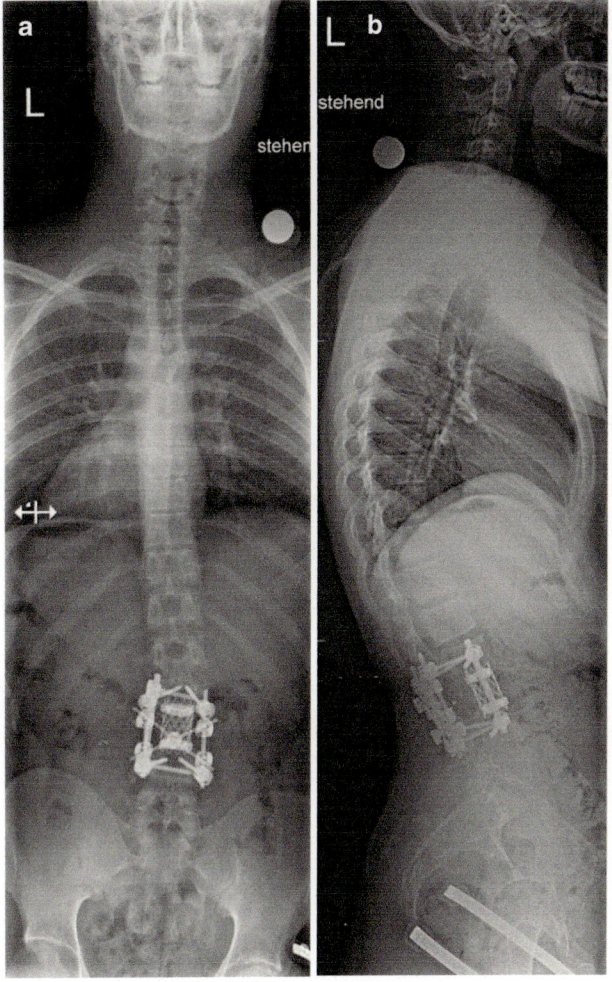

Fig. 51.24 Radiographs 12 years postoperatively in anterior-posterior (**a**) and lateral (**b**) view, Case 4

References

1. Fisher C, Keynan O, Boyd M, et al. The surgical management of primary tumors of the spine. Spine. 2005;30:1899–908.
2. Enneking WF. A system of staging musculoskeletal neoplasms. Clin Orthop. 1980;204:9–24.
3. Ibrahim A, Crockard A, Antonietti P, et al. Does spinal surgery improve the quality of life for those with extradural (spinal) osseous metastases? An international multicenter prospective observational study of 223 patients. J Neurosurg Spine. 2008;8(3):271–8.
4. Tomita K, Kawahara N, Kobayashi T, et al. Surgical strategy for spinal metastases. Spine. 2001;26(3):298–306.
5. Fisher CG, DiPaola CP, Ryken TC, et al. A novel classification system for spinal instability in neoplastic disease: an evidence-based approach and expert consensus from the spine oncology study group. Spine. 2010;35:E1221–9.
6. Tomita K, Toribatake Y, Kawahara N, Ohnari H, Kose H. Total en bloc spondylectomy and circumspinal decompression for solitary spinal metastasis. Paraplegia. 1994;32(1):36–46.

Magnetically Controlled Growing Rod

52

Jacques D. Müller-Broich

52.1 Introduction and Core Message

Magnetically controlled growing rods (MAGEC™) are intended to treat children with a progressive scoliosis during growth, when conservative treatment has already failed or missed and curve progression is expected not to be sufficiently preventable with bracing or corset therapy. MAGEC™ therapy is mainly intended to treat, but not limited to, early-onset scoliosis (EOS), which is defined by a cobb angle of more than $10°$ under the age of 10 years [1]. MAGEC™ is an abbreviation for "**M**agnetic **E**xpansion **C**ontrol." Patient selection and preoperative planning is crucial to reducing complication rates, requiring a thorough understanding of the technical features and capabilities of the device [2] as well as knowledge of child growth development. In comparison to traditional growth-modulating spinal systems, the MAGEC Rod System prevents frequent open surgical lengthening procedures, which are replaced by outpatient clinic interventions when the MAGEC™ construct is lengthened with an external, percutaneous, electromagnetic remote-control device. Those lengthening procedures of a few millimeters are very well tolerated by the children and their families and are almost pain-free [3]. Reducing the number of surgical procedures leads naturally to a decrease in a significant number of surgical complications (e.g., infections). Still the MAGEC™ system has complications due to the complexity of spinal deformity, health status of the children, surgical technique, and also device-related adverse or even serious device-related adverse events [4]. Main advantage is that the frequent lengthening procedures are nonsurgical.

J. D. Müller-Broich (✉)
Department of Orthopedics (Friedrichsheim), University Hospital Frankfurt am Main, Frankfurt am Main, Germany
e-mail: jdmbii@web.de

52.2 Indications and Contraindications

52.2.1 Indications

The indication for a surgical procedure with the MAGEC™ rod system is correction and stopping of spinal deformity, enhancing the remaining expected spinal growth as well as the thoracic volume in early-onset scoliosis (EOS). Once acceptable spinal growth and thoracic capacity have been achieved, conversion to definitive scoliosis surgery/fusion should be considered.

- Child age > older than 2 years.
- Severe and progressive disease with risk of progression of the deformity.
- Pulmonary insufficiency (thoracic insufficiency) with risk of respiratory failure.
- Failed conservative treatment (bracing/casting).
- Cosmetic deformation (relative indication).

The surgical technique and exact positioning of the MCGR vary due to multiple factors such as etiology of the scoliosis, age, vertebral growth, segmental dysmorphism or malformation of vertebrae, thoracic deformities, presence of hyper- or hypokyphosis, and of course the nature of the scoliotic deformity. Hughes et al. demonstrated impressively in a survey that there is little consensus among pediatric spine surgeons regarding treatment of EOS [5]. Therefore, every case must be carefully assessed individually as long as common guidelines do not exist. The standardization of etiologies and description of implants by the International Congress on Early Onset Scoliosis and Growing Spine (ICEOS) has helped to simplify the scientific exchange [1, 6]. Rib-, spine-, and pelvis-based anchoring locations are available for proximal and distal fixation of the MCGR and are well known as they are the same as for TGR. Anchor methods (rib, spine, pelvis) [7], such as hooks, screws, and laminar bands/clamps, have been described in several technical descriptions.

Placement of the anchors is subject to the preferred surgical technique (freehand, percutaneous (MIS), navigation, robotics).

Choosing the level of the anchoring site might be influenced by the fact that different senior pediatric surgeons use the principle of the last substantially touched vertebra (LSTV) as lowest instrumented vertebra (LIV) to avoid an increase in curvature below the level of instrumentation (distal adding on) [8, 9].

To avoid the rebound effect by an improperly contoured kyphosis in the proximal end causing proximal junctional kyphosis, the natural kyphosis of the spine should be mirrored. Still, this will only partially prevent PJK as it is multifactorial.

52.3 Contraindications

A major contraindication is the necessity of MRI postoperatively during further treatment (e.g., Tethered cord). While the MRI itself does not harm the construct or patient, the signals are disturbed/altered in the area of the actuators and MRI stronger than 1.5 Tesla should not be used due to the forces evolving with stronger electromagnetic fields. Reduced patient compliance for follow-up visits and continued treatment is a contraindication. Firm patient guidance is very important.

52.4 Technical Prerequisites (Fig. 52.1 Nuvasive)

Rod diameters available: 4.5 mm, 5.0 mm, 5.5 mm, and 6.0 mm (Fig. 52.1).

Actuator lengths available in 70 mm/90 mm with 28 mm and 48 mm of distraction capacity. Total undistracted rod length is 470 mm.

Number of rods used—single or double rod use possible. Variability of anchors proximal and distal to ribs, laminae, pedicels, sacrum/ilium via screw, hooks, bolts/clamps.

External remote control (ERC—2)—allows for independent or simultaneous distraction mode (Figs. 52.2 and 52.3).

Preoperative planning and definition of remaining growth potential, expected curve progression.

Screw length and size (small stature of children), cannulated/percutaneous versus open/freehand technique versus Navigation.

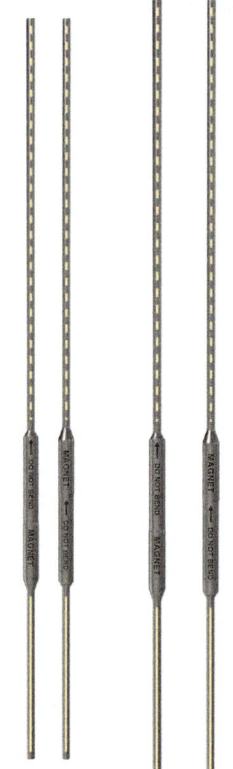

Courtesy of NuVasive, Inc.

Fig. 52.1 Magec rod

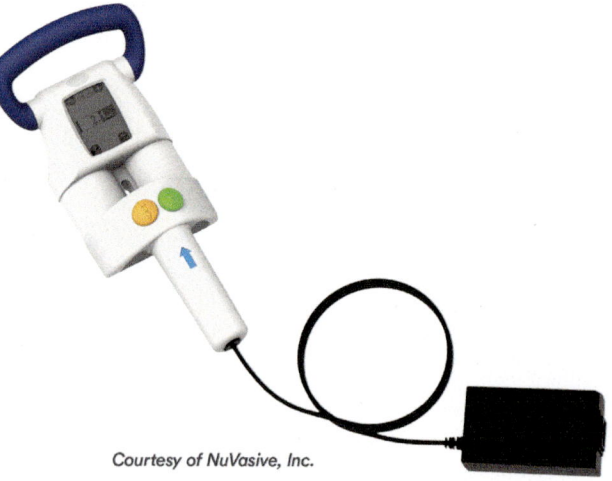

Courtesy of NuVasive, Inc.

Fig. 52.2 External remote control 2

Mobile C-arm for 2D view at least or better for imaging control via fluoroscopy during surgery when using freehand technique.

Navigation and 3D scan optional—Radiation exposure of the young children should be reduced to the minimum.

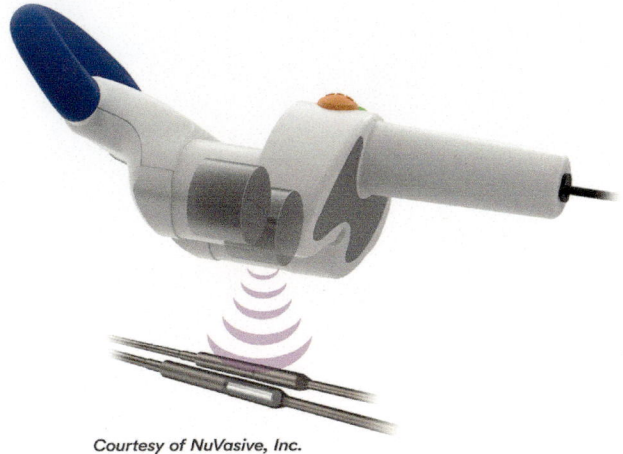

Courtesy of NuVasive, Inc.

Fig. 52.3 ERC 2 projecting magnetic field to MAGEC rod percutaneously

Neuromonitoring (if desired)—Proper planning and pro-active interdisciplinary case discussion with anesthesiologists, neuromonitoring technicians/electrophysiologists, and surgeon are important and should be carried out several times prior to surgery.

Availability of bed at pediatric ICU should be cleared before surgery and reconfirmed at the day of surgery prior to initiation of narcosis.

52.5 Surgical Technique

- Patient is placed in a prone position with special attention to correct padding avoiding soft tissue damage or skin burns by fluid dissipation under surgery.
- Surgery is carried out under general anesthesia.
- When neuromonitoring is desired, the use of narcotics such as muscle relaxants or inhalation of narcotics needs to be avoided as such substances may impede correct signaling.
- Team-Time out is carried out. Special attention must be paid to indication, patient history, comorbidities, esti-mated blood loss, length of surgery, antibiotic regime and expected problems during the course of surgery need to be addressed. Technical issues such as neuromonitoring, availability and sterility of instruments, and implants are checked. Brief explanation of the surgical plan and fall-back options should conclude the discussion.
- Skin incision sites are identified (under fluoroscopy if necessary). Anatomical landmarks are marked with a water-resistant felt marker. (pelvis, spinous process, c7-Sacrum plumb line) and the incision sites are checked for plausibility.

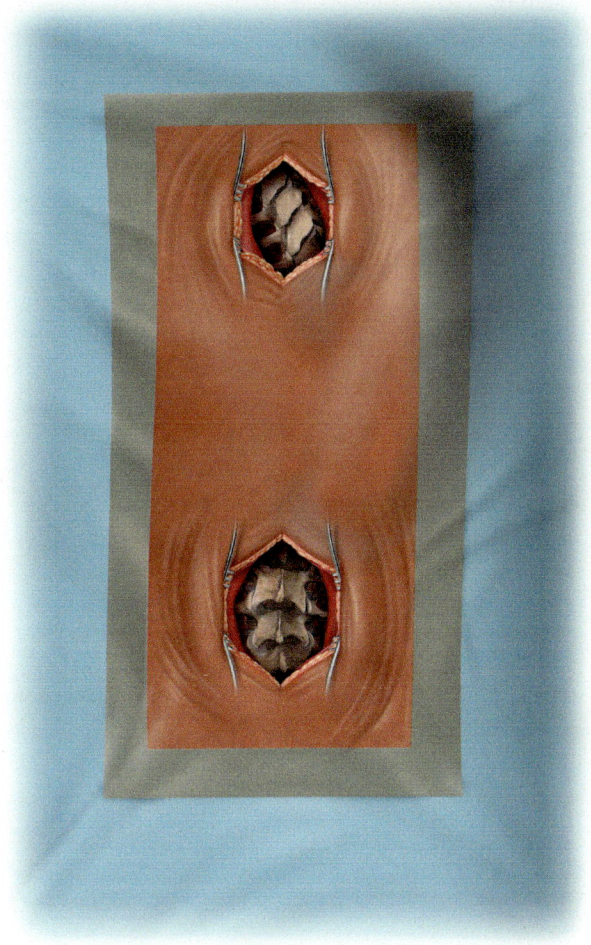

Courtesy of NuVasive, Inc.

Fig. 52.4 Open surgical approach: proximal and distal midline incisions

- For a classic open surgical approach, skin midline incision is carried out. Coagulation of subcutaneous vessels with electrocautery reduces blood loss and improves visibility.
- The spinous process are identified and the fascia thoraco-lumbalis is opened longitudinally directly adjacent to the bone. Electrocautery is then used to prepare the pedicle entry points subperiosteally to reduce blood loss. Hooks or retractors are used as desired (Fig. 52.4).
- Screw placement with the appropriate length and size is carried out. In our freehand technique, we prefer marking the screw slots with k-wires and check them fluoroscopi-cally prior to screw insertion.
- Neuromonitoring with dynamic pedicle probing and screw testing is also a regularly used technique to avoid negative outcomes.
- Adapting a no touch technique for the periosteum of the adjacent segments and facet joints as well as avoiding

extensive soft tissue damage around the planned anchor
locations will certainly foster a beneficial outcome
although reliable data is not available. (Frequent occurrence of segmental fusion adjacent to the targeted locations in our own experience has been iatrogenic and
complicate the conversion to definitive scoliosis surgery).

- For a less invasive approach, we suggest the usage of cannulated screws. Skin midline incision is carried out as
described above. Instead of direct incision of the fascia
thoraco-lumbalis, a modified Wiltse approach incising the
fascia 2–3 cm lateral to the midline longitudinally is possible and marking of the pedicle entry points via K-wire or
even Yamshidi needles for a transpedicular approach is feasible. The advantage is less soft tissue damage in the treated
and adjacent segments. But when fusion is desired at the
anchoring segment(s), the advantage is reduced (Fig. 52.5).

- When the anchoring elements are in place, subfascial
preparation from the two entry sites tunneling the fascia
thoraco-lumbalis is carried out by a blunt surgical instrument (Fig. 52.6).

- A silicone tube is attached at one site and pulled through
the channel. It is later used to insert the MCGR at the
desired entry and guides it subfascially avoiding soft tissue damage.

- When the rod is primarily inserted via the silicone tube,
the appropriate length and curvature are marked and estimated. (If possible, the insertion of the rod is not needed
when length and curve might be estimated sufficiently by
the surgeon).

- Usage of standard and offset rod need to be planned
before surgery (Fig. 52.7). Special attention needs to be
taken to place the actuators at the correct level before cutting the rod (Fig. 52.8).

- The rod is then taken out and cut to the appropriate length
and bend with the proper curvature. I advise to add 1–3 cm
at both ends to allow for proper bending of the rods and
account for the final lengthening procedure. Contouring
of the rod should be carried out with at least one centime-
ter of distance to the actuator in order to prevent intrinsic
construct off-axis loading.

- Each rod must be tested prior to final placement only after
rod cutting and contouring has been completed. The manual distractor is mounted on the actuator, the rod is marked
at the distraction position: 4 rotations to the left should be
applied to distract/check the actuator and 3 rotations to the
right will retract the rod to the starting position (Fig. 52.9).

- For the final tightening procedure after rod placement, we
have an assistant pulling the patient at the armpits cranially and another assistant who fixes the patient at the pelvis. With this technique, we objectively achieve an
improved correction/lengthening of the spine prior to
final tightening of the screws. Appropriate team
communication is important for this step, which has to be
adapted to the individual patients' situations. Application

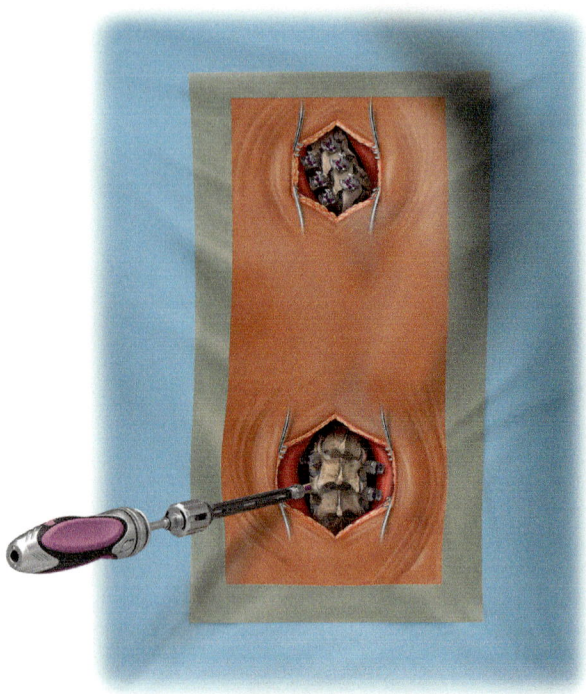

Courtesy of NuVasive, Inc.

Fig. 52.5 Surgical approach levels should be planned preoperatively
in order to reduce soft tissue involvement

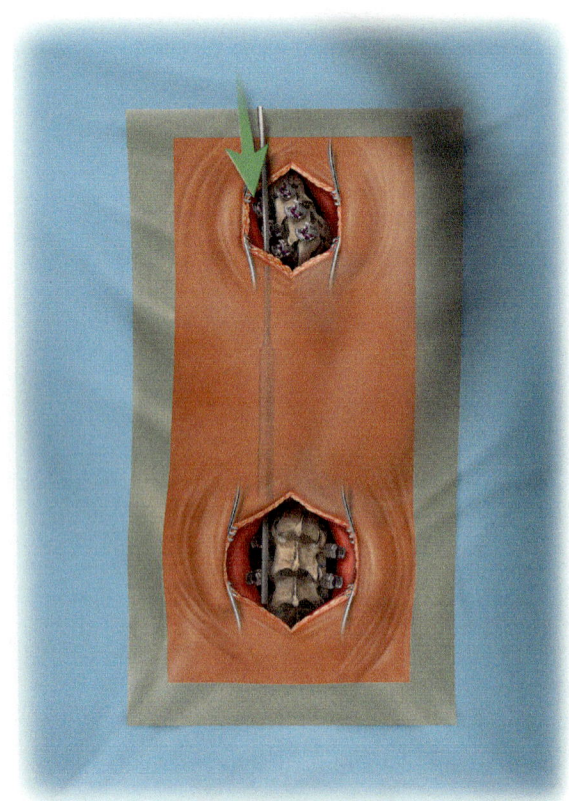

Courtesy of NuVasive, Inc.

Fig. 52.6 Rod placment via a subfascial tunneling technique. A silicone tube is a powerful guiding tool for frequent insertions

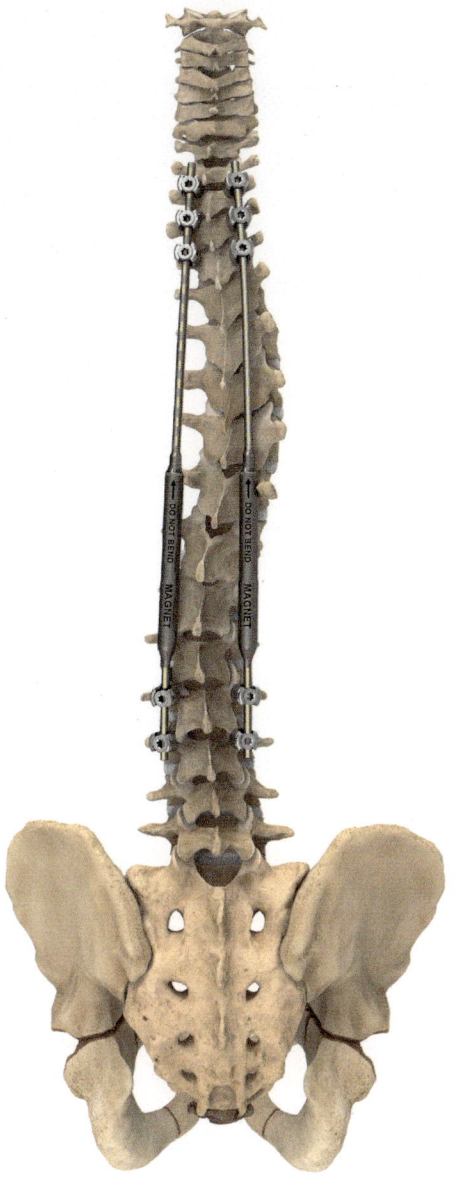

Courtesy of NuVasive, Inc.

Fig. 52.7 Positioning of actuators at insertion planning with a saw bone model

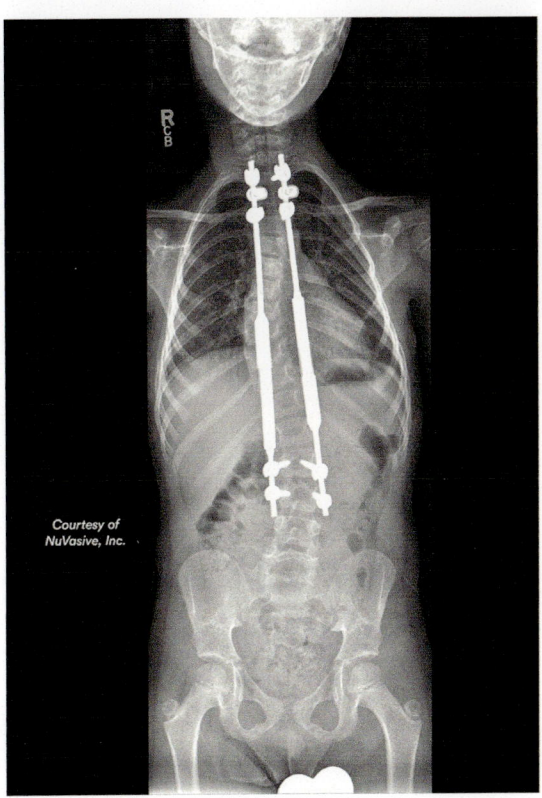

Fig. 52.8 Actuator location of standard and offset rod in x-ray

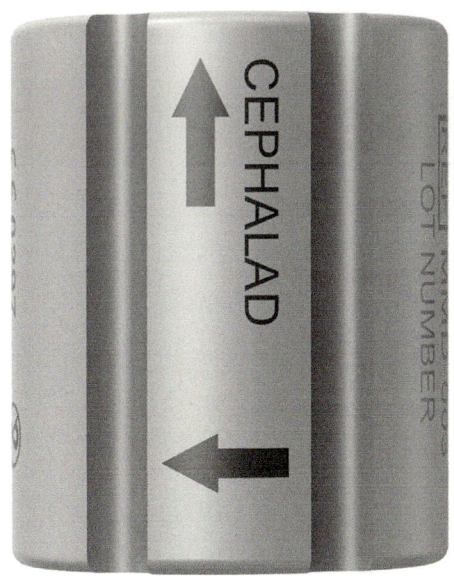

Courtesy of NuVasive, Inc.

Fig. 52.9 Manual distractor for actuator mechanism testing prior to final rod insertion

of a rod clamp and a distraction retractor facilitate the procedure (Figs. 52.10 and 52.11).

- Also special attention to the orientation of the contoured rod ends prior to final tightening of the set screws is of great importance.
- After final tightening of the set screws, a MEP/SSEP check is carried out and compared to the baseline.
- Fascial, subcutaneous, and skin closure follow. In usual settings, a wound drain is not necessary. Sterile dressings are applied.

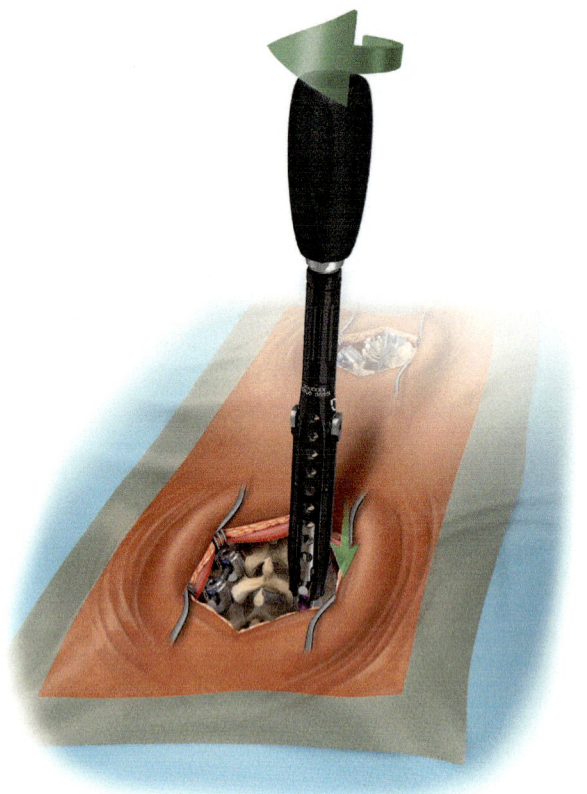

Courtesy of NuVasive, Inc.

Fig. 52.10 Rod reduction tool to insert rod into screw head

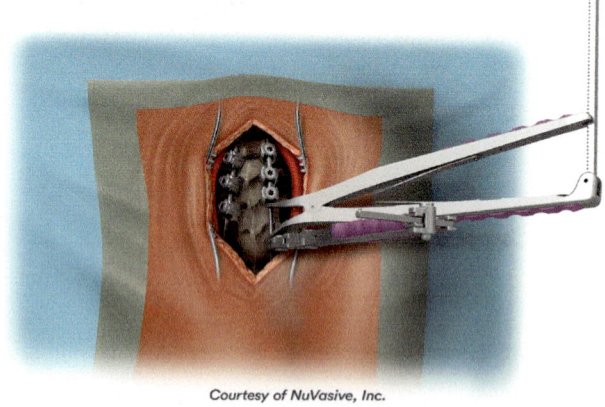

Courtesy of NuVasive, Inc.

Fig. 52.11 Distraction with aid of rod clamp as abutment

52.6   Revision Concepts

In double rod constructs, external distraction depends on the implanted rod types. While the standard rod has the magnet positioned at the caudal end, distracting the rod cranially, the offset rod has the magnet positioned at the cranial end of the actuator. Therefore, the external remote control (ERC) is

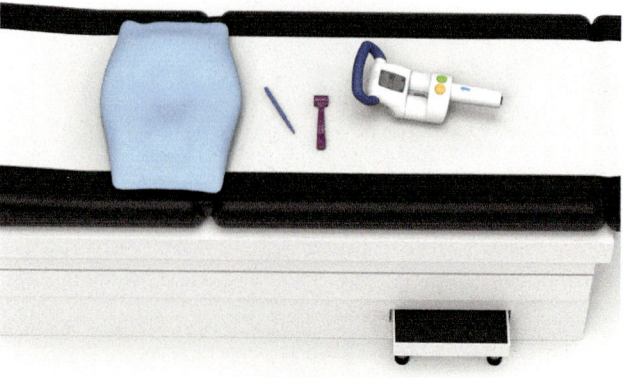

Courtesy of NuVasive, Inc.

Fig. 52.12 Tools for rod distraction. (Felt marker, magnetic wand, ERC 2 controller)

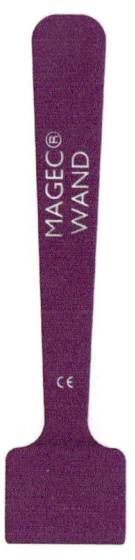

Courtesy of NuVasive, Inc.

Fig. 52.13 Magnetic wand for magnetic actuator field location

able to distract the rod independently from another, which might be helpful at curve control and correction. Finding of the magnetic areas through the skin is simplified by the use of a magnetic wand (Figs. 52.12 and 52.13). The skin is marked with a felt marker and the ERC-2 is directed onto this mark to properly couple with the actuator in order to distract either one or both rods (Fig. 52.14).

Usually, the children are positioned in a comfortable lying prone position over a cushion or blanket or in a lateral decubitus position in order to relax the intrinsic tension of the rod system (Figs. 52.15 and 52.16), but they may also sit in a relaxed upright position, for example, on their parents' lap (Figs. 52.17, 52.18, and 52.19). Two principal techniques to determine the amount of distraction

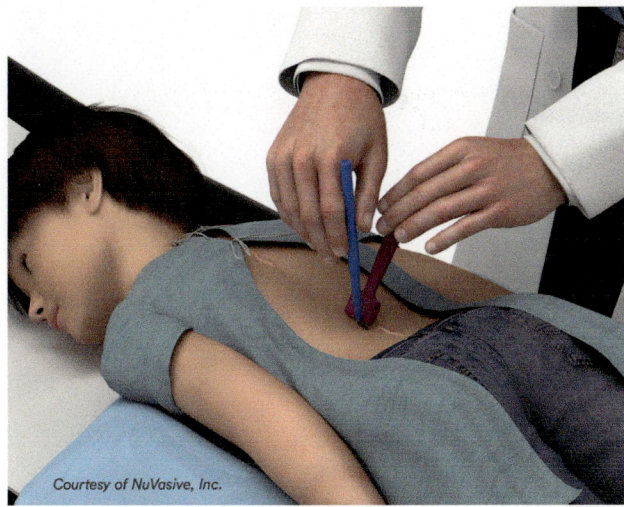

Fig. 52.14 Marking of the skin over the magnetic actuator

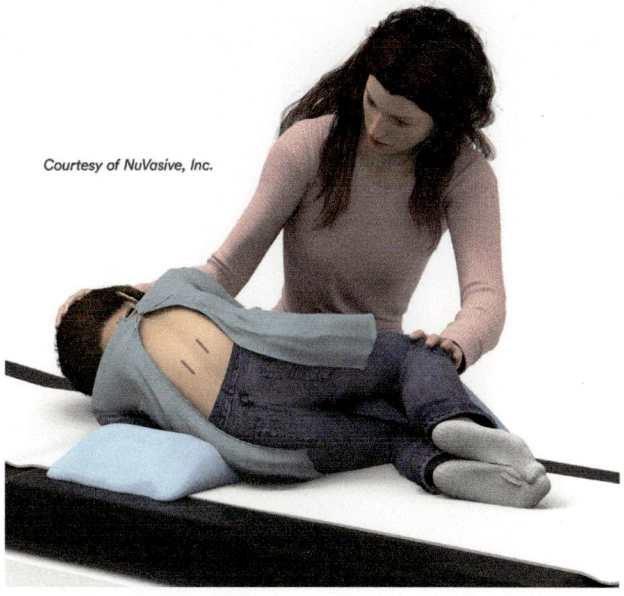

Fig. 52.16 Lateral decubitus position to off-load intrinsic forces of the transport mechanism

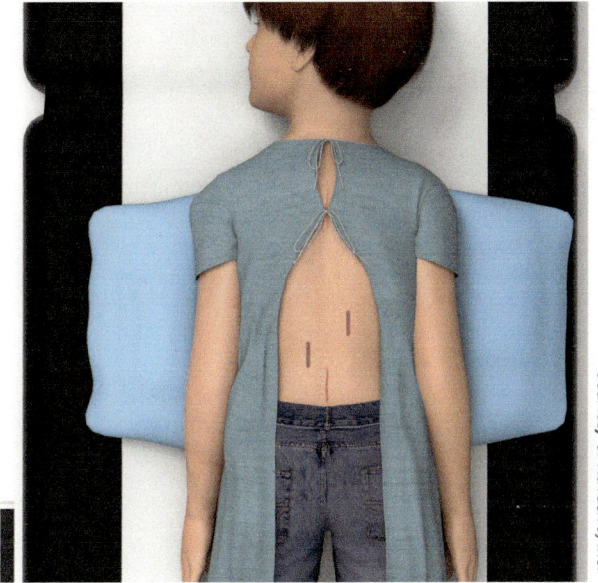

Fig. 52.15 Positioning of child in comfortable prone position with blanket or cushion with marks to position the ERC 2

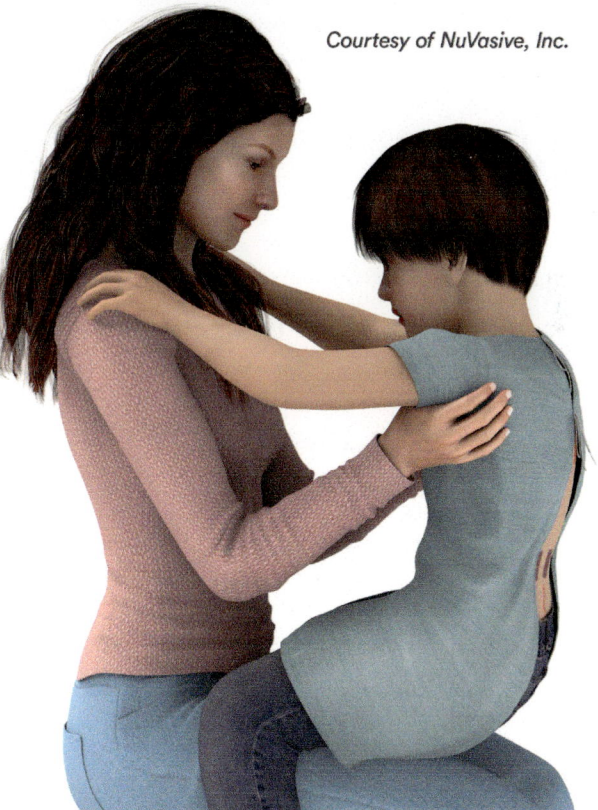

Fig. 52.17 Parental assistance with child sitting on lap to off-load transport mechanism

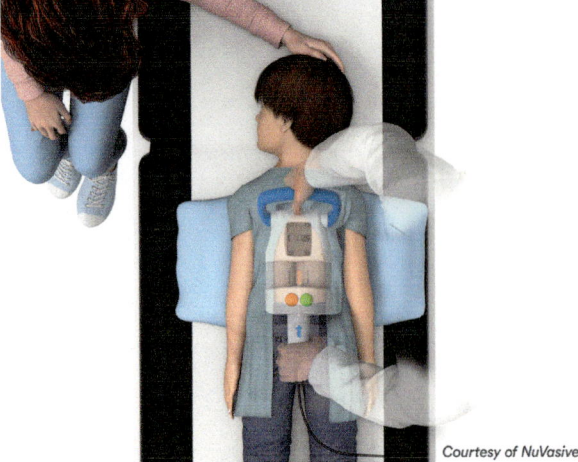

Courtesy of NuVasive, Inc.

Fig. 52.18 Rod distraction with ERC 2 device in prone position

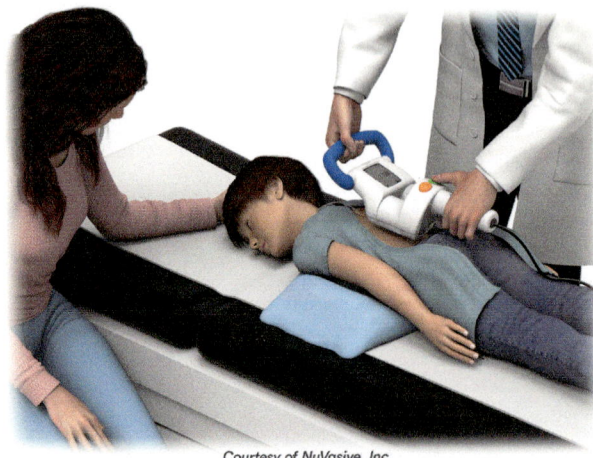

Courtesy of NuVasive, Inc.

Fig. 52.19 Rod distraction with ERC 2 device in prone position

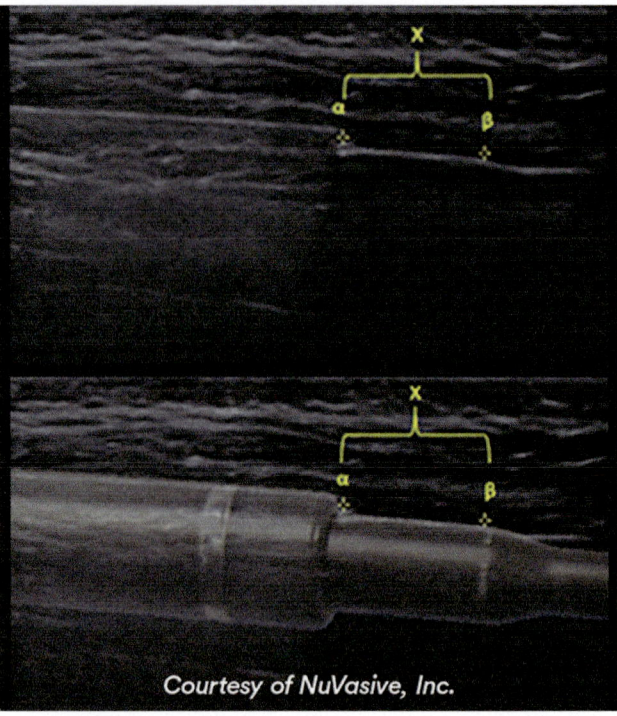

Courtesy of NuVasive, Inc.

Fig. 52.20 Ultrasound image for length control of distraction

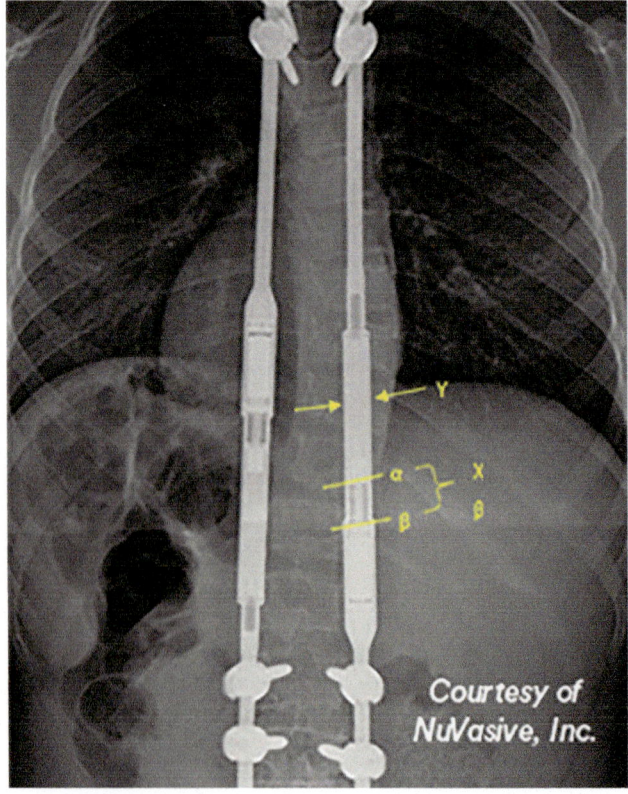

Courtesy of NuVasive, Inc.

Fig. 52.21 X-ray image for length control of distraction. Rod diameter is used as conversion factor in rule of proportion.

are described in literature. One is the clunk technique with maximum distraction at each elongation procedure with the ERC-2 in the outpatient clinic setting. Due to the axial overload of the actuator components, an audible noise (clunk) occurs and is also palpable through the skin. The second technique relies on expected spinal growth charts (DiMeglio et al.) for the calculation of the distraction parameters in comparison to a normal population using child age and weight. It is called tail-gating technique (TGT) [10]. Control of the lengthening is carried out via X-ray or ultrasound, and the length is documented (Figs. 52.20 and 52.21).

52.7 End of MAGEC Therapy

At the end of the spinal growth phase, when the patients reach skeletal maturity, a growth-modulating rod technique such as the MAGEC™ rod system loses its relevance leaving the risk of severe complications if not removed.

Skeletal maturity can be judged by radiological signs of the hand [11, 12] and pelvis. (Risser sign).

Balsano et al. [2] described disastrous developments after the end of the lengthening period with MAGEC treatment after primarily achieving acceptable results with an removal and observation strategy. The MAGEC rods were removed at skeletal maturity and within a very short time, the curves progressed almost doubling the Cobb angle at the time of removal of the rods. Consequently, the patients were treated with definitive scoliosis correction. Still, the available data on the management of EOS after MAGEC therapy upon reaching skeletal maturity is scarce and controversial. Our recommendation is to remove the rods and apply definitive scoliosis correction in a single stage approach.

Definitive scoliosis correction after MAGEC™ therapy should also be planned carefully. Due to autofusion processes, bony and soft tissue release, need for implant removal, and anchor revision where necessary, resources need to be allocated for complex revision surgery and not just normal idiopathic scoliosis surgery. The need for multilevel osteotomies to correct sagittal and coronal imbalances as well as rotational deficits and thoracoplasties in order to regain segmental flexibility are very frequent in my own experience.

52.8 Tips and Tricks

- Protection of proximal instrumented vertebra—use of universal clamps/ 6 screws /3 vertebra.
- Corset therapy for partial correction with MAGEC™ rods—shorter instrumentation/saving segments.
- Avoidance of PJK—increased bending of the proximal part to reach estimated kyphosis (Avoidance of rebound effect).
- Critical validation of the remaining growth potential—when curve progression is expected but vertebral/spinal growth is not expected to exceed 2 years, the larger curve progression might be accepted for a later surgery in order to avoid a growth-modulating surgery with MAGEC™ rods. It may lead to preventable complications while the procedure is not absolutely necessary and impeding later definitive surgery.
- Outpatient organization—scheduling of the MAGEC™ expansion dates at a regular follow-up date (e.g., every 4 months) for every patient at the same day will show children and their families that they are not alone with this kind of therapy and may support psychological relief.

52.9 Complications

Due to the complexity of spinal deformity in EOS, several complications have been reported while using the EOS System. Complication rates vary in literature and are subject to high variabilities due to the heterogeneity of the etiology of EOS, age, surgical method/center, and rod type used.

A common complication in traditional growing but also MAGEC rods is proximal anchor failure with pullout of hooks or screws [13].

Single rod constructs are more susceptible to rod breakage than dual rod constructs and were more frequent with the early MAGEC rod types and though addressed by the manufacturer as also the frequent breakage of the actuator pin.

It also led to the development of a further 5.0 mm rod with greater implant strength. Implant associated complications regarding failure to distract the system or breaking of components such as the rod itself or the actuator pin as well as abrasive circumferential markings, metallosis (titanium debris) with chronic inflammatory soft tissue cellular infiltration are frequently reported. Also, endcap sealing dysfunctions are under continuous investigation. In a laboratory investigation, Rushton et al. [14, 15] found a negative correlation of force produced to time in vivo and documented a relationship of off-axis loading leading to a asymmetric abrasion of the rods causative for titanium metallosis.

In a larger systematic review, Thakar et al. [16] reviewed clinical complications and radiological outcomes including 196 patients from 15 different studies. He noted a complication rate of 44.5% (rod or anchoring failure 10.6%, revision surgery 33%, implant failure 11.7%).

The design of the MAGEC™ rod with an unbendable actuator demands most frequently to place the actuator at the level of the flat thoraco-lumbar junction or the thoracic spine. Its intrinsic forces flatten out the flexible spine and lead to a flat back or hypokyphotic proximal thoracic spine. This is not always tolerable to the proximal part of the spine and kyphotic forces lead to an increasing proximal junctional kyphosis, a so-called rebound effect [17]. Actions to avoid this may include increased proximal rod end curving, usage of a smaller actuator, and placement of the actuator at the lowest possible position. Male, syndromic, hyperkyphotic, and younger (<5 years of age at the time of surgery) children have a higher incidence of PJK [16]. In a larger study of proximal anchor fixation by Meza et al. [13], it was documented that spine-based fixation was superior to rib based fixation with respect to deformity correction. A greater proximal anchor density led to improved major curve correction at 2 years. Higher anchor density (+5 anchors) in the proximal zone did not protect from proximal anchor complication. Helenius et al. suggested a lower risk of wound infections due to less surgical interventions in

MCGR treatment compared to TGR treatment [5]. In an analysis by Teoh et al. [17], it was shown that MCGR had a lesser risk of deep wound and superficial wound infection than TGR.

References

1. Bai J, Chen K, Wei Q, et al. Selecting the LSTV as the lower instrumented vertebra in the treatment of Lenke types 1A and 2A adolescent idiopathic scoliosis: a minimal 3-year follow-up. Spine. 2018;43(7):E390–8.
2. Balsano M, Spina M. Idiopathic early-onset scoliosis treated with MAGEC rods: what to do after the lengthening period is over? Int J Spine Surg. 2020;14(5):847–51.
3. Cheung JP, Cahill P, Yaszay B, et al. Special article: update on the magnetically controlled growing rod: tips and pitfalls. J Orthop Surg. 2015;23(3):383–90.
4. El-Hawary R, Akbarnia BA. Early onset scoliosis - time for consensus. Spine Deform. 2015;3(2):105–6.
5. Helenius IJ. Standard and magnetically controlled growing rods for the treatment of early onset scoliosis. Ann Transl Med. 2020;8(2):26.
6. Hughes MS, Swarup I, Makarewich CA, et al. Expert consensus for early onset scoliosis surgery. J Pediatr Orthop. 2020;40(7):e621–8.
7. Inaparthy P, Queruz JC, Bhagawati D, et al. Incidence of proximal junctional kyphosis with magnetic expansion control rods in early onset scoliosis. Eur Spine J. 2016;25(10):3308–15.
8. Joyce TJ, Smith SL, Rushton PRP. Analysis of explanted magnetically controlled growing rods from seven UK spinal centers. Spine. 2018;43(1):E16–22.
9. Kov ST, Bunger C, Li H, et al. Lengthening of magnetically controlled growing rods caused minimal pain in 25 children: pain assessment with FPS-R, NRS, and r-FLACC. Spine Deform. 2020;8(4):763–70.
10. Mardare M, Kieser DC, Ahmad A, et al. Targeted distraction: spinal growth in children with early-onset scoliosis treated with a tailgating technique for magnetically controlled growing rods. Spine. 2018;43(20):E1225–31.
11. Sanders JO, Browne RH, McConnell SJ, et al. Maturity assessment and curve progression in girls with idiopathic scoliosis. J Bone Joint Surg Am. 2007;89(1):64–73.
12. Sanders JO, Khoury JG, Kishan S, et al. Predicting scoliosis progression from skeletal maturity: a simplified classification during adolescence. J Bone Joint Surg Am. 2008;90(3):540–53.
13. Meza BC, Shah SA, Vitale MG, et al. Proximal anchor fixation in magnetically controlled growing rods (MCGR): preliminary 2-year results of the impact of anchor location and density. Spine Deform. 2020;8(4):793–800.
14. Williams BA, Matsumoto H, McCalla DJ, et al. Development and initial validation of the classification of early-onset scoliosis (C-EOS). J Bone Joint Surg Am. 2014;96(16):1359–67.
15. Qin X, Sun W, Xu L, et al. Selecting the last "substantially" touching vertebra as lowest instrumented vertebra in Lenke type 1A curve: radiographic outcomes with a minimum of 2-year follow-up. Spine. 2016;41(12):E742–50.
16. Thakar C, Kieser DC, Mardare M, et al. Systematic review of the complications associated with magnetically controlled growing rods for the treatment of early onset scoliosis. Eur Spine J. 2018;27(9):2062–71.
17. Teoh KH, Winson DM, James SH, et al. Magnetic controlled growing rods for early-onset scoliosis: a 4-year follow-up. Spine J. 2016;16(4 Suppl):S34–9.

Suggested Reading

Rushton PRP, Smith SL, Forbes L, et al. Force testing of explanted magnetically controlled growing rods. Spine. 2019;44(4):233–9.
Rushton PRP, Smith SL, Kandemir G, et al. Spinal lengthening with magnetically controlled growing rods: data from the largest series of explanted devices. Spine. 2020;45(3):170–6.
Thompson W, Thakar C, Rolton DJ, et al. The use of magnetically-controlled growing rods to treat children with early-onset scoliosis: early radiological results in 19 children. Bone Joint J. 2016;98-B(9):1240–7.
Tsirikos AI, Roberts SB. Magnetic controlled growth rods in the treatment of scoliosis: safety, efficacy and patient selection. Med Devices. 2020;13:75–85.

Part VII

Anterior Lumbar Spine

Overview of Surgical Techniques and Implants

53

Karsten Wiechert

53.1 Introduction and Core Message

The concept of anterior surgery of the lumbar spine has been well established for decades and addresses all forms of anterior column pathology. There are numerous surgical techniques, most of them standardized, serving specific surgical needs depending on pathology, specific anatomical considerations, and the specific implant to be used. The surgical techniques used for the anterior lumbar spine involve combinations of anterior or anterolateral access (open, miniopen, or percutaneous) with various forms of instrumentation (plate-screw systems, rod-screw systems, interbody fusion devices, vertebral body replacement devices, artificial disk, and nucleus replacement systems).

53.2 Approaches

53.2.1 Classic Open Access

- Thoracolumbar access (transpleural-retroperitoneal T9–L5 as described by Hodgson [1]).
- Thoracolumbar access with double thoracotomy T4–L5.
- Retroperitoneal-extrapleural access T11–L5 as described by Mirbaha [2].
- Retroperitoneal anterolateral lumbar spinal access L2–5.
- Transperitoneal or retroperitoneal access to the lumbosacral junction L4–S1 [3].

These access routes are usually highly invasive. They are used mainly in ventral corrective fusion surgery performed to treat scoliotic and kyphotic deformities and in tumor surgery.

K. Wiechert (✉)
Schön Klinik Munich Harlaching, Spine Center "Am Michel", Hamburg, Germany
e-mail: praxis@ruecken-zentrum.de

53.2.2 Miniopen Access Techniques

There are numerous standardized minimally invasive techniques for reaching the lumbar spine with sufficient exposure of the relevant structures to reach the corresponding pathologies and provide treatment. They are all characterized by limited or minimal surgical trauma and make use of existing anatomical pathways. Most of the techniques allow sufficient exposure of the target structure (disk space, vertebral body/bodies). Anterior miniopen access techniques use various retractor systems, for example, SynFrame (Synthes) [4], Activ-O (Aesculap). These allow the access routes to be kept as small as possible and the surrounding tissue to be preserved more effectively. Even reconstructive procedures or vertebral body replacements in the lumbar area can be performed using an anterolateral approach. With the aid of endoscopes, it is possible to carry out an instrumented procedure either entirely or partially by endoscopic means, especially anterior interbody fusion [5]. However, some authors instead favor minimalized access without endoscopy (so-called MiniALIF) (ALIF—Anterior Lumbar Interbody Fusion) [6, 7]. Percutaneous procedures are also available. Among the most commonly used are the following:

- MiniALIF anterolateral approach L2–L5.
- Miniopen midline approach L2–S1.
- Pararectal approach L3–S1.
- ALPA—AnteroLateral transPsoatic Approach.

53.2.2.1 MiniALIF Anterolateral Approach to L2–L5

The MiniALIF approach was first described by Mayer [7]. Its key steps are precise positioning, marking of target projection onto the skin, and a completely blunt dissection of the muscular planes, the peritoneal sac, and exposure of the disk space. It is an entirely universal technique and exposes the disk space and the vertebral bodies. In some cases, the rib cage may restrict access so that certain modifications are necessary. The single steps of the technique are completely standardized, the complications spectrum limited. The MiniALIF technique may be seen as the current gold standard in anterolateral approaches to the lumbar spine [7].

53.2.2.2 Miniopen Midline Approach to L1–S1

This technique is based on the same surgical principles as the anterolateral approach. With the advent of total disk replacement, however, a need for a precise midline placement of the disk prosthesis gained utmost importance. This approach plays a vital role in facilitating minimally invasive surgery in such cases. The planes of the abdominal wall are bluntly dissected and the peritoneal sac exposed. The technique allows for retroperitoneal dissection as well as for transperitoneal exposure of the anterior circumference of the lumbar spine. The approach is easily expandable if necessary and works for the levels L1 to the sacrum. While mono- and bisegmental approaches can easily be carried out, exposure may present limitations for multisegmental surgery.

53.2.2.3 Pararectal Approach to L2–S1

This approach employs the anatomical pathway lateral to the rectus abdominis muscle. The lumbar spine can be reached safely and elegantly even in multilevel procedures, and there are no limitations on the type of lumbar reconstruction possible. However, midline implantations such as in TDR (total disk replacement) are not ideal because of anatomical and tissue restraints.

53.2.2.4 AnteroLateral transPsoatic Approach (ALPA)

This approach focuses on a strict lateral approach to the lumbar motion segment and was originally described for implantation of nucleus replacement devices. After blunt dissection of the planes of the abdominal wall, the psoas fibers are exposed and transected up to the disk space. Special attention needs to be given to the fibers of the lumbosacral plexus. The use of neuromonitoring devices is therefore advocated for this approach.

53.2.3 Endoscopic Approaches

There are numerous descriptions of endoscopic techniques for reaching the lumbar spine. A balloon-assisted extraperitoneal technique through an anterolateral approach dissects the peritoneal plane. Critical attention needs to be given to moving the iliac vessels in order to preserve them as the potential for vascular injury is obvious. On the technical side, it must be mentioned that progress during endplate preparation can be nicely monitored with an endoscope. However, a steep learning curve, some medicolegal considerations with regard to general surgical training in access surgery, and some limitations in implants and devices have kept these techniques to a niche in anterior spine surgery in the orthopedic and neurosurgical areas.

53.3 Implants

The implants fulfilling certain tasks in specialized techniques on the lumbar spine are almost without number. This overview can only cover general properties of implants and does not attempt to address every aspect. General implant categories in anterior surgery of the lumbar spine are the following:
- Intersomatic fusion implants.
- Total disk replacement devices.
- Vertebral body replacements.
- Anterior rod systems.
- Anterior tension plates.

53.3.1 Intersomatic Fusion Implants

This implant category plays a major role in anterior spine surgery. It can be divided into several subgroups, each serving a specific need:
- Intervertebral cages.
- Stand-alone implants/cages with additional forms of fixation.
- Nucleus replacement devices.
- Total disk replacement devices.

53.3.1.1 Intervertebral Cages

These cages are placed in the specially prepared intervertebral disk space and are designed to facilitate fusion of the motion segment. There is a multitude of shapes and designs on the market. The key requirements of these implants are a large contact area for even load distribution and an open-structure facilitating bony ingrowth and subsequent solid bony fusion. It is also important that the design and material are compatible with imaging methods so that fusion status can be assessed. Stable primary fixation of the implant in the vertebral endplate is another important requirement. Most of the intervertebral cages are box-shaped with differences in materials (titanium, PEEK, tantalum) [8]. Some have lordotic angulations; others adapt to the anatomic curvature of the lumbar endplates. Generally, the intersomatic implants used for anterior procedures cover a larger percentage of the endplates than those used for posterior implantation. The radiological results for specific implants may be assessed in the individual literature.

53.3.1.2 Stand-Alone Implants

The surgical trauma of classic 360° fusion techniques has led to the development of alternatives providing equal biomechanical stability. Minimally invasive anterior approaches involve a standardized surgical technique with a defined risk profile. The stand-alone implants, which incorporate additional fixation with cortical screws and biomechanical tests, showed comparable stability to 360° fusion techniques [9–11]. Anterior stand-alone implant types without fixation show a lack of stability during extension and lateral bending of the motion segment due to incomplete or complete removal of the anterior longitudinal ligament [12, 13]. A combination with anterior plating is necessary to provide anterior tension band stability and additional stiffness in lateral bending and torsional movements.

53.3.2 Nucleus Replacement

The trend in restoring motion and stabilization of the motion segment has led to several nucleus pulposus replacement technologies. Prevention of disk space collapse has been a key goal of nucleus replacement devices. These can be implanted through an anterior, posterolateral, or posterior approach. They replace the nucleus and try to mimic its biomechanical properties with regard to axial load and compressive strength, as well as hydration properties. The core material consists of elastic polymers. However, use of most devices is limited to strict study protocols. Long-term results are not yet available.

53.3.3 Total Disk Replacement

Total disk replacement devices are playing an increasingly popular and important role in managing degenerative conditions of the lumbar spine. Their implantation is carried out through an anterior midline or anterolateral approach with special attention to precise implant placement in the midline. The midline total disk implantation may pose a surgical challenge especially at the L4/L5 level due to the position of the venous bifurcation. This potential for complications has led to the development of modified implants and oblique implantation techniques. Precise placement of the total disk device with regard to the center of rotation and the midline may, however, be equally challenging.

There are numerous design concepts in clinical use. These include constrained, semiconstrained, and unconstrained designs with differing bone-implant interfaces, articulating surfaces, and centers of rotation. The medium- and long-term superiority of one concept over the other has not yet been proven. However, it has been clinically shown that the devices as such are effective in preserving motion and giving acceptable clinical results. Those implants accounting for the majority of clinical use worldwide are made of alloys and covered with titanium, which limits the postoperative MRI compatibility. Another challenge for the coming years is posed by the revisability of the implant.

Early studies show a very high risk of potentially life-threatening complications in revision of total disk replacement. The group of implants in current use can still be considered "first generation."

53.3.4 Vertebral Body Replacement

Numerous indications require the removal of the vertebral body. In the lumbar spine, they generally fall into the categories traumatic deformity, tumors and metastases, and infections. Typically, the vertebral body replacements play a key role in a 360° segmental reconstruction with added posterior instrumentation. While the surgical strategy is determined by the underlying indication, reconstruction of the vertebral body generally has the same goals: primary stability and restoration of spinal alignment in all three planes [14]. The implants generally consist of modular elements. Endplates provide secure anchorage and ingrowth into the adjacent bone, as well as lordotic angulations required for proper sagittal alignment. Depending on their main part, vertebral body replacements can be grouped into fixed size and expandable implants. A typical example for the first group is surgical titanium mesh (as used for Harms' cages). The implant is sized intraoperatively and impacted into the gap to be bridged. This implantation may compromise the preliminary segmental correction by a posterior instrumentation in the respective indications. Examples of expandable cages are Synex (Synthes) [15] and Hydrolift (Aesculap) implants. The modular implants are assembled, placed in the gap created by removal of the vertebral body, and mechanically expanded after precise placement. This greatly facilitates sagittal correction. Depending on the indication, posterior instrumentation may be added. The surgical principles employed in use of these implants follow the same guidelines in the lumbar spine as in the thoracic spine (see the relevant chapter in this volume).

53.3.5 Single/Double Rod Systems, Anterior Plates [16]

While posterior instrumentation is associated with a certain degree of surgical trauma in 360° fusions, anterior instrumentation plays an important role in stabilizing the motion segment without the necessity of transpedicular screw placement. The indications include idiopathic scoliotic deformity, traumatic kyphotic deformity, and reconstruction of the motion segment following partial or total vertebrectomy. The implants consist of small anchoring plates fixed with conventional or hollow screws and a single or double rod system. The anterior plates generally have a trapezoid

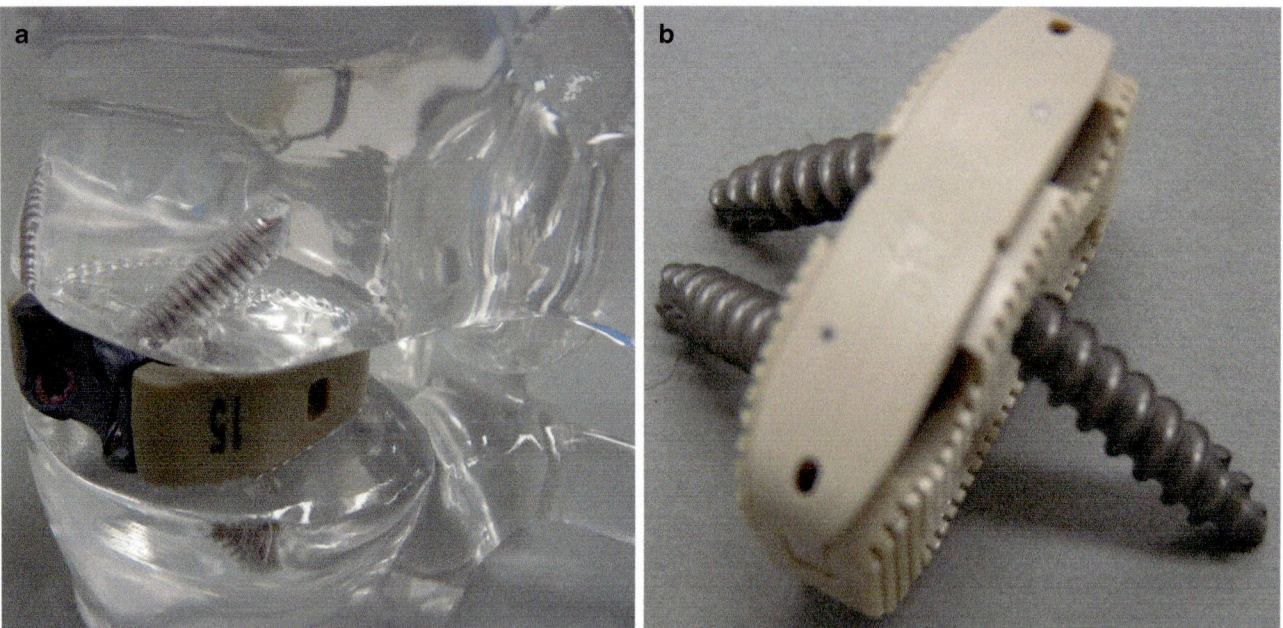

Fig. 53.1 (**a**) Synfix (Synthes) on spine model at L5/S1 level and (**b**) a comparable implant Sovereign (Medtronic)

shape and cover different sizes. Their indication spectrum is the same as those for rod systems except for deformity correction in idiopathic scoliosis. The instrumentations are carried out through an anterolateral approach exposing the lateral surface of the motion segments. In deformity correction, the endplates and anchoring plates are fixed to the motion segment, and the rods play a key role in finalizing the correction. However, in segmental reconstruction, the implant is placed first, correction is archived, and the plate or rod system is added subsequently to facilitate fusion in the archived segmental angulations. Biomechanically, equal results to a 360° fusion can be obtained with all implants with special focus on angular stability and transfer of axial load. Anterior tension band plates constitute a subgroup of anterior plates. They are used in addition to an anterior intervertebral instrumentation in spinal fusion and are placed in the anterior midline to restore the stabilizing moment provided by the resected anterior longitudinal ligament. They increase the maximal stability more in flexion and extension than in axial rotation or lateral bending. The plates cover a single motion segment and are fixed with diverging screws in the upper and lower vertebra. With biomechanically comparable results, the anterior tension band plates can make posterior transpedicular instrumentation unnecessary and archive similar fusion rates. Examples of anterior plates or anterolateral plates are the Unity Lumbosacral Fixation System (Blackstone Medical) for L5–S1, Pyramid (Medtronic) and TSLP L5–S1 (Synthes) (see Figs. 53.1, 53.2, 53.3, 53.4 and 53.5).

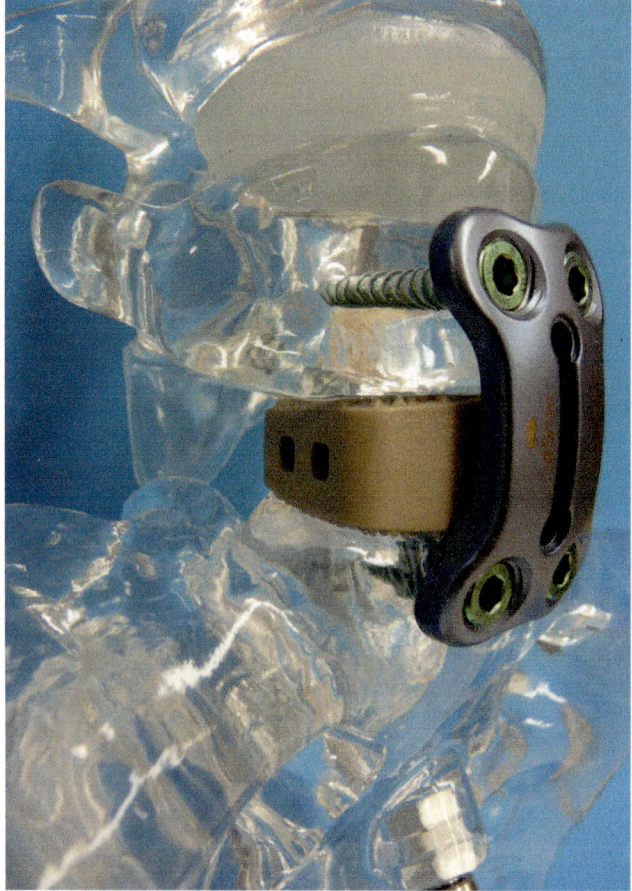

Fig. 53.2 Anterior TSLP plate (Synthes) with ALIF cage L5/S1 on a spine model

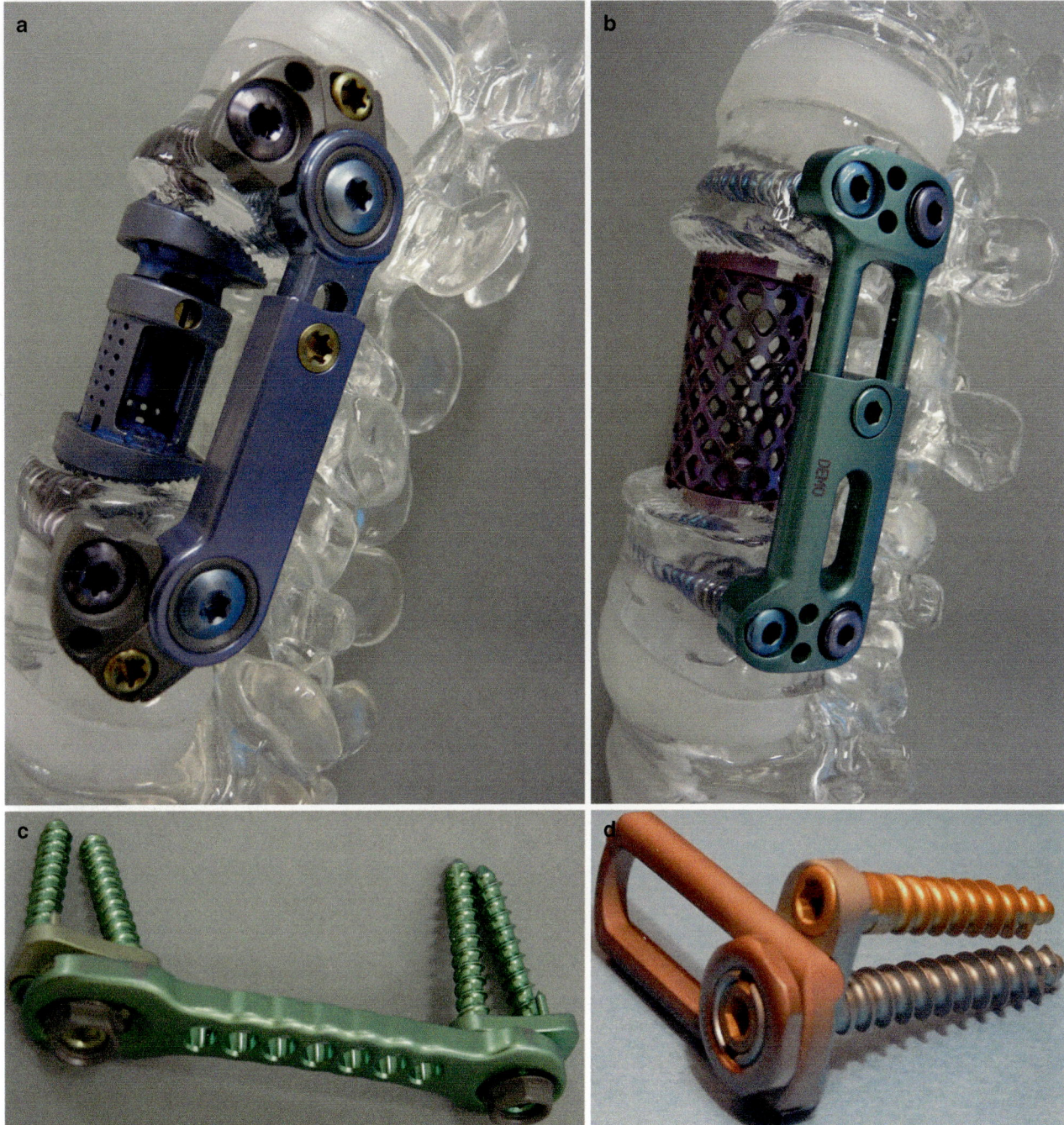

Fig. 53.3 Anterolateral plates (**a**) (Synthes), and (**b**) (Synthes), (**c**) Vantage (Medtronic), (**d**) MACS (Aesculap)

53.4 Special Techniques

One special technique recently introduced is the AxiaLIF technique to provide transvertebral placement of a screw axial to the vertebral body [17]. The indications include disk degeneration at the lumbosacral or the two lowermost lumbar levels. It is advocated that, through a percutaneous approach in the prone position, a presacral axial hole is drilled through the sacrum and the L5 vertebra. Subsequently, a device to curette the disk space and the endplate is introduced, bone graft is placed, and the modular screw is placed to facilitate distraction and fusion. While some studies show equal biomechanical results to ALIF, independent medium- and long-term results are yet to be seen. The risk for potentially lethal complications such as intestinal damage and infection is described and is again pointed out hereby.

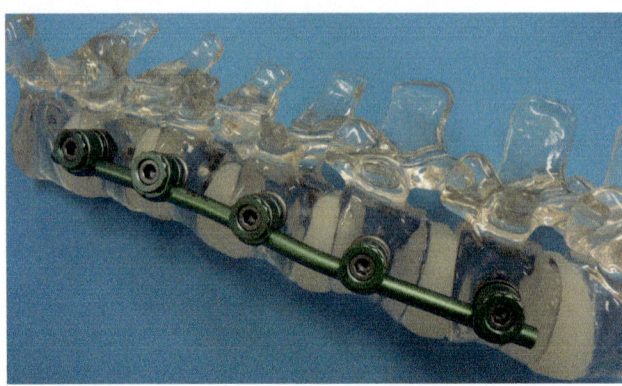

Fig. 53.4 Anterior rod-screw system USS ventral (Synthes)

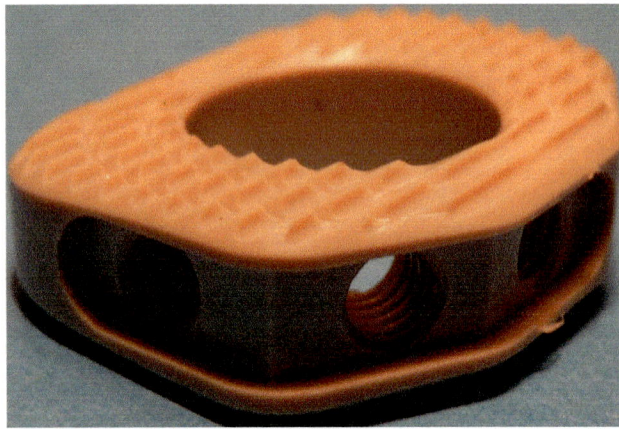

Fig. 53.5 ALIF cage A-Space (Aesculap)

References

1. Hodgson AR. Anterior surgical approaches to the spinal column. Baltimore, MD: Advances in orthopedics, Williams & Wilkens; 1974.
2. Mirbaha MM. Anterior approaches to the thoraco-lumbar junction of the spine by retroperitoneal extrapleural technic. Clin Orthop. 1971;91:12–8.
3. Bauer R, Kerschbaumer F, Poisel S. Orthopädische Operationslehre, vol. Band I. Stuttgart/Thieme, New York: Wirbelsäule; 1991.
4. Aebi M, Steffen T. Synframe: a preliminary report. Eur Spine J. 2000;9:44–50.
5. Zuckerman JF, Zdeblick TA, Bailey SA, et al. Instrumented laparoscopic spinal fusion. Preliminary results. Spine. 1995;20:2029–34.
6. Dewald CJ, Millikan KW, Hammerberg KW, et al. An open minimally invasive approach to the lumbar spine. Am Surg. 1999;65:61–8.
7. Mayer HM, Wiechert K. Ventrale Fusionsoperationen an der Lendenwirbelsäule Mikrochirurgische Techniken. Orthopade. 1998;27:466–76.
8. Spruit M, Falk RG, Beckmann L, et al. The in vitro stabilisation effect of polyetheretherketone cages versus a titanium cage of similar design for anterior lumbar interbody fusion. Eur Spine J. 2005;14:752–8.
9. Cain MJ, Schleicher P, Gerlach R, et al. A new stand alone ALIF device: biomechanical comparison with established fixation methods. Spine. 2005;30:2631–6.
10. Vieweg U, Liner M, Neurauter A, et al. Biomechanical study of a stand-alone cage TOPAZ for the lumbar spine with and without additional posterior fixation. Eur Spine J. 2006;15:1561–2.
11. Weber J, Vieweg U. Anterior lumbale interkorporelle Fusion (ALIF) mit einem stabilisierenden Cage. Z Orthop Ihre Grenzgeb. 2006;144:40–5.
12. Pellise F, Puig O, Rivas A, et al. Low fusion rate after L5-S1 laparoscopic anterior lumbar interbody fusion using twin stand-alone carbon fiber cages. Spine. 2002;27:1665–9.
13. Ray CD. Ray threaded titanium cages for stand-alone lumbar interbody fusions: 6-years follow up study. In: Kaech DL, Jinkins JR, editors. Spinal restabilisation procedures. Boston, MA/London: Amsterdam/Elsevier; 2002. p. 121–33.
14. Dvorak MF, Kwon BK, Fischer CG. Effectiveness of titanium mesh cylindrical cages in anterior column reconstruction after thoracic and lumbar vertebral body resection. Spine. 2003;28:902–8.
15. Vieweg U. Vertebral body replacement system Synex in unstable burst fractures of the thoracic and lumbar spine. J Orthop Traumatol. 2007;8:64–70.
16. Thalgott JS, Kabins MB, Timlin M. Four years experience with the AO anterior thoraco-lumbar locking plate. Spinal Cord. 1997;35:286–91.
17. Marotta N, Cosar M, Pimenta L, et al. A novel minimally invasive presacral approach and instrumentation technique for anterior L5-S1 intervertebral discectomy and fusion: technical description and case presentations. Neurosurg Focus. 2006;20(1):E9.

Anterior Lumbar Interbody Fusion (ALIF) Using Bone or Cage

54

Karsten Wiechert and Uwe Vieweg

54.1 Introduction and Core Message

First described in 1998 by Mayer [1], the classic mini-ALIF technique still sets the standard for modern anterior access surgery to the lumbar spine. Its universal use is owed in part to a very standardized, stepwise surgical technique resulting in a short learning curve. Another important factor is its complete applicability for the majority of indications requiring anterior lumbar spine surgery. The original publications on the classic mini-ALIF technique actually describe two different techniques: the minimally invasive anterolateral retroperitoneal approach to the L2/3, L3/4, and L4/5 segments and the anterior trans- or retroperitoneal midline approach to L5/S1 (L4/L5).

54.2 Indications

- Degenerative disk disease.
- Degenerative or isthmic spondylolisthesis after posterior instrumentation.
- Failed back surgery syndrome including pseudarthrosis.
- Fractures.
- Posttraumatic kyphotic deformity.
- Spondylitis/spondylodiscitis.

K. Wiechert (✉)
Schön Klinik Munich Harlaching, Spine Center "Am Michel",
Hamburg, Germany
e-mail: praxis@ruecken-zentrum.de

U. Vieweg
Department of Conservative and Surgical Spine Therapy with
Interdisciplinary Spinal Deformities Centre and Rummelsberg
Sectional Center, Hospital Rummelsberg,
Schwarzenbruck, Germany
e-mail: uwe.vieweg@sana.de

54.3 Contraindications

- Absolute contraindications to this technique do not exist. However, special caution needs to be exercised in cases with previous extensive retroperitoneal surgery or radiation.

54.4 Technical Prerequisites

Where an anterior approach is used, conditions in the hospital must meet a variety of technical requirements such as availability of appropriate positioning aids, standby facilities for general and vascular surgery, and a complication management plan for cases of intra-abdominal injury. The approach requires appropriate instruments—especially with regard to length (bipolar forceps, hemoclips)—and suitable implants. Preoperative planning must include clarification of the locations of blood vessels, especially when access is exclusively anterior. CT angiography of the pelvic blood vessels can provide the necessary information. A conventional AP and lateral X-ray overview shows the situation of the iliac crest with regard to the L4/5 level. It should be ensured that appropriate X-ray-transparent operating tables, a C-arm for intraoperative X-ray procedures, and Xenon lamps for better illumination are available. Adjustable operating tables and positioning aids facilitate anterior access in the Trendelenburg or da Vinci position and are also helpful for ventrolateral access (Fig. 54.1). For both techniques, a frame-mounted retractor system is helpful (SynFrame, Synthes; activ O retractor, Fig. 54.2, Aesculap; or Miaspas, Fig. 54.3, Aesculap), especially if the surgery is carried out without an assistant [2]. The type of approach can be selected according to the anatomical situation, the position of the major vessels, and the indication: lateral retroperitoneal approach, pararectus approach, midline retroperitoneal approach, or midline transperitoneal approach (see Fig. 54.4a, b).

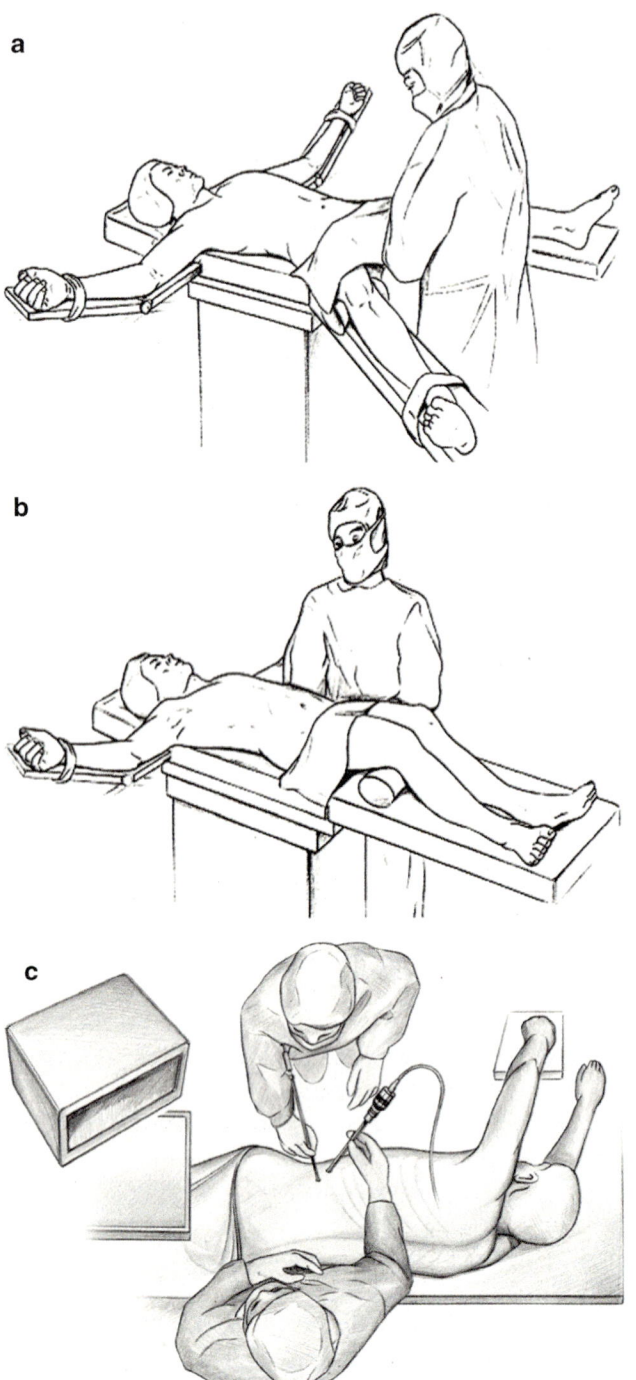

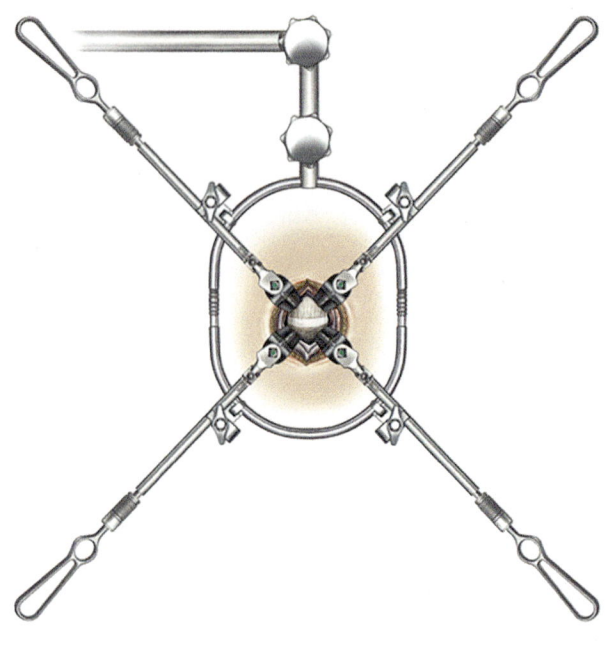

Fig. 54.2 Activ O retractor (Aesculap). (With permission of Aesculap AG, Tuttlingen, Germany)

Fig. 54.1 Different positioning: Da Vinci position for L5/S1 (**a**), conventional supine position for lower lumbar spine (**b**), and lateral position for ventrolateral access to the lumbar spine, here with endoscopic assistance (**c**). (With permission of Aesculap AG, Tuttlingen, Germany)

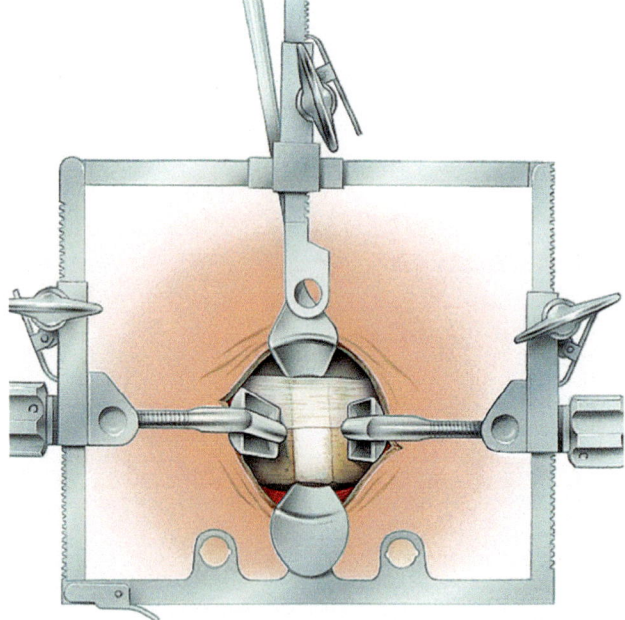

Fig. 54.3 Miaspas ALIF retractor (Aesculap). (With permission of Aesculap AG, Tuttlingen, Germany)

54.5 Planning, Preparation, and Positioning

54.5.1 Anterior Midline Retro- or Transperitoneal Approach

Anterior midline access is best carried out in the da Vinci position (see Fig. 54.1a). In total disk replacement surgery,

the lumbar spine may not be extended. In the anterior midline approach, a thorough preoperative assessment of the vascular anatomy is highly recommended, especially with regard to anatomic variations and projection of the bifurcations in relation to the target disk space. In the anterior midline approach, the projection of the disk space needs to be marked in lateral fluoroscopy as well as the midline.

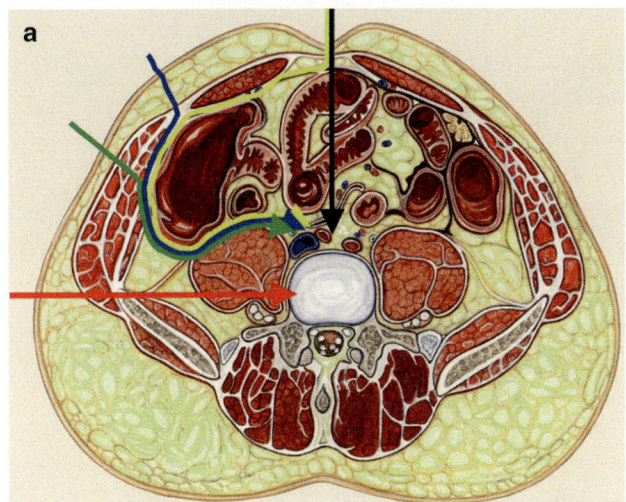

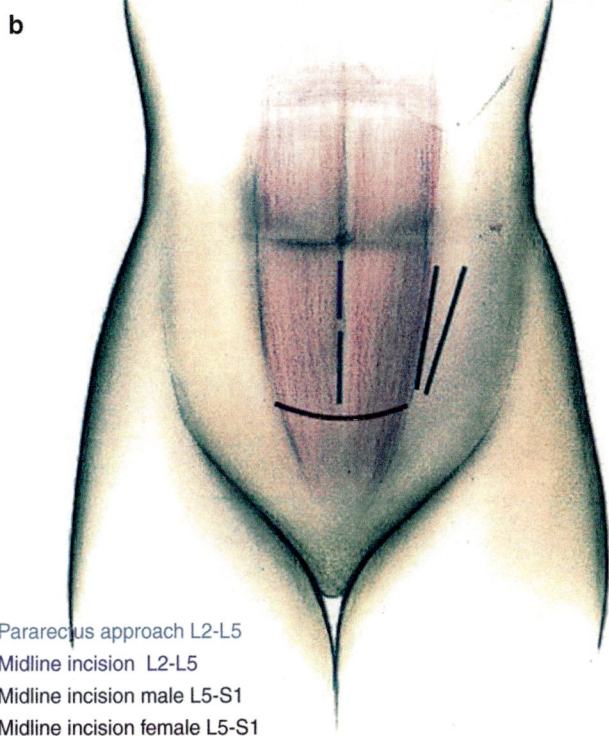

Pararectus approach L2-L5
Midline incision L2-L5
Midline incision male L5-S1
Midline incision female L5-S1

Fig. 54.4 Different anterior lumbar access routes (**a**) (*yellow* midline retroperitoneal approach, *black* midline transperitoneal approach, *blue* pararectal retroperitoneal approach, *green…red..?* -) and the different skin incisions for the various access routes (**b**). (With permission of Aesculap AG, Tuttlingen, Germany)

54.5.2 Lateral Retroperitoneal Approach (L2/3, L3/L4, L4/L5)

The lumbar segments L2/3, L3/4, and L4/5 are reached by a retroperitoneal approach from the left side. For the lateral retroperitoneal approach, the patient is placed in on his or her right side with the operating table tilted backward depending on the level to be fused. The higher lumbar levels require a posterior tilt of approximately 40°, while the lower levels (L4/5) require approximately 20°

and L3/4 30° of posterior tilt in the axial plane. Dissection of the fibers of the psoas muscle is facilitated if the table is angulated to create a right-sided lateral bend. This also increases the costo-iliac distance. If the left leg is positioned with the knee extended, the tension on the psoas fibers increases, facilitating dissection. The anterolateral approach requires some planning with regard to the rib cage and the iliac crest. If the eleventh rib covers the L2/3 disk space, a more anterior skin incision is necessary. In the lateral approach, it is recommended that the disk space level and the center of the disk space be marked on the skin. The skin incision should obliquely cross the center of the disk space.

54.6 Surgical Technique

54.6.1 Approaches

54.6.1.1 Anterior Midline Approaches (L5/S1)
- A midline approach is recommended for the L5/S1 level. Either Pfannenstiel's incision or a linear midline incision may be used (see Fig. 54.4b).
- The projection of the disk space needs to be marked in lateral fluoroscopy as well as the midline. For monolevel fusion surgery, a skin incision approximately 5 cm in length is usually sufficient (see Fig. 54.5), depending on the underlying pathology.
- A linear incision is made in the anterior fascia of the rectus abdominis muscle a few millimeters paramedially (see Fig. 54.6).
- A blunt instrument is used to push the peritoneum away in a medial direction, first from the rear surface of the muscle and then from the lateral abdominal wall (see Fig. 54.7).
- In the anterior midline approach, the dissection is carried out preperitoneally, generally to the left side. The psoas muscle is identified and the anterior edge exposed. Sometimes, the arcuate line needs to be incised for easy exposure. The ureter and the peritoneal sac are then mobilized over the midline.
- Epigastric blood vessels should be coagulated and dissected if necessary.
- The ureter and the presacral plexus are carefully mobilized and retracted together with the peritoneum (coagulation should be avoided).
- The medial sacral vessels are ligated and dissected in the bifurcation of the major vessels (see Fig. 54.8).
- Important landmarks are the lateral edge of the anterior longitudinal ligament, the sympathetic plexus, and the lateral edge of the left common iliac vein (especially in L4/5).
- After X-ray verification of the correct target level, the retractor is put in position, and the disk space is prepared for fusion (see Fig. 54.9a, b).

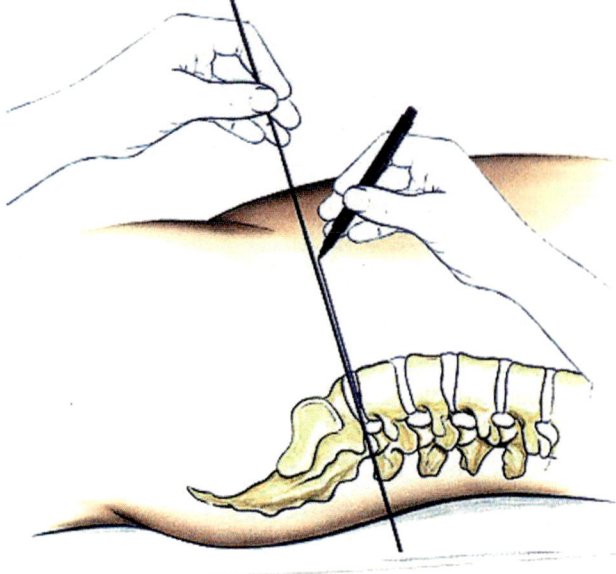

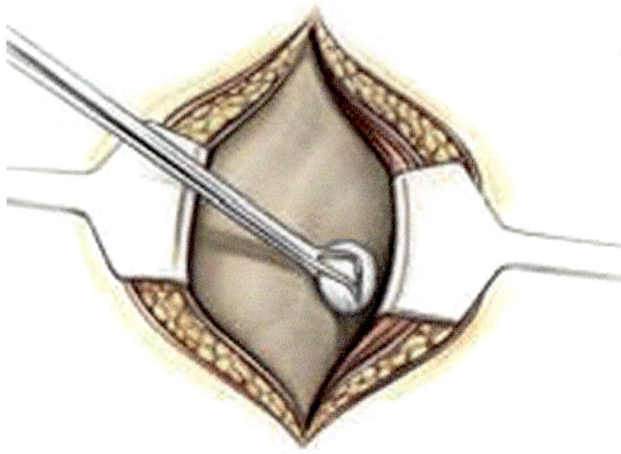

Fig. 54.7 A blunt dissection is used to push the peritoneum away in a medial direction, first from the rear surface of the muscle and then from the lateral abdominal wall. (With permission of Aesculap AG, Tuttlingen, Germany)

Fig. 54.5 The skin incision is marked under X-ray control so that the incision lies along the extended line of the intervertebral space. (With permission of Aesculap AG, Tuttlingen, Germany)

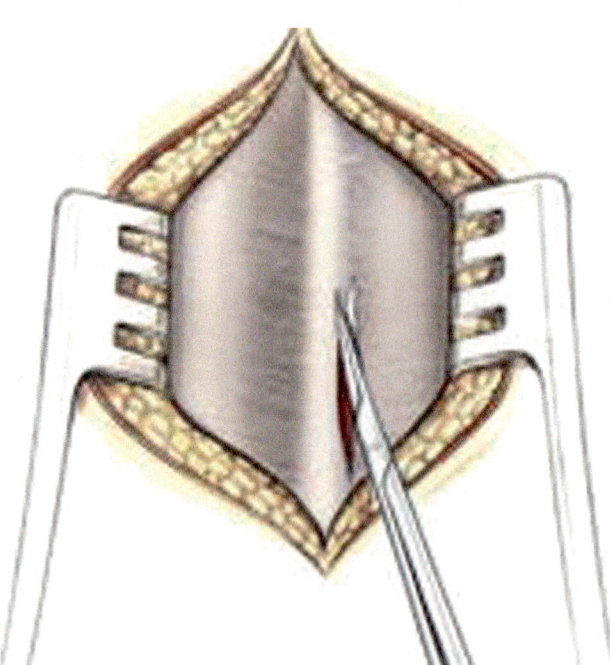

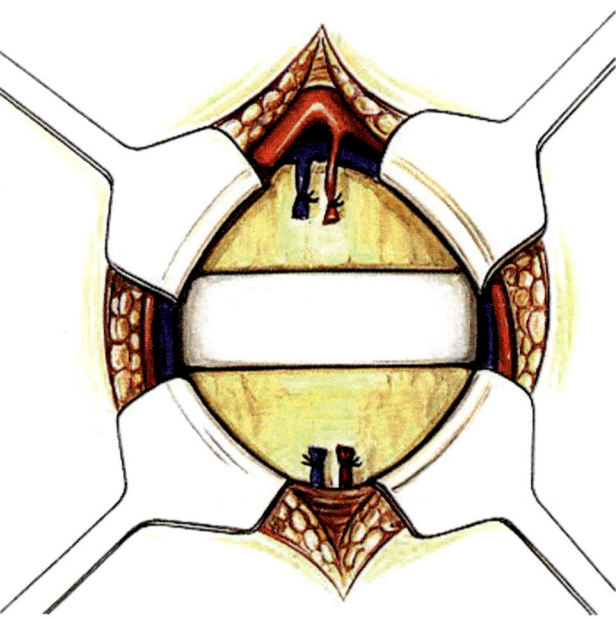

Fig. 54.8 Ligation and dissection of the medial sacral vessels in the bifurcation. (With permission of Aesculap AG, Tuttlingen, Germany)

Fig. 54.6 Linear incision of the anterior fascia of the rectus abdominis muscle. (With permission of Aesculap AG, Tuttlingen, Germany)

- The muscle fascia is dissected longitudinally where the muscles meet at the lateral margin of the rectus abdominis muscle.
- A blunt instrument is used to push the peritoneum away from the abdominal wall while monitoring the epigastric vessels.
- The ureter is mobilized and moved away from the operating site together with the peritoneum.
- The ventrolateral spine is exposed at the anterior margin of the psoas muscle.
- The vessels supplying the neighboring segment are ligated and dissected, including the ascending lumbar vein if the

54.6.1.2 Anterior Pararectal Approach L2/3, L3/4, L4/5

The anterior pararectus approach is considerably easier in the upper lumbar region of the spine but carries a higher risk of segmental denervation of the abdominal muscles.

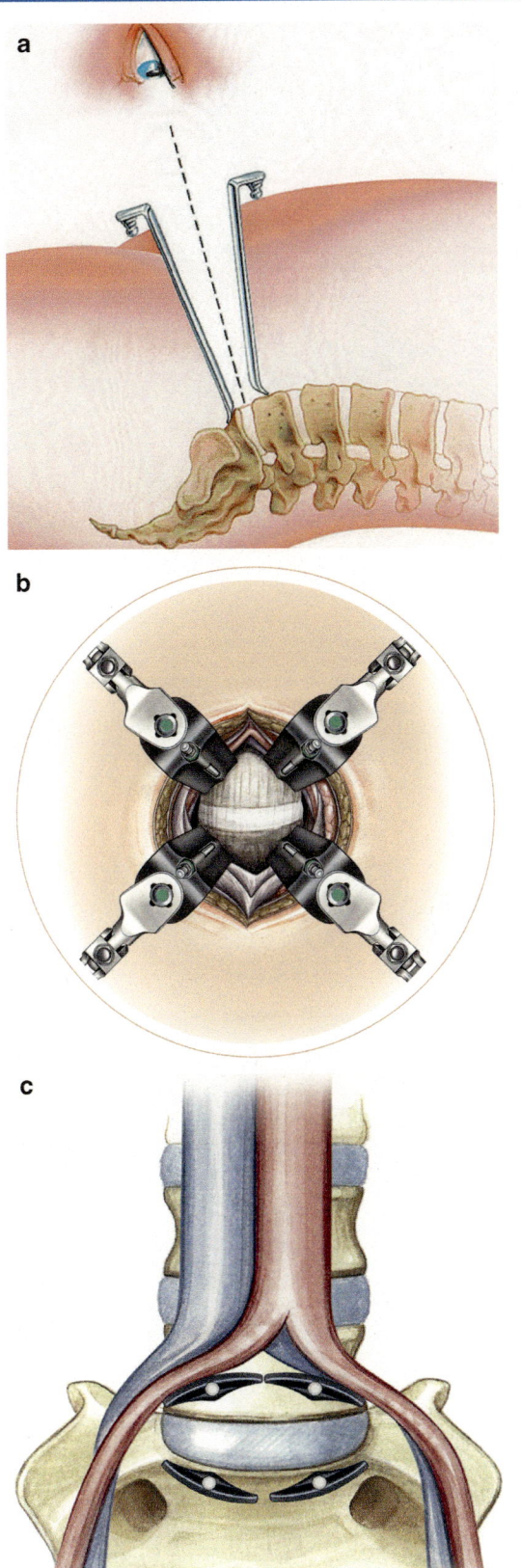

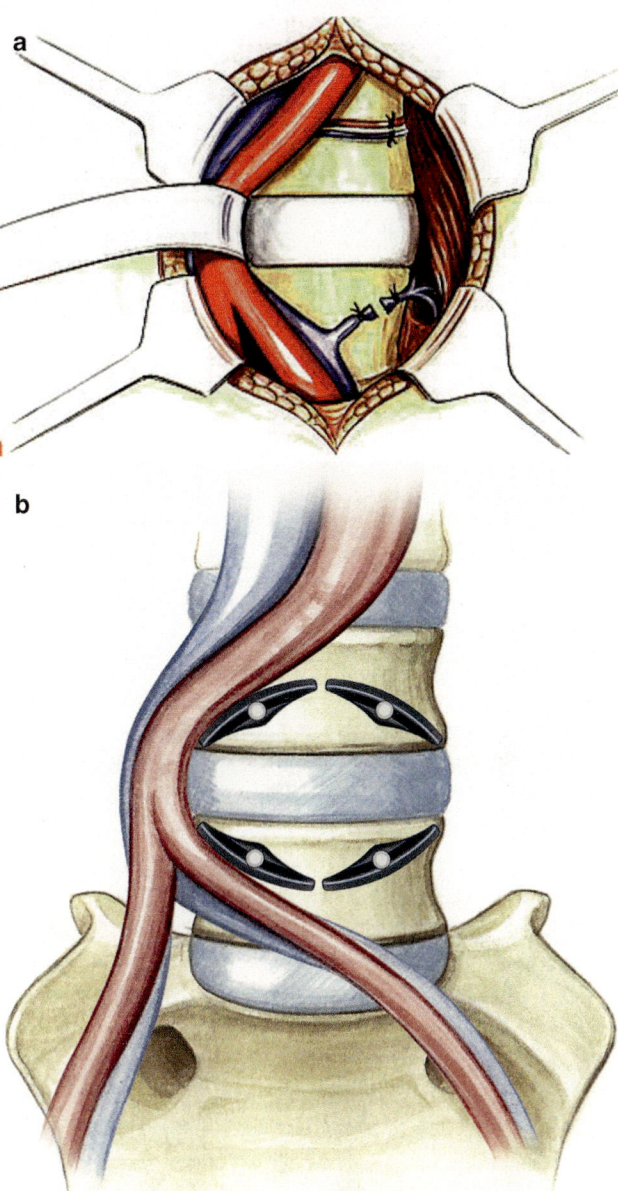

Fig. 54.10 (**a**) The neighboring segment vessels are ligated and dissected, including the ascending lumbar vein for the approach to the L4/5 segment. (**b**) Preferred retractor placement for exposure of anterior circumference of the disk space. (With permission of Aesculap AG, Tuttlingen, Germany)

L4/5 segment is being approached, so that the major vessels can be mobilized to the opposite side (see Fig. 54.10).

- The sympathetic nerve is mobilized in a lateral direction.
- *Note*: In the midline marking process, the lateral inclination of the operating table may have to be adjusted to compensate for any possible turning of the patient caused by retraction of the muscles and abdominal organs.

Fig. 54.9 Placement of the retractor blades, (**a**) lateral view, (**b**) AP view, (**c**) preferrable relation between retractors and the vascular bifurcations

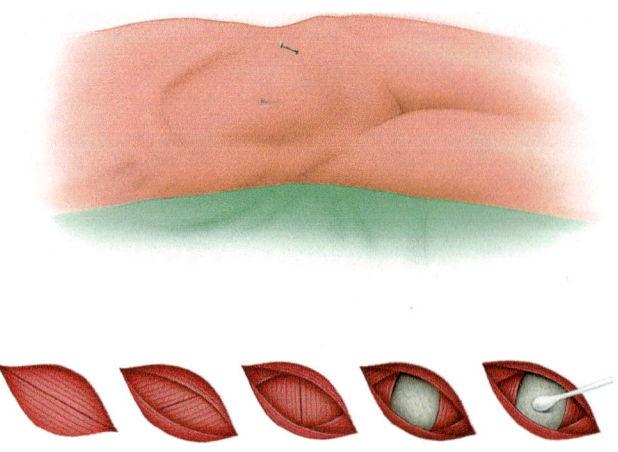

Fig. 54.11 Splitting approach—each muscle layer is dissected in the direction of its fiber orientation. (With permission of Aesculap AG, Tuttlingen, Germany)

54.6.1.3 Lateral Approaches

- In the lateral approach, skin marking of the disk space level and the center of the disk space is recommended, with the skin incision obliquely crossing the center of the disk space.
- A 5–8-cm skin incision is centered above the projection of the center of the disk space in an oblique direction parallel to the fibers of the external oblique abdominal muscles.
- The lateral approach involves a blunt split of the three abdominal wall muscle sheaths, blunt preparation down to the psoas muscle, and exposure of the anterior edge of the psoas muscle.
- Each muscle layer (external oblique, internal oblique, transverse abdominal muscle) is dissected in the direction of its fiber orientation (see Fig. 54.11).
- Care must be taken to preserve the branches of the intercostal nerves 10–12 as well as the iliohypogastric/ilioinguinal nerves, which occasionally cross the surgical field between the layers of the internal oblique and transverse abdominal muscle.
- The transverse abdominal muscle should be split as far as possible to avoid opening of the peritoneum. There is more retroperitoneal fat tissue beneath the lateral part of the transverse muscle. Moreover, the peritoneum adheres more to the inner wall of the medial part of this muscle.
- The retroperitoneal space is enlarged by careful, blunt dissection with cottonoids and Langenbeck retractors.
- The psoas muscle is identified as a first anatomical landmark (Fig. 54.12).
- The paravertebral tissues including the ureter and the vascular bundle are gently retracted toward the midline using the blunt hooks. They are incised and sharply dissected from the lateral circumference of the disk space (see Fig. 54.13). Usually, the lateral border of the left common vein can be identified.

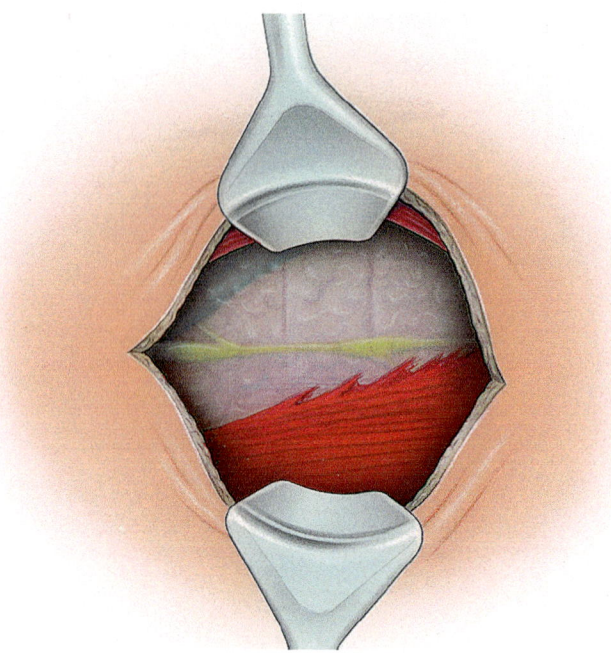

Fig. 54.12 Identification of the psoas muscle. (With permission of Aesculap AG, Tuttlingen, Germany)

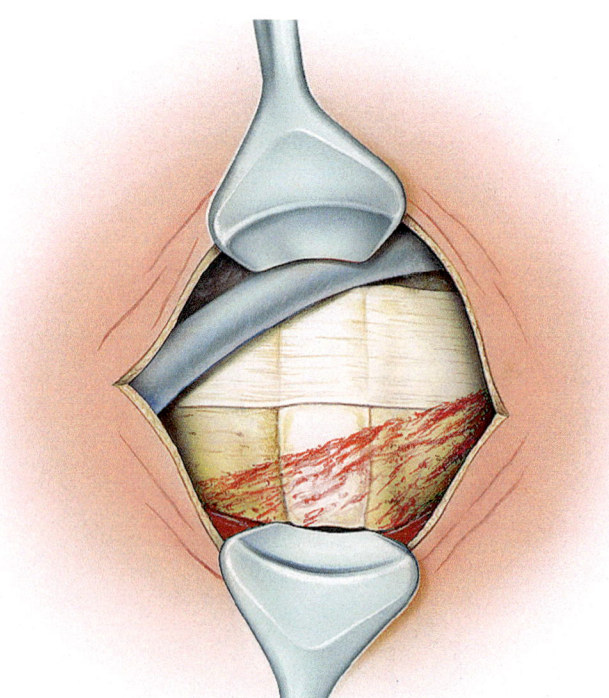

Fig. 54.13 The paravertebral tissue, including the ureter and the vascular bundle, is gently retracted from the midline using blunt hooks. (With permission of Aesculap AG, Tuttlingen, Germany)

- Dissection should be performed very carefully from the ventrolateral aspect of the vertebral bodies. The segmental vessels of the vertebral body inferior to the disk space can be exposed (see Fig. 54.14).

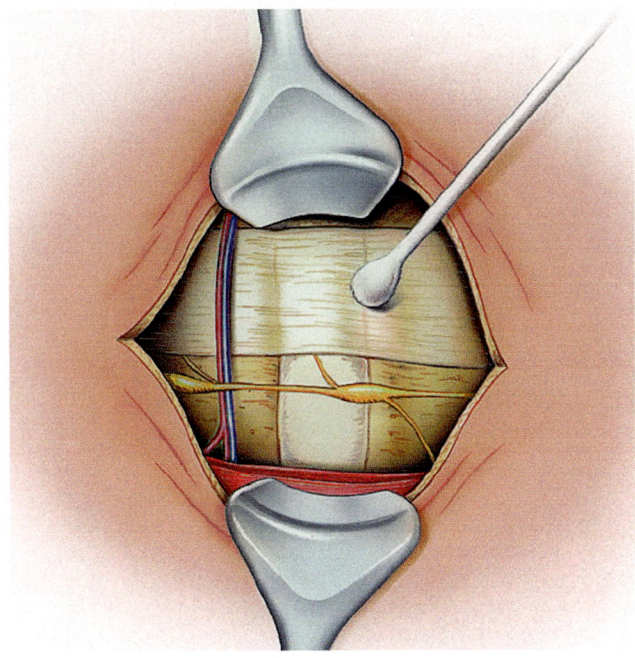

Fig. 54.14 Exposure of the segment vessels of the vertebral body inferior to the disk space

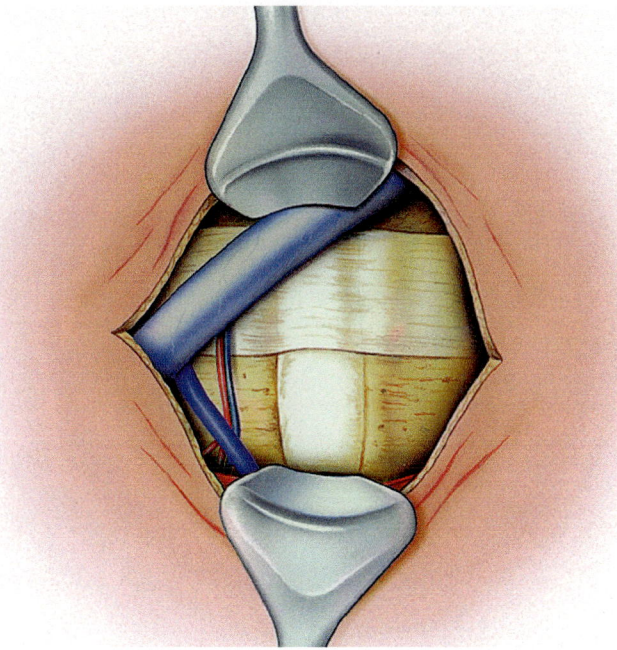

Fig. 54.15 At L4/5, the ascending lumbar vein may obstruct the inferior lateral angle of the surgical field and needs to be ligated with endoclips and dissected. (With permission of Aesculap AG, Tuttlingen, Germany)

- The segmental vessels of the inferior vertebral bodies need to be ligated with endoclips and then cut and dissected from the vertebral surface.
- However, dissection is rarely necessary at the L3/4 and L2/3 levels. At L4/5, the ascending lumbar vein may obstruct the inferior lateral angle of the surgical field and needs to be ligated with endoclips and dissected (see Fig. 54.15).
- Dissection should not be extended posterior to the pedicle entrance in order to avoid irritation of the lumbar nerve roots.
- The disk space level is verified under fluoroscopic control.
- The spatial orientation of the disk space is then identified by cutting the annulus fibrosus parallel to the vertebral endplates.

54.6.2 Interbody Fusion and Instrumentation

Instrumentation is completely unlimited in the mini-ALIF approach. Any intervertebral cages or bone grafts for spinal fusion can be used without specific considerations relating to the approach [3–5]. Any other type of anterior interbody fusion, including those using homograft or allografts, should be possible with this approach.

54.6.2.1 Interbody Fusion with Autologous Iliac Bone Graft

- With a drill guide, the anterolateral cortex of the adjacent vertebral bodies is drilled in a strictly vertical direction to create the holes for the distraction screws.

- The entry point is about 5–8 mm from the intervertebral space at the lateral border of the anterior longitudinal ligament.
- The drill has a safety range of 10 mm and penetrates only the anterolateral cortex of the vertebral body. Then specially designed anchoring screws are inserted (see Fig. 54.16).
- A retractor frame is put in place. A sharp muscle blade is attached laterally to deflect the psoas muscle, whereas a blunt vascular blade is inserted medially to retract the retroperitoneal vessels (see Fig. 54.17a, b).
- Discectomy and preparation of the graft bed. The endplates are carefully removed with chisels (see Fig. 54.18).
- The subchondral bone is smoothed with a high-speed drill (see Fig. 54.19).
- The height and depth of the iliac crest graft needed are measured with sliding callipers (see Figs. 54.20 and 54.21).
- A tricortical bone graft is harvested through a separate small incision over the lateral iliac crest on the same side. The bone graft is also taken from the middle part of the iliac crest. It is removed using a double saw blade, which can be adjusted to the size of the bone graft. The graft is removed with the help of a graft cutter.
- A small hole is drilled into the graft, which is then mounted onto a graft holder and impacted into the intervertebral space (see Fig. 54.22).

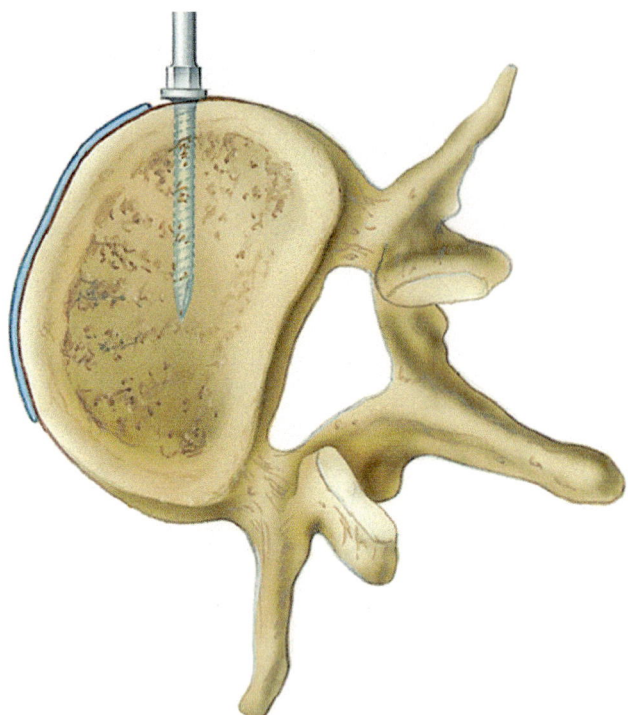

Fig. 54.16 Insertion of specially designed anchoring screws. (With permission of Aesculap AG, Tuttlingen, Germany)

54.6.2.2 Interbody Fusion with ALIF Cage Implantation

- The disk space is cleared using disk knives, rongeurs, curettes, and bone curettes. Angled instruments are available for the lateral approach. Then bone rasps are used to refresh the cartilage endplates (see Figs. 54.23 and 54.24).
- Determination of implant size using trial implants (see Fig. 54.25). Trial implants are available in heights from 9 to 19 mm in 2-mm increments. The insertion instrument and depth stop are assembled. Before the trial implant is attached, the depth stop must be turned forward to the first line on the depth scale. The trial implant is inserted with the T-handle, and the depth stop is set as appropriate for the implant position. For easier removal of the trial implant, we recommend that the T-handle be replaced with a slap hammer.
- The cage can be filled with bone or bone replacement material in a packing block. The second insertion instrument is preadjusted according to the defined depth stop position. The cage is inserted and corrected with the impactor if necessary (see Fig. 54.26).

a

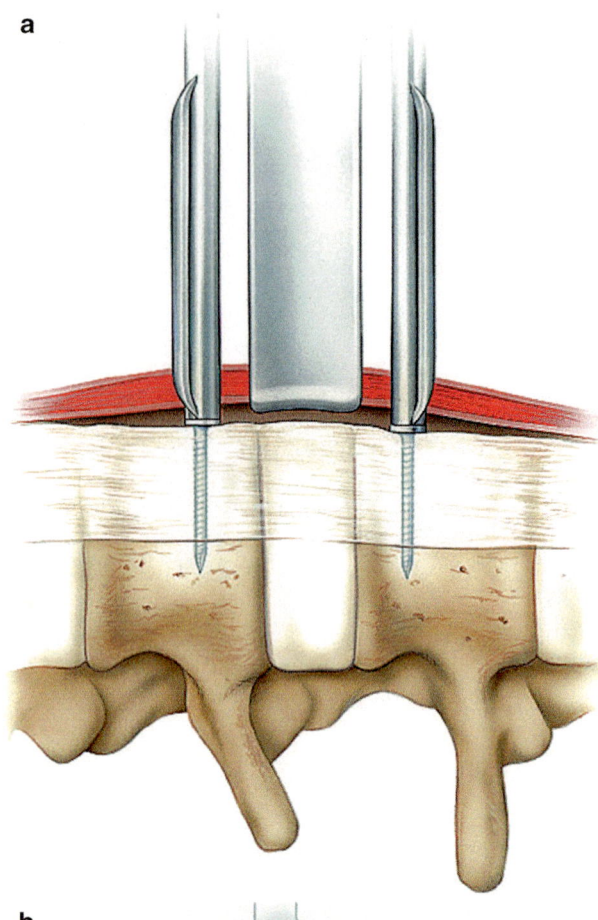

b

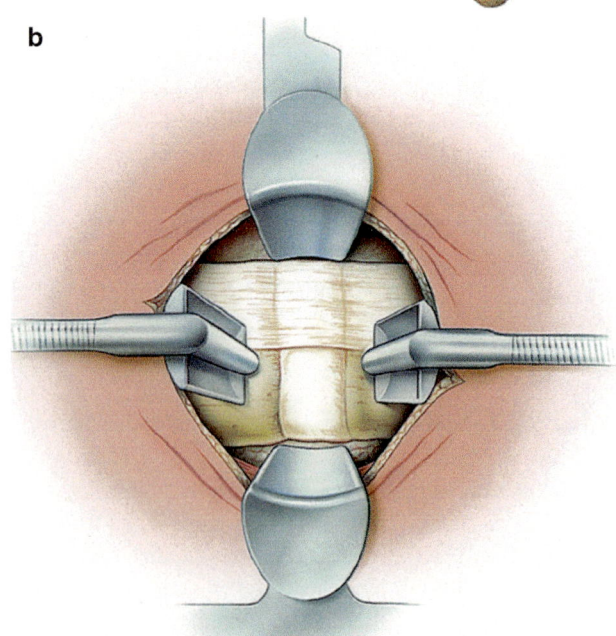

Fig. 54.17 Positioning of the retractor blades in the lateral (**a**) and AP (**b**) view

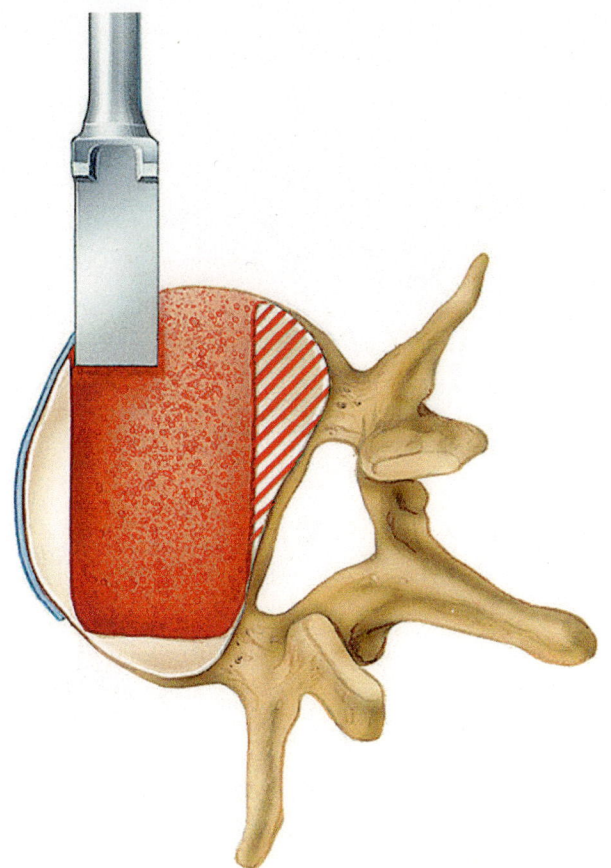

Fig. 54.18 Careful removal of the endplates with chisels. (With permission of Aesculap AG, Tuttlingen, Germany)

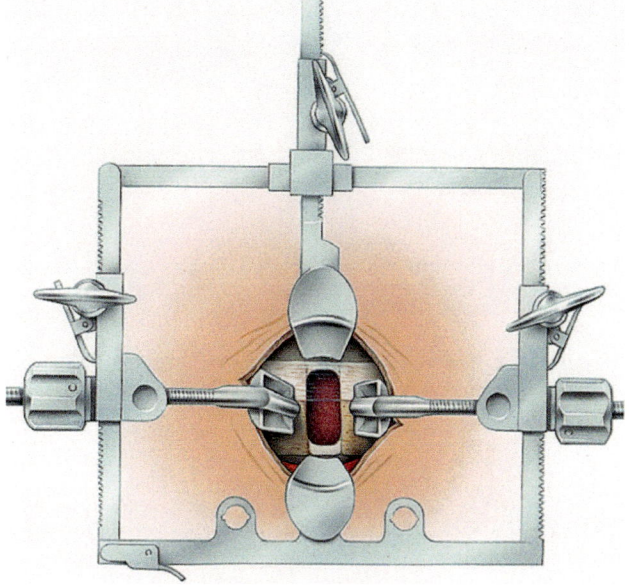

Fig. 54.20 Intraoperative situation after discectomy with Miaspas retractor in position. (With permission of Aesculap AG, Tuttlingen, Germany)

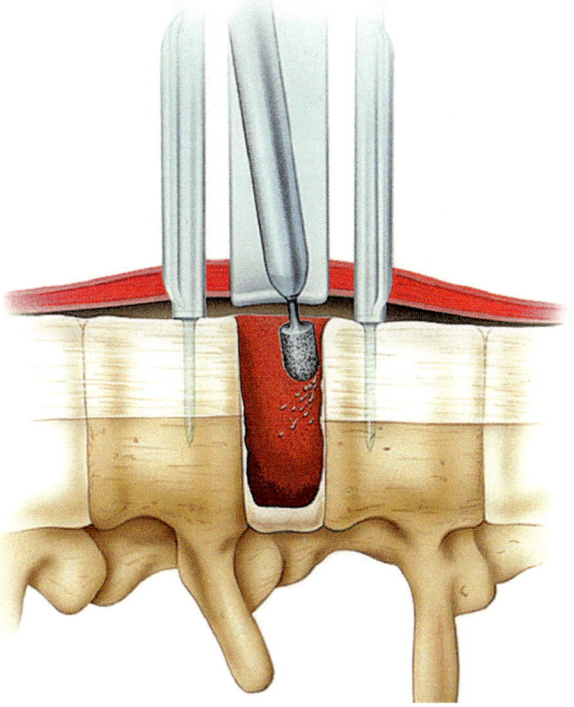

Fig. 54.19 The subchondral bone is smoothed with a high-speed drill. (With permission of Aesculap AG, Tuttlingen, Germany)

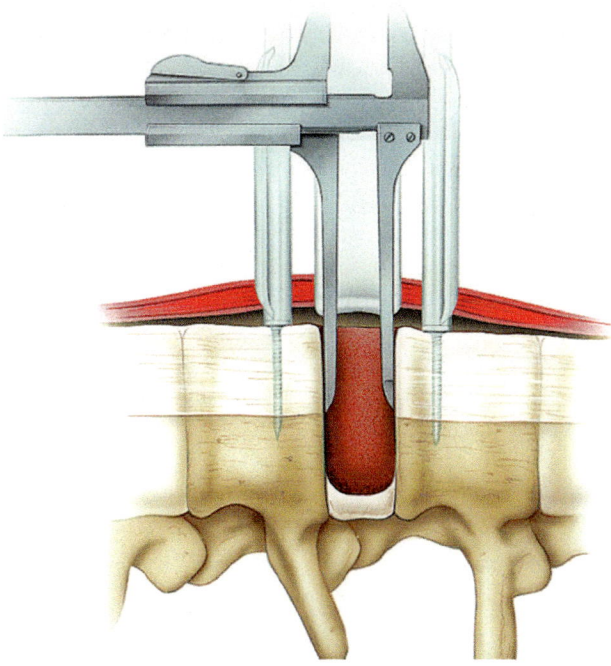

Fig. 54.21 Measurement of the height and depth of the iliac crest graft. (With permission of Aesculap AG, Tuttlingen, Germany)

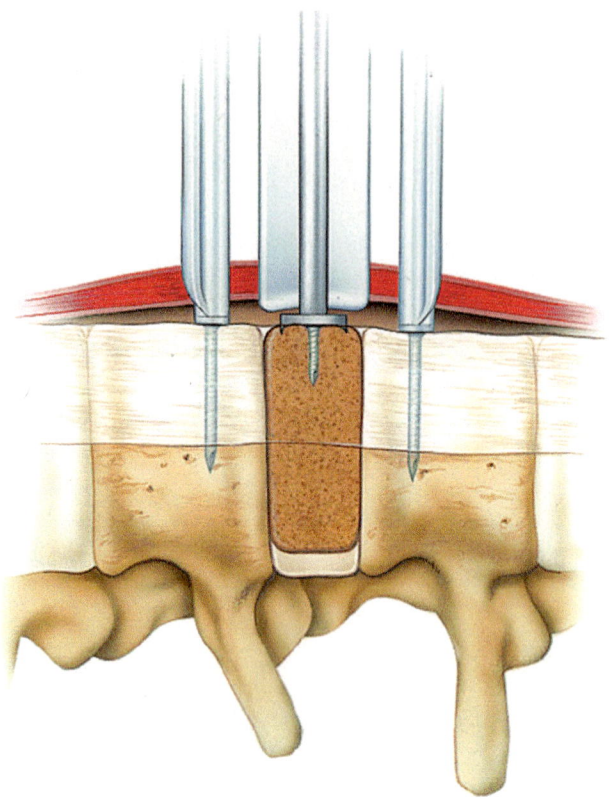

Fig. 54.22 Impaction of the bone piece with a graft holder into the intervertebral space. (With permission of Aesculap AG, Tuttlingen, Germany)

54.6.2.3 Anterior and Anterolateral Plating

Various systems are available to stabilize the anterior or anterolateral lumbar spine. They include plate-screw systems (e.g., TSLP, Synthes; MACS, Aesculap; Pyramid, Medtronic), rod-screw systems (e.g., VentroFix, Synthes), and cages with an integrated plate (e.g., SynFix, Synthes). For a less invasive procedure, it is essential that a retractor system (e.g., activ O, Aesculap; SynFrame, Synthes) be used for anterior and anterolateral plating of the lumbar spine. The preparation and fixing of the retractor blades make instrumentation much easier. For example, the blades of the activ O retractor are placed at the cranial and caudal ends of the segment and fixed with pins. The other blades hold the abdominal viscera and the psoas muscle to the side (see

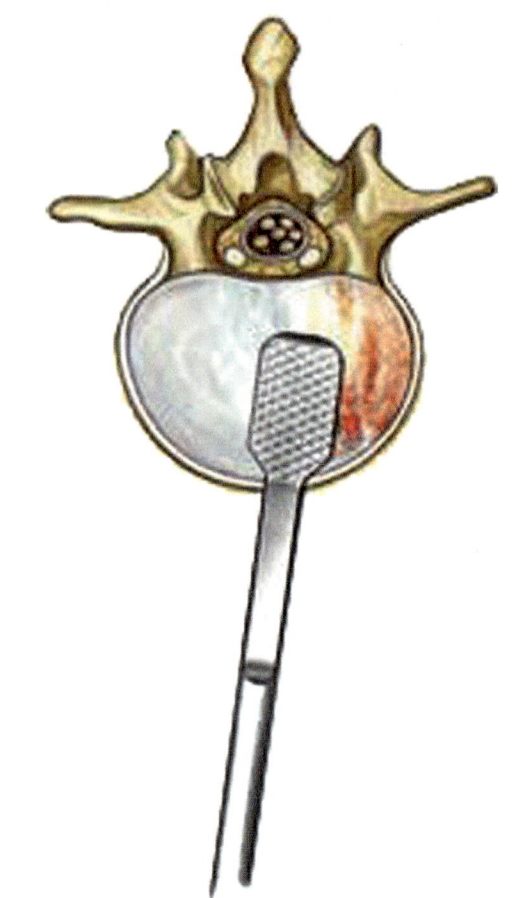

Fig. 54.23 Cleaning of the disk space using disk knives, rongeurs, curettes, and bone curettes. Then bone rasps are used to refresh the cartilage endplates. (With permission of Aesculap AG, Tuttlingen, Germany)

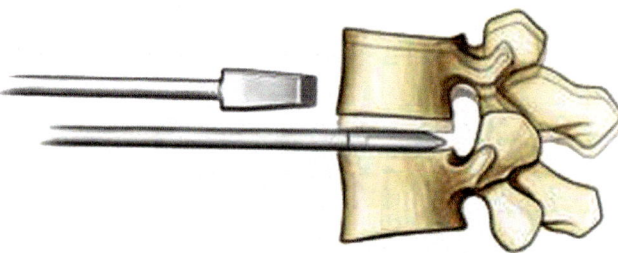

Fig. 54.24 After discectomy, a distractor should be inserted horizontally and then rotated. (With permission of Aesculap AG, Tuttlingen, Germany)

Fig. 54.25 Determination of implant size using trial implants. The trial implant is inserted with the slap hammer. (With permission of Aesculap AG, Tuttlingen, Germany)

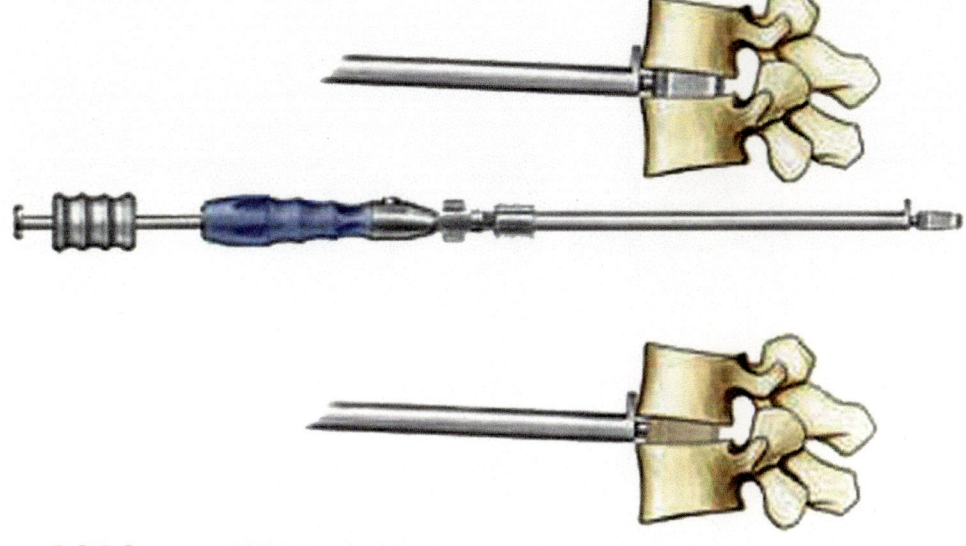

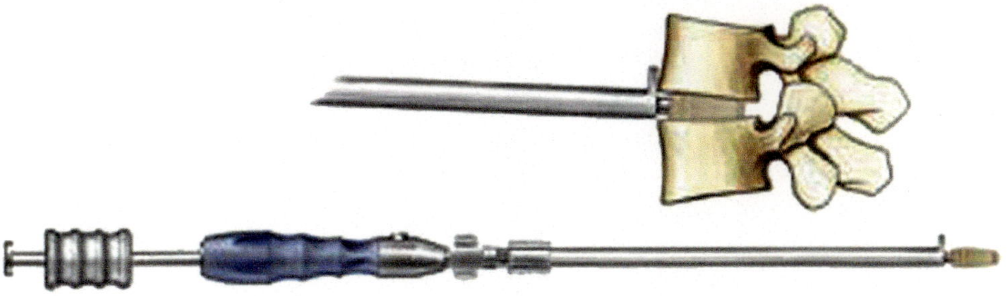

Fig. 54.26 The cage is inserted and corrected with the impactor. (With permission of Aesculap AG, Tuttlingen, Germany)

Fig. 54.27a, b). With the aid of the retractor blades, the psoas muscle is pushed from ventral to dorsal. The authors do not recommend direct entry through the psoas muscle as in the transmuscular XLIF approach. The use of the TSLP (Synthes) is made easier by temporary fixation pins. The appropriate plate is fixed to the ventral spine with the pins. After intraoperative X-ray checks of the position of the plate with respect to the spine, the plate is anchored at a stable angle using four screws [6–8]. The access route can be kept smaller when cages with an integrated plate (SynFix, Synthes; Topaz, Ulrich) are used. The operating time is reduced, because some of the instrumentation steps are rendered unnecessary.

54.7   Tips and Tricks

- A preoperative color-coded 3D CT angiogram is recommended in all cases where the vascular anatomy cannot be precisely identified or where there seem to be anatomic variations.
- Once the patient has been positioned, it is mandatory that an X-ray check of the target level be carried out in two planes prior to surgery.
- Sometimes, the operating table or its base obscures the visual plane. A preoperative check after the final tilt can save trial-and-error X-rays during the operation, thereby reducing radiation exposure for patient and surgeons.

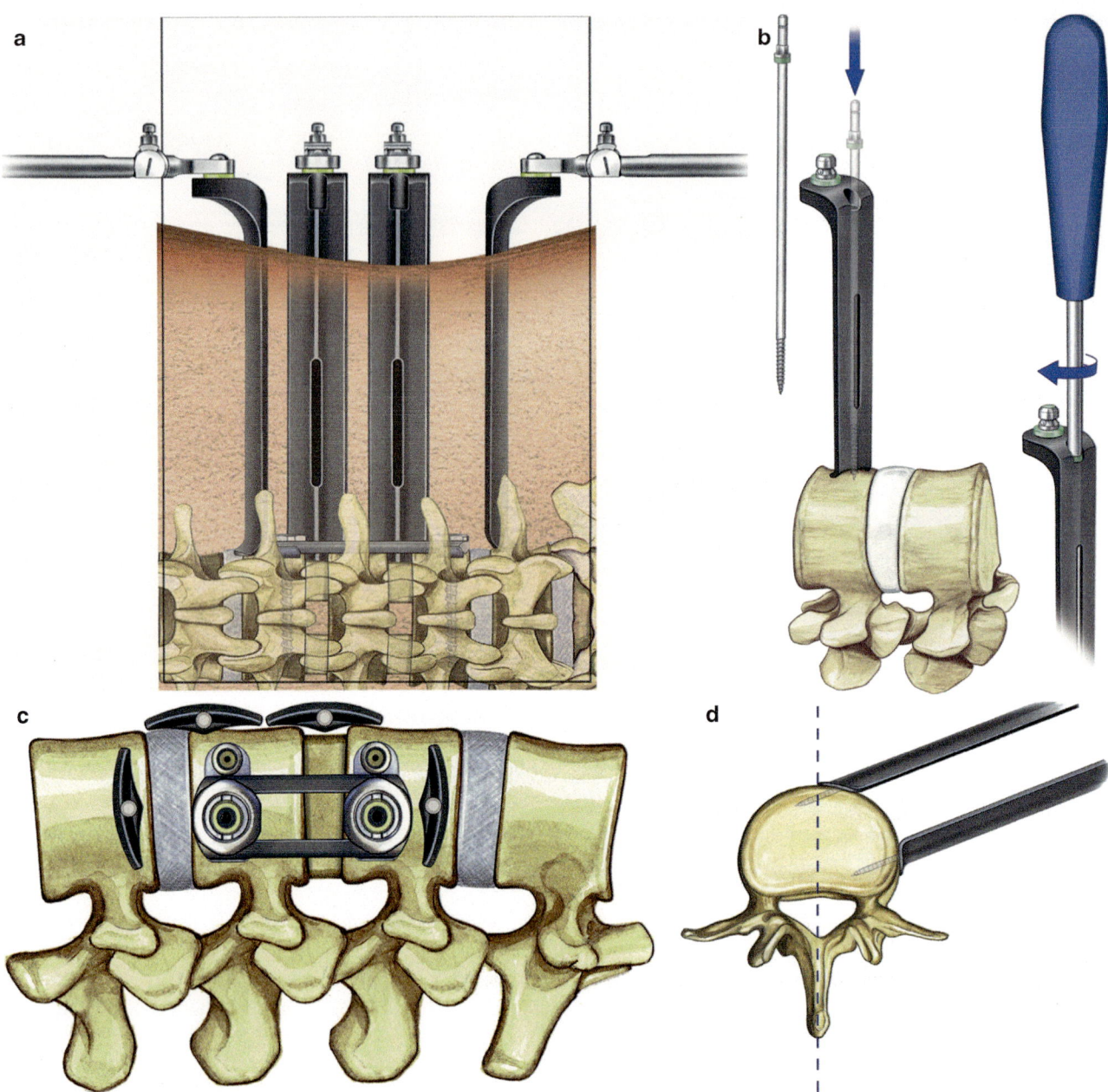

Fig. 54.27 (**a–d**) Ventrolateral plating of the lumbar spine using a retractor system (activ O, Aesculap). Retractor blades are positioned at the cranial and caudal ends of the segment and fixed with pins. The other blades hold the abdominal viscera and psoas muscle to the side

References

1. Mayer HM, Wiechert K. Ventrale Fusionsoperationen an der Lendenwirbelsäule. Mikrochirurgische Techniken Orthopade. 1998;27:466–76.
2. Aebi M, Steffen T. Synframe: a preliminary report. Eur Spine J. 2000;9:44–50.
3. Dvorak MF, Kwon BK, Fischer CG. Effectiveness of titanium mesh cylindrical cages in anterior column reconstruction after thoracic and lumbar vertebral body resection. Spine. 2003;28:902–8.
4. Thalgott JS, Giuffre JM, Klezl Z, Timlin M. Anterior lumbar interbody fusion with titanium mesh cages, coralline hydroxyapatite, and demineralised bone matrix as part of a circumferential fusion. Spine J. 2002;2:63–9.
5. Spruit M, Falk RG, Beckmann L, et al. The in vitro stabilisation effect of polyetheretherketone cages versus a titanium cage of similar design for anterior lumbar interbody fusion. Eur Spine J. 2005;14:752–8.
6. Cain MJ, Schleicher P, Gerlach R, Pflugmacher R, et al. A new stand alone ALIF device: biomechanical comparison with established fixation methods. Spine. 2005;30:2631–6.
7. Vieweg U, Liner M, Neurauter A, et al. Biomechanical study of a stand-alone cage TOPAZ for the lumbar spine with and without additional posterior fixation. Eur Spine J. 2006;15:1561–662.
8. Weber J, Vieweg U. Anterior lumbale interkorporelle Fusion (ALIF) mit einem stabilisierenden Cage. Z Orthop Ihre Grenzgeb. 2006;144:40–5.

Total Lumbar Disk Replacement

55

Christoph J. Siepe

55.1 Introduction and Core Messages

Fusion of lumbar motion segments for the treatment of intractable low-back pain (LBP) has been associated with a variety of negative side effects. Perceived disadvantages such as accelerated adjacent level morbidities, iatrogenic superior segment facet joint violation, symptomatic complaints from facet, and sacroiliac joints or facet joint hypertrophy with consecutive narrowing of the spinal canal have previously been reported [1–12]. In an attempt to avoid these previously published and fusion-related negative side effects, a variety of new motion preserving technologies including total lumbar disk replacement procedures (TDR) have been introduced. This chapter outlines the technique of TDR with ProDisc II (Synthes, Paoli, PA; Fig. 55.1).

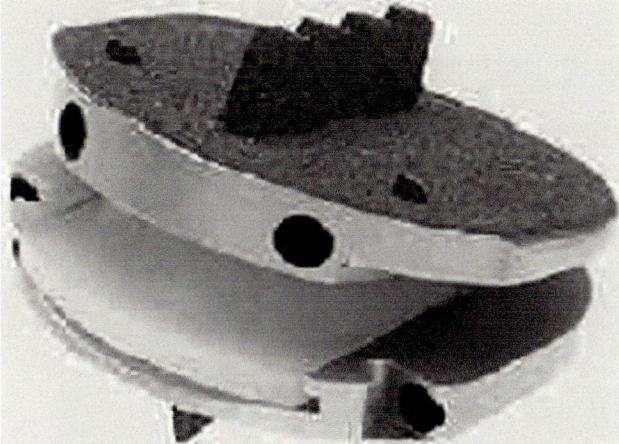

Fig. 55.1 Total lumbar disk replacement with a modular, ball-and-socket-type prosthesis (ProDisc II, Synthes, Paoli, PA). The convex polyethylene inlay is locked into the bottom endplate (© by Synthes)

55.2 Indications

The primary indication for TDR is the treatment of predominant and intractable LBP from lumbar degenerative disk disease (DDD) with or without Modic changes. Favorable outcomes have similarly been reported in candidates following previous minimally invasive discectomy as well as in candidates with DDD and accompanying central to mediolateral disk herniations with predominant LBP [13]. The procedure can be performed mono- or bisegmentally. However, inferior results must be expected in multilevel procedures [14]. Although technically more challenging, highest satisfaction rates have been reported for TDR at the level above the lumbosacral junction, while TDR performed at the lumbosacral junction similarly revealed satisfactory results [14]. Due to increasing and additive destabilizing effects [15–17], the authors do not recommend to perform TDR for more than 2-level pathologies.

55.3 Contraindications

Stringent preoperative decision making is crucial in order to achieve satisfactory outcomes following TDR. The commonly agreed-upon indications and contraindications for this procedure have been thoroughly outlined previously [13, 18–23]. Due to an extensive list of contraindications, which have previously been published, it is estimated that only about 3–5% of fusion candidates are potential candidates for TDR [18, 20]. The most common contraindications include the following:

- Central or lateral spinal stenosis.
- Predominant radiculopathy.

C. J. Siepe (✉)
Schön Klinik München Harlaching, Spine Center, Academic Teaching Hospital and Spine Research Institute of the Paracelsus Medical University (PMU, Salzburg, AU), Munich, Germany
e-mail: csiepe@schoen-kliniken.de

- Facet joint arthrosis/symptomatic facet joint complaints.
- Spondylolysis/spondylolisthesis.
- Spinal instability (iatrogenic/altered posterior elements, e.g., following laminectomy).
- Major deformity/curvature deviations (e.g., scoliosis).
- Metabolic bone disease (e.g., manifest osteoporosis/osteopenia).
- Previous operation with severe scarring and radiculopathy.
- Compromised vertebral body (irregular endplate shape).
- Previous/latent infection.
- Metal allergy.
- Spinal tumor.
- Posttraumatic segments.

55.4 Technical Prerequisites

The disk spaces are approached through means of a miniopen laparotomy using a retroperitoneal approach [24, 25].

Technical prerequisites include the following:

- Radiolucent and adjustable operating table.
- X-ray.
- Access equipment for retroperitoneal approach (i.e., retractor blades, retractor frame).
- Monitoring of oxygen saturation in the left lower extremity with pulse oximeter attached to the left toe.

55.5 Planning, Preparation, and Positioning

- For preoperative planning, it is recommended to analyze the corridor line to the disk space, the sacral tilt, and the vascular anatomy on preoperative X-ray (standing lateral images) as well as on sagittal and axial MRI images (Fig. 55.2a, b).
- The patient is placed in a supine position; the surgeon is positioned in between the legs of the patient (Fig. 55.3).

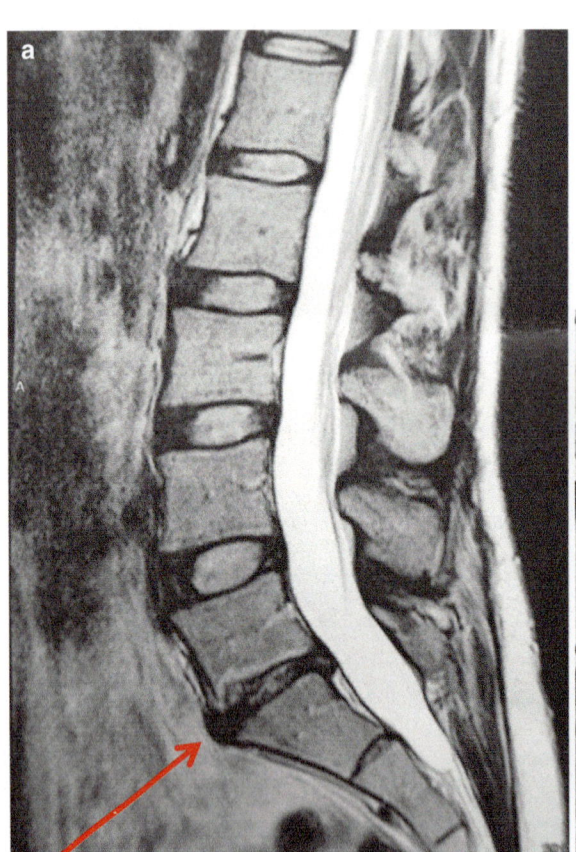

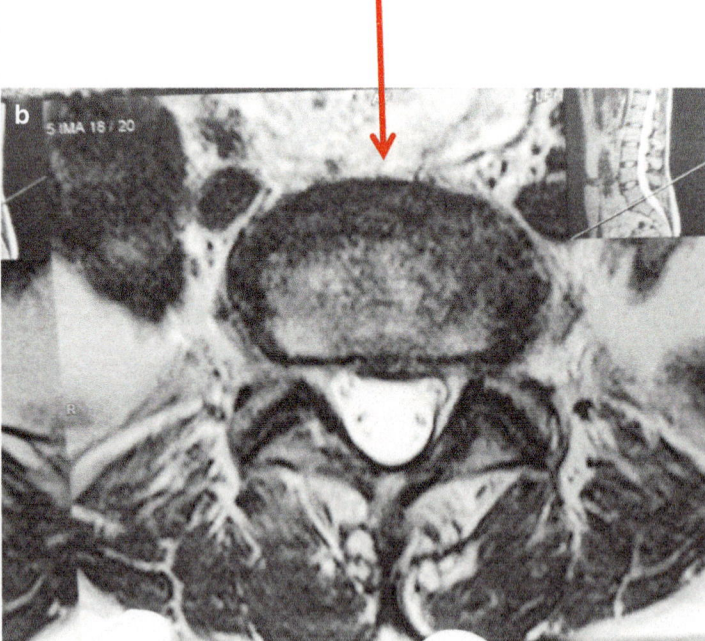

Fig. 55.2 MRI images of an adequate, "perfect" candidate for total lumbar disk replacement with single-level degenerative disk disease. The arrow delineates the projected access corridor to the disk space L5/S1. (**a**) Demonstrates a regular sagittal alignment, which facilitates an anterior approach to the disk space L5–S1. (**b**) Demonstrates a large-access corridor ("safe zone," *arrow*) to the disk space L5–S1 without the need of extensive mobilization of the iliac vessels or the vascular bifurcation. The axial images furthermore serve to exclude any advanced degenerative changes in the facet joints. Preoperative fluoroscopically guided spine infiltrations are helpful in an attempt to rule out any clinically relevant facet or sacroiliac joint complaints

- The corridor line to the disk space (lateral X-ray fluoroscopy), the anterior midline (AP fluoroscopic control), as well as the skin incision are marked on the patient's skin surface (Fig. 55.4a, b).
- For TDR at the lumbosacral junction, the table is slightly tilted in a head-down position to alleviate the access as well as the preparation toward the disk space.
- Any kind of lumbar hyperextension on the operating table should be avoided.

55.6   Surgical Technique

55.6.1   Approach

- Midline horizontal skin incision across the target region. For bisegmental TDRs at the last two lumbar motion segments, the surgeon can either choose to perform a horizontal skin incision in between the two target disk spaces, or alternatively opt for an oblique skin incision.

Fig. 55.3 The patient is positioned in a supine position (Modified da Vinci position). The surgeon is positioned in between the legs of the patient (© by Synthes)

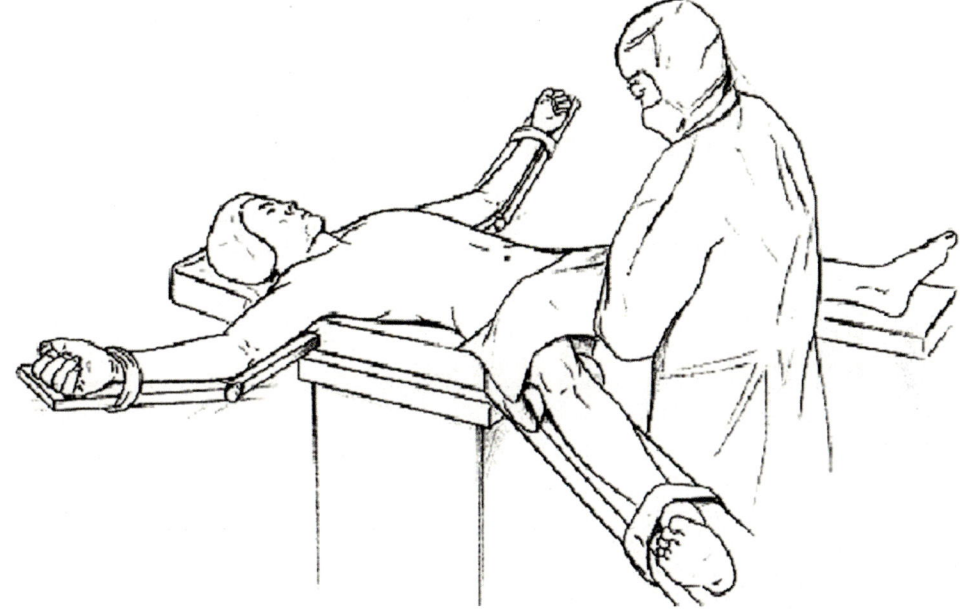

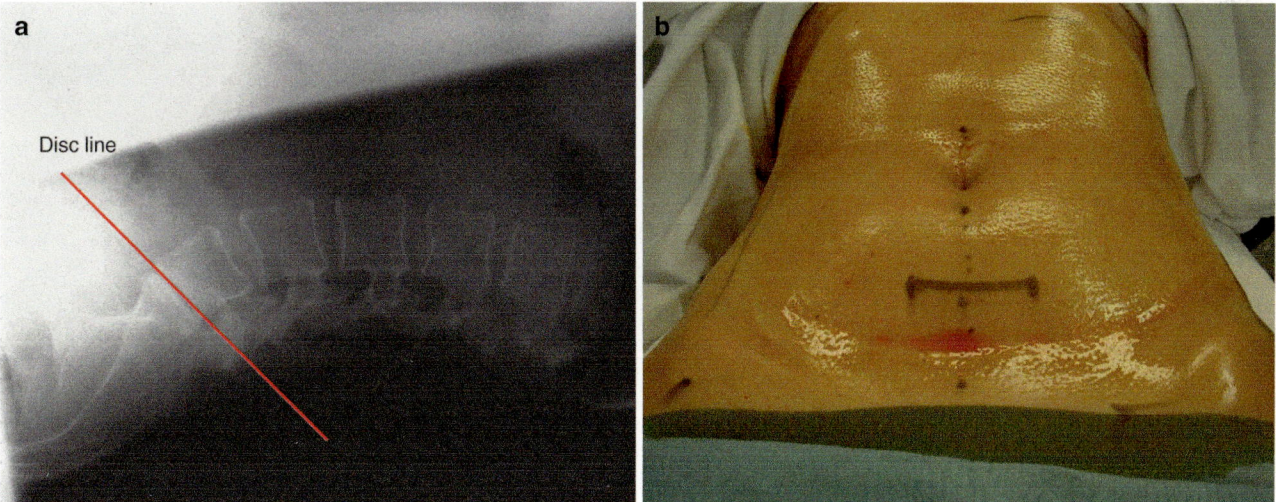

Fig. 55.4 The projection of the disk line (**a**) as well as the anatomic midline are marked on the patient's skin surface (**b**) under lateral fluoroscopic control

- Subcutaneous preparation and longitudinal incision of the linea alba.
- Levels above the lumbosacral junction should be approached via a left retroperitoneal approach due to the vascular anatomy of the prevertebral vessels.
- For TDRs at L5/S1, a right retroperitoneal approach is recommended in order to enable anterior midline access to upper lumbar levels, that is, if another TDR procedure is intended at a later stage.
- Exposure of the linea arcuata and dissection in a craniolateral direction should be performed after the peritoneal sac has been identified and bluntly mobilized away from the fascia.
- The preparation is continued medially, exposing the psoas muscle as well as the iliac vessels adjacent to the medial border of the M. psoas. The ureter is identified and carefully protected behind retractors.
- For TDRs at the level L4/5 or above, exposure and identification of the ascending lumbar vein is recommended. Ligation of the ascending lumbar vein may be required to avoid intraoperative vascular complications in this area before mobilization of the major prevertebral vessels [26].
- Exposure and identification of the disk space.
- Intraoperative fluoroscopic control should confirm the adequate level as well as the precise midline marking of the spine in the AP view. Previous studies have reported that the medial border of both pedicles may be used as a more reliable anatomic landmark for precise midline identification in comparison to the projection of the spinous processes.
- At L5/S1, the median presacral vessels should be identified and ligated. In the majority of cases, bipolar coagulation is sufficient; otherwise, clipping of the vessels may be required.
- Blunt lateral mobilization of the prevertebral vessels. The vessels are retracted laterally with self-retaining retractors, which are mounted to an operating frame, attached to the operating table.

55.6.2 Preparation of the Disk

- Excision of the anterior annulus is followed by a complete discectomy.
- Meticulous endplate preparation. Care should be taken not to violate the integrity of the cortical endplates.
- Distraction of the disk space (Fig. 55.5a, b). Previous biomechanical studies have recommended to leave the PLL intact wherever possible. In cases of advanced stages of disk space collapse, however, it may be required to partially

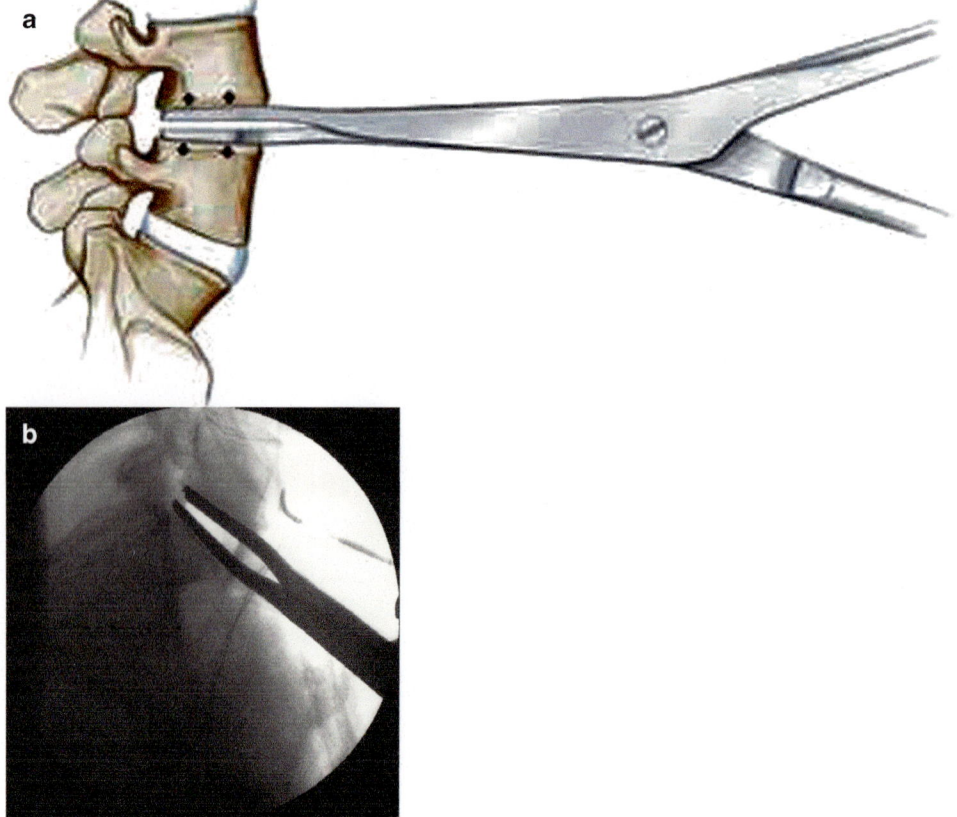

Fig. 55.5 (**a**) Following a complete discectomy, distraction of the collapsed segments can be achieved with a straight or curved spreader forceps (© by Synthes). (**b**) Intraoperative verification of the disk space distraction under image intensifier

resect or incise the posterior annulus as well as the posterior longitudinal ligament (PLL) in order to achieve adequate disk space height restoration. Posterior osteophytes should be removed meticulously in order to facilitate an adequate posterior implant positioning (Fig. 55.7).

55.6.3 Instrumentation

- Insertion of a trial implant (Fig. 55.6a, b).
- An adjustable stopper, which is attached to the insertion device, prevents excessive posterior placement of the trial implant.
- The metallic implant endplates should cover the largest possible surface area of the adjacent vertebral bodies.
- Overdistraction of the disk space should be avoided. In the majority of cases, an implant height of 10 mm is sufficient.
- Similarly, avoid excessive lordosis of the implant. The prostheses tend to shift into a more lordotic position postoperatively, which may result in a segmental hyperlordosis and possible impingement of the facet joints [27–31]. In general, 6° of overall implant lordosis is sufficient. Less than 6° implant lordosis may be chosen in selected cases. For TDRs performed at the lumbosacral junction, it may be advisable to shift some of the lordosis to the caudal endplate, particularly in patients with a steeper sacral inclination.
- Confirmation of adequate trial implant positioning in both AP and lateral plane with X-ray (Fig. 55.6a, b). The implant should be precisely positioned in the midline. Posterior implant positioning is crucial. The posterior projection of the prosthesis should be in line with the posterior wall of the adjacent vertebral bodies. In order to achieve adequate posterior implant positioning, removal of posterior osteophytes may be required (Fig. 55.7).
- The keel bed is prepared with custom-made chisel instruments, which are available in 10, 12, and 14 mm

heights, respectively. The chisel device is securely guided through openings along the midline of the trial implant (Fig. 55.8a). The trial implant serves as a guide for the chisel and sets the direction and the chisel depth (Fig. 55.8b). The chisel cut should be checked under image intensifier (Fig. 55.8c).

- Trial implant and chisels are left in place until the implant is fully assembled ex vivo to avoid bleeding following their removal from the cancellous bone.
- The trial implant is removed and replaced by the actual endplates of the implant, which are mounted to the insertion device. The bottom endplate is locked to the inserter by turning the inserter arms (Fig. 55.9). Previous chiseling of the keels serves as guidance for adequate implant insertion. Posterior implant positioning is confirmed

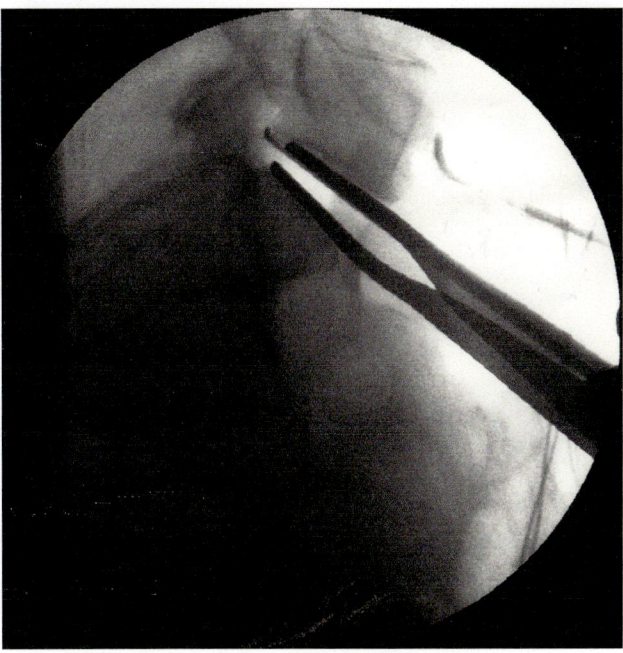

Fig. 55.7 Intraoperative removal of posterior osteophytes

Fig. 55.6 Insertion of the trial implant. A strict midline positioning of the implant should be confirmed under AP fluoroscopic control (**a**). Lateral X-ray images should confirm the largest possible prosthesis surface area as well as an adequate posterior positioning of the implant (**b**). An adjustable stopper, which is attached to the insertion device, prevents excessive posterior placement of the trial implant (© by Synthes)

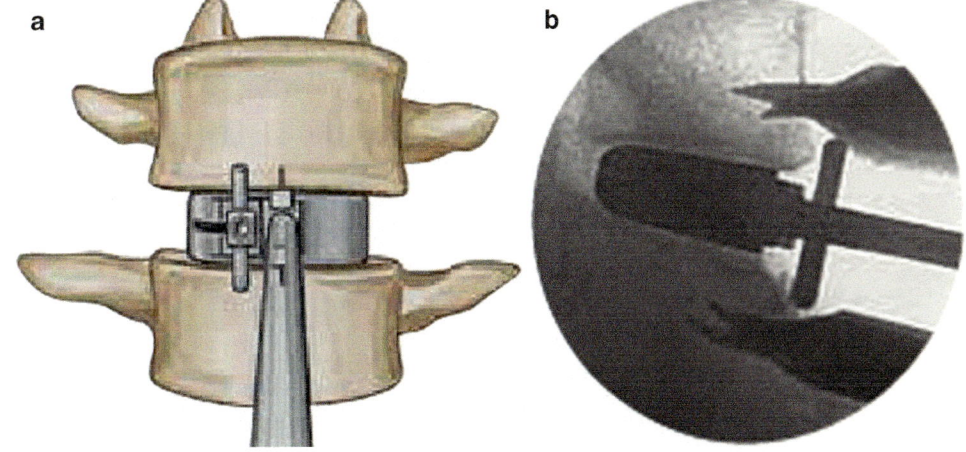

Fig. 55.8 Preparation of the keel bed. The chisel device is securely guided through openings along the midline of the trial implant (**a**). The trial implant serves as a guide for the chisel and sets the direction and the chisel depth (**b**). The chisel cut should be checked under image intensifier (**c**)

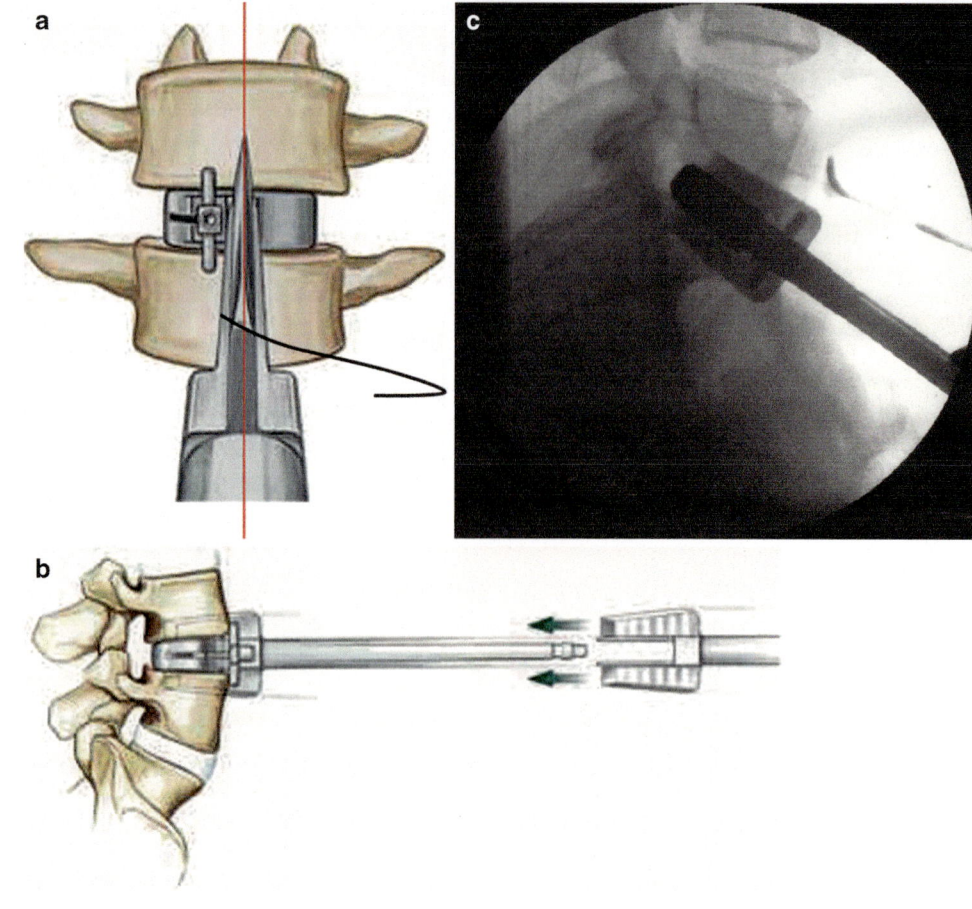

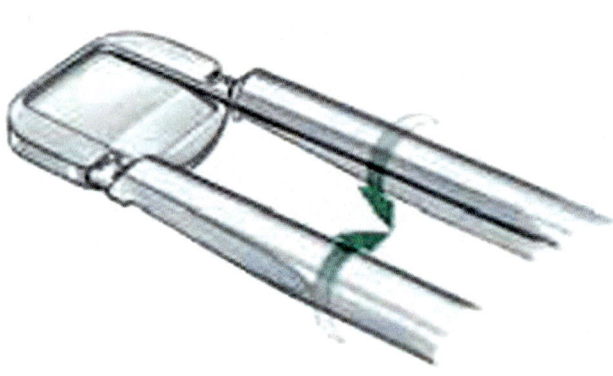

Fig. 55.9 Connection and locking between the bottom implant end-plate and the inserter arms

under lateral fluoroscopic control. Care should be taken that no surrounding soft tissues are impinged during the process of implant insertion. This step is furthermore preformed without segmental distraction.

- The insertion device now serves to guide the UHMWE-PE (ultrahigh-molecular-weight polyethylene) inlay into the caudal endplate. The PE inlay is inserted into the slots of the insertion device ("dome up"). An adequately sized and corresponding distracter is attached to the inserter. The wing nut is used to screw the distracter down to the mechanical stop. During this process, the PE inlay should be easily advanced. Excessive resistance may be a sign of inlay impingement, which should be strictly avoided.
- This process is finalized with a "pusher," until the inlay easily snaps into the caudal endplate. This is usually confirmed by a "click" sound. Macroscopic inspection must confirm that the anterior border of the inlay as well as the caudal endplate is in line with no visible steps or gaps between both components.
- Removal of all insertion instruments and final X-ray control to confirm adequate implant positioning (Fig. 55.10a, b).
- Careful removal of the retractor blades and final inspection of the operating site to confirm that no intraoperative complications, that is, from vascular structures or the ureter, have occurred.
- Insertion of a drain is generally not required.
- Closure of the linea alba, subcutaneous tissue adaptation, as well as skin closure.

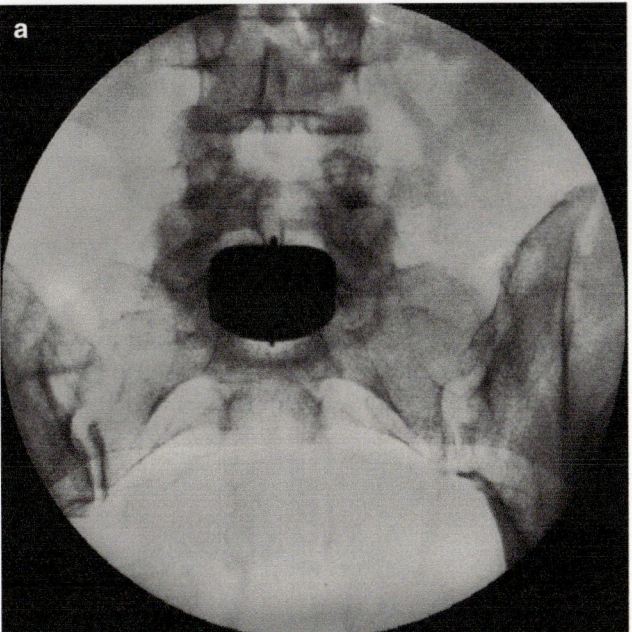

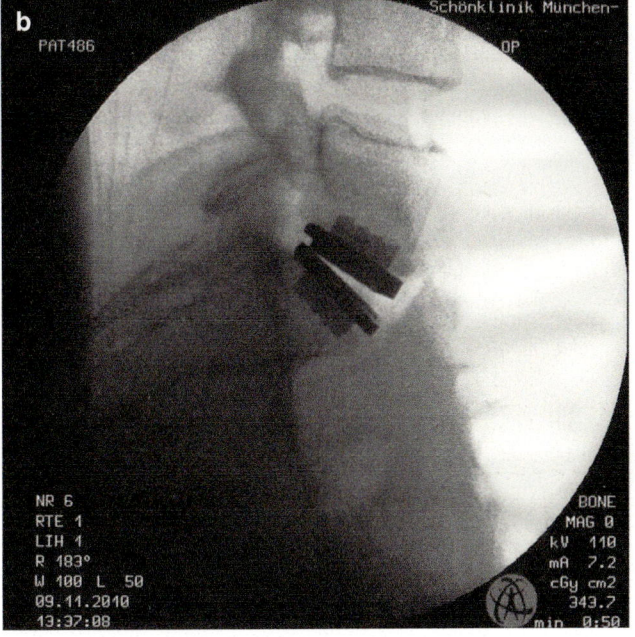

Fig. 55.10 Final AP (**a**) and lateral (**b**) fluoroscopic images demonstrate an adequate implant positioning in both planes

55.7 Postoperative Care

During the immediate postoperative period, supervision of wound healing, regular checkups of the abdomen, as well as the neurological status are paramount and regularly monitored. The patients are generally discharged within a few days following the operative intervention.

One of the advantages of TDR in comparison to fusion candidates is an early, brace-free mobilization of the patients,

as well as an early resumption of sporting and professional activities. The postoperative treatment and mobilization regime in patients with an uneventful intraoperative TDR procedure has been outlined previously [32]:

- Mobilization from the first postoperative day.
- External stabilization/brace not required.
- Early resumption of physical activities is encouraged on a moderate level in noncontact sports (e.g., swimming, cycling) within the first 6–12 weeks following a short rehabilitation period.
- Solid osteointegration of the implants allows for further load increase and participation in preoperative sporting activities from 3 to 6 months postoperatively.
- In an uneventful postoperative course, participation even in highly demanding physical contact sports/extreme sports has been shown to be accessible and may be resumed from 4 to 6 months postoperatively.

55.8 Complications and Pitfalls

55.8.1 Surgery-Related Complications

- Injury to ureter and vascular lesions (high risk in TDR revision surgery).
- Deep vein thrombosis and arterial pulmonary embolism.
- General surgery-related complications such as postoperative ileus, retroperitoneal hematoma, lymphocele, seroma, or urinoma [33].
- Infections.
- Retrograde ejaculations/sexual dysfunction [34].
- Postsympathectomy-related complaints.

55.8.2 Implant-Related Complications

- Implant subsidence/dislocations.
- PE extrusions.
- Postoperative pedicle or isthmus fractures.
- Spinal cord and/or nerve root injury.
- Persisting complaints from facet and iliosacral joints.

55.9 Tips and Tricks

- For all TDRs at the level L4/5 and above and for selected cases of TDRs at the lumbosacral junction, 3-dimensional CT color-coded reconstruction of the prevertebral vessels provides valuable information about the vascular topography (Fig. 55.11) [13, 35]. In selected cases, the vascular anatomy can pose a contraindication against TDR.
- Avoid hyperextension of the lumbar spine on the operating table.

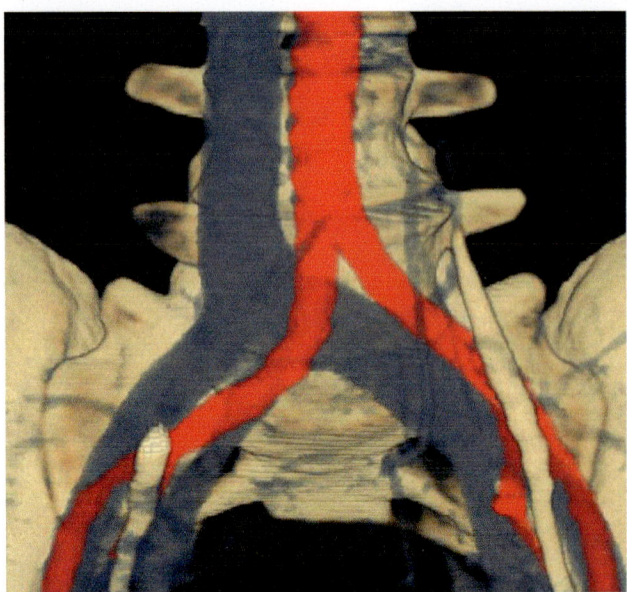

Fig. 55.11 Color-coded, 3D-CT angiography with a reconstruction of the prevertebral vessels

- Carefully prevent and avoid any kind of soft tissue impingement during the process chiseling, trial implant, or implant placement.
- When bleeding from the epidural venous plexus is encountered, it can be managed by the use of hemostatic agents such as Floseal® (Baxter).
- In cases of TDR above the lumbosacral junction, or all cases of TDR at the lumbosacral junction, which required significant mobilization of vascular structures, it is advisable to attach a Gore© membrane to the anterior circumference of the disk space, behind the prevertebral vessels. In cases of anterior TDR revision surgery later than 2 weeks after the primary intervention, which has been associated with a high rate of intraoperative vascular lesions [36], the membrane may facilitate better mobilization of the vascular structures due to avoidance of scar tissue formation between the vascular structures and the anterior circumference of the vertebral body.
- A variety of oblique disk replacement implants have recently been developed. The availability of these oblique implants reduces the risk of vessel mobilization in comparison to TDRs that require a straightforward, midline implantation. These oblique disk replacement implants can therefore be recommended for TDRs performed at the level above the lumbosacral junction in selected cases.

References

1. Gillet P. The fate of the adjacent motion segments after lumbar fusion. J Spinal Disord Tech. 2003;16:338–45.
2. Goulet JA, Senunas LE, DeSilva GL, et al. Autogenous iliac crest bone graft. Complications and functional assessment. Clin Orthop Relat Res. 1997;339:76–81.
3. Kumar MN, Jacquot F, Hall H. Long-term follow-up of functional outcomes and radiographic changes at adjacent levels following lumbar spine fusion for degenerative disc disease. Eur Spine J. 2001;10:309–13.
4. Lee CK. Accelerated degeneration of the segment adjacent to a lumbar fusion. Spine. 1988;13:375–7.
5. Park P, Garton HJ, Gala VC, Hoff JT, et al. Adjacent segment disease after lumbar or lumbosacral fusion: review of the literature. Spine. 2004;29:1938–44.
6. Umehara S, Zindrick MR, Patwardhan AG, et al. The biomechanical effect of postoperative hypolordosis in instrumented lumbar fusion on instrumented and adjacent spinal segments. Spine. 2000;25:1617–24.
7. Katz V, Schofferman J, Reynolds J. The sacroiliac joint: a potential cause of pain after lumbar fusion to the sacrum. J Spinal Disord Tech. 2003;16:96–9.
8. Maigne JY, Planchon CA. Sacroiliac joint pain after lumbar fusion. A study with anesthetic blocks. Eur Spine J. 2005;14:654–8.
9. Ha KY, Lee JS, Kim KW. Degeneration of sacroiliac joint after instrumented lumbar or lumbosacral fusion: a prospective cohort study over five-year follow-up. Spine. 2008;33:1192–8.
10. Moshirfar A, Jenis LG, Spector LR, et al. Computed tomography evaluation of superior-segment facet-joint violation after pedicle instrumentation of the lumbar spine with a midline surgical approach. Spine. 2006;31:2624–9.
11. Shah RR, Mohammed S, Saifuddin A, et al. Radiologic evaluation of adjacent superior segment facet joint violation following transpedicular instrumentation of the lumbar spine. Spine. 2003;28:272–5.
12. Cardoso MJ, Dmitriev AE, Helgeson M, et al. Does superior-segment facet violation or laminectomy destabilize the adjacent level in lumbar transpedicular fixation? An in vitro human cadaveric assessment. Spine. 2008;33:2868–73.
13. Siepe CJ, Mayer HM, Wiechert K, et al. Clinical results of total lumbar disc replacement with ProDisc II: three-year results for different indications. Spine. 2006;31:1923–32.
14. Siepe CJ, Mayer HM, Heinz-Leisenheimer M, et al. Total lumbar disc replacement: different results for different levels. Spine. 2007;32:782–90.
15. McAfee PC, Cunningham BW, Hayes V, et al. Biomechanical analysis of rotational motions after disc arthroplasty: implications for patients with adult deformities. Spine. 2006;31:152–60.
16. Sariali EH, Lemaire JP, Pascal-Mousselard H, et al. In vivo study of the kinematics in axial rotation of the lumbar spine after total intervertebral disc replacement: long-term results: a 10–14 years follow up evaluation. Eur Spine J. 2006;15:1501–10.
17. Ching AC, Birkenmaier C, Hart RA. Short segment coronal plane deformity after two-level lumbar total disc replacement. Spine (Phila Pa 1976). 2010;35:44–50.
18. Huang RC, Lim MR, Girardi FP, et al. The prevalence of contraindications to total disc replacement in a cohort of lumbar surgical patients. Spine. 2004;29:2538–41.
19. McAfee PC. The indications for lumbar and cervical disc replacement. Spine J. 2004;4:177S–81S.
20. Wong DA, Annesser B, Birney T, et al. Incidence of contraindications to total disc arthroplasty: a retrospective review of 100 consecutive fusion patients with a specific analysis of facet arthrosis. Spine J. 2007;7:5–11.
21. Chin KR. Epidemiology of indications and contraindications to total disc replacement in an academic practice. Spine J. 2007;7:392–8.
22. Blumenthal S, McAfee PC, Guyer RD, et al. A prospective, randomized, multicenter Food and Drug Administration investigational device exemptions study of lumbar total disc replacement with the CHARITE artificial disc versus lumbar fusion: part I:

evaluation of clinical outcomes. Spine. 2005;30(1565–1575):discussion E1387–E1591.

23. Zigler J, Delamarter R, Spivak JM, et al. Results of the prospective, randomized, multicenter Food and Drug Administration investigational device exemption study of the ProDisc-L total disc replacement versus circumferential fusion for the treatment of 1-level degenerative disc disease. Spine. 2007;32:–1155, 1162; discussion 1163

24. Mayer HM, Wiechert K. Microsurgical anterior approaches to the lumbar spine for interbody fusion and total disc replacement. Neurosurgery. 2002;51:S159–65.

25. Mayer HM, Wiechert K, Korge A, et al. Minimally invasive total disc replacement: surgical technique and preliminary clinical results. Eur Spine J. 2002;11(Suppl 2):S124–30.

26. Jasani V, Jaffray D. The anatomy of the iliolumbar vein. A cadaver study. J Bone Joint Surg Br. 2002;84:1046–9.

27. Cakir B, Richter M, Kafer W, et al. The impact of total lumbar disc replacement on segmental and total lumbar lordosis. Clin Biomech (Bristol, Avon). 2005;20:357–64.

28. Liu J, Ebraheim NA, Haman SP, et al. Effect of the increase in the height of lumbar disc space on facet joint articulation area in sagittal plane. Spine. 2006;31:E198–202.

29. Rohlmann A, Zander T, Bergmann G. Effect of total disc replacement with ProDisc on intersegmental rotation of the lumbar spine. Spine. 2005;30:738–43.

30. Siepe CJ, Hitzl W, Meschede P, et al. Interdependence between disc space height, range of motion and clinical outcome in total lumbar disc replacement. Spine. 2009;34:904–16.

31. Adams MA, Roughley PJ. What is intervertebral disc degeneration, and what causes it? Spine. 2006;31:2151–61.

32. Siepe CJ, Wiechert K, Khattab MF, et al. Total lumbar disc replacement in athletes: clinical results, return to sport and athletic performance. Eur Spine J. 2007;16:1001–13.

33. Patel AA, Spiker WR, Daubs MD, et al. Retroperitoneal lymphocele after anterior spinal surgery. Spine (Phila Pa 1976). 2008;33:E648–52.

34. Flynn JC, Price CT. Sexual complications of anterior fusion of the lumbar spine. Spine. 1984;9:489–92.

35. Datta JC, Janssen ME, Beckham R, et al. The use of computed tomography angiography to define the prevertebral vascular anatomy prior to anterior lumbar procedures. Spine. 2007;32:113–9.

36. Brau SA, Delamarter RB, Kropf MA, et al. Access strategies for revision in anterior lumbar surgery. Spine. 2008;33:1662–7.

Extreme Lateral Interbody Fusion (XLIF)

56

Valentin Quack, Uwe Vieweg, and Philipp Kobbe

56.1 Introduction and Core Messages

In 2006, Ozgur et al. first presented the extreme lateral interbody fusion (XLIF) [1]. XLIF is a minimally invasive spinal fusion procedure that achieves interbody fusion using a retroperitoneal approach through the psoas major muscle. Lateral interbody fusions were designed to restore and maintain disk height, restoration of lordosis, and widening of the neuroforamen by indirect decompression [2–4]. During the XLIF procedure, indirect decompression of the neural elements and improved intervertebral stability can be achieved through ligamentotaxis, in which a large cage spanning the width of the vertebral body is placed to restore the disk space height [5, 6], avoiding the large anterior vessels and the bowel [4, 7]. Furthermore, XLIF does not require direct intervention to the nerve tissue or the epidural venous plexus, thereby reducing intraoperative blood loss. Additionally, it minimizes soft tissue injury, enables less postoperative pain, abbreviates length of hospital stay, and allows fast return to daily activities [8–10]. In general, the technique can be applied between T5 and L5 [4, 11]. For lumbar segments, neuromonitoring is mandatory to protect the iliolumbar plexus during the psoas passage [4, 12]. High fusion rates of more than 90% are reported in the literature [13, 14]. To support the cage and improve the fusion rate, either a minimally invasive dorsal instrumentation or a lateral screw-plate system can be implanted. In general, the stand-alone variant is practiced for degenerative cases. Regarding the indication and the surgical options for segmental restoration, the XLIF technique is comparable to anterior or anterolateral and open lateral interbody fusion.

V. Quack (✉) · P. Kobbe
Department of Trauma and Reconstructive Surgery, University Clinic RWTH Aachen, Aachen, Germany
e-mail: vquack@ukaachen.de

U. Vieweg
Department of Conservative and Surgical Spine Therapy with Interdisciplinary Spinal Deformities Centre and Rummelsberg Sectional Center, Hospital Rummelsberg, Schwarzenbruck, Germany

56.2 Indications [4, 5, 8, 13, 15]

Indications are as follows:

- Degenerative disk disease (DDD)
- Degenerative spondylolisthesis
- Degenerative scoliosis
- Nonunions
- Incomplete burst fractures (AOSpine A3)
- discitis or vertebral osteomyelitis (without active infection)
- Postlaminectomy instability

56.3 Contraindications

Any generally accepted contraindication to fusion are the following:

- Systemic infection
- Osteoporosis
- Significant comorbidities
- The level L5-S1
- Lumbar deformities with > 30° rotation
- Degenerative spondylolisthesis grade 3 or higher
- Need for direct posterior decompression through same approach (Second posterior microdecompression not contraindicated)

56.4 Technical Prerequisites

The following instruments are required:

- Radiolucent bendable surgical table C-arm
- Access system with light source
- XLIF instruments (long instruments, e.g., rongeurs and punches)

© Springer-Verlag GmbH Germany 2023
U. Vieweg, F. Grochulla (eds.), *Manual of Spine Surgery*, https://doi.org/10.1007/978-3-662-64062-3_56

56.5 Patient Positioning

The patient is positioned on a radiolucent bendable surgical table in a direct lateral right-sided decubitus position (90°), perpendicular to the table, with the trochanter directly positioned over the table break and with legs and knees slightly bent. This configuration increases the space between iliac crest and ribs, especially relevant when accessing thoracolumbar junction or L4-L5 level. The ideal positioning is confirmed by **fluoroscopy**, ensuring that when at 0°, the C-arm provides a true anteroposterior (AP) image, and when at 90°, a true lateral image. It is substantial that the lateral fluoroscopic images show both **vertebral** plateaus and superior pedicles aligned, presented as a single line, and that the AP image reveals the spinous processes in a middle position, and pedicles as circumferences.

It is substantial that the lateral fluoroscopic images show both **vertebral** plateaus and superior pedicles aligned, presented as a single line, and that the AP image reveals the spinous processes in a middle position, and pedicles as circumferences.

56.6 Planning of the Skin Incision

A fluoroscopic height localization with topographic projection of the corresponding intervertebral disk on the skin is carried out in the strict lateral position with the aid of, for example, a K-wire. The intervertebral disk and the adjacent vertebral bodies are marked onto the skin and the incision is planned according to the number of levels to be treated. We prefer the one-incision-technique.

56.7 Approach

Several studies have investigated the location of the neural structures in the psoas muscle. For this purpose, Guérin et al. divided the disk space into 4 zones (1 anterior to 4 posterior). Based on their cadaveric studies, they recommend positioning of the retractor at the level of L1/2 in zones 2 and 3, L2-L4 zone 3, and L4/5 in zone 2 [16]. A comparable classification was published by Uribe et al. [17]. However, Banagan and colleagues concluded that based on their study, there is no absolute safe zone and they would recommend either direct visualization of the nerve and/or the use of neuromonitoring [12]. In the segment L4/5, there is the greatest risk of a neurological damage [18].

56.8 Technique

56.8.1 Lateral Retroperitoneal Access

After skin asepsis, a longitudinal skin incision, approximately 3–5 cm, is made over the marked disk space. Following dissection of the subcutaneous fat layer, the fascia of the oblique externus muscle is opened. The oblique externus, the oblique internus, and the transverse abdominis muscle are now bluntly dissected with the fingertip to develop the fascia under the transverse abdominis muscle. Once this fascia is opened, the retroperitoneal space can be entered with the finger and blunt dissection, with dorsal to anterior movement of the fingertip, is performed until the psoas muscle is reached. The index finger will now safely guide all dilators up to the psoas muscle, protecting abdominal structures (Fig. 56.1).

56.8.2 Psoas Traverse

The first dilator is placed upon the junction of the posterior third and the anterior two-thirds of the disk, as confirmed by AP and lateral fluoroscopy. Then, the fibers are gently separated by the initial blunt dilator with concomitant EMG monitoring for assessing the closeness to the lumbar plexus and allowing determining the proximity of neural structures

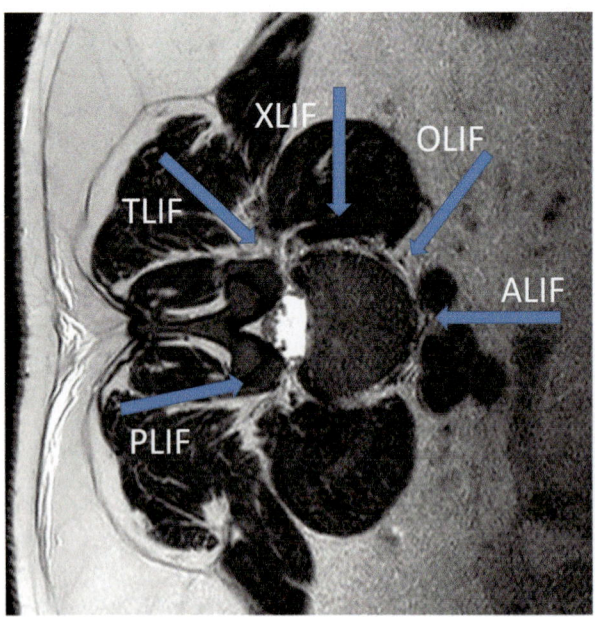

Fig. 56.1 Possible approaches to the lumbar spine. *TLIF* transforaminal lumbar interbody fusion, *PLIF* posterior lumbar interbody fusion, *OLIF* oblique lateral interbody fusion, *ALIF* anterior lumbar interbody fusion

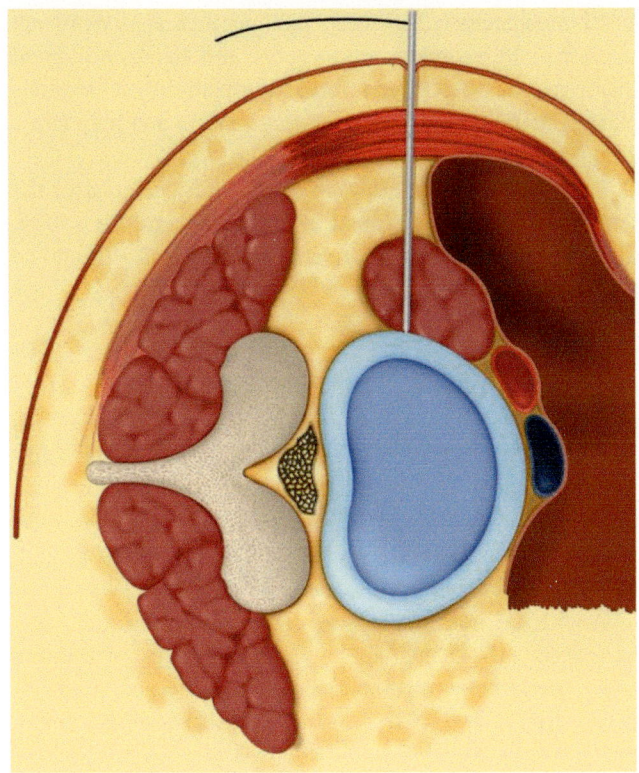

Fig. 56.2 Initial Dilatator is placed on the disk using EMG monitoring. Fluoroscopy is used to confirm the adequate location

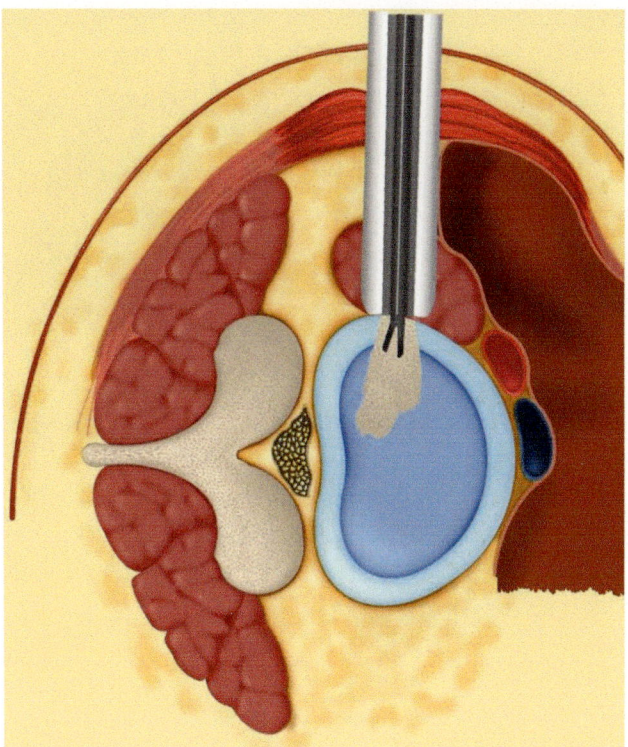

Fig. 56.3 The dilators in sequence are placed over the previous, always checking the EMG, until the final placement of the retractor. The disk is then partially removed. The annulus on the opposite side should be opened

that are adjacent to the surgical field by using a probe (Fig. 56.2). The dilator must be rotated in position to determine proximity and spatial distribution of nerves. The dilators in sequence are placed over the previous, always checking the EMG, until placement of the last retractor. After confirming the ideal position by fluoroscopy, the blades of the retractor are inserted. Depending on the retractor system used, the blades may be further stabilized after opening by the insertion of pins and visualization of the area of interest is improved by a light source clipped on the retractor blade. Retractor opening must be minimized in order to prevent lack of blood flow to the nerves of the plexus and prevent plexopathies due to compression. Now bipolar can be used to achieve disk visualization. The disk is now incised with a knife, and an annulotomy is performed (Fig. 56.3). Using the disk preparation instruments, both endplates are prepared and the annulus on the opposite side is also released. This is critical to achieve the best possible distraction of the disk space, proper coronary alignment, placement of a large implant, and herewith also the best pos-

sible indirect decompression. After adequate preparation of the disk space, the cage can be inserted (Fig. 56.4). Some hyperlordotic cages are available on the market, which can achieve additional optimization of the sagittal alignment. Particular care should be taken to ensure that the cage is inserted well anteriorly. The position of the cage is now checked fluoroscopically in true lateral and AP images. If the position of the cage is satisfactory, there is now the option of additional stabilization by inserting a lateral plate or the percutaneous insertion of a transpedicular screw-rod system in the lateral or a prone position. Prone positioning certainly has the disadvantage that time is lost due to repositioning and renewed skin asepsis. If a lateral plate is used, this certainly has the advantage that no additional skin incision has to be made and no repositioning has to be performed. The plate size is selected depending on the disk space height and centered over the disk space with an insertion instrument. Depending on the plate, it is then fixed with screws, if necessary, after preparing the screw holes with an awl or a tap. Plate and screw placement is carried out under fluoroscopic control.

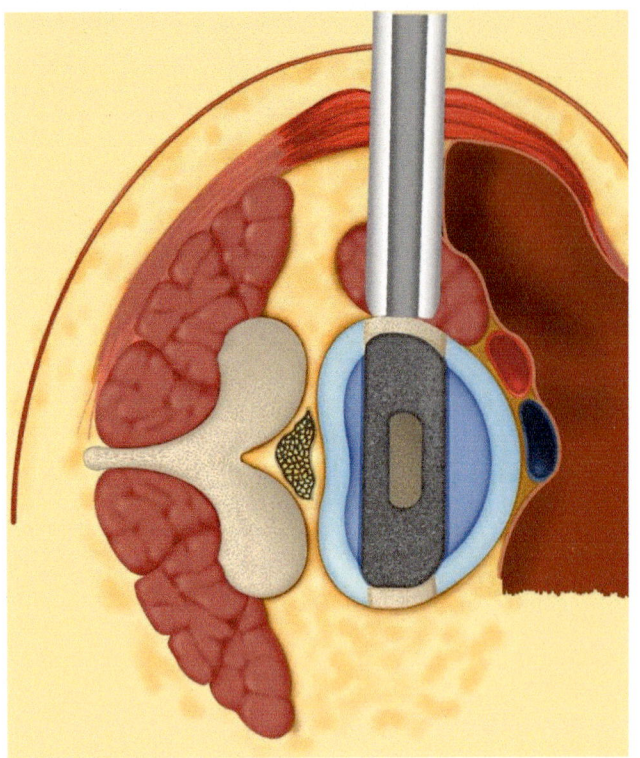

Fig. 56.4 After adequate preparation of the disk space, the cage can now be inserted. The adequate position of the cage is confirmed fluoroscopically

Biomechanically, however, the lateral plate systems are inferior to the pedicle screw systems, although overall good fusion rates are described [13, 14]. Furthermore, voluminous plate systems may irritate the psoas muscle and may cause chronic pain.

Hereafter occurs the lavage of the situs, removal of the retractor system, and wound closure in layers (Fig. 56.5). After mobilization of the patient, a standing X-ray should be taken as a control before discharge (Fig. 56.6).

56.8.3 Complications

XLIF includes a disproportionate increase in the neurological complications of spinal surgery versus other constructs, that is, plexus injuries 13.28%, sensory deficits 0–75% (permanent in 62.5%), motor deficits 0.7–33.6%, anterior thigh pain 12.5–25%, and sympathectomy 4–8%.

Additional nonneurological complications include cage subsidence (10–13.8%), major vascular injuries up to 0.4%, bowel perforation, malpositioning of the cage, nonunion (7.5%), and failure to decompress stenosis [19–22].

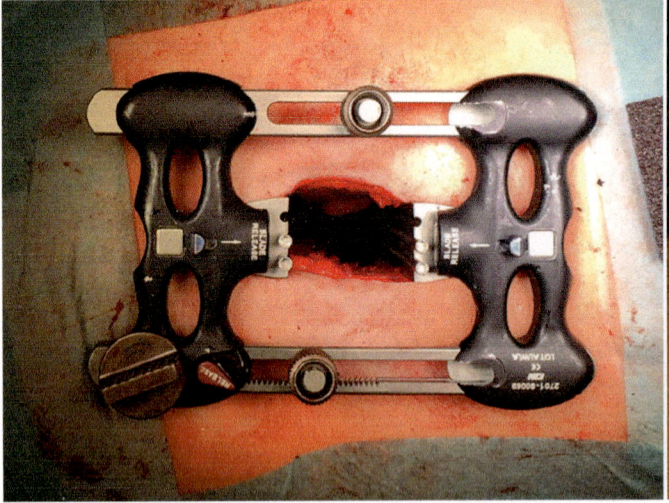 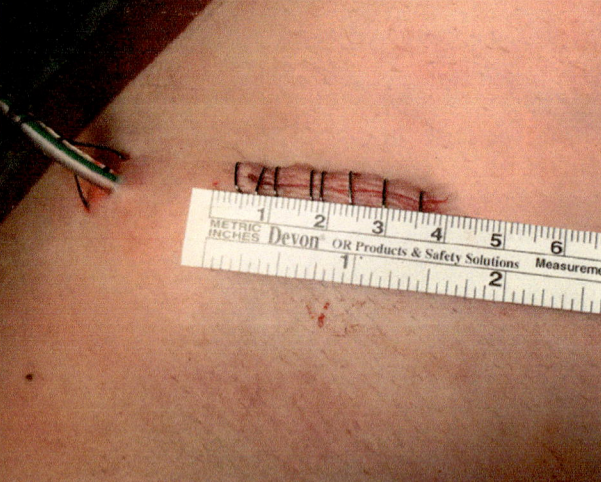

Fig. 56.5 Left: Intraoperative position of the retractor. Right: Wound closure with staple suture. The use of a drain is not always necessary

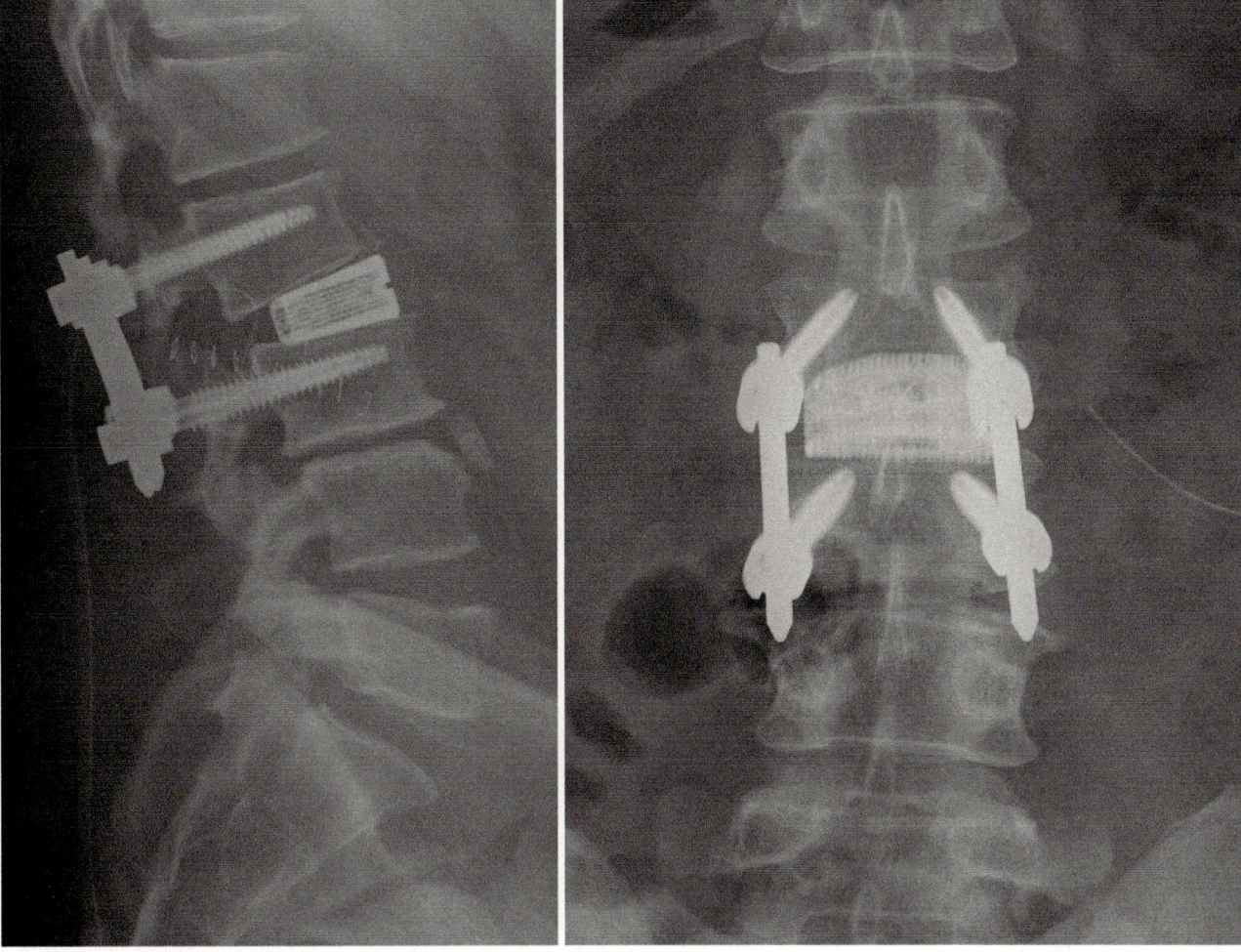

Fig. 56.6 Postoperative radiographs after XLIF L2/3 and minimally invasive dorsal instrumentation

References

1. Ozgur BM, Aryan HE, Pimenta L, Taylor WR. Extreme Lateral Interbody Fusion (XLIF): a novel surgical technique for anterior lumbar interbody fusion. Spine J. 2006;6:435–43.
2. Acosta FL, Liu J, Slimack N, et al. Changes in coronal and sagittal plane alignment following minimally invasive direct lateral interbody fusion for the treatment of degenerative lumbar disease in adults: a radiographic study. J Neurosurg Spine. 2011;15:92–6.
3. Alimi M, Hofstetter CP, Tsiouris AJ, et al. Extreme lateral interbody fusion for unilateral symptomatic vertical foraminal stenosis. Eur Spine J. 2014;24(Suppl 3):346–52.
4. Quante M, Halm H. Extreme lateral interbody fusion: indication, surgical technique, outcomes and specific complications. Orthopade. 2015;44:138–45.
5. Caputo AM, Michael KW, Chapman TM, et al. Extreme lateral interbody fusion for the treatment of adult degenerative scoliosis. J Clin Neurosci. 2013;20:1558–63.
6. Oliveira L, Marchi L, Coutinho E, Pimenta L. A radiographic assessment of the ability of the extreme lateral interbody fusion procedure to indirectly decompress the neural elements. Spine. 2010;35(26 Suppl):S331–7.
7. Berjano P, Gautschi OP, Schils F, Tessitore E. Extreme lateral interbody fusion (XLF): how I do it. Aca Neurochir. 2015a;157:547–51.
8. Patel VC, Park DK, Herkowitz HN. Lateral transpsoas fusion: indications and outcomes. Sci World J. 2012;2012:893608.
9. Scherman DB, Rao PJ, Phan K, Mungovan SF, et al. Outcomes of direct lateral interbody fusion (DLIF) in an Australian cohort. J Spine Surg. 2019;5(1):1–12.
10. Young-Hoon K, Kee-Yong H, Kee-Won R, et al. Lumbar interbody fusion: techniques, pearls and pitfalls. Asian Spine J. 2020;14(5):730–41.
11. Meredith DS, Kepler CK, Huang RC, Hegde VV. Extreme lateral interbody fusion (XLIF) in the thoracic and thoracolumbar spine: technical report and early outcomes. HSS J. 2013;9:25–31.
12. Banagan K, Gelb D, Poelstra K, et al. Anatomic mapping of lumbar nerve roots during a direct lateral transpsoas approach to the spine: a cadaveric study. Spine (Phila Pa 1976). 2011;36(11):E687–91.
13. Berjano P, Langella F, Damilano M, et al. Fusion rate following extreme lateral lumbar interbody fusion. Eur Spine J. 2015b;24(Suppl 3):369–71.
14. Li H, Zhang R, Shen C. Differences in radiographic and clinical outcomes of oblique lateral interbody fusion and lateral lumbar interbody fusion for degenerative lumbar disease: a meta-analysis. BMC Musculoskelet Disord. 2019;20(1):582.

15. Regan C, Kang JD. The role of the minimally invasive extreme lateral interbody fusion procedure for complex spinal reconstruction. Oper Tech Orthop. 2013;23:28–32.

16. Guérin P, Obeid I, Bourghli A, et al. (2011) The lumbosacral plexus: anatomic considerations for minimally invasive retroperitoneal transpsoas approach. Surg Radiol Anat. 2012 Mar;34(2):151–7.

17. Uribe JS, Arredondo N, Dakwar E. Defining the safe working zones using the minimally invasive lateral retroperitoneal transpsoas approach: an anatomical study. J Neurosurg Spine. 2010;13(2):260–6.

18. Kepler CK, Sharma AK, Huang RC, et al. Indirect foraminal decompression after lateral transpsoas interbody fusion. J Neurosurg Spine. 2012;16:329–33.

19. Epstein NE. Extreme lateral lumbar interbody fusion: do the cons outweigh the pros? Surg Neurol Int. 2016a;7(Suppl 25):S692–700.

20. Epstein NE. More nerve root injuries occur with minimally invasive lumbar surgery, especially extreme lateral interbody fusion: a review. Surg Neurol Int. 2016b;7(Suppl 3):S83–95.

21. Epstein NE. More nerve root injuries occur with minimally invasive lumbar surgery: let's tell someone. Surg Neurol Int. 2016c;7(Suppl 3):S96–S101.

22. Epstein NE. Incidence of major vascular injuries with extreme lateral interbody fusion (XLIF). Surg Neurol Int. 2020;11:70.

Part VIII

Posterior Lumbar Spine

Overview of Surgical Techniques and Implants

Uwe Vieweg

57.1 Introduction and Core Messages

Posterior lumbar spine surgery uses various access routes (midline, lateral, far-lateral paracoccygeal) and can employ classic open, miniopen (microscopic or video assisted), or percutaneous access techniques. Decompression operations can be performed by using these access methods, and there are various possibilities of instrumentation as can various forms of instrumentation. The implants are divided into the following groups: rigid systems (internal fixator systems such as rod-screw or screw-plate systems, screws, pedicle screw-hook systems, cages, and spacers for interbody fusion); different dynamic or semirigid systems; and so-called nonfusion systems (pedicle-based systems, interspinous spacers, facet replacements). The following are types of posterior stabilization systems available: tulip screw–type systems, side-loading systems, and plate systems. For the interbody fusion, there are cages in titanium as well as in PEEK on the market. Also, there are implants for the motion preservation available. The spectrum of those implants rises from dynamic pedicle screw systems, interspinous spacers, and facet replacement implants.

U. Vieweg (✉)
Department of Conservative and Surgical Spine Therapy with Interdisciplinary Spinal Deformities Centre and Rummelsberg Sectional Center, Hospital Rummelsberg, Schwarzenbruck, Germany
e-mail: uwe.vieweg@sana.de

57.2 Approaches (see Fig. 57.1)

- *Midline posterior approach*

  A midline approach to the lumbar region is most frequently used for posterior lumbar spine surgery. The exposure of the deeper layer of muscles, however, is imprecise and can entail substantial tissue damage and blood loss. Besides providing access to the cauda equina and the intervertebral disks, the midline approach can expose the posterior elements of the spine: the spinous processes, laminae, facet joints, and pedicles. The midline approach can be extended proximally and distally. The skin incision is made straight along the midline, even in scoliosis cases. For fusion cases, the incision should be one to two segments longer than the section to be fused. The preparation has to be performed strictly subperiosteally to preserve the blood vessels and nerves, which supply the muscles, and to prevent bleeding. In this approach technique, the lumbar spine is prepared from cranial to caudal.

- *Mediolateral posterior approaches*

  The paramedian approach, as well as the intermuscular Wiltse approach, allows a good exposure of the nerve roots at the lumbar levels [1]. The Wiltse technique is a paramedian approach to the lumbosacral junction. Unlike a midline incision, where the exposure is created by cutting through the muscle planes, a Wiltse approach utilizes a blunt dissection of the muscles, this means between the fascial planes of the multifidus and longissimus muscles to create the exposure. In the 1960s, Wiltse et al. described the sacrospinalis-splitting approach to the lumbar spine [2]. This procedure was accomplished by making a paraspinous incision through the deep fascia and developing

U. Vieweg, F. Grochulla (eds.), *Manual of Spine Surgery*, https://doi.org/10.1007/978-3-662-64062-3_57

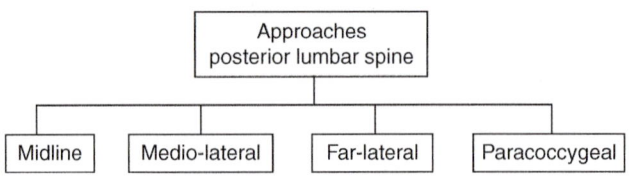

Fig. 57.1 Approaches for the posterior lumbar spine

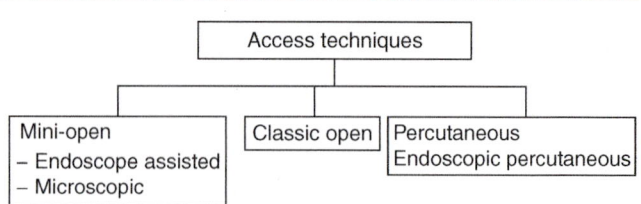

Fig. 57.2 Access techniques

the plane between the multifidus and longissimus muscles. A paramedian skin incision is made to perform the transmuscular approach.

The intramuscular Wiltse approach allows the surgeon to approach the spine in a less invasive way in comparison to a midline incision. It is known as a miniopen approach, invasive because it preserves the posterior musculature of the spine and it is performed unilaterally. In 1953, Watkins described a far-lateral approach, a route between the erector spinae (iliocostalis) and the quadratus lumborum, which requires some resection of the ilium for proper muscle reflection. Another option is the lateral intramuscular planar approach to the lumbar spine described by Newman [3].

- *Transforaminal approach*

    The transforaminal approach to the L5–S1 interspace provides a minimally invasive corridor through which discectomy and interbody fusion can safely be performed. It may provide an alternative route of access to the L5–S1 interspace in those patients who have unfavorable anatomy for, or contraindication to, the traditional open anterior approach to this level [4].

57.3 Access Techniques (see Fig. 57.2)

The access techniques used can be subdivided into classic open, miniopen, and percutaneous techniques. The access routes can be made considerably smaller if special retractors are used [5]. These include MLD-retractor, Caspar retractor (Aesculap); METRx or Quadrant (Medtronic); and ProView Minimal Access Portal System (Blackstone Medical) MaXcess (Nuvasive). These techniques are subsumed under the heading of miniopen access. To optimize visualization, especially in minimally invasive and less invasive spine surgery, either an operating microscope or an optic is used. The techniques are referred to with reference to the visualization method employed (microscopic or

video assisted) [5, 6]. Combinations of percutaneous, microscopic, endoscopic, and miniopen access techniques can be used (see Fig. 57.2) [6].

57.4 Implants (see Fig. 57.3)

57.4.1 Rigid Systems

- Screws and pins

    For the posterior approach, there are several translaminar screws or translaminar pins (ECF Peek from Signas) available. This translaminar pin is a further development of the translaminar facet screw fixation (TLPF). The implantation is performed by using a percutaneous paracoccygeal approach. A reduction and stabilization of minor spondylolisthesis can be achieved by direct screwing as described by Buck [7].

    With a special-designed interbody fusion device (AxiaLIF), a transsacral approach can be achieved, for example, with the transsacral screw of TranS1.

    Examples: Multiple fragment screw–translaminar screw, transsacral screw (TranS1 Inc.) and ECF PEEK translaminar pin (Signus). Using a percutaneous paracoccygeal approach, axial fluoroscopically guided interbody fusion (AxiaLIF) is possible with a special transsacral screw (TranS1 Inc.) [4]. Translaminar pin fixation (TLPF) is a further development of translaminar facet screw fixation (TFSR). Compression and stabilization of minor spondylolisthesis can be achieved by direct screwing, as described by Buck [7].

- Hook-screw systems

    Example: Hook-screw construct described by Morscher [8].

    This surgical procedure is to reconstruct and stabilize the fractured pars interarticularis in minimal spondylolytic spondylolisthesis. It allows compression of the defect without crossing the defect with the screw. Direct repair is indi-

Fig. 57.3 Implants for the posterior lumbar spine

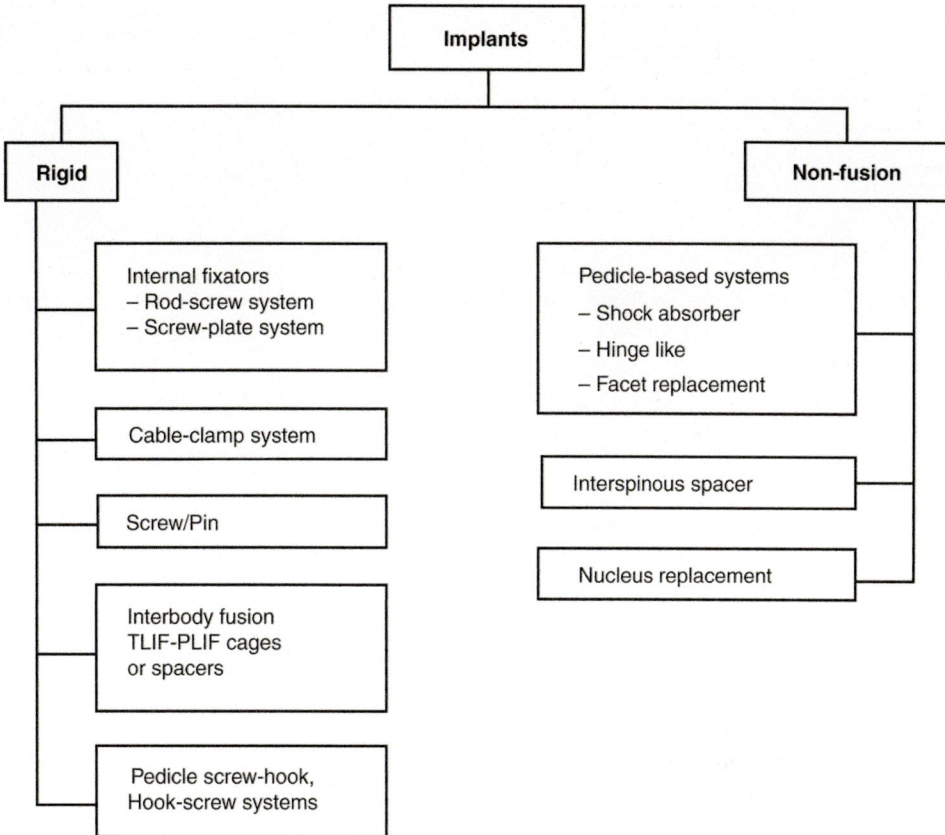

cated only in the absence of disk degeneration. After the age of 25 years, this procedure should not be carried out.

• Internal fixator (screw-rod or screw-plate systems)

Dorsal stabilization procedures employ transpedicularly positioned implants with stable angle fixation. From the internal fixator as described by Dick, further development led to the fixator described by Kluger and the Universal Spine System USS (Synthes) and MOSS System (DePuy). The rigid internal fixator systems can be grouped into different types according to their design details, for example, top-loading and side-loading systems, polyaxial screw, monoaxial screw, reduction screws, augmentation screws, and cannulated screws [9, 34].

57.4.1.1 Internal Fixator Systems for Open Implantation (Current and Older Systems)

Examples: TSRH (Texas Scottish Rite Hospital) 3D Spinal Instrumentation (Medtronic), CD HORIZON LEGACY (Medtronic), MOSS-MIAMI Family (DePuy), SFS Spinal Fixation System (Blackstone Medical), Monarch Spine system (Zimmer Spine), ST 360° Spinal Fixation System (Zimmer Spine), Synergy Spinal System (Interpore Cross International), USS-Universal Spinal System (Synthes), Click'X (Synthes) (see Fig. 57.4), SOCON (Aesculap), Silhouette Spinal Fixation System (Zimmer Spine), Sequoia (Zimmer Spine), Instinct Java (Zimmer Spine), Xia (Stryker), ConKlusion (Signus), SSE Spine System Evolution (Aesculap), and S^4 Spinal System (Aesculap) (see Fig. 57.5).

57.4.1.2 Systems for Less Invasive Percutaneous Implantation

Silverbolt (VertiFlex), CD Horizon Longitude System (Medtronic), CD Horizon Sextant System I/II (Medtronic), Pathfinder (Zimmer Spine), MANTIS (Stryker), SpheRx (Nuvasive), SpiRIT (Synthes), ProView, ICON (Blackstone Medical), and Expedium Viper (DePuy Spine).

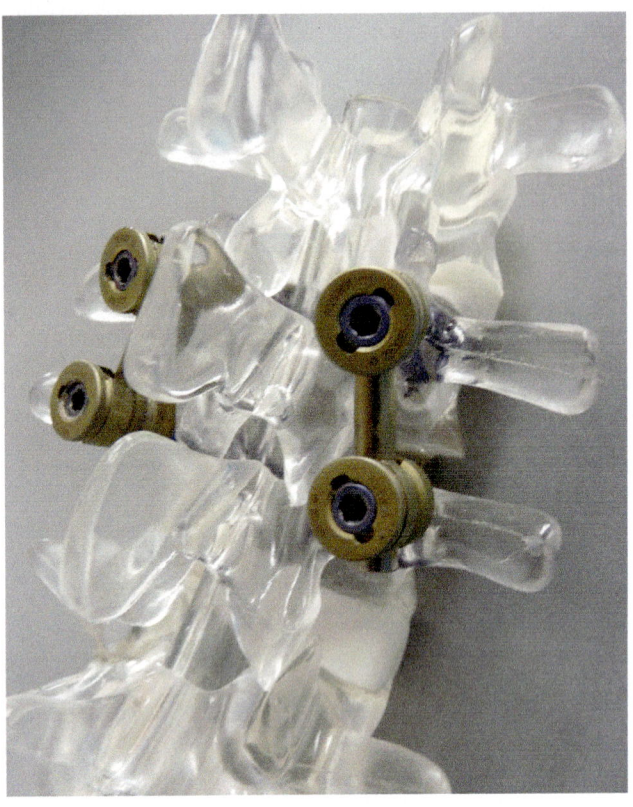

Fig. 57.4 Click'X, internal fixator system (Synthes)

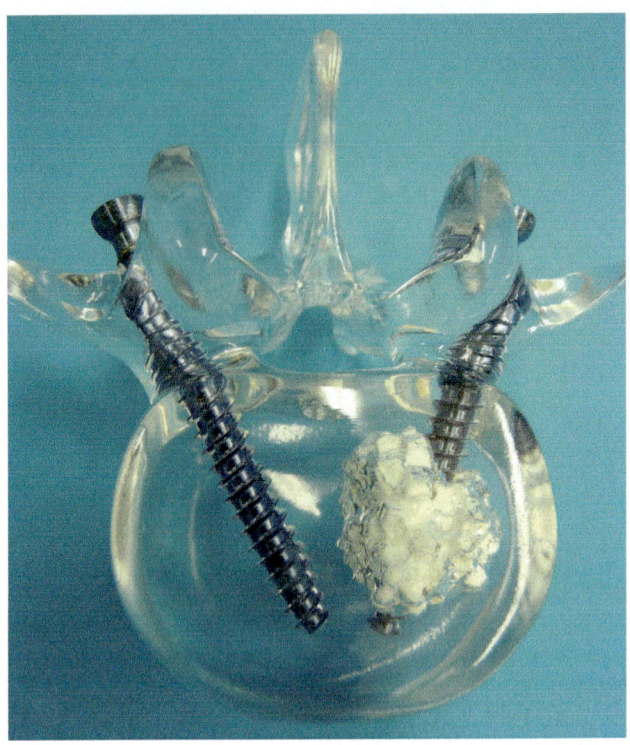

Fig. 57.6 Cannulated pedicle screw click'X for augmentation (Synthes)

57.4.1.3 Pedicle Screw Systems for Augmentation

SOCON (Aesculap), S^4 Spinal System (Aesculap), and Click'X (Synthes) (see Figs. 57.4 and 57.6)

- Cable-clamp systems
  Example: Universal Clamp System (Zimmer Spine)
- The universal clamp is a polyester band passed under the lamina and connected to a rod by a titanium clamp. This is an alternative for replacing screws and hooks for thoracolumbar spinal diseases.
- Screw-plate systems
  Monarch plate or rod system (DePuy Spine)
  It is about a combination of pedicle bolt and in-line polyaxial screw technology. Modular polyaxial washers can be added to provide an angulation at any position.
  Example: Monarch plate or rod system (DePuy Spine)
- Rod-cable systems
  Luque rod and rectangle with wire fixation (Surgicraft), ISOLA (DePuy Spine).
  It is used in deformity cases and employs screws, wires, slotted connectors, hooks, and rods to correct the thoracolumbar spine.
  Examples: Luque rod and rectangle with wire fixation (Surgicraft), ISOLA (DePuy Spine)
- Interbody implants (cages, spacers)
  – *Titanium net cylinders*
  Examples: Harms titanium net cylinder (DePuy Spine), SynMesh (Synthes)
  NGage Surgical Mesh System (Blackstone Medical)

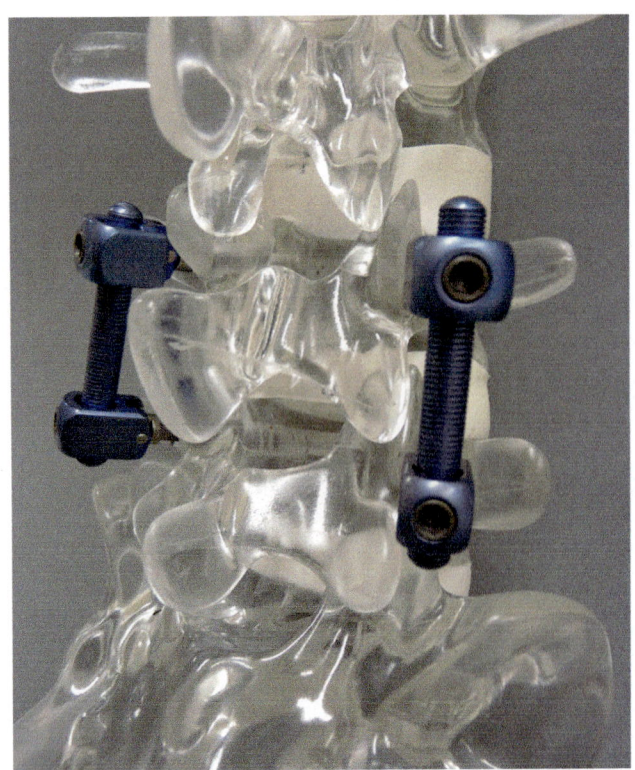

Fig. 57.5 Cosmic internal fixator (Ulrich) with mobile (hinged) screwhead

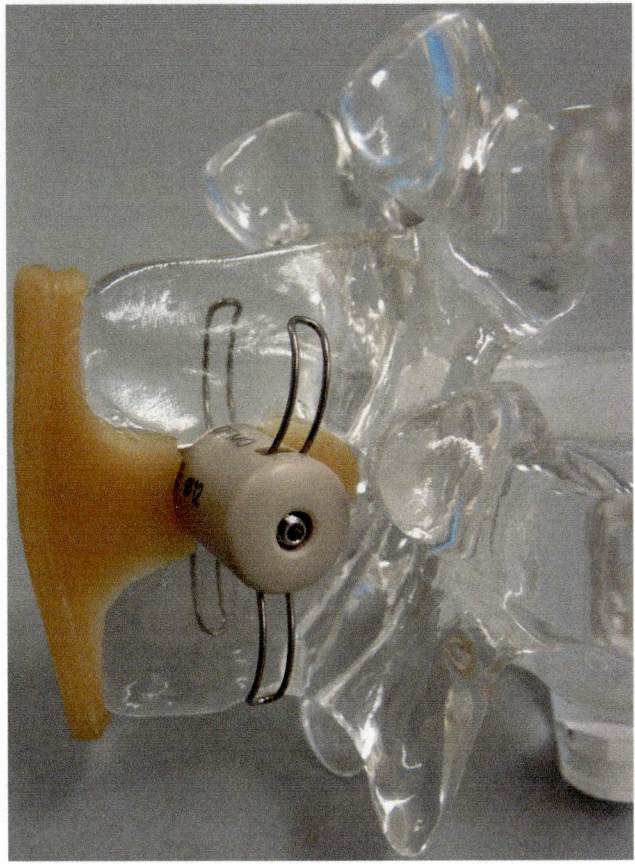

Fig. 57.7 Inspace (Synthes)

- *PLIF Cages* (box like)
  Examples: Ardis PEEK implant (Zimmer Spine), Trabecular Metal PLIF (Zimmer Spine), OIC Cage (Stryker), ProSpace PEEK or titanium cages/spacers (Aesculap), Tetris PEEK (Signus), and Pillar PL (Blackstone Medical).
- *TLIF* cages (kidney-shaped design)
  Trabecular Metal TLIF and TraXis TLIF Peek (Zimmer Spine), CAPSTONE (Medtronic), Devex/Leopard (DePuy Spine), Mobis PEEK (Signus), Pillar TL (Blackstone Medical), and T-Space (Aesculap).

57.4.1.4 Semirigid or Dynamic Systems (Nonfusion Systems)

Semirigid or dynamic types of instrumentation for motion preservation have been developed for the lumbar spine. Dynamic stabilization describes the treatment method employed to achieve stabilization by maintaining the disk with controlled motion of the segment [10]. The implants for dynamic stabilization are either fixed in the pedicle or secured between the spinous processes.

Nucleus replacements, which are implanted posteriorly, are another option.

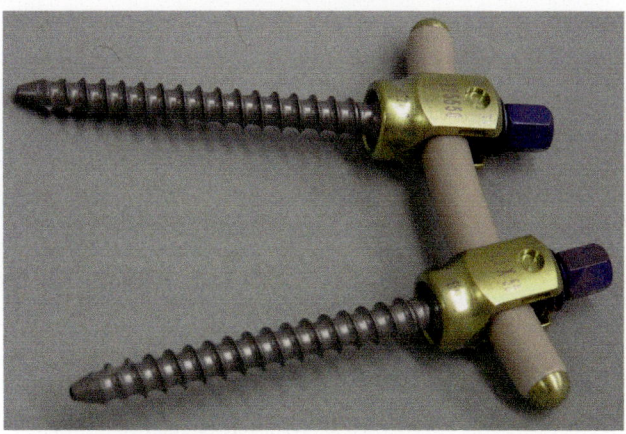

Fig. 57.8 Semirigid PEEK rod system (Medtronic)

- Interspinous implants
  Examples: The principle of implanting a spacer between adjacent spinous processes was used by Knowles to relieve the posterior annulus in patients with disk herniation [11].

  Most implants act in the sagittal plane to inhibit extension. They cause a reduction in lordosis of the motion segment [12], which is visible on X-rays and a reduction in pressure within the disk, thus reducing the load on the facet joint surfaces [13]. They also cause an increase in the subarticular diameter and a widening of the neural foramina. The Wallis implant, for example, is made of polyetheretherketone (PEEK). In addition, the implant includes two ligaments made of woven Dacron that are wrapped around the spinous processes and fixed under tension to the blocker. The Wallis interspinous implant is fixed to the spine by two polyester bands looped around the proximal and distal spinous processes [1, 14]. The DIAM (Medtronic) was designed to dynamically support the vertebrae while at the same time maintaining distraction of the foramina. Other recently developed dynamic stabilization systems are the X-Stop interspinous process decompression system (St. Francis Medical Technologies), the Coflex (Paradigm Spine), and Inspace (Synthes) (see Figs. 57.7 and 57.8).

  However, there exist today no international contents about indications for interspinous devices. Actually, there are controversies about effectiveness of interspinous devices.
- Pedicle screw–based systems
  Examples: Graf Band (SEM Co.), Dynesys (Zimmer Spine), Cosmic (Ulrich Medical), Isobar TTL (Scient'x), and TOPS—Total Posterior Arthroplasty device (Implant).

  Dynamic stabilization with pedicle screw–based systems presents an alternative to instrumented immobilization and relief of spine segments [2]. The Graf Band, which first became available in 1992, was the first pedicle screw–based system [10].

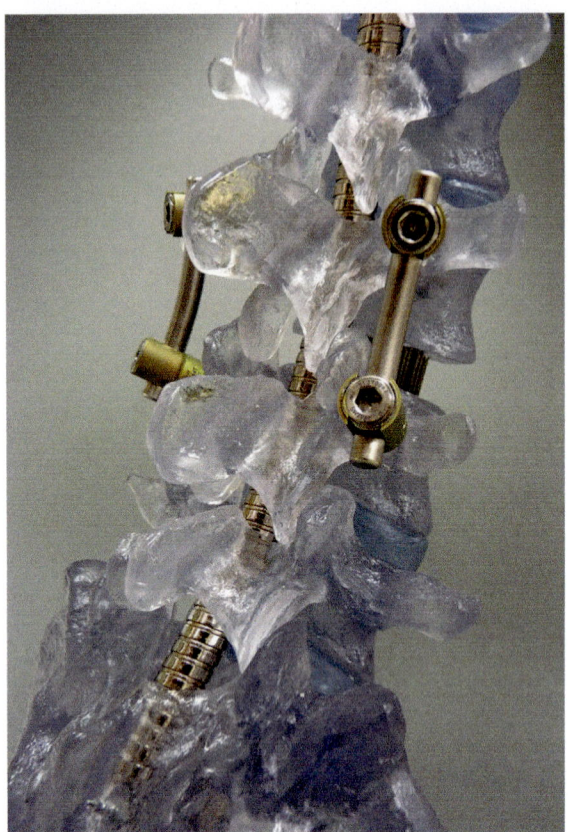

Fig. 57.9 Rigid S⁴ internal fixator (Aesculap)

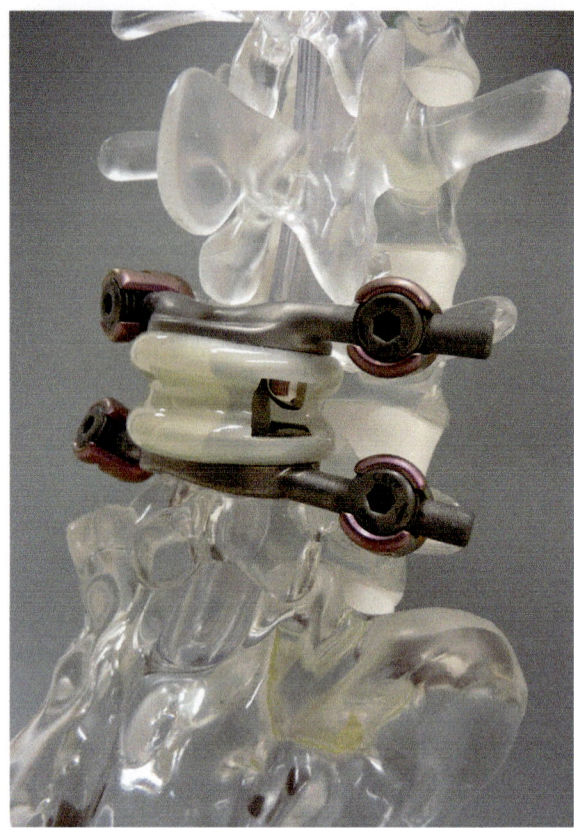

Fig. 57.10 TOPS—total posterior arthroplasty device (Implant)

The Dynesys Dynamic Stabilization System (DSS) (Zimmer Spine) was developed by Dubois [15]. Extensive scientific results have been published for Dynesys [16]. Figure 57.8 demonstrates a semirigid PEEK rod system. The cosmic system (see Fig. 57.9) is a stable and nonrigid system. The screw features a hinged joint between the head and threaded part, which causes the load to be shared between the implant system and the anterior vertebral column. Other options are facet replacement devices, which are designed to replace degenerative facet joints with a prosthetic implant like the TOPS—Total Posterior Arthroplasty device (Implant) (see Fig. 57.10).

- Nucleus replacements

    Examples: Prosthetic Disk Nucleus (PDN) (Raymedica) and DASCOR Disk Arthroplasty System (Disk Dynamics).

    Some nucleus replacement devices can be implanted using a dorsal access route, for example, PDN (Raymedica) or, in part, DASCOR (Disk Dynamics). The PDN devices are constructed from two components: an inner copolymer hydrogel pellet and an outer, superstrong woven jacket of high-molecular-weight polyethylene fibers [17].

References

1. Vialle R, Harding I, Charosky D, et al. The paraspinal splitting approach: a possible approach to perform multiple intercosto-lumbar neurotisations: an anatomic study. Spine. 2007;32:631–4.
2. Wiltse LL, Bateman JG, Hutchinson RH, et al. The paraspinal sacrospinalis-splitting approach to the lumbar spine. J Bone Joint Surg Am. 1968;50:919–26.
3. Newman EW. Lateral intramuscular planar approach to the lumbar spine and sacrum. Technical note. J Neurosurg Spine. 2007;7:270–3.
4. Aryan HE, Newman CB, Gold JJ, et al. Percutaneous axial lumbar interbody fusion (AxiaLIF) of the L5-S1 segment: initial clinical and radiological experience. Minim Invasive Neurosurg. 2008;51:225–30.
5. Roh SW, Kim DH, Cardoso AC, et al. Endoscopic foraminotomy using MED system in cadaveric specimens. Spine. 2000;25:260–4.
6. Foley KT, Smith MM. Microendoscopic discectomy. J Neurosurg. 1997;3:301–7.
7. Buck JE. Direct repair of the defect in spondylolisthesis. J Bone Joint Surg Br. 1970;52:432–7.
8. Morscher E, Gerber B, Fasel J. Surgical treatment of spondylolisthesis by bone grafting and direct stabilization of spondylolysis by means of a hook screw. Arch Orthop Trauma Surg. 1984;103:175–8.
9. Kluger P. Das Fixateurprinzip an der Wirbelsäule. In: Stuhler T, editor. Fixateur externe—fixateur interne. Berlin: Springer; 1989.
10. Grevitt MP, Gardner AD, Spilsbury J, et al. The Graf stabilisation system: early results in 50 patients. Eur Spine J. 1995;4:169–75.

11. Whitesides TE Jr. The effect of an interspinous implant on intervertebral disc pressures. Spine. 2003;28:1906–7.
12. Lindsey DP, Swanson KE, Fuchs P, et al. The effect of an interspinous implant on the kinematics of the instrumented and adjacent levels in the lumbar spine. Spine. 2003;28:2192–7.
13. Wilke HJ, Magerl F, Nelter S, et al. (2000) Biomechanical in vitro comparison of translaminar pins versus translaminar screws for instrumentation of spinal segments. Poster, Eurospine.
14. Korovessis P, Repantis T, Zacharatos S, et al. Does Wallis implant reduce adjacent segmental degeneration above lumbosacral instrumented fusion? Eur Spine J. 2009;18:830–40.
15. Stoll TM, Dubois G, Schwarzenbach O. The dynamic neutralization system for the spine: a multi-center study of a novel non-fusion system. Eur Spine J. 1999;11(Suppl 2):S170–8.
16. Grob D, Benini A, Junge A, et al. Clinical experience with the Dynesys semirigid fixation system for the lumbar spine. Surgical and patient-oriented outcome in 50 cases after an average of 2 years. Spine. 2005;30:324–31.
17. Ray CD. The PDN prosthetic disc-nucleus device. Eur Spine J. 2002;11(Suppl 2):S137–42.

Microsurgical Intra- and Extraspinal Discectomy

58

Luca Papavero

58.1 Introduction and Core Messages

With the landmark report in the New England Journal of Medicine in 1934, the two American surgeons William Jason Mixter and Joseph Seaton Barr finally clarified the pathomechanism of lumbar disk herniation and furthermore, propagated discectomy as the standard therapy [1]. Since then, the surgical procedures were continuously refined. In the late 1970s, the surgical microscope was introduced for spinal surgery almost simultaneously but independently by the neurosurgeons Yasargil and Caspar and by the orthopedic surgeon Williams and so-called microdiscectomy was introduced [2–4]. However, the approach was still the subperiosteal interlaminar inherited from the conventional open discectomy. The "one (route) fits all (disk herniations)" was the golden standard. In 1974, Abdullah describing the surgical technique for 24 cases of "extreme lateral disk herniations" reported: "In a few cases early in the series facetectomy was performed, but this is now avoided when possible" [5]. The extraforaminal approach was born and its technical refinement was described 1984 by Reulen [6]. In 1998, the neurosurgeon Di Lorenzo described the translaminar approach as less invasive route for the removal of cranially extrude disk fragments impinging the exiting root.

The above-mentioned and further refined microsurgical approaches are presented. The intraspinal approaches include the "interlaminar" (ILA) and the "translaminar" (TLA) ones. The interlaminar route is indicated when the extruded disk fragment and/or contained herniation is located between the midline and the medial border of the pedicle (roughly 70%). The translaminar approach is valuable for removing a cranially extruded disk fragment impinging the exiting root. This herniation is commonly within the root canal, that is, between the medial and lateral rims of the pedicle (roughly 20%). The extraspinal approach, or more precisely the transmuscular paraspinal route, deals with disk fragments extruded with at least two-thirds of the volume laterally to the lateral border of the pedicle (roughly 10%). Features common to the tree techniques are (1) a carefully preoperative planning, mostly by MRI, for choosing the most convenient approach; (2) the use of the microscope from skin to skin; (3) the application of soft tissue and facet joint sparing techniques, requiring the insertion of miniaturized retractors; and (4) whenever possible, the solely removal of the offending disk fragment leaving the disk space alone.

58.2 Interlaminar Approach (ILA) [7]

58.2.1 Indications

- All "pure" contained disk herniations and extruded disk fragments between the midline and the medial border of the pedicle. Referring to the disk space, the fragments may be caudally or cranially extruded. In the latter case, the translaminar approach is more selective.
- Disk herniations combined with central/recess stenosis or with asymptomatic segmental instability.
- Recurrent disk herniations.

L. Papavero (✉)
Clinic for Spine Surgery, Schoen Clinic Hamburg, Hamburg, Germany
e-mail: lpapavero@schoen-kliniken.de

© Springer-Verlag GmbH Germany 2023
U. Vieweg, F. Grochulla (eds.), *Manual of Spine Surgery*, https://doi.org/10.1007/978-3-662-64062-3_58

58.2.2 Contraindications

- Disk herniations which bulk is located laterally to the lateral border of the pedicle.

58.2.3 Technical Requirements

- Intraoperative fluoroscopy.
- Microscope. Following features are useful: long holding arm of the *stative* in order to place the micro behind the surgeon, "in front" stereoscopic oculars, powerful illumination (e.g., 300 W Xenon), and external video-line for ORP.
- Positioning device allowing reduction of lumbar lordosis (e.g., Wilson frame, Fig. 58.1).
- Small retractor to be introduced through a 2–3-cm skin incision.
- Microsurgical instruments, better if bayoneted (Fig. 58.2).
- Optional: high-speed drill with angled handpieces, cutting *burrs*, and diamond dust–coated *burrs*.

58.2.4 Preparation, Planning, and Positioning

- *Plain X-rays in AP and lateral view*: Optional in first surgery cases, provided that the MRI investigation encloses a coronal slice (scoliosis!). Obligatory (1) in recurrent disk surgery for evaluating the bone defect (2) whenever the MRI leads to suspect a bony abnormality (spina bifida, defect of the pars interarticularis).
- *MRI*: the first choice investigation! *Sagittal slices*: contained disk herniation (DH) or extruded fragment? Caudal or cranial fragment dislocation (suitable for translaminar approach)? Midvertebral body herniation (on halfway

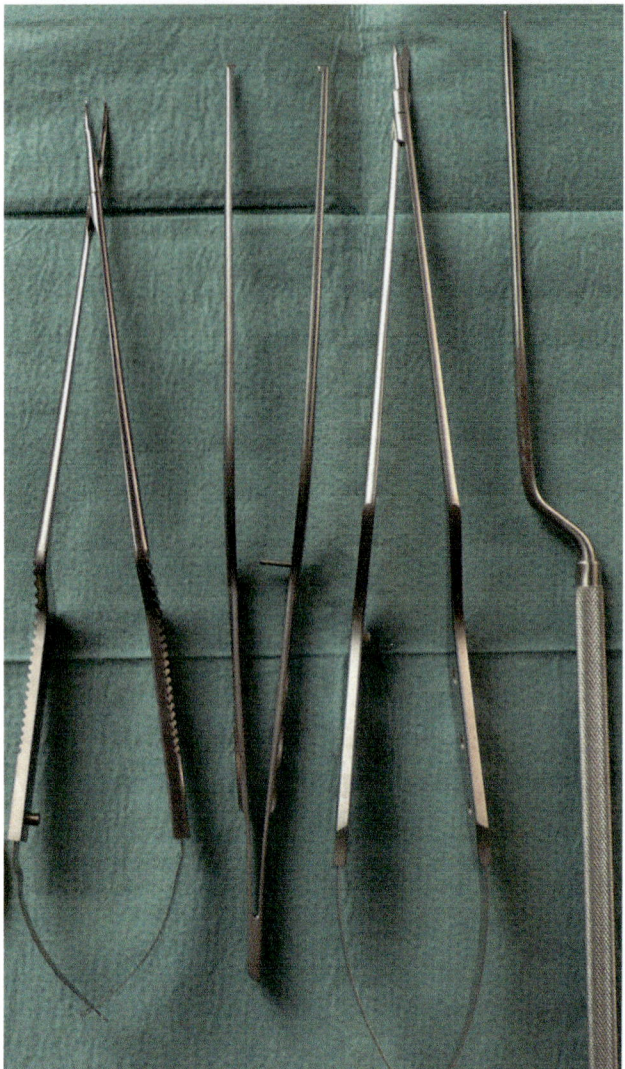

Fig. 58.2 Bayoneted instruments prevent the fingers from obstructing the microsurgical field

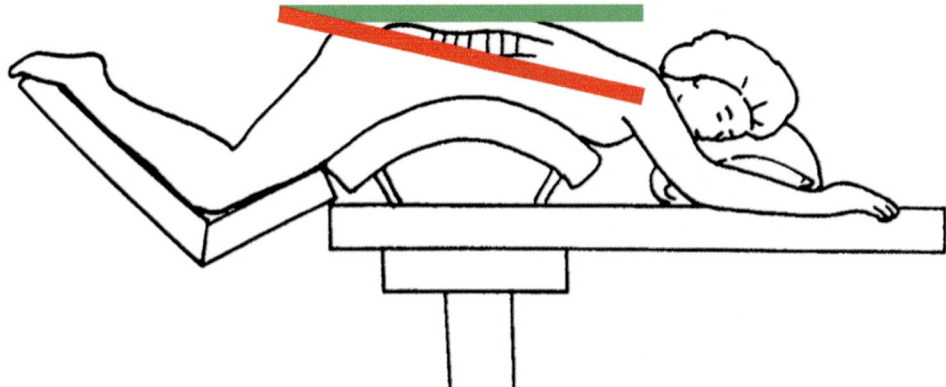

Fig. 58.1 Wilson frame: note that the lumbar spine should be parallel to the floor and straightened. Hip, knee, and ankle are only moderately flexed. Positioning for the translaminar approach should consider that the lumbar laminae "dive" (red line), therefore tilting the table a bit head-up wards will bring the laminae in a horizontal plane (green line): this makes drilling of the translaminar hole easier

between two disk spaces)? Foraminal slice: black neuroforamen? Extraforaminal slice: disk fragment still apparent? *Axial slices*: intra-axillary disk fragment? How much of the DH is underneath the thecal sac, intraforaminal, or extraforaminal? Pseudomeningocele in recurrent disk surgery? *Coronal slices*: which approach for combined intra- and extraforaminal DH? *Gadolineum*: amount of scar tissue on the way to and into the spinal canal? Differentiation between recurrent DH and scar tissue?

- *CT-scan*: second choice whenever MRI is contraindicated or not available. Disco-CT (discography + CT): helpful in suspected extraforaminal DH. CM-enhanced CT: indicated for recurrent disk, differentiation between intraforaminal DH versus neurinoma.
- *Myelography*: as third option.
- We recognize that several positionings could provide good clinical results, especially with experienced ORP. The features of our favorite positioning are described below:
  - The patient is placed prone on the Wilson frame. Advantages: hip and knee joints are not flexed, especially important in obese patients! The lordosis of the lumbar spine can be reduced as required by increasing the height of the arches. The distance between the arches can be adjusted according to the size of the patient in order to allow a free hanging abdomen (Fig. 58.1).
  - The head is positioned into the ProneView mask (manufacturer: Dupaco, Oceanside, California, USA). Eyes, nose, and chin are protected: the anesthesiologist is enabled to check them anytime by a mirror (Fig. 58.3)!
  - For safety reasons, the patient is secured with a belt on the gluteal area: this becomes helpful when the OR table has to be tilted away from the surgeon, for example, in dealing with extraforaminal disk herniations (EFDHs).
  - The OR table is tilted to get the lumbar spine parallel to the floor.

- *X-ray labeling*: A 2–3-cm skin incision does not allow a "seek and find" surgery. Therefore, the correct X-ray labeling of the surgical target area is of paramount importance.
- The needle is always inserted contralateral to the intended surgical side in order to avoid subcutaneous or intramuscular hematoma and off the midline in order to prevent CSF leakage. The needle is perpendicular to the target area (and to the floor): soft tissue dissection is easier straightforward down! Even small oblique deviations can lead to the wrong level, especially in obese patients.
- The needle should point to the equator of the target disk. With increasing experience, it may point to the extruded disk fragment.

58.2.5 Surgical Technique

The interlaminar space can be approached via a subperiosteal (SP) or a transmuscular (TM) route. Although the use of the microscope "skin to skin" is optional, its advantages will be quickly appreciated dealing with a miniaturized surgical corridor. The most relevant steps are described below: single-shot antibiotic (e.g., cephazoline, 2 g) 30 min before skin incision.

- *Skin* (SP and TM): 2-cm incision, 5 mm off the midline.
- *Fascia*: semicircular incision toward the midline. Five holding sutures on the medial lip secured to a clamp with weights (SP). Straight incision with one holding suture on each side (TM).
- *Muscle*: (SP) Retraction of the paravertebral muscles with a hand-held retractor from the interspinal ligament. Sharp dissection of the rotators from the lower rim of the superior lamina and from the facet joint capsule. Insertion of a miniaturized Caspar-type speculum-counter-retractor system ("Piccolino," manufacturer: Medicon, Tuttlingen, Germany, Fig. 58.4a).

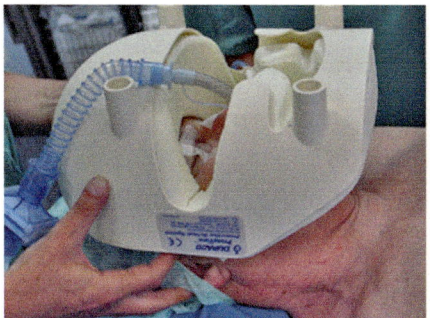 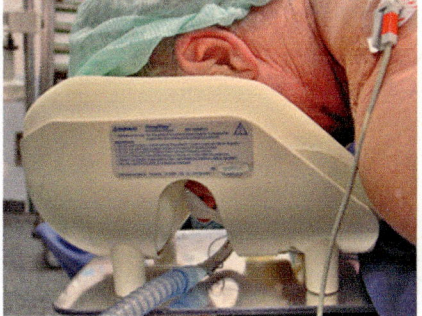 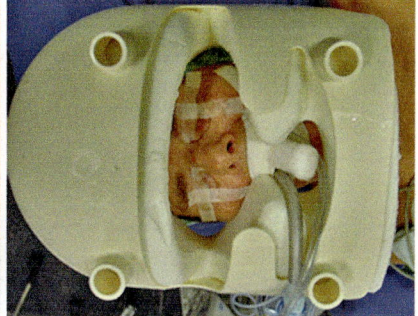

Fig. 58.3 The mask fits to the face before turning the patient (*left*), patient prone with the mask resting on a mirror (*center*), mirror for checking eyes, nose, chin, and airways (*right*)

Fig. 58.4 (**a**)
Miniaturized speculum,
(**b**) miniaturized forceps
(*black*), and (**c**) flat sucker

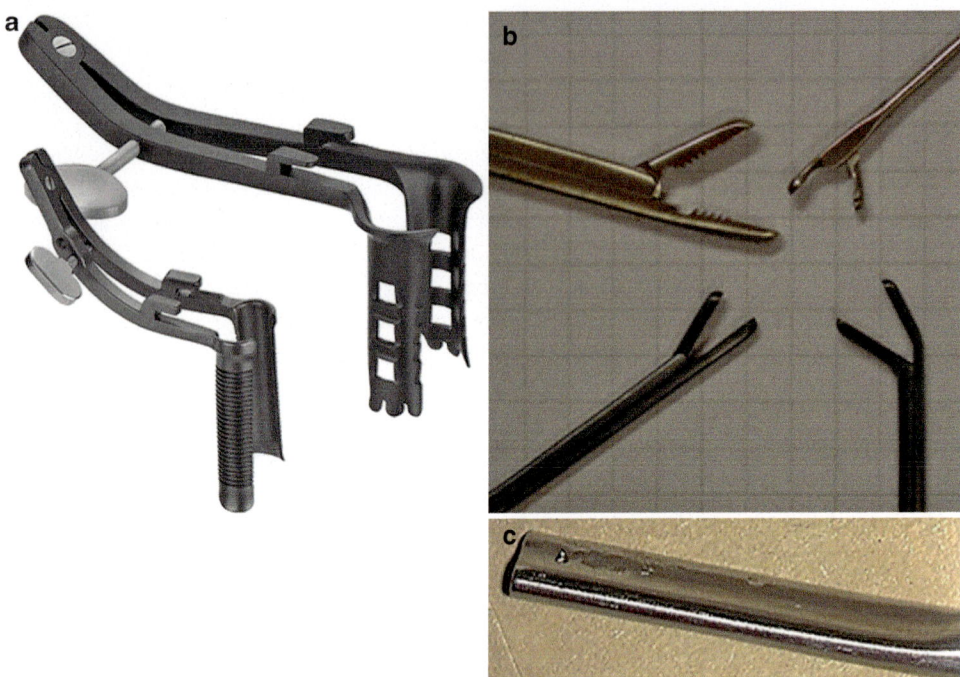

- (TM) Blunt splitting with the index finger until the lami-nofacet junction can be palpated. Opening of the muscular corridor with miniaturized hand-held retractors or with a dilator. Insertion of an expandable tubular retractor ("Microdisc XS," manufacturer Medicon, Tuttlingen, Germany) with 15 mm diameter. The tube is secured with a "snake," a self-holding arm, to the OR table (Figs. 58.5 and 58.6).
- *Interlaminar space*: from this step onward, the surgical technique is identical. The lower rim of the cranial lamina, the medial border of the facet joint, and the yellow ligament should be the area of interest. A fluoroscopic control of the level is performed. Following a lateral flavectomy or flavotomy with suspension sutures, the epidural fat is exposed. The medial border of the inferior articular process is undercut or drilled off until the lateral border of the root is palpated.
- *Epidural dissection*: up-down dissection of the epidural fat performed with a microdissector and a flat sucker (so-called mole-technique, Fig. 58.4c), along with prudent bipolar coagulation of veins, opens the access to the root-DH complex.
- *Management of the DH*: the local anatomy will dictate the necessary steps. Usually, a gentle separation of the cleavage plane between root and disk material is accomplished first. In our experience, the root retraction is performed intermittently with the flat sucker instead of with a conventional root retractor. Free disk fragments are removed with miniaturized forceps (manufacturer:

Medicon, Tuttlingen, Germany, Fig. 58.4b). If indicated, the annulus is split bluntly with the dissector, and further disk material is removed. In the authors' experience, additional discectomy is performed in 20–30% of the cases.
- *Closure*: the disk space, when opened, is rinsed with Ringer solution. The opening of the annulus is closed with a collagen sponge coated with fibrinogen and thrombin (TachoSil, manufacturer: Behring, Marburg, Germany). The epidural fat is mobilized in order to cover the root. Careful hemostasis goes along with closure by layers.

58.2.6 Postoperative Care

The patient is encouraged to leave the bed 6 h after surgery. Sitting is allowed starting from the first postoperative day. Physiotherapy starts the morning after surgery. Hospital staying is usually 3 days.

58.2.7 Complications

The literature lists several "generic" complications such as deep venous thrombosis, pulmonary embolism, urinary infections, missed pathology, retroperitoneal vessel injury, and postoperative segmental instability, which fortunately became more than exceptional events.

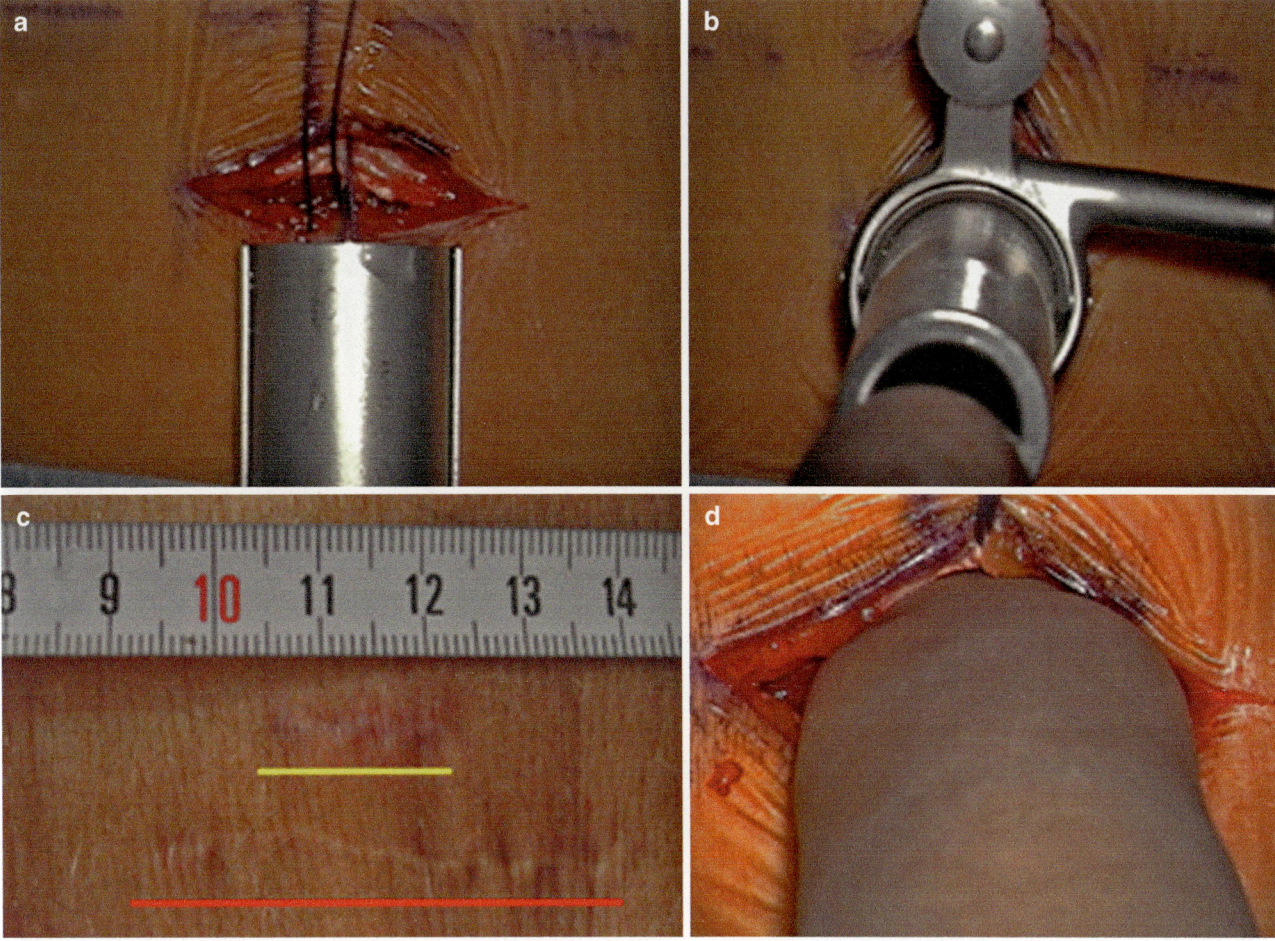

Fig. 58.5 Transmuscular approach: (**a**) 20-mm skin incision, blunt muscle splitting with a dilator (**b**) or with the index finger (**d**), (**c**) scar of transmuscular approach (*yellow line*) for a recurrent disk following previous conventional subperiosteal approach (*red line*)

However, even the refined microsurgical techniques are still burdened by complications such as root injury (0.5%), dural tears (1.5%), spondylodiscitis (>1%), and "recurrent DH" (5%).

58.3   Translaminar Approach (TLA) [8–12]

58.3.1 Indications

- Cranially extruded disk fragments pushing the exiting root against the lower rim of the pedicle. Usually, they are also located intraforaminally (Fig. 58.7a, b).
- Recurrent cranially extruded disk fragments of disk herniations previously addressed by an interlaminar approach.

58.3.2 Contraindications

- Severe spinal canal stenosis and spina bifida, lack of an adequate lamina.
- In case of a foraminal DH, the bulk of the fragment should be between two lines, marking the medial and lateral borders of the superior facet: disk material located more laterally should be approached through a paraspinal approach.

58.3.3 Technical Requirements

- The same as for ILA.
- A must: drill with angled handpieces, cutting *burrs*, and diamond dust–coated *burrs*.

Fig. 58.6 Close-up view (**a**) of the expandable tubular retractor in situ; the tubular retractor is fixed with a self-holding adjustable arm, "the snake" (**b**), and intraoperative fluoroscopy of the closed (**c**) and opened (**d**) tube

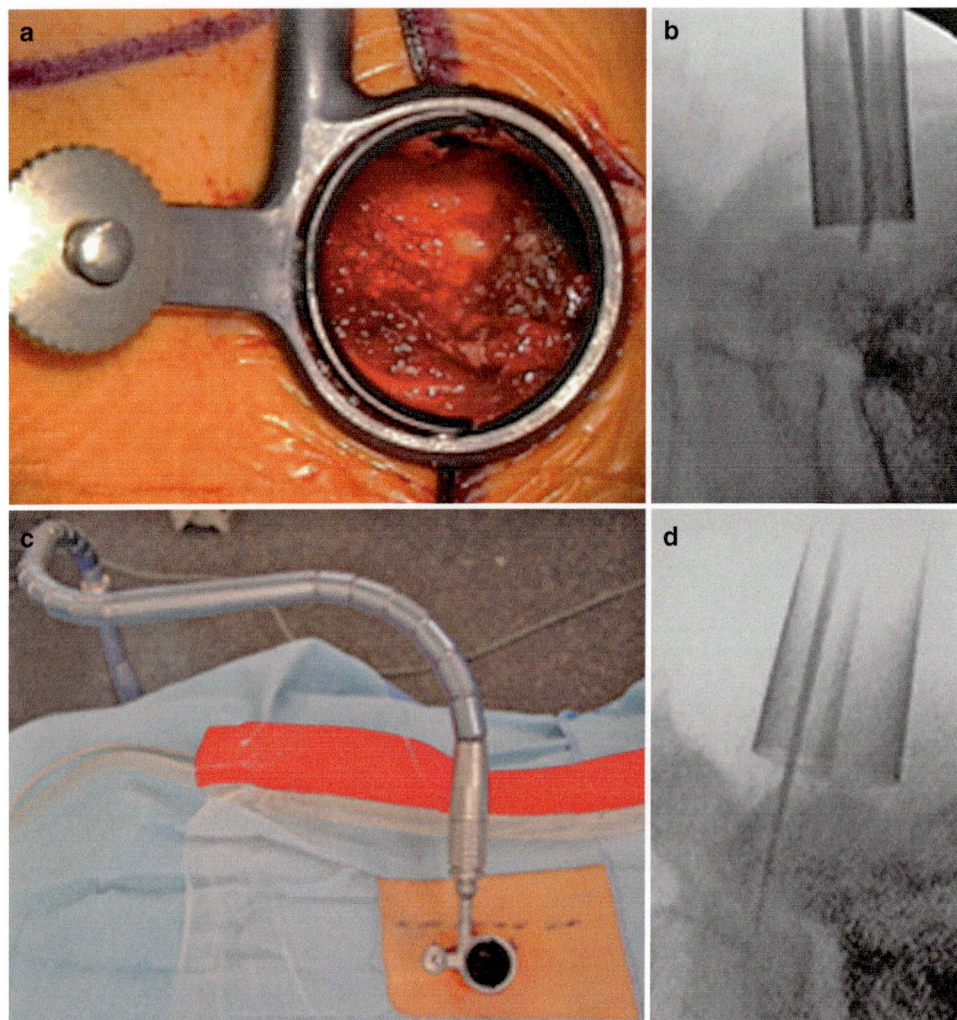

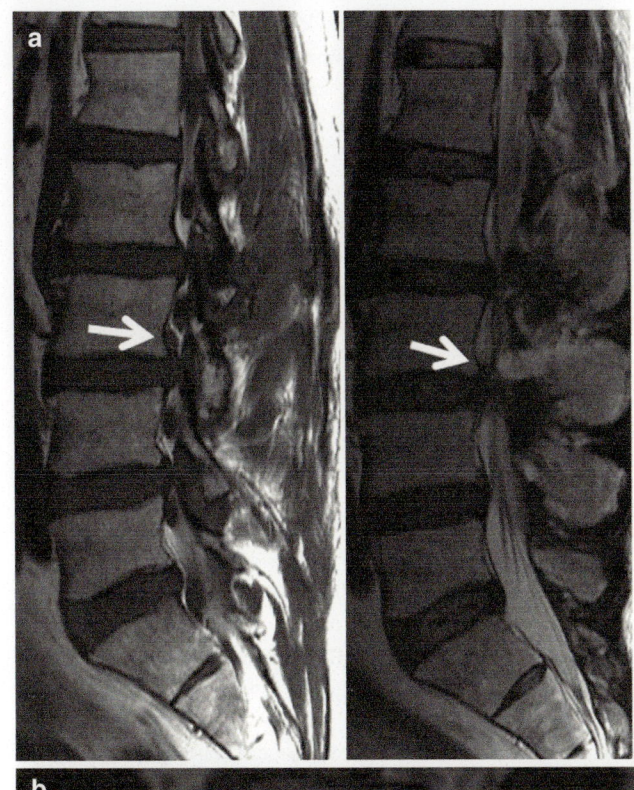

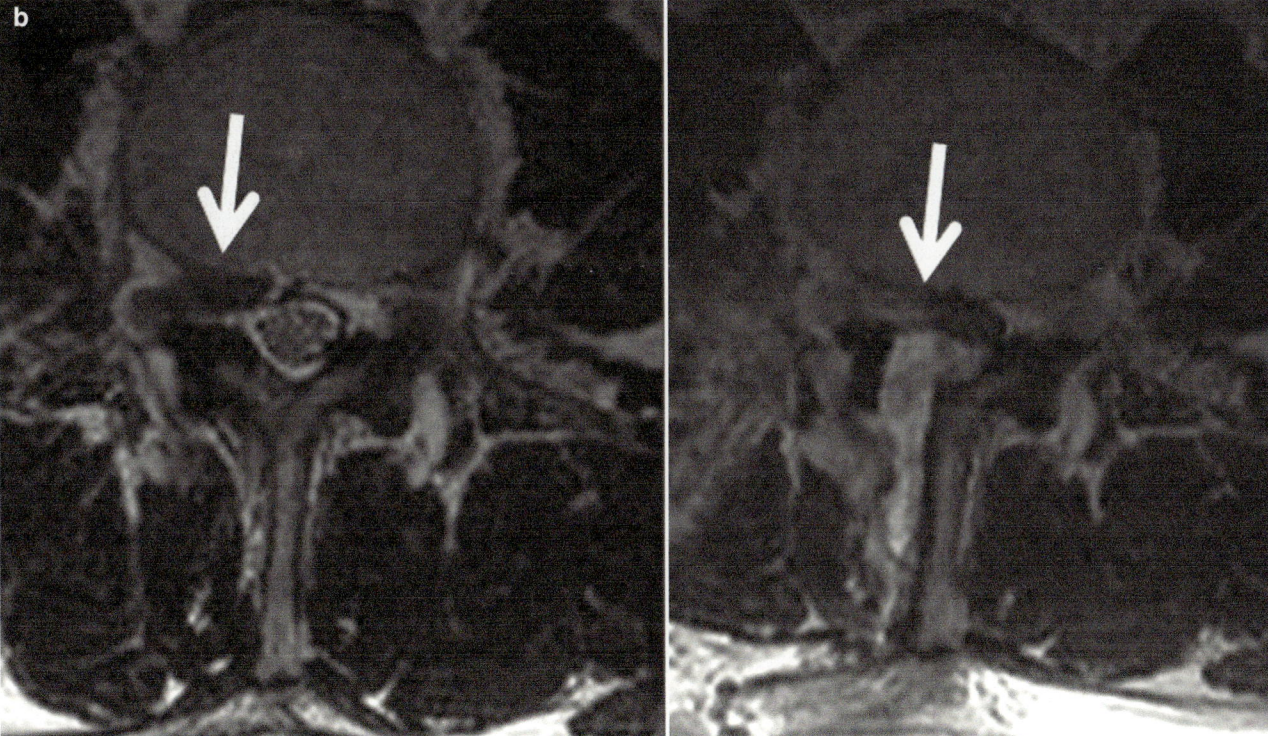

Fig. 58.7 (**a**) Cranially extruded disk fragment L3/L4 (*arrow*, *left*), which has been removed via a translaminar approach (*arrow*, *right*). (**b**) The axial slice shows that the disk fragment (*arrow*) impinges the exiting L3 root on the right side (*left*). The postoperative picture confirms the removal through the lamina (*right*)

58.3.4 Preparation, Planning, and Positioning

- *MRI*: *sagittal slices*: measure the distance between upper border of the disk space and cranial rim of the fragment! The translaminar hole will be centered on the halfway of this distance. *Axial slices*: look at how much of the bulk of the DH is underneath the thecal sac and how much is lateral of it or even intraforaminal. The translaminar hole is centered on the lateral border of the thecal sac.
- Same positioning as for ILA.
- Important: the target lamina should be parallel to the floor! This may require to tilt the OR table a little bit head upward. The advantages of a horizontal target lamina are twofold: the placement of the retractor blade and the drilling of the hole become easier (Fig. 58.1).
- *X-ray labeling*: the needle should point to the maximum bulk of the DH, which is usually halfway between the upper border of the target disk space and the lower rim of the cranial pedicle.
- At the beginning of the learning curve, the upper border of the target disk space and the lower rim of the cranial pedicle may be labeled separately and the skin incision centered in between (Fig. 58.8).

58.3.5 Surgical Technique

The lamina can be approached via a subperiosteal (SP) or a transmuscular (TM) route. The soft tissue approach mirrors exactly that to the interlaminar space and has been already described. Remember that the width and the overlapping of the lamina in relation to the disk space increase in the caudal-cranial direction, whereas the width of the isthmus decreases. This means that the translaminar hole will be more medially and more ovale-shaped in the cranial direction (Fig. 58.9).

- *Lamina*: irrespective of the kind of speculum used, the lateral border of the lamina should be visible underneath the retractor valve. A dissector is placed onto the lamina where the bulk of the DH is suspected and a fluoroscopic control is performed. At this point, the lamina should have been tilted parallel to the floor so that the cutting burr can be held more easily perpendicular to the lamina. With slow circular movements, a round- (L5) or oval-shaped (L4 and cranially) hole of about 10 mm in diameter is performed (Fig. 58.10). Three layers, "white" (outer cortical bone), "red" (spongy bone), and "white" (inner cortical bone), will be drilled off. For the sake of safety, the inner cortical bone should be drilled with a diamond burr. Remarks: (1) At least 3 mm of the lateral border should be spared in order to avoid a fracture of the pars interarticularis (Fig. 58.11). (2) Usually, the translaminar hole is located just cephalad to the cranial insertion of the yellow liga-

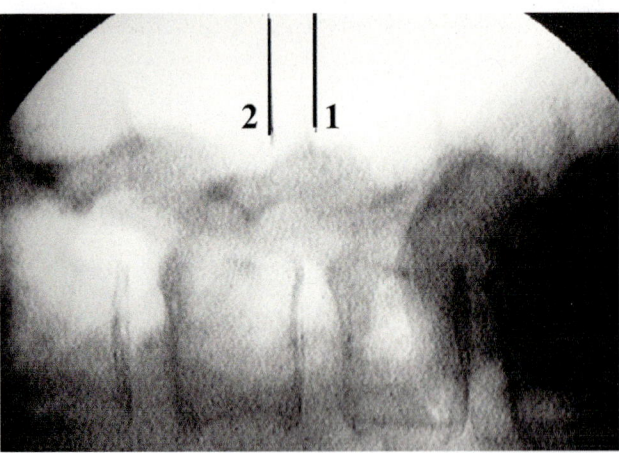

Fig. 58.8 Intraoperative fluoroscopy: the needle (1) points to the upper rim of the target disk, whereas the needle (2) points to disk fragment just underneath the lower rim of the cranial pedicle

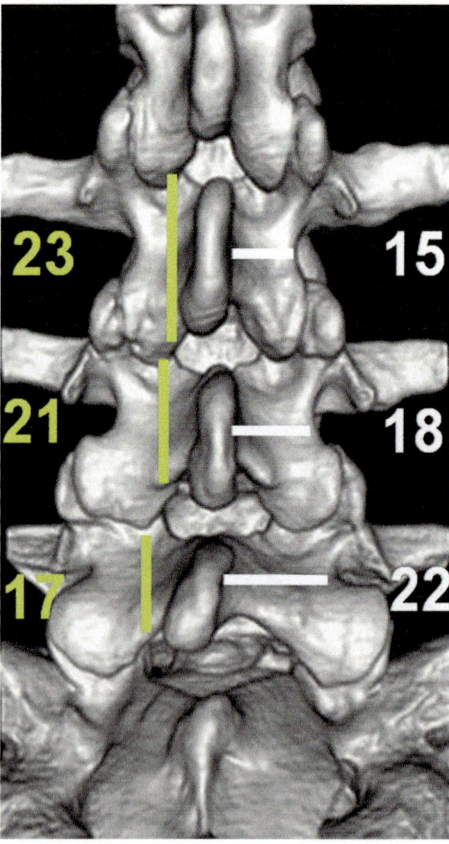

Fig. 58.9 *Yellow numbers*: length of the lamina; *black numbers*: width of the lamina

ment. So, after removal of the thin shell of inner cortical bone with small punches, epidural fat will appear.

- *Epidural dissection*: up and down dissection of the fat along the lateral border of the thecal sac. That should be continued cranial up to the axilla of the exiting root.

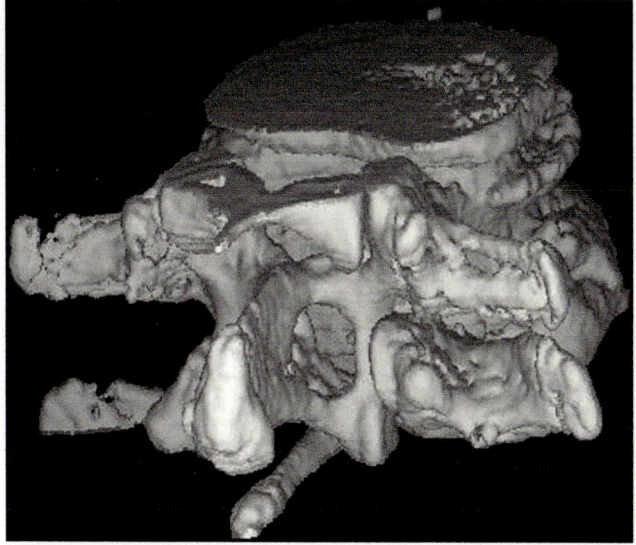

Fig. 58.10 Postoperative 3D-CT, which shows a translaminar hole L3 on the right side

- *Management of the DH*: Usually, an extruded or subligamentous disk fragment/s can be mobilized. After decompression, the root slips caudally into the visible field (Fig. 58.12). The root canal is probed with a double-angled hook. If an extensive annular perforation is detected, the disk space should be cleared. In our experience, that was required in merely 20% of the cases. The rate of recurrence was 7%.

- *Closure*: Gelfoam soaked with long-acting steroid to fill in the hole is optional, but it should be avoided if the disk space has been cleared.

- *Postoperative care*: same as for ILA.

58.3.6 Complications

Tilting of the OR table in order to direct the lamina quite parallel to the floor minimizes the risk of wrong level surgery.

The particularly thin axillary dura should be handled very carefully during dissection of adherent disk fragments. Due to the narrow access, gluing a patch on accidental durotomy is the best solution.

Although not a complication, enlarging the hole to conventional laminotomy becomes necessary whenever a significant annular perforation is detected on the caudal half of the disk space, especially at the L5/S1 level.

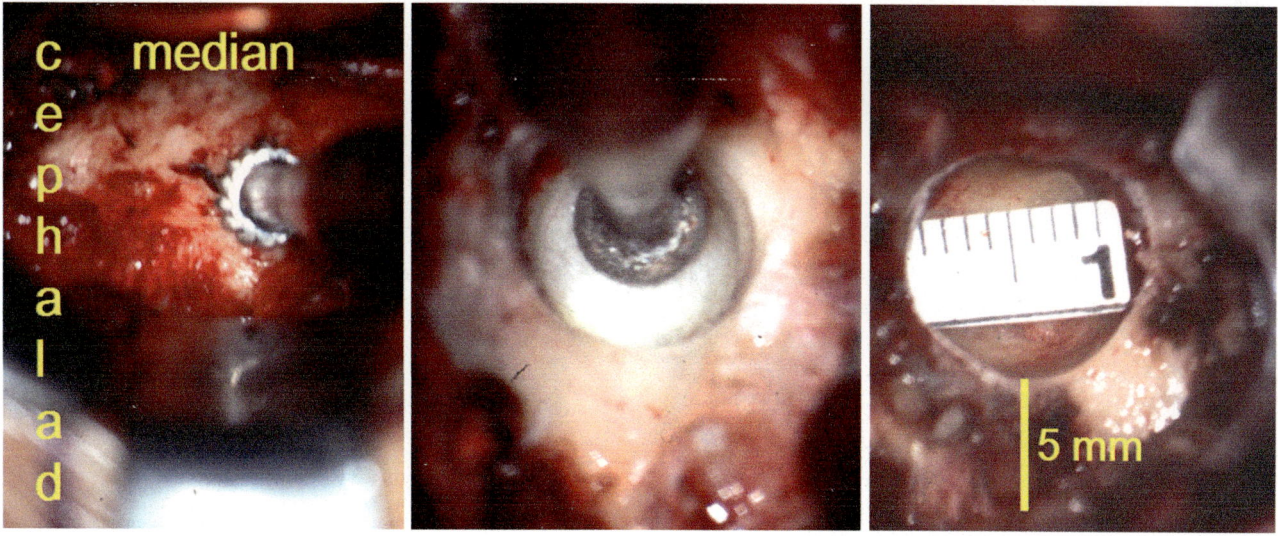

Fig. 58.11 The superficial cortical bone of the lamina is drilled off with a cutting burr (*left*), the inner cortical bone with a diamond dust–coated burr (*center*), keep at least 3 mm safety zone at the lateral border of the pars interarticularis (*right*)

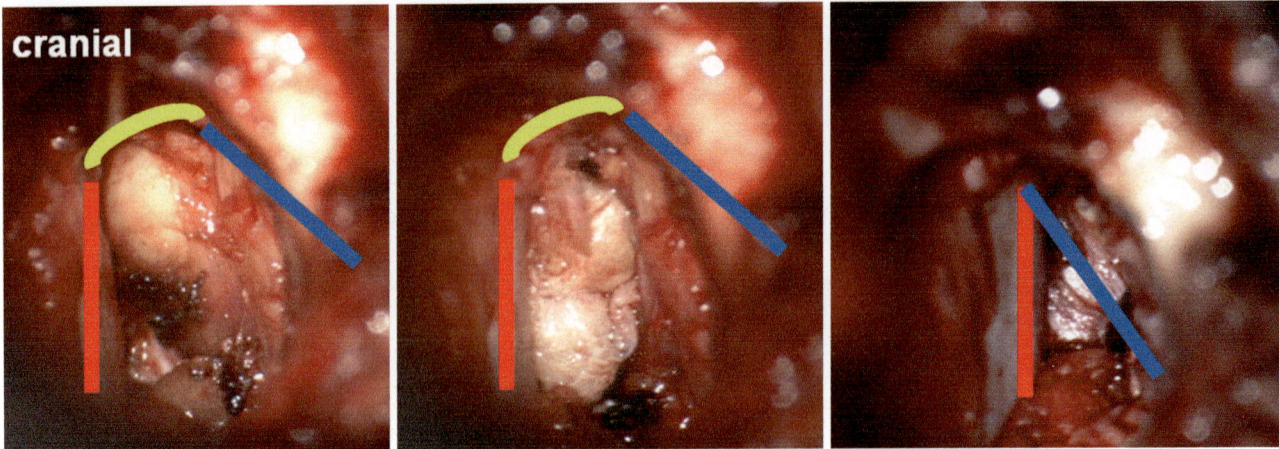

Fig. 58.12 Epidural dissection on the *right side*: the intra-axillary disk fragment pushes the root upward to the lower rim of the pedicle (*left*); the epidural capsule has been removed from the DH (*center*); after the removal of the space occupying disk fragment, the root becomes visible in the surgical field (*left*). *Red line*: lateral border of the thecal sac; *yellow line*: axilla of the exiting root; *blue line*: lower border of the exiting root

58.4 Extraforaminal Approach (EFA)
[6, 13, 14]

58.4.1 Indication

- Disk fragment located at least two-thirds lateral to the pedicle.

58.4.2 Contraindication

- Foraminal disk herniations located more than two-thirds inside the root canal.

58.4.3 Technical Requirements

- The same as for TLA.

58.4.4 Preparation, Planning, and Positioning

- MRI: sagittal slices: cave! Usually, they are not scanned lateral enough, that is, lateral to the root canal, and miss the EFDH. Axial slices: compare the amount and distribution of the extraforaminal fat tissue on both sites. Coronal slices: although rarely performed, they are of invaluable help to show the spatial relationship among exiting root, root canal, and extraforaminal compartment (Fig. 58.13).
- Same positioning as for ILA.

- For safety reasons, the patient should be belted on the gluteal region: the OR table has to be tilted 20–30° away from the surgeon in order to get a better oblique view of the extraforaminal compartment. Especially, obese patients may risk to "roll over" on their own fat.
- *Lateral view* (*X-ray labeling*): insert a spinal needle one finger's breadth lateral to the spinous process, perpendicularly to the skin, and projecting toward the lower border of the affected disk space. Draw a horizontal line at this level (A). Switch the C-arm into the AP-view: Two horizontal lines are drawn: (1) the lower border of the affected disk space should be identical with the previous marking in the lateral view (A) and (2) the lower border of the transverse process above the affected disk (B). Two vertical lines are also drawn: (1) the midline (row of the spinous processes) (C) and (2) a line about 4 cm off to the midline, marking the lateral boundary of the pedicle above and below the affected disk (D). The distance between the two horizontal lines (AB) is the skin incision and will be 3–4 cm in length and about 4 cm paramedian (Fig. 58.14).

58.4.5 Surgical Technique

- The transmuscular blunt splitting approach to EFDH at the level L4/L5 or more cranially can be performed with an expandable tubular retractor or with a miniaturized speculum combined with medial and lateral counterretractor blades (Fig. 58.15). At the level L5/S1, the author

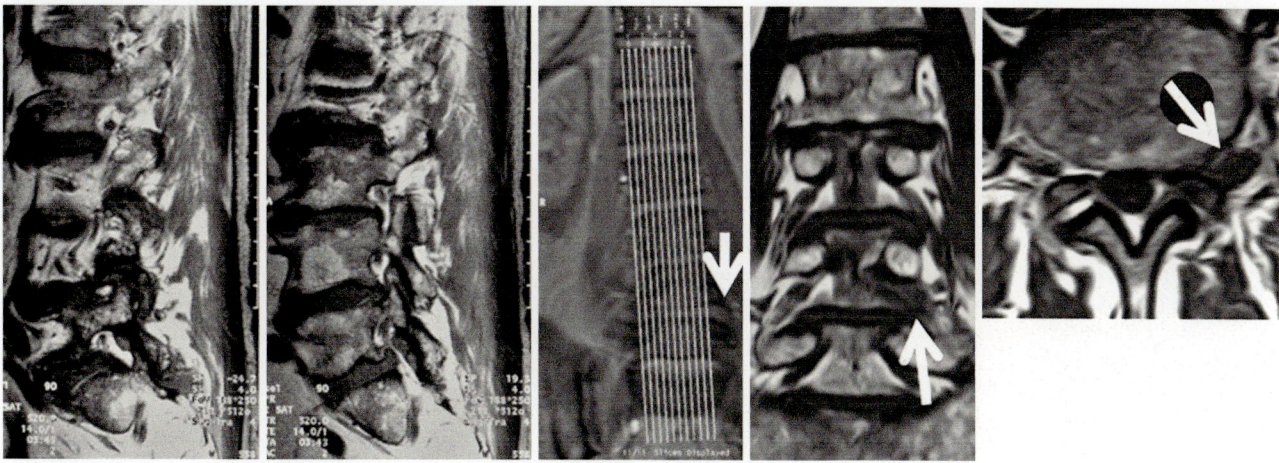

Fig. 58.13 (From *left to right*) Inapparent paramedian slices due to faulty scanning (*center*) omitting the extraforaminal areas, especially on the *left side* (*arrow*); the coronal view shows that the left-sided L4 root is severely impinged by an extraforaminal DH (*arrow*). The disk fragment is also clearly visible on the axial slice (*right, arrow*): compare the different distribution of the extraforaminal fat

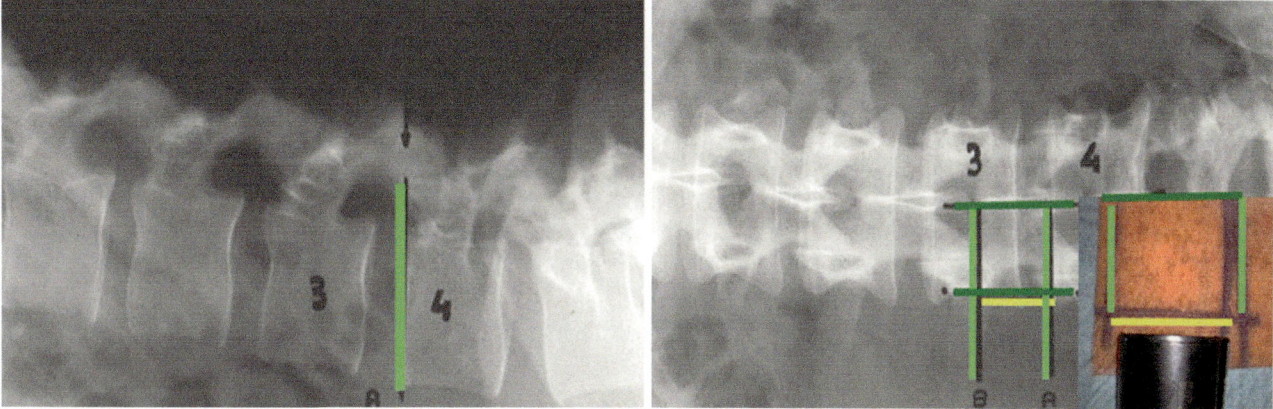

Fig. 58.14 Labeling of the lines of reference on the intraoperative lateral (*Left*) and AP (*right*) view

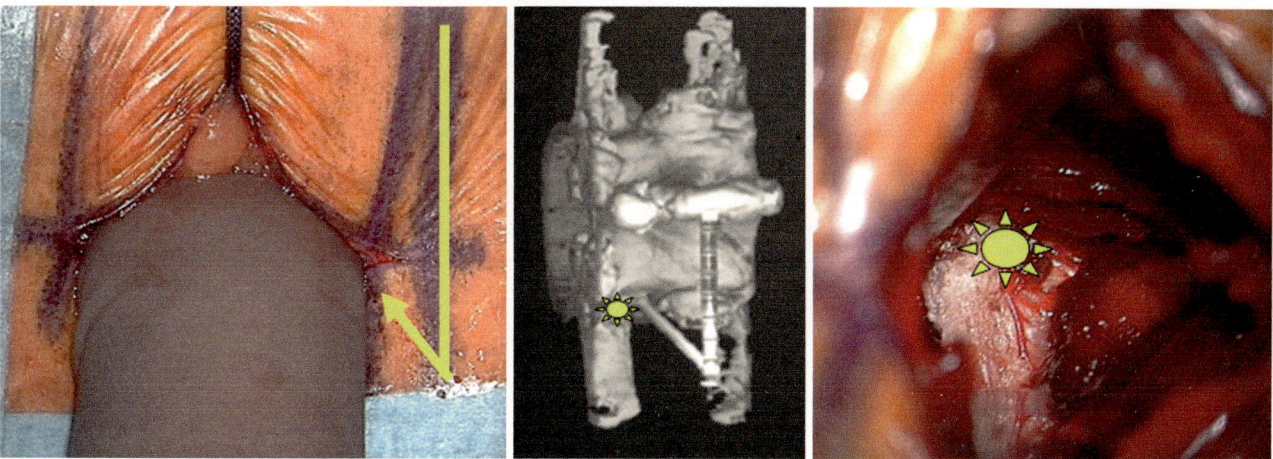

Fig. 58.15 Blunt splitting of the muscles pointing to the medial third of the transverse process cranial to the target disk (*left*), 3D-CT depicting the access (*center*), target point (*asterisk*) of the transverse process (*right*)

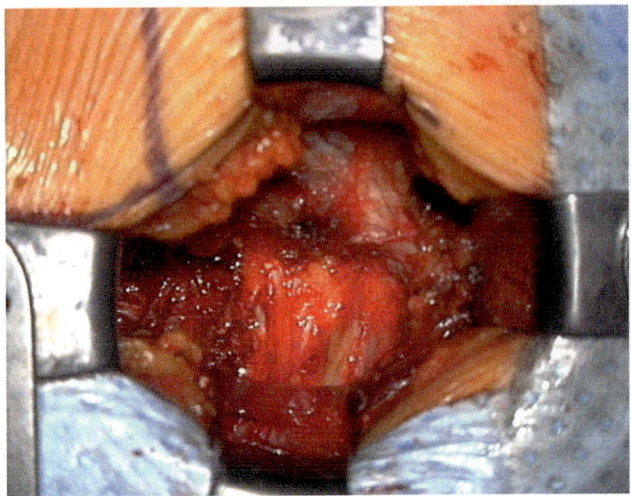

Fig. 58.16 Surgical field to approach L5/S1 on the *left side*: the upper blade rests on the facet joint, the left one on the transverse process L5

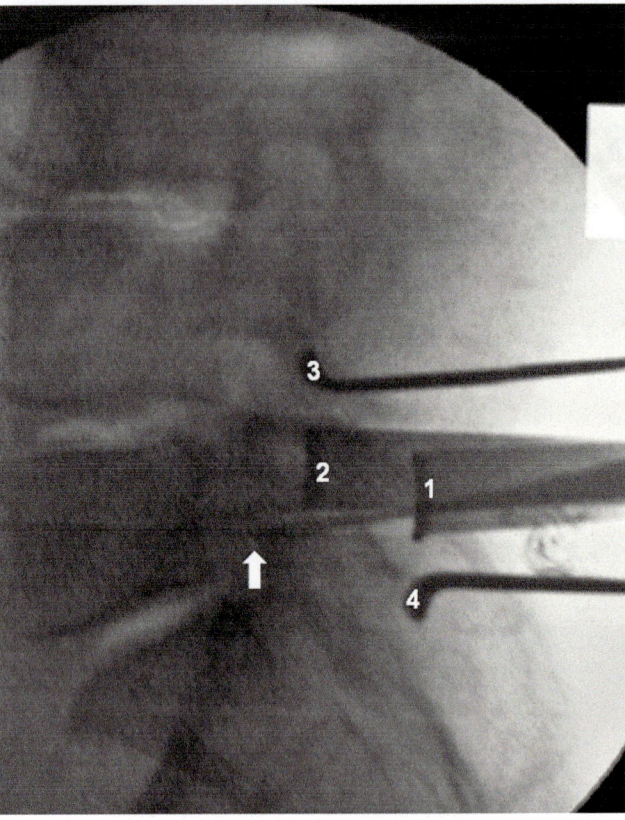

Fig. 58.17 Intraoperative fluoroscopic control L5/S1: (1) medial blade on the facet joint, (2) lateral blade, (3) cranial blade a bit cephalad to the transverse process L5, (4) blade on the ala sacri, dissector pointing to the DH (*arrow*)

recommends the use of two counterretractors inserted perpendicular to each other. That allows to choose four blades of different lengths matching with the following structures: facet joint (medial), transverse plane (lateral), transverse process (cranial), and ala (caudal) (Figs. 58.16 and 58.17). Furthermore, the use of the microscope "skin to skin" is advised.

- *Skin*: 3 cm in length, 4 cm off the midline.
- *Transmuscular route*: after incision of the fascia of m. erector spinae, the muscle is dissected bluntly using the index finger along the cleavage plane between the multifidus and the longissimus muscle (Fig. 58.15). If this fibrous separation cannot be palpated, the muscle is split downward to the medial third of the transverse processes. The selected retractor is then introduced so that the tips rest firmly on the lower half of the upper transverse process and on the upper half of the lower one. The lateral surface of the pars interarticularis represents the medial border of the surgical exposure. A fluoroscopic check at this point of the procedure is essential (Fig. 58.18).
- *Extraforaminal compartment*: tilting the OR table by 15–20° away from the surgeon gives a better view of the area lateral of the pedicle. Drilling off bone is usually not necessary, except in the case of an extremely hypertrophied facet joint or at the L5/S1 level. The medial half of the intertransverse muscle is incised and pushed laterally, thereby exposing the intertransverse membrane, also called the "intertransverse ligament." After its incision, the fat surrounding the nerve appears. Because of the proximity of the nerve, the accompanying vessels, and DH, the sucker should also be used as a nerve retractor. However, beware of an excessive retraction of the dorsal ganglion in order to minimize the incidence of postoperative burning dysesthesias! Branches of the radicular artery should be dissected carefully and spared whenever possible. The accompanying veins can be cauterized if they hinder the access to the disk fragment.
- *Management of the DH*: Typically, we find the nerve and the ganglion pushed laterally and cranially by the mostly free disk fragment. As a rule, removal of the fragment alone is sufficient. If an extensive perforation of the annulus is evident, clearing of the disk space should be considered. After probing the root canal with a double-angled blunt hook for residual fragments, the nerve may be covered with a Gelfoam soaked with crystalline steroid.
- *Closure*: placing a drain is optional and, in our experience, seldom necessary. Musculature requires no suturing.
- *Special considerations for the L5/S1 level*: because of the particular anatomical relationship among disk space, transverse process L5, and ala, the microsurgical muscle-splitting approach at the lumbosacral level should be practiced by a surgeon who is already familiar with the technique at the more cranial levels. Repeated intraoperative fluoroscopic checks may also be necessary. If difficulties should arise, switching to the conventional "macroapproach" should be considered.
- *Postoperative care*: as previously described.

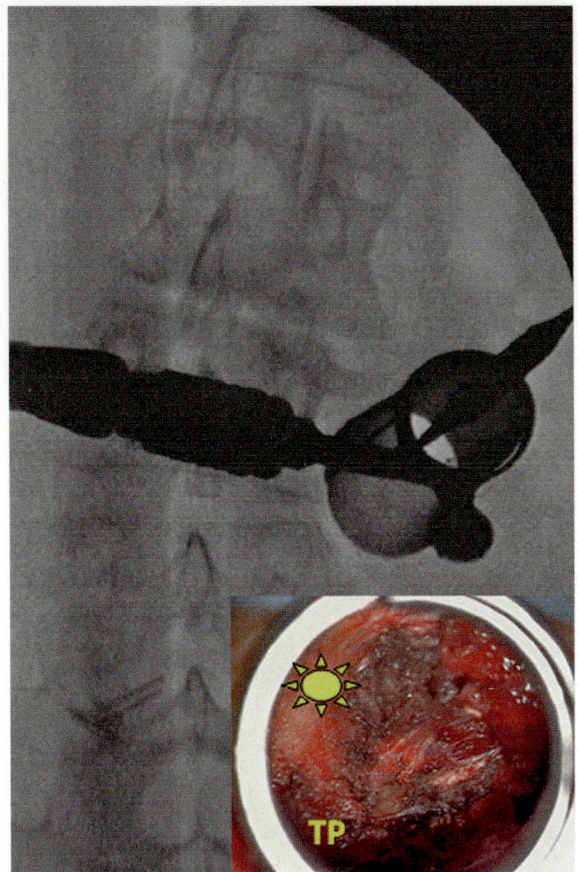

Fig. 58.18 Intraoperative fluoroscopic control in AP view for approaching a left-sided extraforaminal DH L3/L4. Note the concave curve of the degenerative scoliosis. Close-up view of the medial third of the transverse process (*asterisk*) (*bottom right*)

58.4.6 Complications

Reflex sympathetic dystrophy occurs in 1–2% of the patients, mostly within 1 week after surgery, especially at the L5/S1 level. It is characterized by burning discomfort of the shiny leg, which becomes very sensitive to touch. Due to the intracanalicular location of the ganglion, every manipulation of the nerve in the extraforaminal compartment stretches the ganglion, which may cause postoperative causalgic disturbances. Therapy: codeine, sympathetic block (Marcaine 1%), and physiotherapy.

References

1. Mixter WJ, Barr JS. Rupture of the intervertebral disc with involvement of the spinal canal. N Engl J Med. 1934;211:210–2015.
2. Caspar W. A new surgical procedure for lumbar disc herniation causing less tissue damage through a microsurgical approach. Adv Neurosurg. 1977;4:74–7.
3. Yasargil GM. Microsurgical operation of herniated lumbar disc. Adv Neurosurg. 1977;4:81–5.
4. Williams RW. Microlumbar discectomy: a conservative approach to the virgin herniated lumbar disc. Spine. 1978;3(2):175–82.
5. Abdullah AF, Ditto EW, Byrd EB. Extreme-lateral lumbar disc herniations: clinical syndrome and special problems of diagnosis. J Neurosurg. 1974;41(2):229–34.
6. Reulen HJ, Pfaundler S, Ebeling U. The lateral microsurgical approach to the "extracanalicular" lumbar disc herniation. A technical note. Acta Neurochir. 1987;84:64–7.
7. Mayer HM. Lumbar disc herniations: the microsurgical interlaminar, paramedian approach. In: Mayer HM, editor. Minimally invasive spine surgery. Heidelberg: Springer; 2005. p. 284–96.
8. Di Lorenzo N, Porta F, Onnis G, et al. Pars interarticularis fenestration in the treatment of foraminal lumbar disc herniation: a further surgical approach. Neurosurgery. 1998;42:87–90.
9. Bernucci C, Giovanelli M. Translaminar microsurgical approach for lumbar herniated nucleus pulposus (HNP) in the "hidden zone": clinical and radiologic results in a series of 24 patients. Spine. 2007;32(2):281–4.
10. Papavero L. Lumbar disc herniations: the translaminar approach. In: Mayer HM, editor. Minimally invasive spine surgery. Heidelberg: Springer; 2005. p. 304–14.
11. Soldner F, Helper BM, Wallenfang T, et al. The translaminar approach to canalicular and cranio-dorsolateral lumbar disc herniations. Acta Neurochir. 2002;144:315–20.
12. Vogelgesang JP. The translaminar approach in combination with a tubular retractor system for the treatment of far cranio-laterally and foraminally extruded lumbar disc herniations. Zentralbl Neurochir. 2007;68(1):24–8.
13. Papavero L. Lumbar disc herniations: the extraforaminal approach. In: Mayer HM, editor. Minimally invasive spine surgery. Heidelberg: Springer; 2005. p. 297–303.
14. Tessitore E, de Tribolet N. Far-lateral lumbar disc herniation: the microsurgical transmuscular approach. Neurosurgery. 2004;54(4):939–42.

Microsurgical Decompression

59

Frank Grochulla

59.1 Introduction and Core Messages

Degenerative lumbar spinal canal stenosis is a frequent disease of the "aging spine," leading to mono- or bilateral leg symptoms that are often described as spinal claudication [1–3]. The primary goal in treatment is to relieve the patients' leg symptoms. Surgery for lumbar spinal stenosis is generally accepted when conservative treatment has failed or if progressive neurological deficits occur [4]. In the past, laminectomies are considered to be the treatment of choice in lumbar spinal stenosis without instability [3, 5, 6]. Due to the risk of destabilization after laminectomy, limited approaches and less invasive techniques for decompression have been proposed by several authors [7–10]. Today, laminotomy under microscopic guidance is the preferred surgical technique in lumbar spinal stenosis presenting without additional deformity or segmental instability. During the past decade, approaches and techniques for laminotomy have been modified in different manners. In this chapter, the ipsilateral interlaminar approach for microsurgical decompression of the ipsilateral and contralateral spinal canal in the so-called over-the-top technique is described.

59.2 Indications

- Acquired degenerative central and lateral spinal canal stenosis with clinical symptoms (e.g., spinal claudication), verified by MRI or CT scan
- Failed conservative treatment
- No symptoms/signs for segmental instability

59.3 Contraindications

- Unstable lumbar degenerative scoliosis
- Spondylolisthesis grade I or higher with dominant low-back pain
- Severe and/or dominant low-back pain
- Absolute contraindications for general anesthesia

59.4 Technical Prerequisites

- Microscope
- Microsurgical instruments (e.g., Bayonet-shaped instruments)
- Tubular retractor system (e.g., Caspar retractor)
- High-speed drill
- Fluoroscopy

59.5 Planning, Preparation, and Positioning

The patient is placed prone for this procedure on a Wilson frame or alternatively placed on a special operating table in the knee-chest position (mecca position) (see Fig. 59.1). In this positioning, the abdomen is free, thus relieving pressure on the abdominal venous system and decreasing venous backflow into the spinal canal through Batson plexus. Furthermore, the amount of lumbar lordosis is decreased, and the interlaminar spaces are widened. Thus, it is easier to enter the spinal canal for decompression.

F. Grochulla (✉)
Metropol Medical Center, Clinic for Orthopedics, Trauma Surgery and Spinal Surgery, Nuremberg, Germany
e-mail: frank.grochulla@mmc-nuernberg.de

© Springer-Verlag GmbH Germany 2023
U. Vieweg, F. Grochulla (eds.), *Manual of Spine Surgery*, https://doi.org/10.1007/978-3-662-64062-3_59

447

Fig. 59.1 (**a**) Knee-chest (mecca) position, situation in the OR and illustration (**b**), and as an alternative prone positioning (**c**)

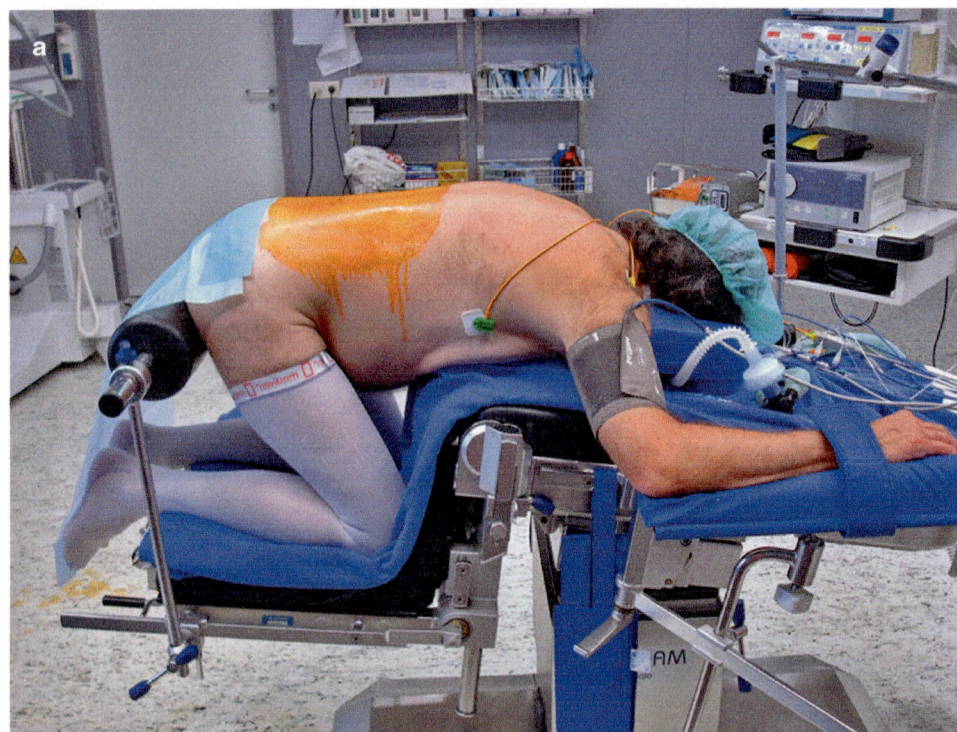

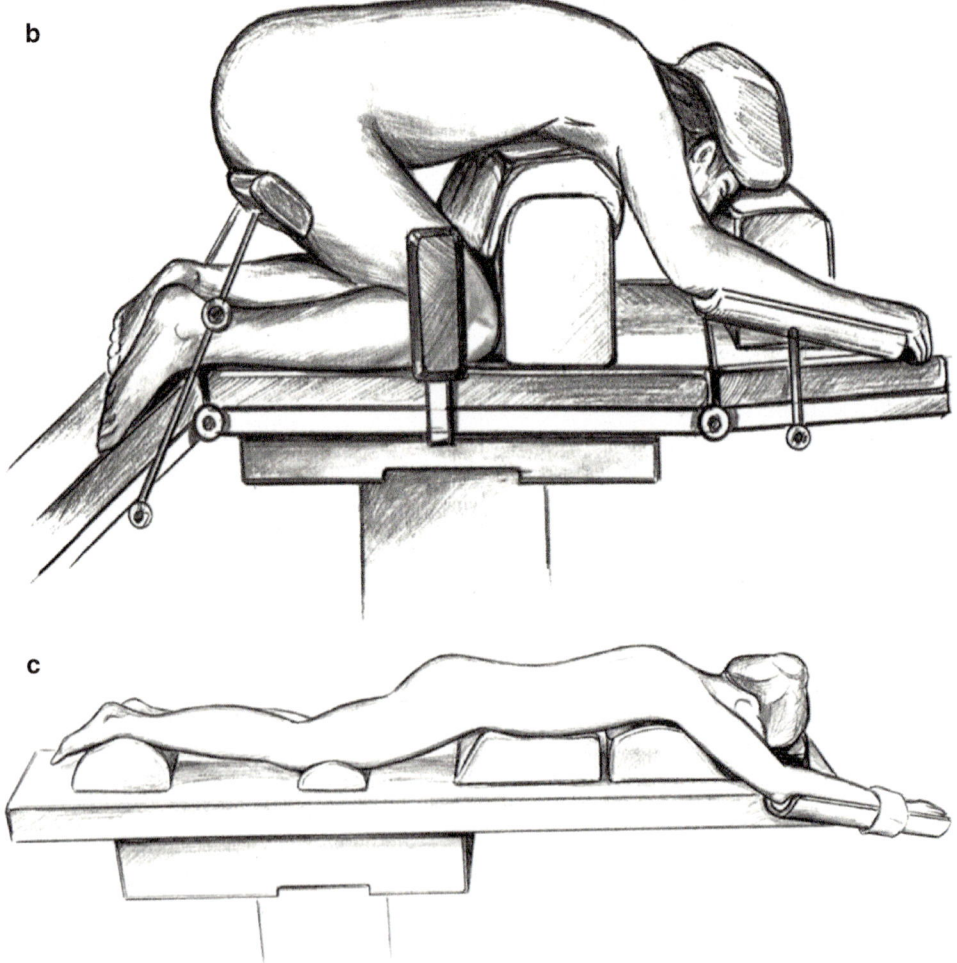

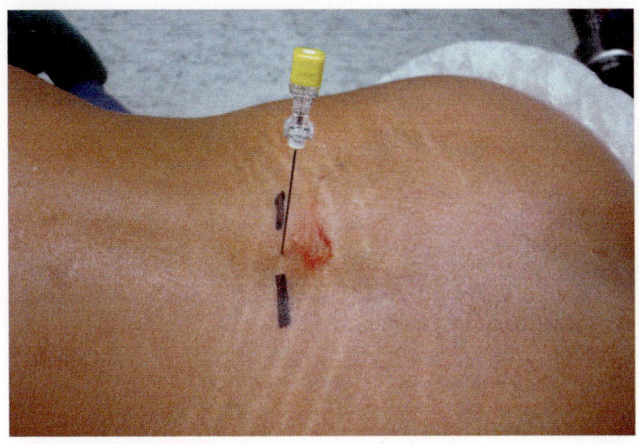

Fig. 59.2 The target level is localized with an inserted needle under lateral fluoroscopy control

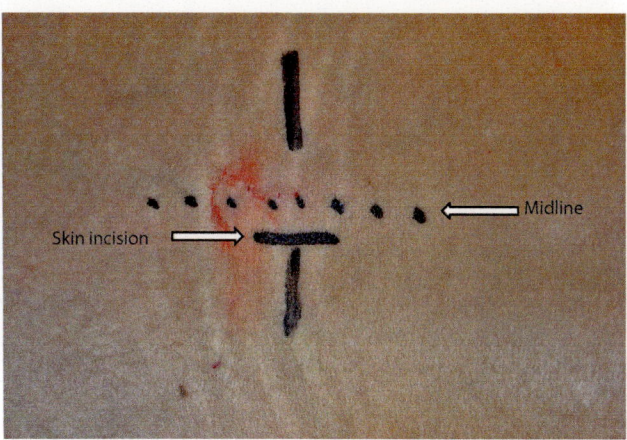

Fig. 59.3 Skin incision 5–10 mm lateral to the spinous process on the affected side and typically 2–3 cm in length for one level

For positioning, some special aspects have to be considered in (mostly elderly) patients with acquired spinal canal stenosis: patients can have limited mobility of the joints (shoulder, hip, knee) and of the cervical spine (avoid head rotation!).

Localization: The target level(s) is localized with an inserted needle under lateral fluoroscopy control, and the approach is planned and marked (see Fig. 59.2). It is important to place the superficial approach exactly over the lumbar segment of interest because of the limited extent of the microsurgical approach.

59.6 Surgical Techniques

- The author recommends the application of the surgical microscope from the beginning of the surgical procedure.
- The skin incision is up to 5–10 mm lateral to the spinous process on the affected side and typically 2–3 cm in length for one level. In the presence of bilateral symptoms, a left-sided approach is preferred for right-handed surgeons.
- A semicircular paramedian incision is made in the thoracolumbar fascia. The length of this incision can be longer than the skin incision (see Fig. 59.3).
- Subperiosteal dissection of the paravertebral muscles is carried out, and a self-retraining speculum retractor (Caspar, Aesculap,- or metrx retractor, Medtronic) is inserted (see Fig. 59.4). It is necessary to control the force of the retractor during surgery to avoid pressure necrosis of the surrounding cutaneous and musculature tissue.
- The laminae of the adjacent vertebrae and the interlaminar space are exposed.

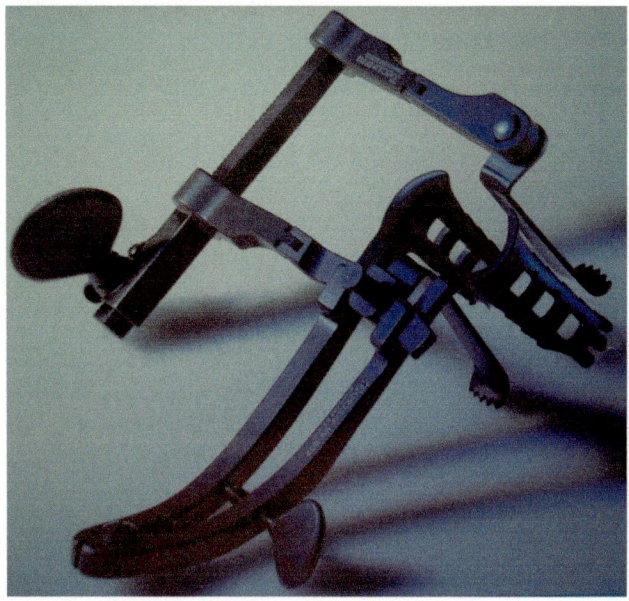

Fig. 59.4 Caspar tubular retractor system

- With a high-speed burr (see Fig. 59.5a, b), the decompression of the ipsilateral spinal canal is started with the removal of lower half of the cephalad lamina until the origin of the ligamentum flavum is exposed (see Fig. 59.6). The ligamentum flavum will be seen to thin out at the cephalad lamina and is detached from the lamina with a dissector. At this point, epidural fat and the dura can be identified (see Fig. 59.7). The extension of the interlaminar space is completed by resection of the cephalad part of the caudal lamina and by resection of a portion of the medial part of the facet joint (medial facetectomy).
- After complete exposure of the ipsilateral ligamentum flavum, it can be removed with rongeurs. Adhesions of the dura to the ligamentum flavum are dissected carefully in order to avoid dural laceration.

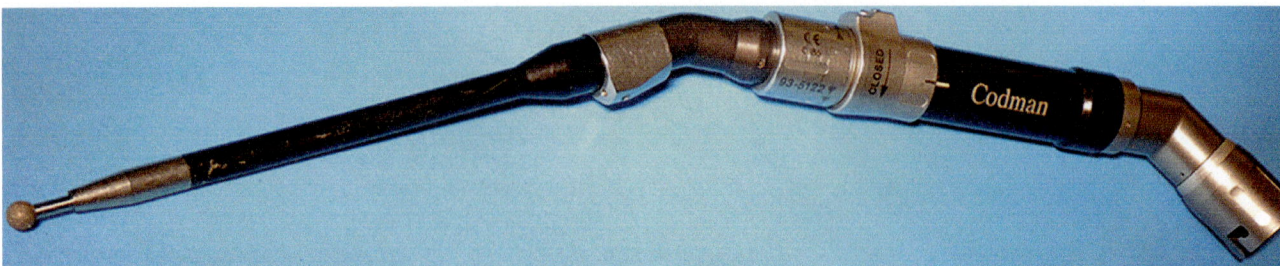

Fig. 59.5 Angular handpiece for high-speed drill

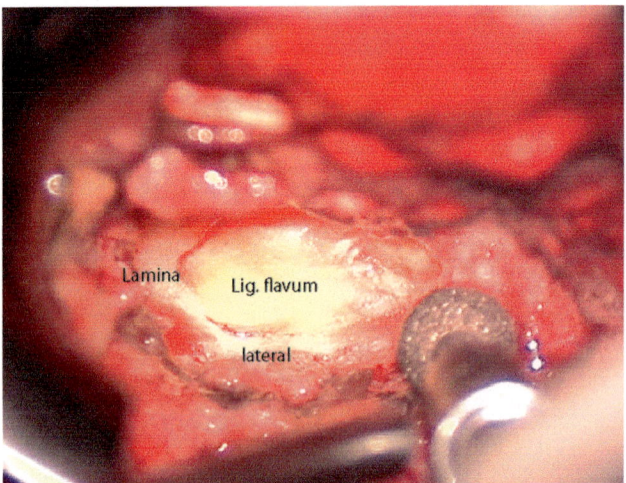

Fig. 59.6 Partial removal of the lamina and exposure of the ligamentum flavum

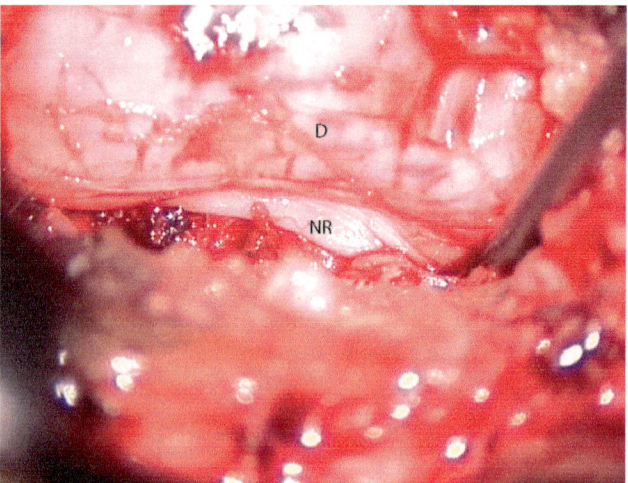

Fig. 59.8 Exposure of dura and nerve root after ipsilateral decompression. *D* dura, *NR* nerve root

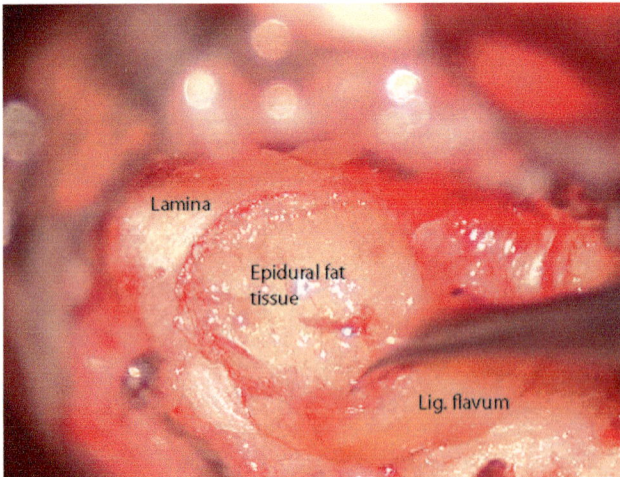

Fig. 59.7 The ligamentum flavum is detached from the lamina with a dissector. Epidural fat and the dura can be identified

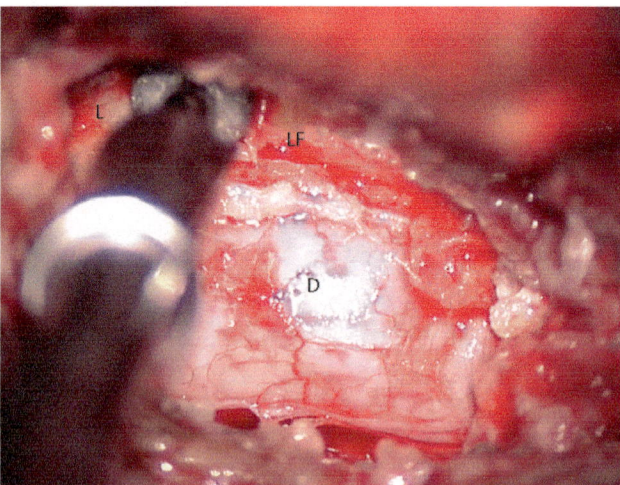

Fig. 59.9 Undercutting of the lamina with a high-speed burr. *L* lamina, *LF* ligamentum flavum, *D* dura

- An adequate ipsilateral subarticular decompression has been accomplished when the medial part of the pedicle and the lateral border of the nerve root are identified—and when the traversing nerve root can be easily mobilized (Fig. 59.8).

- The contralateral decompression is initiated by a tilting of the table away from the surgeon, and the microscope is adjusted to obtain a clear field of vision across the midline. Utilizing a high-speed burr, the undercutting of the adjacent laminae and the part of the base of the spinous process is performed (Fig. 59.9).

- The next step is the resection of the contralateral ligamentum flavum and the subarticular decompression until the lateral border of the dura and the medial border of the contralateral inferior pedicle are identified. In cases with severe stenosis, the dura should be separated from the ligamentum flavum with blunt dissection before resection to avoid cerebrospinal fluid leak.
- The adequate decompression should be checked with a blunt probe.
- Check the bone margins with a blunt dissector to be certain that no sharp bony spicules remain (which can penetrate the dura postoperatively).
- Meticulous hemostasis and wound closure.

59.7 Postoperative Care

- Bed rest for 6 h in supine position with elevated chest (30°) to elevate lumbar CSF pressure for compression of epidural veins.
- We recommend bracing only in cases with more than two-level decompression.

References

1. Berney J. Epidemiology of narrow spinal canal. Neurochirurgie. 1994;40:174–8.
2. Verbiest H. A radicular syndrome from developmental narrowing of the lumbar vertebral canal. J Bone Joint Surg Br. 1954;36-B:230–7.
3. Verbiest H. Pathomorphologic aspects of developmental lumbar stenosis. Orthop Clin North Am. 1975;5:177–96.
4. Amundsen T, Weber H, Nordal HJ, et al. Lumbar spinal stenosis: conservative or surgical management? A prospective 10-year study. Spine. 2000;25:1425–35.
5. Herkowitz HN, Kurz LT. Degenerative lumbar spondylolisthesis with spinal stenosis. A prospective study comparing decompression with decompression and intertransverse process arthrodesis. J Bone Joint Surg Am. 1991;73:802–8.
6. Silvers HR, Lewis PJ, Ash HL. Decompressive lumbar laminectomy for spinal stenosis. J Neurosurg. 1993;78:695–701.
7. Hopp E, Tsou PM. Postdecompression lumbar instability. Clin Orthop Relat Res. 1988;227:143–51.
8. McCulloch JA. Microsurgery for lumbar spinal canal stenosis. In: McCulloch JA, Young PH, editors. Essentials of spinal microsurgery. Philadelphia: Lippincott-Raven; 1998. p. 453–86.
9. Poletti CE. Central lumbar stenosis caused by ligamentum flavum: unilateral laminotomy for bilateral ligamentectomy. Preliminary report of two cases. Neurosurgery. 1995;37:343–7.
10. Senegas J, Etchevers JP, Vital JM, et al. Recalibration of the lumbar canal, an alternative to laminectomy in the treatment of lumbar canal stenosis. Rev Chir Orthop Reparatrice Appar Mot. 1988;74:15–22.

Endoscopic Lumbar Disk Surgery

60

Sebastian Ruetten

60.1 Introduction and Core Messages

Minimally invasive techniques can reduce tissue damage and its consequences. Endoscopic operations are now considered standard in certain areas. The most common full endoscopic technique for patients with lumbar disk afflictions is the posterolateral transforaminal operation. Laser and bipolar radiofrequency current can be used. Removal of intra- or extraforaminal disk herniations is technically possible. Resection of herniations within the spinal canal—in the sense of a retrograde removal from intradiscal through the existing annulus defect—has been described. Nevertheless, difficulties in the resection of herniated discs located within the spinal canal cannot always be completely ruled out. Using the lateral transforaminal access, the spinal canal can be more sufficiently reached under continuous visualization. Even so, the bony borders of the foramen and the exiting nerve may limit mobility and thus the resection of dislocated disk material. In addition, the pelvis and abdominal organs may hinder access. Thus, there may be limitations for the transforaminal procedure. The full endoscopic interlaminar access was developed to enable operation of pathologies outside the indication spectrum for the transforaminal procedure. The combination of new operative accesses with the technical advances now enables for the first time a full endoscopic procedure with visual control, which is equal to conventional operations when the indication criteria are heeded. Basically, the transforaminal procedure has more limitations than the interlaminar, but at the same time, it is less tissue traumatic.

60.2 Indication

60.2.1 General Indications

The indication for operation corresponds to current valid standards [1]. The greatest experience has been gained in the therapy of herniated discs and lateral spinal canal stenoses [2–6]. Existing secondary pathologies, such as instabilities, must possibly be treated at the same time with other procedures. The following indications are currently unequivocal (Figs. 60.1, 60.2, and 60.3):

- Sequestered or nonsequestered lumbar disk herniations, independent of localization
- Recurrent disk herniations after conventional or full endoscopic operations
- Lateral bony and ligamentary spinal canal stenoses
- In special cases, cysts of the zygapophyseal joint
- In special cases, positioning of implants in the intervertebral space
- In special cases, intervertebral debridement and draining in spondylodiscitis

60.2.2 Indication for Transforaminal Approach

All intra- and extraforaminal disk herniations are taken as indications for the transforaminal approach. In disk herniations within the spinal canal, the following inclusion criteria must be heeded due to the limited mobility [3–6]:

- Sequestration toward cranial maximal to the start of the pedicle above, toward caudal maximal to the middle of the pedicle below the level in question

S. Ruetten (✉)
Department of Orthopädic Surgery, Center for Spine Surgery and Pain Therapy, Center for Orthopaedics and Traumatology, St. Anna-Hospital, Herne, Germany
e-mail: spine-pain@annahospital.de;
spine-pain@elisabethgruppe.de

© Springer-Verlag GmbH Germany 2023
U. Vieweg, F. Grochulla (eds.), *Manual of Spine Surgery*, https://doi.org/10.1007/978-3-662-64062-3_60

Fig. 60.1 Posterolateral
transforaminal approach

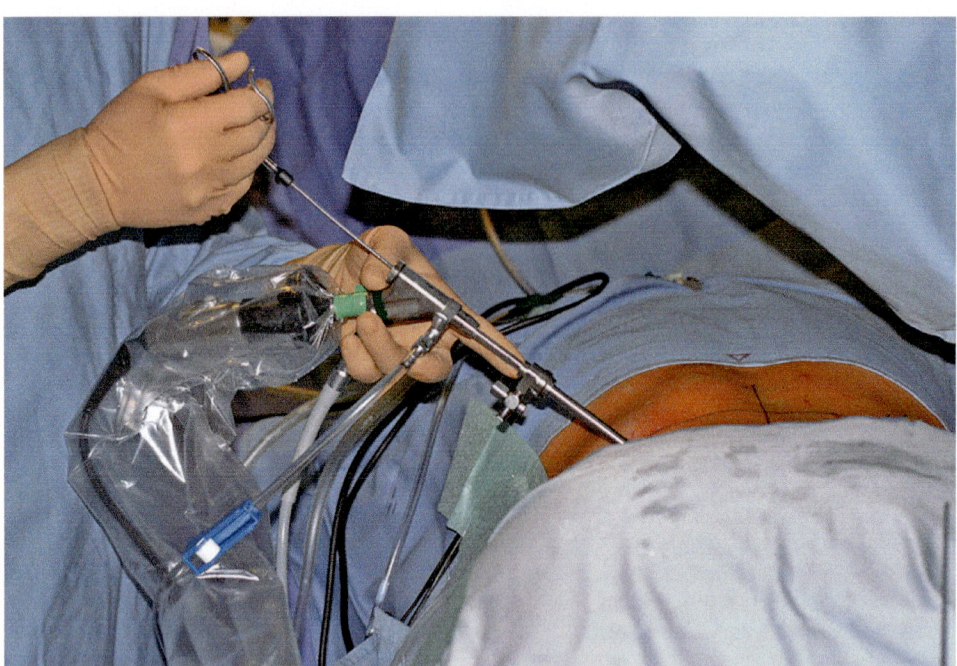

Fig. 60.2 Lateral
transforaminal approach

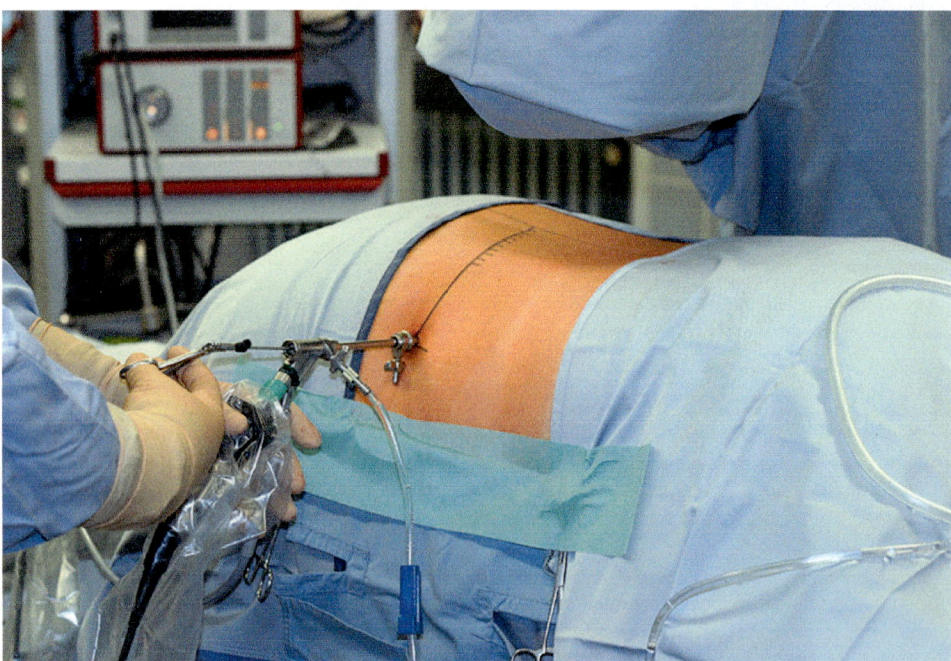

- In orthograde lateral ray path, pelvic overlay of the level in question maximal to the middle of the pedicle

    Note: In lateral spinal canal stenoses, the craniocaudal extension should reach maximal from the upper edge of the pedicle below to the lower edge of the pedicle above the level in question. In applying the usually necessary lateral approach, the access pathway may not be shifted by abdominal structures. This is especially to be heeded in the levels cranial to L3/4. If the finding is not entirely clear, a single

abdominal CT scan should be made through the disk for evaluation and preoperative planning.

60.2.3 Indication for Interlaminar Approach

- All disk herniations located within the spinal canal, which cannot be operated technically in the transforaminal approach because of the criteria cited, are taken as indications for the interlaminar approach [2–5].

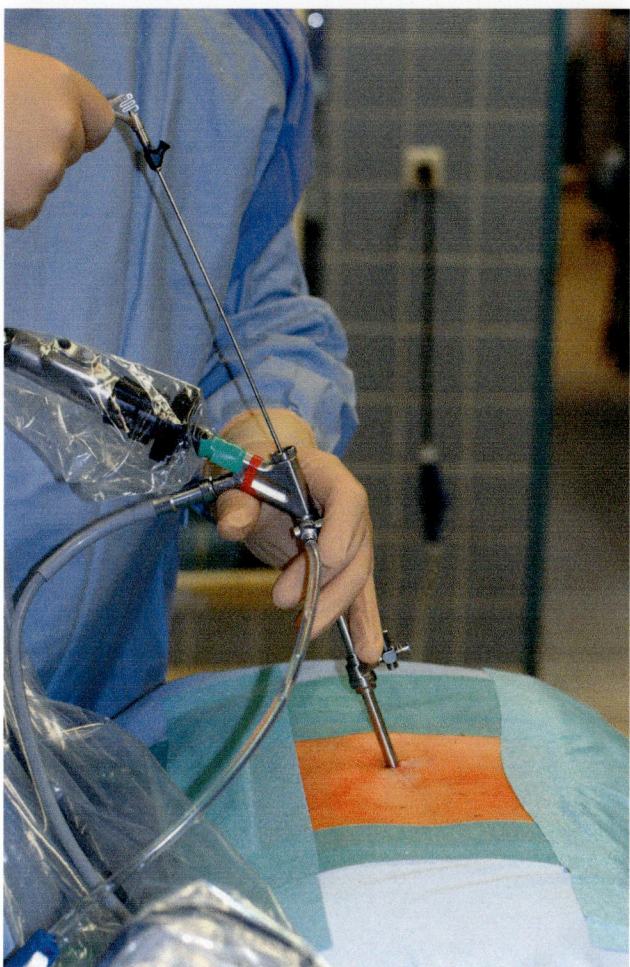

Fig. 60.3 Interlaminar approach

60.3   Contraindications

- All criteria, which generally apply as contraindications to decompressing operations, taking into consideration the specific technical possibilities and the inclusion criteria of each surgical procedure, are considered contraindications.

60.4   Technical Prerequisites

An X-ray permeable, electrically adjustable operation table and a C-arc are necessary. In addition to the surgical instruments and optics, general equipment for endoscopic operations under fluid flow are needed, such as monitor, camera unit, light source, documentation system, fluid pump, shaver system, or radio-frequency generator. Equipment available for arthroscopy or endoscopy can be used.

60.5   Planning, Preparation, and Positioning

As with all microsurgical techniques, the intraoperative procedure must be planned preoperatively based on imaging findings. The goal is to perform the resection of spinal canal structures as sparingly as possible depending on the pathology. Full endoscopic operations can usually be performed under general anesthesia. This is more comfortable for both the patient and the surgeon, enables positioning as needed, and also makes extensive work within the spinal canal possible. The operations are performed with the patient in prone position on an X-ray permeable table, under orthograde radiological control at two levels. The patient lies on a hip and thorax roll to relieve the abdominal and thoracic organs. The operation table can be adjusted intraoperative lumbar either lordotic or kyphotic depending on the anatomy and pathology. A single-shot antibiosis is applied for infection prophylaxis.

60.6   Operating Technique

60.6.1 Transforaminal Approach [3–6]

- First, the skin incision is localized. The goal is to reach the spinal canal as tangentially as possible. At levels L4/5 and L3/4, in lateral ray path, the dorsal line of the descending facet usually serves as the boundary, which should not be crossed toward ventral. To avoid injury to abdominal organs, a single abdominal CT scan through the individual disk should be made for evaluation and preoperative planning, especially in the cranial levels when findings are not unequivocal. Depending on the scan, an individual, less lateral approach should be selected.
- A 1.5-mm atraumatic spinal needle is inserted through the skin incision orthograde to the disk space in the target area (Fig. 60.4). After a 0.8-mm target wire is inserted and the cannula removed, the cannulated dilator is inserted.
- The target wire is removed, and the 7.9-mm operation sheath with beveled opening is pushed through the dilator (Figs. 60.5 and 60.6). From this point on, decompression is made under visualization and continuous irrigation with isotonic saline without any special additives.
- Further entry into the epidural space, which may be required, is made under visual control. If the bony diameter of the foramen does not permit passage, the foramen is widened with a burr and instruments.
- If the position of the exiting nerve is not clear, for example, in intra- or extraforaminal herniation or foraminal stenosis, an extraforaminal access is created on the caudal

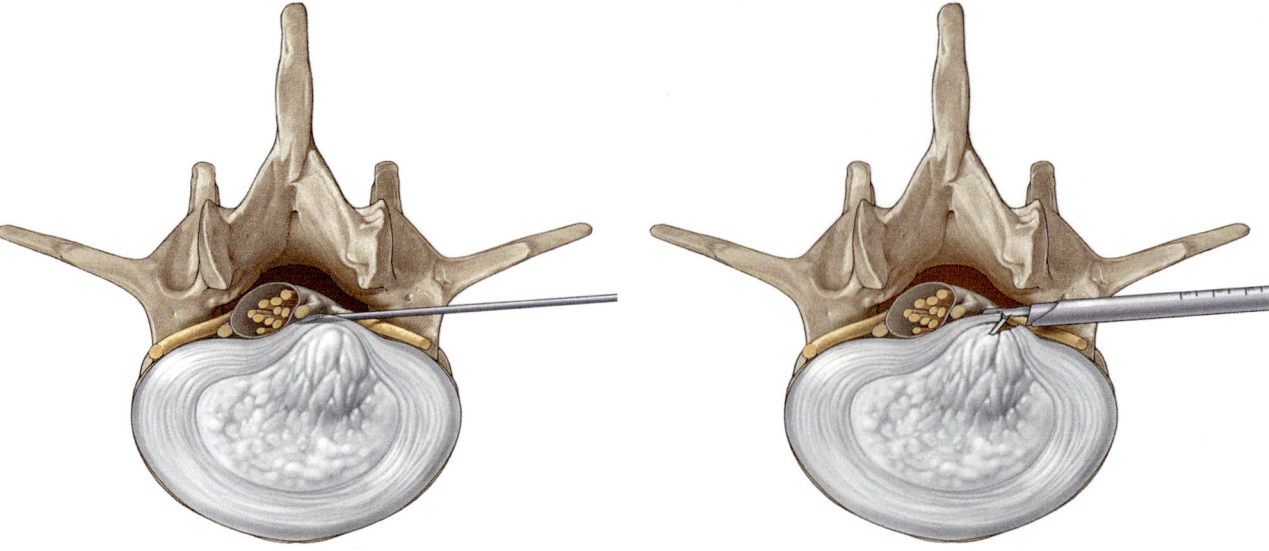

Fig. 60.4 Example of the end position of the operation sheath *AP* in the spinal canal

Fig. 60.6 Full endoscopic transforaminal operation

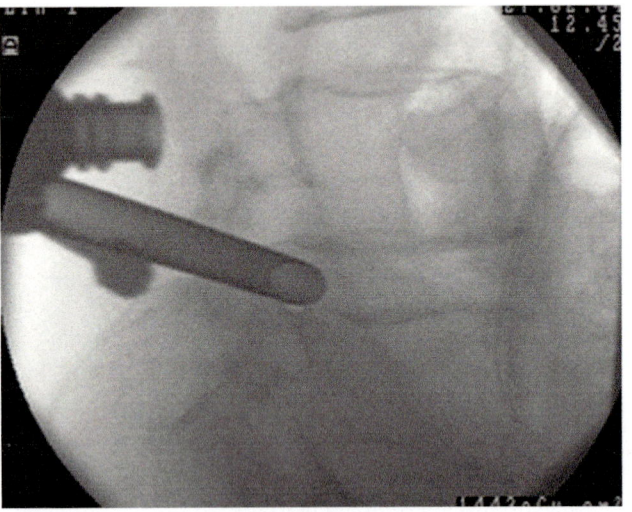

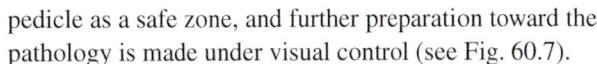

Fig. 60.5 The opening of the operation sheath is in the epidural space

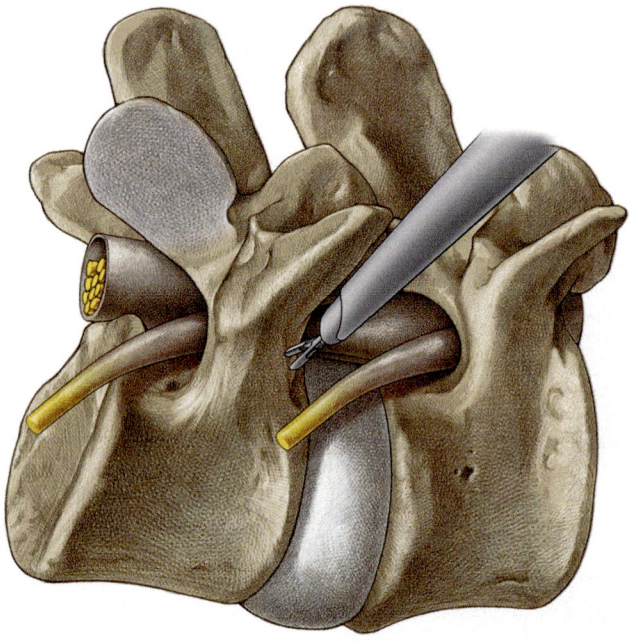

Fig. 60.7 Start of the extraforaminal operation on the caudal pedicle outside the foramen

pedicle as a safe zone, and further preparation toward the pathology is made under visual control (see Fig. 60.7).
- The precise performance of decompression depends on the finding in each case.

60.6.2 Interlaminar Approach [2–5]

- The skin incision is made as medial as possible over the interlaminar window. The craniocaudal localization depends on the findings of the pathology in question.
- The dilator is inserted bluntly on the lateral edge of the ligamentum flavum or on the descending facet of the zygapophyseal joint.

- The 7.9-mm operation sheath with beveled opening is inserted via the dilator in the direction of the ligament (see Fig. 60.8).
- From this point on, the further procedure is performed under visualization and continuous irrigation with isotonic saline solution without any special additive. To reach the spinal canal, the ligamentum flavum is incised lateral to ca. 3–5 mm.
- The further procedure is enabled by the elasticity of the ligament (see Figs. 60.9 and 60.10).

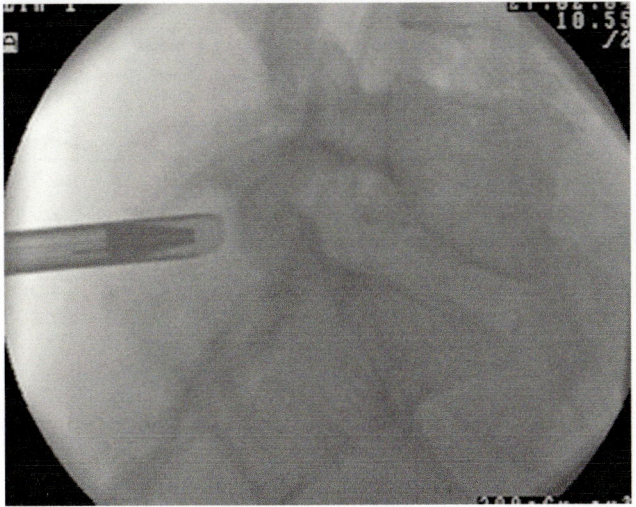

Fig. 60.8 Inserted dilator with operation sheath

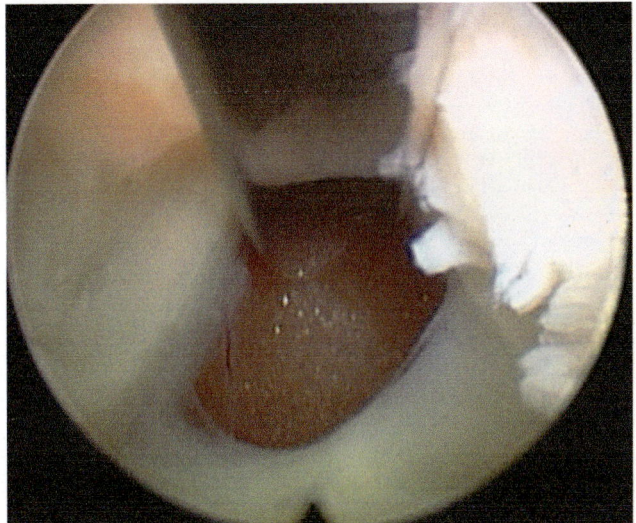

Fig. 60.9 Lateral incision of the ligamentum flavum

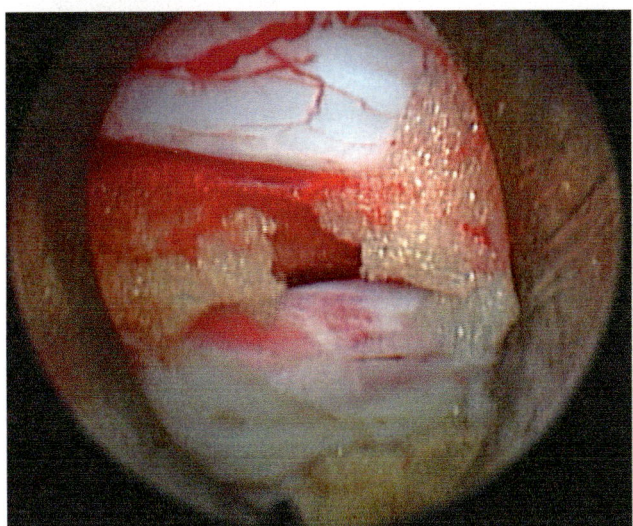

Fig. 60.10 Identification of the anatomical structures

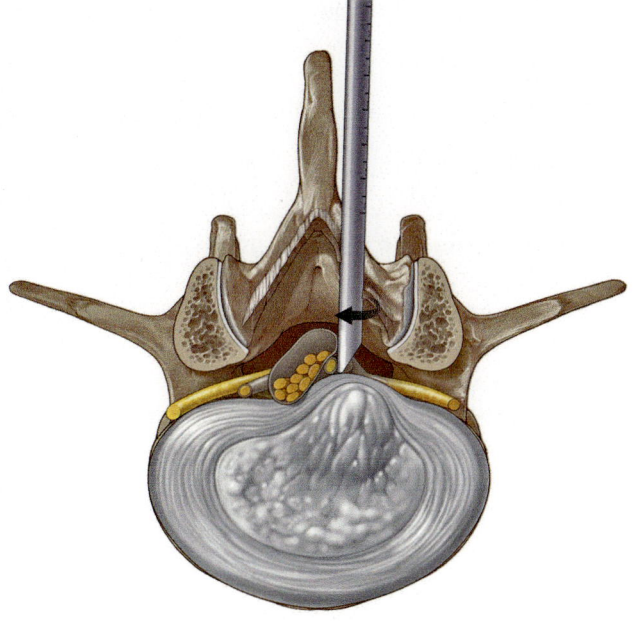

Fig. 60.11 Rotation of the operation sheath

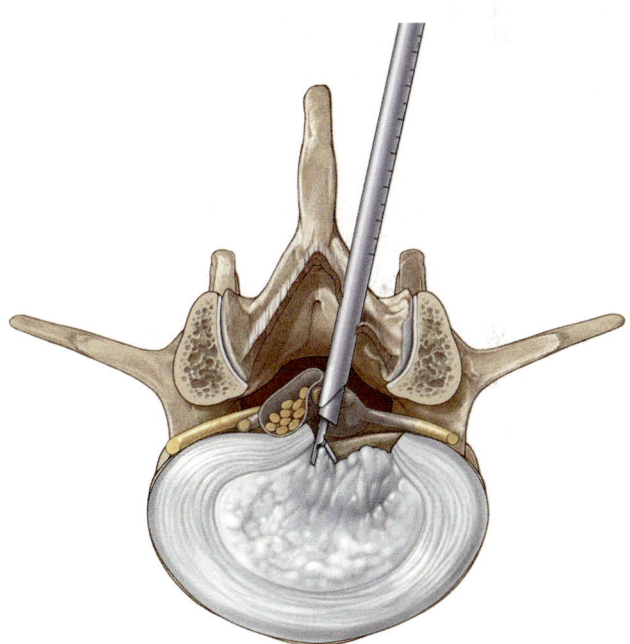

Fig. 60.12 Full endoscopic interlaminar operation

- The operation sheath with beveled opening can be used as a second instrument by rotation and serves, for example, as a nerve hook in shifting the neural structures toward medial (see Figs. 60.11 and 60.12).
- If the bony diameter of the interlaminar window does not permit passage or in the operation of a spinal canal stenosis, the window is enlarged using a burr and instruments.
- In cases of clearly dislocated sequesters, which cannot be completely reached from a level without more extensive

bone resection, consideration can be given to creating another access later via the neighboring interlaminar window.

- The precise performance of the decompression depends on the findings in each case.

60.7 Possible Complications

Possible complications during microsurgical procedures are known, and there are numerous publications [7–10]. A minimally invasive procedure can reduce the complication rate, though statistically, it cannot be completely avoided [11, 12]. In principle, all of the complications are possible, which are known in conventional operating procedures [2–6]. With respect to the full endoscopic procedures, it must be emphasized that a one- or two-sided switch to an open procedure may be necessary for the therapy of a complication. Especially, endoscopic suture of a dural injury is technically not possible. Theoretically, in long operating times and overlooked blockage of the outflow of irrigation fluid, the consequences of increased pressure within the spinal canal and the attached and neighboring structures cannot be completely ruled out. In the interlaminar approach, a long-lasting and uninterrupted excessive retraction of the neural structures with the working sheath toward medial must be avoided or made only intermittently in order to avoid the risk of neurological damage. In the transforaminal approach, the risk of injury to the exiting nerves cannot be completely ruled out. In using the lateral access, it must be ruled out that abdominal organs block the path of access. Especially during the learning curve, experience has shown that there is an increased risk that complications will occur, as is the case in any new technique.

References

1. Andersson GBJ, Brown MD, Dvorak J, et al. Consensus summary on the diagnosis and treatment of lumbar disc herniation. Spine. 1996;21:75–8.
2. Ruetten S, Komp M, Merk H, et al. Surgical treatment for lumbar lateral recess stenosis with the full-endoscopic interlaminar approach versus conventional microsurgical technique: a prospective, randomized, controlled study. J Neurosurg Spine. 2009;10:476–85.
3. Ruetten S, Komp M, Merk H, et al. Recurrent lumbar disc herniation following conventional discectomy: a prospective, randomized study comparing full-endoscopic interlaminar and transforaminal versus microsurgical revision. J Spinal Disord Tech. 2009;22:122–9.
4. Ruetten S, Komp M, Merk H, et al. Full-endoscopic interlaminar and transforaminal lumbar discectomy versus conventional microsurgical technique: a prospective, randomized, controlled study. Spine. 2008;33:931–9.
5. Ruetten S, Komp M, Merk H, et al. Use of newly developed instruments and endoscopes: full-endoscopic resection of lumbar disc herniations via the interlaminar and lateral transforaminal approach. J Neurosurg Spine. 2007;6:521–30.
6. Ruetten S, Komp M, Godolias G. An extreme lateral access fort the surgery of lumbar disc herniations inside the spinal canal using the full-endoscopic uniportal transforaminal approach—technique and prospective results of 463 patients. Spine. 2005;30:2570–8.
7. Ramirez LF, Thisted R. Complications and demographic characteristics of patients undergoing lumbar discectomy in community hospitals. Neurosurgery. 1989;25:226–31.
8. Rompe JD, Eysel P, Zollner J. Intra- and postoperative risk analysis after lumbar intervertebral disk operation. Z Orthop Ihre Grenzgeb. 1999;137:201–5.
9. Stolke D, Sollmann WP, Seifert V. Intra- and postoperative complications in lumbar disc surgery. Spine. 1989;14:56–9.
10. Wildfoerster U. Intraoperative complications in lumbar intervertebral disc operations. cooperative study of the spinal study group of the German Society of Neurosurgery. Neurochirurgica. 1991;34:53–6.
11. Schick U, Doehnert J, Richter A, et al. Microendoscopic lumbar discectomy versus open surgery: an intraoperative EMG study. Eur Spine J. 2002;11:20–6.
12. Weber BR, Grob D, Dvorak J, et al. Posterior surgical approach to the lumbar spine and its effect on the multifidus muscle. Spine. 1997;22:1765–72.

Translaminar Screw Fixation

61

Stefan Schären

61.1 Introduction and Core Messages

Translaminar screws (TLSs) were developed by F. Magerl in 1980 as an evolution to the transarticular screws first published by D. King in 1948 and later modified by H. Boucher in 1959 [1–3]. Compared to these precursors, TLSs have a longer trajectory in bone blocking the facet joints as setscrews more efficiently [4, 5]. Since the screw directory runs tangentially to the exiting nerve root, the risk for injury is minimal. Compared to pedicle screws, TLS yields inferior biomechanical stability especially in flexion and rotation [6, 7]. With pedicle screws nowadays being the gold standard for posterior instrumentation, TLS remains an elegant and cost-effective method for selected cases. The translaminar screw fixation is a safe and effective method for posterior stabilization of one or two motion segments. It is mostly used supplementary to anterior fusion techniques and can effectively stabilize one or two motion segments in conjunction with anterior instrumentation [8, 9]. This technique is contraindicated in anterior column defect.

61.2 Indications

Stabilization in degenerative disorders with mainly intact posterior elements:

- Posterior fusion of one or two motion segments from T12 to S1
- Supplementary to anterior interbody fusion

- In combination with pedicle instrumentation for long-range fusion (see Fig. 61.1)

61.3 Contraindications

- Missing posterior elements, for example, after laminectomy
- Missing anterior support, for example, fracture and tumor
- Fusion of three and more levels
- Severe osteoporosis

61.4 Technical Prerequisites

Fluoroscopy, positioning device (e.g., Relton Hall frame), 4.5-mm cortical screws in various lengths (usually 45–55 mm), preferably in titanium for better MRI compatibility (e.g., Synthes GmbH, Solothurn, Switzerland), long 3.2-mm drill and drill sleeve, and long tab. Alternatively, carbon/PEEK pins can be used (Signus GmbH, Alzenau, Germany) (see Fig. 61.2).

61.5 Surgical Technique

61.5.1 Approach

A standard midline posterior approach is performed with subperiosteal exposure of the spinous processes, laminae, and transverse processes. The joint capsules of the motion segments to be fused are resected, and the bony elements are thoroughly cleaned using a chisel. In order not to compromise the bony elements, which are important for the TLS, a formal decortication should not be performed. In case of spinal stenosis or disk hernia, decompressive laminotomy or discectomy is added, preserving the lamina.

S. Schären (✉)
Department of Orthopaedic Surgery/Spine, University Hospital, Basel, Switzerland
e-mail: sschaeren@uhbs.ch

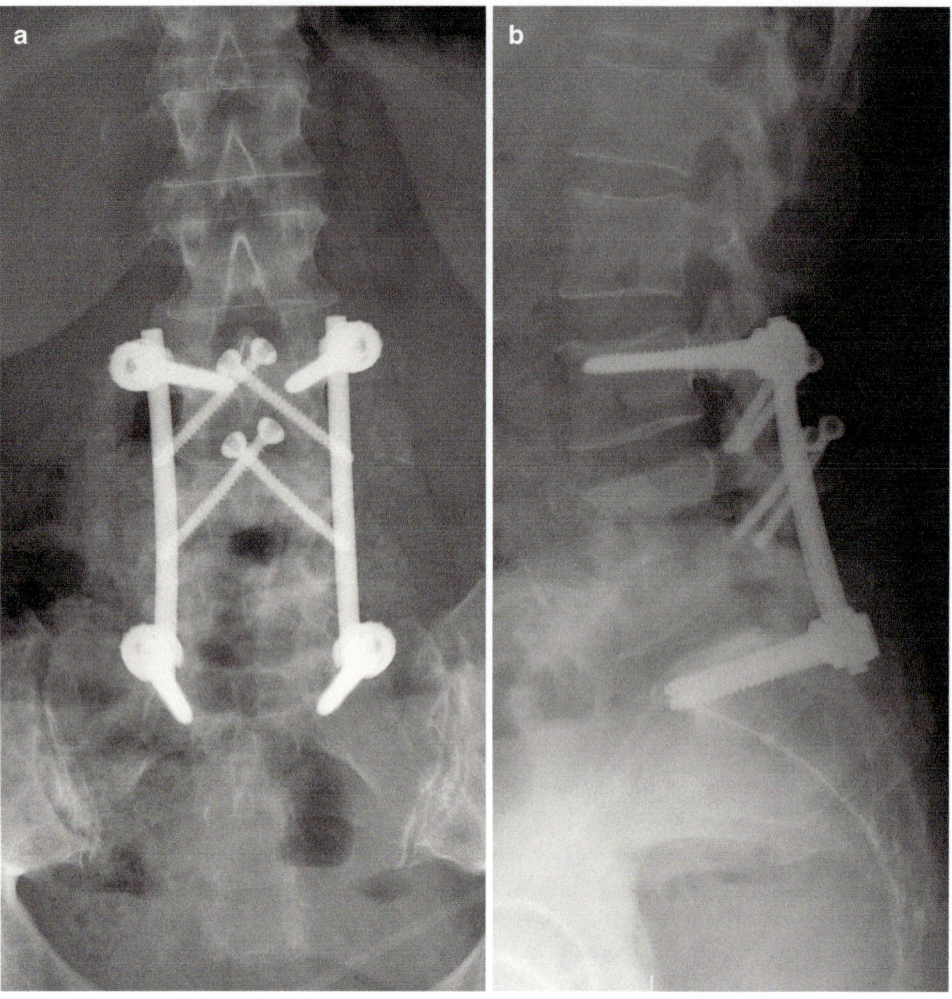

Fig. 61.1 (**a**, **b**) A 47-year-old woman with candida spondylodiscitis L4/5 with severe destruction of the adjacent end plates was treated with posterior transpedicular stabilization L3/S1, anterior debridement, and fusion L4/5 using iliac crest autograft followed by antimycotic treat-

ment. Translaminar screws L3/4 and L4/5 were used, avoiding the insertion of transpedicular screws penetrating into the infected vertebral bodies of L4 and L5. AP and lateral radiographs 24 months postoperatively show solid fusion and stable implants

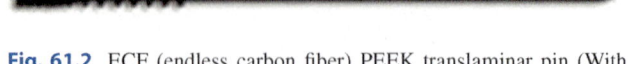

Fig. 61.2 ECF (endless carbon fiber) PEEK translaminar pin (With permission from Signus GmbH, Alzenau, Germany)

61.6 Instrumentation

- The first screw hole is drilled starting cranially from the base of the spinous process aiming toward the inferior border of the opposite transverse process. The drill subcortically passes the contralateral lamina, crosses the facet joint, and penetrates the cortex of the transverse process (Fig. 61.3).

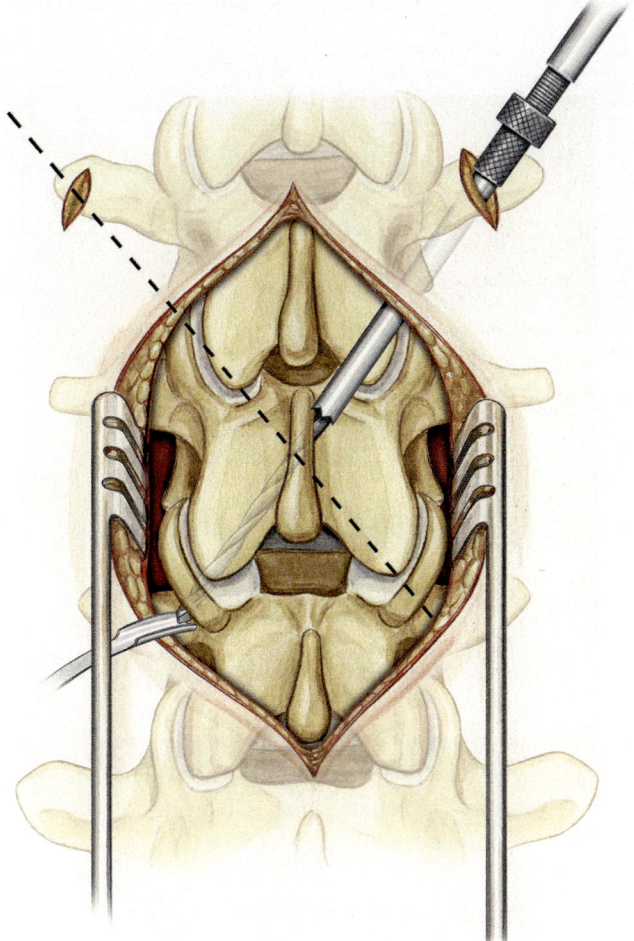

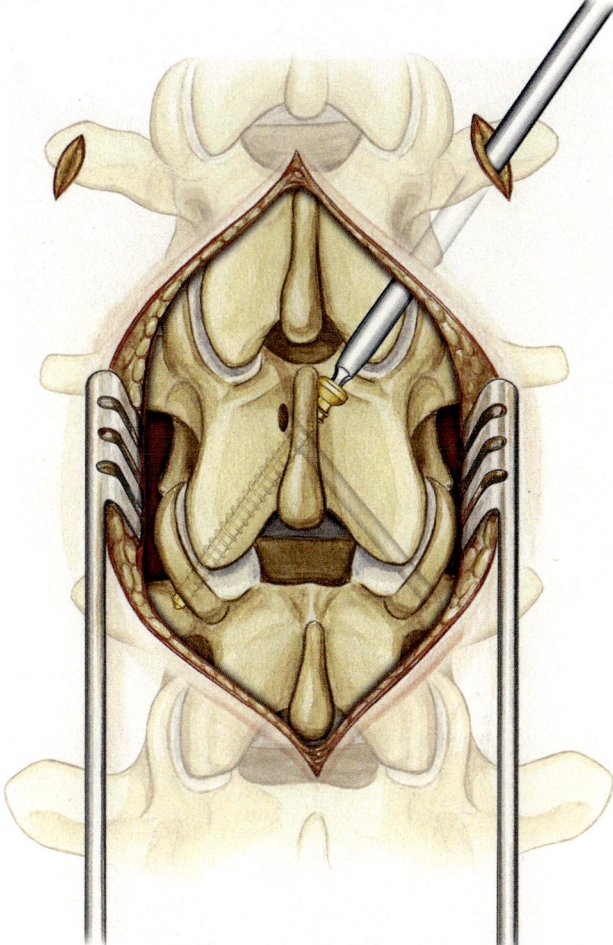

Fig. 61.4 Insertion of the 4.5-mm cortical screw of appropriate length

Fig. 61.3 Direction of a long 3.2-mm drill bit, protected with a drill sleeve

- After measuring the screw length, the hole is tabbed shortly across the facet joint taking care not to penetrate the outer cortex.
- The corresponding 4.5-mm titanium cortical screw is inserted until the screw head has contact with the spinous process (Fig. 61.4).
- The second screw hole is drilled running posterior to the first screw through the opposite lamina.
- After measuring and tabbing, a second screw is inserted (Figs. 61.5, 61.6, and 61.7).

- In case of posterior fusion, the posterior elements are covered with bone graft (e.g., from the iliac crest).

61.7   Tips and Tricks

- In the event of a deep situs and abundant soft tissues, it is possible to drill and insert the screw percutaneously using a troikar system.

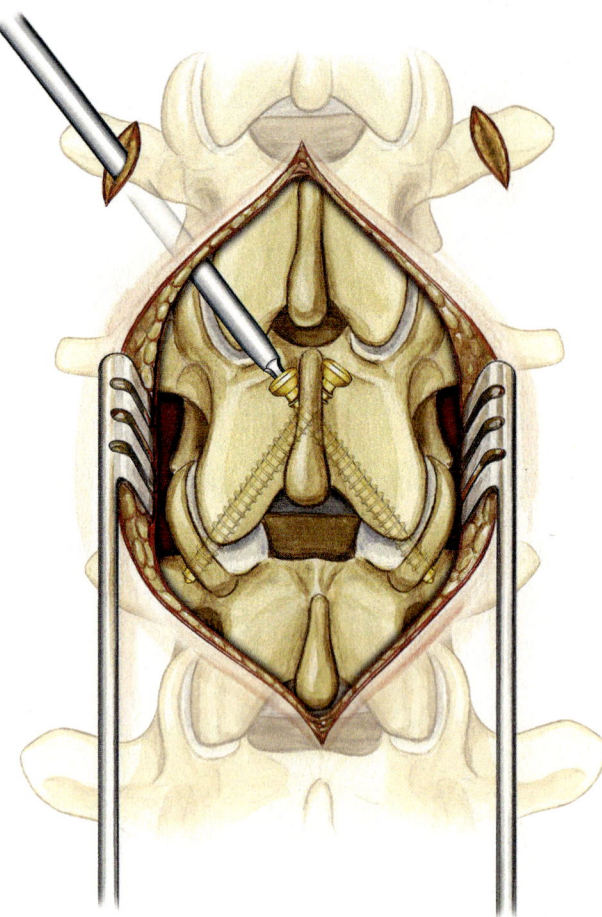

Fig. 61.5 Insertion of the second translaminar screw

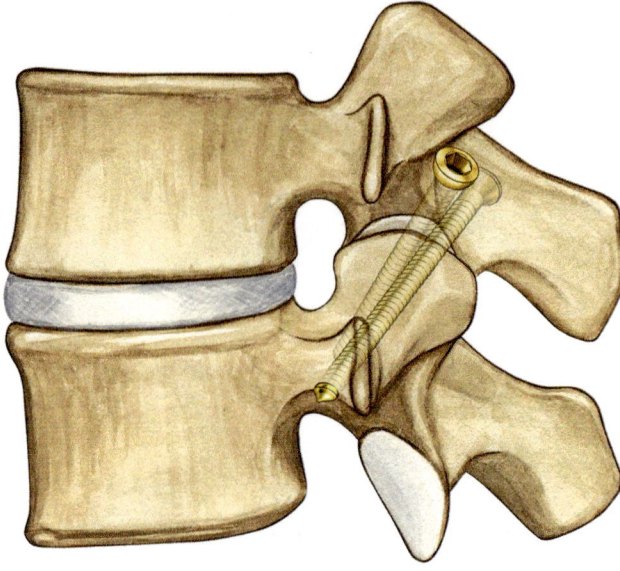

Fig. 61.7 Lateral view of the two-inserted screws

- Similarly, in case of anterior fusion, a minimized posterior approach can be performed, exposing only the spinous process, lamina, and facet joint, and inserting the screws percutaneously.

References

1. Boucher H. A method of spine fusion. J Bone Joint Surg. 1959;41-B:248–59.
2. King D. Internal fixation for lumbosacral fusion. Am J Surg. 1944;66:357–61.
3. Magerl F. Verletzungen der Brust- und Lendenwirbelsäule. Langenbecks Arch Chir. 1980;352:427–33.
4. Jeanneret B, Kleinstück F, Magerl F. Translaminar screw fixation of the lumbar facet joints. Oper Orthop Traumatol. 1995;4:37–53.
5. Montesano PX, Magerl F, Jacobs RR, et al. Translaminar facet joint screws. Orthopedics. 1988;11:1393–7.
6. Heggenes MH, Esses SI. Translaminar facet joint screw fixation for lumbar and lumbosacral fusion. A clinical and biomechanical study. Spine. 1991;16S:266–9.
7. Kandziora F, Schleicher P, Scholz M, et al. Biomechanical testing of the lumbar facet interference screw. Spine. 2005;30:E34–9.
8. Phillips FM, Cunningham B, Carandang G, et al. Effect of supplemental translaminar facet screw fixation on the stability of stand-alone anterior lumbar interbody fusion cages under physiologic compressive preloads. Spine. 2004;29:1731–6.
9. Rathonyi GC, Oxland TR, Gerich U, et al. The role of supplemental translaminar screws in anterior lumbar interbody fixation: a biomechanical study. Eur Spine J. 1998;7:400–7.

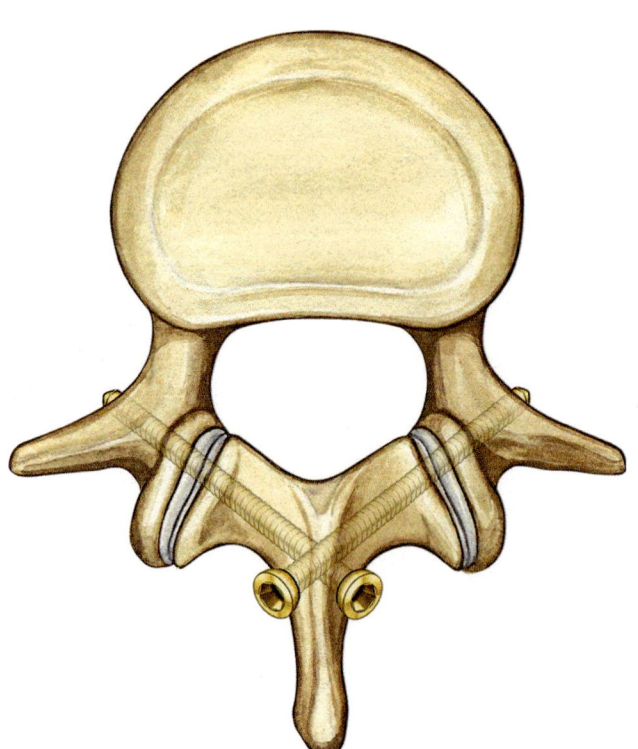

Fig. 61.6 Screws seen in the axial plane

Vertebroplasty and Kyphoplasty

62

Khalid Saeed, Edward Bayle, and Bronek Boszczyk

62.1 Introduction and Core Messages

Vertebroplasty and kyphoplasty are described including indications, contraindications, surgical technique, and complications. Both vertebroplasty and kyphoplasty achieve good pain relief in appropriately selected patients with osteoporotic compression fractures and those with spinal metastases, multiple myeloma, and some traumatic fractures as discussed further in the chapter. The main technical point to remember is never to cross the projection of medial pedicle cortex in AP view before posterior vertebral wall has been reached in the lateral view.

K. Saeed (✉)
Department of Spinal Surgery, New Cross Hospital, The Royal Wolverhampton Hospitals NHS Trust, Wolverhampton, UK
e-mail: drksaeed@hotmail.com

E. Bayle
Department of Spinal Surgery, The Centre for Spinal Studies and Surgery, Queens Medical Centre, University Hospital NHS Trust, Nottingham, UK

B. Boszczyk
The Centre for Spinal Studies and Surgery, Queens Medical Centre, University Hospital NHS Trust, Nottingham, UK
e-mail: Boszczyk@gmx.net

62.2 Indications

- Painful osteoporotic vertebral compression fractures (VCFs), which have failed conservative treatment or show unacceptable progressive collapse. Patients most likely to benefit have fractures that demonstrate bone marrow edema on MRI or radiotracer uptake on a nuclear medicine bone scintigram. Two recent randomized trials have concluded that they found no beneficial effect of vertebroplasty as compared with a sham procedure in patients with painful osteoporotic vertebral fractures [1, 2].

- Vertebral metastases with painful pathological fractures unsuitable for curative resection. Patients with spinal metastases and multiple myeloma can be treated with vertebral augmentation, and a biopsy can be obtained at the same time [3].

- Traumatic fractures
  Balloon kyphoplasty is principally suitable for treatment of vertebral fractures that have a localized fragmented zone within the spongiosa and a kyphotic deformity or for treatment of endplate impression fractures. These criteria are met by fractures of type A1.1 (endplate impression fracture), A1.2 (wedge fracture), and A3.1 (incomplete burst fracture) [1, 3–7] (see Fig. 62.1a–d). According to current knowledge, split fractures (A2), burst fractures (A3.2), and complete burst fractures (A3.3) are not suitable for balloon kyphoplasty, as the splitting component of these fractures cannot be stabilized by the augmentation. However, a complete burst fracture type A3.3 must be distinguished from an osteoporotic collapse of a vertebral body type A1.3 as the latter is suitable for balloon kyphoplasty, as the endplates are hardly fragmented or not fragmented at all, unlike in a complete burst fracture.

© Springer-Verlag GmbH Germany 2023
U. Vieweg, F. Grochulla (eds.), *Manual of Spine Surgery*, https://doi.org/10.1007/978-3-662-64062-3_62

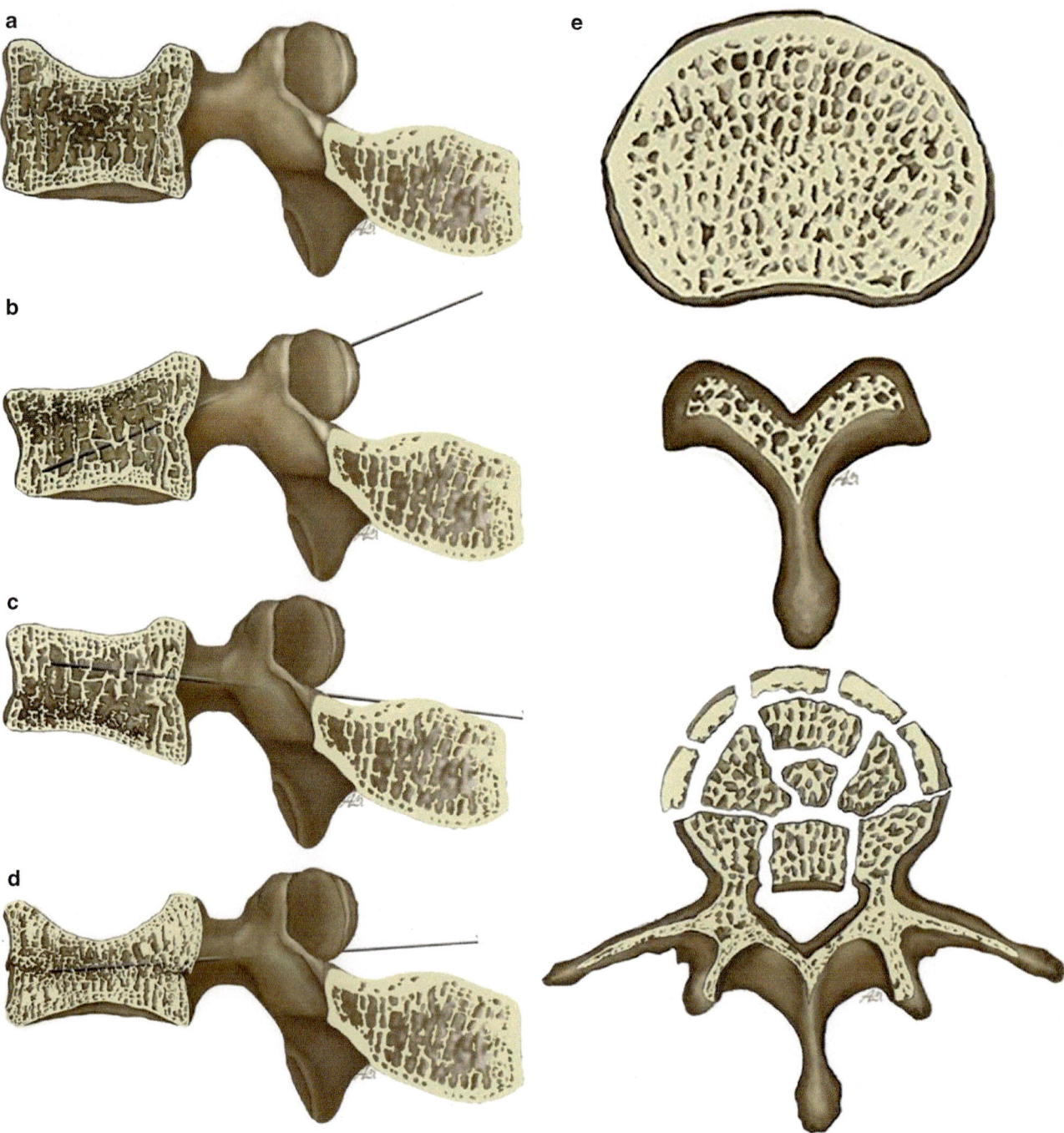

Fig. 62.1 Schematic drawing of various fracture types and the appropriate needle trajectories. (**a**) Endplate impression fracture A1.1. (**b**) Superior wedge fracture A1.2.1. (**c**) Inferior wedge fracture A1.2.3. (**d**) Vertebral body collapse A1.3. (**e**) Axial views of an incomplete burst fracture below the level of the pedicles (*upper image*) and at the level of the pedicles (*lower image*) demonstrating disruption of the posterior wall only at the level of the pedicles

- Vertebral hemangiomas
  VP is an effective treatment option in this category if the pain is the main presenting feature. It is not suitable for cases with neurological deficit [8]. VP can achieve pain relief as well as stabilization, reducing the risk of secondary vertebral collapse. This treatment must be reserved only in vertebral hemangiomas, which are symptomatic and resistant to common conservative treatments, with radiological evidence of aggressiveness and/or epidural extension [6].

  Balloon kyphoplasty (KP) is indicated if vertebral height restoration or cavity formation is the aim, for example, in correcting the kyphotic deformity associated with osteoporotic VCFs, or traumatic vertebral fractures as mentioned before in the indications section or for situations where cavity formation might help, for example, in difficult indications for tumourous lesions. In order to achieve this aim, procedure should be performed relatively early on after the fracture (literature recommending periods of under 3 weeks to under 3 months).

62.3 Contraindications

- Coagulation disorders.
- Patient unfit for general anesthetic or local anesthetic with sedation or unable to lie prone on the operating table for the duration of the procedure.
- Pregnancy (relative contraindication).
- Hypersensitivity to cement components.
- Local infection.
- Relative: pulmonary hypertension (exacerbation through fat embolism).
- Neurological compromise through posterior wall fracture or tumor mass extension.
- Precaution: posterior wall disruption (increased leakage rate).
- Adequate preoperative imaging is also an essential prerequisite to do the procedure and if for some reason, the relevant landmarks cannot be visualized on AP and lateral imaging, then it is not possible to proceed.

62.4 Technical Prerequisites Planning, Preparation, and Positioning

Preoperative workup should include MR scan with STIR sequences (fat suppression sequences that identify edema) for proper identification of the painful vertebral level, and clinical and radiological correlation is required as the collapsed vertebra may not always be the source of the pain and the pathology may reside in another noncollapsed vertebra. A chest X-ray is essential as well to count the ribs when dealing with thoracic spine. Adequate imaging quality and proper positioning of the patient on the table is essential, and before draping the patient, one must ensure that appropriate landmarks can be seen on AP and lateral fluoroscopy. On AP image, pedicles should be seen to lie in the upper lateral quadrant of the vertebral body; spinous processes should lie midway between the pedicles, and both the endplates and the posterior wall must come to lie parallel (superimposed so that double image is eliminated) on the AP and lateral images.

The procedure can be performed either under general anesthetic or with local anesthetic and sedation depending on patient's/anesthetist's/surgeon's preference and anticipated duration of procedure. The patient is positioned prone on pillows on a radiolucent operating table. A single C-arm fluoroscopy is usually used, which can be easily switched between AP and lateral orientation, although some surgeons prefer biplanar imaging with two image intensifiers.

62.5 Surgical Technique

62.5.1 Vertebroplasty

- After prepping and draping, under image intensifier in AP view, and after local anesthetic infiltration, transverse 1–2-cm stab incisions are made over the entry points, which, in the lumbar spine, is over the tip of the transverse process and, in the thoracic spine, for the extrapedicular approach, is immediately superior to the costal angle of the relevant rib [4] (see Fig. 62.2).
- The entry point can be adjusted also based on the fact whether unilateral or bilateral approach is being done and how much convergence is required (in unilateral approach, more convergence is required and hence more lateral starting point on the skin).
- Central placement of the needle usually results in sufficient cement distribution in the smaller vertebrae of the thoracic spine.
- The vertebral body can be either directly penetrated by the Jamshidi needle or first Kirschner (K)-wires are placed into the relevant vertebral bodies and then Jamshidi needle can be passed over the K-wires.
- The vertebrae can be accessed through transpedicular approach in lumbar spine and transcostovertebral approach in the thoracic spine [4].
- Once K-wire is advanced 2–2.5 cm into the pedicle without breaching the medial cortex on the AP view, switch to lateral view to see if the posterior vertebral cortex has been penetrated.
- If the needle/K-wire is in the vertebral body, then this can be advanced further and converged more at this stage. One must never breach the medial pedicle cortex on AP view without penetrating the posterior vertebral cortex on the lateral view. Jamshidi needles are then passed over the K-wires.
- Once the surgeon is satisfied with the position of the Jamshidi needles, that lateral image is saved on the screen as a reference image (this helps identify leakages through comparing the current image with the reference image without cement).
- Cement is mixed and, when of appropriate consistency, injected under live screening, (lateral view) watching for

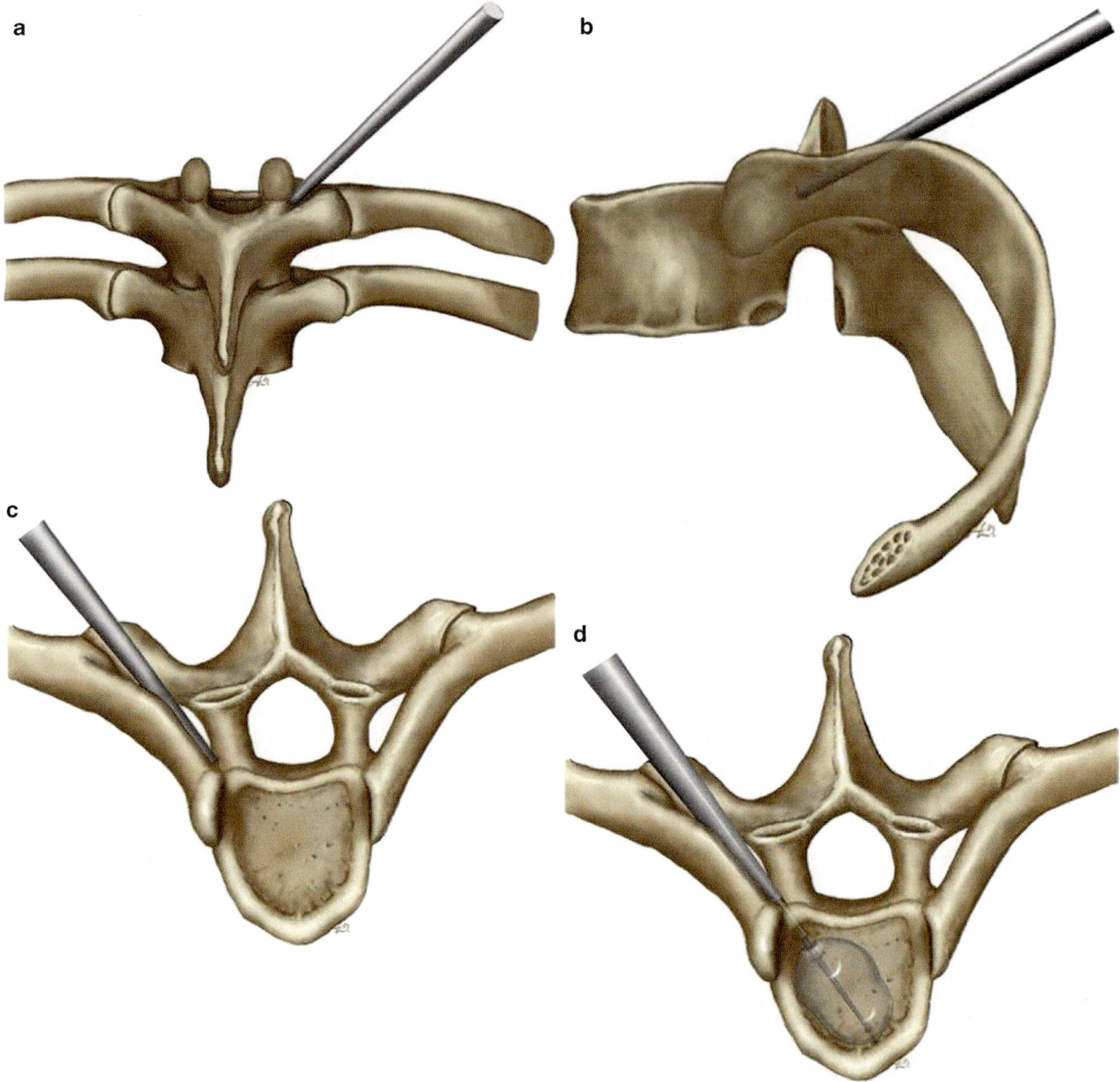

Fig. 62.2 Drawing of the transcostovertebral placement of the bone biopsy needle with the tip just penetrating the lateral pedicle at its base. In the view from posterior (**a**), the needle passes above the transverse process and meets the pedicle at the craniolateral circumference. The lateral view (**b**) confirms the placement of the tip of the needle close to the base of the pedicle. In an axial view (**c**), the needle is seen to pass through the costovertebral gap, between the neck of the rib and the lateral pedicle circumference, toward the base of the pedicle (**d**) balloon inflated within the vertebral body

any leak either posteriorly into the spinal canal or anteriorly into the veins.

- *Note*: We try not to exceed 20–30 mL of cement injection in one sitting because of the risk of fat embolism resulting in pulmonary hypertension. Close collaboration with the anesthetist is essential, and if the cardiorespiratory state is compromised, injection should stop. Also, if there is any leakage of cement into canal or vessels, injection should be aborted.

62.5.2 Balloon Kyphoplasty

- The relevant anatomy (pedicles, posterior vertebral wall, endplates, spinous processes, etc.) should be clearly identifiable on image intensifier before proceeding.
- In KP, it is essential to place the balloon in an optimum position in the middle of the vertebral body to achieve best possible reduction of the fracture without injuring the lateral margins of the vertebral body.

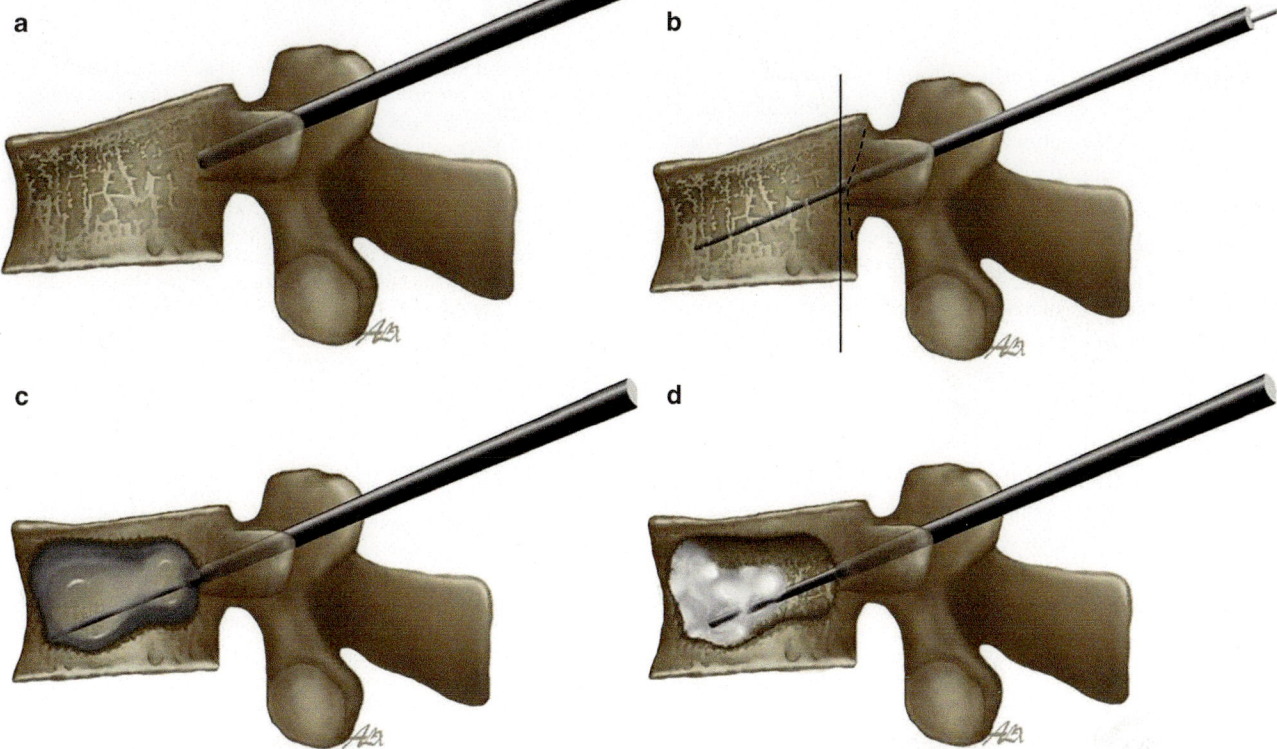

Fig. 62.3 Lateral view of balloon kyphoplasty (**a**). The tip of the working cannula lying just within the posterior vertebral cortex (**b**), the K-wire and then the drill passed to the anterior third of the vertebral body where balloon is going to be sited (**c**). Balloon seen inflated and see the height restoration (**d**) cement being injected into the cavity created by the balloon

- The principles and tool introduction are similar to the technique for PV described earlier.
- The K-wire is inserted first on AP view so that the needle tip appears to lie just outside the pedicle ring on AP view when bone contact is made. It is then advanced so that it does not breach the medial pedicle cortex on AP view until it penetrates the posterior vertebral wall on the lateral view.
- On AP view, tip of the needle should not cross the midline. On lateral view, K-wire is advanced to the anterior third of the vertebral body.
- Jamshidi needle is passed over the K-wire.
- Bone biopsy can be taken with the biopsy bone filler, and a hand drill bit can be used to drill the area where the balloon is going to lie and smoothen the bone edges.
- A special curette can be used as well; the angle at the tip can be changed to 30°, 60°, and 90°. Then, Jamshidi needle is withdrawn and working cannula passed over the K-wire, the tip of the cannula lying only about 3 mm ventral to the posterior wall of the vertebra (to give space for the balloon) (see Fig. 62.3).
- Bilateral approach is used and balloons are then passed bilaterally so that they lie in the middle next to each other, making sure that both markings of the balloons should lie outside the working cannula (Fig. 62.3).

- The balloons are then simultaneously inflated keeping an eye on the pressure and the volume of the balloon and also frequently checking with imaging.
- The inflation of the balloons is continued until the maximum volume or maximum pressure is reached or the pressure keeps dropping indicating that further elevation of the endplate is not possible.
- Cement is then mixed, and once of appropriate viscosity, balloons are deflated and removed and the cavity in the bone filled with bone cement using bone fillers through the working cannulae under live fluoroscopy.
- The bone fillers and the working cannulae are removed once the cement is fully hardened and stab incisions are sutured.
- Final AP and lateral images are obtained.

62.6   Complications and Their Avoidance

Listing all the possible complications is beyond the scope of this chapter; however, few salient learning points are mentioned: Both PV and KP are deceptively "easy" techniques and should only be performed by properly trained surgeons who can also deal with complications, for example, able to do open surgery (decompression/stabilization), if needed.

Cement leakage: Cement should be viscous enough before injecting. Good-quality imaging is essential to recognize the leaks at the very early stage. In difficult cases where fluoroscopy is suboptimal, CT-guided procedure combined with fluoroscopy can be done. Cement with an adequate radiopacity must be used.

Pulmonary emboli: Both VP and KP procedures will expel a volume of marrow equal to that of the cement injected. Although this is asymptomatic in most patients, those with pre-existing pulmonary disease, for example, COPD, are particularly at risk and should be monitored accordingly. They should be informed of the high risk preoperatively and amount of cement injected in one sitting should be limited in such patients.

Disk space leaks: In case of large leaks into the disk space, consideration should be given to augmenting the adjacent vertebra or careful follow-up of this, as there has been some speculation that this leads to higher incidence of adjacent vertebral fracture.

Acknowledgments Illustrations courtesy of spinegraphics@gmx.net.

References

1. Buchbinder R, Osborne RH, Ebeling PR, et al. A randomized trial of vertebroplasty for painful osteoporotic vertebral fractures. N Engl J Med. 2009;361:557–68.
2. Kallmes DF, Comstock BA, Heagerty PJ, et al. A randomized trial of vertebroplasty for osteoporotic spinal fractures. N Engl J Med. 2009;361:569–79.
3. Mendel E, Bourekas E, Gerszten P, Golan JD. Percutaneous techniques in the treatment of spine tumors: what are the diagnostic and therapeutic indications and outcomes? Spine (Phila Pa 1976). 2009;34(22 Suppl):S93–100.
4. Boszczyk BM, Bierschneider M, Hauck S, et al. Transcostovertebral kyphoplasty of the mid and high thoracic spine. Eur Spine J. 2005;14:992–9.
5. Jensen ME, Evans AJ, Mathis JM, et al. Percutaneous polymethylmethacrylate vertebroplasty in the treatment of osteoporotic vertebral body compression fractures: technical aspects. AJNR Am J Neuroradiol. 1997;18:1897–904.
6. Guarnieri G, Ambrosanio G, Vassallo P, et al. Vertebroplasty as treatment of aggressive and symptomatic vertebral hemangiomas: up to 4 years of follow-up. Neuroradiology. 2009;51:471–6.
7. Magerl F, Aebi M, Gertzbein SD, et al. A comprehensive classification of thoracic and lumbar injuries. Eur Spine J. 1994;3:184–201.
8. Acosta FL Jr, Dowd CF, Chin C, et al. Current treatment strategies and outcomes in the management of symptomatic vertebral hemangiomas. Neurosurgery. 2006;58(2):287–95.

Transpedicular Stabilization with Internal Fixation in the Thoracolumbar and Lumbar Spine

63

Robert Morrison and Uwe Vieweg

63.1 Introduction and Core Messages

The preparation of the pedicle requires knowledge of the following points: anatomical structures marking the entry point, pedicle orientation, and desired screw length. Performing an adequate preoperative planning (radiographs, CT-scan) and planning of the instrumentation based on these diagnostics are elemental for a good surgical result. The instrumentation of the lumbar spine allows stabilization and reduction using the posterior implants. For biomechanical reasons, an additional anterior procedure can be necessary to achieve a lasting stability.

63.2 Indications

- Fractures of the thoracolumbar or lumbar spine
- Degenerative disorders
- Tumors or infections of the spine

63.3 Contraindications (Relative)

- Osteopenia and osteoporosis
- Ongoing infection within the instrumented vertebra
- Poor medical condition of the patient

63.4 Technical Prerequisites

Fluoroscopy, special cushions (e.g., Wilson Frame), internal fixator (rod-screw system) or screw plate system, and radiolucent operating table.

63.5 Planning, Preparation, and Positioning

Preoperative measurement includes the pedicle diameter and especially the transverse diameter. This can be done either with AP radiographs or, more correctly, with a CT scan. If the transverse diameter is large enough to carry the screws, the preoperative planning can take place. The correct *entry point* can be found after identifying the necessary landmarks. These include the facet joint with its boarders and the transverse process. (*Note*: Intraoperatively, the entry point is

R. Morrison (✉)
Spine & Scoliosis Center, Asklepios Klinik Bad Abbach, Germany
e-mail: dr.r.morrison@googlemail.com

U. Vieweg
Department of Conservative and Surgical Spine Therapy with Interdisciplinary Spinal Deformities Centre and Rummelsberg Sectional Center, Hospital Rummelsberg, Schwarzenbruck, Germany
e-mail: uwe.vieweg@sana.de

Table 63.1 Average pedicle diameters and angulations within the lumbar spine. Adapted from Olsewski et al. [1]

Vertebra	Gender	Transversal pedicle diameter (mm)	Transversal angle of the pedicle (°)	Inclination angle of the pedicle (°)
L1	M	9.5	7	5
	F	7.7	5	6
L2	M	9.6	7	6
	F	7.9	6	5
L3	M	11.7	8	6
	F	9.6	7	6
L4	M	14.7	11	6
	F	12.5	10	7
L5	M	21.1	17	5
	F	18.4	18	8

located in the lateral half of the oval area of the pedicle in the AP fluoroscopy.) This also includes measuring the transverse diameter of the pedicles (illustrated in Table 63.1). The *orientation of the pedicle* can be gauged in lateral radiographs or, even more precise, using CT-Scans (sagittal reconstructions for the cranial-caudal angle and coronary scans for the lateral deviation as illustrated in Table 63.1). The *pedicle length* also shows great variations. The correct screw length cannot be gauged intraoperatively in lateral fluoroscopy, as the anterior cortex has a convex shape. When deciding for a screw length, one must keep in mind that 60% of the pullout force is achieved in the pedicle and 15–20% additionally in the cancellous bone of the vertebra body. So, the screw is rather chosen too short than too long!

63.5.1 Anatomical Specifications of the Thoracolumbar and Lumbar Spine

- Large pedicle diameter (average 8 mm in L1 to 18 mm in L5). Avoid using too small screws. The screw diameter should be 75–80% of the transverse pedicle diameter.
- Often, degenerative changes of the facet joints make it difficult to identify the proper entry point.
- Plain radiographs in two planes are enough to plan the instrumentation, if there are not any severe degenerative changes.

The patient is placed in a prone position with cushioning of the body parts in contact with the table. The definitive positioning depends on the case to be treated. In the case of decompression, the lumbar spine should be slightly kyphotic for an easier approach to the canal. On the other hand—in case of fractures—depending on the habits of the surgical team, extension/traction can be added. The patient should always be positioned in a lordotic position to ease the reduction. In scoliosis surgery,

as there is no spinal canal decompression, the patient is placed directly in the lumbar lordotic position. In cases of decompression and reduction surgery (e.g., spondylolisthesis), decompression can be realized in a kyphotic position with flexion of the hips of up to 60°. To avoid the risk of arthrodesis in a kyphotic position, the extension of the legs may be performed during the surgery. Whatever the position chosen, there are always certain rules to respect:

- Avoid abdominal compression to decrease the pressure in the epidural veins.
- Positioning of the shoulders and elbows flexed with cubital nerve protection.
- Flexion of the knees to relax the sciatic nerves.
- Rest position of the head with eye protection and straight cervical spine.
- Follow the basic rules of prone position surgery.
- Cushioning of body parts in contact with the table.

63.6 Surgical Technique

63.6.1 Approach

- *Open access via a midline incision*: The incision should be one or two segments longer than the intended length of fusion. The subcutis is dissected to the fascia, and wound retractors are applied. The fascia is detached on both sides of the spinal processes using a diathermy knife close to the bone. The paraspinal structures are retracted with a raspatory. The muscles are retracted to expose the ends of the costal processes.
- *Alternative, paraspinal approach*: Two paramedian skin incisions are made two fingerbreadths laterally to the spinous processes. The fascia of the iliocostal muscles is split longitudinally. Blunt dissection through the muscles until the vertebral joint is palpated. Implementation of the retractor.

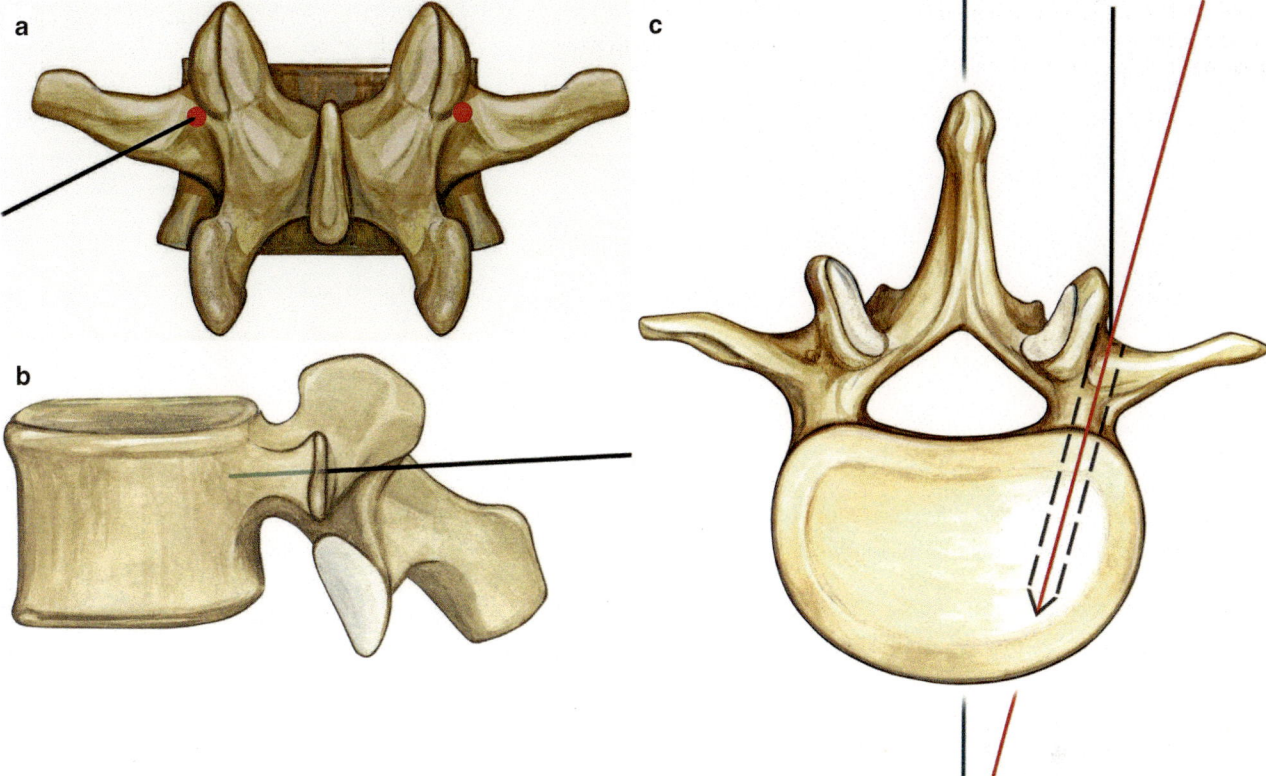

Fig. 63.1 *Converging screw placement* (**a**, **b**). The anatomical landmark for converging screw placement is the transverse process (processus costarius). These *lines* are close to the midline of the transverse process (slightly above in the upper lumbar spine). The orientation of the trocar must be strictly in the longitudinal axis of the pedicle.

Usually, an angle of about 15–25° to the sagittal plane is chosen for the lumbar spine (With permission from Aesculap AG, Tuttlingen, Germany [2]). *Standard screw placement* (**c**). In the so-called straightforward technique described by Roy Camille, the entry point is the downward projection of the posterior articular process 1 mm below the joint [3]

- *Percutaneous technique*: Marking of the entry points on the skin using fluoroscopy. Minimally invasive percutaneous approach to each pedicle. Marking of the intended screw position using K-Wires.

63.6.2 Instrumentation

63.6.2.1 Lumbar Spine

Entry point/trajectory: The entry point can be found at the intersection of the vertical line along the lateral edge of the superior articular process and the horizontal line through the middle of the transverse process. The bony crest on the entry point for the pedicle screw can be removed with a rongeur or, alternatively, with a high-speed drill; the subcortical cancellous bone of the pedicle entrance is exposed. The opening of the pedicle is then enlarged with a sharp center punch under lateral control to verify the correct entry point, and the sagittal angle or drilling of the pedicle is then performed with gentle pressure using a universal trocar or the adjustable trocar step by step under fluoroscopic control.

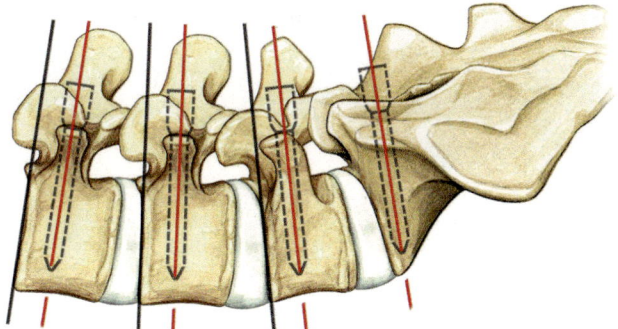

Fig. 63.2 For easier rod placement, the screws should be placed in one line and parallel to the upper endplates

- To detect the correct entry point, the "processus costarius" is a good landmark (see Fig. 63.1a–c) [4].
- Within the lumbar spine, the screws will have an increasing convergence toward the midline (10° in L1 to 20° in L5). The screws should be placed parallel to the superior endplate (see Fig. 63.2) [2].
- The pedicle is opened with a pedicle awl, followed by consecutive deepening with a pedicle trocar. The length of the

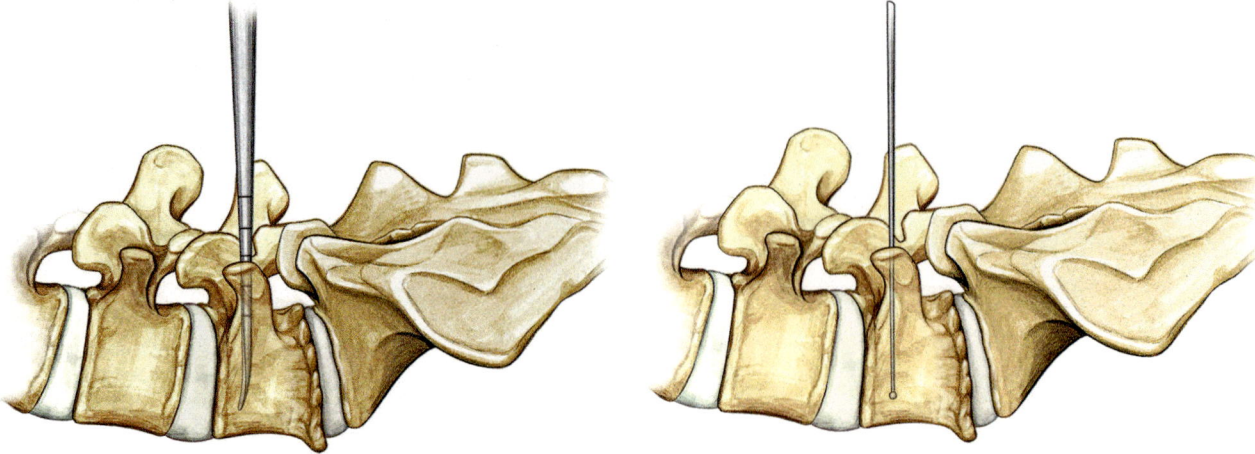

Fig. 63.3 The opening of the pedicle is then enlarged with a sharp center punch first under AP control for the entry point and then under lateral control to verify the correct sagittal angle

Fig. 63.4 Following the preparation of the screw hole, the channel can be checked using a dissector or pedicle sonde to disclose possible perforations of the pedicle wall

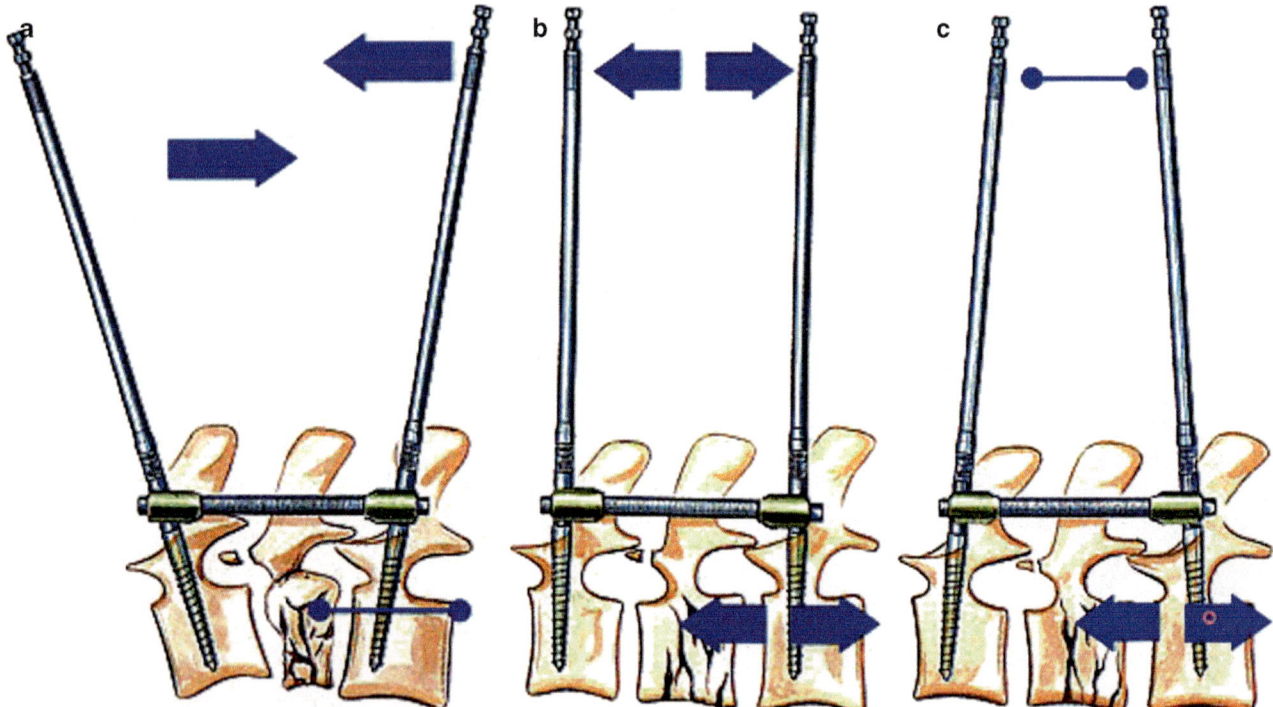

Fig. 63.5 (**a–c**) Repositioning examples ((**a**) repositioning, (**b**) parallel distraction, (**c**) lordosation) with a pedicle screw system (With permission from Aesculap AG, Tuttlingen, Germany)

screw can be seen on the side of the trocar. To verify the intact pedicle walls, the walls of the canal can be tested with a ball-tipped pedicle probe (see Figs. 63.3 and 63.4).

- The pedicle screw systems allow movements/corrections in three directions, individually or combined, during the repositioning procedure: compression, angulation (see Fig. 63.5a, c), distraction (see Fig. 63.5b).

63.7 Sacrum

63.7.1 Entry Point/Trajectory

The entry point of the segment S1 is located on a vertical line along the lateral wall of the superior facet and right on the inferior border of the facet joint. Due to degenerative

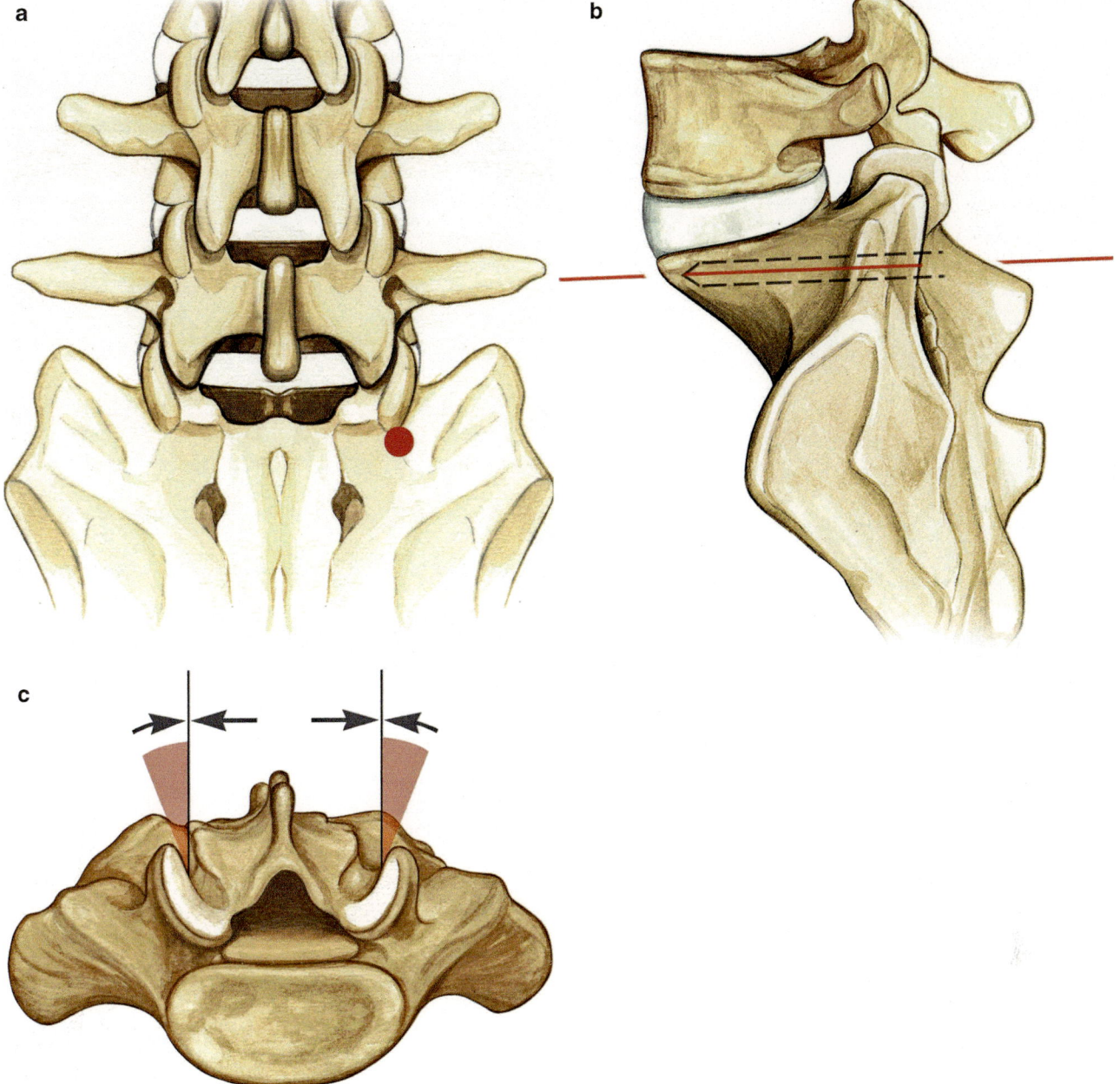

Fig. 63.6 (**a–c**) Preparation of the sacrum. The entry point for the converging screw channels in the sacrum is about 5 mm inferior and 10 mm lateral to the inferior border of the facet of S1

changes, the identification of the exact entry point is sometimes quite difficult. A partial resection of the inferior facet of L5 is helpful in these cases.

There are two different trajectories in the sacrum:

- The most common is the trajectory aiming at the anterior corner of the promontorium with a 15–20° convergence of the screws. Superior strength of fixation is achieved by bicortical fixation of the screws along the pedicle axis in this "safe zone" (see Fig. 63.6b).

- The alternative safe zone is found in an angle of 45° deviation, aiming the screws toward the sacroiliacal joint. In this case, the screws should be no longer than 45 mm to avoid interference with the SI joint.

The sacrum has particular anatomical properties. Here, the values for the pullout strength are reversed, with anterior cortical fixation being responsible for 60%. Therefore, careful purchase of the anterior cortex is sometimes necessary for optimal fixation.

63.8 Tips and Tricks

- Start out by marking the entry points with K-wires or short pins using the fluoroscopy in the AP direction!
- For easy rod placement, the screws should be placed in one line and parallel to the upper endplates; the insertion depth should be the same for all pedicle screws to achieve aligned screw heads (see Fig. 63.2).
- Using pedicle markers, the screw channels can be checked under lateral X-ray control.

References

1. Olsewski JM, Simmons EH, Kallen FC, et al. Morphometry of the lumbar spine: anatomical perspectives related to the transpedicular fixation. J Bone Joint Surg Am. 1990;71:541–9.
2. Weinstein JN, Spratt KF, Spengler D, et al. Spinal pedicle fixation: reliability and validity of roentgenogram-based assessment and surgical factors on successful screw placement. Spine. 1988;13:1012–8.
3. Roy-Camille R, Saillant G, Mazel C. Plating of thoracic, thoracolumbar, and lumbar injuries with pedicle screw plates. Orthop Clin North Am. 1986;17:147–59.
4. Ebraheim NA, Rollins JR, Xu R, et al. Projection of the lumbar pedicle and its morphometric analysis. Spine. 1996;21:1296–300.

Correction of Degenerative Scoliosis with Polyaxial Internal Fixator and Intercorporeal Fusion with TLIF and PLIF Cages

64

Uwe Vieweg and Robert Morrison

64.1 Introduction and Core Messages

The degenerative scoliosis is the so-called de novo scoliosis. It is a form of secondary scoliosis in elderly patients (patients >65 years), as a result of gradual disk degeneration with a lateral deviation and rotated vertebral bodies. Surgical correction using a polyaxial internal fixation represents a possible treatment of a degenerative scoliosis. The correction is performed step by step using polyaxial pedicle screws, intercorporeal fusion (generally using TLIF at the caudal level), a correction of the scoliosis using PLIF cages (box-like) following the resection of the facet joints, and an intercorporeal fusion using a TLIF cage (banana-like or kidney-shaped cage), again at the cranial end. The remaining malposition is corrected by restoration of the lumbar lordosis and the derotation of the vertebras using the prebent rods [1–7].

64.2 Indications

- Degenerative scoliosis >20°, with a significant progression of the scoliosis
- Persistent back pain and or leg pain that interferes with activities of daily living
- Failed conservative therapy and neurological deficits

64.3 Contraindications

- Severe osteoporosis, osteopenia, or osteomyelitis
- Poor psychological or medical situation of the patient

64.4 Technical Prerequisites

Fluoroscopy, special cushions (e.g., Wilson Frame), polyaxial screw system with cross connectors, PLIF and TLIF cages, distraction forceps, cell saver, radiolucent operating table, and bone grinder.

64.5 Planning, Preparation, and Positioning

Extensive radiological diagnostics such as conventional radiographs, functional radiographs (flexion, extension, lateral bending), MRI, and determination of the bone density are elemental. The lumbar myelography is a centerpiece of

U. Vieweg (✉)
Department of Conservative and Surgical Spine Therapy with Interdisciplinary Spinal Deformities Centre and Rummelsberg Sectional Center, Hospital Rummelsberg, Schwarzenbruck, Germany
e-mail: uwe.vieweg@sana.de

R. Morrison
Spine & Scoliosis Center, Asklepios Klinik Bad Abbach, Germany
e-mail: dr.r.morrison@googlemail.com

the diagnostics, as it shows the extent of the stenosis. These findings combined help to specify the extent of the instrumentation and the type as well as the location of the decompression. They are also elemental in planning the intercorporeal fusion and reconstruction of the intervertebral height. During the operation, the patient is in a prone position on a radiolucent operating table. Different positioning systems can be used (Wilson frame, chest rolls, Relton hall frame, Hasting frame, Heffington frame). The patient should be positioned to minimize intra-abdominal pressure and thereby avoid venous congestion and excess intraoperative bleeding. The incision is planned using the fluoroscopy.

64.6 Surgical Technique

64.6.1 Approach

- A midline posterior approach to the spine is performed with subperiosteal exposure of the posterior elements down to the transverse processes. For improved tissue protection and in order to use a smaller skin incision, a subcutaneous lumbar retractor system is advisable (see Figs. 64.1 and 64.2).
- The exposure of the spinous process should extend to at least one additional level above and below the levels to be instrumented. Care must be taken not to disrupt the facet joint capsules of the joints above and below the intended fusion segments.

64.6.2 Instrumentation

- Using the awl or Steinmann nail, the cortex is penetrated under fluoroscopy. The trajectory angle is determined preoperatively. Use the ball-tipped probe to make sure the pedicle is intact under fluoroscopy. The pedicle entry point is intersected by the vertical line that connects the lateral edges of bony crest extension of the pars interarticularis and the horizontal line that bisects the middle of the transverse process. Subsequently, transpedicular implantation of the polyaxial screws is carried out (see Fig. 64.3).
- After pedicle screw insertion, the superior and inferior articular processes of the caudal facet joint (in the most cases on the convex site) are resected with a high-speed drill and a Kerrison punch, and the intervertebral disk space is exposed. The disk is then resected subtotally using angled rongeurs, shavers, and curettes. After preparation of the end plates, the anterior part of the disc space

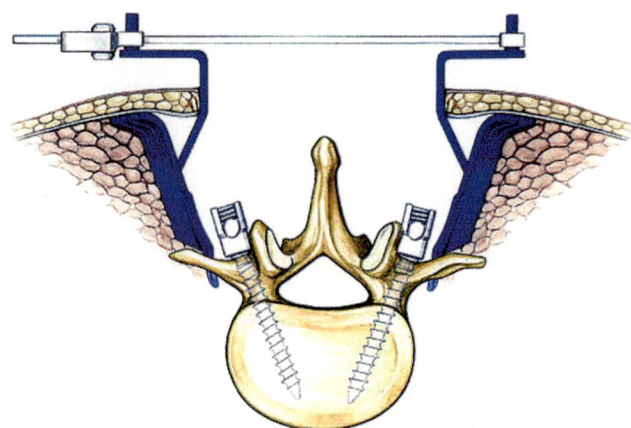

Fig. 64.1 Placement of the subcutaneous lumbar retractor system (SLR, Aesculap AG, Tuttlingen) in an axial view to reduce hematomas and postoperative pain. (With permission from Aesculap AG, Tuttlingen, Germany)

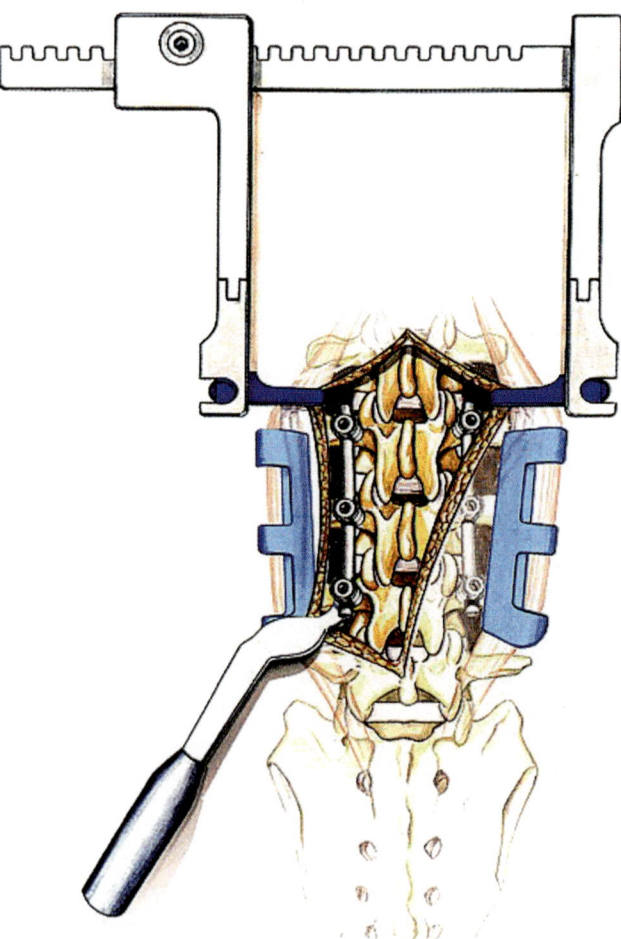

Fig. 64.2 Smaller skin incision with the SLR to reduce the operative trauma. (With permission from Aesculap AG, Tuttlingen, Germany)

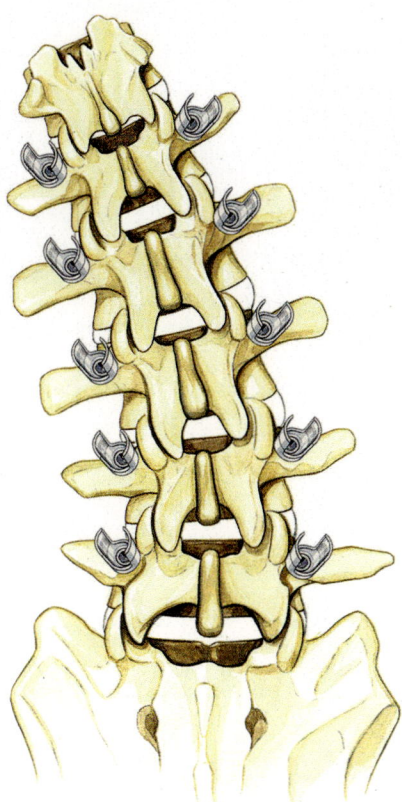

Fig. 64.3 Extensive instrumentation from L1 through L5 using a polyaxial internal fixateur. (With permission from Aesculap AG, Tuttlingen, Germany)

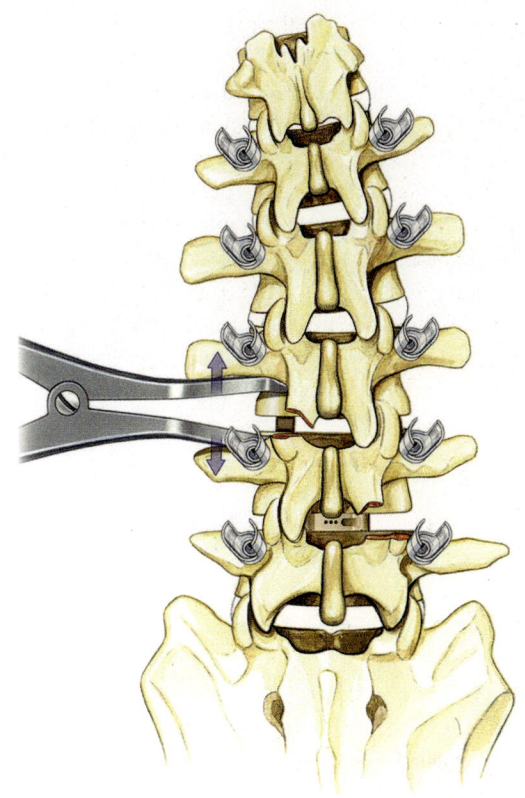

Fig. 64.5 Straightening of the scoliosis in the segment L3/4 by distracting the intervertebral space using a distraction forceps placed underneath the screw heads. Then, a PLIF cage is placed into the space. (With permission from Aesculap AG, Tuttlingen, Germany)

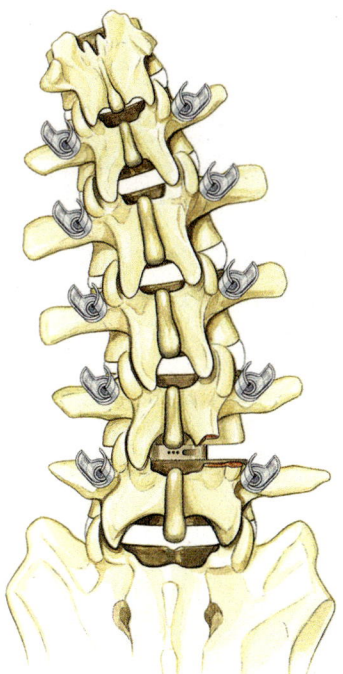

Fig. 64.4 First step of the correction by performing an intercorporeal fusion using TLIF technique on the left side in the caudal segment (L4/5). (With permission from Aesculap AG, Tuttlingen, Germany)

is packed with autologous bone. A curved PEEK cage specially designed for the TLIF technique is also filled with autologous bone and inserted into the disk space (see Fig. 64.4).

- Now, the next facet joint on the concave site is resected using a high-speed drill and a Kerrison punch. The disk space is distracted with angulated distraction forceps. This distraction and the implantation of an additional interbody cage (PLIF) reconstruct the disc space (see Figs. 64.5 and 64.6).
- The cranial disk space is resected coming from the contralateral side. Here, we also recommend a reconstruction using the TLIF technique described above (see Fig. 64.7).
- The appropriate-sized rod is bent to match the sagittal contour of the spine using the rod bender. Place the rod into the screws, and then lock it in place with the setscrews. By using this specific screw design with the removable tabs, an additional correction can be achieved (lordosis, reposition of a spondylolisthesis as well as a derotation) (see Fig. 64.8a, b).

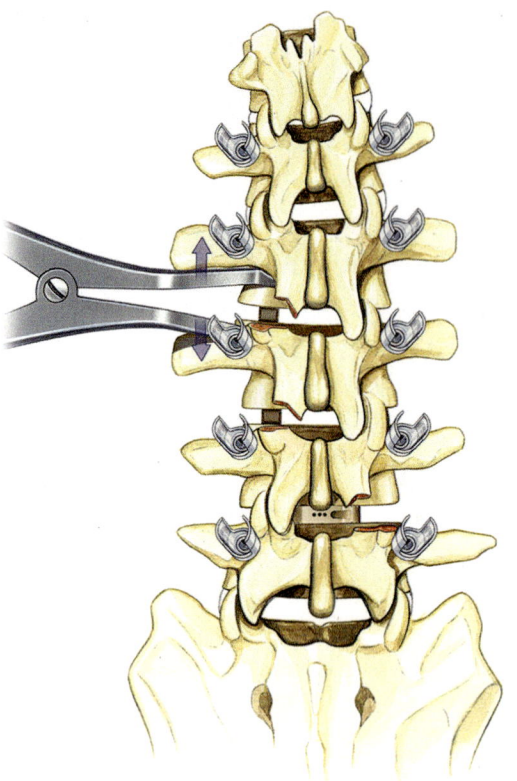

Fig. 64.6 Next step is the same procedure in the segment L2/3. (With permission from Aesculap AG, Tuttlingen, Germany)

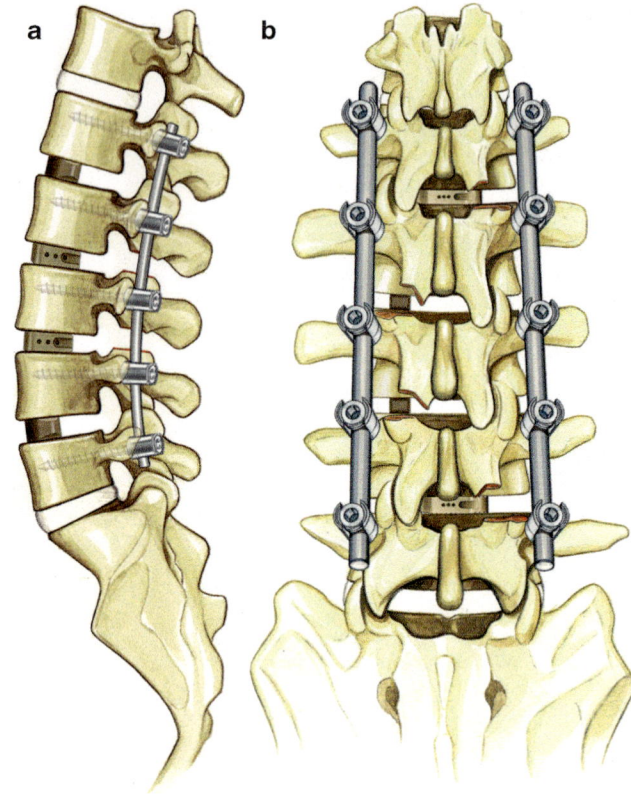

Fig. 64.8 (**a, b**) Additional correction of the lumbar lordosis and derotation using an accordingly bent rod. (**a**) lateral (**b**) AP view. (With permission from Aesculap AG, Tuttlingen, Germany)

64.7   Tips and Tricks

- Pedicle screw augmentation for the upper and lower ends of the instrumentation.
- Note the sagittal balance, not only the anterior Cobb angle.
- Note the junction regions with instrumentation of lower thoracic spine (T10, T11, T12) or with S1 with or without a ilium screw.
- Position the fluoroscopy to where it is parallel to the instrumented segment; the end plates of the vertebra will be depicted as parallel lines.
- Guide pins are available and can be used to mark the pedicle before the pedicle screws are implanted. This allows a perfect pedicle screw placement.

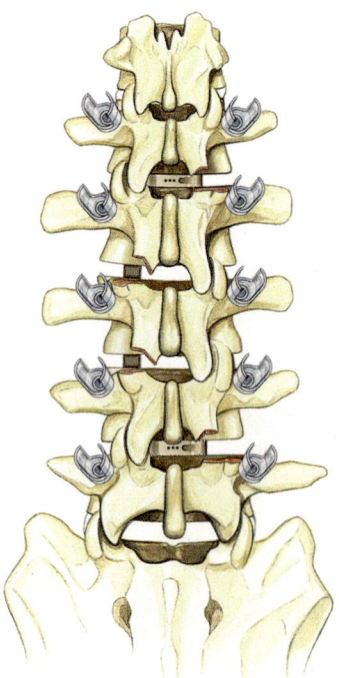

Fig. 64.7 To complete the correction, a TLIF cage is placed into the segment L1/2, coming from the left side. (With permission from Aesculap AG, Tuttlingen, Germany)

References

1. Aebi M. The adult scoliosis. Eur Spine J. 2005;14:925–48.
2. Akbarnia BA, Ogilvie JW, Hammerberg KW. Debate: degenerative scoliosis: to operate or not to operate. Spine. 2006;9(Suppl):S195–201.
3. Bradford DS, Tay BK, Hu SS. Adult scoliosis: surgical indications, operative management, complications and outcome. Spine. 1999;24:2617–29.
4. Glassman SD, Bridwell K, Dimar JK. The impact of positive sagittal balance in adult spinal deformity. Spine. 2005;30:2024–9.
5. Daffner SD, Vaccaro AR. Adult degenerative lumbar scoliosis. Am J Orthop. 2003;32:77–82.
6. Dick W, Widmer H. Degenerative Lumbalskoliose und Spinalkanalstenose. Orthopade. 1993;22:232–42.
7. Tribus CB. Degenerative lumbar scoliosis: evaluation and management. J Am Acad Orthop Surg. 2003;11:174–83.

Correction of Spondylolisthesis

Uwe Vieweg

65.1 Introduction and Core Messages

The goals of surgical treatment of spondylolisthesis are as follows: decompression of neuronal structures, stabilization of spondylolytic instability, reduction of slippage, restoration of the disk height, and restoration of the sagittal alignment [1, 2]. With the appropriate instruments, it is possible to instrument a single compartment and, in most cases, to completely reduce the spondylolisthesis. This technique allows an instrumented monosegmental slippage reduction of low- and middle-grade isthmic spondylolisthesis via fusion with a polyaxial internal fixator, titanium spacer, and cross-link connector.

65.2 Indications

- Spondylolytic spondylolisthesis Meyerding grade I–III (IV) L5/S1 and L4/L5
- Significant progression of the slip spondylolisthesis
- Persistent back pain and/or leg pain that interferes with activities of daily living
- Failed conservative therapy
- Neurological deficits [1–5]

65.3 Contraindications

- Reduction should not be attempted in patients with spondyloptosis.
- Osteoporosis, osteopenia, or osteomyelitis.
- Poor psychological and/or poor general medical state of the patient [1–5].

65.4 Technical Prerequisites

Fluoroscopy, positioning device (e.g., Wiltse frame), adequate implants, and instruments with the following technical requirements:
- Simultaneous correction of translation and slip angle.
- Reduction with single-level fusion and sparing adjacent healthy vertebrae.
- Reduction of the listhetic vertebral body along the same curved displacement route. This minimizes interference with anatomical structures and eliminates the neurological deficits that typically result from initial overdistraction of an already stretched nerve root.

U. Vieweg (✉)
Department of Conservative and Surgical Spine Therapy with Interdisciplinary Spinal Deformities Centre and Rummelsberg Sectional Center, Hospital Rummelsberg, Schwarzenbruck, Germany
e-mail: uwe.vieweg@sana.de

Fig. 65.1 The S⁴ SRI spondylolisthesis reduction instrument (SRI) has a *right* and a *left* component. Each has two pedicle screw attachments. One attaches to the cephalad vertebral screw that will be repositioned and the other to the caudal vertebral screw. (With permission from Aesculap AG, Tuttlingen, Germany)

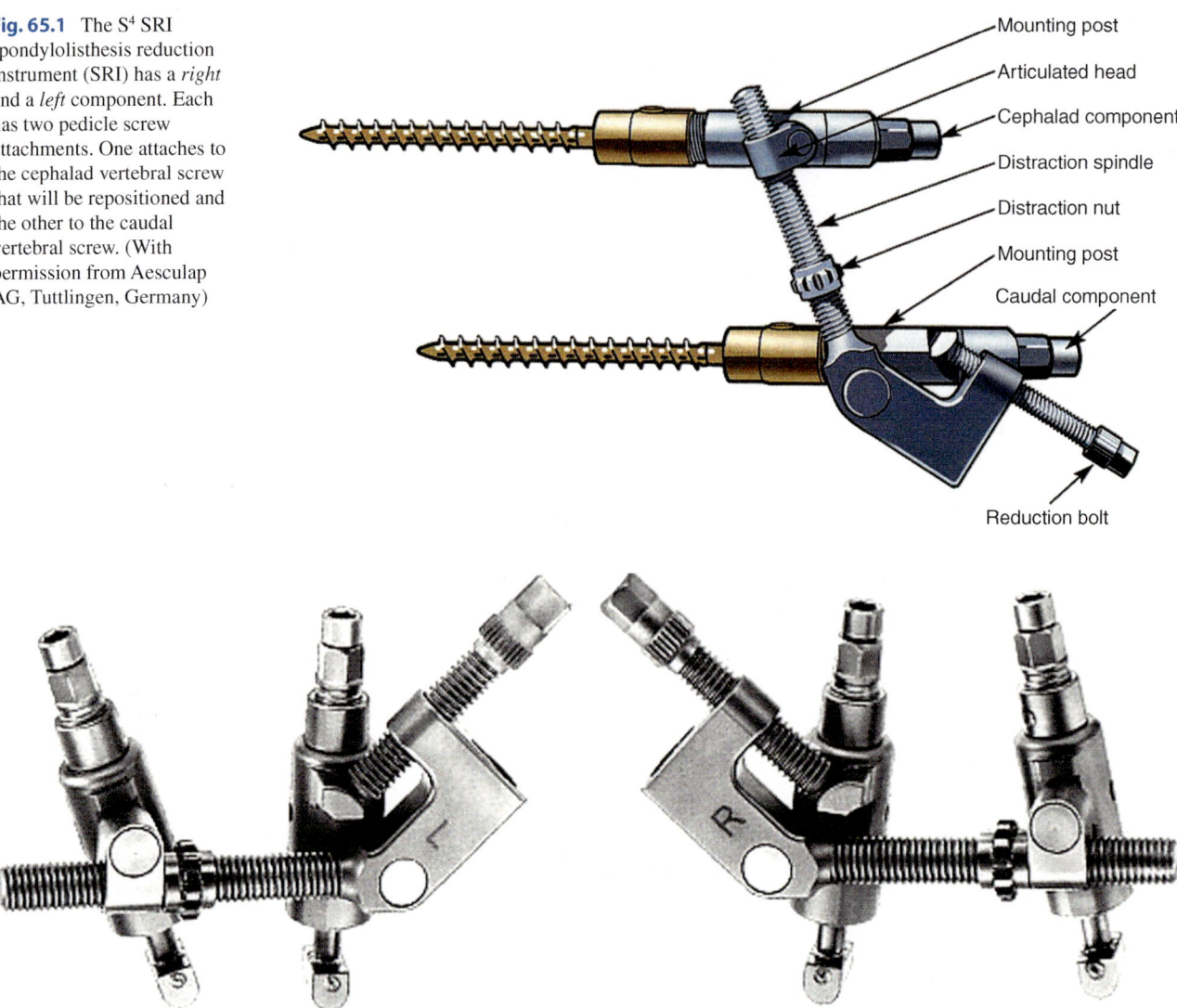

Mounting post
Articulated head
Cephalad component
Distraction spindle
Distraction nut
Mounting post
Caudal component

Reduction bolt

Fig. 65.2 The *right* and the *left* component of the S⁴ SRI. (With permission from Aesculap AG, Tuttlingen, Germany)

The S⁴ SRI = spondylolisthesis reduction instrument is one possible method of reducing a spondylolisthesis (see Figs. 65.1 and 65.2). Other possibilities are Krypton (Ulrich, Ulm, Germany), TSRH 3D Plus MPA (Medtronic, USA), Xia (Stryker, USA), Pathfinder (Abbott Spine, USA), SOCON (Aesculap, Tuttlingen, Germany), and USS Click'X (Synthes, Umkirch, Germany).

65.5 Planning, Preparation, and Positioning

Prior to surgery, the patient's X-rays are reviewed to access pedicle diameter, length, and orientation. Knowledge of normal pedicle anatomy is essential for proper placement of pedicle screws, especially in L5. The patient is positioned prone on a radiolucent operating table. The abdomen is permitted to hang freely. The hips are extended to enhance lumbar lordosis.

65.6 Surgical Technique

65.6.1 Approach

A midline posterior approach to the spine is performed with subperiosteal exposure of the posterior bony elements to the level of the transverse processes. On the lateral side, the posterior segments are exposed including the facet joints. (Access to L5/S1 should generally be made large enough to ensure reliable instrumentation.)

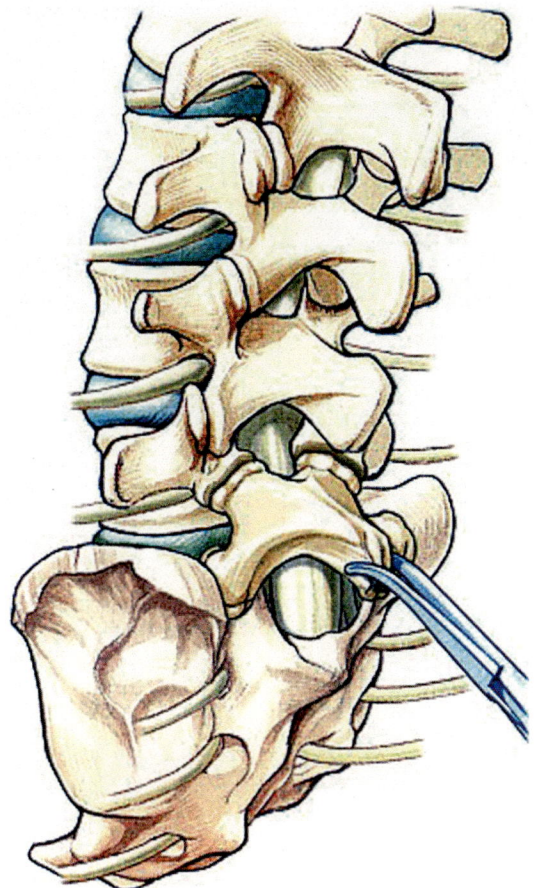

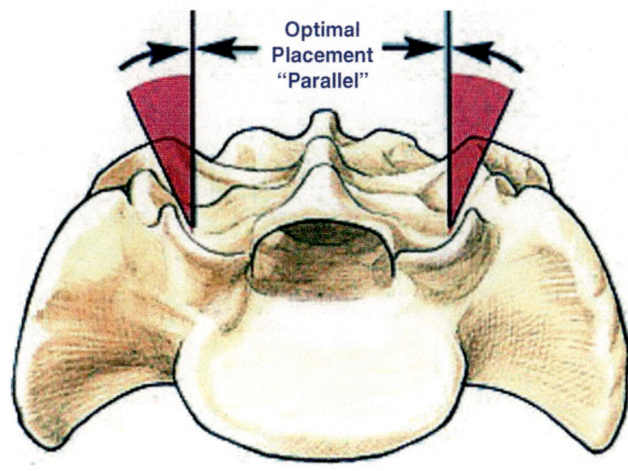

Fig. 65.4 Optimal parallel placement of the pedicle screws in the sacrum. (With permission from Aesculap AG, Tuttlingen, Germany)

Fig. 65.3 Standard Gill procedure. (With permission from Aesculap AG, Tuttlingen, Germany)

65.6.2 Instrumentation

- Perform a standard Gill procedure (see Fig. 65.3).
- Using the awl, the cortex is penetrated under C-arm control. The drilling angle is determined. Use the ball-tipped probe to make sure the pedicle is intact.
- Screws in the sacrum are best placed parallel to its superior end plate and as parallel to each other as possible (see Fig. 65.4, see pedicle access, pedicle preparation, and screw placement, Chap. 46).
- Place the caudal screws so that they are parallel to the cephalad vertebra screws in both planes. This differs from the standard convergent manner (see Fig. 65.5).
- *An alternative technique—instrumentation with polyaxial screws—allows a standard convergent positioning and easier attaching of the S^4 SRI.*
- In the case of an L5/S1 reduction, the chosen length at S1 should achieve bicortical purchase. In most cases, this is 45 mm in length and 7 mm diameter.
- During the decompression, perform a complete resection of the pars interarticularis defects to fully decompress the exiting nerve roots. This may include removal of the Gill fragment.

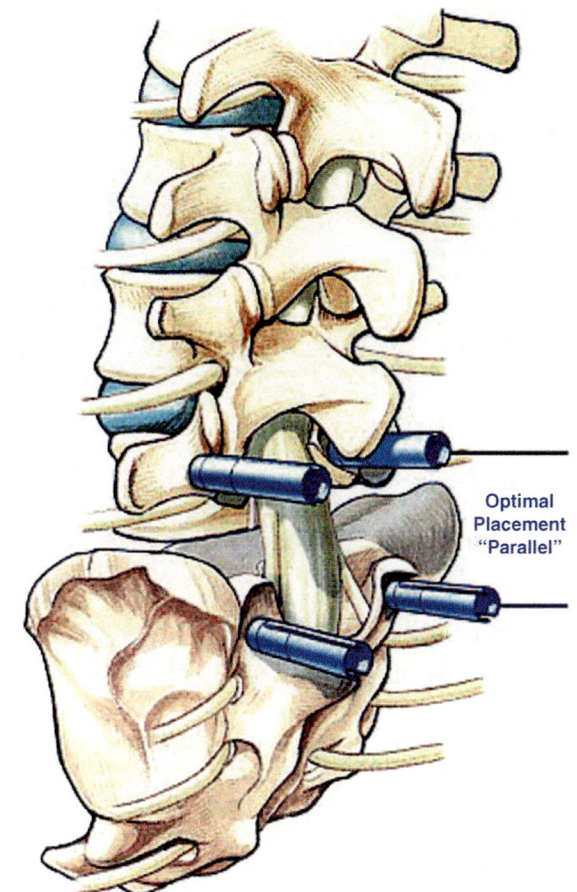

Fig. 65.5 Parallel placement of the caudal vertebral screws to the cephalad vertebra screws in both planes and complete decompression of the exiting nerve roots. (with permission from Aesculap AG, Tuttlingen, Germany)

- Perform a complete resection of the residual superior articular processes in preparation for the PLIF. A wide decompression allows access to the intervening disk space, lateral to the thecal sac.

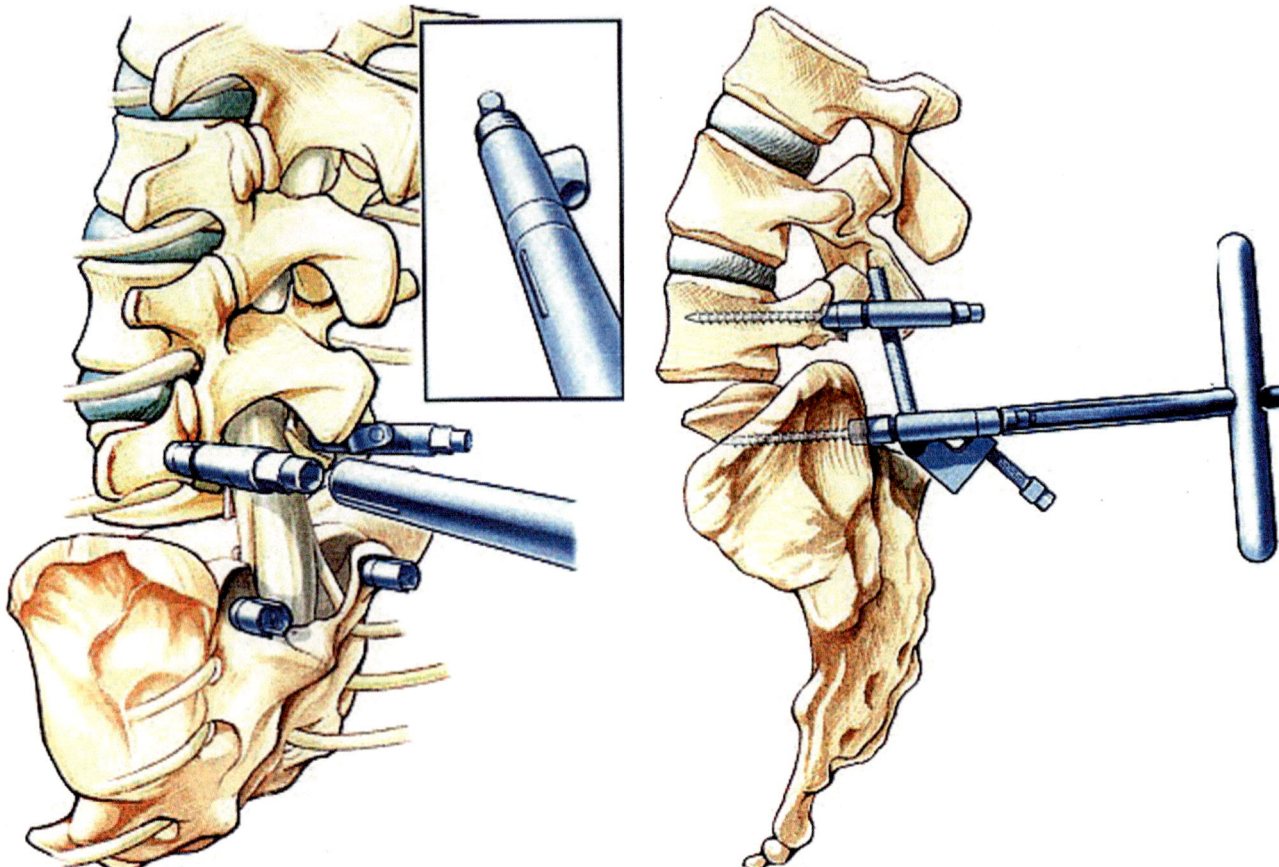

Fig. 65.6 Insert the mounting post into the tulip of the screw and finger tighten. Attach the cephalad component first. (With permission from Aesculap AG, Tuttlingen, Germany)

Fig. 65.7 The instrument is attached and positioned properly. Tighten the caudal and cephalad components using the T-handles. (With permission from Aesculap AG, Tuttlingen, Germany)

- On the caudal components, make sure the distraction nuts are of a point of minimal distraction (toward the most caudal position of the S⁴ SRI).
- On the caudal components, make sure the reduction bolts are backed out to the point of minimal reduction.
- Attach the cephalad component first (see Fig. 65.6).
- Insert the mounting post into the tulip of the screw and finger tighten (Fig. 65.7).
- The caudal components are labeled "R" for right and "L" for left. For alternative placement of SRI medially to the pedicle screws, (see Figs. 65.8 and 65.9).
- Ensure that the articulated head is positioned inferiorly and insert the distraction spindle (caudal component) into the articulated head of the cephalad component. At the same time, insert the mounting post into the tulip of the pedicle screw of the caudal vertebra and finger tighten.
- Once the instrument is attached and positioned properly, tighten the caudal and cephalad components using the T-handles.

- Hold the smaller inner T-handle and use it to apply countertorque while tightening with the larger outer T-handle.
- The mounting post on polyaxial screws should be tightened enough to lock slightly the polyaxial head.
- The mounting post on monoaxial screws needs to be tightened enough to cover the break-off tabs and part of the screw head.
- Using the distraction forceps, slowly spread the SRI device to achieve the desired distraction. Then, lock the distraction nut on the threaded distraction spindle (see Fig. 65.10).
- Using the larger outer T-handle on the reduction bolt, turn clockwise to carefully reduce the spondylolisthesis under fluoroscopy control (see Fig. 65.11).
- Monitor the nerve root tension during reduction. Typically, a decrease in the nerve root tension will be observed.
- Remove the SRI from one side if required to provide room to work and perform a routine PLIF (TLIF). If the decompression is great enough, the SRI can be left in place.

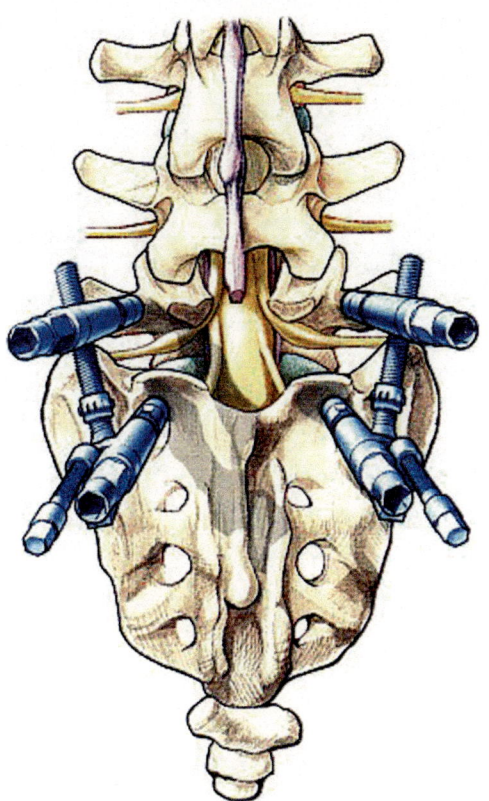

Fig. 65.8 Lateral placement of the reduction instrument. (With permission from Aesculap AG, Tuttlingen, Germany)

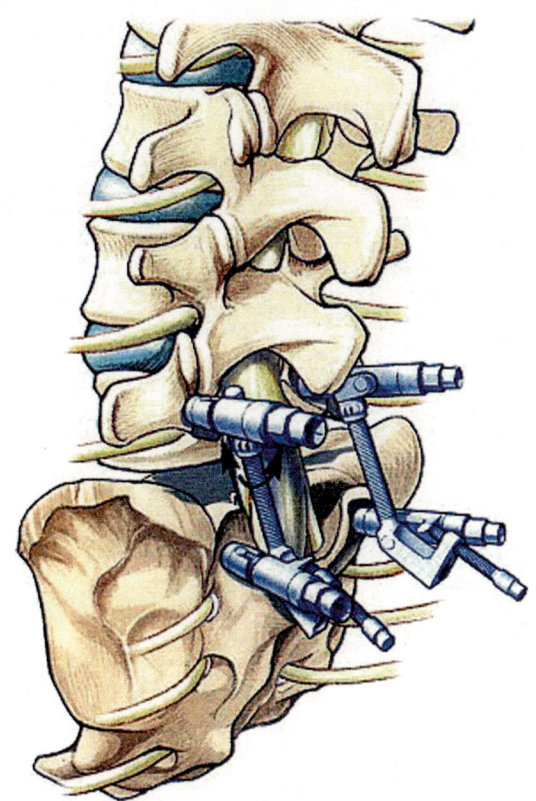

Fig. 65.10 First perform distraction with spreading of the SRI device with distraction forceps or with the distraction nut. Then, lock the distraction in place with the distraction nut on the threaded distraction spindle. (With permission from Aesculap AG, Tuttlingen, Germany)

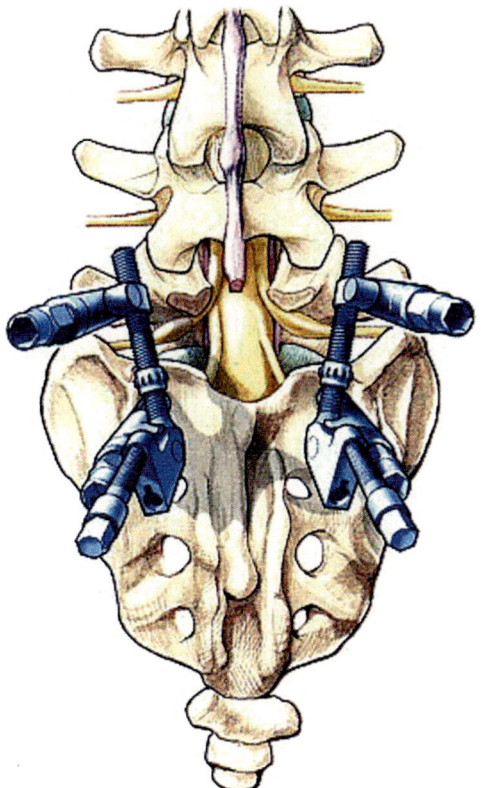

Fig. 65.9 Medial placement of the reduction instrument (alternative). (With permission from Aesculap AG, Tuttlingen, Germany)

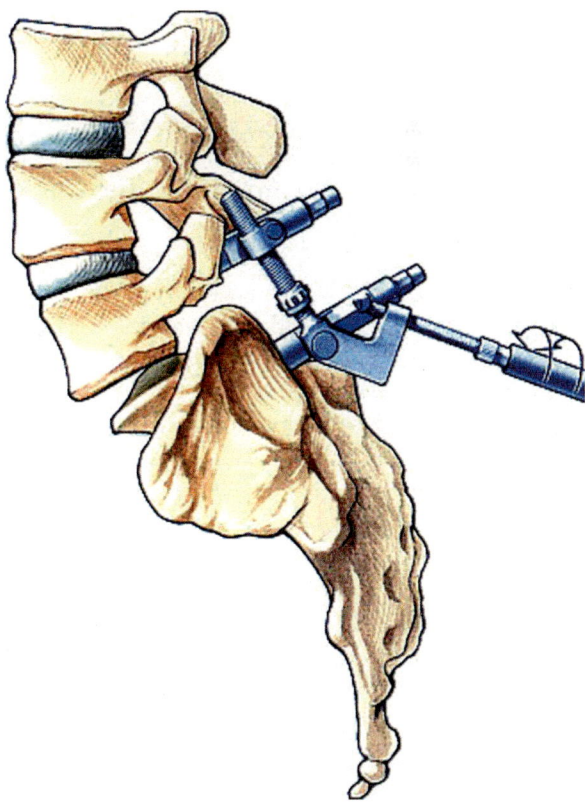

Fig. 65.11 Reduction progress using the larger outer T-handle. (With permission from Aesculap AG, Tuttlingen, Germany)

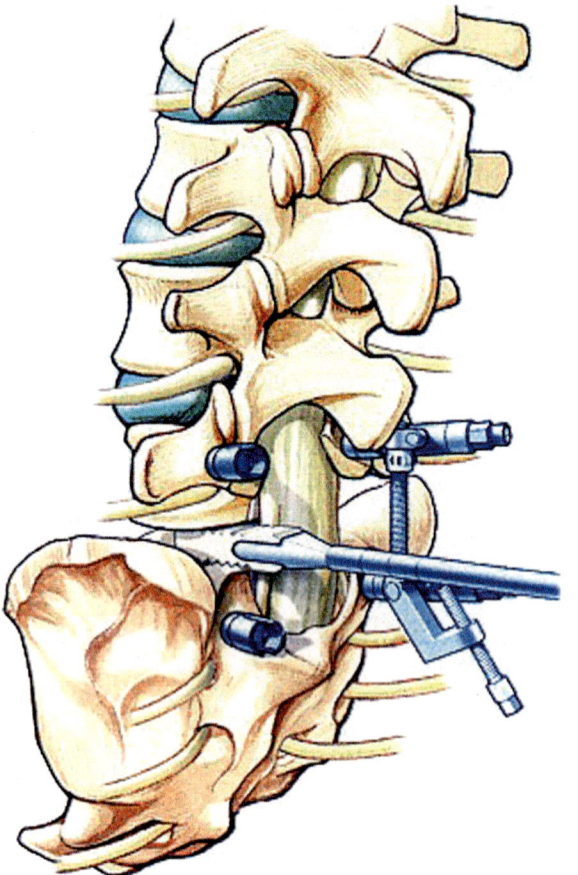

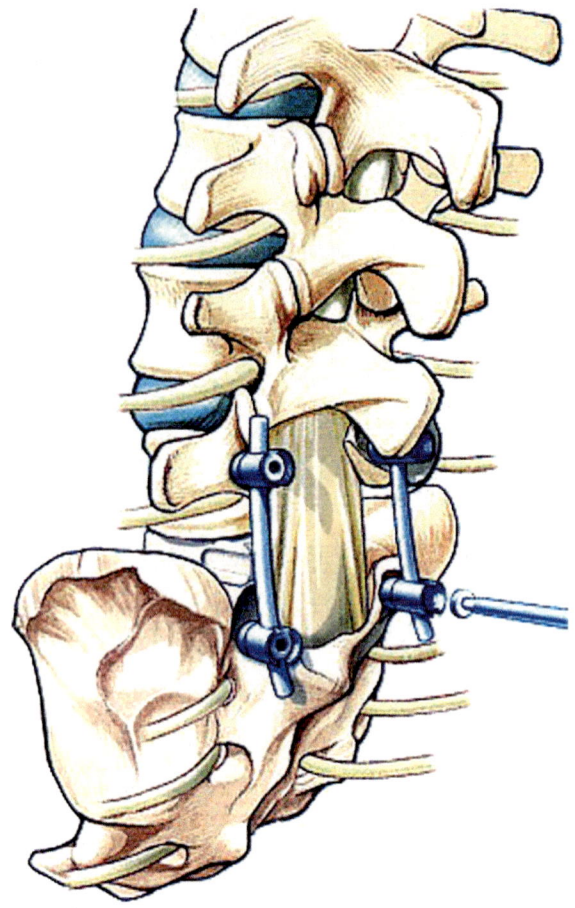

Fig. 65.12 Interbody fusion with PLIF cage. (With permission from Aesculap AG, Tuttlingen, Germany)

Fig. 65.13 Placement of the rod and locking into place with setscrews. (With permission from Aesculap AG, Tuttlingen, Germany)

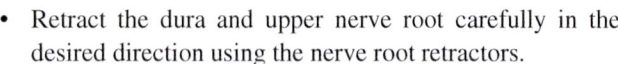

- Retract the dura and upper nerve root carefully in the desired direction using the nerve root retractors.
- Besides retracting, the nerve root retractor provides protection for the surrounding tissues during the following operative steps.
- In order to make room for the insertion of the distractor of the PLIF instruments, resection of disk material is now carried out using rongeurs and forceps on both sides of the disk.
- The PLIF implant (see Prospace Titan Spacer) should be inserted in the disk space 2–3 mm beyond or anterior to the rear edge of the vertebral body (Fig. 65.12).
- During insertion of the spacer or cage, the provided retractor can be used to ensure that the dura and nerve roots are carefully protected.
- Position the rod, and then lock in place with the setscrews (Figs. 65.13 and 65.14).

65.7 Tips and Tricks

- In the event that the space lateral to the pedicle screws is not sufficient for introduction of the distraction spindle, both SRI components (right/left) can also be transposed laterally.
- Medial placement of the reduction instruments is the preferred method. This usually allows for easier reduction and less soft tissue impingement from the device itself. Lateral placement sometimes allows an easier interbody placement, but can make the reduction maneuver more difficult.
- In order to avoid breaking of the tab during reduction, make sure to fully tighten the SRI device to the pedicle screw prior to performing the reduction.
- Prepare the small pedicle L5 with cannulated instruments and use cannulated screws in L5.

Fig. 65.14 (**a**) Lateral radiological X-ray of a spondylolytic spondylolisthesis at L5/S1, (**b**) lateral postoperative radiograph after repositioning with the S⁴ SRI and interbody fusion with the PLIF cage

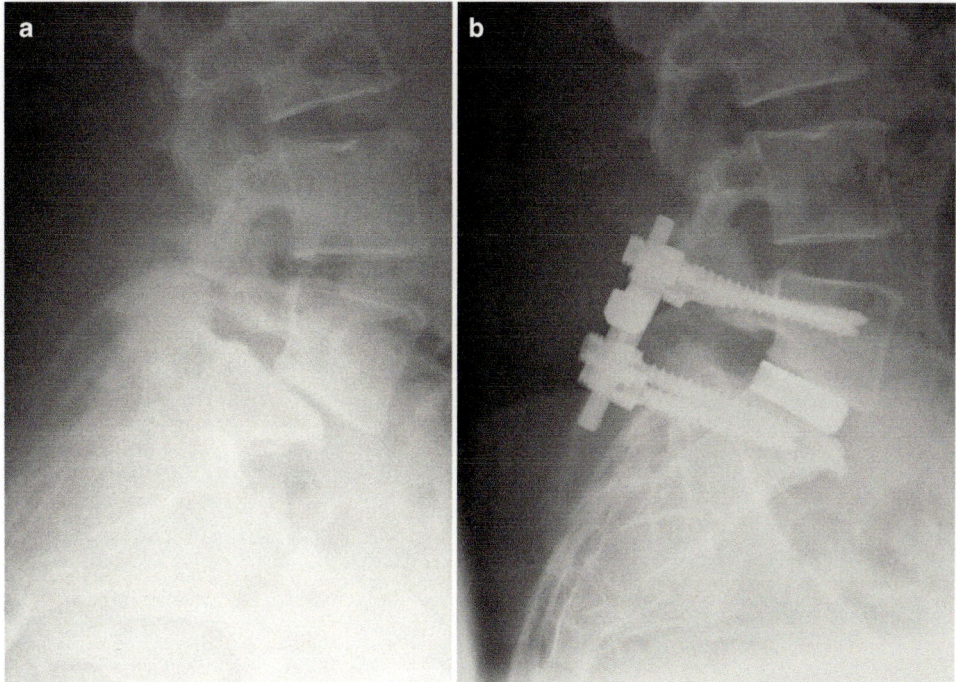

References

1. Harrington PR, Dickson JH. Spinal instrumentation in the treatment of severe progressive spondylolisthesis. Clin Orthop. 1976;117:157–63.
2. La Rosa G, Germano A, Conti A, et al. Posterior fusion and implantation of the SOCON-SRI system in the treatment of adult spondylolisthesis. Neurosurg Focus. 1999;7(6):E2.
3. La Rosa G, Cacciola F, Conti A, et al. Posterior fusion compared with posterior interbody fusion in segmental spinal fixation for adult spondylolisthesis. Neurosurg Focus. 2001;10(4):E9.
4. Majcher P, Fatyga M, Skwarcz A. Internal fixation systems in the surgical treatment of spondylolisthesis. Ortop Traumatol Rehabil. 2000;30:65–8.
5. Periasamy K, Shah K, Wheelwright EF. Posterior lumbar interbody fusion using cages, combined with instrumented posterolateral fusion: a study of 75 cases. Acta Orthop Belg. 2008;74:240–8.

Transforaminal Lumbar Interbody Fusion

Stefan Kroppenstedt and Uwe Vieweg

66.1 Introduction and Core Messages

Interbody fusion performed by placing spacers or graft materials via a transfacetar route is named transarticular lumbar interbody fusion (TLIF). TLIF is typically performed via a unilateral approach and can be performed via a standard open approach with a midline lumbar incision or in a less invasive miniopen fashion). Because the TLIF approach uses a unilateral facetectomy, it is typically combined with screw fixation (see Fig. 66.1). Advantages compared to bilateral PLIF are as follows: contralateral facet joint and posterior laminar arch are preserved, and iatrogenic contralateral scar formation is eliminated. Further, exposure of the disk space requires less or no medial dural retraction.

This can be particularly advantageous in the face of scarring after prior surgery and in the thoracolumbar area, where the myelon restricts the retraction of the thecal sac. Other potential advantages are less bleeding and a shorter operation time. Compared to bilateral PLIF, TLIF has potentially the following disadvantages. In case of high-grade spondylolisthesis, extended segmental mobilization may be necessary to achieve a proper reduction. This can be done worse. Although contralateral decompression via undercutting is possible, it is technically more challenging. Since for TLIF generally one cage is used theoretically, the risk for cage migration and loss of correction is higher compared to bilateral PLIF using two cages, and thereby having a larger cage contact area to only approach an additional posterior decompression is possible in the bone face.

S. Kroppenstedt (✉)
Department of Spinal Surgery, Center of Orthopedic Surgery, Sana Hospital Sommerfeld, Kremmen, Germany
e-mail: s.kroppenstedt@sana-hu.de

U. Vieweg
Department of Conservative and Surgical Spine Therapy with Interdisciplinary Spinal Deformities Centre and Rummelsberg Sectional Center, Hospital Rummelsberg, Schwarzenbruck, Germany
e-mail: uwe.vieweg@sana.de

66.2 Indications

The indications and contraindications for TLIF are similar to those for posterior lumbar interbody fusion (PLIF).

- Degenerative diseases from the thoracolumbar area down to S1
- Degenerative pathologies that require complete facetectomies
- Isthmic spondylolisthesis
- Pseudoarthrosis after posterolateral fusion

Fig. 66.1 Illustration of the transarticular or transforaminal interbody fusion (TLIF). (**a**) Preserved facet joint (**b**) resected facet joint

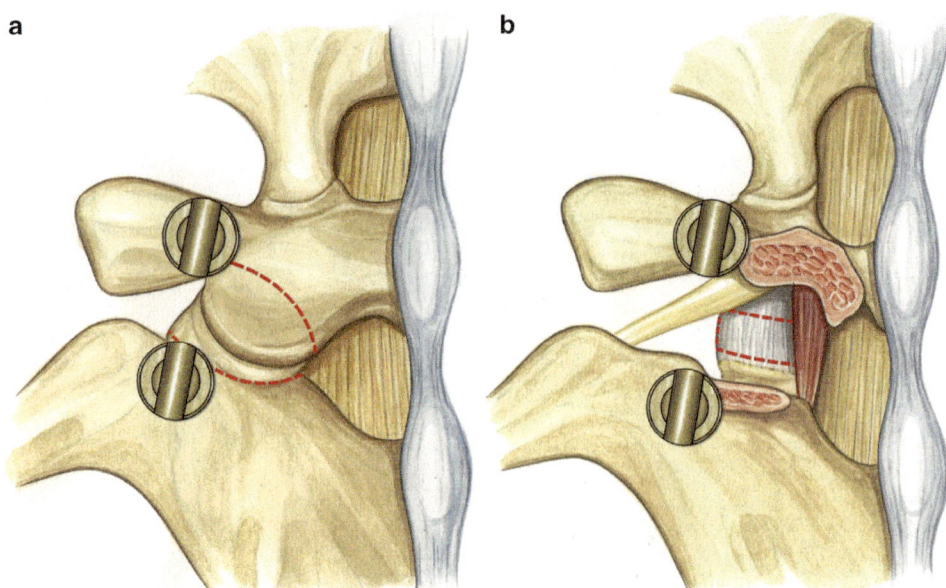

66.3   Contraindications

- High angulation of the level L5/S1
- Destruction of the end plates

66.4   Technical Prerequisites

Fluoroscopy, positioning device (e.g., Wiltse frame), adequate implants (e.g., kidney-shaped or banana-designed PEEK or titanium cages or spacer; see Fig. 66.2), and different instruments (Fig. 66.3a–c).

66.5   Planning, Preparation, and Positioning

The patient is positioned prone on a radiolucent operating room table with chest and hip rolls/pillows in order to enhance lumbar lordosis and to permit the abdomen to hang freely. For L5–S1 fusions, the operating table is moved in 20–30° of reverse Trendelenburg to allow the surgeon to have a more convenient view into the L5–S1 disk space. The level of the incision is verified fluoroscopically.

66.6   Surgical Technique [1–4]

66.6.1   Approach

A midline posterior approach to the spine is performed with subperiosteal exposure of the posterior bony elements to the level of the transverse processes.

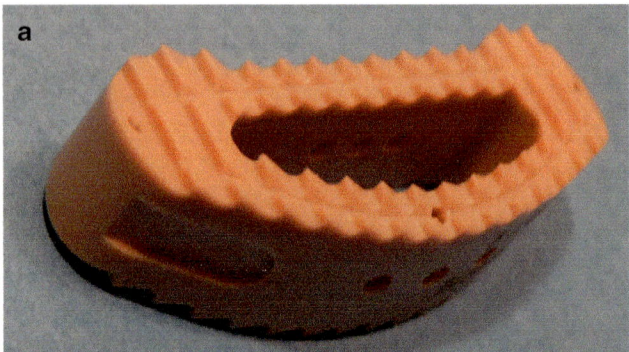

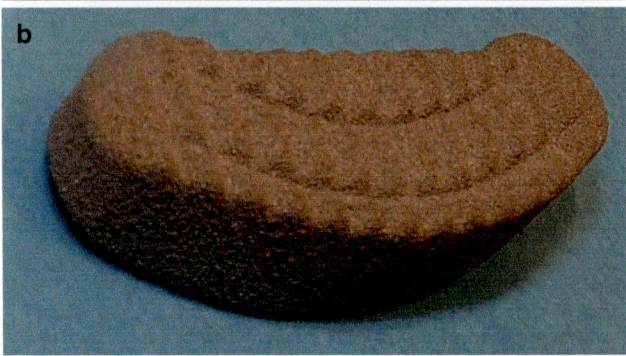

Fig. 66.2 Different TLIF cages T-Space PEEK (**a**) and titanium allow (**b**) (Aesculap AG, Germany)

66.6.2 Instrumentation

66.6.2.1   Pedicle Preparation
- The pedicle is instrumented using clinical and radiological landmarks.
- The pedicle screw entry points (junction of the midpoint of the transverse process with the lateral facet) are identified and marked under fluoroscopy.

Fig. 66.3 (**a–e**) Different TLIF instruments: angled bone curette (**a**), angled curette (**b**), and trial implant (**c**)

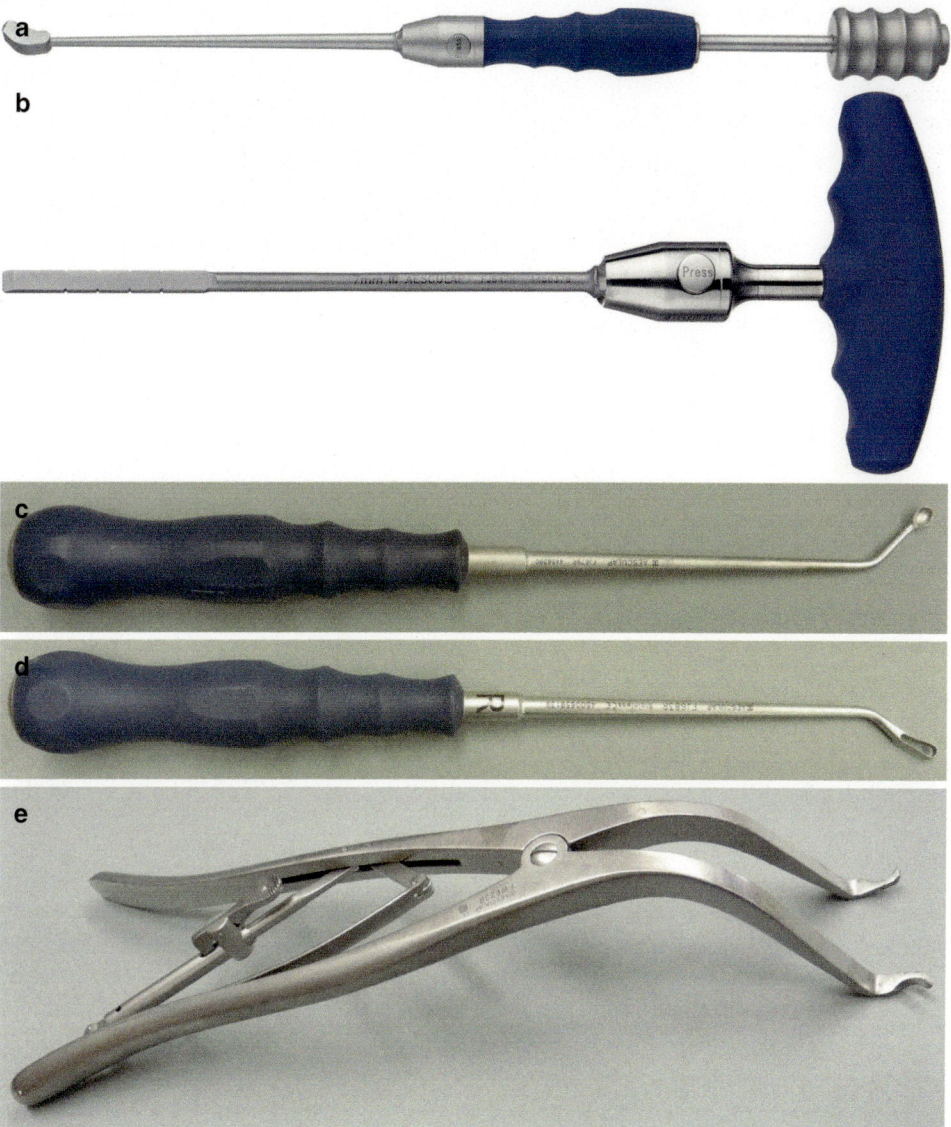

- The pedicles are probed and tapped, and screws are inserted on the side ipsilateral to the decompression.

66.6.2.2 Decompression and End Plate Preparation

- On the symptomatic side, a total facetectomy is performed using a combination of osteotomes, Kerrison rongeurs, and a high-speed burr.
- Using a big bone rongeur, the top of the facet joint is removed until the gap of the facet joint is clearly seen. This is of importance for the later use of the osteotome.
- With an osteotome, the inferior articular facet is removed (Fig. 66.4). The direction of the osteotome is from medial to lateral and from cranial to caudal orienting on the gap of the facet joint. Care must be taken not to break the pedicle or to injure the intraspinal structures.

- Using bone rongeurs, Kerrison punches, and/or a drill, the superior articular facet is removed (Fig. 66.1a, b). Care must be taken not to injure the exiting nerve root.
- The working corridor is the space defined by the thecal sac medially, exiting nerve root superiorly, and pedicle wall inferiorly. Care should be taken to protect the exiting and traversing nerve root during the remainder of the surgery.
- The annulotomy and discectomy is performed in the standard technique with standard pituitary rongeurs.
- Distraction and if necessary removal of the posterior lip of both end plates open a wider window to the posterolateral disk space and thereby facilitates extensive disk excision.

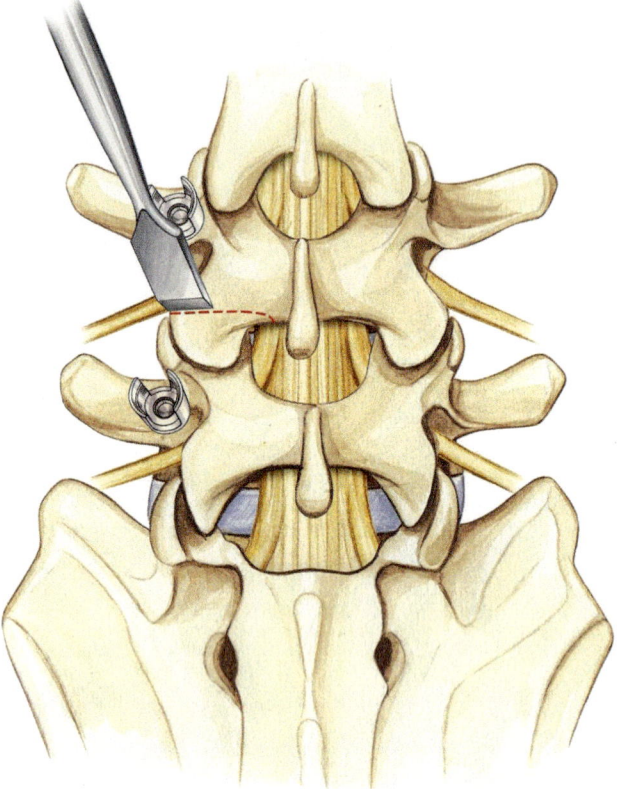

Fig. 66.4 Using a big bone rongeur, the top of the facet joint is removed until the gap of the facet joint is clearly. With an osteotome, the inferior articular facet is removed. The direction of the osteotome is from medial to lateral and from cranial to caudal orienting on the gap of the facet joint

- Special-angled rongeurs, bone curettes, shavers, and rasps aid in cleaning of the disk space and end plates from the cartilaginous surface (Fig. 66.5a–d).
- Special care should be taken not to penetrate the anterior part of the annulus with the curettes in order to avoid vascular injury.

66.6.2.3 Interbody Fusion
- The desired restoration of the natural disk height can be set using distractors. They are available in heights from 7 to 17 mm in 2-mm increments (see Fig. 66.6).
- In addition to the osteoinductive graft material, a structural interbody spacer should be placed in the interbody space to maintain intervertebral body and neuroforaminal height and sagittal balance.

- Depending on the shape of the end plates and the spinal profile, it has been our practice to use either boomerang or rectangular spacers in case of TLIF. For example, in case of segmental kyphosis, we prefer to position a rectangular cage laterally at the affected side.
- The appropriate size of the spacer is selected using specifically designed trials.
- Before placement of a cage, milled local autograft from the facet joint (and lamina) is inserted into the disk space using a special funnel or a syringe (see Fig. 66.7).
- After autograft insertion, the cage is inserted under distraction into the intended position. Distraction can be achieved by placing a spreader under the screw heads of the ispi- or contralateral pedicel screws. Placement of a lamina spreader at the base of the spinous process is a further option in case of a midline approach.
- Using a boomerang cage, it is impacted until it is completely inside the disk space and then it is gradually rotated into position using an impactor (Fig. 66.8). If the cage is already in midline position and further anterior placement is needed, a hockey-stick-shaped impactor is placed onto the concave surface of the cage in order to push the cage straight anterior.
- After the cage is placed, the distraction is released and the rods are attached and fixed.
- A further option is the placement of a translaminar facet screw from the ipsilateral side. If lumbar lordosis needs to be restored, mild compression of the screws can be performed before final fixation of the rods. Overdo of the pedicle screw compression may create a contralateral foraminal stenosis. A standard closure in layers is performed (Fig. 66.9).

66.7 Tips and Tricks

- Cage position is an important factor to avoid cage migration. Mapping the structural properties of the lumbosacral vertebral end plates has shown that the rigidity of the end plates varies significantly. In general, the strongest region is located posterolaterally, just in front of the pedicles, with more than twice the strength of the central end plate. Due to difficulties in preparation of the anterior end plates and especially in case with anterior lips, it is often very difficult to position a boomerang cage on the anterior cortical ring. Thus, contrary to a rectangular cage, a frequent position of a boomerang cage is in the "weaker" anterior-central end

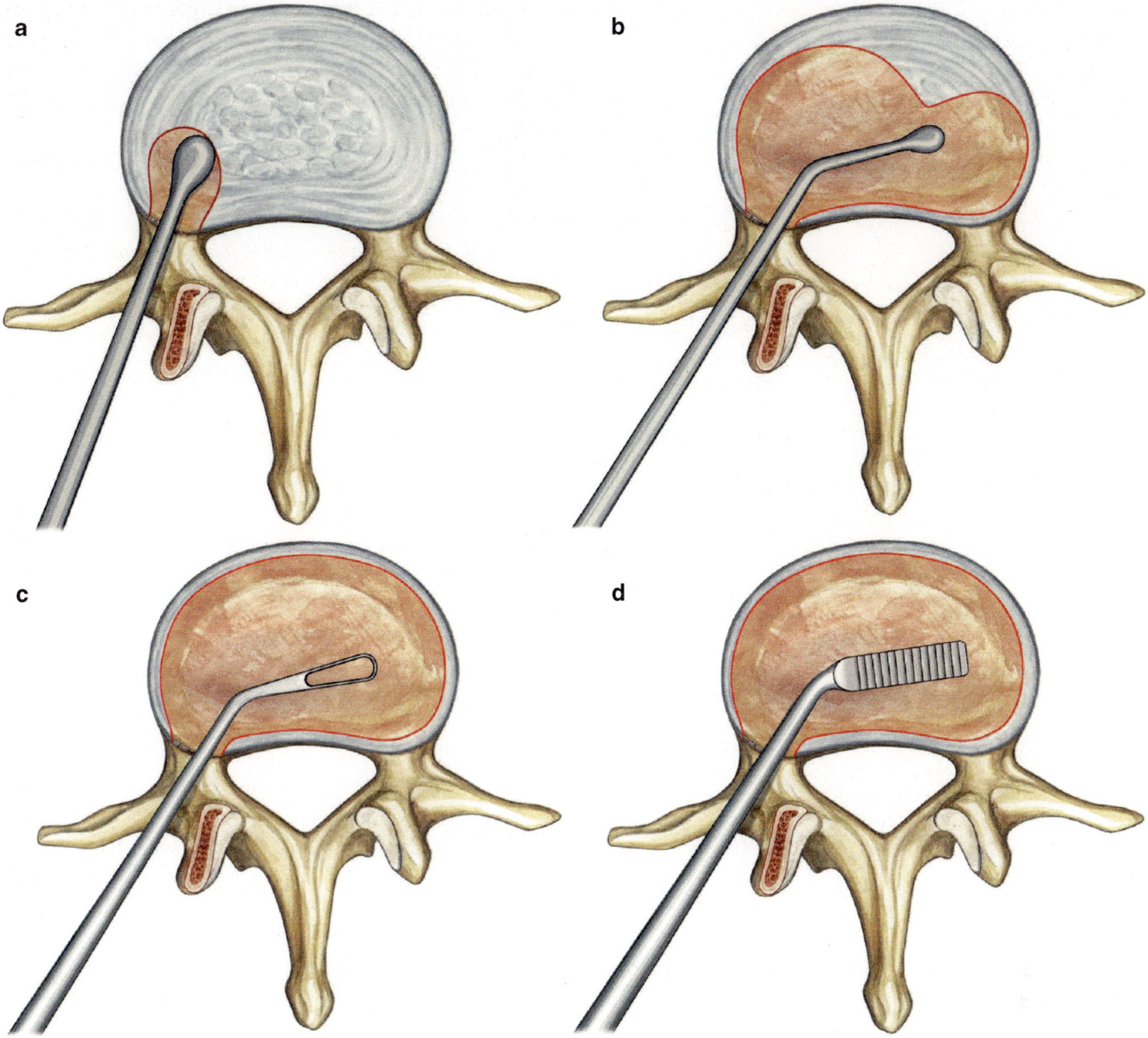

a

b

c

d

Fig. 66.5 Disk space and end plate preparation (**a–d**)

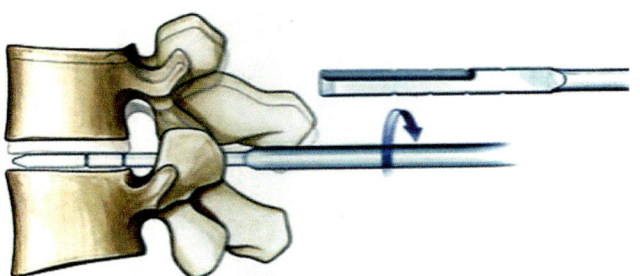

Fig. 66.6 Restoration of the disk height using a distractor

plate region. If this fact is associated with a higher rate of cage migration, associated loss of correction has so far not been investigated in the clinical setting. Using a long rectangular cage might overcome this potential problem.

• If too much autograft is packed ventrally into the disk space, adequate anterior positioning of a boomerang cage might not be possible. If it is intended to place an rh-BMP-2 sponge into the disk space, the sponge should be placed into the anterior disk space before cage placement to avoid inducing of heterotopic bone formation near the dura mater.

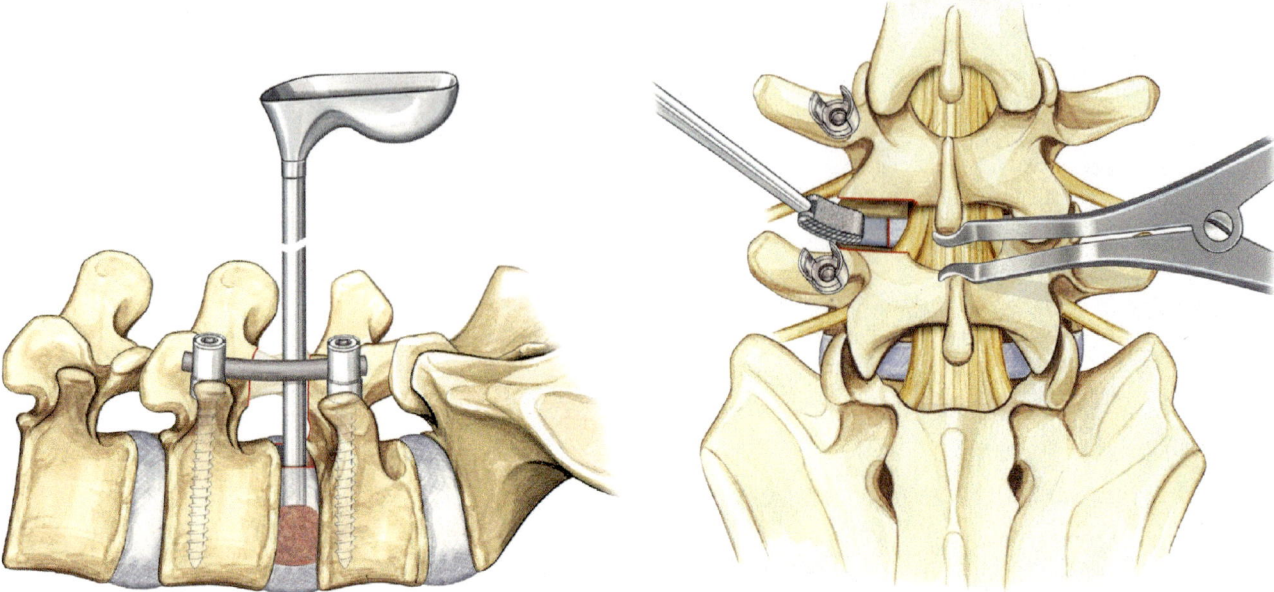

Fig. 66.7 Insertion of cancellous bone graft or bone substitute into the disk space using a funnel

Fig. 66.8 Introduction under interspinous distraction of a boomerang cage (TLIF Cage) with an implant holder into the disk space. Alternatively, distraction with an angled distraction forceps over the ipsilateral side fixed on the pedicle screws

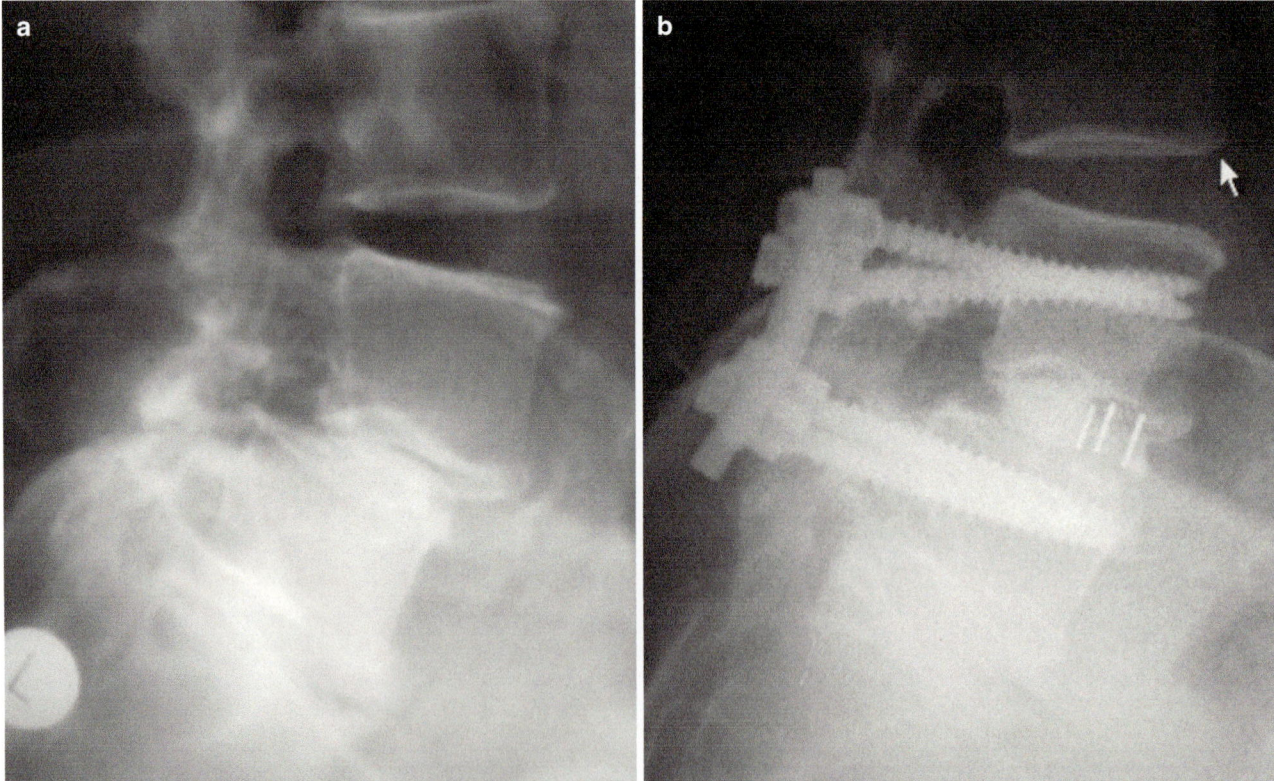

Fig. 66.9 X-ray of a patient with a spondylolisthesis L4/L5 (**a**), postoperative final construct with bilateral pedicle screws and TLIF cage and additional bone substitute (anterior, posterior, and inside the cage) (**b**, **c**); CT scans: level L4 (**d**), disk space level L4 (**e**) and level L5 (**f**)

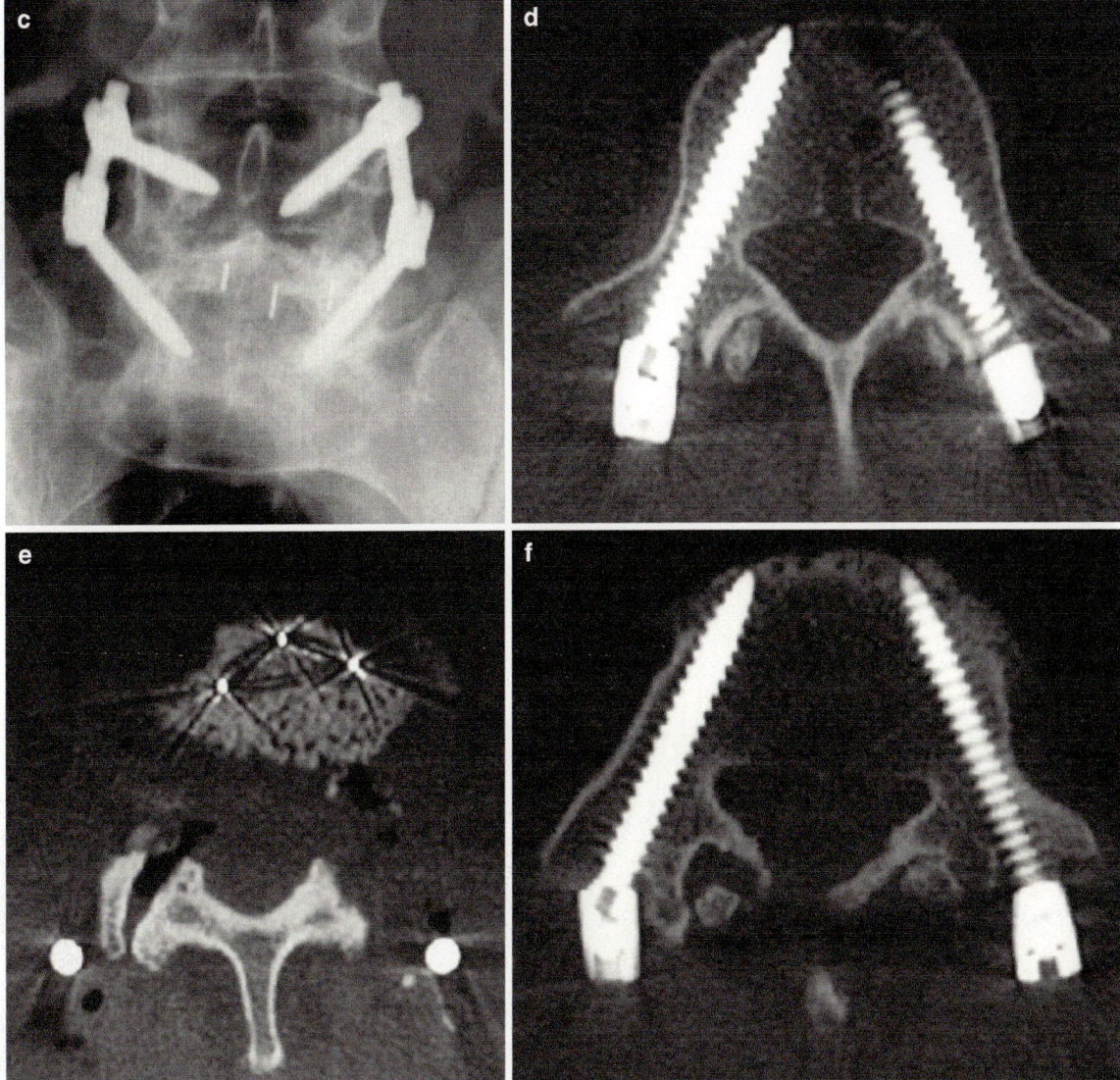

Fig. 66.9 (continued)

References

1. Rosenberg WS, Mummaneni PV. Transforaminal lumbar interbody fusion: technique, complications, and early results. Neurosurgery. 2001;48:569–74.
2. Mummaneni PV, Rodts GE. The mini-open transforaminal lumbar interbody fusion. Neurosurgery. 2005;57:256–26.
3. Dhall SS, Wang MY, Mummaneni PV. Clinical and radiographic comparison of mini–open transforaminal lumbar interbody fusion with open transforaminal lumbar interbody fusion in 42 patients with long-term follow-up. J Neurosurg Spine. 2008;9:560–5.
4. Hackenberg L, Halm H, Bullmann V. Transforaminal lumbar interbody fusion: a safe technique with satisfactory three to five year results. Eur Spine J. 2005;14:551–8.

Cement Augmentation of Pedicle Screw Fixation

67

Jürgen Nothwang

67.1 Introduction and Core Messages

Reduced bone quality is a particular problem of spine surgery in older elderly people. To force up anchorage of pedicle screws as well as pull-out strength, greater stability and fatigue resistance either a bigger diameter of (augmentable) screws [1] or cement augmentation [2] are sufficient tools. Different techniques are described, but under scientific aspects, none could be determined as obviously superior [3]. In principle, augmentation of the screw can be achieved using three different techniques: [4] cement insertion through cannulated pedicle screws with slots (either open or minimally invasive), or [5] vertebroplasty/kyphoplasty followed by insertion of the pedicle screw into the cement (either open or minimally invasive). Several aspects in cemental techniques have to be respected, so as cement volume, timing of cementing, screw type, augmentation technique, and cement materials [1, 6]. Knowing about the advantages of cement augmentation, we should always be aware of the cement-related complications, which may occur in pedicle augmentation techniques [7]. Meanwhile, new cement materials are introduced [8, 9] to avoid the respectable drawbacks of PMMA cement, for example, tissue damage due to polymerization temperature of more than 70 °C. For instance calcium phosphate converts into hydroxyapatite, and has, due to osteoconductivity and osteoinductivity, a high capability for bone remodeling and osteointegration [10] and, in the case of biomechanical testing, shows same pull-out strength as PMMA [11].

But all new cement materials have the disadvantage of a lower viscosity during injection compared to PMMA, which potentially increases the risk of extravasation. Furthermore, the biggest disadvantage is that they require 24 h for curing and therefore do not provide enhanced fixation at the time of surgery. Whether light activation of a certain length with the hands on controlled surgeon-determined polymerization opens new and safe opportunities for augmentation is still to be proved in studies.

67.2 Indications

- Osteoporosis or history of osteoporosis treatment
- Past osteoporotic fracture
- Decrease of bone mineral density to $\leq$80–100 mg/cm^3
- Rarification of trabecular pattern in CT-scan
- Need for multisegmental stabilization in older patient
- Multilevel osteolytic destruction of the vertebral bodies (i.e. multiple myeloma, plasmocytoma, NHL)
- Revision surgery of a previous implant
- Systemic diseases causing a deterioration in bone quality (M. Cushing, diabetes type I, rheumatoid arthritis, anorexia, primary and secondary hyperparathyroidism, hyperthyroidism, medication)
- Para-tetraplegia

67.3 Contraindications

- Reduced general condition of the patient: pulmonary and cardiac risk factors (ASA $\geq$ IV, NYHA IV)
- Allergy to radiopaque cement
- Severe pre-existing deformity with high degree of osteoporosis of the whole vertebral column
- Pulmonary deficiencies with severe disturbance of vascularization, ventilation, or pre-existent pulmonary embolisms

J. Nothwang (✉)
Rems-Murr-Klinik Schorndorf, Department for Trauma Surgery and Orthopedics, Schorndorf, Germany
e-mail: juergen.nothwang@rems-murr-kliniken.de

© Springer-Verlag GmbH Germany 2023
U. Vieweg, F. Grochulla (eds.), *Manual of Spine Surgery*, https://doi.org/10.1007/978-3-662-64062-3_67

Fig. 67.1 Augmentable cannulated
monoaxial pedicle screw (SOCON, Aesculap)

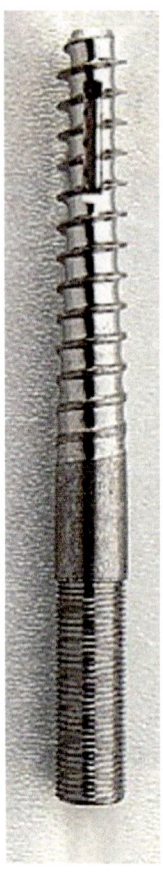

67.4 Technical Prerequisites

- Fluoroscopy, radiolucent operating table (In multilevel stabilization—i.e., de novo scoliotic deformity—a slidable operating table is helpful.).
- Cannulated pedicle screws with slots or holes (see Figs. 67.1 and 67.2a).
- For the minimally invasive technique, cannulated instruments are essential.
- Connection device for cement delivery (see Figs. 67.2b, c and 67.3) to the pedicle screw (Luer lock connector).
- Radiopaque low viscosity slow setting cement.
- Trocars for cannulation and vertebroplasty augmentation.
- As alternative kyphoplasty set with ballons

67.5 Basic Biomechanical Messages

- The strength of the vertebrae decreases with age with a definite relationship between failure stress and vertebral bone quality. Basically, the mean thickness of vertical trabeculae is preserved with age and the mean horizontal thickness of trabeculae decreases. Additionally, the mean distance between horizontal trabeculae and between vertical trabeculae increases. Both aspects are leading to a dramatic loss of bone strength [11].
- In bone matrix, the amount of glycosaminoglycans (GAGs) with its major subtype chondroitin sulfate decreases with age and may lead to significant reduction in the tissue-level toughness of bone. The loss of bound water with aging is in great part attributable to the loss of GAGs in bone matrix with increasing age [12].
- A 25% decrease in bone quality results in a decrease of more than 50% in the strength of a vertebra.
- There is a high correlation between the risk of screw loosening and the density of the bone [13, 14]. The quality of the bone is more important than the design of the pedicle screws. Below a critical bone density ($\leq$80–100 mg/cm^3), early loosening of the screws is to be expected. Clinical trials confirmed these biomechanical results [14, 15].
- Reduced bone mineral density must be addressed in early endplate failure under axial load. Below 40 years of age, the functional spine unit can bear about 8000 N (1800 lbf) of compressive load. Between 40 and 60 years, the strength decreases to 55% of this value, and above 60 years, it decreases to 45% [16].
- Compression forces generated by various loading conditions affect the end plates of the vertebral bodies more than the vertebral walls. Load related fatigue of the end plate is an important cause of cut out of pedicle screws and adjacent level disease.
- By using 2–3 cm^3 cement to augment a screw, we can increase the strength to greater than that of larger diameter screws in normal density bone. (~1600 N) [1, 17, 18].
- In biomechanical tests, cement augmentation of pedicle screws in reduced bone quality has been proved to increase

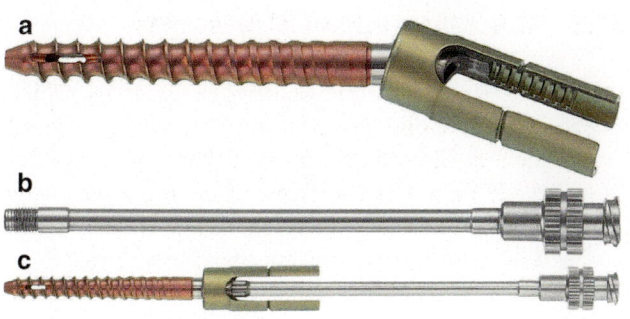

Fig. 67.2 Cannulated polyaxial pedicle screw for cement augmentation (**a**) (S4, Aesculap) with delivery cannula (**b**) and connected to the pedicle screw (**c**)

the pull-out strength of the pedicle screws [1, 19, 20] as well as the fatigue strength of augmented screws in fatigue tests [14, 21]. Erforderliche Parameter fehlen oder sind falsch.Erforderliche Parameter fehlen oder sind falsch [22].

- Clinical studies confirm the biomechanical results of cement augmentation and indicate high levels of reliability and safety [20, 21]. Nevertheless, pedicle screw augmentation techniques bear similar risks of extravertebral cement dislocation and pulmonary embolism [23, 24] as it is known for vertebro- or kyphoplasty procedures.

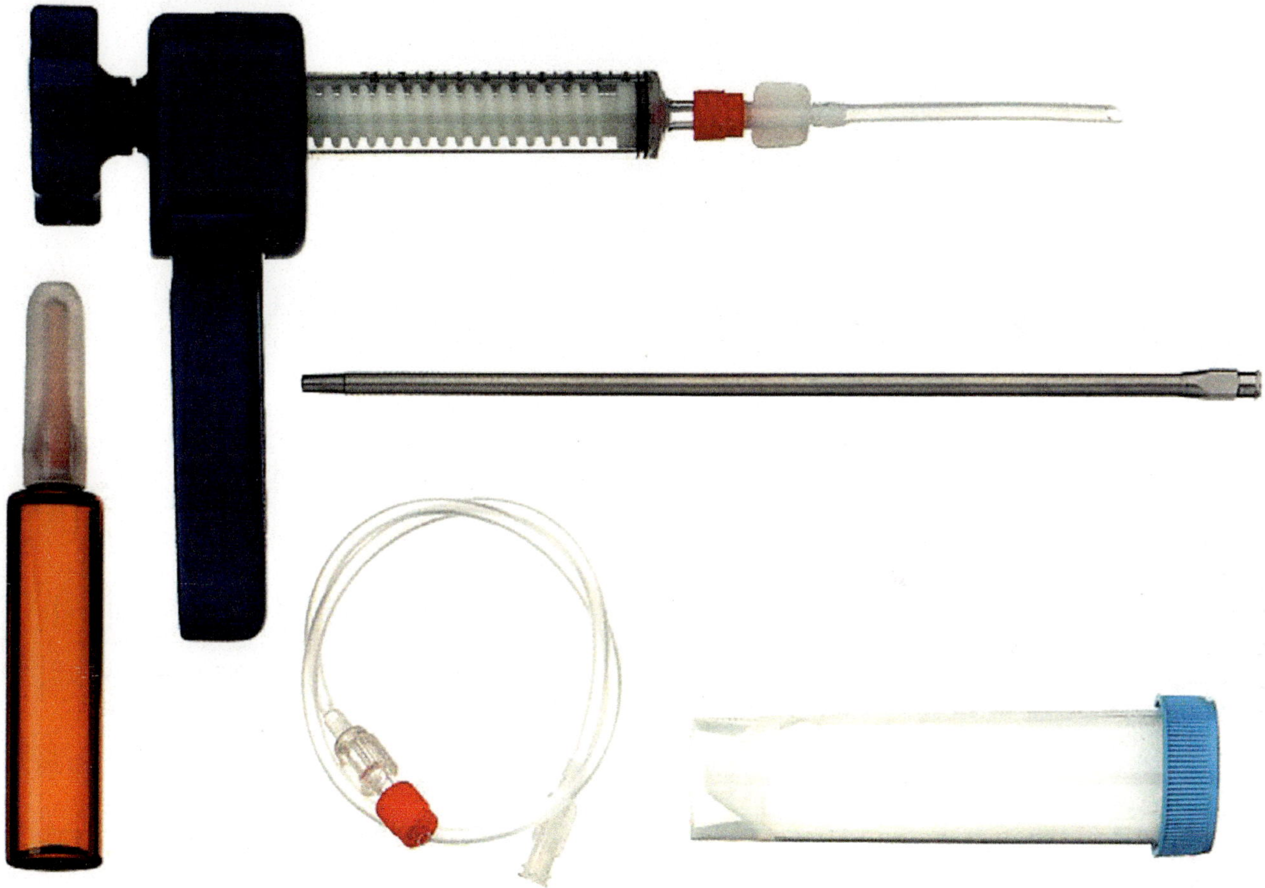

Fig. 67.3 Application set for pedicle screw augmentation (Aesculap)

67.6   Planning, Preparation, and Positioning

- Knowledge about bone mineral density or verified osteoporosis is helpful.
- Preoperative x-rays and CT-scans are analyzed to evaluate the diameter and direction of the pedicles and the integrity of the vertebral wall.
- Patient lies in a prone position (Figs. 67.4, 67.5, 67.6, 67.7, 67.8, and 67.9).

- The position of the pedicles should be verified preoperatively by fluoroscopy. Especially in higher thoracic spine, it is mandatory to verify both planes of the spinal column free from superpositions.
- The peduncular shape is exposed symmetrically with the spinous processes in the midline. The end plates should be free from double contours.
- Navigation tools might support the precision of pedicle screw application (Figs. 67.10).

Fig 67.4 Positioning of the patient

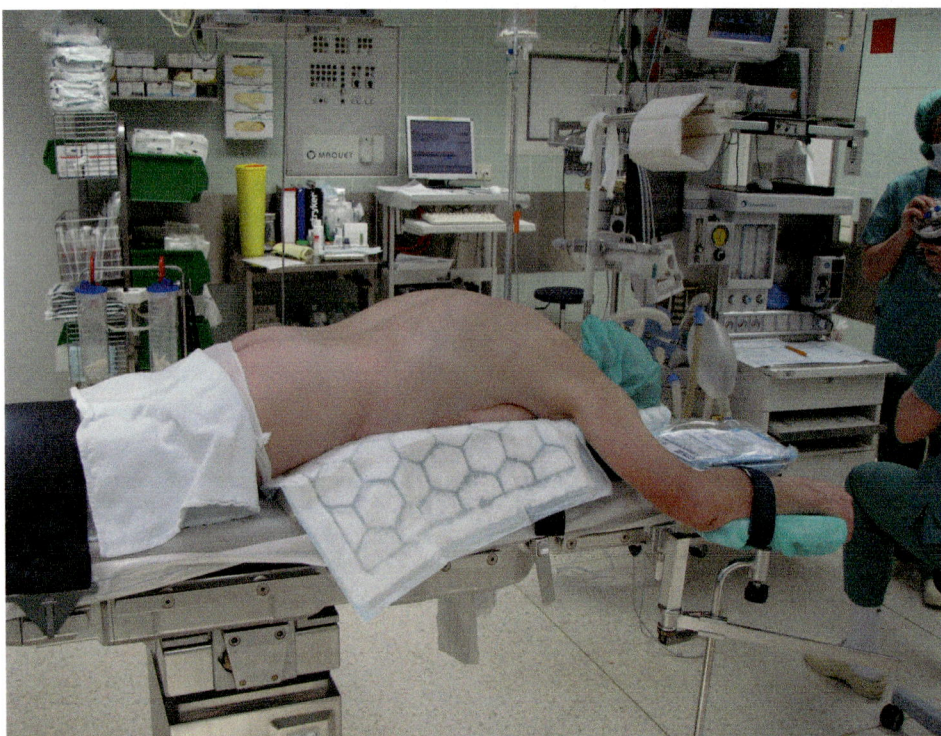

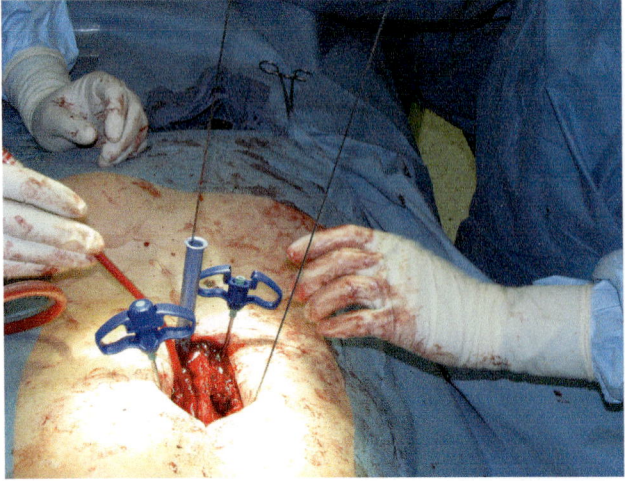

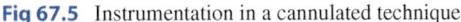

Fig 67.5 Instrumentation in a cannulated technique

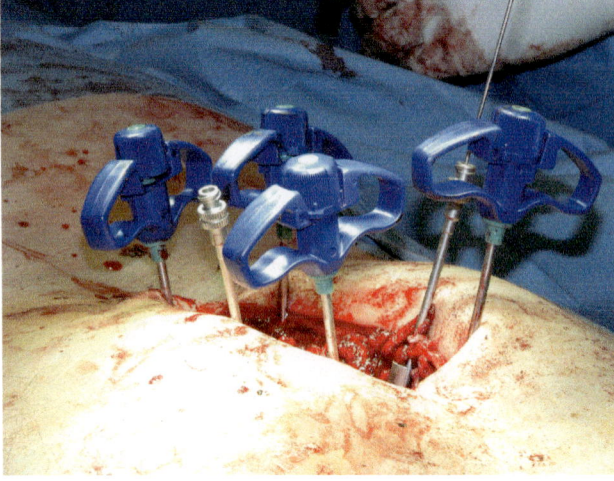

Fig 67.6 Adaption of the connector guided by the K-wire instrumentation in a canulated technique

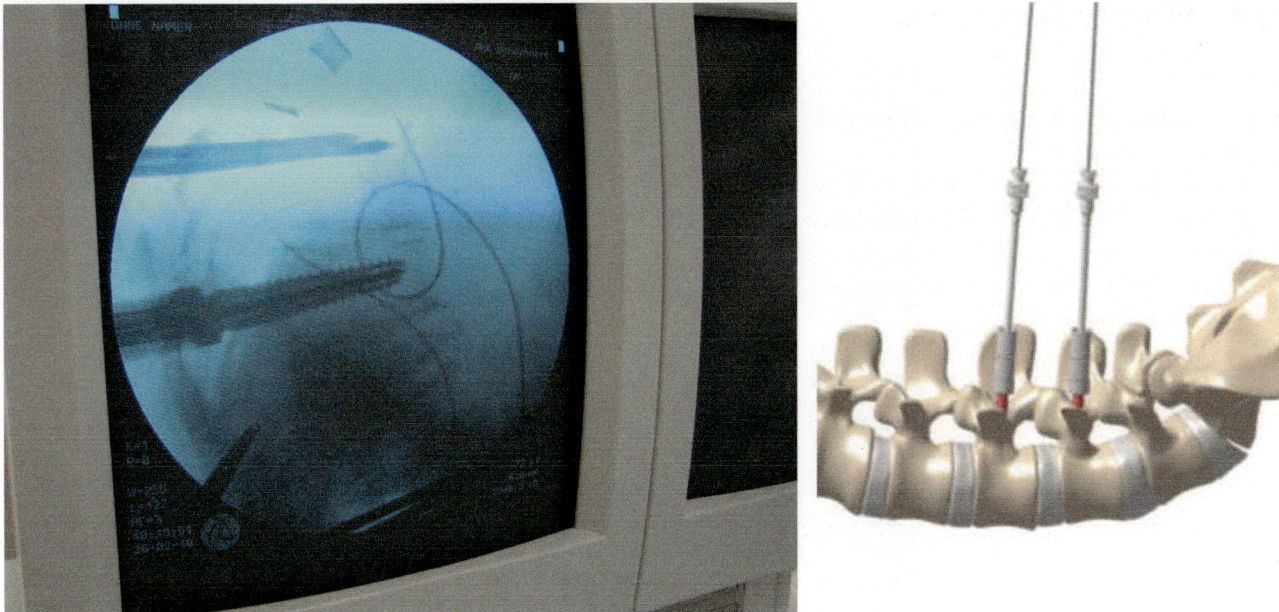

Fig. 67.7   Jamshidi-Needles and slot screw with K-wire: schema and X-ray-imaging

Fig 67.8 Jamshidi-
Augmentation-Technique and
X-ray-Imaging

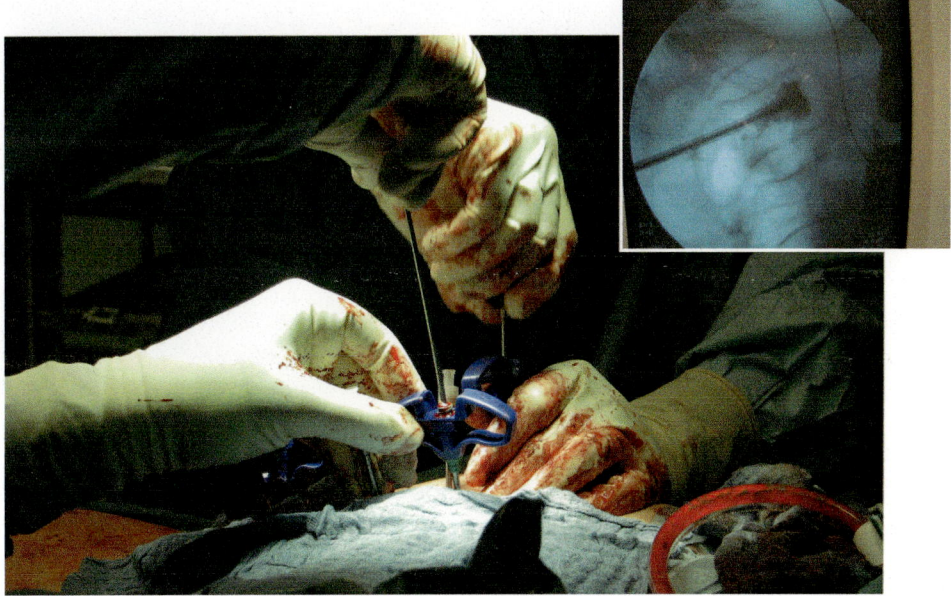

Fig 67.9 Slot-Screw-
Augmentation-Technique and
X-ray-Imaging

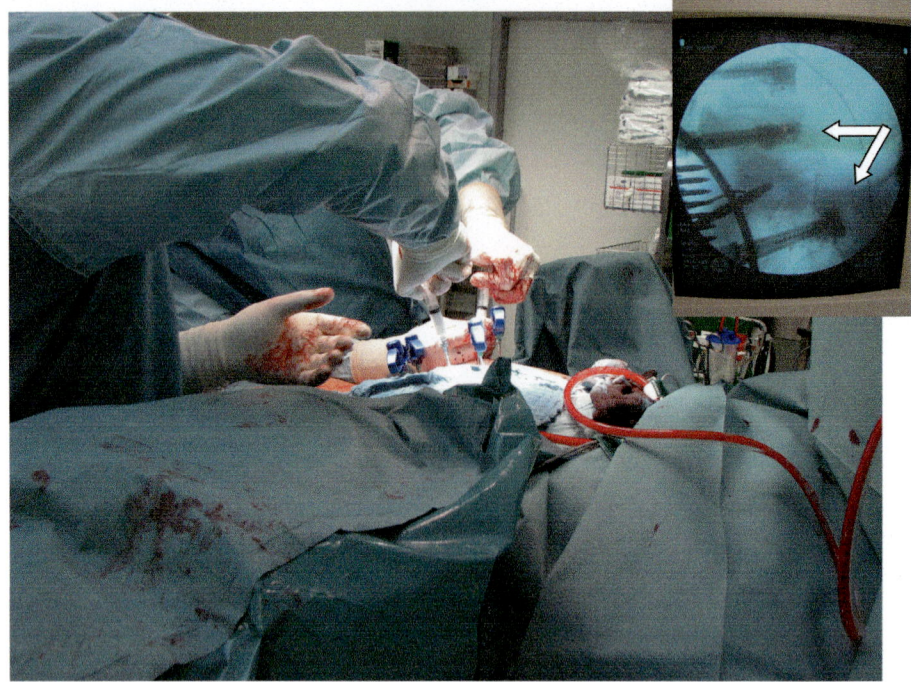

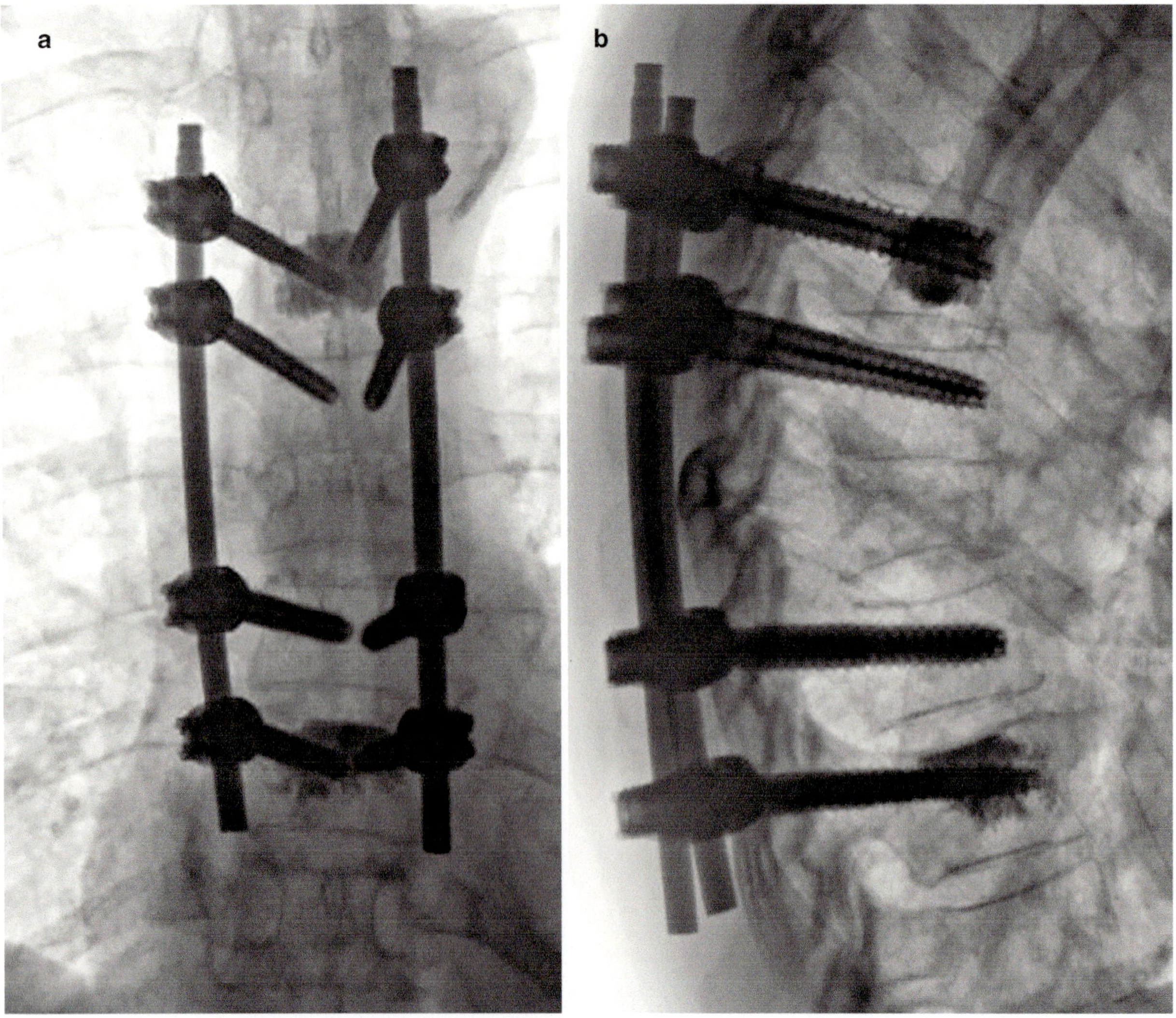

Fig. 67.10 Postoperative x- rays in ap (**a**) and (**b**) lateral view after pedicle screw instrumentation and additional pedicle screw augmentation

67.7 Operating Technique

67.7.1 Approach

The skin incision depends on the surgical technique chosen. To avoid the risk of higher blood loss especially in older patients, percutaneous minimally invasive instrumentation techniques are becoming more and more important. In our experience, they have also influenced the assessment of the risks to the patient arising from the anesthetic and the operation.

67.7.2 Minimally Invasive Technique

- We use the same technique as for vertebro- or kyphoplasty: the skin incision is at the lateral border of the pedicle.
- The incision should have a length of 10 mm to provide enough space for the holding device of the pedicle screws and later insertion of the rod.
- Blunt dissection of the soft tissue leads to the cross section of transverse process and facet joint.
- For subsequent steps, the soft tissue should be protected by a sleeve.

67.7.3 Open Procedure

- Under fluoroscopic control, we mark the beginning and end point of the planned extent of instrumentation.
- The midline incision has to respect these endpoints and should allow the instrumentation of the pedicles without stressing the skin.
- The preparation then follows the typical steps as already described in previous chapters.
- A blunt retractor exposes the field of operation.

67.8 Instrumentation I: Minimally Invasive Technique

67.8.1 Trocar Technique

- When the trocar has reached the lateral border of the pedicle, the lateral cortex is opened.
- The trocar is inserted toward the medial border of the pedicle using a.p. imaging.
- To confirm the ideal positioning of the trocar within the pedicle, we recommend a "Scottie dog projection" to the facet joints when a.p. instrumentation has finished.
- In the lateral plane, the trocar should penetrate a little way past the posterior margin of the vertebral body.

- Preferring a ballon kyphoplasty-technique, the ballon is expanded and than removed, comparable to typical kyphoplasty.
- Having ensured the correct position, the trocar can be replaced with a long-threaded wire.
- With a soft tissue dilator, the access to the pedicle should be expanded.
- The pedicle is opened toward its entrance into the vertebral body with a tap. In self-taping screws, this step is not mandatory. In facet joint hypertrophy, taping supports easy screw application.
- The tap is removed and the trocar is again inserted at least into the first third of the vertebral body.
- The length of the screws (i.g. 45–50 mm) should be measured and prepared by the operating nurse.
- The low viscosity cement is prepared. The right moment for application of the cement is comparable to the viscosity characteristics for vertebro- or kyphoplastic cement application.
- The trocar is filled with cement. The cement is then injected into the vertebral body under controlled conditions using the inserter. Usually at most 2–3 cm^3 is required for each side.
- **Attention: Avoid cement extrusion into the disK and spinal canal. Stop cement insertion if cement flow into a vessel is observed**.
- The threaded wire is inserted through the trocar and the trocar can be removed.
- Then the prepared screws can be inserted along the threaded wires.

67.8.2 Direct Screw Augmentation

- New pedicle screw designs allow cement to be delivered after the cannulated and perforated pedicle screws have been positioned.
- (Advantage: more stable connection between the cement and the pedicle screws through the side opening holes or slots of the screw.) [6]
- After insertion of the screws, a connector is fixed to the pedicle screw and the cement is injected into the screw.
- The cement flow and anchorage must be observed using fluoroscopy.
- **Attention:** Do not perforate the anterior cortex of the vertebral body. Do not allow cement to enter the central vertebral vein, which leads directly into the spinal canal. Because of reduced bending stability, polyaxial screws are not suitable for bisegmental four-point fixation. If polyaxial screws are preferred in bisegmental stabilization, we recommend a 6-point anchorage to increase rotatory stability and reduce the bearing loads for each screw.

67.8.3 Open Procedure

- The entrance point on the pedicle is identified and the pedicle is then opened and penetrated using an awl or trocar. Correct positioning must be checked with fluoroscopy.
- The integrity of the pedicle must be confirmed using the ball tip probe.
- The subsequent steps are as for the trocar or direct screw application technique described above.
- Noncannulated screws can be inserted into the tapped pedicle canal.
- In open approaches, cannulated pedicle screws allowing direct cement injection are preferred. The screws must not perforate the anterior cortex.
- The low viscosity cement can be inserted with an adapter device and a Luer lock connection. A cement gun is helpful.
- **Attention:** Following the line of least resistance, the cement leaves the screw first through the most proximal lateral holes (beware: central vein and posterior venous sinusoids). If there is a slot in the screw, the valve effect is lower. The distribution of the cement seems to be better, but the risk of central cement leakage still remains. In our experience, the safest position of the screws is close to the anterior wall. The cement distribution and positioning are quite different between the cementing in a Jamshidi punch technique and pedicle screw augmentation through slots. Keep in mind that even under high caution [25] cement augmentation techniques includes a respectable rate of complications. In an own one year investigation of 39 cases with 100 augmented pedicle instrumentations, the rate of complications due to cement application reached 15% and included paravertebral cement extrusion, lung embolism, and, in 2 cases, temporary radicular deficiency.

67.9 Tips and tricks

- For cement application, the pedicle screws must be perfectly seated. For instrumentation and cement insertion, fluoroscopic control is essential. If possible, simultaneous fluoroscopy in both planes provides maximum safety.
- In simultaneous instrumentation, we choose a more lateral skin incision to the lateral border of the peduncular shape (i.a. 2 cm more lateral) to compensate traction effects of the skin and to achieve a higher degree of convergence.
- Tapping should only extend as far as the pedicle root and should not be continued into the vertebral body. The trocar for cement delivery should then be anchored in the cancellous bone of the anterior vertebral body. This prevents the cement from flowing along the tapped canal toward the pedicle [19].

- The time of cement application often depends on individual experience and special knowledge of the cement being used. It is likely that this problem can be solved in future with the help of a viscometer, which is provided by several companies. It must, of course, be remembered that these viscometers are normally calibrated to the cement of the particular company.
- Looking at the failure mode of screw anchoring, the failure is more likely to be at the bone-cement interface in "soft" cement and the screw-cement interface for "hard" cement. This indicates that integration of the screw threads and surrounding trabecular bone is superior in "soft" PMMA cement [1, 5].
- In our experience, the trocar insertion technique is the safest method of controlling the flow of cement. After pushing the inserter into the trocar, the distribution of the cement can be followed under fluoroscopy. Nevertheless, some authors reported higher pull-out and fatigue strength for in situ screw technique than for prefilled technique [19, 21] and described lower risks of cement leakage [26]
- If there are any doubts concerning the precise position of the trocar, it can be checked in relation to the 45° "Scottie dog projection." Especially in L5 with a very lateral pedicle entrance, this fluoroscopic control is helpful to confirm correct pedicle penetration.
- In cases of generalized decrease of bone mineral density due to osteoporosis or tumor diseases (plasmocytoma, multiple myeloma, NHL), the spine surgeon should consider prophylactic adjacent level vertebroplasty.
- In accordance with the traditional rules governing the treatment of spinal deformities, instrumentation should not terminate within the apex of the kyphotic or scoliotic deformity to avoid progression of the deformity and adjacent level collapse. This so-called windshield-wiper effect (cutting-out of the screws through the cranial endplate) is typically observed in clinical practice and due to cranial-caudal cyclic loading of the screws.
- The design of the pedicle screw fenestrations (number and position of fenestration) seems to influence fixation strength [26].

References

1. Bostelmann R, Keiler A, Steiger HJ, et al. Effect of augmentation techniques on the failure of pedicle screws under cranio-caudal cyclic loading. Eur Spine J. 2017;26:181–8.
2. Kiner DW, Wybo CD, Sterba W, et al. Biomechanical analysis of different techniques in revision spinal instrumentation: larger diameter screws versus cement augmentation. Spine. 2008;33(24):2618–22.

3. Becker S, Chavanne A, Spitaler R, et al. Assessment of different screw augmentation techniques and screw designs in osteoporotic spines. Euro Spine J. 2008;17:1462–9.

4. Chang MC, Liu CL, Chen T. Polymethylmethacrylate augmentation of pedicle screws for osteoporotic spinal surgery: a novel technique. Spine. 2008;33(1):317–24.

5. Hoppe S, Keel MJB. Pedicle screw augmentation in osteoporotic spine: indications, limitations and technical aspects. Eur J Trauma Emerg Surg. 2017;43:3–7.

6. Sun H, Liu C, Chen S, et al. Effect of surgical factors on the augmentation of cementinjectable cannulated pedicle screw fixation by a novel calcium phosphate-based nanocomposite. Front Med. 2019;13(5):590–601.

7. Bai B, Kummer F, et al. Augmentation of anterior vertebral body screw fixation by an injectable, biodegradable calcium phosphate bone substitute. Spine. 2001;15(26):2679–83.

8. Kobayashi H, Fujishiro T, Belkoff SM, et al. Long-term evaluation of a calcium phosphate bone cement with carboxymethyl cellulose in a vertebral defect model. J Biomed Mater Res A. 2009;88(4):880–8.

9. Gao M, Lei W, Wu Z, et al. Biomechanical evaluation of fixation strength of conventional and expansive pedicle screws with or without calcium based cement augmentation. Clin Biomech. 2011;26(3):238–344.

10. Mosekilde L. Age-related changes in vertebral trabecular bone architecture—assessed by a new method. Bone. 1988;9(4):247–50.

11. Wang X, Hua R, Ashan A, Ni Q, et al. Age-related deterioration of bone toughness is related to diminishing amount of matrix glycosaminoglycans (GAGs). J BMR PLUS. 2018;2(3):164–71.

12. Weiser L, Huber G, Sellenschloh K, et al. Insufficient stability of pedicle screws in osteoporotic vertebrae: biomechanical correlation of bone mineral density and pedicle screw fixation strength. Eur Spine J. 2017;26:2891–7.

13. Weiser L, Huber G, Sellenschloh K, et al. Time to augment? Impact of cement augmentation on pedicle screw fixation strength on bone mineral density. Eur Spine J. 2018;27:1964–71.

14. Okuyama K, Abe E, Suzuki T, et al. Influence of bone mineral density on pedicle screw fixation, a study of pedicle screw fixation augmenting posterior lumbar interbody fusion in elderly patients. Spine J. 2001;1:402–7.

15. Perey O. Fracture of the vertebral end plate in the lumbar spine: an experimental biomechanical investigation. Acta Orthop Scand Suppl. 1957;25:1–101.

16. Frankel BM, D'Agostino S, Wang CA. biomechanical cadaveric analysis of polymethylmethacrylate-augmented pedicle screw fixation. J Neurosurg Spine. 2007;7(1):47–53.

17. Folsch C, Goost H, Figiel J, et al. Correlation of pull-out strength of cement-augmented pedicle screws with CT-volumetric measurement of cement. Biomed Tech. 2012;57(6):473–80.

18. Choma TJ, Pfeiffer FM, Swope RW, et al. Pedicle screw design and cement augmentation in osteoporotic vertebrae: effects of fenestrations and cement viscosity on fixation and extraction. Spine. 2012;37:1628–32.

19. Yu BS, Li ZM, Zhou ZY, et al. Biomechanical effects of insertion location and bone cement augmentation on the anchoring strength of iliac screw. Clin Biomech. 2011;26(6):556–61.

20. Kueny RA, Kolb JP, Lehmann W, et al. Influence of the screw augmentation technique and a diameter increase on pedicle screw fixation in the osteoporotic spine: pullout versus fatigue testing. Eur Spine J. 2014;23:2196–202.

21. El Saman A, Meier S, Sander A, et al. Reduced loosening rate and loss of correction following posterior stabilization with or without PMMA augmentation of pedicle screws in vertebral fractures in the elderly. Eur J Trauma Emerg Surg. 2013;5:455–60.

22. Sawakami K, Yamazaki A, Ishikawa S, et al. Polymethylmethacrylate augmentation of pedicle screws increases the initial fixation in osteoporotic spine patients. J Spinal Disord Tech. 2012;25(2):E28–35.

23. Janssen I, Ryang Y-M, Gempt, Jet al (2017) Risk of cement leakage and pulmonary embolism by bone cement-augmented pedicle screw fixation of the thoracolumbar spine Spine J 17: 837–844.

24. Chang MC, Kao HC, Ying SH, Liu CL. Polymethylmethacrylate augmentation of cannulated pedicle screws for fixation in osteoporotic spines and comparison of its clinical results and biomechanical characteristics with the needle injection method. J Spinal Disord Technol. 2013;26–6:305–15.

25. Ulusoy OL, Kahraman S, Karalok I, et al. Pulmonary cement embolism following cement-augmented fenestrated pedicle screw fixation in adult spinal deformity patients with severe osteoporosis (analysis of 2978 fenestrated screws). Eur Spine J. 2018;27:2348–56.

26. Tan QC, Wu JW, Peng F, et al. Augmented PMMA distribution: improvement of mechanical property and reduction of leakage rate of a fenestrated pedicle screw with diameter-tapered perforations. J Neurosurg Spine. 2016;24(6):971–7.

Less Invasive Pedicle Screw Instrumentation of Lumbar Spine Fractures

68

Ulrich Hahn

68.1 Introduction and Core Messages

The distinctive feature of the minimally invasive posterior dorsal instrumentation is not so much the less invasive placement of mono- or polyaxial pedicle screws, but rather the fact that it allows a genuine distraction and lordosis reduction, the real benefit of the procedure described here. However, this minimally invasive reduction requires a special instrumentation and the mandatory use of monoaxial pedicle screws, since only such screws can sustain the preload resulting from the reduction. The goals of the minimally invasive posterior instrumentation with S4 fracture reduction instruments are almost no soft tissue damage, because muscle attachments are not detached, same reduction results as in open procedures, same implants as for open procedures, reduced postoperative pain, shorter operation time, and negligible blood loss.

68.2 Indications

- Anterior compression fractures with kyphosis angle and unstable fractures of the lumbar spine [1]
- Only restricted indication in AO C-type fractures (see contraindications [2])
- Only relative indications in multilevel injuries [3]

68.3 Contraindications

- Severe osteoporosis, osteopenia, or osteomyelitis
- Transverse connector required in cases of rotational instability
- Same contraindications as for open procedures [4, 5]

68.4 Technical Prerequisites

Fluoroscopy, radiolucent operating table, cannulated pedicle screws (S4 Spinal System, Aesculap AG), special fracture reduction instruments (e.g., S4 spinal system with fracture reduction instrument—FRI, Aesculap, see Fig. 68.1). If kyphosis correction is intended, the use of monoaxial fracture screws is required, because only these screws can sustain the preload of the reduction maneuver. There are other devices available for percutaneous dorsal instrumentation (e.g., Sextant, Medtronic), but at the moment, only the FRI device allows genuine fracture reduction.

U. Hahn (✉)
Rems-Murr Schorndorf Hospital, Department of Orthopedics and Traumatology, Schorndorf, Germany
e-mail: u.hahn@ots-praxisklinik.de

© Springer-Verlag GmbH Germany 2023
U. Vieweg, F. Grochulla (eds.), *Manual of Spine Surgery*, https://doi.org/10.1007/978-3-662-64062-3_68

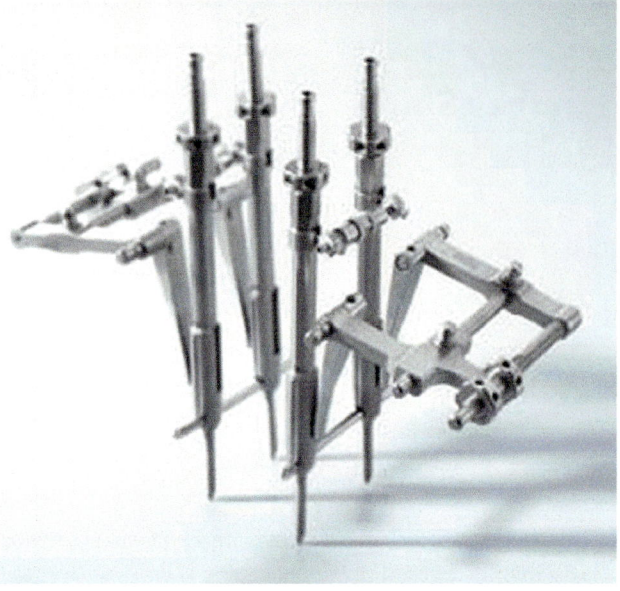

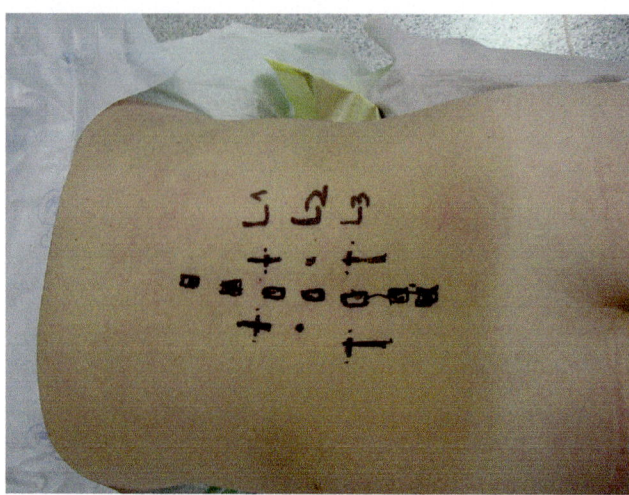

Fig. 68.2 Preoperative fluoroscopy-based planning of the skin incision

Fig. 68.1 S4 fracture reduction instrument (Aesculap AG). (With permission from Aesculap AG, Tuttlingen, Germany)

68.5 Planning, Preparation, and Positioning

During the operation, the patient is in a prone position on a radiolucent operating table. Different positioning systems can be used (Wilson frame, chest rolls, Relton-Hall frame, etc.).

Exact C-arm-controlled planning of the approach is mandatory (see Fig. 68.2).

68.6 Surgical Technique

68.6.1 Approach

- Access is obtained by an incision of the thoracolumbar fascia between the multifidus and the longissimus muscles. The muscles are dissected bluntly only in the fiber direction. As a rule, this procedure can be carried out without bleeding or with minimal blood loss. With the help of an appropriate cannulated guiding device (see Fig. 68.3), the entry point is selected at the junction of the facet and the transverse process.
- Remove the trocar; the K-wire aiming device remains in the pedicle (see Fig. 68.4).

To guide the cannulated pedicle screw, insert the K-wire into the aiming device. As alternative, you can use a K-wire protection sleeve (see Fig. 68.5).

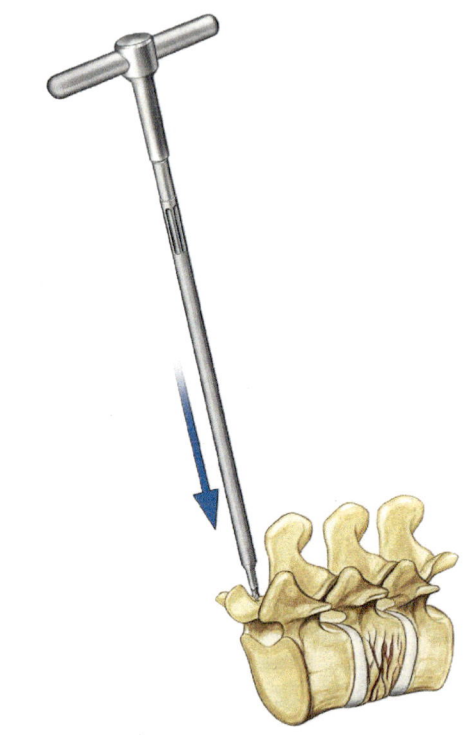

Fig. 68.3 Selection of entry point at the junction of the facet and the transverse process and decortication with cannulated guiding device. (With permission from Aesculap AG, Tuttlingen, Germany)

Note: The Kirschner wire should be inserted so far that its tip represents the end position of the pedicle screw tip.
- You must be absolutely certain that the Kirschner wire is not inserted too far to avoid damaging soft tissue and vessels. Use intraoperative fluoroscopy!

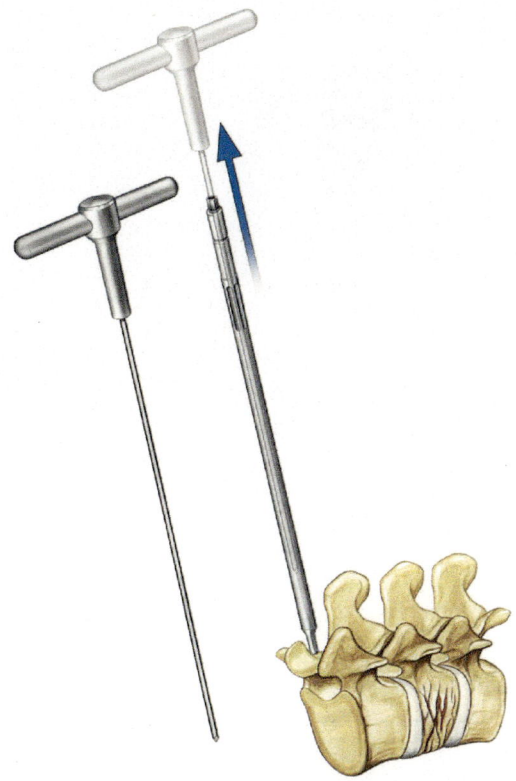

Fig. 68.4 Removal of trocar, the K-wire aiming device remains in the pedicle. (With permission from Aesculap AG, Tuttlingen, Germany)

- Insert dilatation sleeves via the K-wire aiming device to create sufficient space for the pedicle screw (see Fig. 68.6).
- Slide the blue tissue protection sleeve over the dilatation sleeve (see Fig. 68.7).

68.6.2 Instrumentation [1–7]

- If necessary, use a pedicle reamer to further prepare the pedicle (see Fig. 68.8) or, in the case of sclerotic bone, a thread cutter with the appropriate diameter (see Fig. 68.9).
- To determine the length of the screw, insert the screw length-measuring instrument, with the calibration markings turned upward, via the K-wire and place it on the vertebral body with the distal end (see Fig. 68.10). The length of the screw can be read from the markings on the K-wire (see Fig. 68.10).
- Insert the screws with the cannulated screwdriver under fluoroscopy guidance in lateral and anteroposterior projections.
- *Note*: If necessary, after 3–4 turns of the screw, the K-wire should be removed to avoid its rotation and ventral perforation.

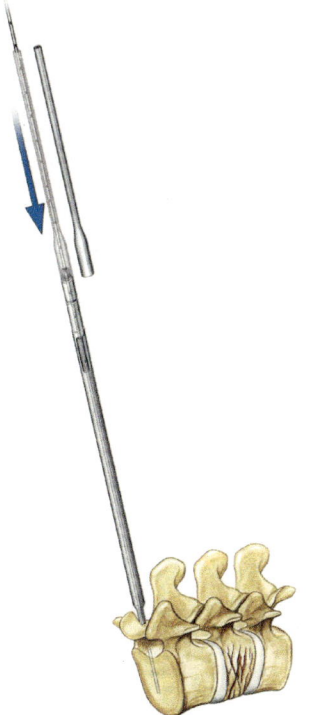

Fig. 68.5 Insertion of K-wire, if necessary, a K-wire protection sleeve is used. (With permission from Aesculap AG, Tuttlingen, Germany)

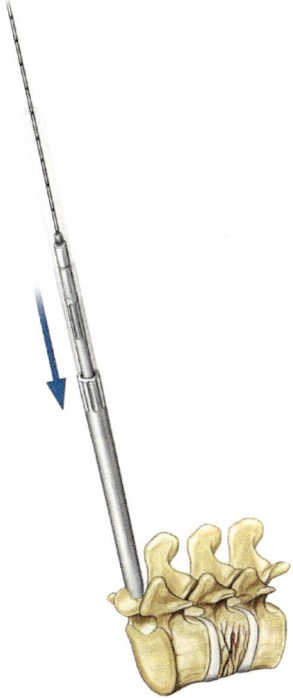

Fig. 68.6 Insertion of dilatation sleeves via the K-wire aiming device. (With permission from Aesculap AG, Tuttlingen, Germany)

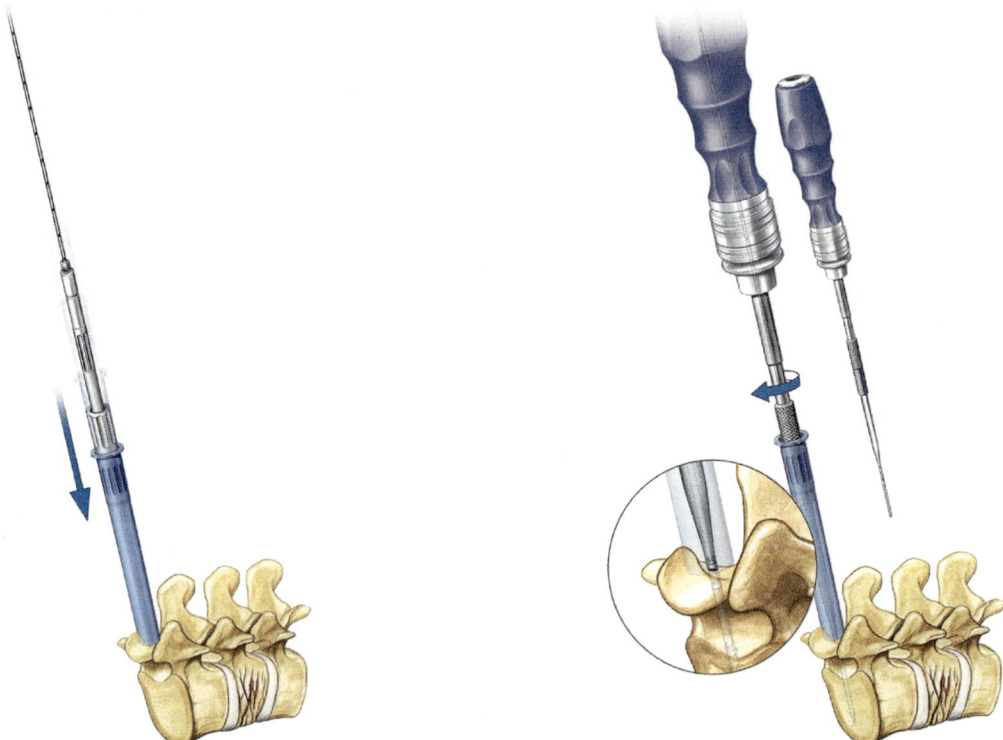

Fig. 68.7 Sliding of the blue tissue protection sleeve over the dilatation sleeve. (With permission from Aesculap AG, Tuttlingen, Germany)

Fig. 68.9 Preparation of pedicle using a thread cutter in the case of sclerotic bone. (With permission from Aesculap AG, Tuttlingen, Germany)

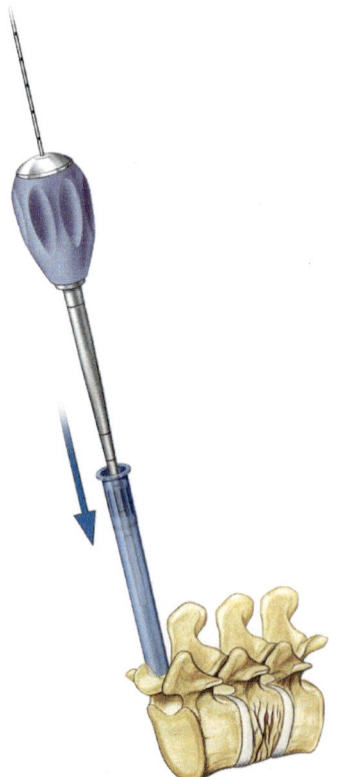

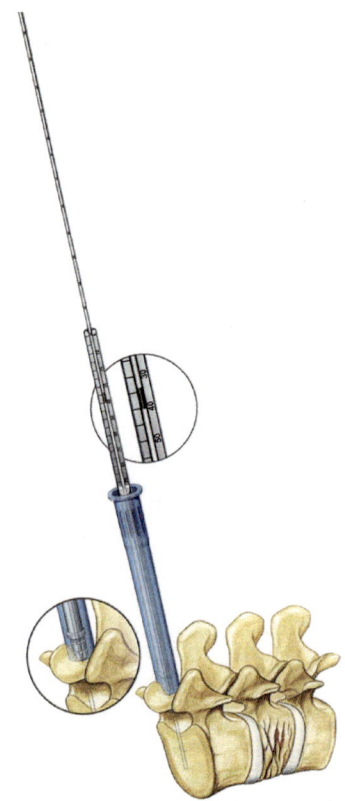

Fig. 68.8 Preparation of pedicle using a pedicle awl. (With permission from Aesculap AG, Tuttlingen, Germany)

Fig. 68.10 Length determination using the cannulated measuring instrument. (With permission from Aesculap AG, Tuttlingen, Germany)

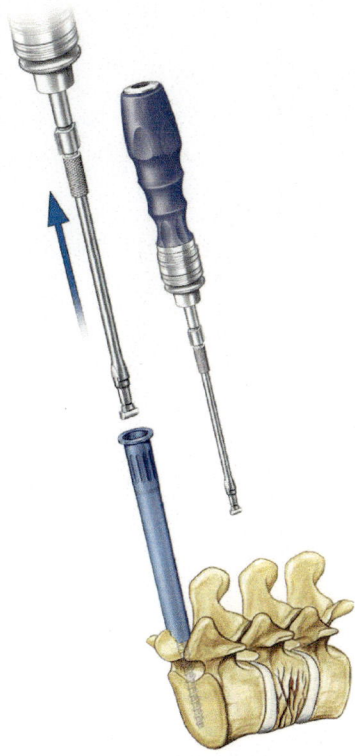

Fig. 68.11 Correct alignment of the screw slot, using the wings of the alignment device. (With permission from Aesculap AG, Tuttlingen, Germany)

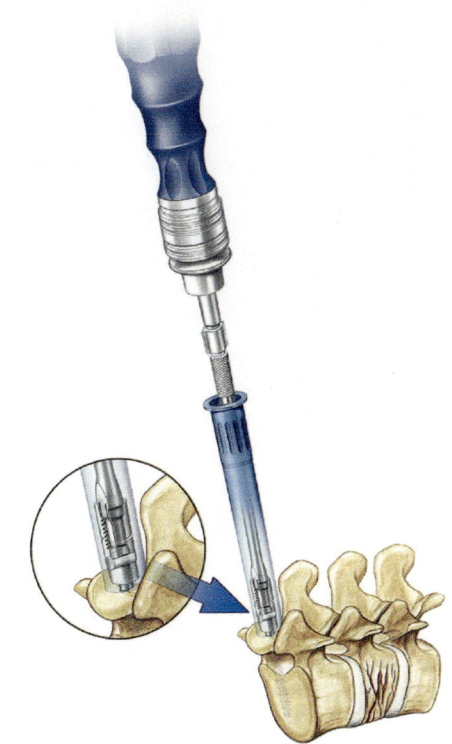

Fig. 68.12 Alternatively, a special alignment device can be used. (With permission from Aesculap AG, Tuttlingen, Germany)

- Align the screw to the cranio-caudal axis. Both sides of the screwdriver must show in the cranio-caudal direction (see Fig. 68.11). If necessary, a special top piece can be used (Fig. 68.12).
- Measure the length of the rod with the rod length–measuring instrument (see Fig. 68.13). If a distraction is necessary, a longer rod should be used accordingly. If you use prebent rods, add ca. 10 mm.
- Then, insert the FRI outer sleeves through the tissue protection sleeves. Align the longitudinal slit of the outer sleeve caudally. Then, remove the protection sleeves and insert the transverse rod with the rod inserter (see Fig. 68.14).
- *Note*: Before placing the FRI outer sleeves, the surgical field can be kept free using a Langenbeck hook; the rod can then be inserted through this aperture (see Fig. 68.15).
- Put the reduction lever in place, the setscrew is received; then insert the construct through the FRI sleeve in the pedicle screw (see Fig. 68.16). Screw the construct as far as it will go into the flanks of the pedicle screw (see Fig. 68.17).

  Note: Make sure the setscrew does not block the rod to avoid blocking the distraction (s. b.). If necessary, loosen the setscrews a quarter of a turn.

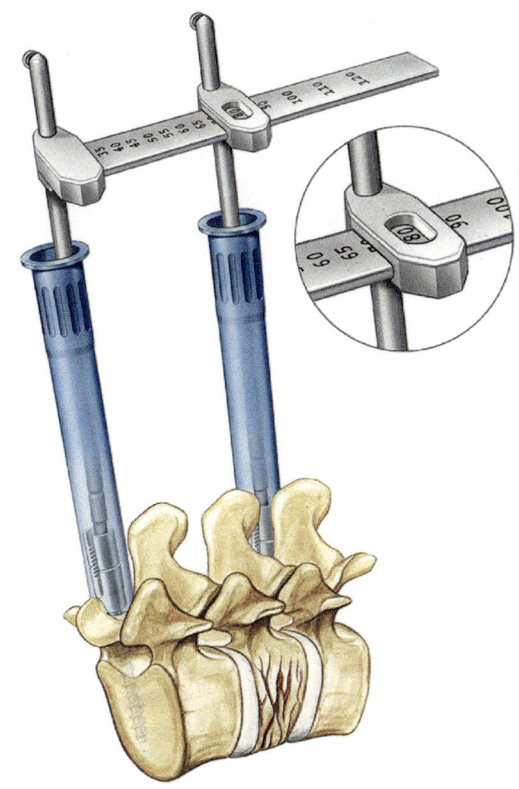

Fig. 68.13 Measurement of rod length with the rod length–measuring instrument. (With permission from Aesculap AG, Tuttlingen, Germany)

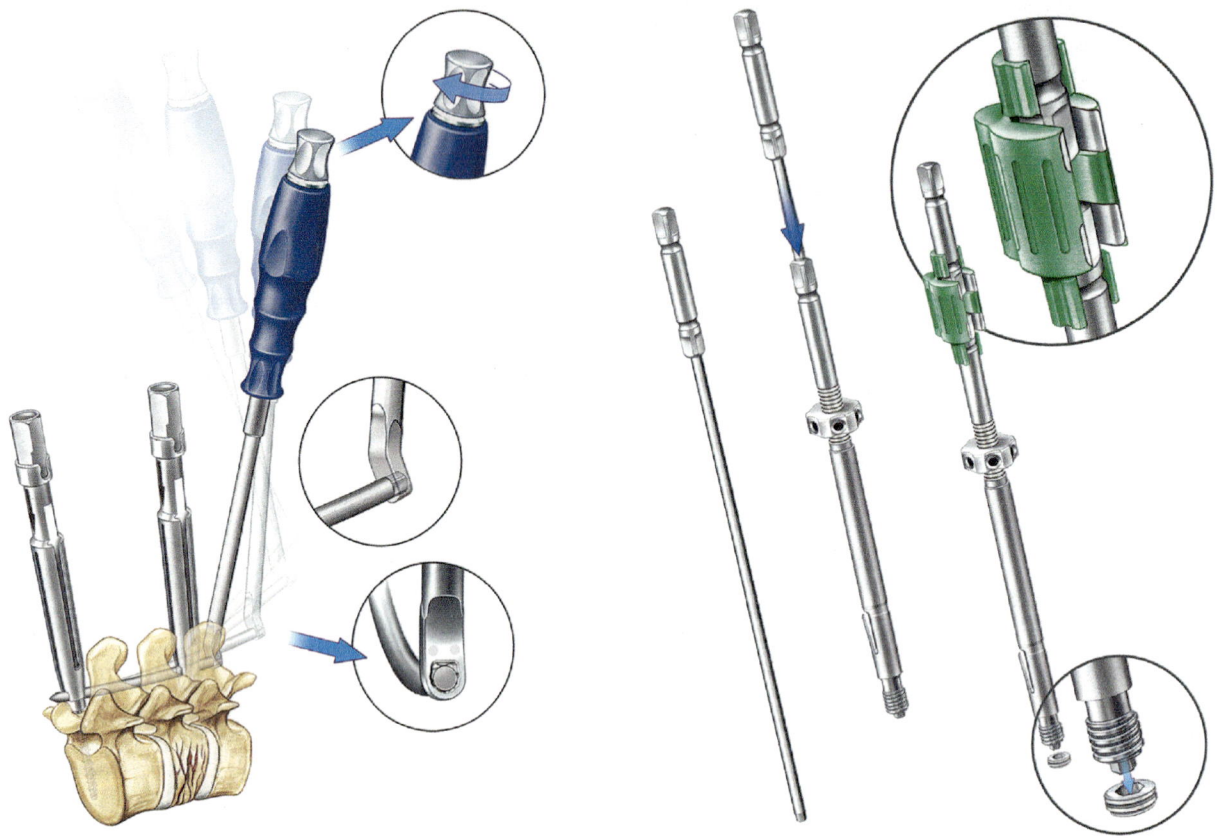

Fig. 68.14 Representation of screw with two Langenbeck hooks. (With permission from Aesculap AG, Tuttlingen, Germany)

Fig. 68.16 Assembly of reduction lever. (With permission from Aesculap AG, Tuttlingen, Germany)

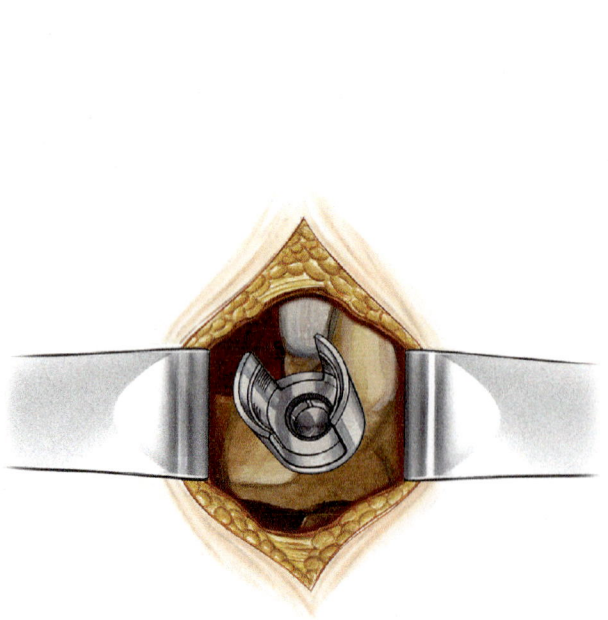

Fig. 68.15 Insertion of rod with rod inserter. (With permission from Aesculap AG, Tuttlingen, Germany)

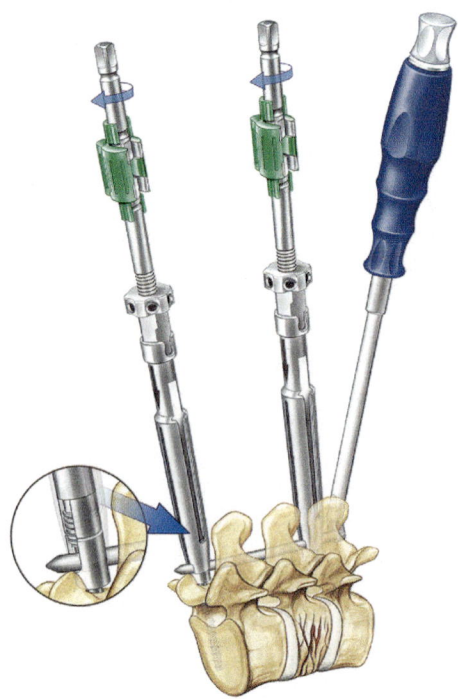

Fig. 68.17 Turning of setscrew down to contact. If necessary, loosen a quarter of a turn. (With permission from Aesculap AG, Tuttlingen, Germany)

Fig. 68.18 (**a**) Installation of distractor and (**b**) reduction of vertebral height. (With permission from Aesculap AG, Tuttlingen, Germany)

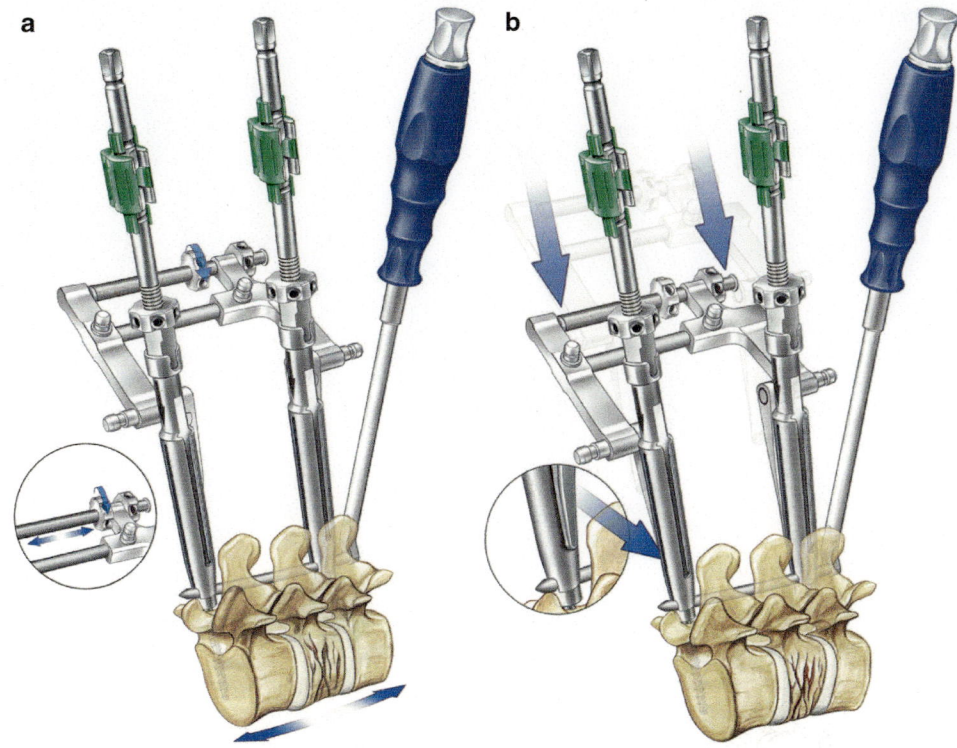

a

b

68.6.3 Reduction

- Now, the installation of the distraction tool follows. The distractor is inserted via the bolt in the guiding groove of the cranial and caudal outer sleeve. The distraction blades must be aligned parallel to the outer sleeves (see Fig. 68.18a, b). The distraction is carried out consecutively (1 surgeon) or simultaneously (surgeon and assistant) under C-arm guidance.
- To reconstruct the natural lordosis, insert the spindle distractor into the corresponding nut and, by activating the control knob, adjust the lordosis under fluoroscopy guidance (see Fig. 68.19a, b).
- Using the regulating screw on the threaded tube, press the rod firmly. You must loosen the regulating crew a quarter of a turn to avoid blocking of the setscrew. Then, tighten up the setscrew with the screwdriver (see Fig. 68.20).
- Remove the screwdriver and unscrew the threaded tube with the ratchet handle (see Fig. 68.21).
- Final tightening of the construct is carried out with a countering instrument and a 10-Nm (90-in/lb) torque wrench (see Fig. 68.22). Finally, the flanks are broken off using the flank breaking forceps (Fig. 68.23).

68.7 Tips and Tricks

- Accurate positioning of patient, carefully aligned anterioposteriorly to the perpendicular line of the room axis, is enormously helpful for the surgeon's spatial orientation and facilitates the initial pedicle screw alignment.
- If the instrumentation "is stuck," then loosen the setscrew or regulating screw little bit.
- If the insertion of prebent rods is planned, then it is helpful to position the cranial pedicle screws at an angle of ca. 10° cranially and the caudal pedicle screws at an angle of ca. 10° caudally.

68.8 Results

The example of an LWK 1 AO-A3.1 fracture shows that, through a minimally invasive procedure, the FRI instrumentation allows to achieve an anatomical reduction in spite of restricted access. It permits a clearly more expeditious postoperative mobilization of the patients while causing them less pain in comparison to the open procedure (Figs. 68.23).

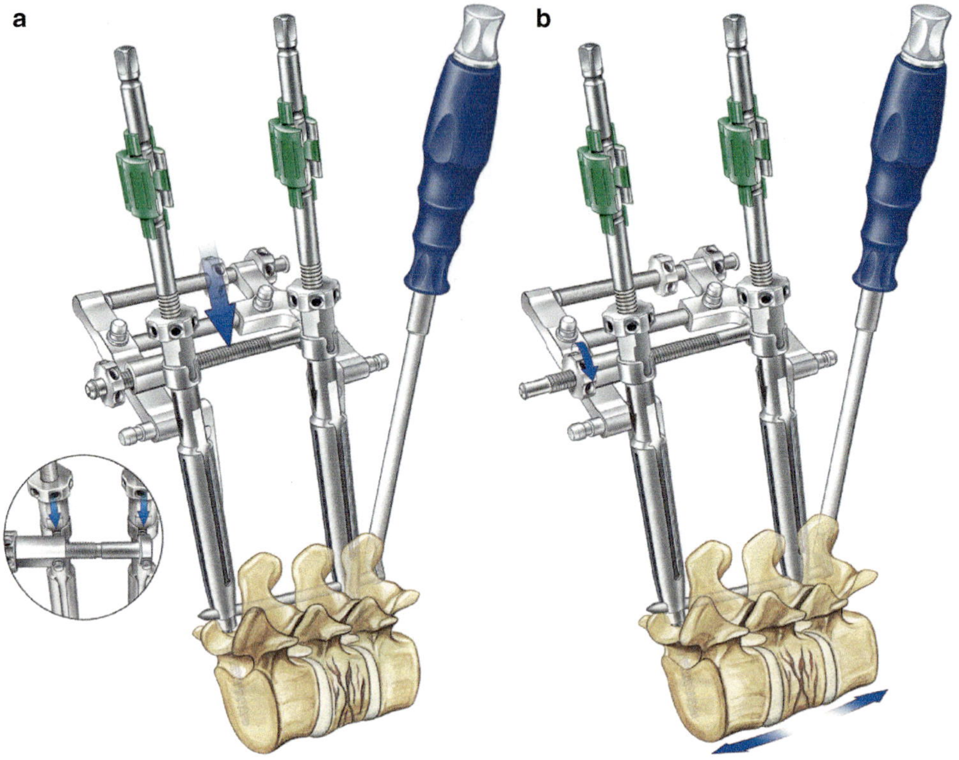

Fig. 68.19 (a, b) Installation of spindle retractor and lordosis reduction. (With permission from Aesculap AG, Tuttlingen, Germany)

a

b

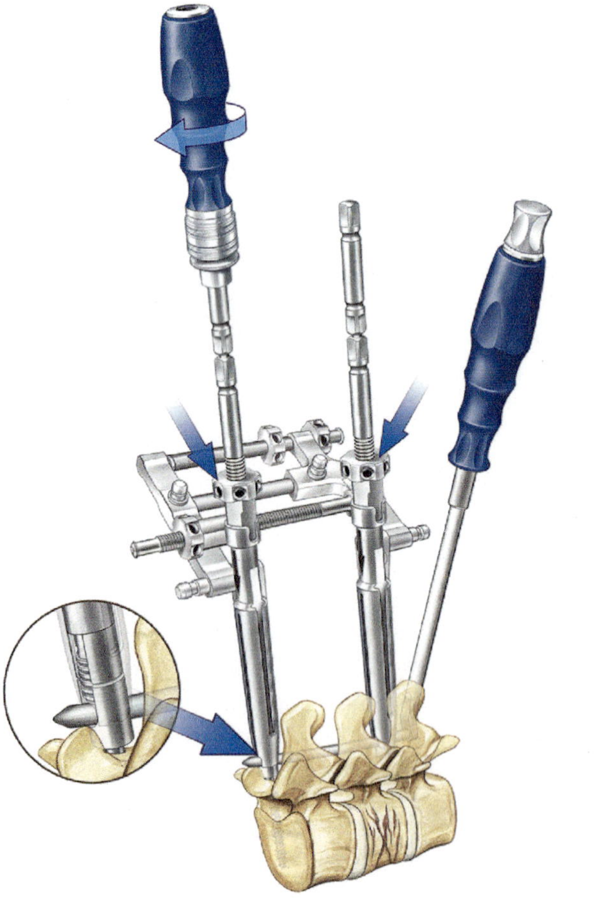

Fig. 68.20 Tightening the regulating screw and loosening a quarter of a turn. Tightening up the setscrew. (With permission from Aesculap AG, Tuttlingen, Germany)

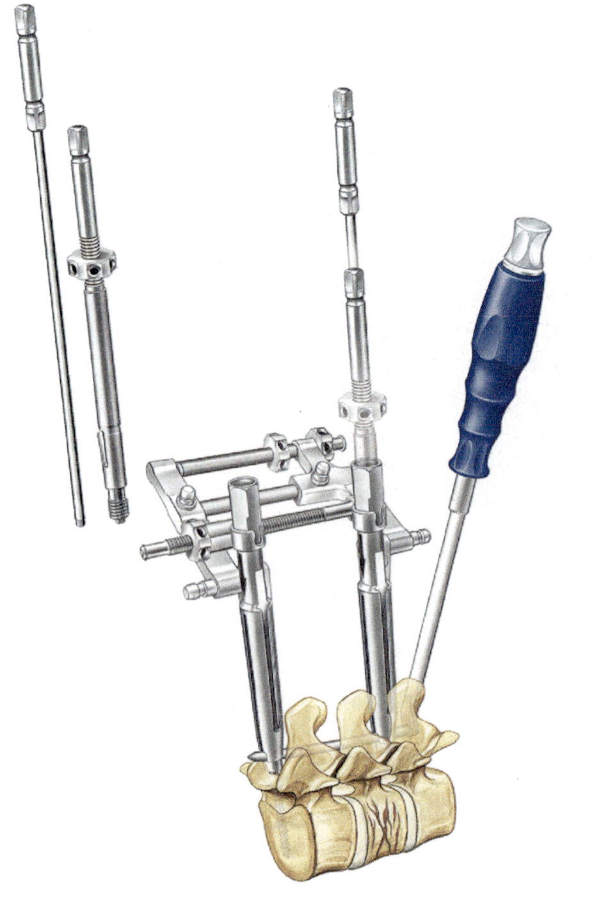

Fig. 68.21 Removal of screwdriver and threaded tubes. (With permission from Aesculap AG, Tuttlingen, Germany)

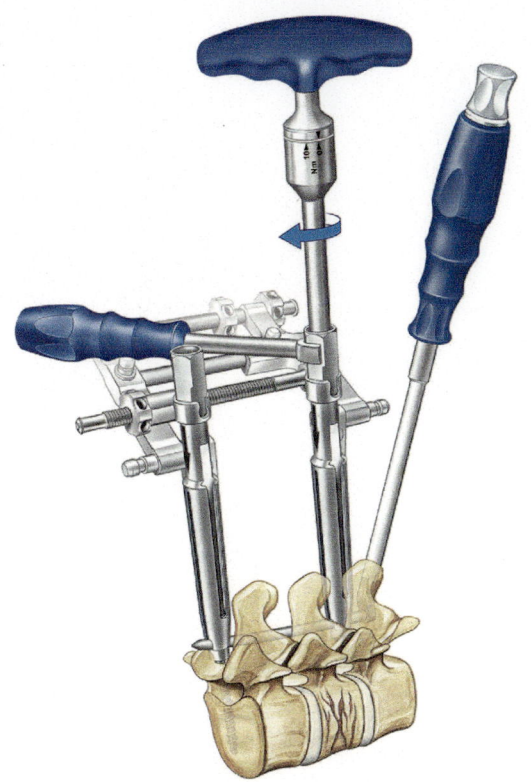

Fig. 68.22 Final tightening with prescribed torque. (With permission from Aesculap AG, Tuttlingen, Germany)

References

1. Foley KT, Gupta SK. Percutaneous pedicle screw fixation of the lumbar spine: preliminary clinical results. J Neurosurg. 2002;97(1 suppl):7–12.
2. Hahn U, Andermahr J, Prokop A, Rehm KE. Minimal-invasive Operationstechniken an der Wirbelsäule. Mediathek der Deutschen Gesellschaft für Chirurgie: Aesculap Akademie; 2006.
3. Palmisani M, Gasbarrini A, Brodano GB, et al. Minimally invasive percutaneous fixation in the treatment of thoracic and lumbar spine fractures. Eur Spine J. 2009;18(suppl 1):71–4.
4. Grass R, Biewener A, Dickopf A, et al. Percutaneous dorsal versus open instrumentation for fractures of the thoracolumbar border. a comparative, prospective study. Unfallchirurg. 2006;109:297–305.
5. Prokop A, Lohlein F, Chmielnicki M, Volbracht J. Minimally invasive percutaneous instrumentation for spine fractures. Unfallchirurg. 2009;112:621–6.
6. Korovessis P, Hadjipavlou A, Repantis T. Minimal invasive short posterior instrumentation plus balloon kyphoplasty with calcium phosphate for burst and severe compression lumbar fractures. Spine. 2008;33:658–67.
7. Merom L, Raz N, Hamud C et al. Minimally invasive burst fracture fixation in the thoracolumbar region. Orthopedics. 2009;32(4).

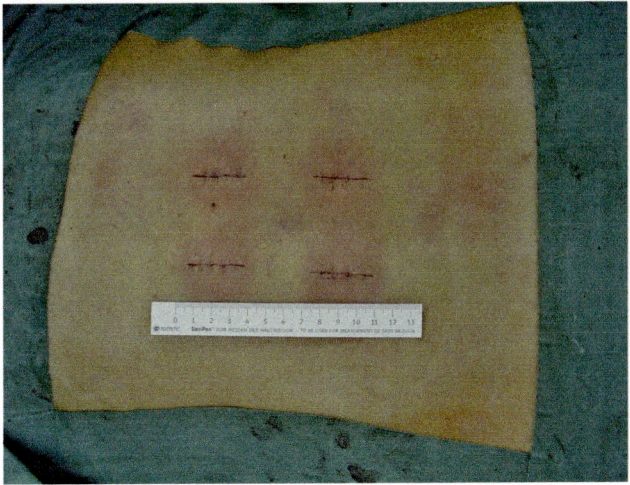

Fig. 68.23 Scars after less invasive transpedicular stabilization

Microsurgical Monosegmental Fusion with Internal Fixator and Transforaminal Interbody Fusion (TLIF)

Uwe Vieweg and Stefan Kroppenstedt

69.1 Introduction and Core Messages

The methods described here (Method I: ipsilateral transpedicular instrumentation and interbody fusion about a lateral paraspinal approach and contralateral percutaneous transpedicular instrumentation, Method II: instrumentation and interbody fusion about both paraspinal lateral approaches) allow the surgeon to perform less invasive spinal instrumentation with short operating time, less blood loss, and small skin incisions. The technique of transforaminal lumbar interbody fusion involves facetectomy, discectomy, and interbody fusion, carried out with the aid of a high-speed drill burr microsurgical instruments, and an operating microscope or endoscope. Patients benefit from reduced trauma, less pain, and shorter hospitalization and recovery times [1–7].

69.2 Indications

- Spondylolisthesis that has not responded, or has responded inadequately, to non-operative treatment of symptoms
- Discogenic low-back pain with or without paresis [1, 2, 4, 6]

U. Vieweg (✉)
Department of Conservative and Surgical Spine Therapy with Interdisciplinary Spinal Deformities Centre and Rummelsberg Sectional Center, Hospital Rummelsberg, Schwarzenbruck, Germany
e-mail: uwe.vieweg@sana.de

S. Kroppenstedt
Department of Spinal Surgery, Center of Orthopedic Surgery, Sana Hospital Sommerfeld, Kremmen, Germany
e-mail: s.kroppenstedt@sana-hu.de

69.3 Contraindications

- Severe spinal canal stenosis
- Higher-grade spondylolisthesis (Meyerding grade III–IV) and deformities
- Absent, fractured, or atrophic pedicles and severe osteopenia that limits secure screw purchase
- Signs of current active infection

69.4 Technical Requirements

C-arm fluoroscope, microscope or endoscope, supporting pads and cushions to aid positioning, radiolucent surgical table, high-speed burr, and retractor systems (METRx X-TUBE MicroDiscectomy Retraction System (Medtronic), MLD retractor system (Aesculap), ProView Minimal Access Portal System (Blackstone), Luxor (Stryker), MIRA (Synthes)). Internal fixator systems (top loading system) with cannulated screws (CD Horizon Sextant I/II and CD Horizon Longitude, Medtronic; S^4 internal fixator or Enovat, Aesculap). Other systems for minimally invasive screw and rod insertion for posterior stabilization are spirit with cannulated screws Click'X (Synthes), REVOLVE Stabilization System (Globus Medical), SpheRx-DBR system (NuVasive), EXPEDIUM and VIPER (DePuy), Silverbolt (Via 4 Spine).

69.5 Planning, Preparation, and Positioning

The patient is placed in a prone position on a radiolucent table under general anesthesia (see Fig. 69.1) and prepared and draped in the conventional manner. The abdomen is permitted to hang freely. The hips are extended to enhance lumbar lordosis. The skin incision is planned under X-ray control with a C-arm fluoroscope using anteroposterior and lateral beam directions. Four needles are placed at the level of the pedicles to ascertain the level (see Fig. 69.2). The Ferguson arrangement

Fig. 69.1 Positioning of the patient. (With permission from Aesculap AG, Tuttlingen, Germany)

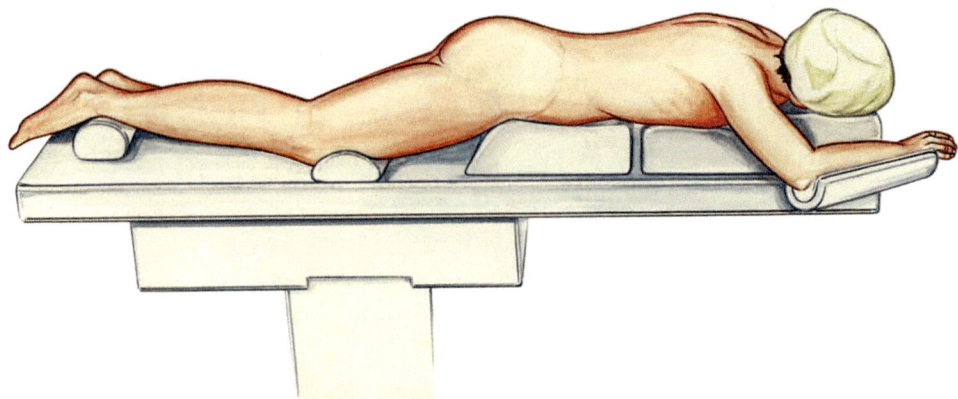

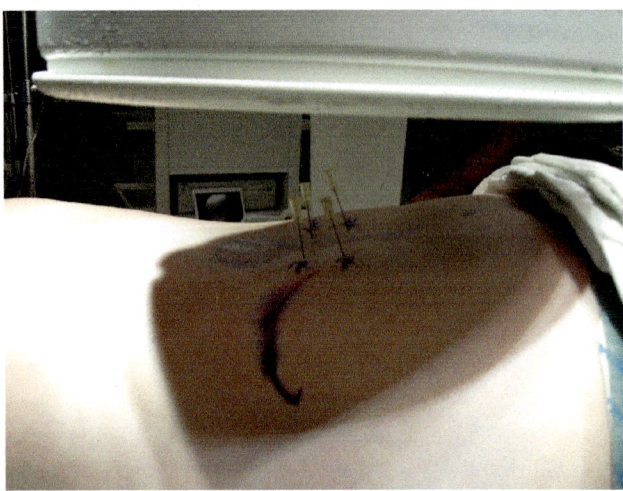

Fig. 69.2 Planning of the skin incision with C-arm fluoroscope

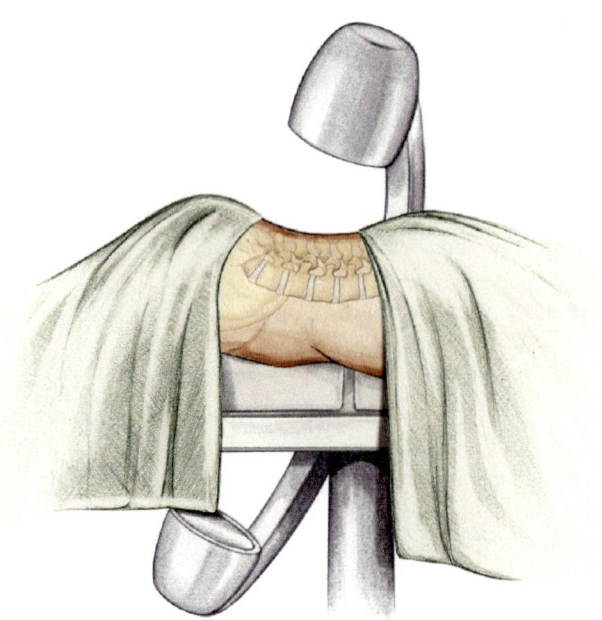

Fig. 69.3 Ferguson arrangement/positioning of the C-arm for the L5/S1 level

provides the best image, focusing correctly on the S1 pedicle (see Fig. 69.3). Biplanar fluoroscopy with two C-arms facilitates safer and easier radiographic assessment (see Fig. 69.4). *Note*: When planning the approach, the spinous processes should appear exactly in the middle between the two pedicles, and the superior end plates should appear exactly parallel when viewed in AP X-rays. Care should be taken to ensure that the superior end plates are also parallel in lateral X-rays.

69.6 Surgical Technique

69.6.1 Method I: Ipsilateral Miniopen and Contralateral Percutaneous Instrumentation [1–3]

69.6.1.1 Miniopen Access

- After radiological planning incisions are made in the skin (4–5 cm long) and the lateral fascia of or over the pedicle.
- The retractor system (METRx, Medtronic) is delivered via the dilatation tubes at approximately the angle at which the pedicle screws are to be inserted.
- The expansion and position of the retractor system are confirmed by imaging.
- A Jamshidi needle is inserted. After locating the entry point on the pedicle, the Jamshidi needle needs to be aligned with the pedicle trajectory. The needle is driven in as far as the anterior edge of the vertebral body. It should not extend beyond the medial edge of the pedicle (see Figs. 69.5 and 69.6a, b). If necessary, the needle must be reinserted and realigned. The position is fixed by slightly pushing the Jamshidi needle into the cortex.
- The pedicle is prepared with the appropriate tap. The tap must correspond to the screw type and diameter.
- The Kirschner wire is replaced with a marker pin or about 3 cm of wire (see Fig. 69.8b).
- The second pedicle is prepared as described above.
- The microscope is swung into place.
- Transforaminal access to the disk is typically performed on the most symptomatic side. The facet is resected with

Fig. 69.4 Using two C-arm fluoroscopes for percutaneous instrumentation

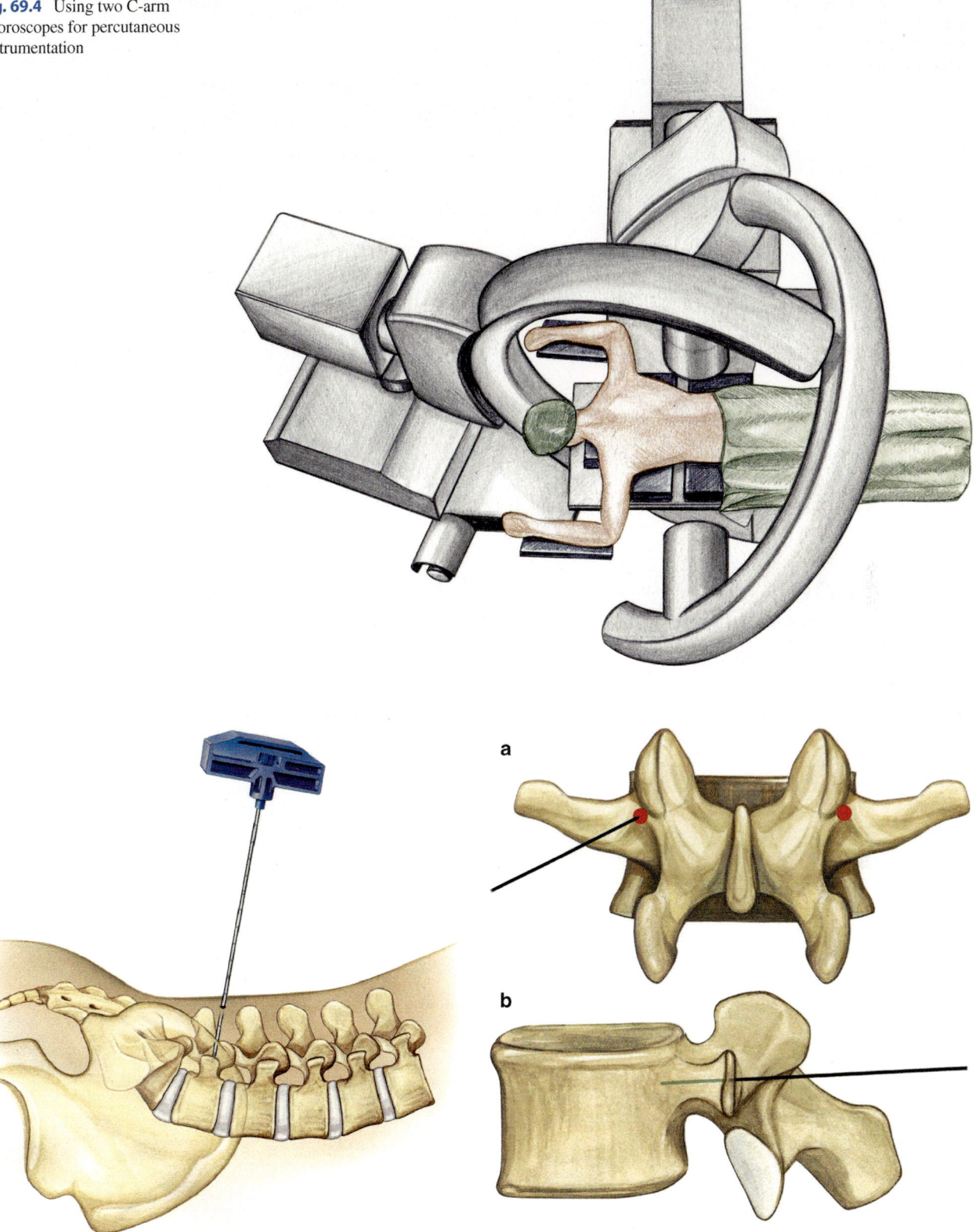

Fig. 69.5 Positioning the Jamshidi needle

Fig. 69.6 AP (**a**) and lateral (**b**) X-ray views of the ideal positioning of the cannula in the pedicle

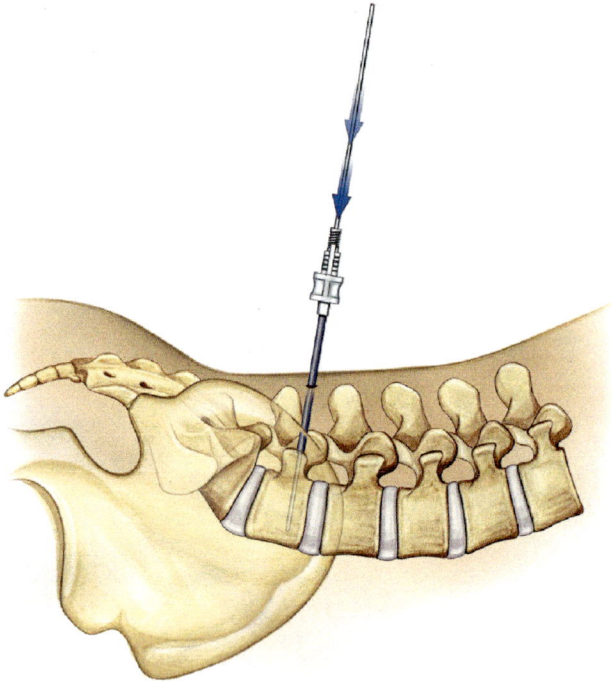

Fig. 69.7 Insertion of the K-wire

a high-speed reamer. *Note*: Bone removal should begin caudally between the two pedicles, directly over the disk space.

- A diamond reamer is then used. This is subsequently replaced with a punch. The nerve roots leaving the vertebra are viewed microscopically.
- The end plate is prepared for interbody fusion.
- Once the disk space has been meticulously prepared, cancellous bone is inserted into the disk space using angled and straight forceps (or a funnel). A cage or spacer is then inserted with autologous bone or bone substitute.
- The marker pin is removed, and the pedicle screws are screwed in. The rod is inserted either using the conventional technique or with a rod inserter (below).

69.6.1.2 Percutaneous Instrumentation of the Contralateral Side

- Skin incisions 1–2 cm long are made, as planned, slightly lateral to the pedicle. Incisions are also made in the fascia to make tissue dilatation easier.
- Using C-arm fluoroscopy, the pedicle is accessed with a Jamshidi needle. The correct entry point should be identified in both AP and lateral X-ray views (see Fig. 69.5).
- After placing the Jamshidi needle at the intersection of the facet and the transverse process, the needle may be driven partially through the pedicle using a hammer. When the Jamshidi needle reaches the medial wall on the AP view, its position needs to be verified in the lateral

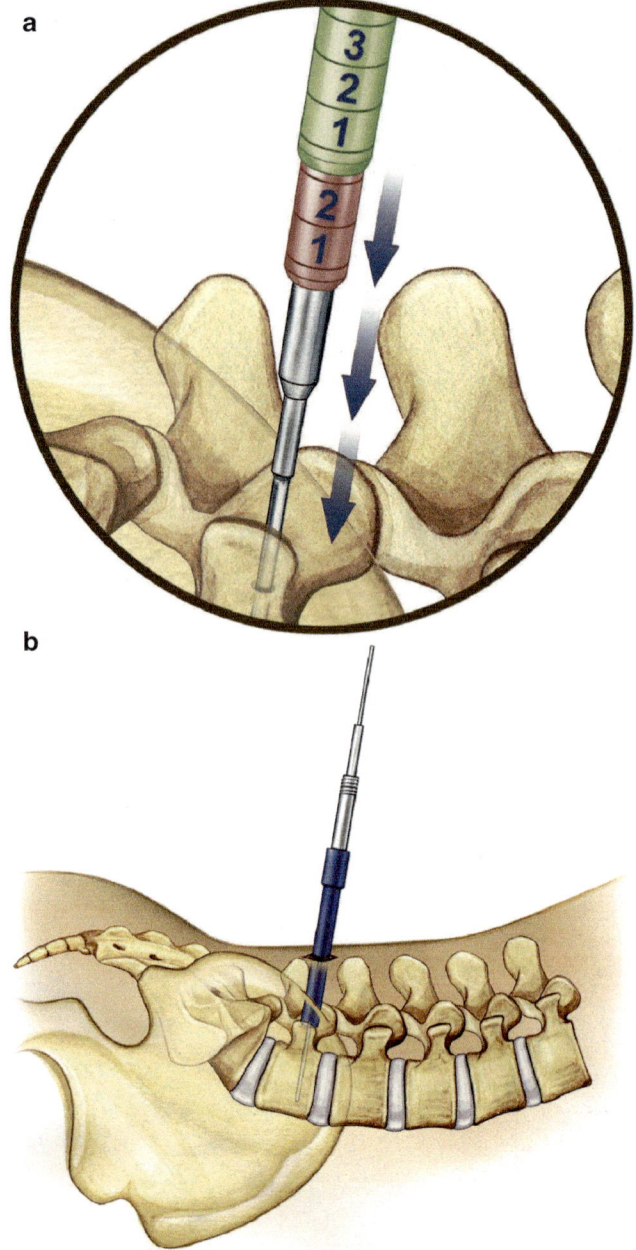

Fig. 69.8 (**a, b**) Insertion of the dilatation sheath

view to ensure that the needle is in the bony canal of the pedicle (see Fig. 69.6a, b).

- The handle and inner trocar are removed from the Jamshidi needle, and a K-wire is inserted. The position of the K-wire is verified with fluoroscopy to ensure that it extends through 2/3 of the vertebral body (see Fig. 69.7). *Note*: During advancement of the K-wire, its progress must be checked using continuous radiological monitoring.
- An incision is made in the skin and fascia around the K-wire. The incision is dilated with dilatation tubes (see Fig. 69.8a, b).

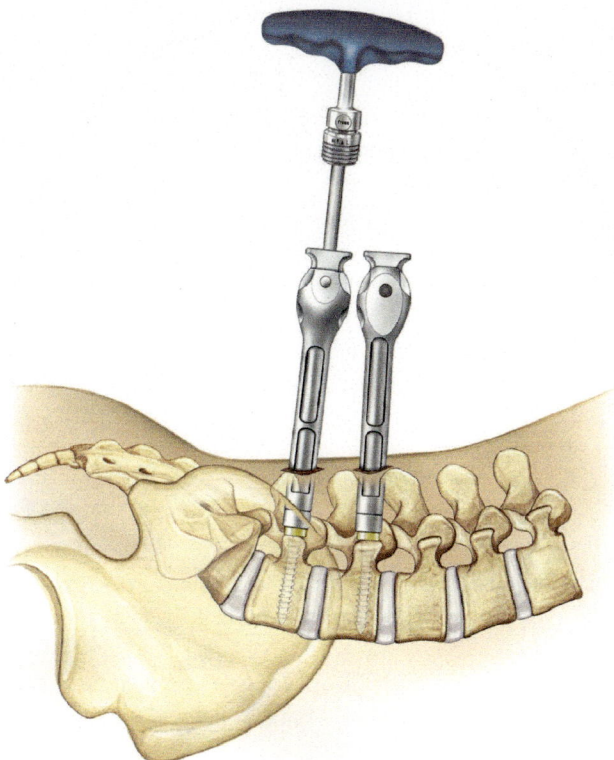

Fig. 69.9 Screwing in the pedicle screws

- The pedicle is prepared by placing an awl over the K-wire or, if the bone is too hard, a tap may be used to prepare the pedicle screw canal. The K-wire must be held in position when removing the awl or tap. *Note*: The axis of the tap must be kept constant to avoid bending the wire. The K-wire must not advance during tapping and must not become displaced when instruments are removed.
- Using the additional extender, the pedicle screws are driven over the K-wire into the prepared pedicle. Fluoroscopy must be used to monitor screw insertion and placement (Fig. 69.9). Once the screw reaches the posterior aspect of the vertebral body, the wire can be removed.
- *Note*: The screw assembly must not be inserted too far. The K-wire must not be allowed to advance.
- The second screw is inserted in the same way. *Note*: After inserting additional bone screws, the heads of the bone screws should be at the same height.
- The extenders are connected.
- The rod inserter is attached.
- A trocar is used to prepare the way through the fascia and muscle (see Fig. 69.10a). The trocar is inserted through a small skin incision and pushed through the muscle, checking its position on the image converter, until it reaches the first screw.

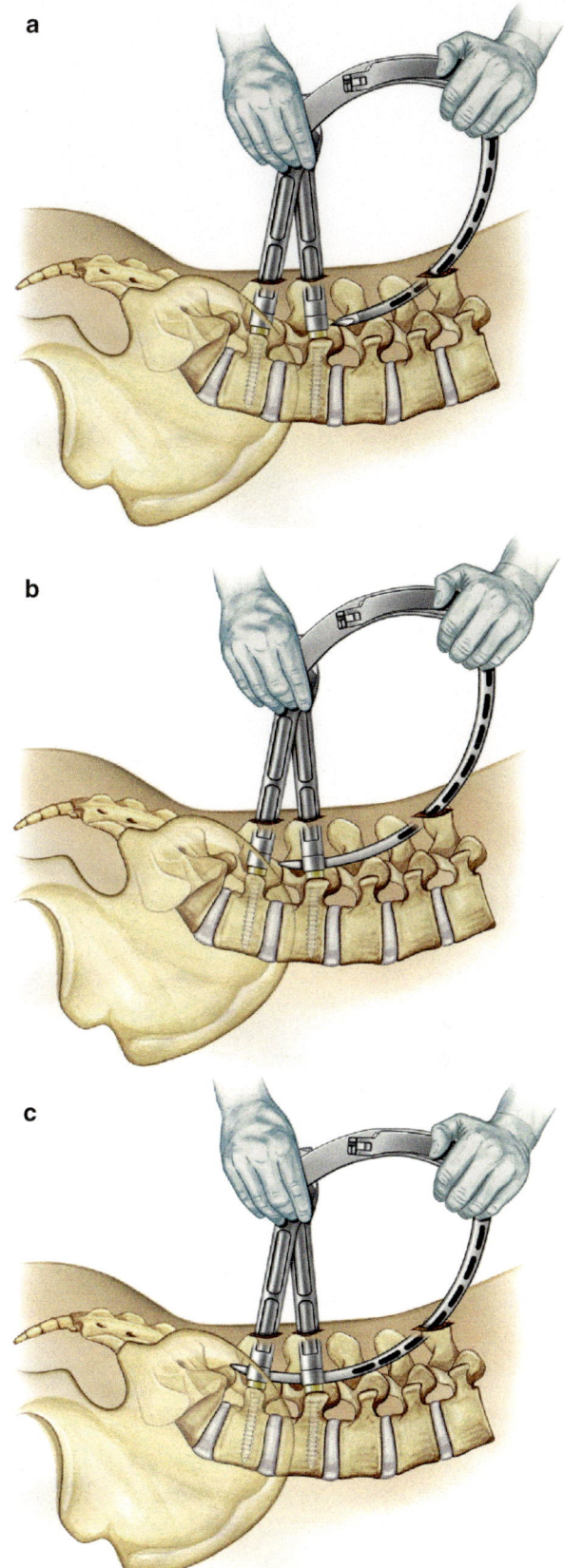

Fig. 69.10 Swinging items into place: trocar (**a**), rod (**b**), and final position (**c**)

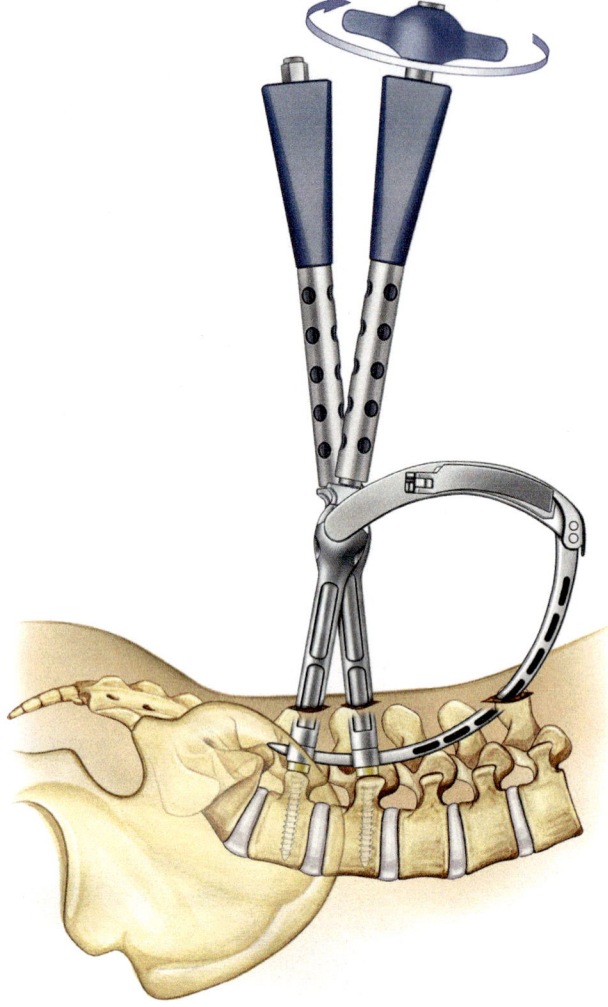

Fig. 69.11 Fixing the setscrews

- A rod-measuring instrument is used to determine the correct rod length.
- Using the rod inserter, the rod is then pushed into the heads of the polyaxial screws (see Fig. 69.10b, c). *Note*: The AP view must also be used to check whether the rod has been inserted into both the screw heads.
- The rod is then fixed with setscrews (see Fig. 69.11). *Note*: Fixation must start with the deepest screw. The firmness of the connection must be checked by pulling on the inserter.

69.6.2 Method II: Less Invasive 360° Fusion About Two Lateral Paraspinal Approaches

- A 4–5-cm skin incision is made approximately 3 cm from the midline, and the fascia is incised and divided (see Figs. 69.12a and 69.21).
- Using the fingers, the muscles are bluntly dissected, and an MLD retractor (Aesculap) is introduced (see

Fig. 69.12b, c). Upon insertion, the retractor exposes portions of the lamina, facet joints, and transverse process.

- *Conventional screw technique with uncannulated screws.*
- Under X-ray control and using a Steinmann nail, the pedicles are drilled open and polyaxial screws (S4 internal system, Aesculap) are then placed transpedicularly (see Fig. 69.13).
- *Cannulated screw technique.*
- After the screw entry point has been determined, the pedicle is accessed. The guiding instrument is inserted at the junction between the facet and the transverse process. The trocar is then removed, leaving the targeting device in the pedicle. The K-wire is inserted to guide the screws. *Note*: Care must always be taken to ensure that the K-wire is not inserted too far.
- The working area must be dilated with the metal dilatation sheath so that the implant screws can be positioned. The dilatation sheath is guided in via the K-wire targeting device.
- The pedicle is prepared by placing an awl over the K-wire or, if the bone is too hard, a tap may be used to prepare the pedicle screw canal.
- Using the additional extender, the pedicle screws are driven over the K-wire into the prepared pedicle.
- The disk space is distracted with angulated distraction forceps.
- After pedicle screw insertion, the superior and inferior articular processes are resected with a high-speed drill and Kerrison punch. In cases of unilateral nerve root compression, the facet joint is resected on that side only.
- The intervertebral disk is exposed and is subtotally resected using angled rongeurs, shavers, and curettes (see Figs. 69.14a, b and 69.15).
- After scraping off the end plates, bone or bone substitute is packed into the anterior part of the disk space. Insertion of a trial to measure the height of the implant (see Fig. 69.16).
- A curved PEEK cage specially designed for the TLIF technique is packed with bone or bone substitute and inserted into the disk space (see Fig. 69.17a–d).
- The tulips heads of the bone screws are aligned using a screw head adjuster to facilitate rod insertion.
- The appropriate rod is loaded into a fixed rod holder.
- A rod is inserted into the heads of the polyaxial screws and fixed with setscrews. The precontoured bullet-nosed rod is inserted.
- The polyaxial head is given 42° angulation to provide optimal and easy rod placement. To reposition the vertebra in cases with spondylolisthesis, the setscrew of the higher pedicle is fixed first. Only then is the setscrew of the lower pedicle fixed. *Note*: Rod position and advancement must be verified using fluoroscopy until fully seated (see Fig. 69.18a).

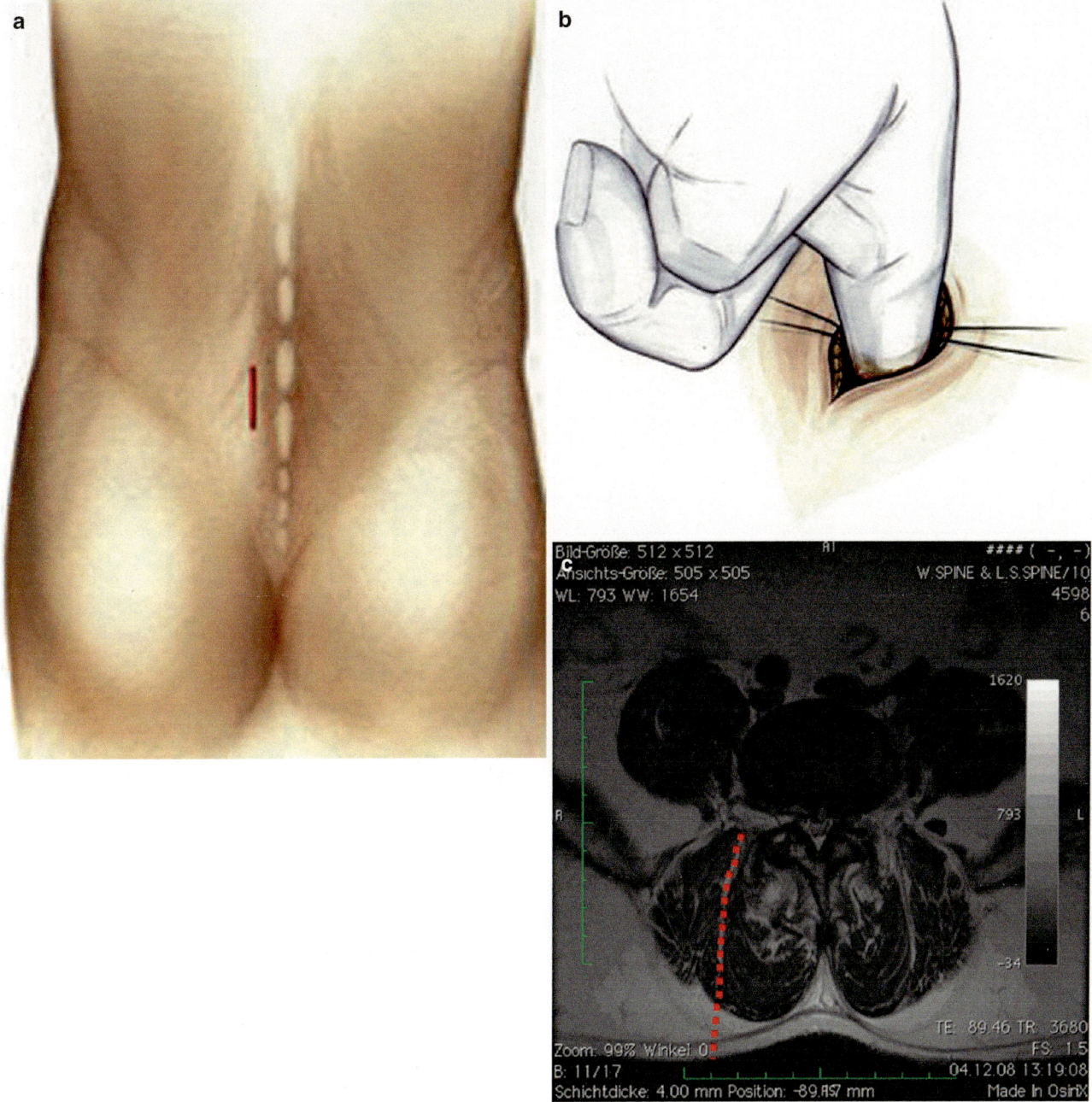

Fig. 69.12 Skin incision about 3 cm from the midline (**a**), separation of muscle fascia, and preparation of muscle using the fingers (**b**), demonstration of the lateral paraspinal approach on an MRI scan (**c**)

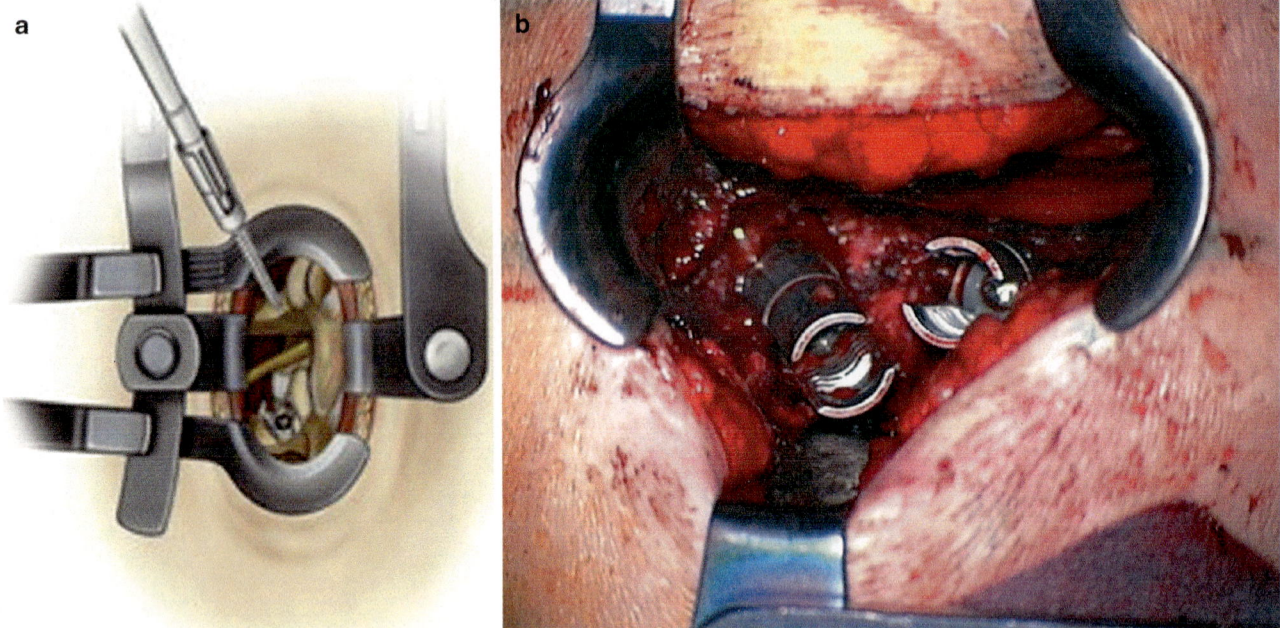

Fig. 69.13 Insertion of MLD retractor and transpedicular positioning of pedicle screws (**a**), intraoperative situation (**b**)

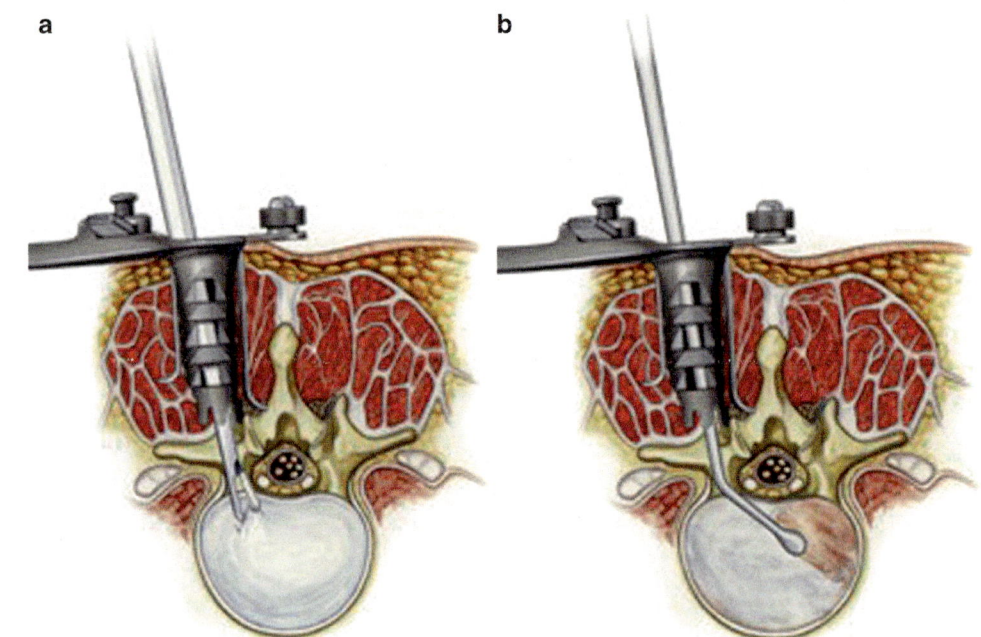

Fig. 69.14 (**a**) Discectomy and debridement of the intervertebral surfaces of the (**b**) vertebral body as far as the contralateral side using angled instruments. (With permission from Aesculap AG, Tuttlingen, Germany)

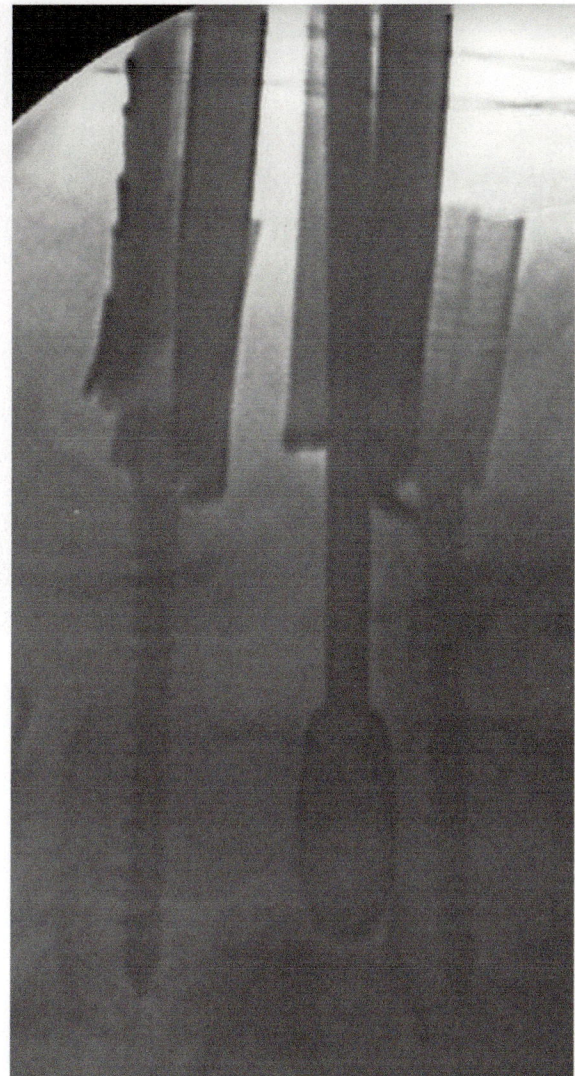

Fig. 69.15 Intraoperative X-ray demonstrates the preparation of the endplates with plate shavers

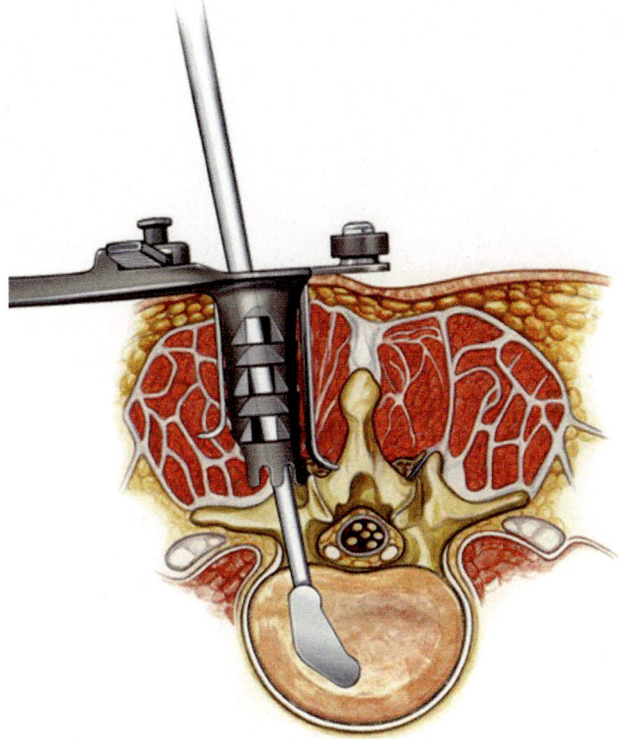

Fig. 69.16 Insertion of a trial to measure the height of the implant. (With permission of Aesculap AG, Tuttlingen, Germany)

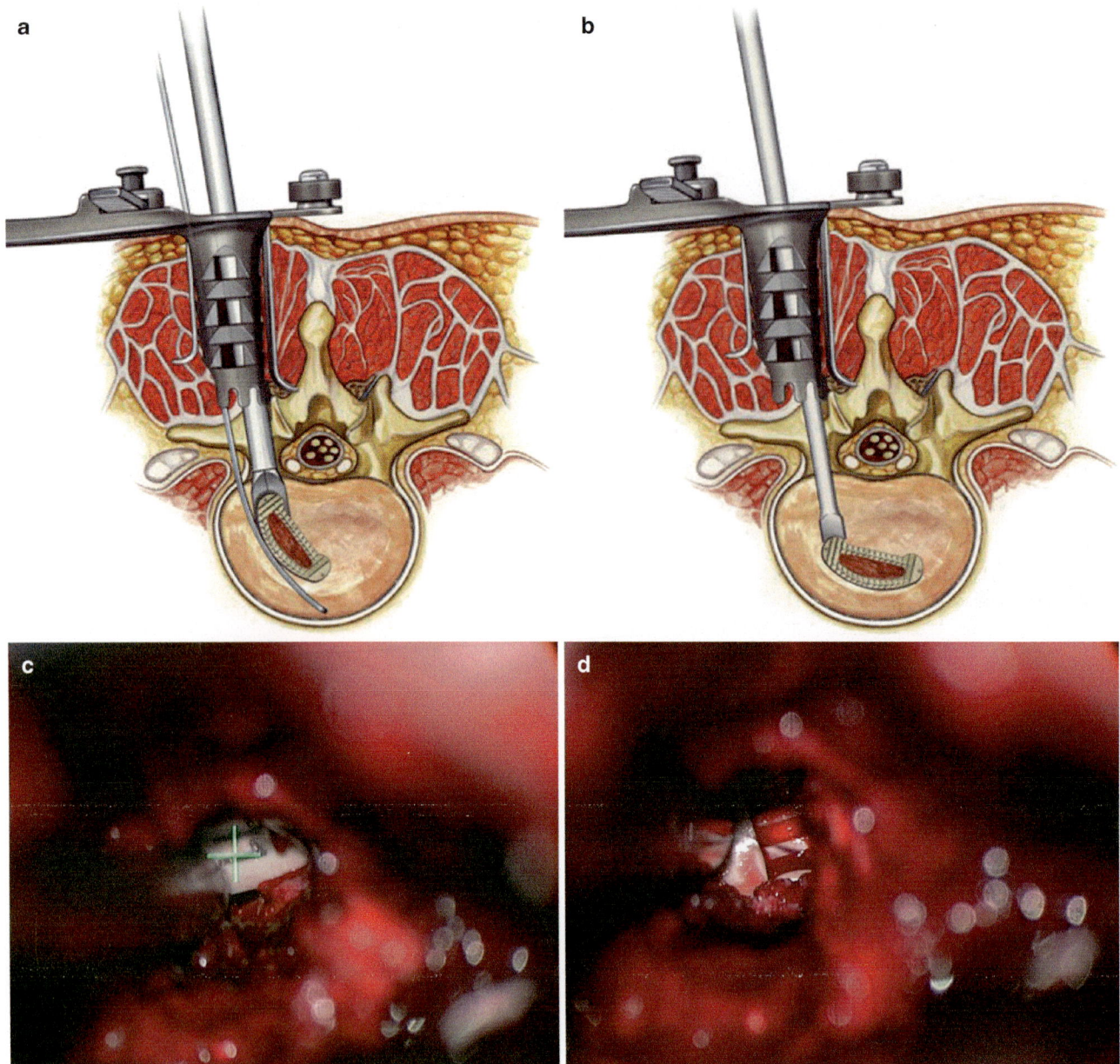

Fig. 69.17 (**a–d**) Insertion of the curved TLIF cage. Bone substitute is packed around the cage (ventrally and dorsally). Turning and final positioning of the cage (intraoperative situation)

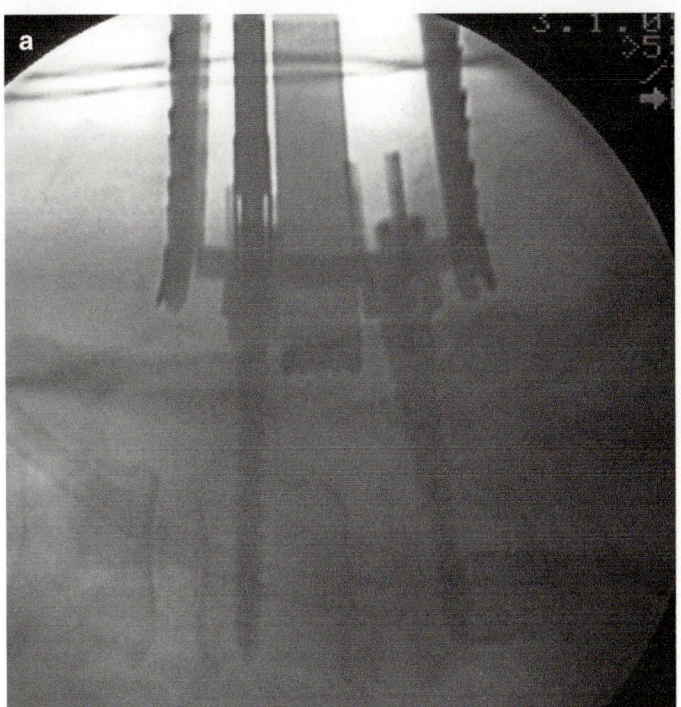

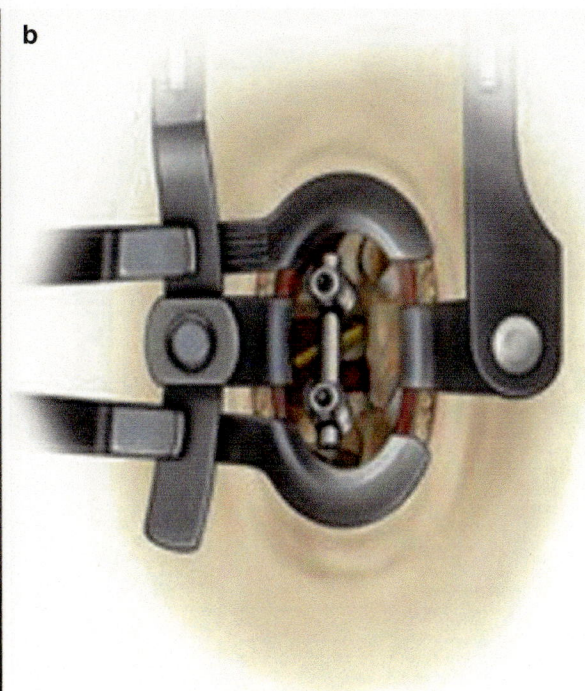

Fig. 69.18 Fixing of the rod (**a**) intraoperative X-ray (**b**) illustration

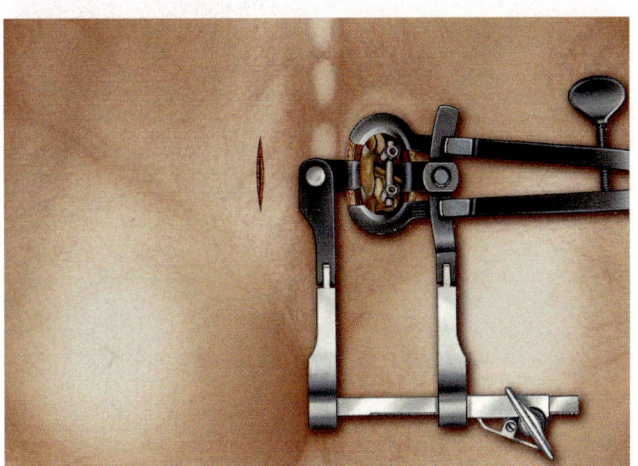

Fig. 69.19 Contralateral pedicle screw instrumentation. (With permission of Aescupap AG, Tuttlingen, Germany)

- After closure of the fascia and skin, an identical procedure is carried out on the contralateral side (see Figs. 69.19, 69.20, and 69.21).

69.7   Tips and Tricks

- The K-wires should remain securely in position throughout the entire procedure and must not slip out before the screws are inserted. The wires are long enough to be held in place by hand during the different surgical steps.
- The tip of the K-wire should be monitored fluoroscopically to ensure that it does not penetrate the anterior wall of the vertebral body.
- The K-wires should be kept parallel to one another during insertion.

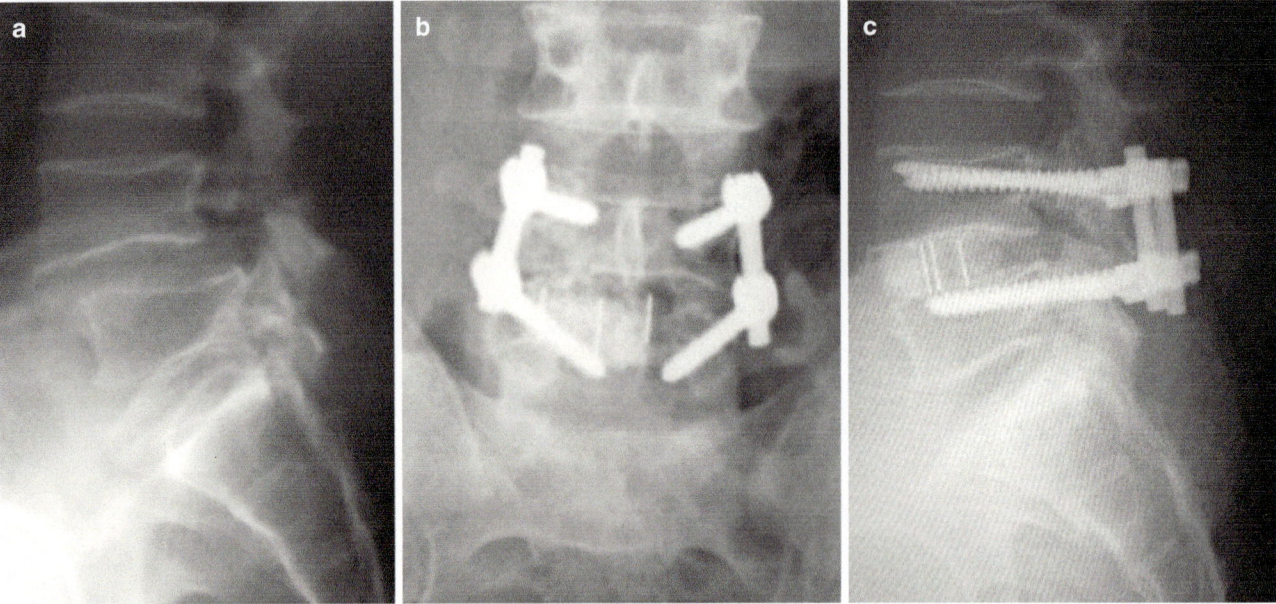

Fig. 69.20 Patient with spondylolytic spondylolisthesis: preoperative X-ray at L4/L5 (**a**) and postoperative AP (**b**) and lateral (**c**) X-rays

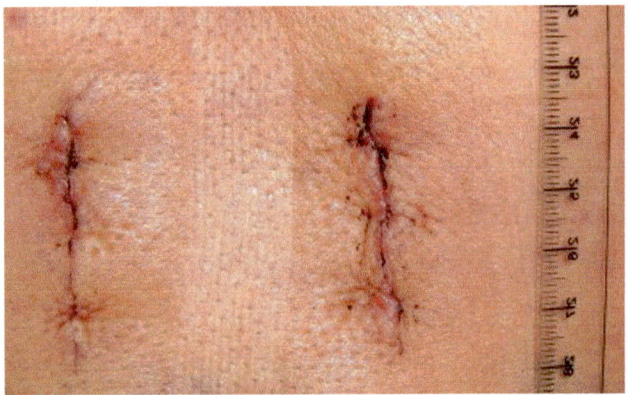

Fig. 69.21 Length of the two scin incision (3–4 cm) postoperatively

References

1. Ge DH, Stekas ND, Varlotta CG, et al. Comparative analysis of two transforaminal lumbar interbody fusion techniques: open TLIF versus Wiltse MIS TLIF. Spine. 2019;44:E555–60.
2. Foley KT, Holly LT, Schwender JD. Minimally invasive lumbar fusion. Spine. 2003;28(Suppl):26–35.
3. Harms JG, Jeszensky D. The posterior lumbar interbody Fusion in a unilateral technique. Oper Orthop Traumatol. 1998;10:90–102. In German
4. Jong JS, Lee SH. Minimally invasive transforaminal lumbar interbody fusion with ipsilateral pedicle screw and contralateral facet screw fixation. J Neurosurg Spine. 2005;3:218–23.
5. Khoo LT, Palmer S, Loich OT. Minimally invasive percutaneous posterior lumbar interbody fusion. Neurosurgery. 2005;51(Suppl 2):166–81.
6. Park Y, Lee SB, Seok SO, et al. Perioperative surgical complications and learning curve associated with minimally invasive transforaminal lumbar interbody fusion: a single-institute experience. Clin Orthop Surg. 2015;7:91–6.
7. Wimmer C, Pfandlsteiner T, Walochnik N. Less invasive spine fusion. A comparison study. Eur Spine J. 2006;10:179–82.

Posterior Lumbar Interbody Fusion with an Interbody Fusion Spacer or Cage

70

Uwe Vieweg and Steffen Sola

70.1 Introduction and Core Messages

Posterior lumbar interbody fusion (PLIF) is a treatment option currently used for degenerative disk diseases [1] and was introduced by Cloward in the 1940s [2]. Interbody fusion probably results in the most stable construction for intersegmental spinal fusion. Anterior column support is provided via a posterior approach, and the disk height is restored in order to open the neural foramen. A PLIF procedure is especially attractive in cases where a posterior approach is needed anyway, for example, for nerve root or spinal canal decompression. Different devices are available including allograft spacers, titanium spacers with or without a Plasmapore coating, tantalum spacers, and titanium or PEEK cages. This chapter describes the posterior technique for implanting an interbody spacer or cage. These implants are used to obtain 360° fusion.

70.2 Indications

- Degeneration of lumbar segments (L2 to sacrum)
- Discogenic low-back pain
- Degenerative spondylolisthesis
- Pseudarthrosis of a posterolateral fusion
- Isthmic spondylolisthesis grade I–II (III)

70.3 Contraindications

- Severe osteoporosis
- Infection
- Severe epidural scarring
- Unstable burst fractures and compression fractures
- Destructive tumors

70.4 Technical Prerequisites

Fluoroscopy, positioning device (e.g., Wilson frame), adequate instruments, and implants to meet the following requirements: primary stability, restoration of natural lordosis, and long-term maintenance of spinal balance. Intersomatic devices: allograft spacers (Vertigraft VG2 PLIF, DePuy Spine; ProSpace spacer, Aesculap; PLIF allograft spacer, Synthes), titanium cages (CONTACT Fusion Cage, Synthes; Ray cage, Surgical Dynamics, LT cage, Medtronic; OIC PL, Stryker), titanium Plasmapore-coated spacers (ProSpace, Aesculap) (see Fig. 70.1a), tantalum spacers (Zimmer Spine), and PEEK cages (ProSpace, Aesculap, see Fig. 70.1b; Plivios, Synthes; Coda, Mercy Health System; Tetris, Signus; Oria Natura/Adonys, Alphatec Spine/ Scient'X; Pezo-P, Ulrich; Luna Cage, Bricon; OIC PL, Stryker; Lumbo-Space PLIF, Intromed).

U. Vieweg (✉)
Department of Conservative and Surgical Spine Therapy with Interdisciplinary Spinal Deformities Centre and Rummelsberg Sectional Center, Hospital Rummelsberg,
Schwarzenbruck, Germany
e-mail: uwe.vieweg@sana.de

S. Sola
Department of Neurosurgery, University of Rostock,
Rostock, Germany
e-mail: solastef@med.uni-rostock.de

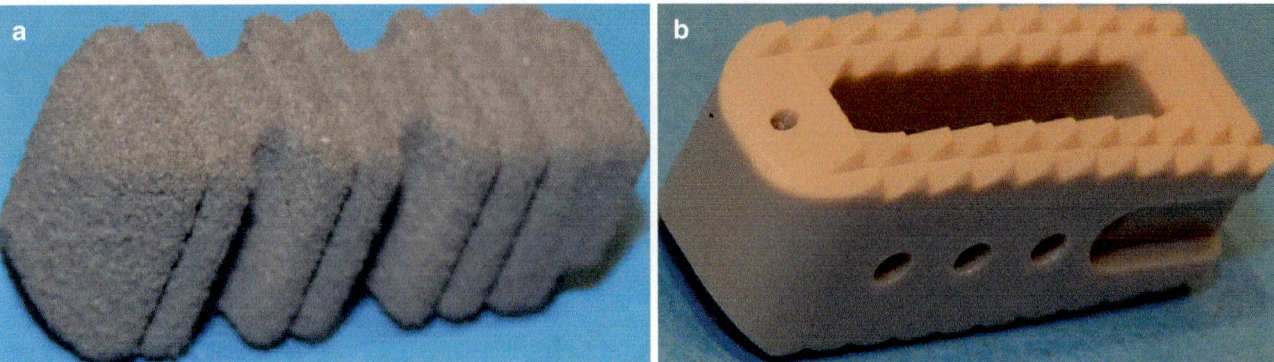

Fig. 70.1 ProSpace titanium spacer with Plasmapore coating (**a**) and ProSpace PEEK cage (**b**). (Aesculap AG, Tuttlingen, Germany)

70.4.1 Plasmapore-Coated Spacer

The heart of the disk implant is a solid core. The core is coated with Plasmapore to increase the area of contact between the implant and the end plates. The implant is made of ISOTAN F, a titanium alloy, which also has a Plasmapore coating. Plasmapore is a well-established pure titanium coating material, which offers an optimal foundation for the ingrowth of bone due to its balanced relationship among pore depth, porosity, and roughness. Plasmapore promotes osteointegration and osteoconduction without requiring additional bone graft material [1].

The aim of the Plasmapore coating is to achieve both primary and secondary stability. The increased surface roughness of the Plasmapore coating, in combination with a posterior fixation device, ensures immediate primary stability of the motion segment. Bone growth into the coating is rapid, owing to the optimal properties of Plasmapore. This results in bone fusion between vertebrae and implant (secondary stability).

70.4.2 PEEK Cages

PEEK stands for polyetheretherketone. The use of PEEK as an orthopedic device material has become increasingly popular in recent years owing to the material's unique combination of characteristics. Its properties include radiolucency, high mechanical strength, biocompatibility, and compatibility with standard sterilization methods. The intrinsic radioscopic transparency of the material gives it permeability on X-rays and CT scans, making it possible to view bone growth adjacent to the implant. Of particular interest is the modulus of elasticity of PEEK, which is 3.6 GPa and thus similar to that of cortical bone. This spe-

cific stiffness encourages load sharing between implant material and natural bone, thereby stimulating bone-healing activity (see Fig. 70.2).

70.5 Planning, Preparation, and Positioning

The patient is placed in a prone position. A radiolucent operating table is recommended to ensure unobstructed intraoperative fluoroscopic visualization in the anteroposterior (AP) and lateral planes. The elbows and knees are appropriately padded. The abdomen must be free. The lumbar spine should be in natural lordosis.

70.6 Surgical Technique

70.6.1 Approach

A midline incision is performed over the levels to be instrumented. The muscle should not be stripped more laterally than the lateral aspects of the facet joints unless posterolateral fusion between transverse processes is planned.

70.6.2 Instrumentation [1–7]

70.6.2.1 With a Plasmapore-Coated Titanium Spacer
- Bone resection
- The bone is resected using an osteotome and Kerrison bone punch to gain access to the intervertebral space. Alternatively, bone can be removed at the joints using a chisel or high-speed burr. The bone that has been removed is stored in a container under gauze to serve as graft material.

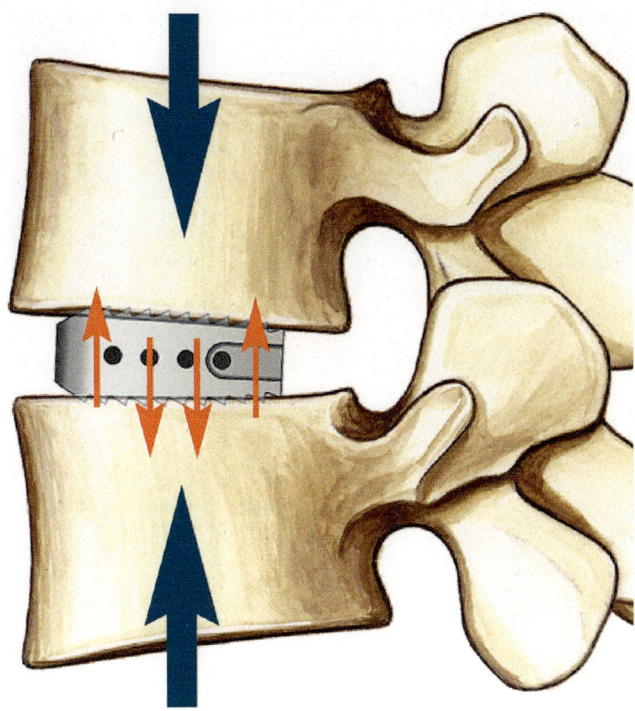

Fig. 70.2 Load sharing between PEEK implant material and natural bone stimulates bone-healing activity. (With permission from Aesculap AG, Tuttlingen, Germany)

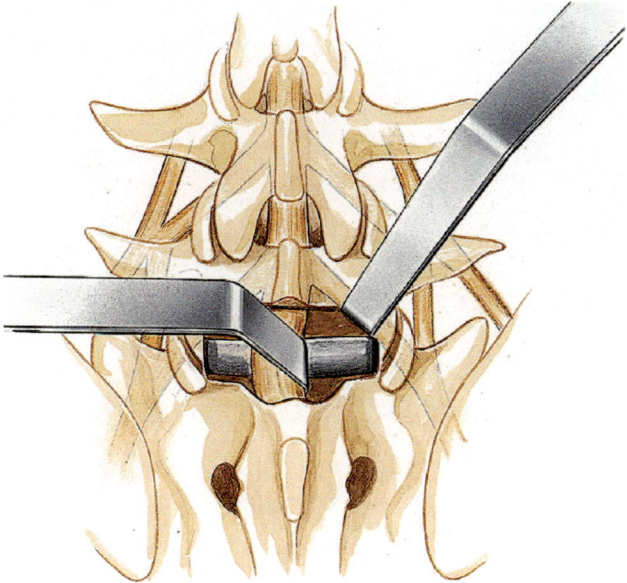

Fig. 70.3 After appropriate laminectomy, the nerve root and dura mater should be protected and the disk sufficiently exposed. Retraction of the dura and upper nerve root with nerve root retractors

- Revealing the disk space
- The dura and upper nerve root are carefully retracted in the desired direction using the nerve root retractors (see Fig. 70.3). Often, large epidural veins need to be cauterized to permit visualization of the posterolateral disk annulus. This must be done carefully, using bipolar cautery to prevent damage to the nerve roots.
- Restoration of disk height
- In order to make room for the insertion of the distractor, the disk material is now resected using rongeurs and forceps. Distraction can be set to the required height using the distractors (see Fig. 70.4). The distractors are inserted one after the other on alternate sides of the disk until the desired distraction is obtained (see Fig. 70.5).
- Clearance of the intervertebral space
- Besides rongeurs and curettes, reamers and rasps can also be used to prepare the intervertebral space. Turning the instrument will remove disk material (see Fig. 70.6). Using the rasps, the cartilaginous end plates are refreshed (see Fig. 70.7). The annulus has to be cleaned out as completely as possible, and the end plates need to be freed from cartilage, taking care not to perforate the bone.
- Preparation of the implant bed

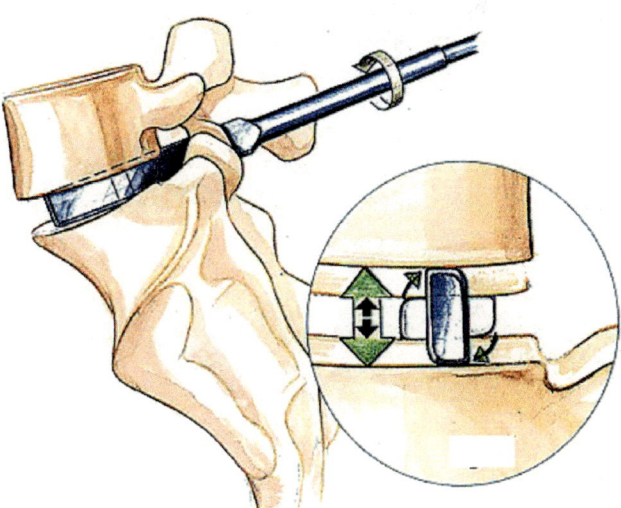

Fig. 70.4 Restoration of the disk height using different distractors. (With permission from Aesculap AG, Tuttlingen, Germany)

- Any unevenness of the borders of the implant bed can be smoothed using the broach. The sharp leading edge of the instrument permits simple bone resection to the dimensions required (see Figs. 70.7 and 70.8). The implant bed is now prepared, and the implant can be inserted.
- Insertion of the cage

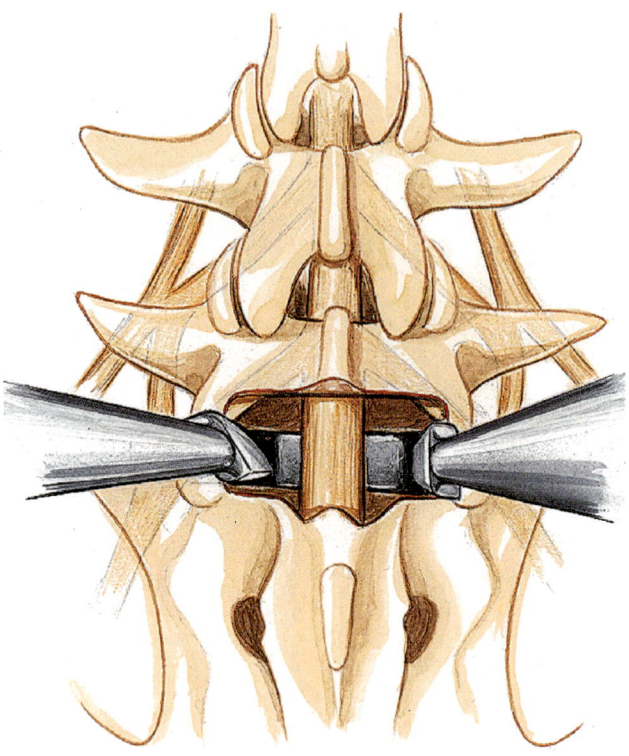

Fig. 70.5 The distractors are inserted one after the other on alternate sides. (With permission from Aesculap AG, Tuttlingen, Germany)

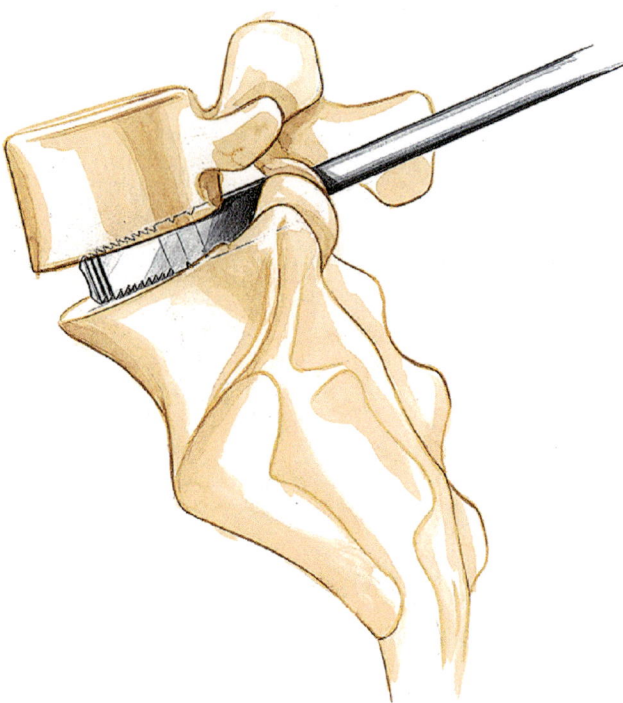

Fig. 70.7 Preparation of the implant bed using a broach. (With permission from Aesculap AG, Tuttlingen, Germany)

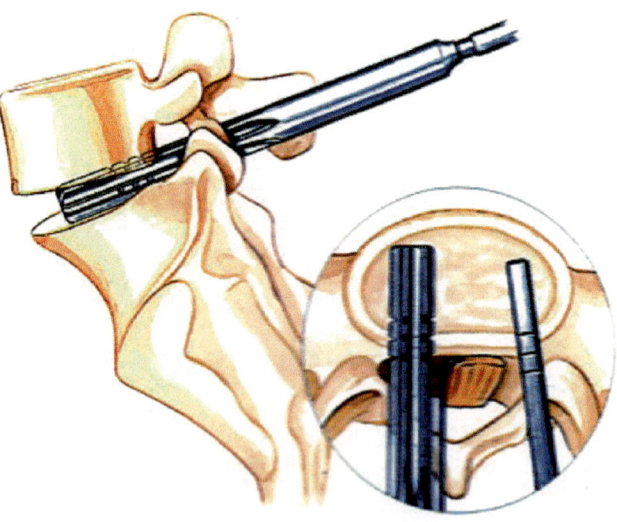

Fig. 70.6 Clearance of the intervertebral space with curettes, reamers, and rasps. (With permission from Aesculap AG, Tuttlingen, Germany)

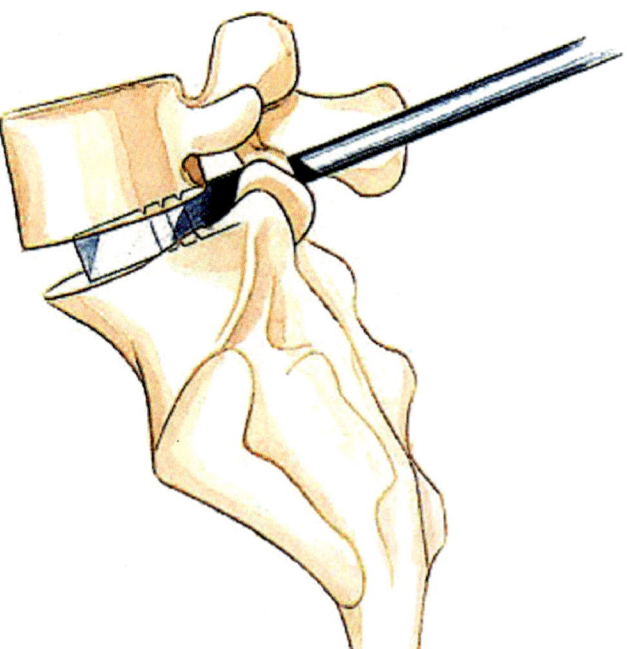

Fig. 70.8 Preparation of the implant bed using a broach. (With permission from Aesculap AG, Tuttlingen, Germany)

- Either a straight implant (0°) or a lordotic implant (5° or 8°) can be used, depending on the particular level and anatomy. The implant is connected to the inserter by engaging the thread using the Allen key connected to the instrument (see Fig. 70.9). The spacer is introduced on the flat side and turned clockwise in order to spread the disk space. The implant is then brought into its final vertical position. The position of the implant can be corrected with the impactor (see Fig. 70.10).

- Insertion on the contralateral side

  The operative steps described above are now repeated for the contralateral side. Bone material can be packed between both implants. Additional posterior stabilization of the segment should be performed (see Figs. 70.10 and 70.11).

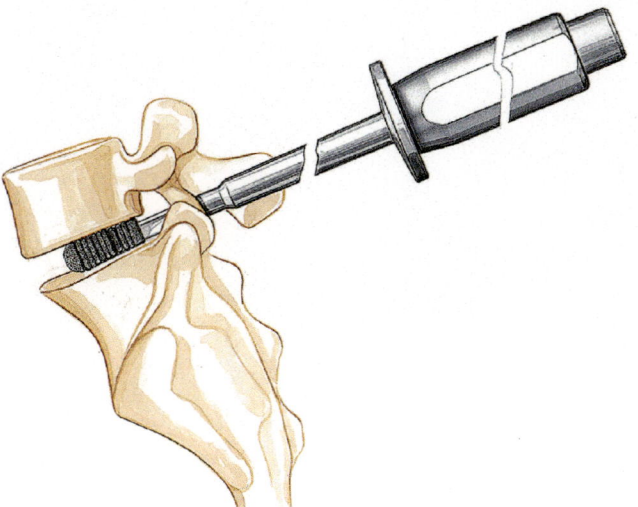

Fig. 70.9 Insertion of the spacer with the insertion instrument and impactor. (With permission from Aesculap AG, Tuttlingen, Germany)

70.6.2.2   With a PEEK Spacer

(Operating steps are comparable to those for the titanium cages.)

- Bone resection
- The bone is resected using an osteotome and a Kerrison bone punch to gain access to the intervertebral space. Alternatively, bone can be removed at the joints using a chisel or high-speed burr.
- Revealing the disk space
- The dura and upper nerve root are carefully retracted in the desired direction using the nerve root retractors (see Fig. 70.3).
- The sharp leading edge of the instrument permits simple bone resection to the dimensions required.
- Restoration of disk height

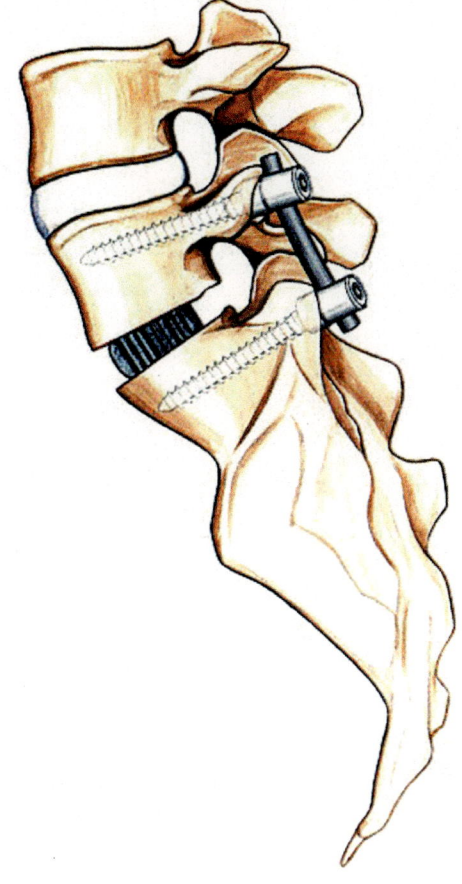

Fig. 70.10 Additional posterior stabilization of the motion segment is necessary

- Distraction can be set to the required height using the distractors (see Figs. 70.11 and 70.12). The distractors are inserted one after the other on alternate sides of the disk until the desired distraction is obtained.
- Clearance of the intervertebral disk

Fig. 70.11 Restoration of disk height using different distractors. Positioning of contralateral distractor. (With permission from Aesculap Ag, Tuttlingen, Germany)

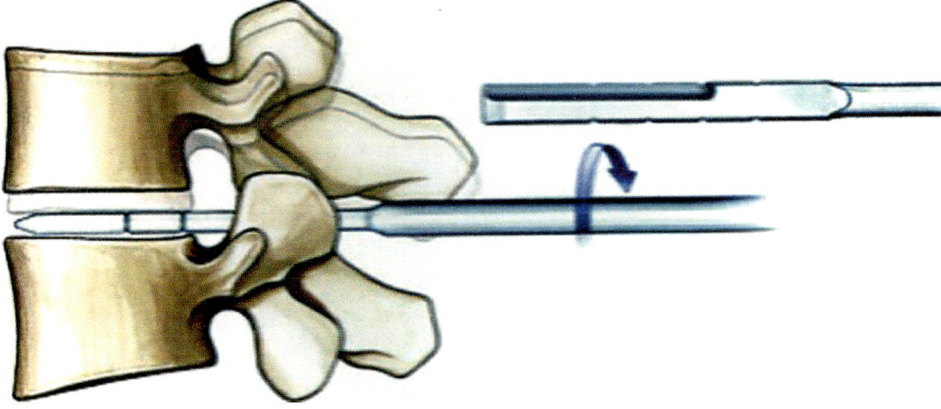

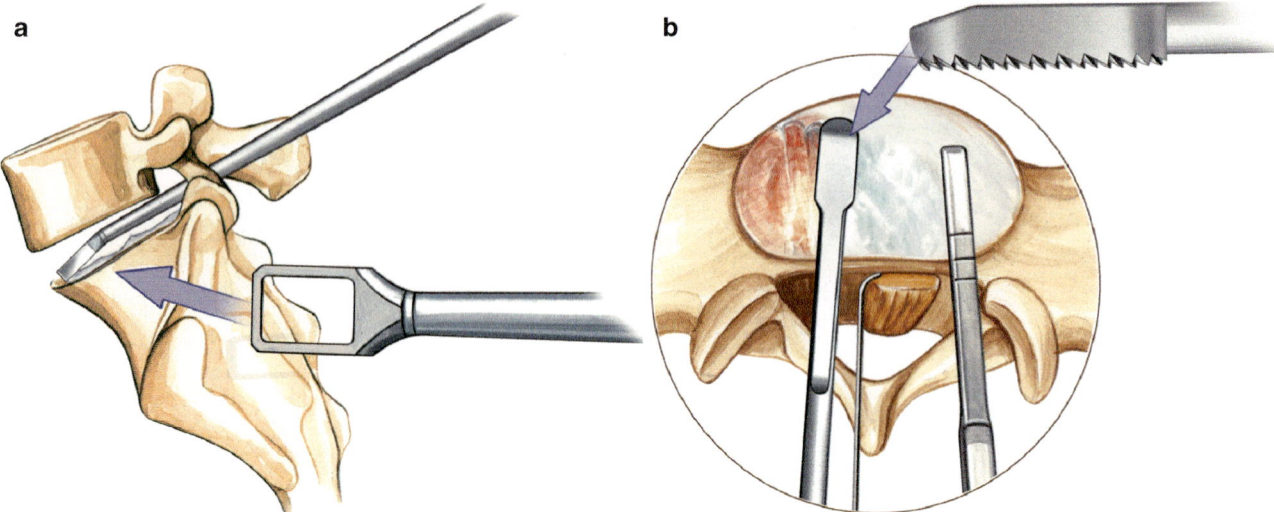

Fig. 70.12 (**a**, **b**) Clearance of the intervertebral space. (With permission from Aesculap AG, Tuttlingen, Germany)

Fig. 70.13 Determination of the implant size using trial implants. (With permission from Aesculap AG, Tuttlingen, Germany)

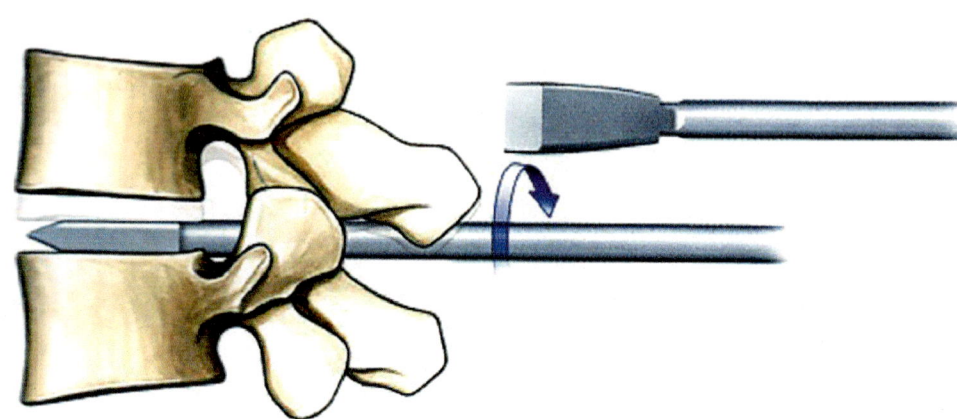

- The disk space is cleared using rongeurs, bone curettes, and rectangular curettes. Bone rasps are used to refresh the cartilaginous end plates (see Figs. 70.12 and 70.13).
- Determination of implant size using trial implants
- Trial implants are available in different sizes and with different angulations. Trial implants are inserted in turn, starting with the smallest size. Each is inserted horizontally and rotated clockwise (see Figs. 70.13 and 70.14). Progressively, taller trial implants are inserted until the required distraction has been achieved. The trial implant now in place indicates the height, angle, and length of the implant to be inserted.
- Insertion of the PEEK cage

- After filling the PEEK implant with bone graft or artificial bone substitute, the implant is clamped to the PEEK insertion instrument (see Figs. 70.14 and 70.15) and inserted in the intervertebral space (see Figs. 70.15 and 70.16). The cage is filled with finely milled autologous bone (the resected bone from the spinous processes and the facet joints will generally be sufficient).
- Insertion on the contralateral side.
- The operative steps described are now repeated for the contralateral side. Bone material can be packed between both implants.
- Posterior stabilization
- Additional posterior stabilization of the segment should be performed.

Fig. 70.14 The implant is clamped to the insertion instrument. (With permission from Aesculap AG, Tuttlingen, Germany)

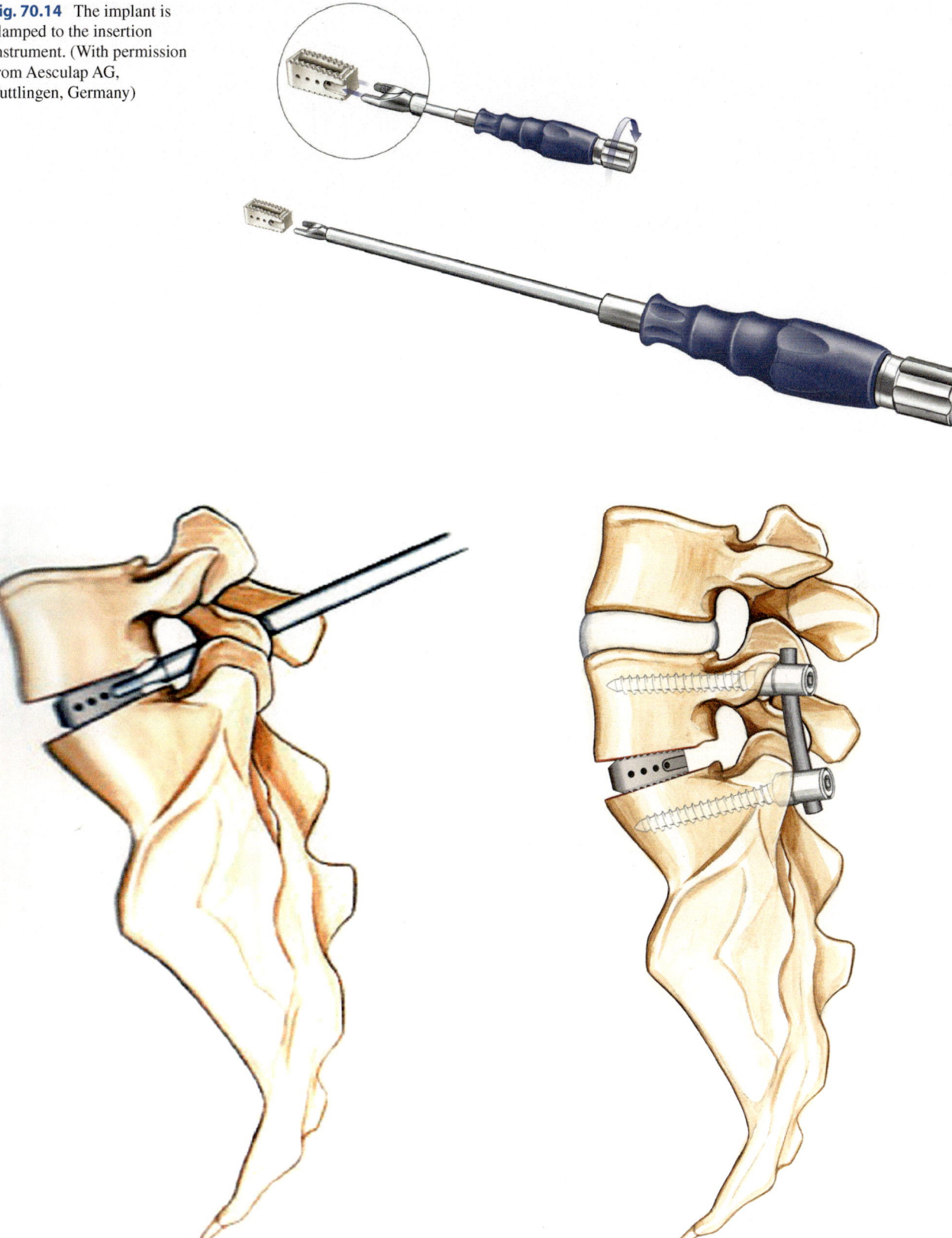

Fig. 70.15 Insertion of the PEEK cage with the insertion instrument. (With permission from Aesculap AG, Tuttlingen, Germany)

Fig. 70.16 Three-column stabilization with anterior column fusion with PEEK cage and posterior column fixation with internal fixator. (With permission from Aesculap AG, Tuttlingen, Germany)

References

1. Bronsard JJ, Tropiano P, Louis C, et al. Three–column spinal fusion using ProSpace intervertebral blocks. In: Kaech DL, Jinkins JR, editors. Spinal restabilisation procedures. Amsterdam: Elsevier Science; 2002. p. 153–70.
2. Cloward RB. Spondylolisthesis: treatment by laminectomy and posterior lumbar interbody fusion. Clin Orthop. 1981;154:74–82.
3. Freemann BJ, Licina P, Mehdina SH. Posterior lumbar interbody fusion combined with instrumented posterolateral fusion: 5 year results in 60 patients. Eur Spine J. 2000;9:42–6.
4. La Rosa G, Germano A, Conti A, et al. Posterior fusion and implantation of the SOCON-SRI system in the treatment of adult spondylolisthesis. Neurosurg Focus. 1999;7(6):E2.
5. La Rosa G, Cacciola F, Conti A, et al. Posterior fusion compared with posterior interbody fusion in segmental spinal fixation for adult spondylolisthesis. Neurosurg Focus. 2001;10(4):E9.
6. Periasamy K, Shah K, Wheelwright EF. Posterior lumbar interbody fusion using cages, combined with instrumented posterolateral fusion: a study of 75 cases. Acta Orthop Belg. 2008;74:240–8.
7. Potel A, Welch WC. Posterior lumbar interbody fusion with metal cages: current techniques. Oper Tech Orthop. 2000;10:311–9.

Palaniappan Lakshmanan and Sashin Ahuja

71.1 Introduction and Core Messages

The goals of treatment of high-grade spondylolisthesis including spondyloptosis are to relieve back pain by stabilizing the segmental instability, to achieve 360° fusion to prevent instability and pseudarthrosis to relieve leg pain by decompressing the neuronal structures, and to minimize risks to neuronal structures by avoiding reduction. Using different methods, a circumferential 360° fusion can be achieved in high-grade spondylolisthesis including spondyloptosis through an all-posterior approach [1–5]. The technique outlined in this chapter employs two transsacral hollow modular anchorage (HMA) screws (Inventors Jean Hupp, Thierry Marnay, Marc Ameil 1995) filled with bone graft and supplemented with posterolateral fusion with pedicle screw instrumentation.

71.2 Indications

- High-grade spondylolisthesis Meyerding grade III–V L5/S1 including spondyloptosis
- Persistent back pain and/or leg pain affecting quality of life
- Failed nonoperative treatment

71.3 Contraindications

- Infection
- Medically unfit for operation and general anesthesia
- Poor bone quality—osteoporosis (poor screw purchase)

71.4 Technical Prerequisites

- Fluoroscopy with live screening
- Radiolucent table
- Patient positioning device's like Wilson's frame, Jackson's table, etc.
- Hollow modular anchorage (HMA) screw (Aesculap Ltd, Tuttlingen) and instrumentation
- Polyaxial pedicle screw system with implants and instrumentation (Figs. 71.1 and 71.2)
- Drill sleeve from any bone drill set

71.5 Planning, Preparation, and Positioning

The patient's X-rays are reviewed to assess the length of the transsacral screw from the posterior body of S1 to the superior corner of the anterior margin of L5 vertebral body on the lat-

P. Lakshmanan (✉)
Sunderland Royal Hospital, Sunderland, UK
e-mail: lakunns@gmail.com

S. Ahuja
University Hospital of Wales, Cardiff, UK
e-mail: sashinahuja@doctors.org.uk

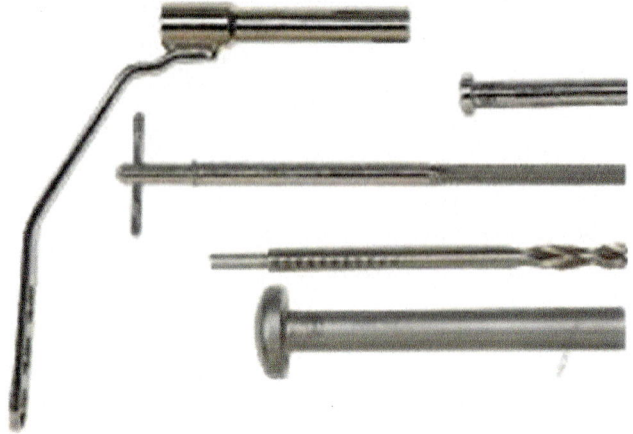

Fig. 71.1 Instruments for transsacral screw fixation. (With permission from Aesculap AG, Tuttlingen, Germany)

Fig. 71.2 Hollow modular anchorage (HMA) screw. (**a**) Fixation nut, (**b**) sleeve, (**c**) locking nut. (With permission from Aesculap AG, Tuttlingen, Germany)

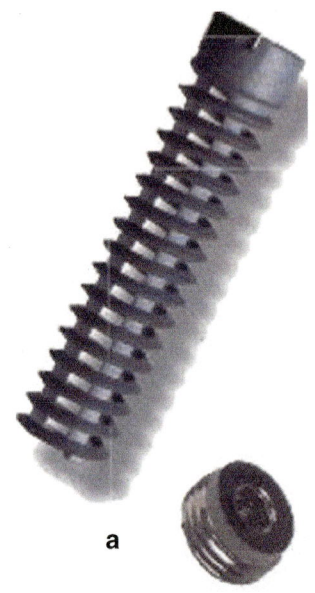

a

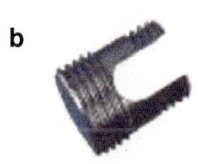

b

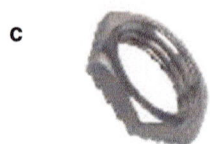

c

anatomy aids the surgeon to decide the proper placement of the pedicle screws in the L4 and S1 vertebral bodies.

The patient is positioned prone under general anesthesia on a radiolucent operating table, and the image intensifier is used to check whether adequate anteroposterior (AP) and lateral imaging of the lumbosacral spine can be obtained. Also, the abdomen should be free to avoid venous impediment.

71.6 Surgical Technique

71.6.1 Approach

The approach is via a posterior midline longitudinal incision approximately from L3 to S2 spinous processes. The posterior elements up to the transverse processes are exposed by subperiosteal elevation of the paraspinal muscles on either side. Care is taken not to disrupt the facet joint of L3/4.

71.6.2 Instrumentation

- Perform adequate decompression by removing the posterior element of L5 with removal of the fibrous tissue around the pars defect. Also, the bony and soft tissue elements compressing the L5 nerve root are removed until the L5 nerve root is completely free under the L5 pedicle (Gill's procedure).
- The posterior part of the sacrum is deroofed, and an extensive posterior spinal decompression is performed to expose the S1 and S2 nerve roots.
- The S1 nerve root and the theca are carefully freed up from any underlying adhesions.
- The S1 nerve root is retracted laterally with a nerve root retractor, while the theca with the rest of the nerve roots is retracted medially. Care is taken not to retract forcefully to avoid postoperative neurological complications.
- During periods of inactivity, the retraction must be released to avoid constant traction on the nerve roots for long periods.
- The entry point on the posterior wall of the body of S1 between the S1 and S2 nerve roots is identified lateral to midline using C-arm and confirmed on the lateral view depending on the angle it penetrates the L5 vertebral body to reach the anterosuperior corner of L5 vertebral body (Fig. 71.3).
- The guide wire is passed using a drill sleeve under image guidance from the posterior wall of S1 vertebral body through the L5–S1 disk space and then into the L5 vertebral body to end 5 mm short of penetrating the anterosuperior corner of L5 vertebral body (Fig. 71.7).

eral view and taking away 1 cm from the measurement. The length and thickness of the pedicle screws at L4 and S1 can be preoperatively determined by reviewing the axial sections of the MRI scans. Further, complete analysis of the pedicular

Fig. 71.3 Decision for a posterior transsacral approach. *Note*: Laminectomy S1/S2 is required to visualize the nerves

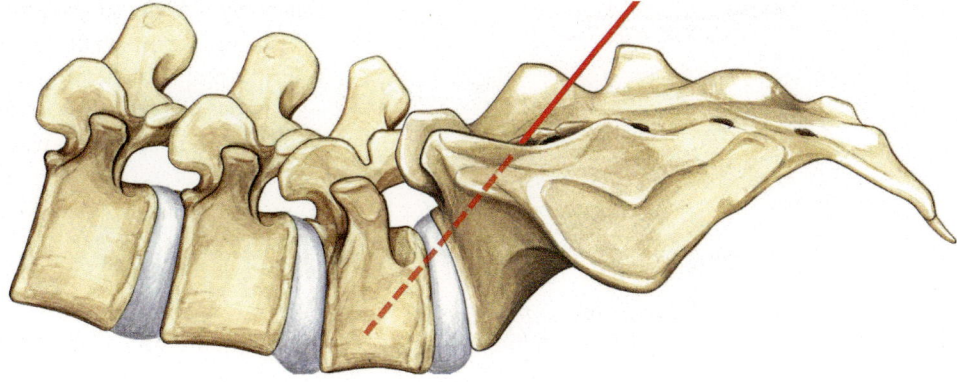

Fig. 71.4 Preparation of the sacrum and the disk L5/S1

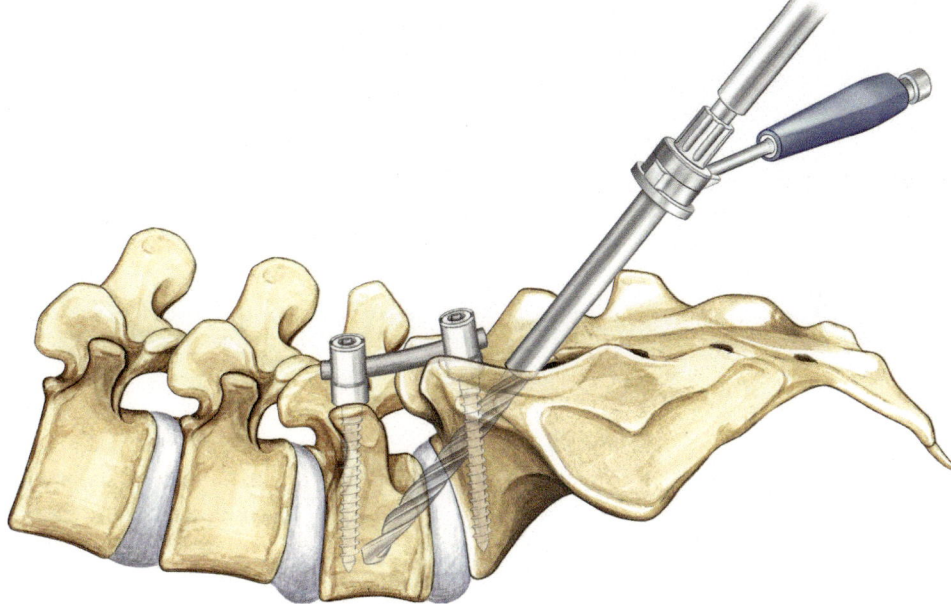

- A cannulated drill is then passed over the guide wire with a drill sleeve in position. To prevent the drill sleeve from slipping, the tip can be buried in the posterior cortex of S1 vertebral body by nibbling away the cortex to avoid catching the dura or the S1 nerve root (Fig. 71.4).
- The drill hole must be tapped adequately depending on the size of the screw chosen. The size of the HMA screw is determined by the size of the sacral vertebra and should be in such a way that two screws on either side can be used with no difficulty.
- A depth gauge is used to find the length of the HMA screw, and the closest available length is used.
- The hollowness in the HMA screw is then filled with cancellous bone graft procured from the posterior elements of the spine during decompression with or without posterior iliac crest bone grafting. It can also be supplemented with bone graft substitutes.
- The screw with the bone graft is then inserted to anchor the L5 on S1 to produce an in situ fixation for high-grade spondylolisthesis including spondyloptosis.

- The same procedure is repeated on the other side to insert another HMA screw parallel to the previous one.
- To supplement the transsacral HMA screw construct, a pedicle screw fixation from L4 to S1 is performed as detailed below (see Figs. 71.5 and 71.6).
- The entry point for the pedicle screw of L4 is identified, and the cortex is nibbled away to show the bleeding cancellous bone.
- The awl is then used to make entry for the pedicular probe. However, in some cases where the anatomy is distorted, C-arm can be used to guide the awl and subsequently the pedicular probe in the appropriate angle both in the AP and lateral planes. A ball-tip probe is then used to confirm the intactness of the walls on all four sides and also the anterior wall. The graduations on the ball-tip probe can give the length of the screw.
- A separate depth gauge can be used to measure the length of the screw up to the anterior cortex of the vertebral body.
- The polyaxial pedicle screw is then inserted in a converging direction.

Fig. 71.5 Implant in place

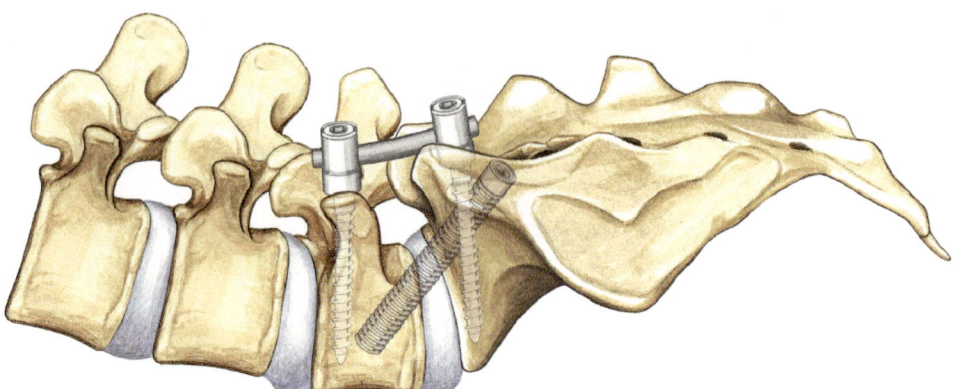

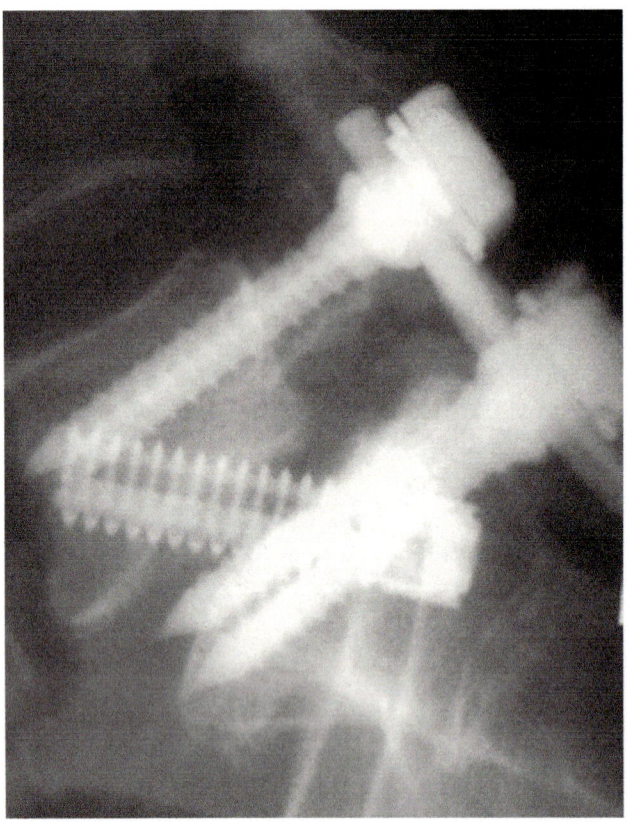

Fig. 71.6 Fusion of the level L5–S1 with internal fixator and HMA screw

- The same technique is repeated on the other side of L4.
- At S1, the pedicle screws are inserted as above, but the screws are aimed toward the promontory of the sacrum, and they are medialized as much as possible. Further, a bicortical purchase is achieved with each sacral screw.
- The transverse processes of the vertebral bodies and the ala of the sacrum are decorticated to act as a bed for the posterolateral bone graft.
- The titanium rods usually >5.5 mm in diameter are contoured and fixed to the pedicle screws using setscrews or grub screws without attempting any reduction.

- The bone graft obtained from the removed posterior elements and/or the posterior iliac crest is packed on either side to give a posterolateral fusion. This can be supplemented with bone graft substitutes if needed.

71.7 Tips and Tricks

- If the posterior body of the sacrum is indenting the dura significantly, then the posterosuperior corner of the sacral dome can be carefully osteotomized or nibbled away to prevent any compression on the dura.
- Care must be taken while drilling over the guide wire, and repeated C-arm pictures are needed, or even live screening is required as there is a potential for the guide wire to be pushed anteriorly inadvertently, which can result in serious injury to the neurovascular structures in the front.
- Also, as the guide wire passes through three cortices (Fig. 71.7) and if the bone is strong, then the guide wire may gently curve. This results in the drill rotating against the guide wire, thereby heating it up and ultimately breaking the guide wire. Hence, we advice to frequently take X-rays while drilling, for smooth passage of the drill over the guide wire (Fig. 71.8).
- If, however, the guide wire breaks inadvertently, then instruments like narrow pituitary rongeur or grasper must be readily available to retrieve the broken part.
- Adequate and appropriate tapping of the HMA screw is needed as otherwise the screw may break while inserting if not adequately tapped.
- If the posterior body of the sacrum is small and looks like it may not take up two HMA screws, then a midline large single HMA screw can be used instead of two HMA screws on either side.
- The HMA screws are not strong enough to use them as stand-alone devices and need posterior supplementation with pedicle screws and posterolateral fusion (Fig. 71.9) as otherwise the HMA screws may break.

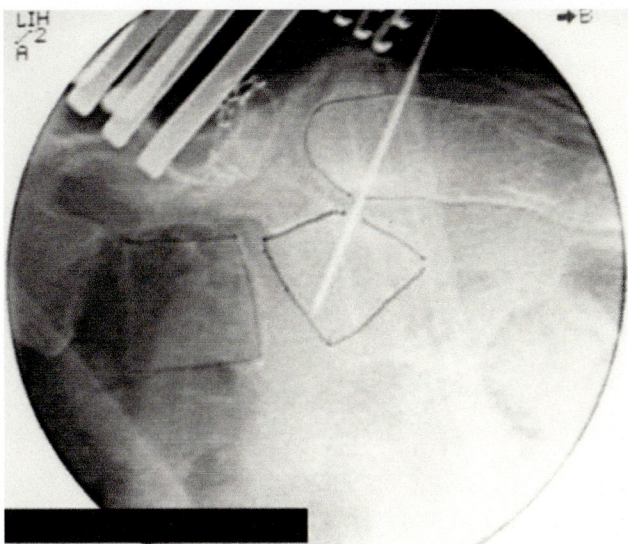

Fig. 71.7 Interoperative X-ray demonstrating the guide wire. The guide wire is passed using a drill sleeve under image guidance from the posterior wall of S1 through L5–S1 disk space

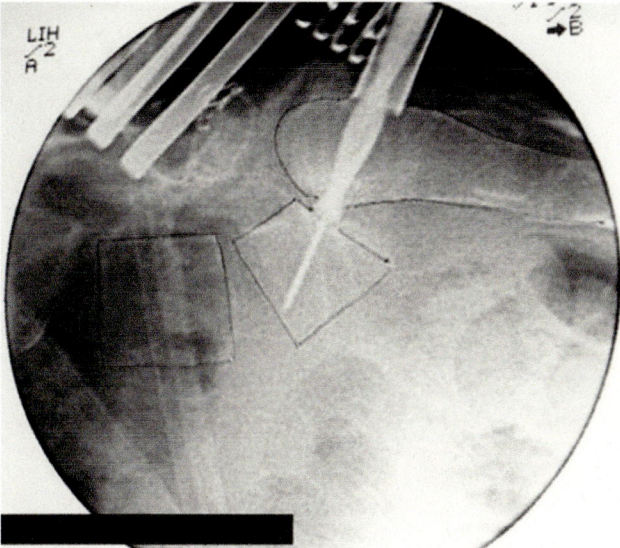

Fig. 71.8 Drill on the guide wire with the drill sleeve

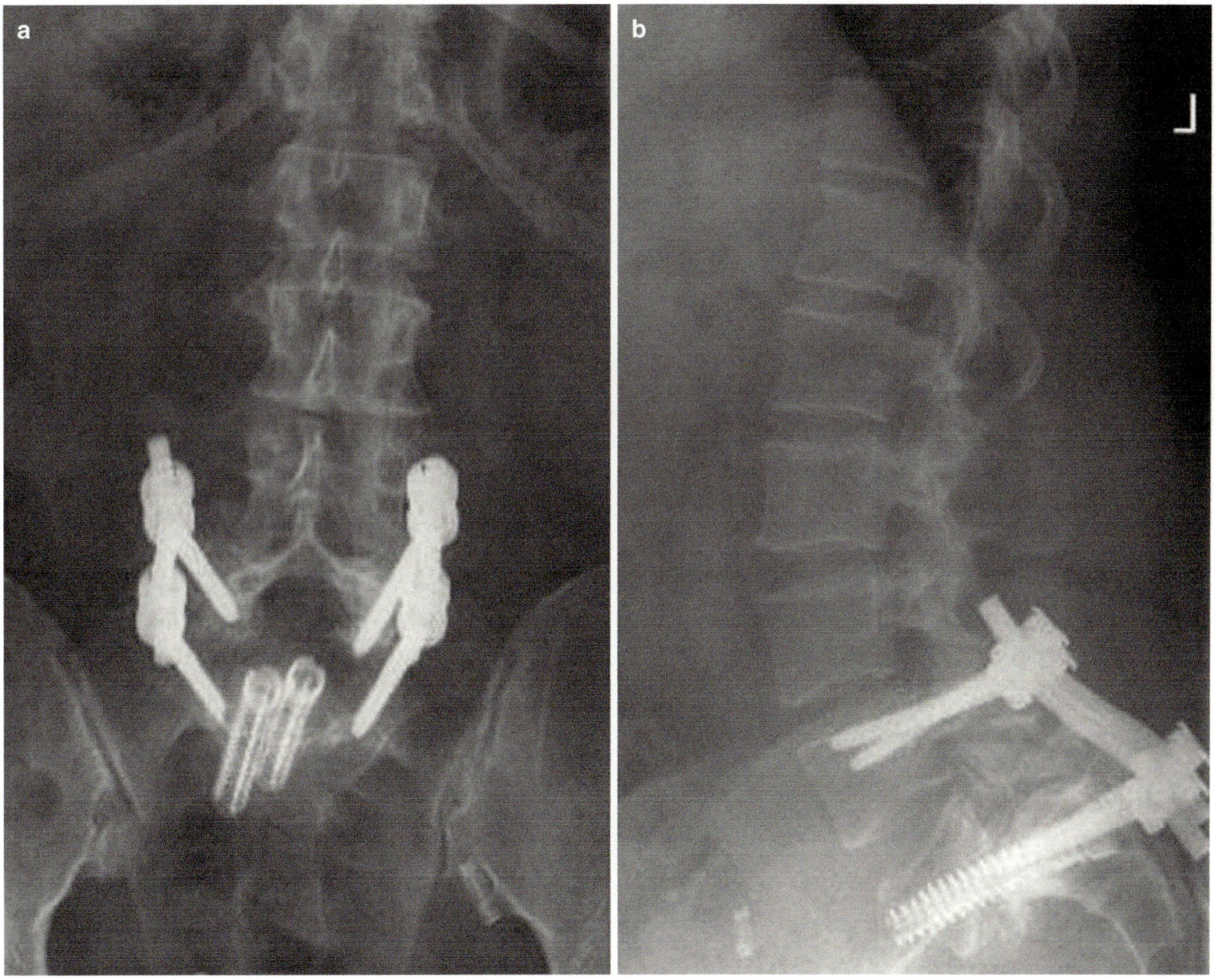

Fig. 71.9 Final postoperative AP X-ray (**a**) and (**b**) lateral view with the 2 HMA screws and pedicle screws

References

1. Bohlman HH, Cook SS. One-stage decompression and posterolateral and interbody fusion for lumbosacral spondyloptosis through a posterior approach. Report of two cases. J Bone Joint Surg Am. 1982;64(3):415–8.
2. Esses SI, Natout N, Kip P. Posterior interbody arthrodesis with a fibular strut graft in spondylolisthesis. J Bone Joint Surg Am. 1995;77(2):172–6.
3. Lakshmanan P, Ahuja S, Lewis M, et al. Achieving 360 degrees fusion in high-grade spondylolisthesis using HMA screws. Surg Technol Int. 2009;18:219–22.
4. Roca J, Ubierna MT, Cáceres E, et al. One-stage decompression and posterolateral and interbody fusion for severe spondylolisthesis. An analysis of 14 patients. Spine (Phila Pa 1976). 1999;24(7):709–14.
5. Whitecloud TS 3rd, Butler JC. Anterior lumbar fusion utilizing transvertebral fibular graft. Spine (Phila Pa 1976). 1988;13(3):370–4.

Percutaneous Pedicle Screw Instrumentation and Pedicle Screw Augmentation with Vertebral Body Stenting (VBS) in Cases with Unstable Osteoporotic Thoracolumbar Fractures

Uwe Vieweg

72.1 Introduction and Core Messages

The management of osteoporotic vertebral fractures in affected elderly patients can be complex because of the presence of comorbidities, lack of functional reserves and cognitive dysfunction [1, 2]. A conservative or surgical approach can be taken for the treatment of fractures of this nature. However, it is difficult to effectively deal with unstable osteoporotic fractures using conservative methods. At the same time, open surgical procedures involving reconstruction of vertebral body height and restoration of the spinal ventral column are generally of more extensive duration and associated with an increased rate of complications and greater loss of blood. In addition, open surgery also leads to extensive damage to dorsal muscles. In view of this, when treatment of unstable osteoporotic fractures is necessary, viable alternatives that can be considered are either the use of a minimal invasive procedure involving percutaneous internal fracture fixation using cement-augmented pedicle screws in combination with a vertebral body stenting system (VBS) or kyphoplasty [3, 4]. Trauma mechanisms differ considerably between older and younger patients. In older patients, low-energy trauma is more common in contrast to high-energy trauma in young patients. Skrzypiec et al. [5] undertook mechanical testing of cadaveric tissues to compare the strength of disks and vertebrae from the same spine in order to determine which are more vulnerable to injury and to determine how their relative vulnerability depends on age and gender. The work group found that the low adaptive potential of intervertebral disks makes them relatively weak in the strengthening spines of young men but relatively strong in the weakening spines of elderly women [5]. This in summary is the theoretical basis for the so-called hybrid technology ("metal plus bone cement") approach adopted in elderly and senile patients [3, 4].

72.2 Indications

An indication for intervention can be based on the old or new AO Spine classification system [6] or preferably, the OF classification [1, 2]. In principle, use of the AO Spine classification is, however, not suitable or at least less suitable in connection with osteoporotic fractures. In spite of this, both classification systems are cited in the following, mainly because the AO Spine system has been longer in use.

72.2.1 Indications Based on the AO Spine Classification

Indications based on the AO Spine classification are
- A3 incomplete burst fracture (see Fig. 72.1a, b),
- A4 complete burst fracture (see Fig. 72.2a–c).

It is a matter of judgement whether intervention of this kind should be initiated in cases of these types of fracture. The fracture gap must not be too large. However, it is relatively often possible to stabilize an A4 fracture using a vertebral body stent (VBS). If this proves unsuccessful, subsequent spinal replacement surgery can be considered and implemented if the clinical status of the patient makes this possible.

U. Vieweg (✉)
Department of Conservative and Surgical Spine Therapy with Interdisciplinary Spinal Deformities Centre and Rummelsberg Sectional Center, Hospital Rummelsberg, Schwarzenbruck, Germany
e-mail: uwe.vieweg@sana.de

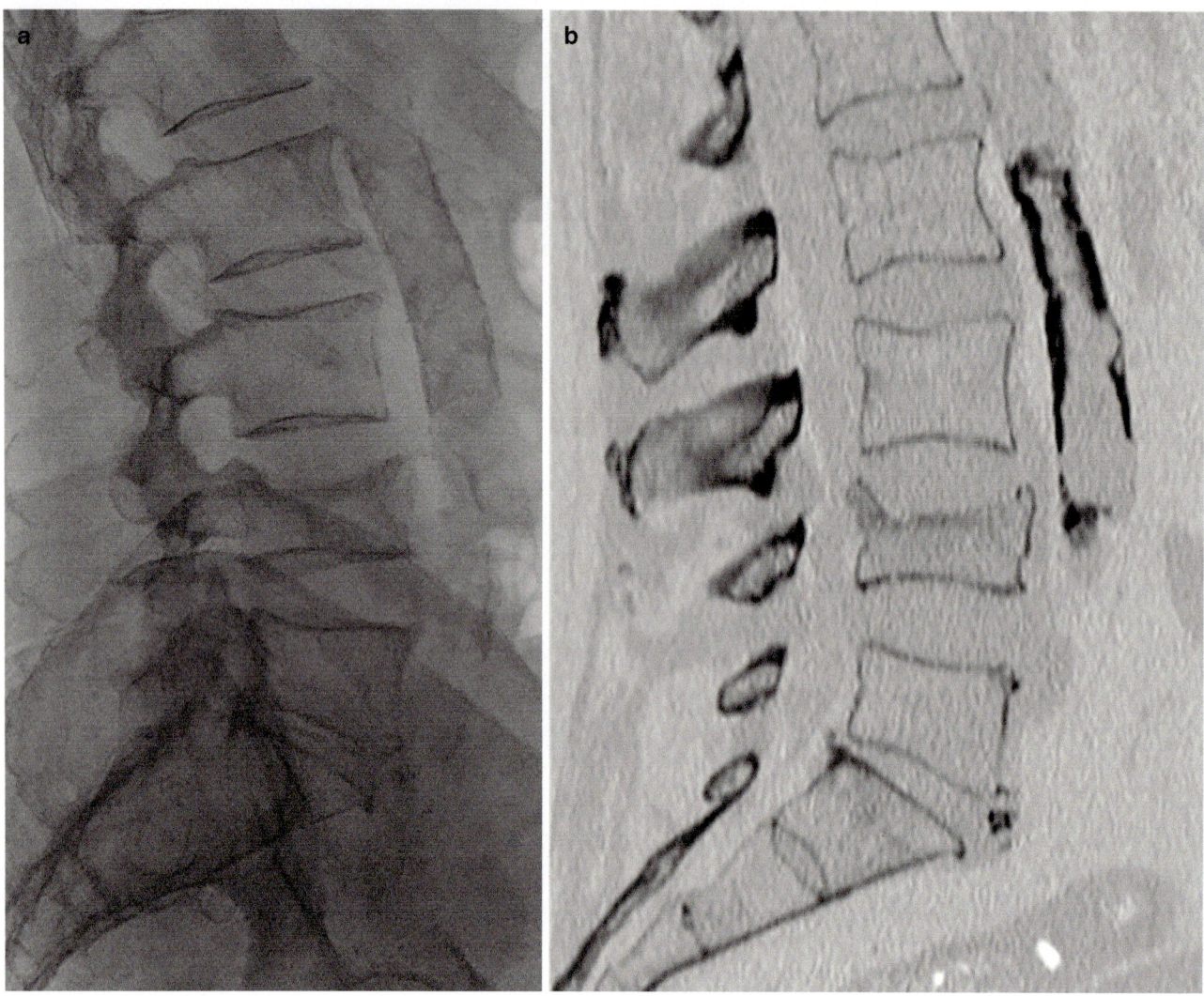

Fig. 72.1 Conventional X-ray lateral view and CT of a 78-year-old male (Case1) with a type A3 fracture (AO Spine classification)/OF 3 (OF classification) in the level L4

72.2.2 Indications Based on the OF Classification [1, 2]

The OF classification system consists of five groups: OF I—no vertebral deformation, vertebral edema; OF 2—deformation with no or minor (<1/5) involvement of the posterior wall, OF 3—deformation with distinct involvement (>1/5) of the posterior wall; OF 4—loss of integrity of the vertebral frame or vertebral body collapse or pincer type fracture; OF 5—injuries with dislocation or rotation. Indications based on the OF classification are as follows:

- OF 3 type fractures (see Fig. 72.1a, b),
- Borderline indications can be OF 4 (see Fig. 72.2a, b) and in some cases OF 2 type fractures.

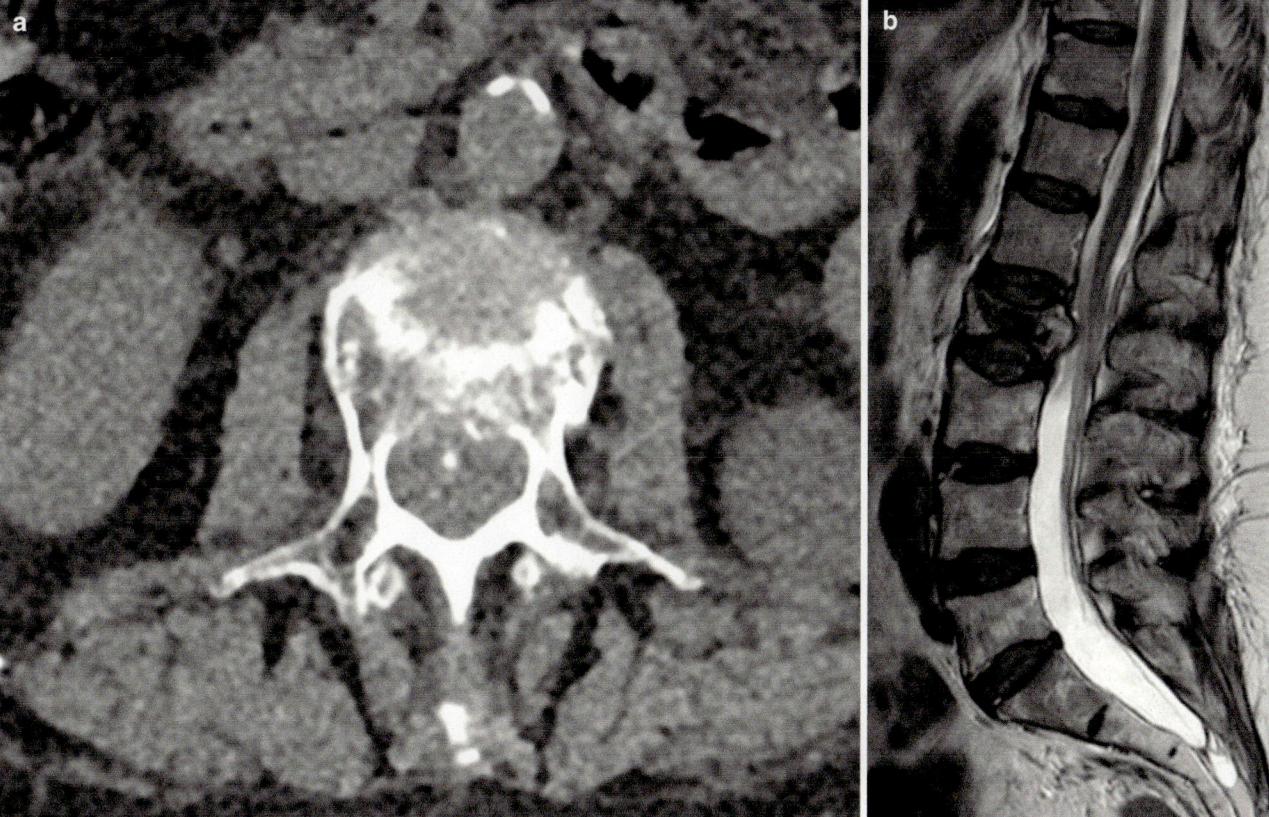

Fig. 72.2 CT (**a**) and MRT (**b**) examinations show a complete burst fracture L2 (AO Spine A4, OF4) from an 83-year-old female (reduced general condition (ASA 4) and immobilizing back pain (VAS-8) without neurological deficits falled from stairs

72.3   Contraindications

The generally accepted relative contraindications for use of the technique (either for the employment of a vertebral body stent or pedicle screw augmentation) are

- Lesions that require definitive reconstruction of the anterior column in open surgery.
- Acute or chronic systemic or local spinal infections.
- The presence of injuries other than C or B injuries as per the AO Spine classification.

72.4   Technical Prerequisites

72.4.1   Preoperative Imaging

The following images/scans are required for diagnosis and planning of the surgical procedure:

- Radiographic images of the thoracic and lumbar spine in two planes.
- CT and MRI scans of the fractured spinal regions (if possible with STIR).

In addition to the classification of the fracture, the positioning and size of the pedicle screws (transpedicular, extrapedicular) and of the VBS required are to be determined on the basis of the above images.

72.4.2   Intraoperative Imaging

Adjustable radiographic equipment should be employed during the whole surgical procedure as all surgical phases need to be monitored in both planes. Suitable for this purpose are two C-arm X-ray machines or a single fully mobile C-arm. The operating table must be such that it allows for suitable positioning of the C-arm for imaging of the surgical site in both planes.

72.4.3   Implants and Bone Cement

72.4.3.1   Percutaneously Implanted Internal Fixation with Augmented Pedicle Screws

In principle, all internal fixation systems that can be implanted by the percutaneous route can be used in this procedure. The system should employ polyaxial screws that allow additional pedicle screw augmentation. Pedicle screw augmentation is necessary to ensure sufficient stability of the construct as a whole [7–9].

72.4.3.2 Vertebral Body Stent [4, 10–14]

Conventional kyphoplasty or even vertebroplasty [3, 4, 15] can also be used, if necessary, to reconstruct and augment a fractured vertebral body. But it is advisable, particularly in cases of complete or incomplete burst fractures, to use a *vertebral body stent* (VBS) as this facilitates reconstruction (see Fig. 72.3a–c); a VBS comes with a corresponding inflation system (see Fig. 72.4). The technique has been described in various publications [4, 10–14]. There are three differently sized vertebral body stent-balloon combinations available (small-maximum volume 4.5 mL, medium-maximum volume 5 mL, large-maximum volume 5.5 mL). We consider it theoretically more possible to reconstruct a vertebral body using a stent and removing outside the gap any disk tissue that has penetrated the fracture. However, there is as yet no definitive medical verification of the efficiency of this concept. VBS systems (see Fig. 72.3b, c) use a specially designed catheter-mounted stent, which can be implanted and expanded inside the vertebral body. On deflation of the balloon, the stent remains in the fractured vertebral body. As a rule, the stent will preserve the corrective reconstruction and will tend to prevent disk tissue re-entering the fracture. The VBS stent provides for height restoration and the cement ensures the stabilization of the vertebral body. Other comparable alternatives are use of the Osseofix or SpineJack systems. These two other systems employ a mechanism that allows a controlled reduction of a vertebral fracture [16]. The VBS, Osseofix, and SpineJack systems represent a further evolution of the kyphoplasty technique [8].

72.4.3.3 Bone Cement

So that all pedicle screws and the stent can be augmented as quickly as possible so that there is sufficient time to deal with all vertebral bodies that need attention, the bone cement must have a specific property; that is, it must retain a suitably fluid viscosity for a relatively long period of time. We recommend utilization of a ready-to-use cement, such as Vertecem V+ (see Fig. 72.5). Of course, other standard bone cements that are designed for use in vertebroplasty or pedicle screw augmentation can also be

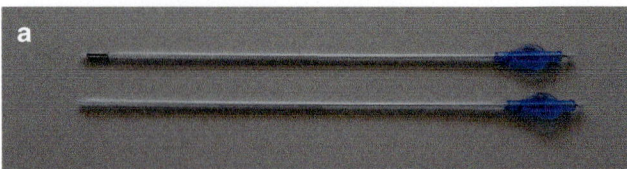
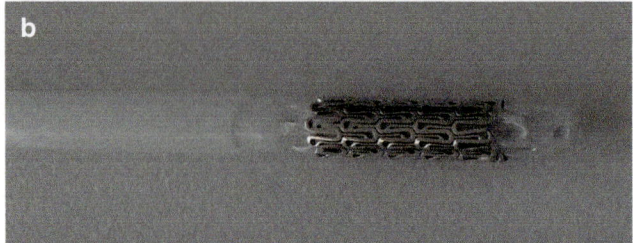
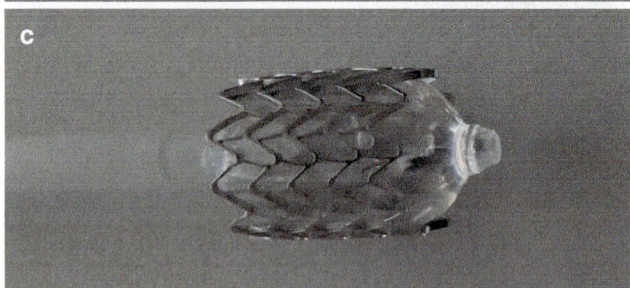
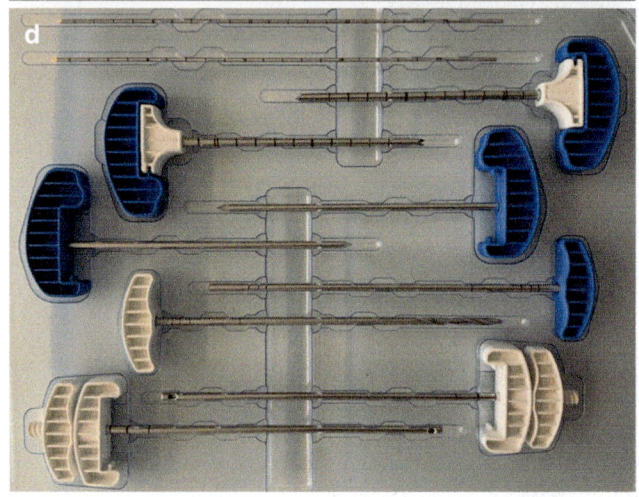

Fig. 72.3 (**a–c**) Vertebral body stent (**a, b**) (VBS) with catheter, guide wire, and VB stent with access kit (**c**) made by DePuy Synthes consisting of injection needle, trocar, cannulated trocar, working sleeve, and borer

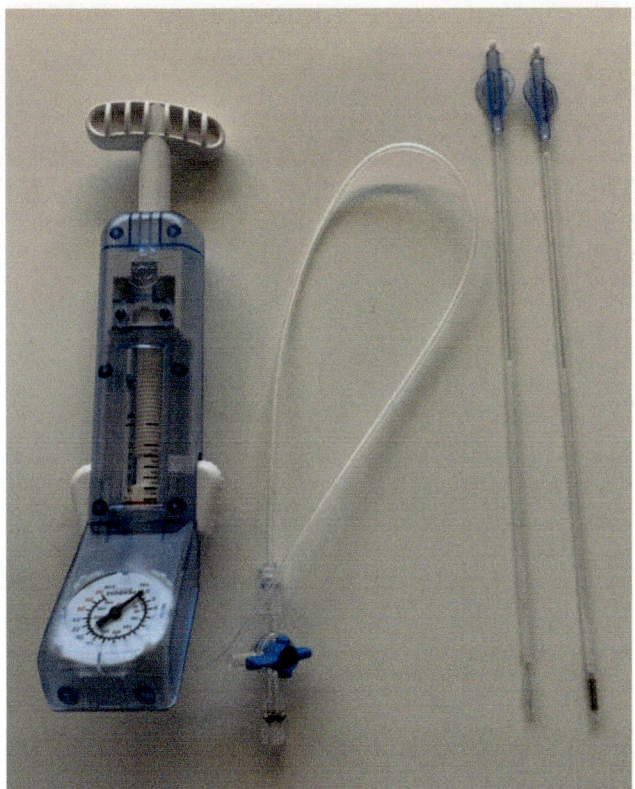

Fig. 72.4 System (DePuy Synthes) for the inflation of the balloon of the vertebral body stent (VBS)

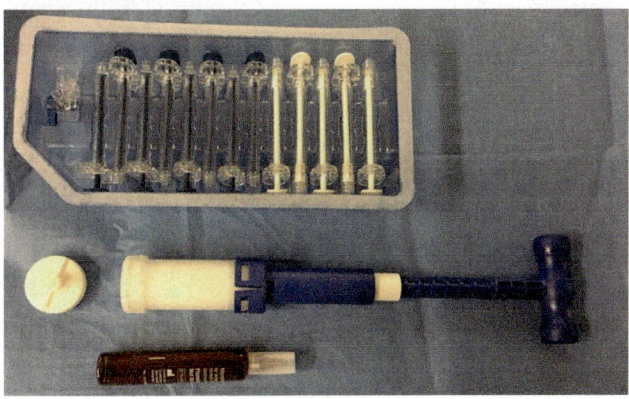

Fig. 72.5 Ready-to-use cement Vertecem V+ Cement Kit (DePuy Synthes)

employed. In many cases, one pack of bone cement is not sufficient if multisegmental reconstruction is required. It is often necessary to use a second and even a third pack.

72.5 Technique

72.5.1 Patient Positioning

- The patient should be positioned prone lying flat on a radiolucent Table. A Jackson Table can be recom-

mended. Confirm the C-arm will allow for easy rotation in the lateral, oblique, and AP positions around the table.

72.5.2 Planning of the Skin Incision

- To be first marked using radiographic monitoring are the intended pedicle sites in the fractured vertebral body and in the vertebral bodies next to the fractured body. Use the C-arm to identify the appropriate levels and to identify the lateral wall of the pedicle. In the AP view, mark the midlines and the connecting lines of the right and left pedicle using a K-wire. Plan each pedicle entry point in a straight line.
- Then mark each transverse process. The point at which lines cross represents the entry point for the Jamshidi needle. ***Note:*** To facilitate and speed up positioning of the Jamshidi needle, each pedicle can be marked with a needle. (see Fig. 72.6).

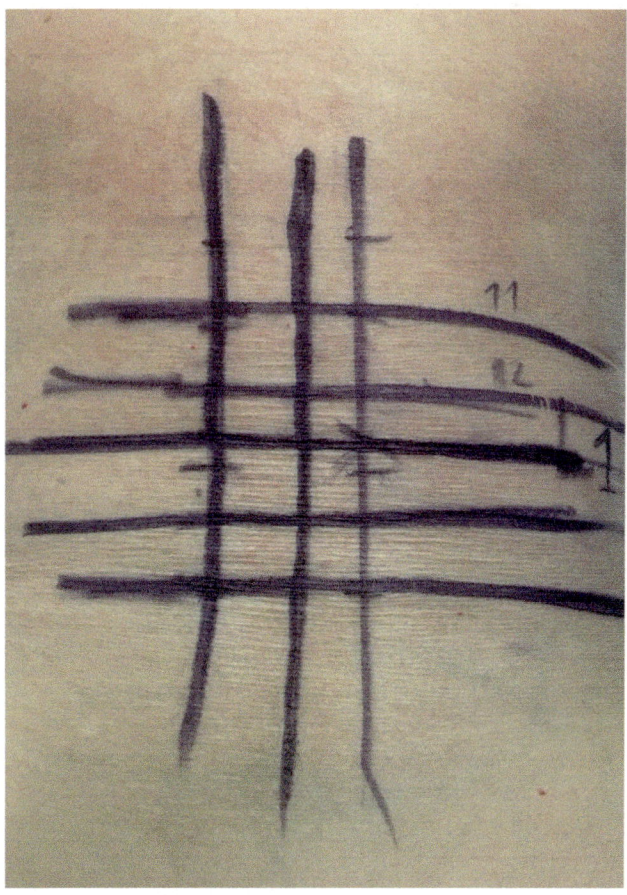

Fig. 72.6 Planning of the instrumentation. Using AP fluoroscopy, place a K-wire longitudinally in the midline and 3 cm from the lateral margins of the pedicles and mark the line on the skin. Place the K-wire perpendicular to the longitudinal line over the center of the pedicle and use a marker pen to a mark it

72.5.3 Jamshidi Needle Placement

- A 1–2 cm long incision is made through the skin and fascia. In general, incisions for transpedicular access should be positioned 1–2 cm to the lateral and up to 1 cm to the cranial side of the pedicle center. Alternatively, this incision can be made later in the area around the K-wires. This means that the incision can be kept smaller.
- Monitoring the procedure in AP and lateral fluoroscopy, advance the Jamshidi needle to the pedicle entry point at the insertion of the facet and transversal process.
- Confirm placement with AP and lateral fluoroscopy to ensure that the Jamshidi needle does not breach the wall of the pedicle.
- Remove the inner stylet of the Jamshidi needle. Remove the guide drain.

72.5.4 Guide Wire (K-Wire) Placement

- Insert the guide wire into the Jamshidi needle. This procedure must be constantly monitored by fluoroscopy to ensure that there is no ventral displacement of the K-wire.
- Place multiple guide wires at each level. The wires can be bent left and right or to the cranial and caudal sides and fixed in place on the patient using tape or better a plastic sleeve (packaging material used for the Jamshidi needle!) (see Fig. 72.7).

72.5.5 Dilatation of Skin, Fascia, and Muscles

- Advance a dilator using the guide wire down to the bone.

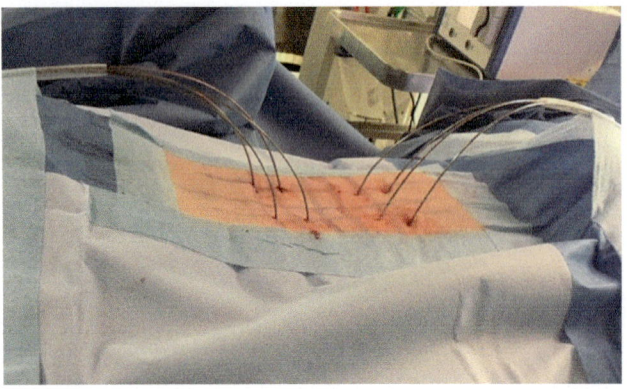

Fig. 72.7 Placement of multiple guide wires (K-wire) at each level. The wires can be bent to the cranial and caudal sides and fixed in place on the patient using tape and plastic sleeve

72.5.6 Pedicle Screw Placement

- Guide the first screw assembly using the guide wire down to the pedicle and insert the polyaxial screw. Pedicle screws can, however, be put in place before and even after the positioning of the VBS.
- Use fluoroscopy to monitor correct placement of screws.
- *Note:* Screw heads should not be fully in contact with bone (to ensure polyaxial adjustment is possible).
- Repeat screw placement at all levels.
- Verify the polyaxial capability of the screws by manipulating the screw extensions.
- Following implantation of the VBS and end positioning, these screws are then used for augmentation with bone cement (described below).

72.5.7 Vertebral Body Stent Placement

- The pedicles of the fractured vertebral body are similarly prepared as in the case of the pedicle screws for the placement of the VBS using trocars (see Fig. 72.8a–c).
- For this purpose, an access kit trocar or a cannulated trocar with guide wire can be employed. If a cannulated trocar is used, a guide wire needs to be first put in place on which the trocar can be positioned. We always use the access kit option. Using this variant, it is possible, if carefully planned, to introduce the system via the existing percutaneous access, in other words, without the need to make another skin incision.
- Following confirmation of the correct positioning of the trocar in fluoroscopy, the stent and balloon are introduced and gradually inflated from 12 to up to 30 bar/atm during fluoroscopy monitoring (see Fig. 72.9).
- The positioning of the VBS must be again reviewed in fluoroscopy and verified in the AP view. The whole of the balloon must sit within the vertebral body and the inflatable components must have passed through the working sleeve. The VBS must be positioned symmetrically to the midline and the anterior wall of the vertebral body and in a sufficiently medial position.
- The catheter with stents should be in a symmetrical paramedial position in the affected vertebral body. Ideally, the distance between the end plate of the fractured vertebral body and stents should be in the region of 5 mm.
- Repeat the procedure on the contralateral side.
- For the repair of complete burst fractures, stents should be in the center of the vertebral body; in the case of cranial burst fractures, they should be positioned more toward the end plate. *Note*: Do not inflate the balloon beyond the maximum recommended volume or pressure; otherwise, there is a risk that the balloon can burst.

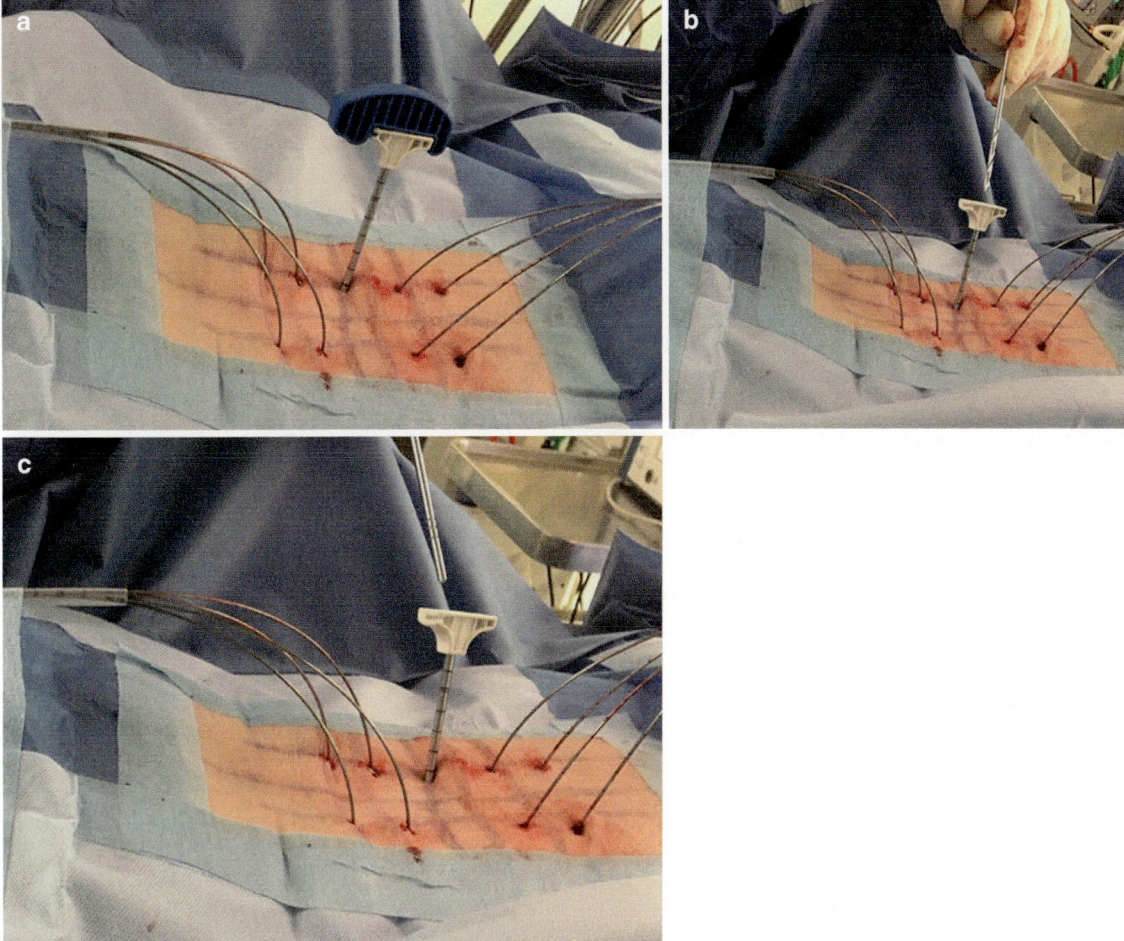

Fig. 72.8 (**a–c**) The pedicles of the fractured vertebral body are prepared using a trocar (**a**). Guide the drill (**b**) and the plunger (**c**) through the working sleeves to create an access channel for the stents

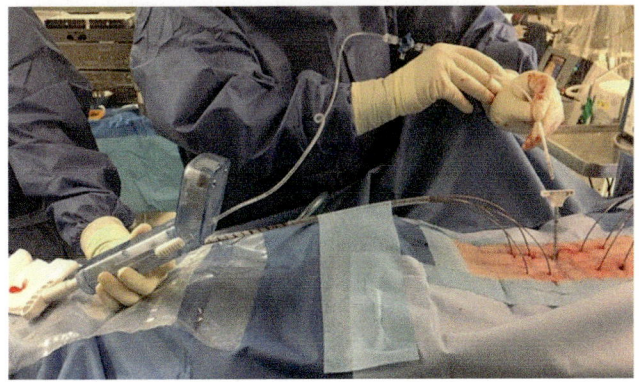

Fig. 72.9 Insertion and inflation of the VBS during fluoroscopy monitoring

- Following reduction of balloon pressure, remove the inflation system and then the balloon. The corresponding stent should remain in the fractured vertebral body.

72.5.8 Augmentation Technique

- It is generally advisable to first successively augment the pedicle screws and then the two stents.
- Augmentation must be continually monitored by means of fluoroscopy. Check to see if there is intraspinal or intravasal escape of bone cement.
- It is possible to optimize the augmentation of pedicle screws by first filling saline in the contralateral pedicle screw; this will be aspirated during application of the bone cement.
- The quantity of bone cement required per VBS will be that specified in accordance with the size of the VBS.
- A special cement application system is used to fill the VBS. By rotating the system's injection needle, which has a lateral outlet, it is possible to alter the direction of flow of the cement.

- **Note:** Ensure that the preparation, injection, and setting time of the cement used are observed. If the application system is removed at too early a point in time from a pedicle screw, cement can penetrate the screw head (see Fig. 72.10). If the injection needle and the working sleeve of a VBS are withdrawn too soon, cement can escape into muscle tissue. On the other hand, if removal of the VBS injection needle is delayed for too long, it may be difficult, if not impossible, to withdraw it.

72.5.9 Rod Introduction

- Using the rod gauge, determine that the rods have the required size.
- Align the openings of the screw extensions and rotate the closed screw extensions so that the arrow faces the open screw extension.
- After removal of the access instruments used for VBS positioning and allowing for setting of the bone cement, the two rods can be introduced.
- The rods must not be positioned above the fascia. The tip of each rod must thus always come to rest over the top of the screw heads.
- Confirm rod placement using the C-arm.
- Using a persuader, gradually insert the rods in the screw heads, fix in place with the setscrews, and tighten these with a torque key. *Note:* Start by tightening the persuader/set screws at the cranial end of a rod. By means of rod movement, it is thus possible to determine that a rod is correctly positioned.

72.6 Complications

- The bone cement must be allowed to set. If the injection needle is removed from the pedicle screws too soon, the cement can leak from the screws (see Fig. 72.10). The connection between rod and screw can thus subsequently be insufficiently stable.
- Intravasal escape of bone cement can relatively frequently occur. However, even if this is radiologically detected, it is generally of little clinical relevance (Figs. 72.11, 72.12, and 72.13).

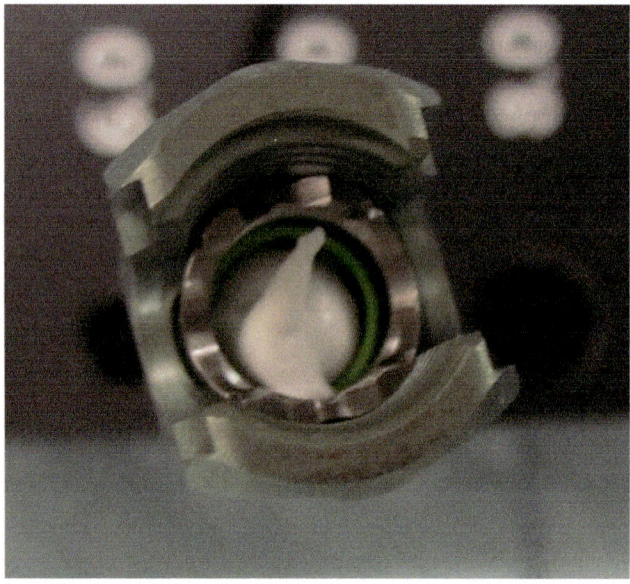

Fig. 72.10 Escape of bone cement from the head of a pedicle screw. If this cement is allowed to remain in place, it will prevent the development of a stable connection between rod and pedicle screw head

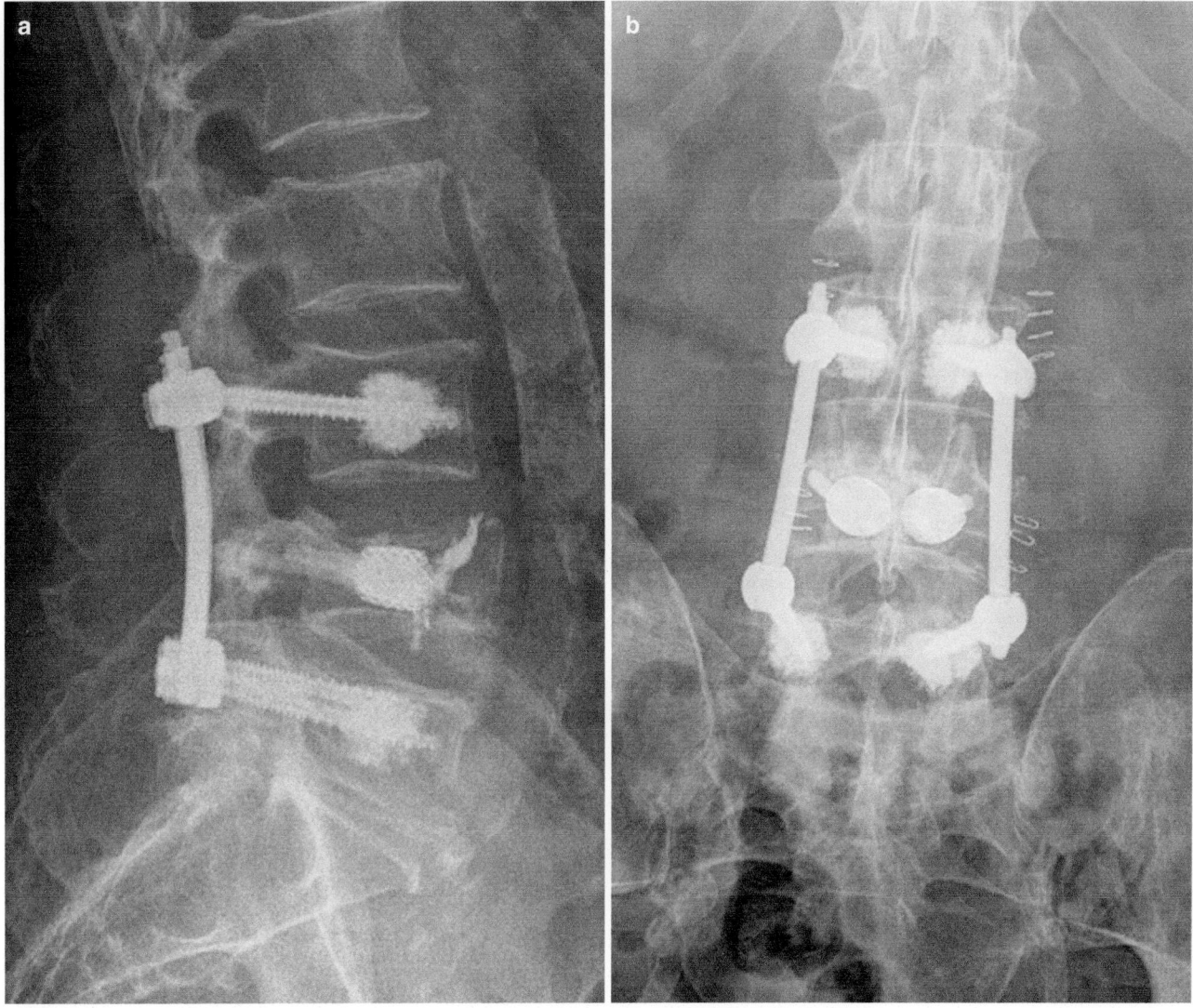

Fig. 72.11 Case 1: Postoperative radiological ((**a**) lateral and (**b**) AP view) result after percutaneous instrumentation of the incomplete burst fracture L4

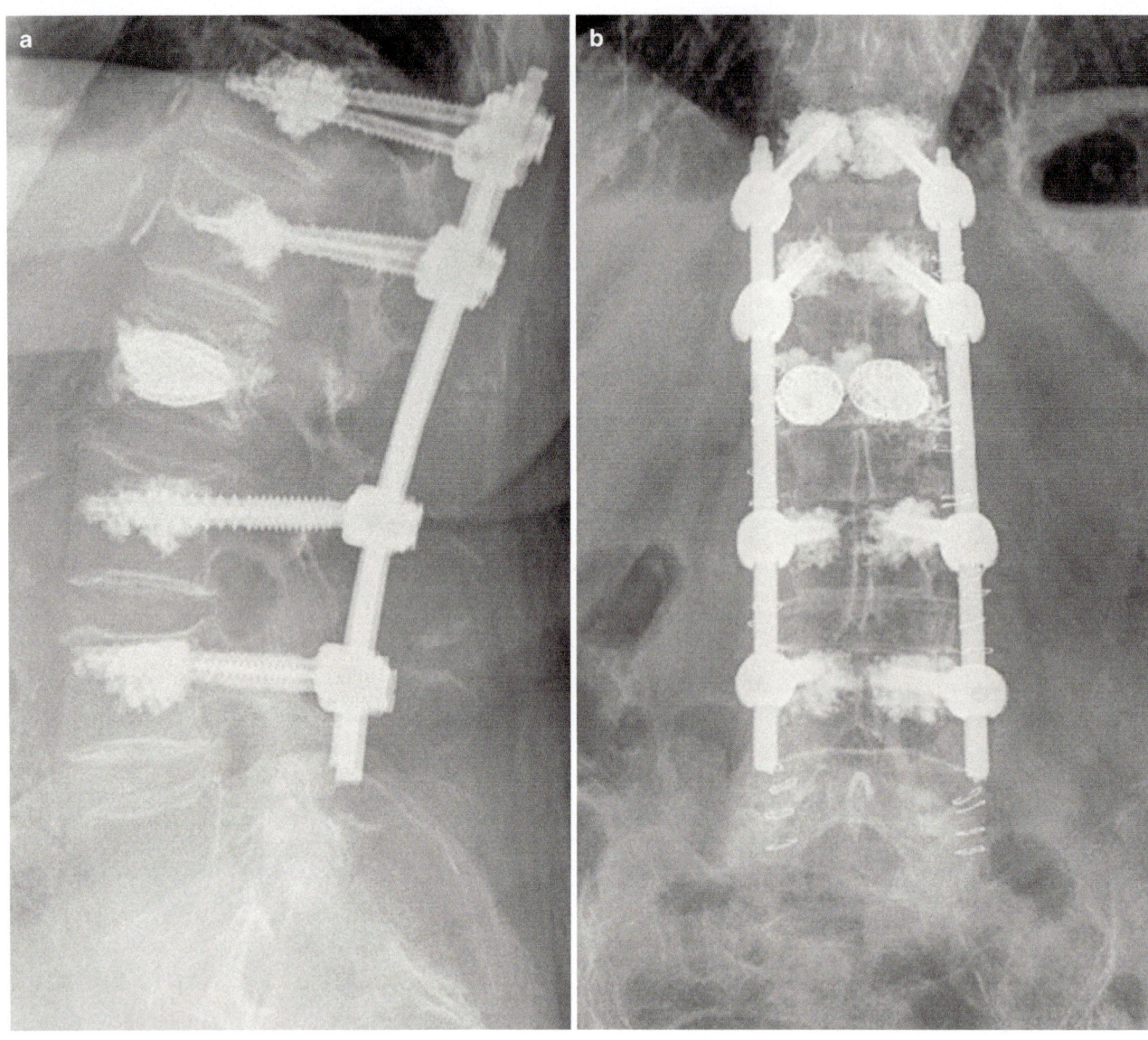

Fig. 72.12 Case 2: Postoperative radiological ((**a**) lateral and (**b**) AP view) result after percutaneous instrumentation with internal fixator Th12/L1 and L3/4, pedicle screw augmentation and vertebral body stenting of the complete burst fracture L2

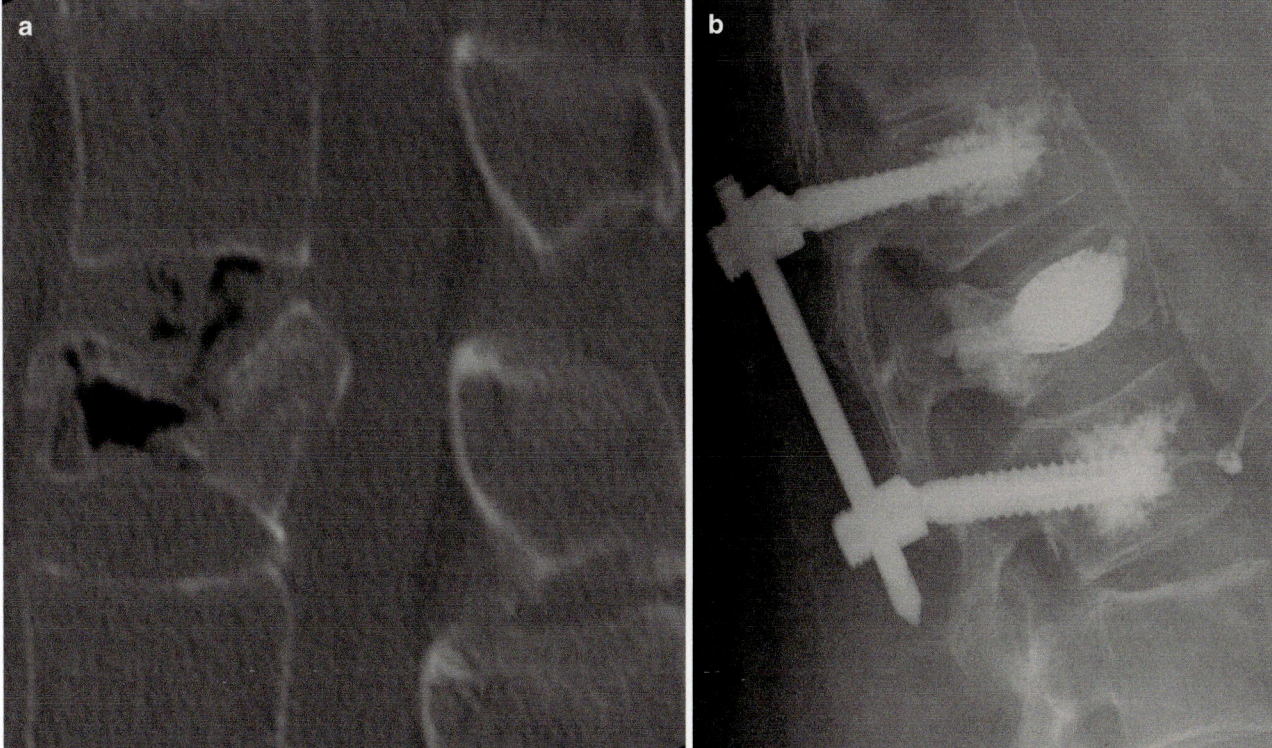

Fig. 72.13 Case 3: (**a**) CT scan of a 79-year-old patient (ASA 4, bronchial asthma, status after acute myocardial infarction 3 months ago, cardiac arrhythmia, status after pacemaker implantation) (**b**) Radiological result after percutaneous instrumentation with internal fixator, pedicle screw augmentation, and perfect reconstruction of the fracture with the vertebral body stent

References

1. Suzuki N, Ogikubo O, Hansson T. The course of the acute vertebral body fragility fracture: its effect on pain, disability and quality of life during 12 months. Eur Spine J. 2008;17:1380–90.
2. Vaccaro AR, Oner C, Kepler CK, et al. AOSpine thoracolumbar spine injury classification system: fracture description, neurological status, and key modifiers. Spine. 2013;38:2028–37.
3. Blondel B, Fuentes S, Metellus P, et al. Severe thoracolumbar osteoporotic burst fractures: treatment combining open kyphoplasty and short-segment fixation. Orthop Traumatol Surg Res. 2009;95(5):359–64.
4. Rotter R, Martin H, Fuerderer S, et al. Vertebral body stenting: a new method for vertebral augmentation versus kyphoplasty. Eur Spine J. 2010;19:916–23.
5. Schnake KJ, Blattert TR, Hahn P, et al. Classification of osteoporotic thoracolumbar spine fractures: recommendations of the spine section of the German Society for Orthopaedics and Trauma. Global Spine J. 2018;8(2):46–9.
6. Magerl F, Aebi M, Gertzbein SD, et al. A comprehensive classification of thoracic and lumbar injuries. Eur Spine J. 1994;3:184–201.
7. Burval DJ, McLain RF, Milks R, Inceoglu S. Primary pedicle screw augmentation in osteoporotic lumbar vertebrae: biomechanical analysis of pedicle fixation strength. Spine. 2007;32:1077–83.
8. Heyde CE, Rohlmann A, Weber U, Kayser R. [Stabilization of the osteoporotic spine from a biomechanical viewpoint]. Orthop. 2010;39:407–416 (in German).
9. Kolb JP, Weiser L, Kueny RA et al. [Cement augmentation on the spine: biomechanical considerations]. Orthop. 2015;44:672–680 (in German).
10. Disch AC, Schmoelz W. Cement augmentation in a thoracolumbar fracture model: reduction and stability after balloon kyphoplasty versus vertebral body stenting. Spine. 2014;39:E1147–53.
11. Fürderer S, Anders M, Schwindling B et al. [Vertebral body stenting. A method for repositioning and augmenting vertebral compression fractures]. Orthop. 2002;31:356–61 (in German).
12. Heini PF, Teuscher R. Vertebral body stenting stentoplasty. Swiss Med Wkly. 2012;142:W3658.
13. Klezl Z, Majeed H, Bommireddy R, John J. Early results after vertebral body stenting for fractures of the anterior column of the thoracolumbar spine. Injury. 2011;42:1038–42.
14. Werner CML, Osterhoff G, Schlickeiser J, et al. Vertebral body stenting versus kyphoplasty for the treatment of osteoporotic vertebral compression fractures: a randomized trial. J Bone Joint Surg Am. 2013;95:577–84.
15. Gu Y, Zhang F, Jiang X, et al. Minimally invasive pedicle screw fixation combined with percutaneous vertebroplasty in the surgical treatment of thoracolumbar osteoporosis fracture. J Neurosurg Spine. 2013;18:634–40.
16. Vannini D, Galzia R, Kazakova A, et al. Third-generation percutaneous vertebral augmentation. J Spine Surg. 2016;2(1):13–20.

Percutaneous Interspinal Process Implantation

73

Uwe Vieweg

73.1 Introduction and Core Messages

Posterior dynamic systems for the lumbar spine could be divided into:

Tension band systems (i.e., Coflex from Paradigm Spine)
Facet joint replacements (i.e., TOPS™ from Premia Spine Ltd) and Interspinous spacer systems (In-Space from DePuy Synthes Company, Aperius™ from Medtronic, and RENEGADE™ from Globus)

The systems were placed between adjacent spinous processes of the lumbosacral spine and are designed to indirectly decompress spinal segments. The percutaneous interspinous spacer systems offer interspinous distraction through a minimally invasive lateral approach allowing the preservation of both ligaments and soft tissue.

73.2 Biomechanical Characteristics of Interspinous Spacers

Biomechanical studies have shown that the devices significantly reduced intradiscal pressure and facet load and prevented narrowing of the spinal canal and neuronal foramen. A number of authors reported a decrease of the axial spinal canal area as well as intervertebral foramen in lumbar extension due to bulging of the disk and thickening of the ligament flavum in both in vitro and in vivo studies [1–3]. Takahashi et al. [4] reported the importance of increased epidural pressure in provoking neurological symptoms in lumbar spinal canal stenosis [2, 4–7]. Biomechanical studies have shown that these implants increase stability in extension and that their insertion between the spinous processes has a segmental distractive effect increasing the size of the spinal canal and foraminal canals without influencing the adjacent levels [8, 3].

73.3 Indications [1, 3, 9, 10]

The intraspinous spacer systems are indicated for treatment of

- Lumbar spinal stenosis (LSS).
- Critical indication is the Baastrup's disease ("kissing spine syndrome").

The percutaneous implantation of an interspinous spacer as an alternative to open microdecompression surgery in carefully selected patients is now seen in a critical light in view of the reported secondary outcomes and the higher reoperation rates [11]. However, this author considers this to be a potentially viable strategy, particularly in cases in which conservative and/or invasive surgical approaches have already failed to produce the desired effect in cases of Baastrup's disease.

73.4 Technical Prerequisites

- X-ray transparent operating table
- C-arm fluoroscopy or other radiographic methods should be utilized throughout surgery to ensure correct implant placement. Radiopaque features are incorporated into all implants to facilitate visualization and
- Suitable implant devices

U. Vieweg (✉)
Department of Conservative and Surgical Spine Therapy with Interdisciplinary Spinal Deformities Centre and Rummelsberg Sectional Center, Hospital Rummelsberg, Schwarzenbruck, Germany
e-mail: uwe.vieweg@sana.de

© Springer-Verlag GmbH Germany 2023
U. Vieweg, F. Grochulla (eds.), *Manual of Spine Surgery*, https://doi.org/10.1007/978-3-662-64062-3_73

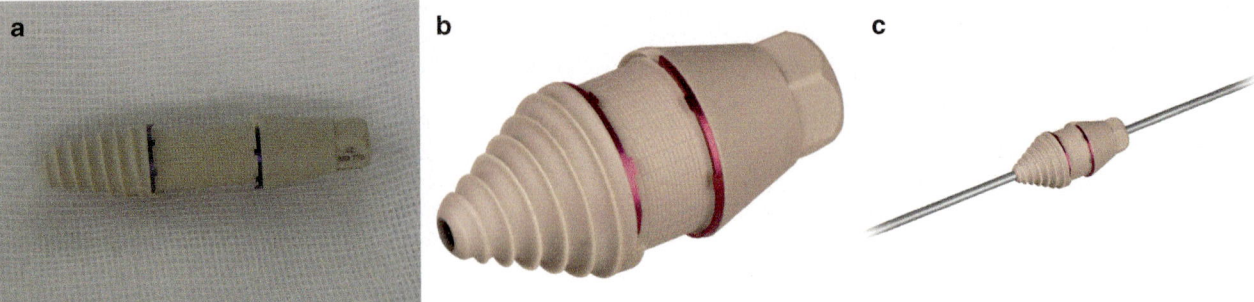

Fig. 73.1 (**a**, **b**) Overview of the implant RENEGADE™ device made from radiolucent PEEK material. The titanium rings are color-coded by height for identification with lateral teeth to provide rotational resistance. The outer contour of the entire shape of the implant is elongated in an ellipse or spindle shape. The implant has to pass through a hole formed in the shaft to insert the guide wire (**c**). (With permission from Globus Medical, Audubon, USA)

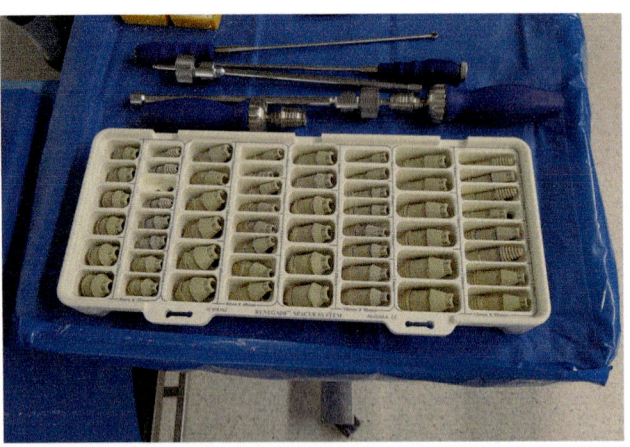

Fig. 73.2 Surgical set with instruments (locator, probe, mini quick connector small handle, implant holder, and flex driver) and the implants in various sizes

- The RENEGADE™ Spacer System from Globus Medical is a PEEK interspinous stabilization device (see Fig. 73.1a–c). The spacers are made from radiolucent PEEK material with titanium rings for an easy radiographic visualization. The system may be implanted in the lumbar spine from L1 to S1. The device is a minimally invasive interspinous process decompression device that can be implanted percutaneously. This system has the four following main features:
- Tapered thread design
- Self-distracts upon implant insertion
- Cannulated for MIS approach
- L5-S1 capable
  RENEGADE™ Spacers are available in different sizes (barrel length: 8 or 16 mm, overall implant length: 35, 45, 55 mm; implant height: 8, 10, 12, 14, 16, 18, 20 mm) (see Fig. 73.2). The principal concept of the implant is a combination of interference screw and interspinous process spacer, which can be inserted percutaneously [12].

73.5 Technique

73.5.1 Patient Positioning

- The patient is positioned prone on a Jackson table (or equivalent) radiolucent frame, with table adjusted to place the patient into flexion. The patient should be positioned in slight flexion to aid in implant sizing (see Fig. 73.3a, b).
- With a K-wire, the level is located under fluoroscopic view.

73.5.2 Approach

The operative area is carefully cleaned, and the locator instrument is used with fluoroscopy to verify lateral position (see Fig. 73.4a–c). After radiographic identification of the surgical level, a 2–3 cm incision is made at the affected level, approximately 15 cm lateral to the midline.

73.5.3 Instrumentation

73.5.3.1 Probe Placement
- The probe is inserted through the incision (see Fig. 73.5a, b).
- The probe is positioned centered between the spinous processes and slightly dorsal to the facet joint.
- The probe is used to puncture the interspinous ligament.
- The supraspinous and interspinous ligaments are preserved throughout the procedure.

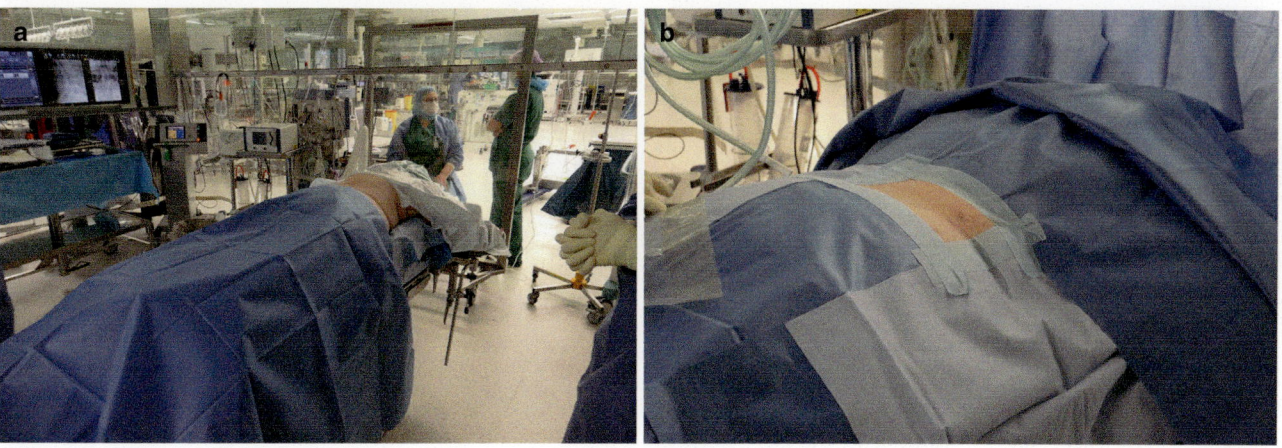

Fig. 73.3 (**a**, **b**) Position of patient (**a**) and situation following exposure and taping of the site of surgery (**b**)

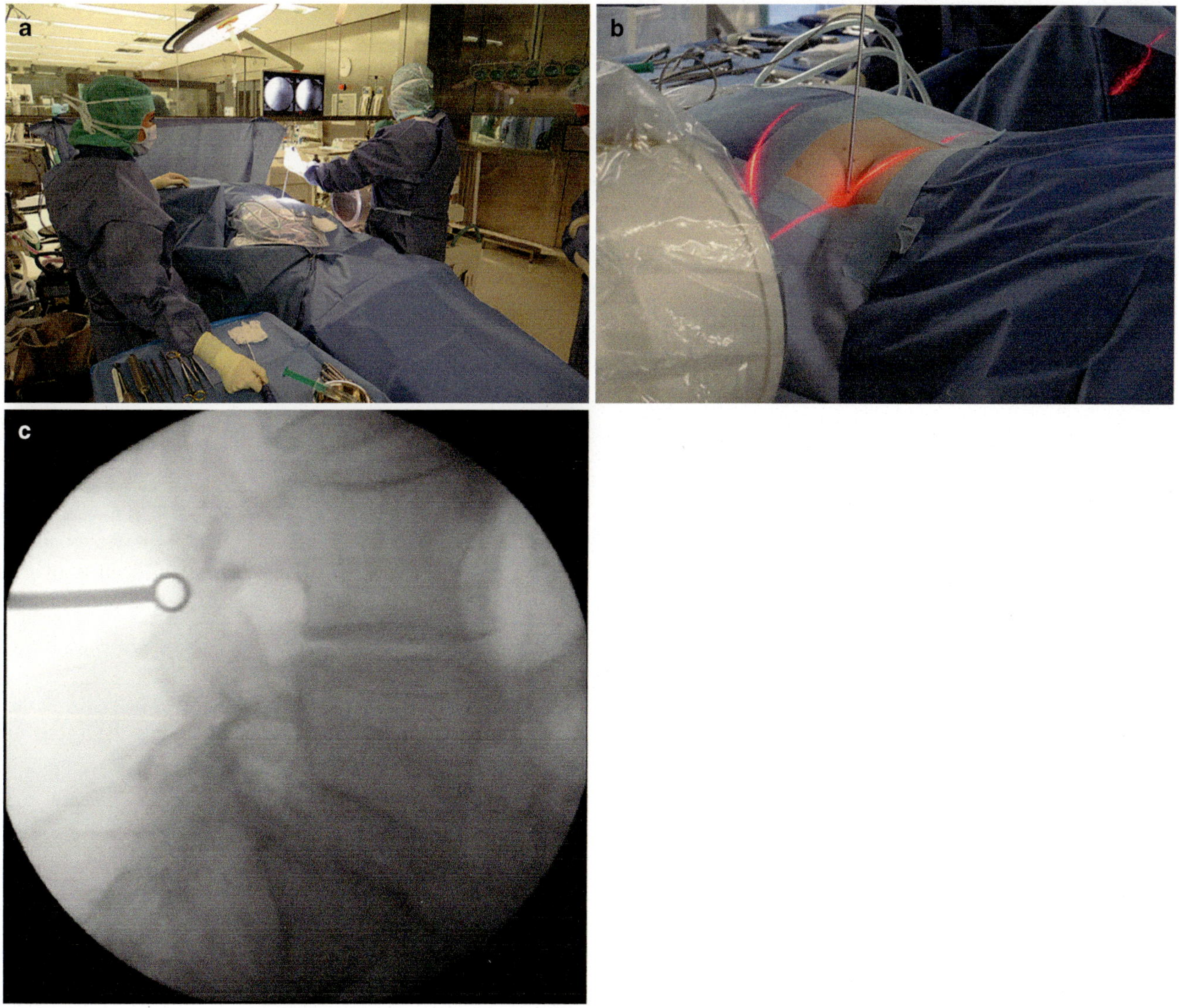

Fig. 73.4 Planning of the skin incision with the locator instrument (**a**, **b**)-intraoperative lateral X-ray (**c**) to verify lateral position

Fig. 73.5 (**a, b**) The probe is inserted through the incision and, using the tip of the probe, the superior and inferior spinous processes are located, as well as the lamina and facet joint

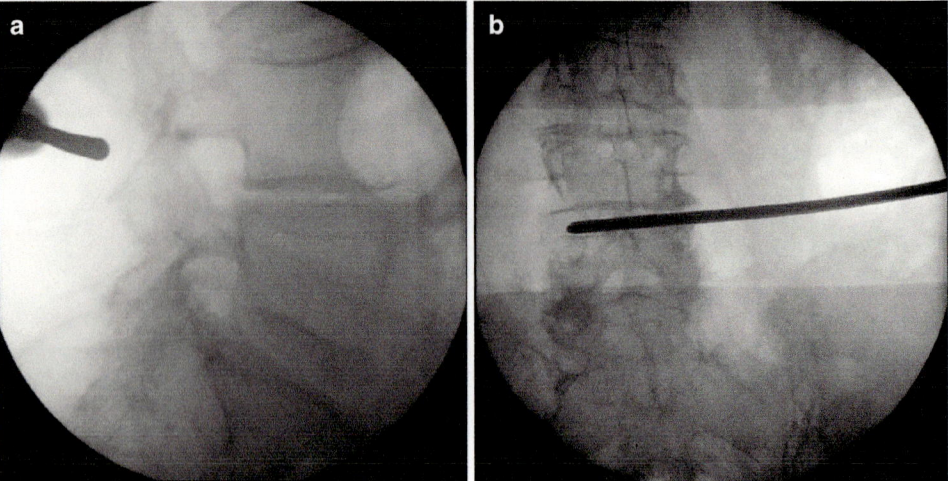

73.5.3.2 Tissue Dilation

- Remove the perforator plug from the probe to allow the K-wire to slide through.
- Attach the mini quick connect small handle to the proximal end of the K-wire.
- With the small handle attached to aid in maneuverability, the K-wire is passed through the probe and into the interspinous space.
- The small handle is then detached from the K-wire and the probe is removed, with the K-wire left in place.
- Insert the 4 mm aluminum cannula through the incision over the K-wire (see Fig. 73.6).
- The cannula should be positioned centered between the spinous processes and slightly dorsal to the facet joints. Slide the 9 mm aluminum cannula over the 4 mm cannula (Fig. 73.7).
- Use the rest of the cannulas to sequentially dilate up, until desired dilation is achieved.
- Once proper dilation is achieved, all internal cannulas are removed, ensuring that the K-Wire stays in place.

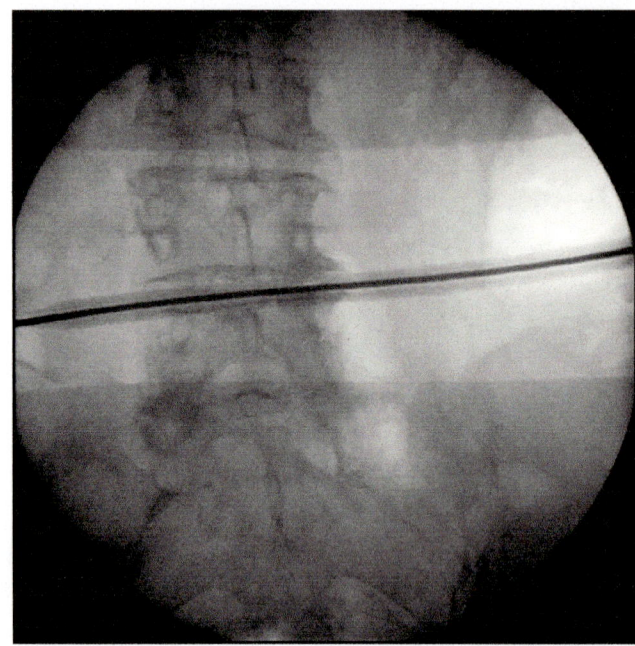

Fig. 73.6 The anteroposterior fluoroscopic image shows the insert of the 4 mm aluminum cannula through the incision over the K-wire

73.5.3.3 Distraction and Sizing

- Start trialing by attaching the 8 mm trial to the straight ratchet handle.
- Slide the trial over the K-wire and through the cannula up to the interspinous ligament (see Fig. 73.8).
- With forward pressure applied, rotate the trial clockwise, advancing the tip into the interspinous space, until in position.
- If a larger height is desired, remove the trial by pulling backward and rotating counterclockwise. Repeat trial insertion and removal until adequate distraction is

achieved and the correct implant height has been determined.
- To determine the appropriate implant length, position the trial tip just past the interspinous ligament. The correct groove can be identified on the trial using fluoroscopy.

73.5.3.4 Implant Insertion

- After determining the appropriate implant size, attach the straight ratchet handle to the implant holder and insert the tip of the driver over the hex form of the implant (see Fig. 73.9).

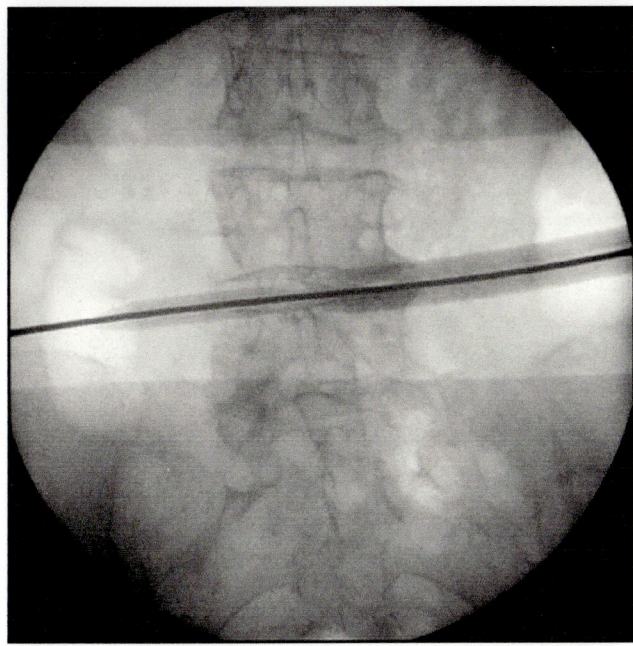

Fig. 73.7 Once proper dilation is achieved, all internal cannulas (9 mm aluminum cannula, 14–19-mm radiolucent cannulas) are removed, ensuring that the K-wire stays in place

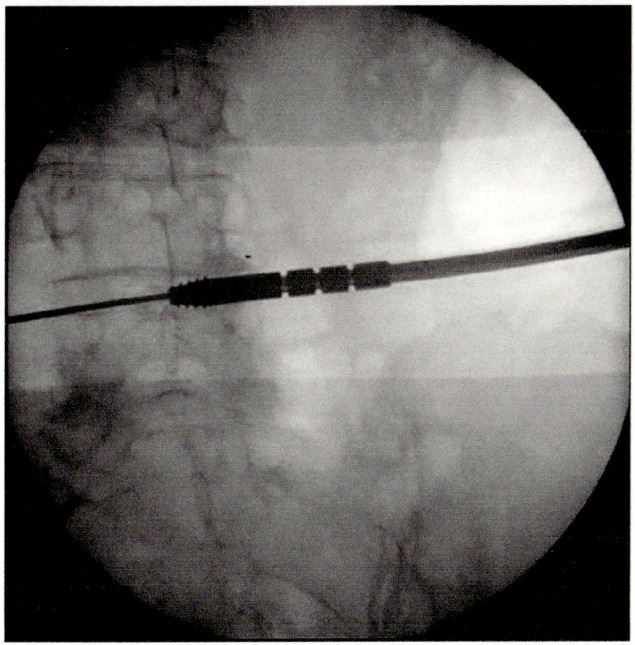

Fig. 73.8 To determine the appropriate implant length, position the trial tip (from 8–20-mm trial) just past the interspinous ligament

- Rotate the thumb wheel of the driver clockwise to connect the implant to the driver. Keeping the K-wire and cannula in place, slide the implant and driver over the K-wire and through the cannula up to the interspinous ligament.

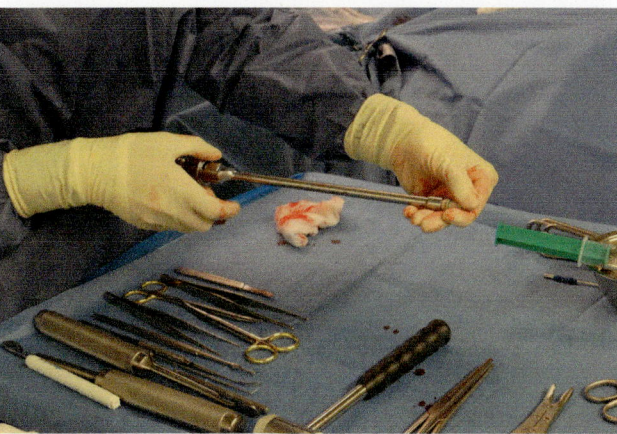

Fig. 73.9 Attach the straight ratchet handle to the implant holder and insert the tip of the driver over the hex form of the implant and rotate the thumb wheel of the driver clockwise to connect the implant to the driver

- Applying forward pressure, rotate the driver clockwise to feed the implant's self-distracting tip into the interspinous space. The spinous processes contact the implant tip during insertion, until the implant is centered in the interspinous space.
- Final implant placement should be confirmed fluoroscopically. Once placement is confirmed, detach the driver from the implant by rotating the thumb wheel counterclockwise. (Fig. 73.10) After removal of the driver, remove all cannulas, followed by the K-wire.

73.5.3.5   L5-S1 Implant Insertion
- The K-wire and flexible implant drivers allow for lateral implantation at the L5-S1 level.
- To determine the sizing at L5-S1, flexible trials should be used in the same manner as standard trials. This allows the trial to pass by the iliac crest without interference.
- After determining the appropriate implant size, attach the Straight Ratchet Handle to the Flex Driver. Insert the tip of the driver over the hex form of the appropriate RENEGADE™ implant. The implant and instrument are loosely connected. Slide the implant and driver over the K-Wire and down the cannula up to the interspinous ligament.
- Applying forward pressure, rotate the driver clockwise to feed the implant's self-distracting tip into the interspinous space. The spinous processes will contact the implant tip during insertion until the implant is centered in the interspinous space.
- Following implant positioning, pull the driver backward to separate from the implant and remove.
- Final implant placement should be confirmed fluoroscopically. Remove the K-wire and cannula.

Fig. 73.10 (**a–c**) Placement of the implant in the interspinous space. (With permission from Globus Medical, Audubon, USA

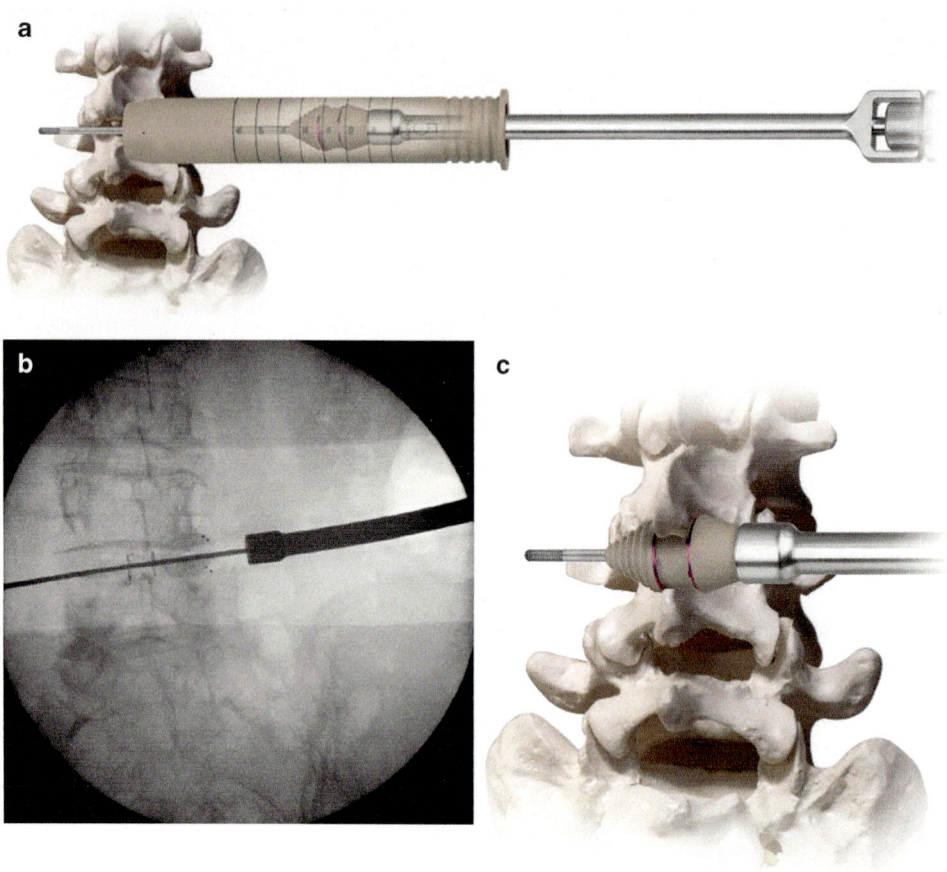

73.5.3.6 Implant Removal

- The implant is removed by reversing the steps of insertion.
- With the straight ratchet handle attached, insert the implant holder to the implant.
- Applying slight forward pressure, rotate the driver slowly until the hex end seats over the implant. The thumb wheel

is rotated clockwise to attach the implant. Remove the implant by pulling backward and rotating the instrument counterclockwise.

- Following implant removal, rotate the thumb wheel counterclockwise to detach the instrument, gently pulling if needed (Fig. 73.11).

Fig. 73.11 (**a, b**)
Postoperative x-ray (**a**—
anterior-posterior, **b**—lateral)
of a 75-year-old female with a
kissing spine in two levels

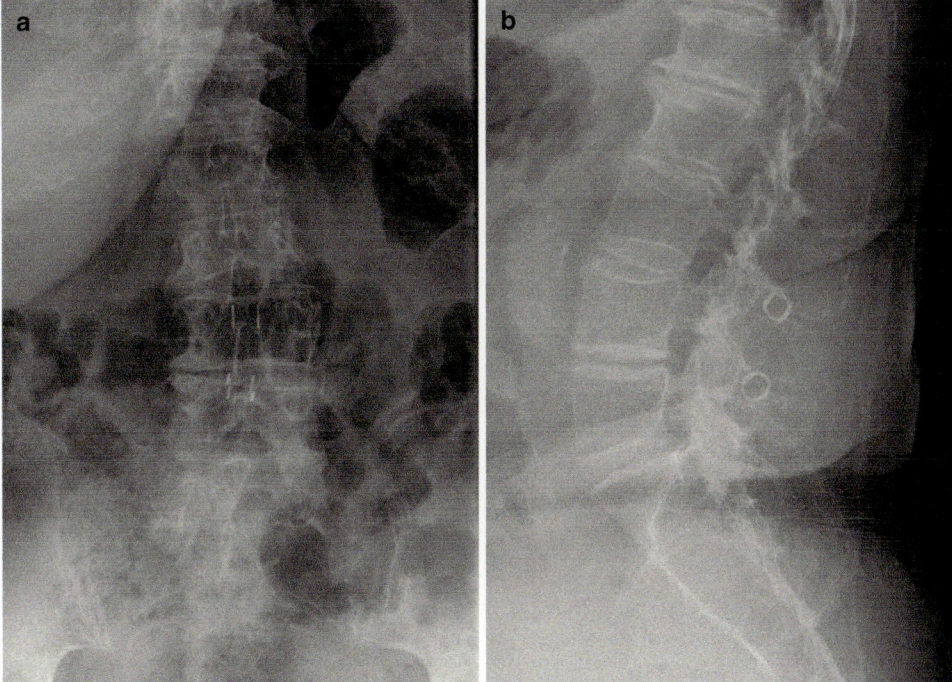

References

1. Bono CM, Vaccaro AR. Interspinous process devices in the lumbar spine. J Spinal Disord Tech. 2007;20:255–61.
2. Chung KJ, Hwang YS, Koh SH. Stress fracture of bilateral posterior facet after insertion of interspinous implant. Spine. 2009;34(10):E380–3.
3. Fransen P. Long-term results with percutaneous interspinous process devices in the treatment of neurogenic intermittent claudication. J Spine Surg. 2017;3(4):620–3.
4. Surace MF, Fagetti A, Fozzato S, et al. Lumbar spinal stenosis treatment with Aperius perclid interspinous system. Eur Spine J. 2012;21(Suppl 1):S69–74.
5. Chung SS, Lee CS, Kim SH, et al. Effect of low back posture on the morphology of the spinal canal. Skelet Radiol. 2000;29:217–23.
6. Fujiwara A, An HS, Lim TH, Haughton VM. Morphologic changes in the lumbar intervertebral foramen due to flexion—extension, lateral bending, and axial rotation: an in vitro anatomic and biomechanical study. Spine. 2001;26:876–82.
7. Parchi PD, Evangelisti G, Vertuccio A, et al. Biomechanics of interspinous devices. Biomed Res Int. 2014;14:839325.
8. Takahashi K, Miyazaki T, Takino T, et al. Epidural pressure measurements: relationship between epidural pressure and posture in patients with lumbar spinal stenosis. Spine. 1995;20:650–3.
9. Beyer F, Yagdiran A, Neu P, et al. Percutaneous interspinous spacer versus open decompression: a 2-year follow-up of clinical outcome and quality of life. Eur Spine J. 2013;22:2015–21.
10. Wilke HJ, Drumm J, Haussler K, et al. Biomechanical effect of different lumbar interspinous implants on flexibility and intradiscal pressure. Eur Spine J. 2008;17:1049–56.
11. Meyer B, Baranto A, Schils F, et al. Percutaneous interspinous spacer vs decompression in patients with neurogenic claudication: an alternative in selected patients? Neurosurgery. 2018;82:621–9.
12. Nishida K, Doita M, Kakutani K, et al. Development of percutaneously removable interspinous process spacer for treatment of posture-dependent lumbar spinal-canal stenosis: preclinical feasibility study using porcine model. Eur Spine J. 2012;21:1178–85.

Overview of the Different Approaches and Different Techniques of the Sacrum and the Sacroiliac Joint

Uwe Vieweg

74.1 Introduction and Core Messages

Surgical interventions on the sacrum and sacroiliac joint are performed in following indications: fractures of the sacrum, sacrum tumors, inflammation of the sacroiliac joint, sacroiliac joint syndrome (SIJS). The approaches to the sacrum are the posterior medial and the anterior approach. The approaches to the sacroiliac joint are the posterior and the posterior lateral, the lateral and the ventral approach. Today we have different sacroiliac joint fusion techniques according to the criteria approach, implant architecture, bone graft delivery, implants material, and insertion.

74.2 Anatomy and Physiology of the Sacroiliac Joint and Sacrum [1–6]

The *sacroiliac joint* is the connection between the ilium and sacrum. The sacroiliac joint is the largest axial joint in the body, with an average surface area of 17.5 cm². The joint's surfaces are flat or planar in early life and as we start walking, the sacroiliac joint surfaces develop distinct angular orientations. The major function of the SI joints is providing stability of the pelvis. Their functions include

- The transmission and dissipation of loads from the trunk to the lower extremities
- Limiting rotation
- Facilitating parturition

U. Vieweg (✉)
Department of Conservative and Surgical Spine Therapy with Interdisciplinary Spinal Deformities Centre and Rummelsberg Sectional Center, Hospital Rummelsberg, Schwarzenbruck, Germany
e-mail: uwe.vieweg@sana.de

The sacroiliac joint exhibits individual variations in terms of size, and in particular in terms of the center of rotation [1]. The sacroiliac joint is partly a symphysis, and partly a synovial joint. The accessory sacroiliac ligaments of the sacroiliac joint comprise the ligamentum sacroiliacale dorsal et ventral as well as the ligamentum sacrospinale, ligamentum sacrotuberale, and ligamentum iliolumbale. These ligaments ensure stability, and certain movement limitations. In addition to these ligaments, the erector trunci, and the fascia thoracolumbalis in particular, also contribute to the stability of the sacroiliac joint. A knowledge of the adjacent muscles is important for surgical procedures. The gluteus maximus muscle attaches to the iliac wing and pulls toward the trochanter and therefore stabilizes as well as influences the sacroiliac joint. The iliopsoas and piriformis muscles are two further major muscles located adjacent to the sacroiliac joint. The piriformis muscle in particular plays an important role in the differential diagnosis of so-called sacroiliac joint syndrome. The fascia thoracolumbalis and the adjacent stomach muscles also influence the stability or imbalance of the sacroiliac joint. The balance among the erector trunci muscle, tractus iliotibialis, ischiocrural muscles, and the gluteus maximus therefore also plays a significant role in the various pathological processes of the sacroiliac joint. The sacroiliac joint allows rocking as well as sliding. Nutation (rocking) of the sacroiliac joint is described as between 0.4 and 4.3°. Its axes are very variable as well as gender-specific. The sacroiliac and accessory ligaments act as a brake on movement. Sacroiliac joints are true synovial joints and thus subject to various forms of arthritis and degenerative processes. The *sacrum* is a complex anatomical structure. The cephalad surface of the body of the first sacral vertebra represents the base of the sacrum. The anterior portion of the first sacral vertebra is the sacral promontory. Posterior to the first sacral vertebra is the triangle-shaped sacral canal. The point lateral and inferior to the S1 facet is the most common entrance for dorsal sacral screw placement. The superior part of the lateral sacral mass is the ala of the sacrum [7]. The ventral aspect of the sacrum is concave in the vertical and horizontal planes (Fig. 74.1) and is smoother than the dorsal aspect. As such, a thorough understanding of the anatomy of the *sacrum* and its relations to the vast array of surrounding structures is of utmost importance. The *sacrum* is formed by fusion of the five sacral vertebral segments and lies between the two iliac bones of the pelvis. The sacrum articulates with the fifth lumbar vertebra by means of an intervertebral joint and two facet joints and with the iliac bones by means of the sacroiliac joints. The sacrum tends to be wedge-shaped in adults, and develops through the fusion of cross vertebrae (sacral vertebrae), originally separate vertebrae, which have grown together. The sacral bone encloses the rear section of the vertebral canal and, together with the two hip bones, forms the pelvic girdle. The sacrum is a large bone of the axial skeleton, formed from the fusion of the S1 through S5 sacral vertebrae. It is triangular in shape and articulates with four other bones: the L5 vertebra, the left and right innominate bones, and the coccyx. The majority of the lateral sacrum is comprised of the sacral portion of the sacroiliac joint, is convoluted in geography, and is covered in articular cartilage. There are three general areas of ligamentous attachment to the sacrum: cranially at the lumbosacral articulation, laterally at the sacroiliac joints, and inferiorly with the sacrospinous and sacrotuberous attachments (Fig. 74.2).

Indications for Surgery on the Sacroiliac Joint and Sacrum

Surgical interventions on the sacrum and sacroiliac joint are performed in the event of the following indications:

- Fractures of the sacrum
- Sacrum tumors
- Inflammation of the sacroiliac joint
- Sacroiliac Joint Syndrome (SIJS)

Different disorders of the sacroiliac joint and sacrum are possible (sacroiliac arthritis like ankylosing spondylitis, sacroiliitis, psoriasis, Reiter's syndrome, septicarthritis, gout and osteoarthrosis, sacroiliac joint syndrome, bone disorders (tumors, fractures of the pelvis). The sacrum is a rare location for spinal metastasis. These lesions are typically large and destructive by the time of diagnosis, making treatment difficult. From limited anterior sacroiliac exposure for benign tumors to combined anterior and posterior approaches for total sacrectomy in the treatment of large sacral chordomas, anterior sacroiliac exposure for benign tumors to combined anterior and posterior approaches for total sacrectomy in the treatment of large sacral chordomas. The ability of mechanical lesions of the sacroiliac joint to cause backache and referred pain to the buttock and posterior leg was first recognized by Goldthwait and Osgood in 1905 [8]. SIJS can occur following a traumatic event or cumulative shear events, or can occur spontaneously [9]. Today we have different sacroiliac joint fusion according to the criteria approach, implant architecture, bone graft delivery, implants material, and insertion (see Table 74.1).

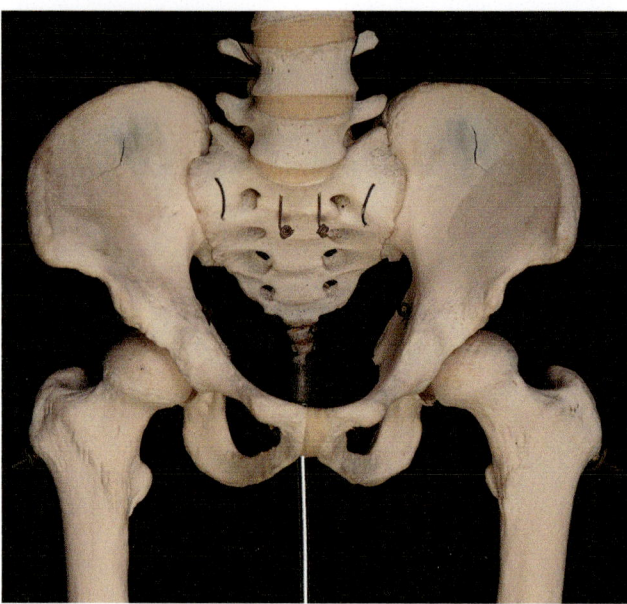

Fig. 74.1 Ventral aspect of the sacrum

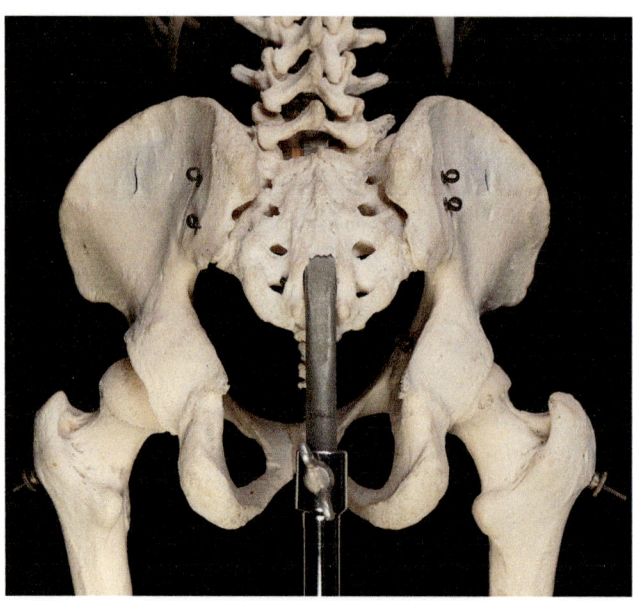

Fig. 74.2 Dorsal aspect of the sacrum with foramen S1, S2, and S3

74.3 Approaches to the Sacrum and Sacroiliac Joint and Different Implants for an Arthrodesis of the Sacroiliac Joint [10–15]

74.3.1 Approaches to the Sacrum

- Posterior medial approach
- Anterior approach

Table 74.1

Product	Manufacturer	Description	Bongraft Option	Principle
Ifuse	SI-Bone	Porouscoated triangular Bolt	No	Transgluteal fixation Percutanous
Simmetry	Zyga Technology	Hollow screw HA coated	Yes	Transgluteal fixation Percutanous
SI-Lok	GLOBUS Medical	Hollow screw HA coated	Yes	Transgluteal fixation Percutanous
SILEX	X-Tant	Hollow screw HA coated	Yes	Transgluteal fixation Percutanous
SAMBA	Orthofix	Hollow screw HA coated	Yes	Transgluteal fixation Percutanous
SIJ-Fuse Screw	Spine Frontier Inc.	Cannulated screw	Yes	Mechanical stabilization Transfixing
Torpedo	Deltacor	Porouscoated turned Dowel	No	Transgluteal fixation Percutanous
DIANA	Signus	Hollow cannulated screw	Yes	Mini-open

74.3.2 Approaches to the Sacroiliac Joint

- Posterior and posterior lateral
- Lateral
- Ventral

74.4 Anterior Approach to the Sacroiliac Joint

The anterior approach is useful for surgical exposure to manage sacroiliac joint dislocations and fractures of the ilium, even extending into the sacroiliac joint. This approach enables direct visualization of the anterior and superior portions of the sacroiliac joint. The anterior approach to the sacroiliac joint allows anterior plates to be positioned accurately across the joint. It also permits the exposure of the inner wall of the ala of the ilium, allowing fixation of associated iliac fractures. The anterior approach allows greater exposure and control than does the seemingly more logical posterior approach, because of the shape of the joint. Anteriorly, the joint is flat and directly available, whereas posteriorly, it is overhung by the posterior iliac crest [4]. The anterior approach to the sacroiliac joint is a reliable, reproducible, and safe approach that can provide direct access to the entire anterior joint and lateral sacral ala. The patient is positioned supine on the operating table, with the option of placing a bump under the ipsilateral buttock. An incision is made along the margin of the iliac crest starting several centimeters proximal and posterior to the anterior superior iliac spine and extending 2–3 cm distal to the anterior superior iliac spine. Once through subcutaneous fat, incise the fascia and periosteum overlying the outer table of the iliac crest, and carry this subperiosteal dissection over the brim of the iliac crest. This, in effect, is dissecting the attachment of the abdominal wall musculature to allow for suitable closure. At this point, the iliacus, whose origin is the inner table of the ilium, is encountered and can be freed from the inner table bluntly. This is often best done using a Cobb elevator and a laparotomy sponge. This dissection is carried all the way to the sacroiliac joint. Several perforating blood vessels will be encountered, which will need to be cauterized or controlled with firm placement of bone wax. This dissection can be carried all the way to the lateral border of the sacral foramina; dissection should not be carried medial to this point, unless necessary, as there is considerable risk of damage to the anterior sacral nerve roots. Cranially, caution should be exercised, as the L5 nerve root can be encountered as it crosses the brim of the sacral ala. Hohmann retractors can be placed directly into the sacrum medially, as long as care is taken not to inadvertently place the point of the retractor into the sacral foramen. Closure is fairly simple, requiring only reapproximation of the abdominal musculature fascia, subcutaneous tissue, and fat. The L5 and L4 nerve roots travel across the sacral ala and lie medial to the sacroiliac joint. The surgeon must be careful when working in this area.

74.5 Lateral Approach to the Sacroiliac Joint

A number of studies have been published regarding minimally invasive surgical (MIS) fusion of the sacroiliac (SI) joint using a lateral transarticular approach. Bloom should be credited with the first attempt to perform a minimally invasive sacroiliac arthrodesis [10]. He described a small straight-line incision based on anatomical landmarks to cut a cylindrical core of bone through the ilium and across the joint into the sacrum. The plug was removed, the opposing cartilage surfaces were excised, and the plug was then reinserted and countersunk, providing a cancellous plug spanning the joint. The modern minimally invasive percutaneous techniques were performed using fluoroscopy or navigation equipment [16, 17]. The procedures are performed through small incisions in the skin on the side of the buttocks. Correct placement of the implants is ensured with real-time images, made available to the surgeon by means of a fluoroscopy. The procedure may be performed in the prone or supine position. Where important are the radiological landmarks in the lateral view, the inlet view and outlet view. With the help of cannulated instruments, the implants, which are also cannulated, are then inserted under radiological control.

74.6 Posterior Open and Posterior Lateral Approach to the Sacroiliac Joint

The posterior lateral open approach for sacroiliac joint arthrodesis was first described by Smith-Petersen [18]. The posterior approach provides access to the posterior ilium, sacroiliac joint, and posterior surface of the sacrum. The posterior open approach to the sacroiliac joint is a simple, safe approach that does not endanger any vital structures. Its uses include open reduction and internal fixation of disruptions of the joint, open reduction and internal fixation of fractures of the ilium near the joint, and treatment of infections of the sacroiliac joint or surrounding bones. For the skin incision, you have to make a curved incision overlying the posterior iliac crest. The skin incision begins proximally enough for fracture access and follows the crest distally to the posterior inferior iliac spine. Alternatively, a straight vertical incision can be made. The subcutaneous tissues is to divide in line with the skin incision until the iliac crest is reached. The gluteus muscles are sharply detached from the ilium and elevated laterally to expose the lateral ilium as needed. During the subperiosteal exposure of the posterolateral ilium, and elevation of gluteal muscles, note the superior gluteal vessels and nerves. SI joint alignment can be assessed by palpation through the greater sciatic notch, with a finger dorsal to the piriformis and anterior to the SI joint.

74.7 Transsacral Interbody Fusion: AxiaLIF

Transsacral Interbody Fusion (AxiaLIF) is a surgical procedure in which the front part of the lumbar spine is fused from below. The method was described for the first time in the literature by Cragg et al. 2004 [8]. The patient is positioned on a radiolucent operation table so that the hips and knees are extended to maximize lordosis. The pre sacral plane is entered through an incision at the level of the paracoccygeal notch. The surgeon makes an incision just above the tailbone. The transsacral fusion surgery applies only to the lower-most disk(s). Blunt finger dissection to the sacrum provides access for placement of a blunt guide pin on the

posterior third of the inferior endplate of the sacrum. After preparation of a 12 mm bony channel in the sacrum, the L5-S1 disk space is entered. Instruments are passed through a tube into the disk space. Disk material is removed, and a fusion graft with or without BMP and the TransS1 screw were placed into and through the disk space. Possible complications include pseudarthrosis, infections, rectocutaneous fistula, and rectal or bowel injuries [19, 20].

References

1. Bakland O, Hansen JH. The "axial sacroiliac joint". Anat Clin. 1984;6(1):29–36.
2. Bellamy N, Park W, Rooney PJ. What do we know about the sacroiliac joint? Semin Arthritis Rheum. 1983;12(3):282–313.
3. Foley BS, Buschbacher RM. Sacroiliac joint pain: anatomy, biomechanics, diagnosis, and treatment. Am J Phys Med Rehabil. 2006;85(12):997–1006.
4. Guo W, Xu WP, Yang RL, Tang XD. The surgical management of sacral tumors. Zhonghua Wai Ke Za Zhi. 2003;41:827–31.
5. Marmor M, Lynch T, Matityahu A. Superior gluteal artery injury during iliosacral screw placement due to aberrant anatomy. Orthopedics. 2010;33(2):117–20.
6. Shuler TE, Boone DC, Gruen GS, Peitzman AB. Percutaneous iliosacral screw fixation: early treatment for unstable posterior pelvic ring disruptions. J Trauma. 1995;38(3):453–8.
7. Varga PP, Lazary A. Chordoma of the sacrum: "en bloc" high partial sacrectomy. Eur Spine J. 2010;19:1037–8.
8. Cragg A, Cal A, Casteneda F, et al. New percutaneous access method for minimally invasive lumbosacral surgery. J Spinal Disord Tech. 2004;17:21–8.
9. Chou LH, Slipman CW, Bhagia SM, et al. Inciting events initiating injection-proven sacroiliac joint syndrome. Pain Med. 2004;1:26–32.
10. Bloom FA. Sacroiliac fusion. J Bone Joint Surg. 1937;19:704–8.
11. Clarke MJ, Dasenbrock H, Bydon, et al. Posterior-only approach for en bloc sacrectomy: clinical Outcomes in 36 Consecutive Patients. Neurosurgery. 2012;71:357–64.
12. Esses SI, Bobsford DJ, Huler RJ, Rauschnig W. Surgical anatomy of the sacrum. A guide for rational screw fixation. Spine. 1991;16(6 Suppl):283–8.
13. Fourney DR, Rhines LD, Hentschel SJ, et al. En bloc resection of primary sacral tumors: classification of surgical approaches and outcome. J Neurosurg Spine. 2005;3:111–22.
14. Smith-Peterson MN. Arthrodesis of the sacroiliac joint. A new method of approach. J Orthop Surg. 1921;3:400–5.
15. Soloman MJ, Tan K, Bromilow RG, et al. Sacrectomy via the abdominal approach during pelvic exenteration. Dis Colon Rectum. 2014;57:272.
16. Al-Khayer A, Hegarty J, Hahn D, Grevitt MP. Percutaneous sacroiliac joint arthrodesis: a novel technique. J Spinal Disord Tech. 2008;21(5):359–63.
17. Sim F. Master techniques in orthopaedic surgery: orthopaedic oncology and complex reconstructions. Philadelphia: Lippincott Williams and Wilkins; 2011.
18. Schwarzer AC, Aprill CN, Bogduk N. The sacroiliac joint in chronic low back pain. Spine. 1995;20:31–7.
19. Lindley EM, McCullough MA, Burger EL, et al. Complications of axial lumbur interbody fusion. J Neurosurg Spine. 2011;15(3):273–9.
20. Siegel G, Patel N, Ramakrishnan R. rectocutaneous fistula and nonunion after TransS1 axial lumbar interbody fusion L5-S1 fiaxtion. J Neurosurg Spine. 2013;19:197–200.

Percutaneous Dorsolateral Fusion of the Sacroiliac Joint

75

Uwe Vieweg, Johannes Keck, and Hannes Moritz

75.1 Introduction and Core Messages

The sacroiliac joint (SIJ) is the largest joint in the human body. It can be subject to extreme shear forces of up to 4800 N [1]. In order to relieve pain in SIJ dysfunction, special implants need to be used that can withstand the extensive stress to which the joint is exposed and sustain the movements required. Surgical insertion of such an implant can be achieved by means of open and minimal invasive techniques in which a dorsal, dorsolateral, or lateral access is created. The Torpedo implant (Deltacor, Germany) (see Fig. 75.1a–c) and the iFuse implant (SI-BONE, USA) (see Fig. 75.2a, b) can be used for the fusion of the SIJ to relieve pain caused by degenerative sacroiliitis or SIJ dysfunction after conservative therapy has proved ineffective. These two implants are both inserted via an identically created lateral percutaneous access. The benefits associated with these implants are the minimal invasive techniques required for implantation and the secondary fixation with the help of the porous surfaces, ensuring that the largest possible surface expanse is available to provide an optimal bond between implant and bone.

75.2 Indications

The main indication for SIJ implant treatment is SIJ dysfunction. Clinical diagnosis of SIJ dysfunction is performed by means of intra-articular injection of a contrast medium with local anesthesia. Physical examination tests for sacroiliac joint dysfunction are the thigh thrust, flexion, abduction, and external rotation (FABER), pelvic gapping (distraction), compression, and the Gaenslen test. As a rule, if at least three of these tests prove positive, it can be assumed that SIJ dysfunction is present [2–6].

75.3 Contraindications

Contraindications are
- Cancer of the sacral or iliac bone
- Infections
- Known metal allergy
- Unstable pelvic fractures with involvement of the SIJ

  In the case of women of childbearing age, the possible consequences for natural childbirth should be discussed.

75.4 Preoperative Planning, Preparation, and Positioning of the Patient

- During preoperative planning, it is advisable to undertake a CT scan of the pelvis in order to exclude the presence of any possible anatomical anomalies, such as sacral dysplasia or lumbosacral transitional vertebrae. An MRI scan of the pelvis and lumbar spine is also recommended to exclude the possibility of spinal pathologies. In addition, precautionary conventional radiology examination of the lumbar and thoracic spine is mandatory.
- Bowel prep is unnecessary.
- Surgery is performed under general anesthesia with the patient in the prone position.

U. Vieweg (✉)
Department of Conservative and Surgical Spine Therapy with Interdisciplinary Spinal Deformities Centre and Rummelsberg Sectional Center, Hospital Rummelsberg, Schwarzenbruck, Germany
e-mail: uwe.vieweg@sana.de

J. Keck · H. Moritz
Clinic for Surgical and Conservative Spinal Therapy with Interdisciplinar Spinal Deformities Centre and Rummelsberg Sectional Center, Rummelsberg Hospital, Schwarzenbruck, Germany

© Springer-Verlag GmbH Germany 2023
U. Vieweg, F. Grochulla (eds.), *Manual of Spine Surgery*, https://doi.org/10.1007/978-3-662-64062-3_75

- The chest of the prone patient should be elevated to slightly bend the hips and relax the SI joint.
- The X-ray transparent operating table must allow correct image adjustment in inlet and outlet projection and for a lateral beam path.
- The X-ray device is to be adjusted so that the beam path is laterally directed into the vertebral disk space and the end plates of segment L5/S1.
- Landmarks are to be recorded on the skin during lateral beam path projection. It must be ensured that there is no visible double contour of the ala line and the sciatic foramen. This will not be possible in the presence of rare pronounced pelvic asymmetry. If the lateral view is correct, there will be superimposition of the greater sciatic notch. The sacral ala line should be clearly visible.
- Three C-arm views are required for surgery (lateral view, outlet view, and inlet view). The outlet and inlet view landmarks are the SI joint, the S1 foramen, S2 foramen, and the inferior endplate L5 and superior endplate S1.

75.5 Technical Prerequisites

- One or two C-arms.
- Commonly used is a Jackson table or a flat imaging table.
- Suitable implant systems (e.g., the Torpedo implant, Deltacor, Germany; iFuse SI-BONE, USA) (see Figs. 75.1 and 75.2) for an insertion via a lateral access.

75.5.1 The Torpedo Implant System (Deltacore, Germany)

This implant system (see Fig. 75.1a–c) is designed to be used for the fusion of the SIJ in degenerative sacroiliitis or painful SIJ dysfunction after failure of conservative therapy. The advantages of the Torpedo system are the facts that only a minimally invasive technique using a lateral access is required for implantation, while the porous SLA surface coating provides for the maximum possible extent of the surface, ensuring subsequent optimal bone fixation of the implant. The CST-Profil®—the conical-spiral-turn form—stabilizes the movement of the SI joint across the plane vertical to the joint surfaces, in other words, in the axial direction of movement of the implant. The implant is available in various sizes. As a rule, two implants are sufficient. In obese patients or in osteoporosis, three implants are advisable.

75.5.2 The iFuse Implant System (SI-BONE, USA)

The iFuse implant system is a triangular titanium implant that is coated with a porous titanium plasma spray (see Fig. 75.2a, b). The triangular shape allows an interference fit that provides immediate stabilization and minimizes micromotion and rotation of the instrumented SIJ. The porous plasma spray coating facilitates biological fixation with bone. The iFuse implant is available in configurations ranging from 30 to 70 mm in length and either 4 or 7 mm in inscribed diameter. The manufacturer recommends placement of at least two to three implants across the SIJ [5, 6].

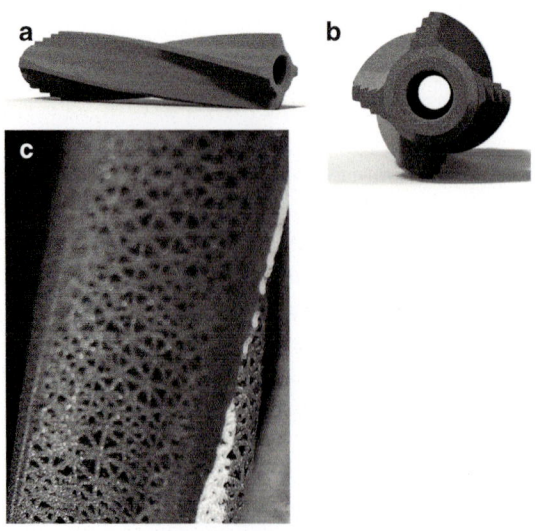

Fig. 75.1 (**a–c**) Lateral (**a**) and top view (**b**) and the porous surface (**c**) of a Torpedo implant (Deltacore, Germany)

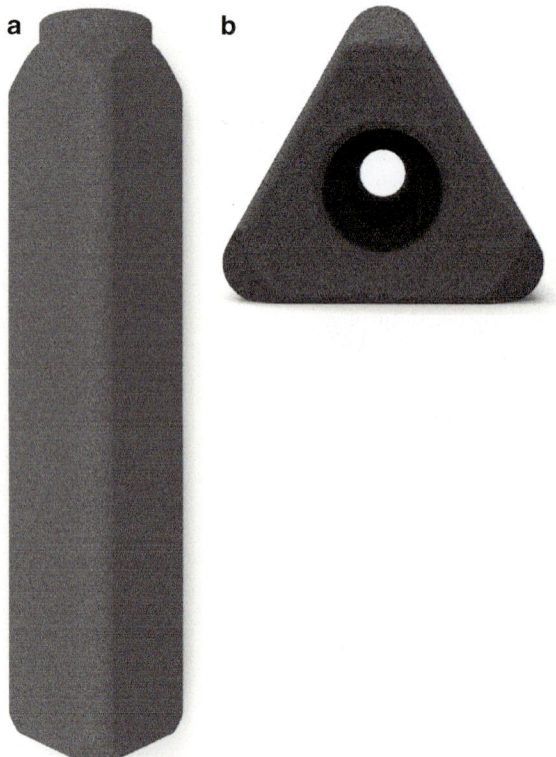

Fig. 75.2 (**a, b**) iFuse (SI-BONE, USA), lateral (**a**) and top view (**b**)

75.6 Technique

75.6.1 Planning of the Skin Incision

- The implantation is performed in prone position of the patient.
- First align the sciatic notches using C-arm "Wig-wag" or swivel. This gets the alignment close. Finalize the alignment by superimposing the left and right alae.
- With an image intensifier in lateral view, the sacrum and the operative landmarks are marked. The safe zone for the entry point of the implants is caudal of the Ala line and between the anterior corticalis and the spinal canal/posterior wall of the sacrum.
- A pin can be used to locate the ala line. A Kirschner wire is employed to show the position of the ala line that is then marked with the pin (see Fig. 75.3a).
- The second mark is made on the skin on the site of the posterior cortex of the sacrum. Make a 3 cm additional mark along the second line starting about 1 cm from the firs (Ala) line. The skin incision is made along this line (see Fig. 75.3c). **Note:** The greater sciatic notch may not be perfectly aligned due to parallax errors; however, the alae are aligned, which is more important.
- In the case of a more obese patient, the posterior sacral line should be positioned about 1–3 cm posterior to the posterior cortical wall depending on the size of the patient.

75.6.2 Skin incision

- A 3–4-cm small skin incision is made. The incision should be at the level of the fascia. The fascial incision is to be perpendicular to the skin incision in line with the underlying muscle fibers. It is necessary to undermine the edges of the fascia to expose the underlying muscle fibers and to facilitate fascial closure.

75.6.3 Initial Pin Placement (see Fig. 75.4a–d)

- For each implant, pass a guide pin/K-wire and soft tissue protector through the muscle fibers ensuring minimal spreading of the fibers.
- The first Kirschner wire should be positioned with a lateral beam path view appropriately set using the c-arm.
- The Kirschner wire should be placed approximately 5 mm to the caudal side of the ala line and inserted approximately 2 cm into tissue (Fig. 75.4d).
- With the inlet view, the image intensifier is tilted caudally by approximately 40° to optimize the visualization of the anterior corticalis of the sacrum. The outlet view is used for the visualization of the sacral neuroforamina, for which the C arm is tilted cranially by approximately 40°.
- The first Kirschner's wire is placed cranial to the S1 neuroforamen (outlet view) between the ventral corticalis of the sacrum and the spinal canal triangle and caudal to the Ala line. The introduction of the Kirschner's wire is continuously monitored with the C arm.
- Now the X-ray beam path is adjusted so that the site of the pin can be reviewed in the inlet/outlet view.
- If possible, the trajectory of the K wire should point toward the center of vertebra S1. The pin should be inserted at a slight angle to avoid the risk of penetrating the sacral canal.
- In the inlet view angle, the pin should be slightly anterior to the sacral canal, but should not penetrate the anterior cortex. In the outlet view, the initial pin should be above the level of S1 foramen.

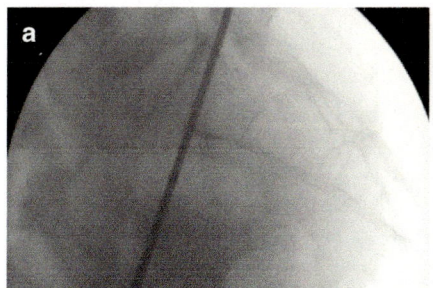 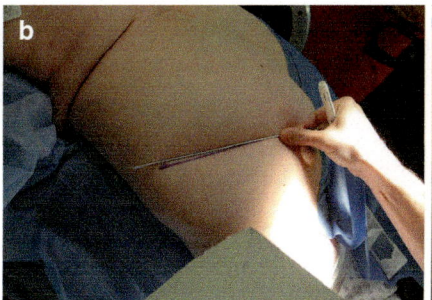 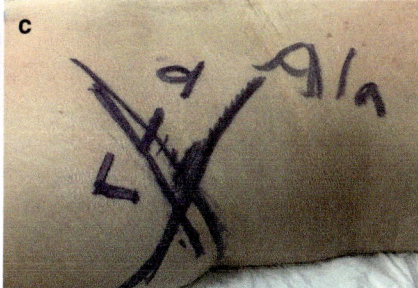

Fig. 75.3 (**a–c**) C-arm-facilitated lateral view of the ala line. Use a K wire to locate the ala line (**a**) and mark skin along the ala line (**b**) and the posterior (d-dorsal) and anterior (v-ventral) sacral wall (**c**)

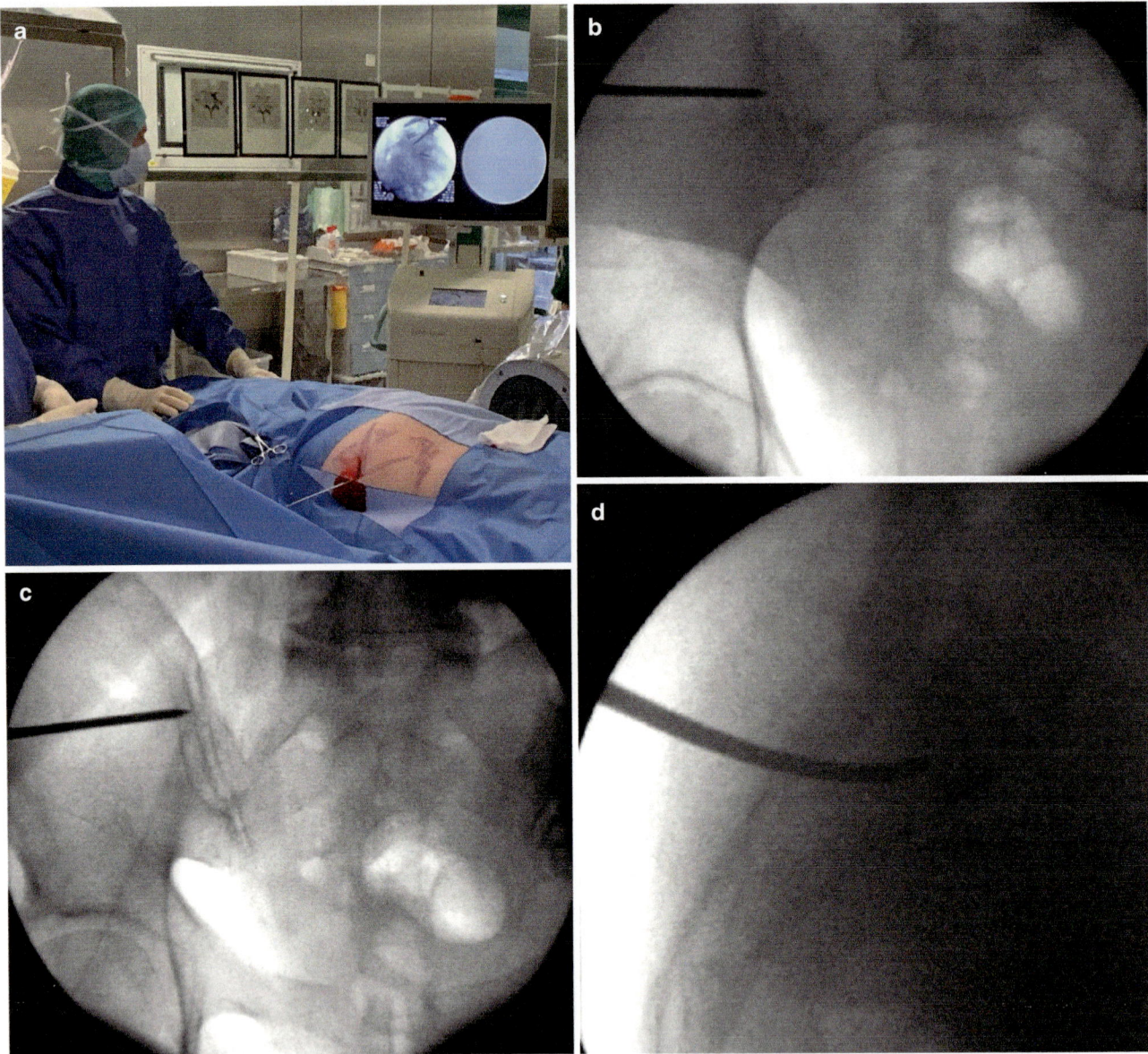

Fig. 75.4 Initial pin placement in the operation room (**a**) and X-ray inlet (**b**), outlet (**c**) and lateral (**d**) views

75.6.4 Placement of the Soft Tissue Protector and Determination of the Required Implant Length

- The soft tissue protector is placed together with a trocar on the guide wire and this is then inserted through the tissue with slight rotation until it comes into contact with the bone (see Fig. 75.5).
- The guide wire can then be used to determine the required length of the implant. Only the K wires designed for use with the system should be employed as the individual components are appropriately coordinated.

  Note: In the case of hard or sclerotic bone, it is advisable to prepare the site for the implant using a drill. The thread former is also positioned on the guide wire and

inserted through the soft tissue protector. Thread drilling should be monitored with the help of X-ray. Drill only a few millimeters beyond the sacral notch into the sacral cortex.

75.6.5 Introduction of the Implant (see Fig. 75.6a–c)

- The implant is inserted with the help of the guide wire through the soft tissue protector.
- The impactor is also inserted into the soft tissue protector. The implant is driven home using the slotted hammer until the impactor comes into contact with the soft tissue protector.

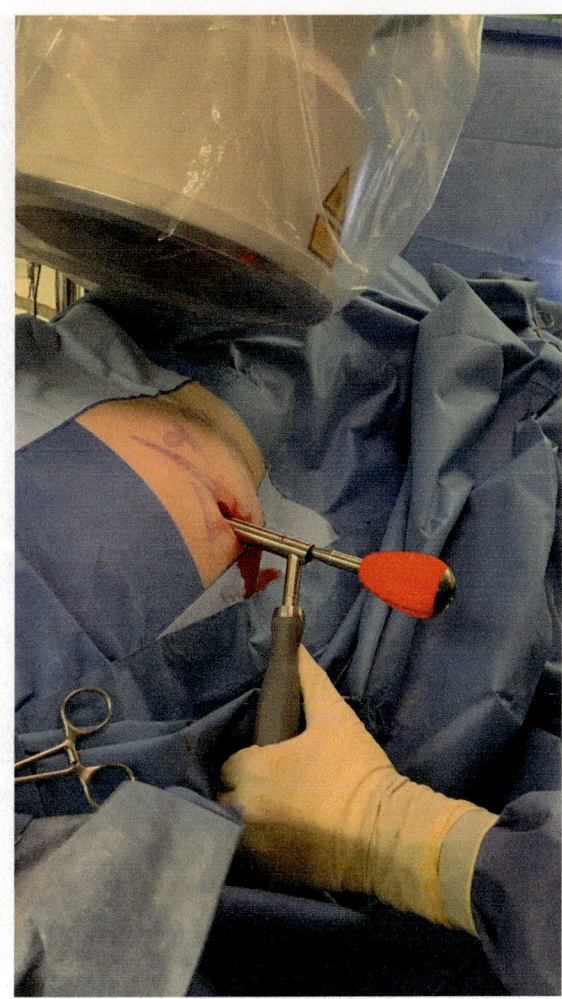

Fig. 75.5 Placement of the soft tissue protector. The soft tissue protector slides over the Steinman pin until bony contact is achieved

- A manual digital review is always necessary following introduction of the implant. The implant should project a few millimeters from the bone.

75.6.6 Introduction of the Second Implant

- It is very important to check the lateral and inlet views for cortical breach and the outlet view for foramen breach. The second pin is positioned with the help of the parallel pin guide (see Fig. 75.7a, b). This insures parallel introduction of the second guide wire and thus the second implant. The clearance of the second implant can be adjusted from 13 to 25 mm in 2-mm increments. Experience has shown that 21 mm clearance is optimal.
- The same procedure as for placement of the first pin and implant is followed, whereby the second pin should as a rule be sited between the S1 and S2 foramina.

75.7 Wound Closure

The fascial incision is then closed with a running suture, followed by routine closure of the subcutaneous tissue and skin. One option that can be considered for the minimization of postoperative pain is the injection of a longer-acting local anesthetic.

75.8 Revision of the Implant

The removal adapter is used if revision of the implant is necessary. The removal adapter is not cannulated, so it is necessary to use your finger to guide the tip of the tool to

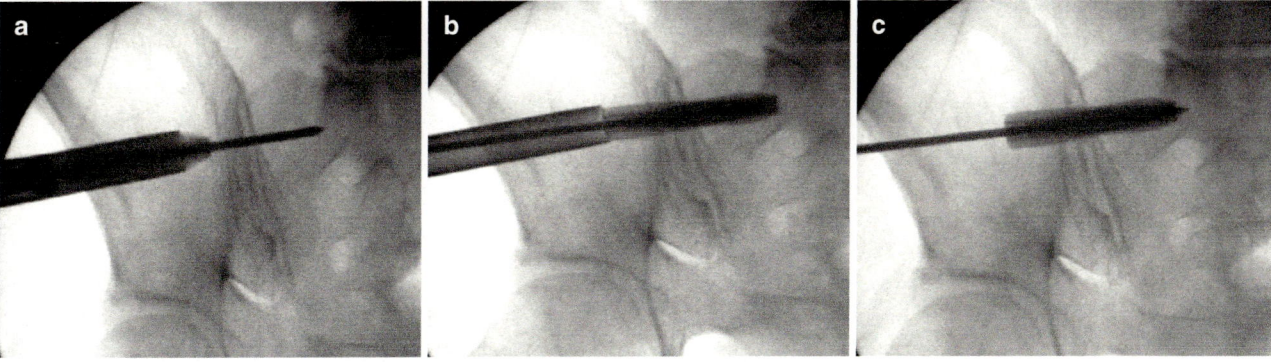

Fig. 75.6 (**a–c**) The implant is inserted with the help of the guide wire through the soft tissue protector

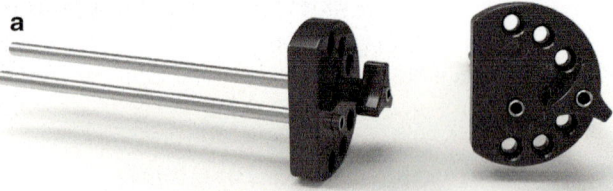

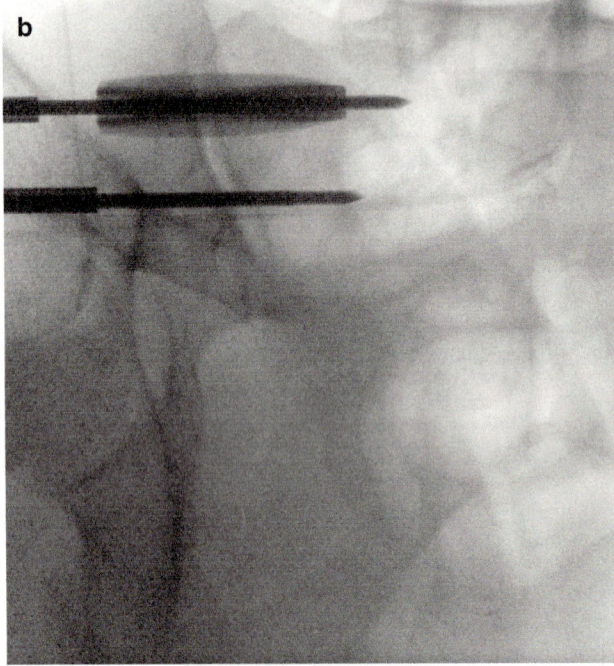

Fig. 75.7 (**a**) Placement of the second pin with the help of the parallel pin guide. The clearance of the second implant can be adjusted from 13 to 25 mm in 2-mm increments. (**b**) Intraoperative situation with a parallel placement of the second pin

the end of the implant requiring adjustment. An intraoperative x-ray (C-arm) will be needed to confirm the location. Attach the slap hammer to the end of the removal adjuster and gently tap until the implant reaches the required depth.

75.9 Postoperative Care

The postoperative treatment contains mobilization with 20-kg partial weight-bearing on the operated side for 3 weeks, instructed walking using crutches by a physiotherapist, then gradually increasing up to full weight-bearing. A thrombosis prophylaxis is recommended until the lower extremity achieves full weight-bearing (Fig. 75.8).

75.10 Complications

Possible complications include
- Infections
- Migration of the implant
- Muscle pain as a result of the alterations to biomechanical status (position of the hip, the legs, and the feet during normal daily activities)
- Irritation of the root nerves
- Metal hypersensitivity or allergy
- Potential complications during vaginal delivery due to impairment of the expansion of the SI joint.

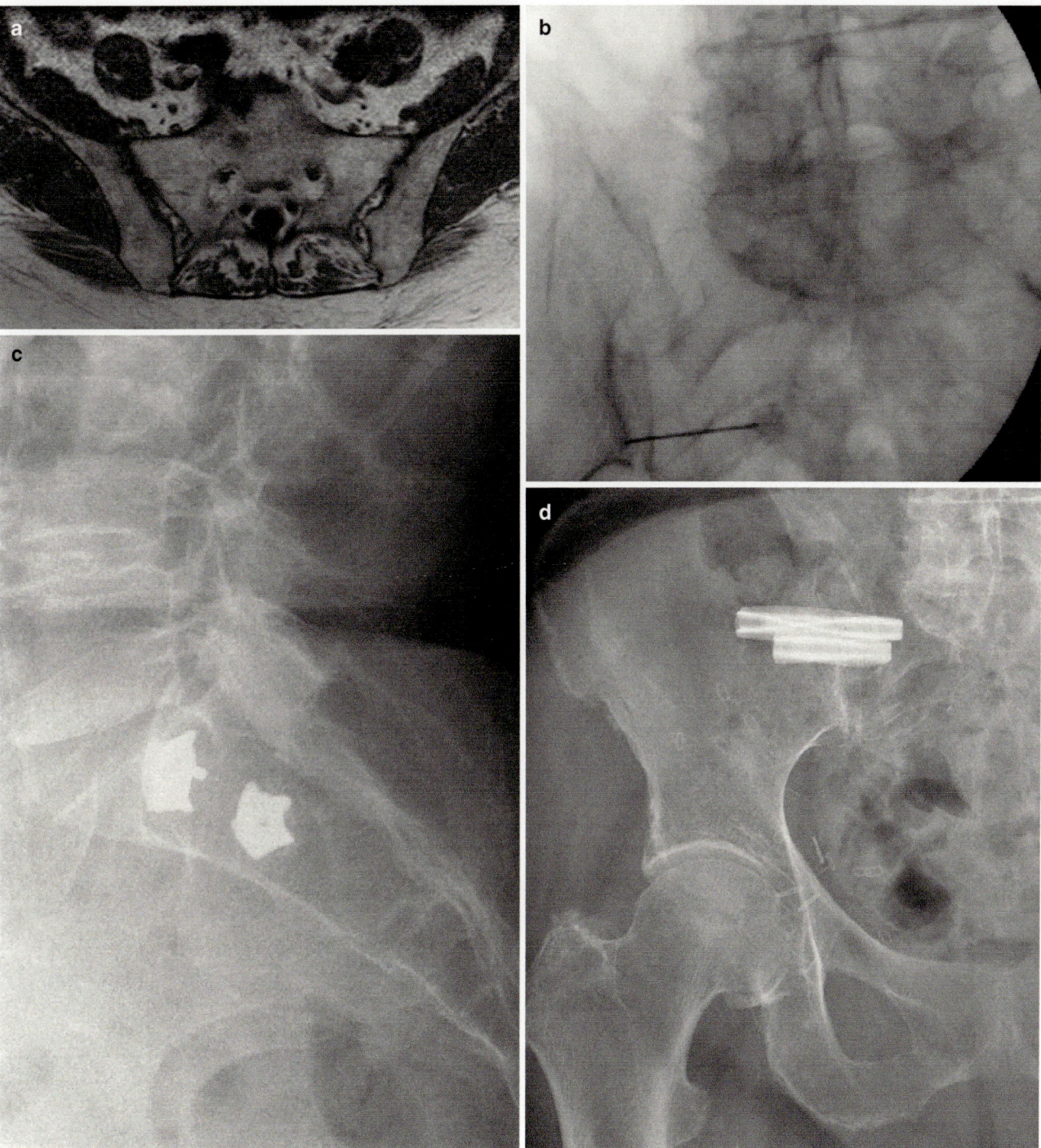

Fig. 75.8 (**a**–**d**) MRI scan (**a**) of an 80-year-old female with failed conservative treatment of SIJ-associated pain. SIJ-associated pain was identified with positive response to SIJ injection with local anesthetic and additional contrast medium (**b**) and positive SIJ provocation tests (SIJ-compression test, distraction test, Gaenslen-test, FABER-Test). The postoperative X-rays documented the instrumentation with two implants (Torpedo implant system) in the lateral (**c**) and AP (**d**) views

References

1. Ha KY, Lee JS, Kim KW. Degeneration of sacroiliac joint after instrumented lumbar or lumbosacral fusion- a prospective cohort study over five-year follow-up. Spine. 2008;33:1192–8.

2. Albert H, Godskesen M, Westergaard J. Evaluation of clinical tests used in classification procedures in pregnancy-related pelvic joint pain. Eur Spine J. 2009;9(2):161–6.

3. Al-Khayer A, Hegarty J, Hahn D, Grevitt MP. Percutaneous sacroiliac joint arthrodesis: a novel technique. J Spinal Disord Tech. 2008;21(5):359–63.

4. Khurana A, Guha AR, Mohanty K, Ahuja S. Percutaneous fusion of the sacroiliac joint with hollow modular anchorage screws: clinical and radiological outcome. J Bone Joint Surg Br. 2009;91(5):627–63.

5. Polly DW, et al. Randomized controlled trial of minimally invasive sacroiliac joint fusion using triangular titanium implants vs non-surgical management for sacroiliac joint dysfunction: 12-month outcomes. Neurosurgery. 2015;77:674–91.

6. Rainov NG, Schneiderhan R, Heidecke V. Triangular titanium implants for sacroiliac joint fusion. Eur Spine J. 2019;28(4):727–34.

Fusion Surgery of the Sacroiliac Joint (DIANA®/NADIA®)

76

Volker Fuchs

76.1 Introduction and Core Messages

In 2009, a new surgical procedure for the fusion of the painful sacroiliac joint (SIJ) was introduced, the so-called Distraction Interference Arthrodesis with Neurovascular Anticipation (DIANA®, SIGNUS® Medizintechnik GmbH, Germany). In 2019 the inventor of the DIANA® method Dr. John Stark improved the implant by adding hydroxyapatite and titanium plasma spray (NADIA®, Ilion Medical®, USA). Several studies demonstrated that applying a pelvic belt or a Hoffmann–Slätis frame over the wing of the ilium might increase the force closure of the SIJ [1–4]. A distraction arthrodesis over the recess is hypothesized to have similar effects, but is placed on the short lever side of the ilium via a posterior approach to the SIJ [5]. Inserting an interference screw in the joint recess between the sacrum and ilium at the level of S2 brings about distraction near the joint and as a result of the accompanying ligamentotaxis, causing a repositioning of the joint surfaces (see Fig. 76.1a, b). The distraction enables primary stabilization of the SIJ culminating in fusion [6] (see Fig. 76.2).

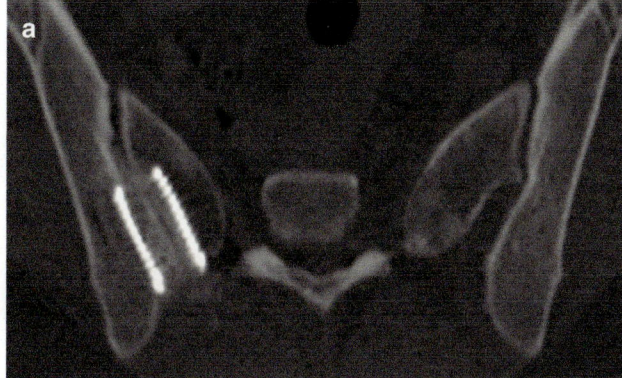

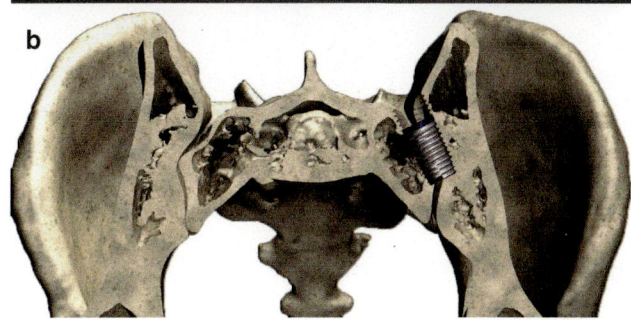

Fig. 76.1 DIANA®/NADIA® implant located in the recess of the SIJ between sacrum and ilium; the cartilaginous part of the SIJ is almost not addressed with the implant. Postoperative CT scan, implant on the right side and distraction of the SIJ (**a**); pelvis model, implant on the left side and distraction of the SIJ (**b**)

76.2 Indications

- Secondary osteoarthritis consistent with adjacent segment degeneration after lumbar/lumbosacral fusion
- Accessory joints (false joints of unknown etiology located in the recess of the SIJ either between the S2-transverse process or more rarely between the S1-transverse process of the sacrum against the ilium on one or both sides)
- Dysplasia of the SIJ

- Repetitive microtrauma of the pelvis with concomitant damage to the interosseous ligaments and/or the cartilage of the SIJ
- Postpartum arthritis of the SIJ
- Posttraumatic arthritis of the SIJ
- Axial spondyloarthritis
- Primary osteoarthritis of the SIJ

76.3 Contraindications

- Multiple prior surgical procedures to the SIJ

V. Fuchs (✉)
Department of Orthopedics, AMEOS Hospital Halberstadt, Halberstadt, Germany
e-mail: dr.v.fuchs@t-online.de

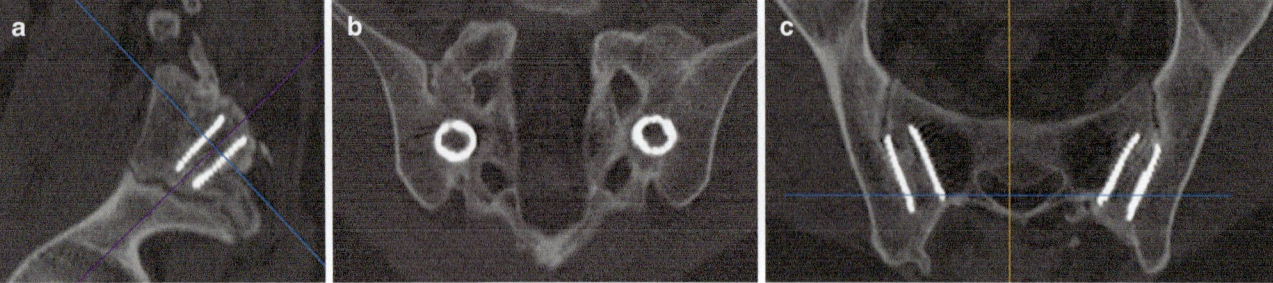

Fig. 76.2 SIJ-fusion on both sides: parasagittal (**a**), sacral coronal (**b**), and para-axial view (**c**)

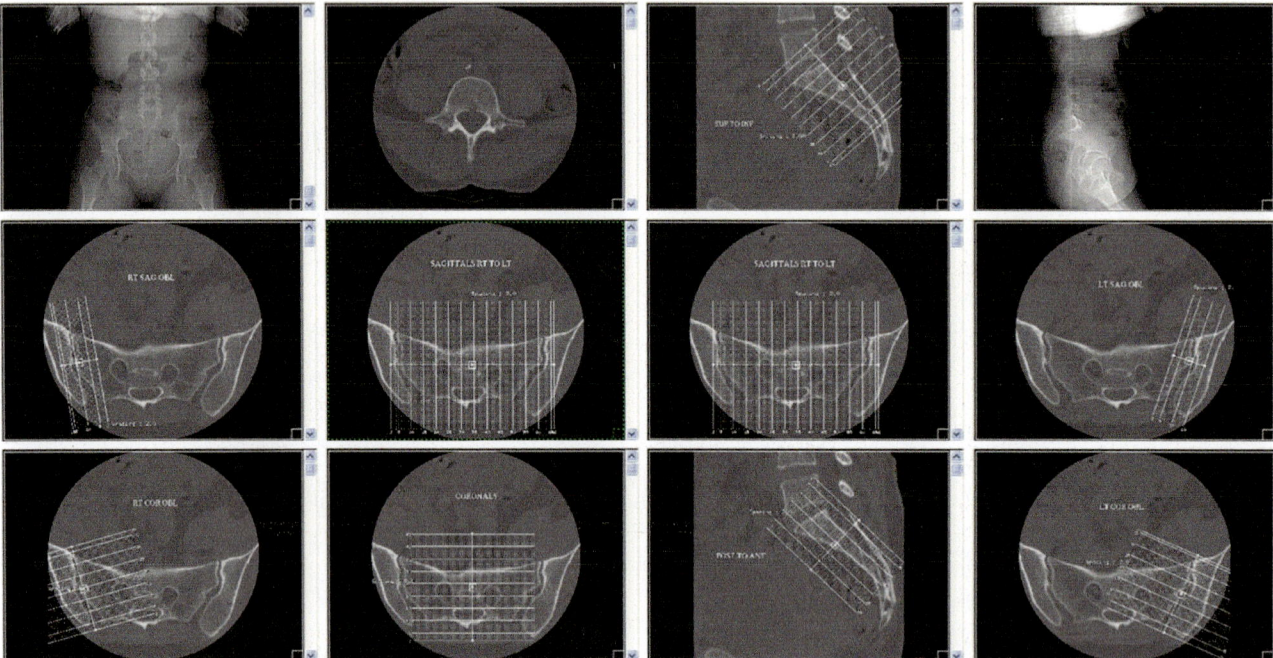

Fig. 76.3 Nine different *reconstructed* planes of the SIJ (from left to right: coronal scout, axial raw data, *para-axial planes*, lateral scout, *parasagittal planes right*, *sagittal planes right* and *left*, *parasagittal* *planes left*, *paracoronal planes right*, *coronal planes*, *sacral coronal planes*, *paracoronal planes left*)

- Fractures and sacral insufficiency fractures
- Bony defects in the area of the recess of the ilium and sacrum following bone graft harvesting
- Presence of a tumor or bacterial infection of the SIJ

- SIGNUS®/Ilion Medical® trays and instruments
- DIANA® implants (13 mm, 15 mm, 17 mm and 19 mm diameter) or NADIA® implants (16 mm and 18 mm diameter)

76.4 Technical Prerequisites

- Adjustable, radiotranslucent operating table (optimal condition: carbon table)
- C-arm
- Microscope
- Angled retractors
- High-speed drill (rosebud)
- Power drill
- Allograft (cancellous bone; 30-45 cc)

76.5 Planning, Preparation, and Positioning

- High-resolution CT-scan of the pelvis (from L4 down to the femoral heads; slice thickness up to max. 2.0 mm) for preoperative planning and reconstruction (see Fig. 76.3)
- Prone position
- C-arm on the ipsilateral side of the pathologic SIJ (see Fig. 76.4)
- Before starting to drape the patient, the C-arm has to be adjusted; ap-view (visibility of superior sacral rim, SIJ,

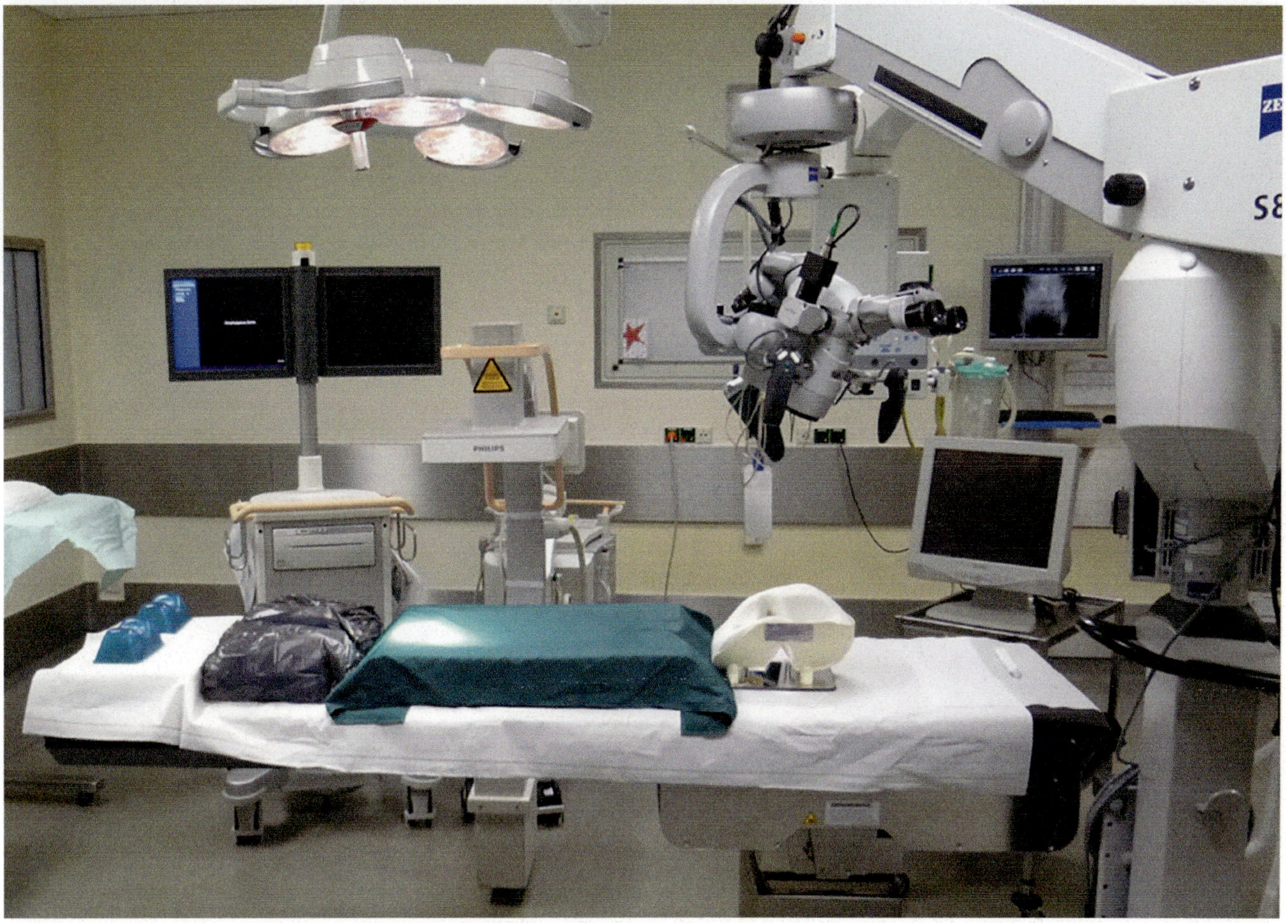

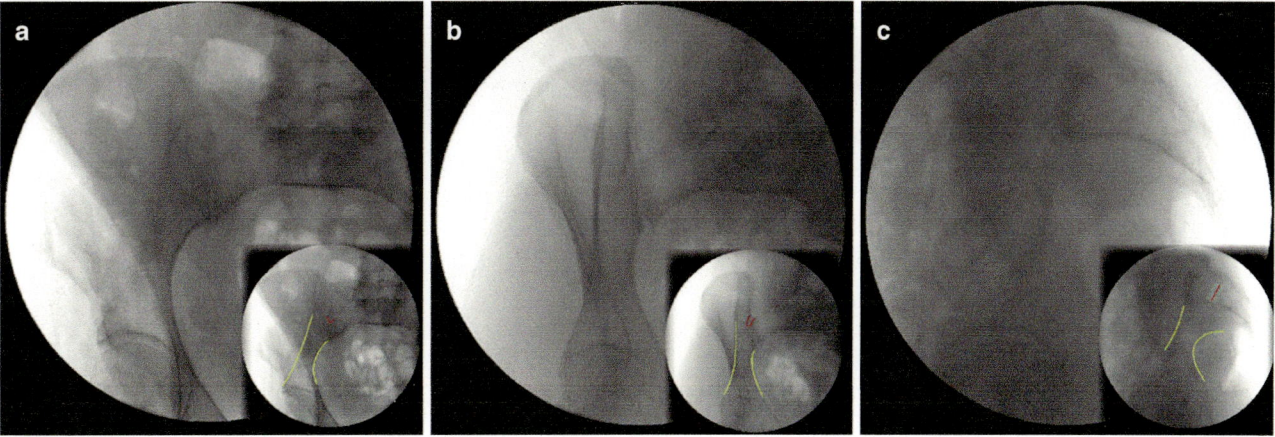

Fig. 76.4 Operative setup for a SIJ fusion with the DIANA®/NADIA® implant (left side)

Fig. 76.5 ap-view (**a**) and oblique view (**b**) with iliac corridor in yellow and bottom of the SIJ recess in red; lateral view with arcuate line and congruent left and right greater sciatic notch in yellow and S1/2 disk space in red (**c**)

and acetabulum), lateral view (visibility of arcuate line, sacrum, and greater sciatic notch), oblique view (visibility of SIJ recess, iliac corridor, and acetabulum); in the lateral view (visibility of sacrum, arcuate line, greater sci-atic notch, acetabulum), the left and right greater sciatic notch have to be congruent; in the oblique view, the C-arm has to be angled according to the orientation of the recess (see Figs. 77.5a–c and 77.6).

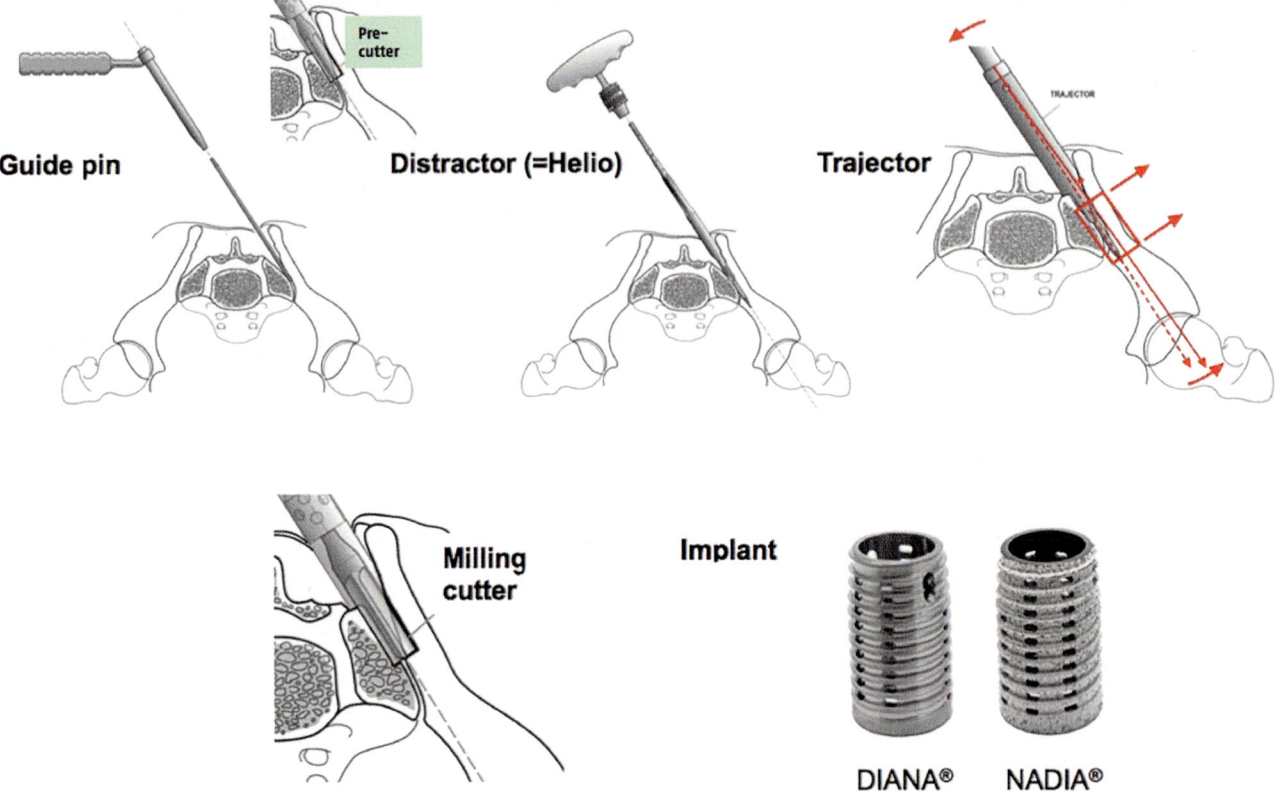

Fig. 76.6 Summary of surgical steps DIANA®/NADIA® operation

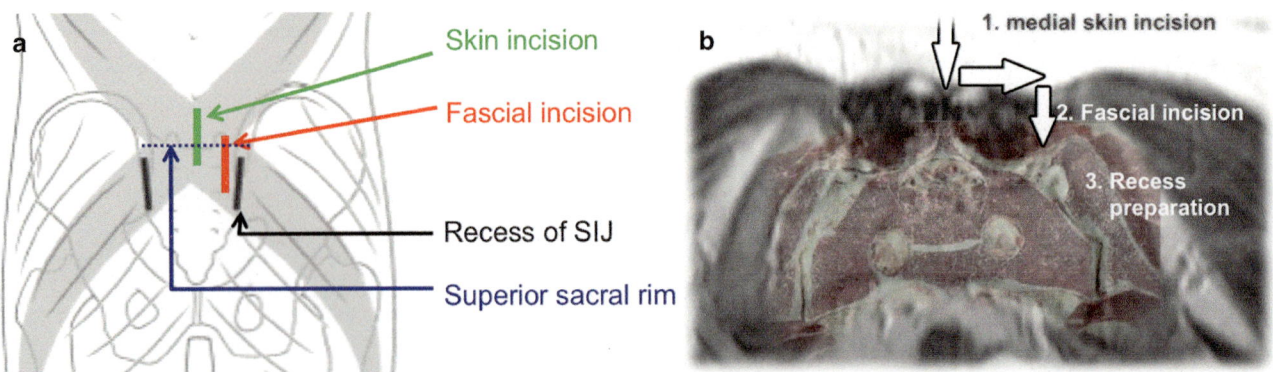

Fig. 76.7 Approach to the recess of the SIJ: ap (**a**) and axial view (**b**)

76.6 Surgical Technique

A dorsal 5–6-cm-long midline approach is used, with the center of the skin incision corresponding to the upper border of the sacrum. The incision is then extended to the thoracolumbar fascia, continuing laterally to the posterior superior iliac spine (PSIS). A lengthwise fascia incision is made 1.5 cm medial to the PSIS and somewhat further caudally than the skin incision but at the same length (see Fig. 76.7a–b).

After blunt retraction of the spinal erectors toward medial, the posterior sacroiliac ligaments are exposed and resected over the recess of the SIJ between the S1 and S2 transverse processes of the sacrum. In a next step, the interosseous ligaments are removed and the cortical surfaces of the ilium and sacrum exposed, along with the posterior joint space opening at the floor of the recess (see Fig. 76.8a–b).

A high-speed drill is used to open the iliac and sacral cortical bones (see Fig. 76.9).

A sharp guide pin is positioned along the weight-bearing axis of the ilium using a C-arm in three predefined planes (see Fig. 76.10a–c).

The individual width of the recess together with additional possible distraction between the ilium and the sacrum

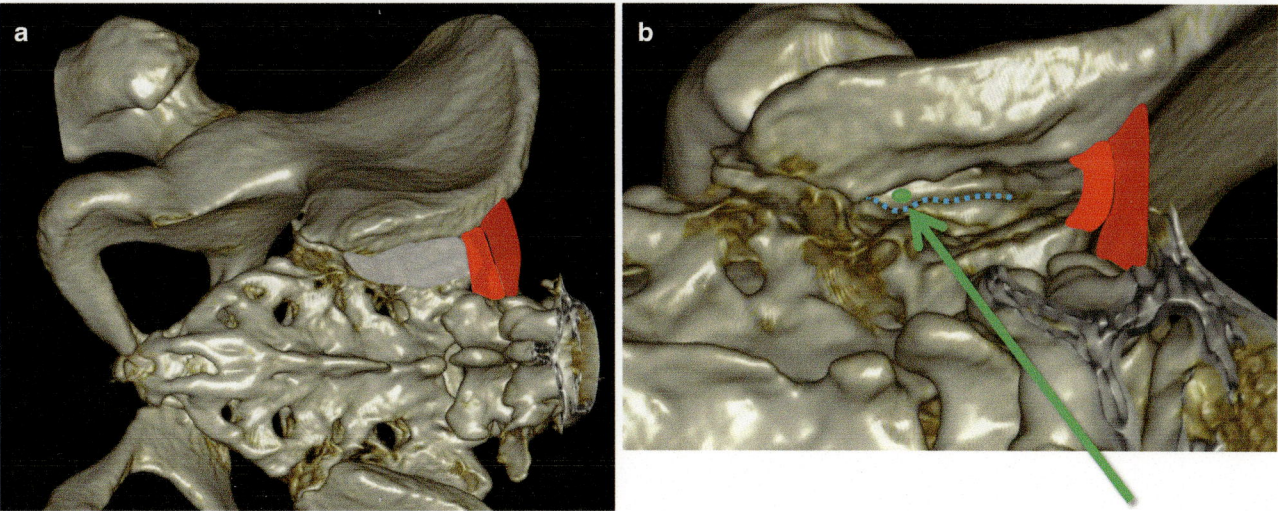

Fig. 76.8 SIJ recess covered by dorsal sacroiliac ligaments in grey (**a**); bottom of the recess with joint line in blue, guide pin (green arrow) and guide pin entry point in green (**b**); cranial sacroiliac and iliolumbar ligaments (red) should remain intact

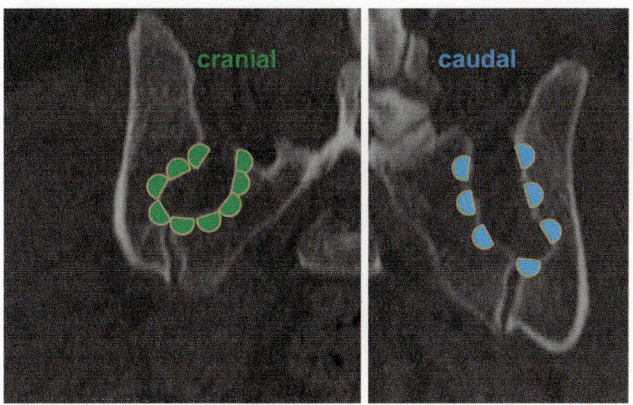

Fig. 76.9 Extent of decortication in the cranial (green) and in the caudal (blue) part of the recess

are acquired with a distraction instrument (=Helio) used to determine the size of the required implant (Figs. 76.11a–c and 76.12a, b).

The Trajector of the same size as the Helio is introduced into the recess with vigorous hammer blows (see Fig. 76.13a, b).

After removal of the Helio, the implant bed is prepared with a Milling cutter (see Fig. 76.13c). Maintaining distraction between ilium and sacrum, the interference screw is inserted through the Trajector into the recess (see Fig. 76.14a–c).

A large quantity of cancellous allograft (30–45 cc) according to the size of the recess is deposited in and around the implant until the recess and the implant are filled completely. A drainage is used before closing the fascia (Fig. 76.2).

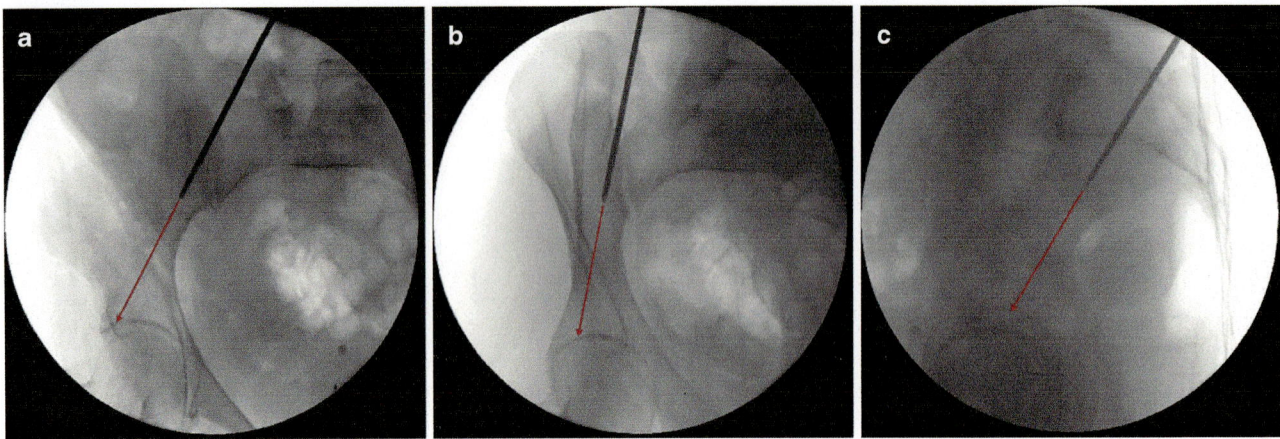

Fig. 76.10 Correct position and trajectory of the sharp guide pin in the ap (**a**), oblique (**b**), and lateral view (**c**)

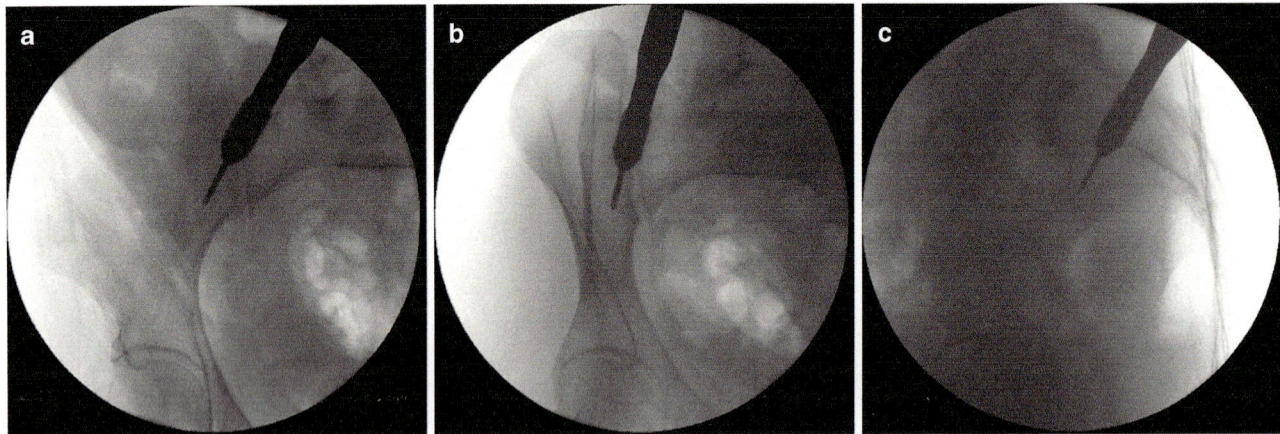

Fig. 76.11 End position of the Helio in the ap (**a**), oblique (**b**), and lateral view (**c**)

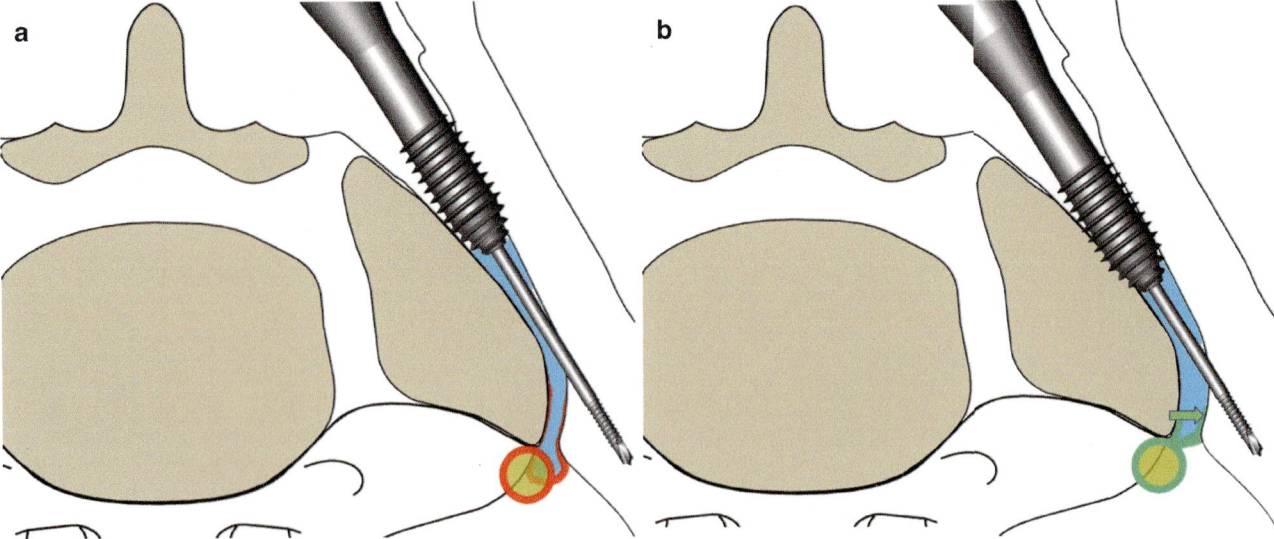

Fig. 76.12 Starting and end position of the Helio before (**a**) and after distraction (**b**) of the SIJ—note the tensioning of the anterior SIJ ligaments (red to green)

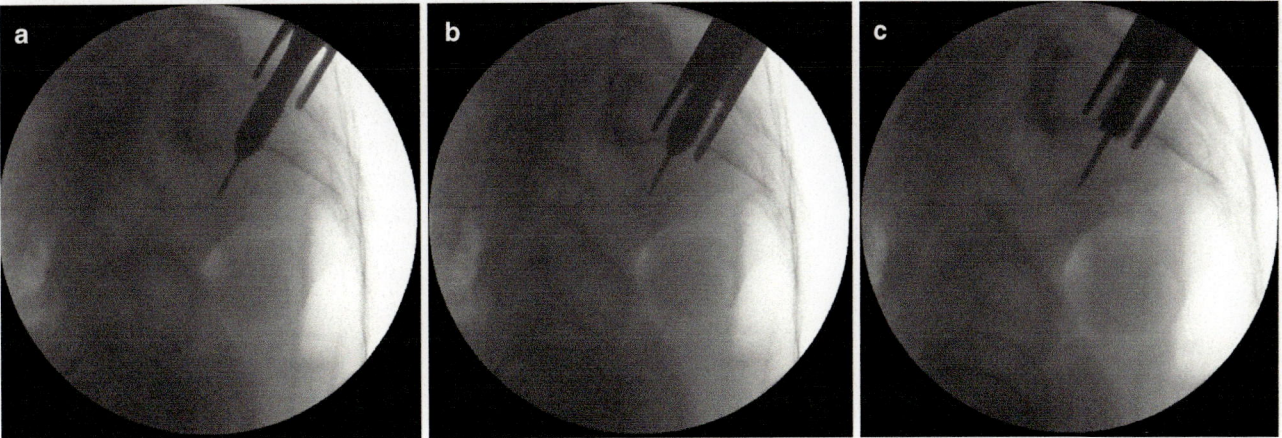

Fig. 76.13 Starting (**a**) and end position (**b**) of the Trajector; end position Milling Cutter (**c**)

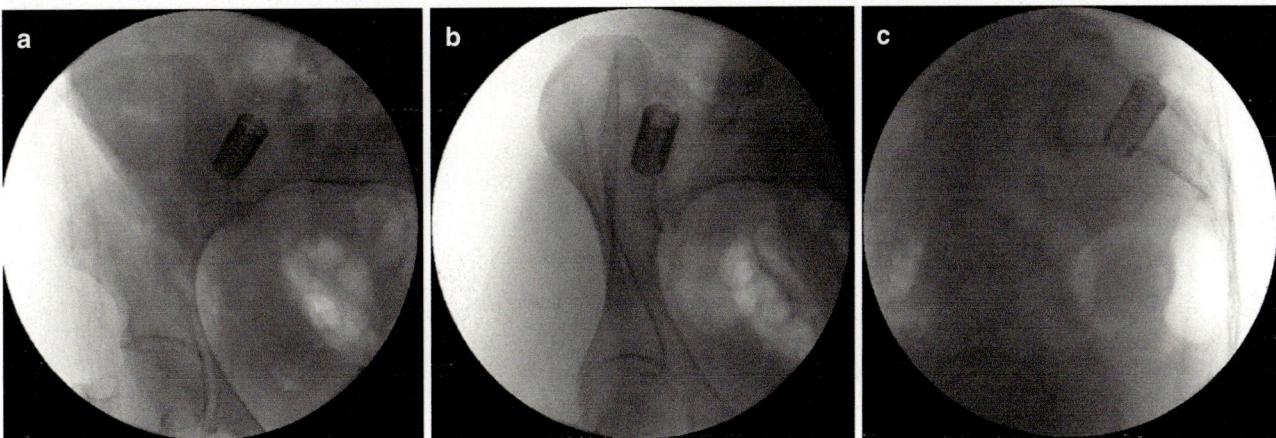

Fig. 76.14 Correct Position of the DIANA®-implant in the ap (**a**), oblique (**b**), and lateral view (**c**)

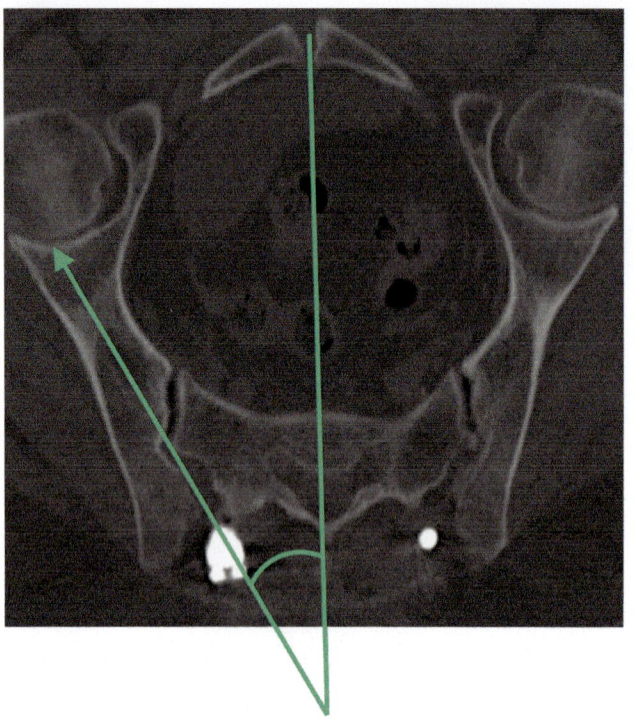

Fig. 76.15 Estimated angle for the oblique C-arm setting; green arrow: trajectory of guide pin and implant. (Note: S1-screw is obstructing the recess and has to be removed)

76.7   Tips and Tricks

- Determine expected angulation of the C-arm for the intraoperative oblique view in preoperative CT-scans and be aware of S1-screws that obstruct the passage into the recess (see Fig. 76.15).
- Use the microscope for the preparation of the recess.
- Prepare thoroughly down to the bottom of the recess without violating the cortical bone of the ilium or sacrum; start with the iliac side (better bone quality).
- Prepare the recess in full extension from cranial to caudal.

- Do not violate the superior sacroiliac ligaments or even the iliolumbar ligaments.
- Visualize the vertical SI-joint line at the bottom of the recess.
- Carefully open the top of the recess with punches to visualize the horizontal joint line.
- Prepare the cavities on the sacral side between the S1 and S2 and also between the S2 and S3 transverse processes.
- Perform a good decortication of the recess to create the best condition for fusion.
- Insert 50% of the bone graft before introducing the guide pin into the recess.
- Point the guide pin toward the center of the acetabular roof in all three views (not to the center of femoral head).
- In case of a narrow recess, use the pre-drill if the smallest Helio does not bite.
- In case of soft bone, do not use the Milling cutter.

References

1. Snijders CJ, Vleeming A, Stoeckart R. Transfer of lumbosacral load to iliac bones and legs. Part 1: biomechanics of selfbracing of the sacroiliac joints and its significance for treatment and exercise. Clin Biomech. 1993;8:285–94.
2. Vleeming A, Buyruk HM, Stoeckart R, Karamursel S, Snijders CJ. An integrated therapy for peripartum pelvic instability: a study of the biomechanical effects of pelvic belts. Am J Obstet Gynecol. 1992;166:1243–7.
3. Damen L, Spoor CW, Snijders CJ, Stam HJ. Does a pelvic belt influence sacroiliac joint laxity? Clin Biomech (Bristol, Avon). 2002;17:495–8.
4. Mens JMA, Damen L, Snijders CJ, Stam HJ. The mechanical effect of a pelvic belt in patients with pregnancy-related pelvic pain. Clin Biomech (Bristol, Avon). 2006;21:122–7.
5. Stark JG, Fuentes JA, Fuentes TI, Idemmili C. The history of sacroiliac joint arthrodesis: a critical review and introduction of a new technique. Curr Orthop Pract. 2011;22(545):557.
6. Fuchs V, Ruhl B. Distraction arthrodesis oft he sacroiliac joint: 2-year results of a descriptive prospective multi-center cohort study in 171 patients. Eur Spine J. 2018;27:194–204.

Percutaneous Iliosacral Screw (ISS) Technique

77

Jörg Böhme, Uwe Vieweg, Johannes Keck, and Hannes Moritz

77.1 Introduction and Core Messages

Osteoporotic lateral fractures with minimal displacement in the area of the anterior pelvic ring can be addressed specifically and successfully by percutaneous iliosacral screw (ISS) fixation. Especially fragility fractures of the pelvis are an important clinical challenge. The primary goal in the treatment of these patients is an early full weight-bearing mobilization, which may be aided by surgical stabilization to decrease pain and facilitate mobility. Percutaneous minimally invasive techniques are indicated for quicker mobilization with fewer possibilities of complications especially for these patients, usually also presenting a number of comorbidities. ISS fixations were first described already in 1913 in Lambotte's textbook "Chirurgie operattoire des fractures" [1]. The percutaneous technique developed by Ebraheim and Duwelius for nondislocated fractures or luxations to be set closed was standardized by Matta/Saucedo and developed further by Rout [2, 3–9]. Based on different preparatory work and on developments over past years, the ISS is now commonly applied for the stabilization of pelvic posterior ring injuries [10]. In respect to the biomechanical limitations faced by the single ISS technique, the dual iliosacral screw technique was developed [11]. ISS are able to restore greater than 80% of pretraumatic static stability of a vertical shear injury in patients with normal bone stock [12]. Some authors suggest the use of cement augmentation of the ISS, because this has been proven to increase pull out strength of screws [13, 14].

77.2 Indications [4, 6, 7, 15–18]

Indications are

- Nondisplaced or minimally displaced unilateral or lateral transalar, transforaminal, or central sacral fractures,
- Weal and osteoporotic bony scaffold of the pelvic,
- Sacral fractures in older patients,
- Pathological fractures or instabilities in cases with lumbosacral metastasis,
- Immobilizing low back pain with radiological proof of a sacral fracture.

Many classifications have been proposed to describe sacral fractures. The sacrum fractures must be classified in relation to the classification of the pelvic fractures. We recommend the AO sacral trauma and the Rommens classification. Other possible classifications would include the Denis (Zone 1: fracture involves the sacral ala lateral to the neural foramina, zone 2: fracture involves the neural foramina, but does not involve the spinal canal zone 3: fracture is medial to the neural foramen, involving the spinal canal (suptype1-4)) or the Roy-Camille classification [6, 7, 19, 20–22]. Sacrum fractures may be differentiated in accordance with the AO sacral trauma classification into types A, B, and C. The hierarchical system of the AO sacral fracture classification includes Type A fractures (lower sacrococcygeal injuries) with no impact on posterior pelvic or spino-pelvic instability, Type B fractures (posterior pelvis injuries) the primary impact is on posterior pelvic stability, and the type C fractures (spino-pelvic injuries

J. Böhme (✉)
Department of Trauma Surgery, Orthopaedics and Specialist Septic Surgery, St. Georg Hospital Leipzig, Leipzig, Germany
e-mail: j.boehme@sanktgeorg.de

U. Vieweg
Department of Conservative and Surgical Spine Therapy with Interdisciplinary Spinal Deformities Centre and Rummelsberg Sectional Center, Hospital Rummelsberg, Schwarzenbruck, Germany
e-mail: uwe.vieweg@sana.de

J. Keck · H. Moritz
Clinic for Surgical and Conservative Spinal Therapy with Interdisciplinar Spinal Deformities Centre and Rummelsberg Sectional Center, Rummelsberg Hospital, Schwarzenbruck, Germany

© Springer-Verlag GmbH Germany 2023
U. Vieweg, F. Grochulla (eds.), *Manual of Spine Surgery*, https://doi.org/10.1007/978-3-662-64062-3_77

with a spino-pelvic instability). Type A may be considered stable, type B rotationally unstable vertically stable, and type C rotationally unstable vertically unstable.

The three types are each subdivided into three further subgroups [10, 15, and] in ascending order according to severity. Transsacral screwing may be applied especially for Type C0 fractures. Types B1 to B3 and other C fractures may be functionally stabilized in combination with additional spino-pelvic care. Classification according to Rommens and Hofmann will be useful especially in cases of fragility fractures of the pelvis (FFP) [7]. Especially fracture type FFP IIb appears to indicate a preferred screwed connection only (FFP II A and C if applicable). Aches in the lower back of older patients may be indicative of sacrum insufficiency fractures.

77.3 Contraindications

Contraindications are

- Displaced or highly unstable sacral fractures.
- Sacral fractures with neurological impairment requiring decompression
- Insufficient fluoroscopic visualization of the anatomical landmarks of the upper sacrum [1].

77.4 Preoperative Planning, Preparation, and Positioning of Patients

- MRI of the pelvis or lumbar spine with short tau inversion recovery (STIR). (see Fig. 77.1)
- A CT of the pelvis is crucial for diagnostic procedure (see Fig. 77.2) and planning safe paths for ISS placement. High-quality pelvic CTs are crucial for planning reduction maneuvers and safe, effective paths for ISS placement.
- A anteroposterior, inlet, and outlet views and lateral radiograph centered on S1 are essential for the preoperative planning and ISS insertion.
- **Inlet image: 40-60°** Cranially tilted beam. The X-ray beam is tilted by 40–60° cranially for inlet imaging. This allows evaluation on the pelvic inlet plane in respect of dorsal and ventral displacement of the pelvis.
- The **outlet image** is based on 30–45° caudally tilted X-ray beams and is indicative of vertical displacement. Since the sacrum will be viewed orthogonally to its ventral plane, it will generally be fully recognizable, with no significant projection errors.

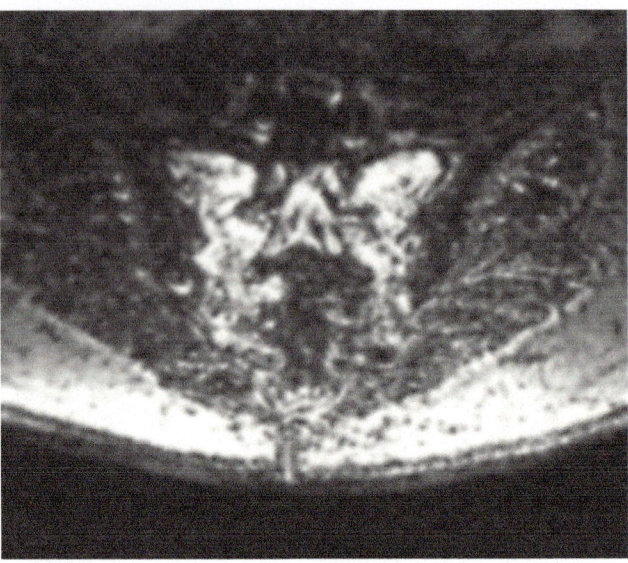

Fig. 77.1 MRT image, axial T2 sequent of a 76-year-old patient with deep lumbar backache showing a bilateral osteoporotic sacral insufficiency fracture

- You have to confirm that the **lateral view** is indeed true, without rotation (101).
- C-arm setup, and resulting images, should be finalized after the patient is anesthetized and positioned.

77.5 Technical Prerequisites

77.5.1 Imaging Techniques

In the literature, the current technique has been modified by combining with different imaging techniques with computer navigation in order to decrease the complication rate.

77.5.2 Implants

Cannulated screws of different designs have proven useful for transsacral screw connections. Cannulated ISSs (e.g., TIS™ screw, Königsee, Germany) (see Figs. 77.3 and 77.4) have lateral perforations at the screw tip to allow controlled discharge of cement into the bone. Screws may be fully or semithreaded to use as adjusting or traction screws. Central cannulation and lateral perforation at the screw tip will allow precise and controlled cementing in osteoporotic bones (Fig. 77.5).

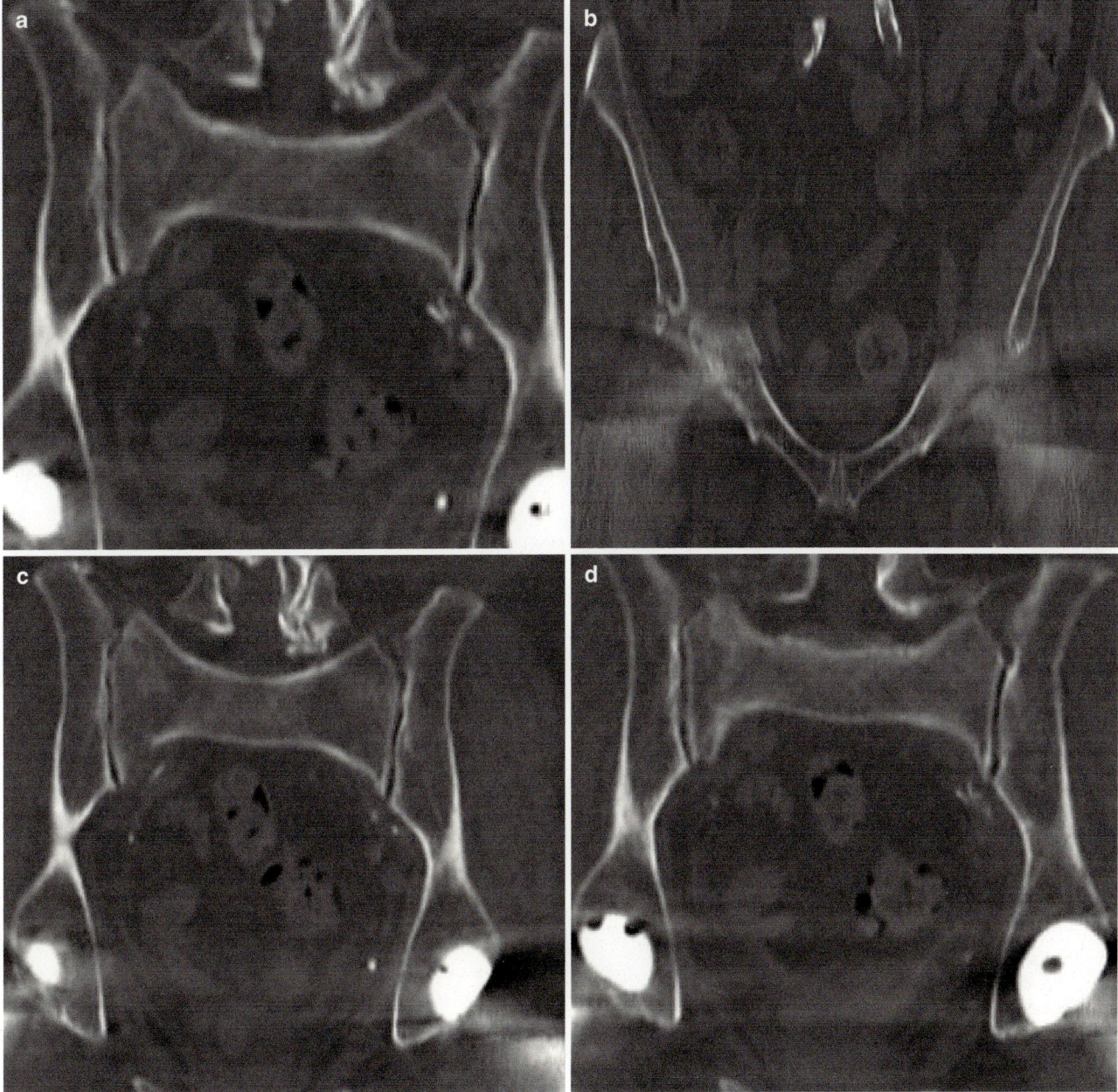

Fig. 77.2 (**a–d**) CT pelvis of an 82-year-old patient with deep lumbar backache with a Rommens IIb osteoporotic fracture on the right-hand side with anterior pelvic ring fracture on the right side

77.6 Technique [1, 8, 9, 18]

77.6.1 Skin Marking

- C-arm setup, and resulting images, should be finalized after the patient is anesthetized and positioned.
- The entry point should be anterior in S1 and inferior to the iliac cortical density, which parallels the sacral alar slope, usually slightly caudal and posterior.

- The safe zone for the entry point of the implants is caudal of the Ala line and between the anterior corticalis and the spinal canal.
- Access planning and access is identical to Chap. 75.

77.6.2 Skin Incision

- A 2–3-cm long incision is made. The underlying tissues are dissected down to bone, with scissors.

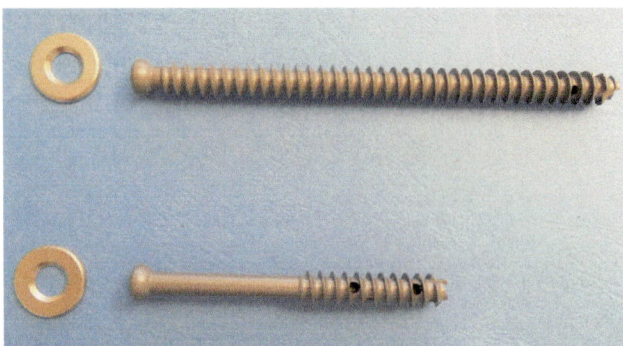

Fig. 77.3 TIS screws and washers with full thread and partial thread (32 mm). Note the cross holes on the tip of the screws

77.6.3 Instrumentation

- A guidewire/K-wire is placed 2–3 mm, or drilled into the planned screw entry point. This is controlled by X-ray on the lateral view (see Fig. 77.6a).
- The guidewire/K-wire position must be controlled radiologically via the inlet and outlet view (see Fig. 77.6a, b).
- The screw length is measured with a gauge suitable for the guidewire (see Fig. 77.7).

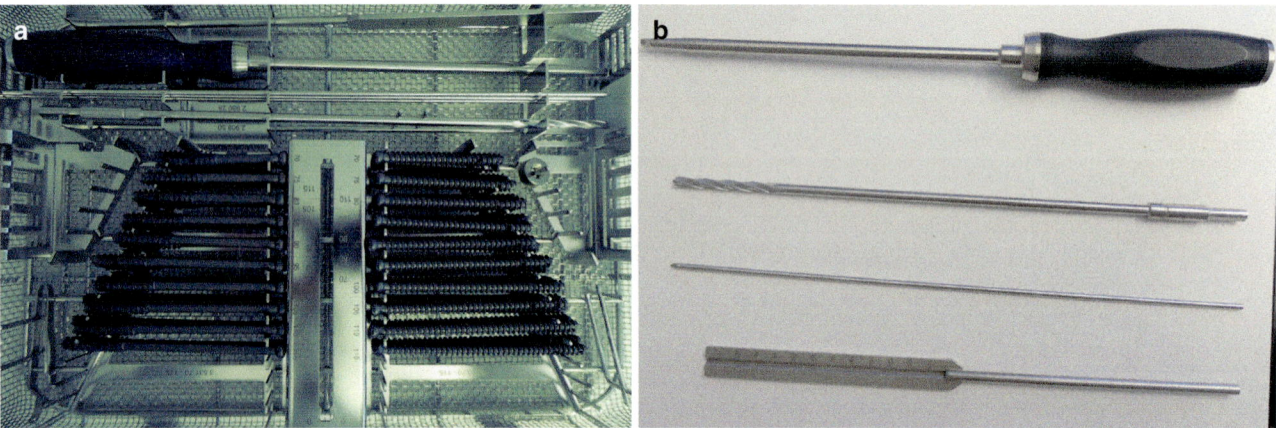

Fig. 77.4 (**a**, **b**) Instruments and implants container (**a**) and the most important instruments (**b**) with cannulated screw driver, drill, K-wire, and measuring instrument for determining the screw length

Fig. 77.5 Patient in supine position after the planning of the skin incision on both sides (**a**) and the skin marker. (**b**) skin marking for planning access based on the radiologically determined Ala line as well as the posterior and anterior borders of the sacrum. The marking for the skin incision is drawn on the back line approximately 2 cm below the ala line

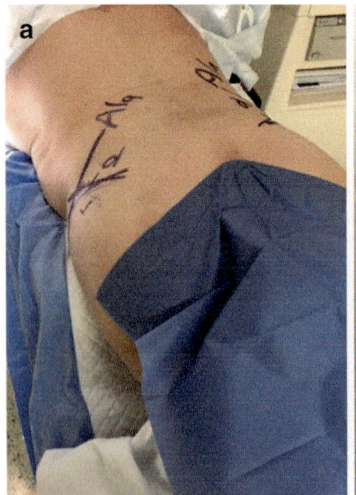

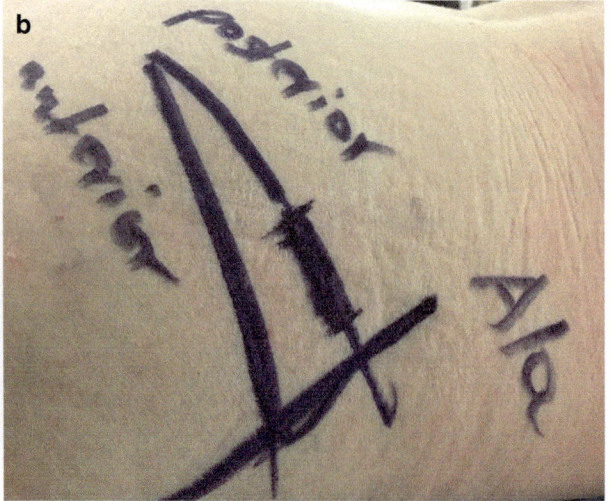

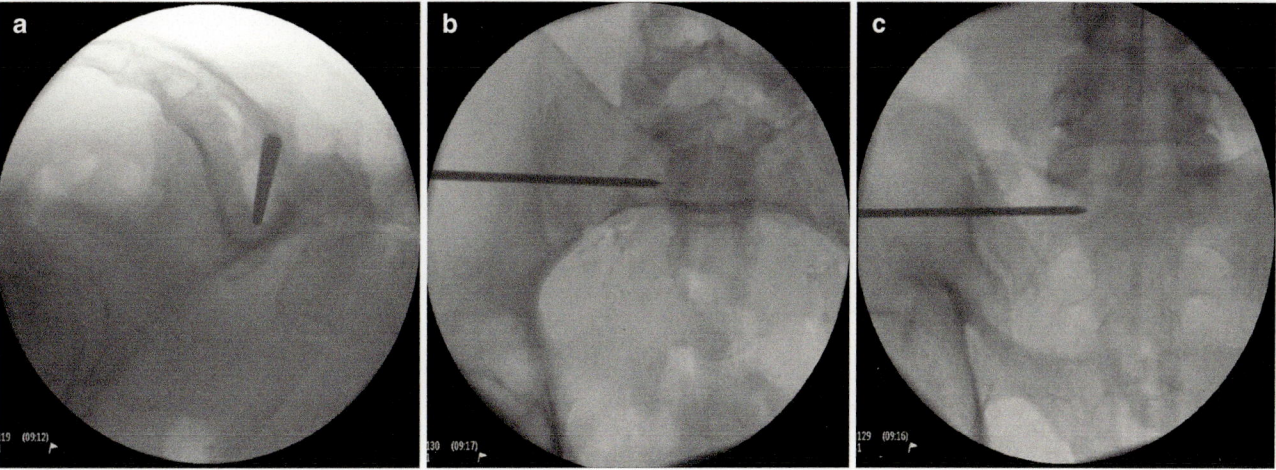

Fig. 77.6 (**a**) The intraoperative x rays showing the guidewire in the lateral (**a**) inlet (**b**) and outlet (**c**) views

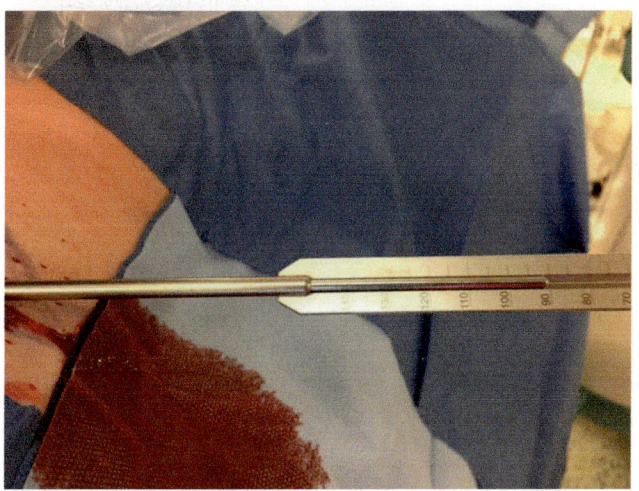

Fig. 77.7 Intraoperative measurement of the screw length with a gauge suitable for the guidewire

- An appropriate screw hole is drilled over the guidewire, which should remain anchored in the bone, if it has been advanced far enough beyond the intended screw tip site.
- In osteoporotic fractures, ISS can be augmented, with cement to increase the stability. Although good preoperative planning, perfect orientation using the C arm or intraoperative computer navigation will allow the screws to be accurately placed, contrast media should be applied prior to the application of cement to avoid contact with the neuroforamen and spinal canal.

77.7 Postoperative Management

- Cryotherapy as needed during inpatient care.
- Patients should use ca. 20 kg partially weight-bearing underarm support to relieve pressure on the surgically treated joint. Physiotherapy instruction will be useful and will also in most cases be strictly indicated.
- No subsequent removal of material will be planned, especially in cases of osteoporotic fracture treatment.

77.8 Complications

77.8.1 Loosening and Nonunion

In patients with osteoporotic bone, however, loosening of the screws frequently is seen [16, 23, 24].

77.8.2 Misplacement, Screw Perforation into Spinal Canal, Screw Perforation into Sacral Neural Foramina

The conventional fluoroscopy-based approach of sacral screw placement can be technically challenging and radiation intense even for experienced surgeons. Screw misplacement rates are reported to range from 2.8 to 29.5% [1, 23]. Neural lesions of L4-L5, S1 roots range between 2 and 15% and superior gluteal artery damage caused by wrong positioning of a screw ranges between 1 and 2% [11].

Fig. 77.8 (**a, b**)
Postoperative X-ray, (**a**)
anteroposterior, and (**b**) lateral
view, after iliosacral screwing
on the right side

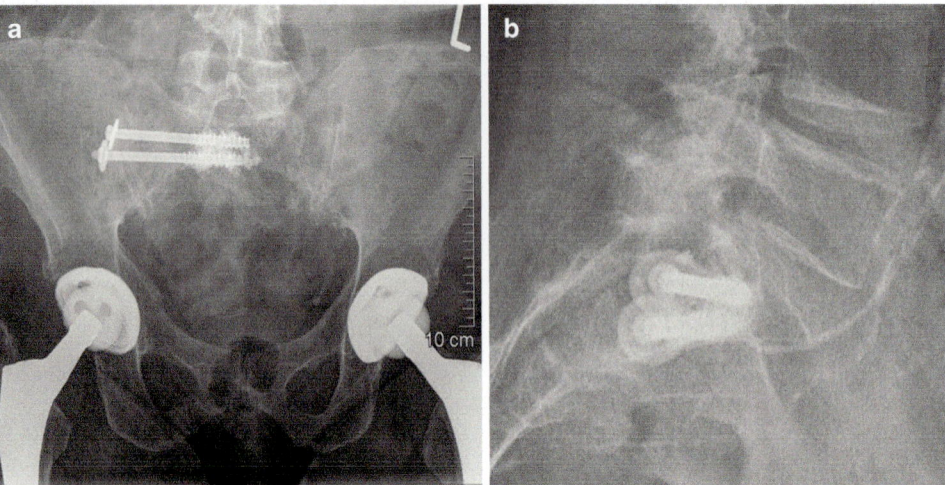

77.8.3 Problems of Wound Healing

Wound healing problems are rare.

The reasons of the different complications are

- Variability in pelvic anatomy,
- Narrowness of the bone corridor to be screw and
- Inadequacies in imaging and surgical technique.
- The fact that intraoperative two-dimensional fluoroscopic guidance of SI screw placement using inlet, outlet, and lateral views in the standard technique has its limitations in the presence of sacral dysmorphism should be taken into account [1] (Figs. 77.8, 77.9, 77.10, and 77.11).

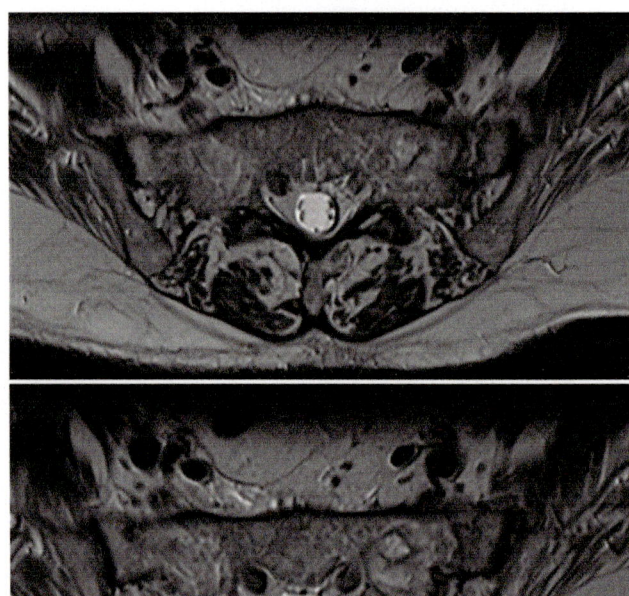

Fig. 77.9 Case 2. MRI of the pelvis (T2, axial view) of a 72 year old female with bilateral sacrum fractures (FFP IVb, u-shaped fracture type)

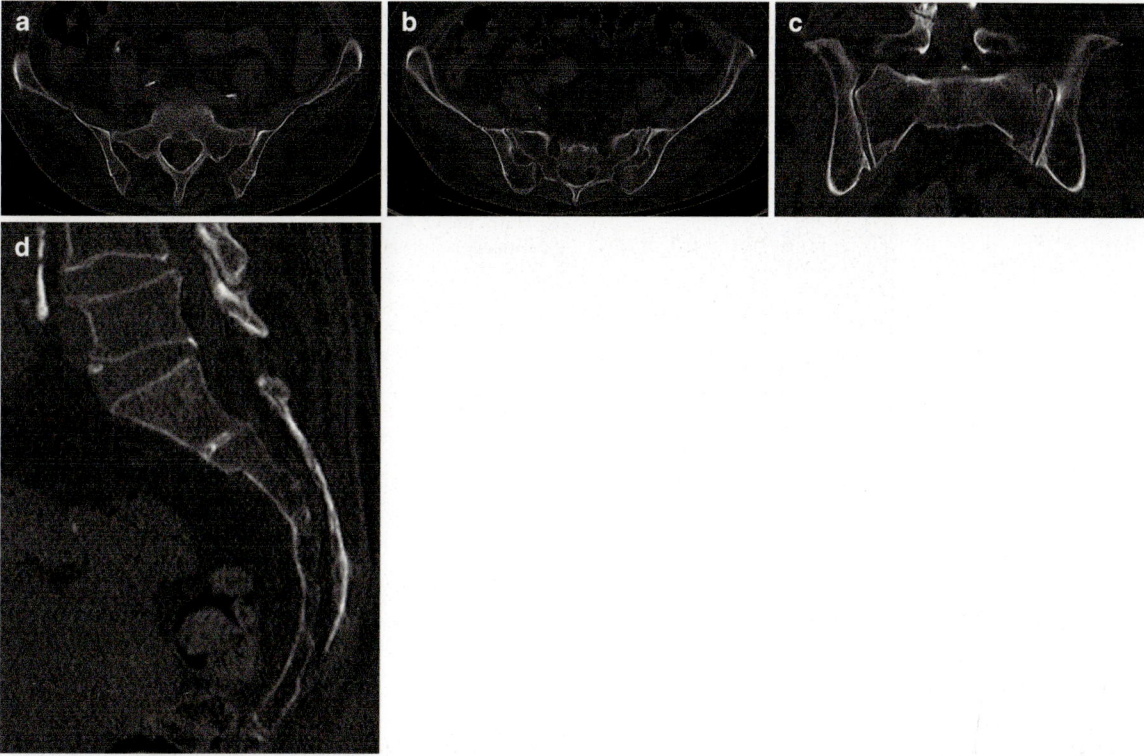

Fig. 77.10 Case 2. CT scans in different axial (**a**, **b**), coronary (**c**), and lateral (**d**) views

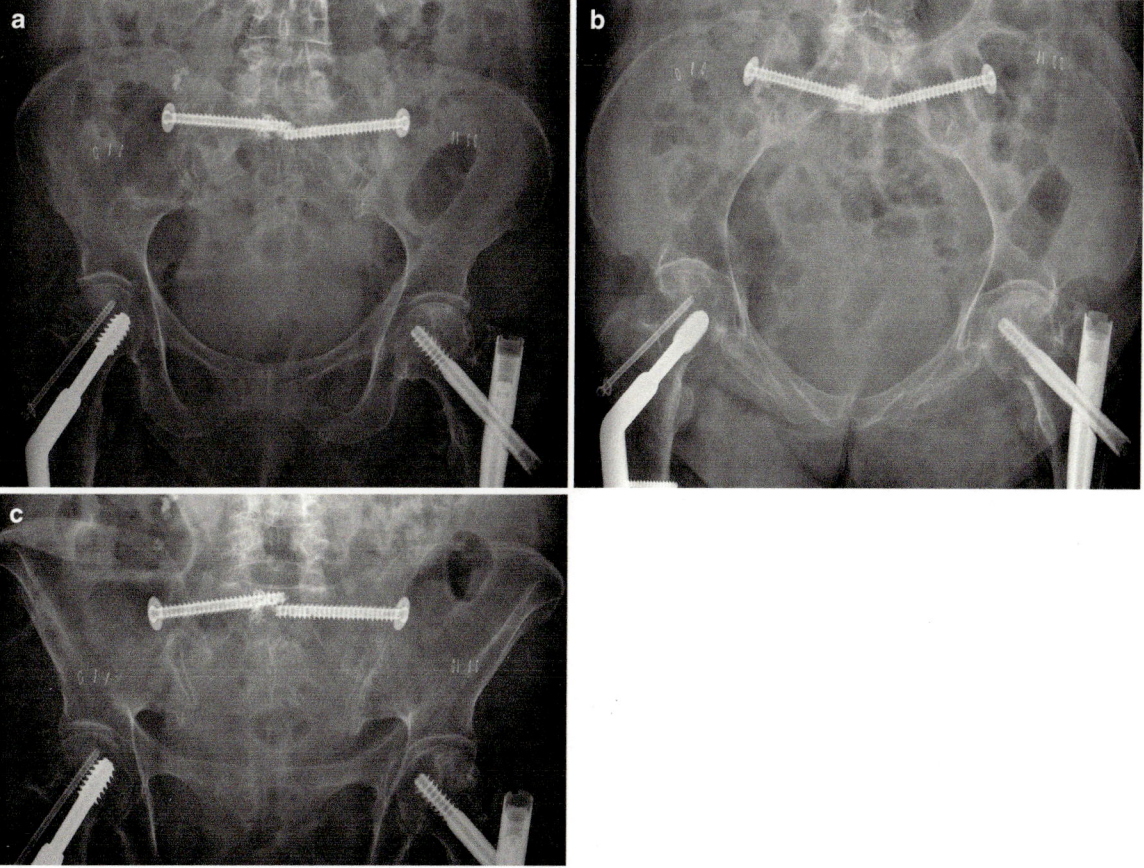

Fig. 77.11 X ray pelvis ap (**a**), inlet (**b**) with bilateral ISS in S1 with cement augmentation (Königsee comp., 7.5 mm cannulated, fully threaded titanium screw)

References

1. Krappinger D, Lindtner RA, Benedikt S. Preoperative planning and safe intraoperative placement of iliosacral screws under fluoroscopic control. Oper Orthop Traumatol. 2019;31:465–73.
2. Matta JM, Saucedo T. Internal fixation of pelvic ring fractures. Clin Orthop Relat Res. 1989;242:83–97.
3. Duwelius PJ, Van Allen M, Bray TJ, Nelson D. Computed tomography-guided fixation of unstable posterior pelvic ring disruptions. J Orthop Trauma. 1992;4:420–6.
4. Ebraheim NA, Rusin JJ, Coombs RJ, et al. Percutaneous computed-tomography-stabilization of pelvic fractures: preliminary report. J Orthop Trauma. 1987;3:197–204.
5. Rommens PM, Arand C, Hofmann A, et al. When and how to operate fragility fractures of the pelvis? Indian J Orthop. 2019;53:128–37.
6. Rommens PM, Hofmann A. Comprehensive classification of fragility fractures of the pelvic ring: recommendations for surgical treatment. Injury. 2013;44:1733–44.
7. Routt ML Jr, Meier M, Kregor PK. Percutaneous iliosacral screws with the patient supine technique. Op Tech Orthop. 1993;3:35–45.
8. Routt ML Jr, Kregor PJ, Simonian PT, et al. Early results of percutaneous iliosacral screws placed with the patient in the supine position. J Orthop Trauma. 1995;9:207–14.
9. Rout ML Jr, Routt ML Jr, Simonian PT, et al. Radiographic recognition of the sacral alar slope for optimal placement of iliosacral screws: a cadaveric and clinical study. J Orthop Trauma. 1996;10:171–7.
10. Alvis-Miranda HR, Farid-Escorcia H, Alcala-Cerra G, et al. Sacroiliac screw fixation: a mini review of surgical technique. J Craniovertebral Junction Spine. 2014;5:2.
11. Yu BS, Zhuang XM, Zheng ZM, et al. Biomechanical advantages of dual over single iliac screws in lumbo-iliac fixation construct. Eur Spine J. 2010;19:1121–8.
12. Comstock CP, van der Meulen MC, Goodman SB. Biomechanical comparison of posterior internal fixation techniques for unstable pelvic fractures. J Orthop Trauma. 1996;10:517–22.
13. Grechenig S, Gansslen A, Gueorguiev B, et al. PMMA-augmented SI screw: a biomechanical analysis of stiffness and pull-out force in a matched paired human cadaveric model. Injury. 2015;46(Suppl 4):125–8.
14. Osterhoff G, Andrew ED, Unno F, et al. Cement augmentation in sacroiliac screw fixation offers modest biomechanical advantages in a cadaver model. Clin Orthop Relat Res. 2016;474:2522–30.
15. Al-Khayer A, Hegarty J, Hahn D, Grevitt MP. Percutaneous sacroiliac joint arthrodesis: a novel technique. J Spinal Disord Tech. 2008;21(5):359–63.
16. Balling H. 3D image-guided surgery for fragility fractures of the sacrum. Oper Orthop Traumatol. 2019;6:499–502.
17. Fuchs T, Freistühler M, Raschke M. Geriatric pelvic fractures. Principles of diagnosis and therapy. Research OUP. 2013;2(5):248–52. (in German).
18. Routt ML Jr. Posterior pelvic ring disruptions: iliosacral screws. In: Wiss DA, Capers CM, Williams CB, editors. Master techniques in orthopaedic surgery. Lippincott Williams & Wilkins; 2006. p. S649–67.
19. Arand M. Verletzungen des Beckens. Mutschler WE Hrsg, Praxis der Unfallchirurgie. Thieme, Stuttgart, pp. S363-367; 1999.
20. Gansslen A, Krettek C. Retrograde transpubic screw fixation of transpubic instabilities. Oper Orthop Traumatol. 2006;18:330–40.
21. Schroeder GD, Kurd MF, Kepler CK, et al. The development of a universally accepted sacral fracture classification: a survey of AOspine and AOTrauma members. Global Spine. 2016;J6:668–94.
22. Takao M, Nishii T, Sakai T, et al. Iliosacral screw insertion using CT-3D-fluoroscopy matching navigation. Injury. 2014;45:988–94.
23. Balling H. Time demand and radiation dose in 3D-fluoroscopy-based navigation-assisted 3D-fluoroscopy-controlled pedicle screw instrumentation. Spine. 2018;43(9):E512–9.
24. Heydemann J, Hartline B, Gibson ME, et al. Do transsacral-transiliac screws across uninjured sacroiliac joints affect pain and functional outcomes in trauma patients? Clin Orthop Relat Res. 2016;474:1417–21.
25. Beaulé PE, Antoniades J, Matta JM. Trans-sacral fixation for failed posterior fixation of the pelvic ring. Arch Orthop Trauma Surg. 2006;126:49–52.
26. Esses SI, Botsford DJ, Huler RJ, Rauschning W. Surgical anatomy of the sacrum. A guide for rational screw fixation. Spine. 1991;6 Suppl:S283–8.
27. Frank M, Dedek T. Percutaneous iliosacral screw placement using a radiolucent drive. Acta Orthop Belg. 2012;78:519–22.
28. Fujibayashi S, Neo M, Nakamura T. Palliative dual iliac screw fixation for lumbosacral metastasis. Technical note J Neurosurg Spine. 2007;7:99–102.
29. Gardner MJ, Routt ML Jr. Transiliac-transsacral screws for posterior pelvic stabilization. J Orthop Trauma. 2011;25:378–84.
30. Hilgert RE, Finn J, Egbers HJ. Technique for percutaneous iliosacral screw insertion with conventional C-arm radiography. Unfallchirurg. 2005;108(954):956–60. (in German)
31. Khurana A, Guha AR, Mohanty K, Ahuja S. Percutaneous fusion of the sacroiliac joint with hollow modular anchorage screws: clinical and radiological outcome. J Bone Joint Surg Br. 2009;91(5):627–63.
32. Lehmann J. Luxation einer Beckenhälfte. Zentralbl Chir. 1934:2149–2152.
33. Marmor M, Lynch T, Matityahu A. Superior gluteal artery injury during iliosacral screw placement due to aberrant anatomy. Orthopedics. 2010;33(2):117–20.
34. Mehling I, Hessmann MH, Rommens PM. Stabilization of fatique fractures of the dorsal pelvis with a trans-sacral bar: operative technique and outcomes. Injury. 2012;43:446–51.
35. Meyer-Burgdorff G. Über BeckenbrÜche. Zentralbl Chir. 1936:1016–8.
36. Heydemann J, Hartline B, Gibson ME, et al. Do transsacral-transiliac screwsacross uninjured sacroiliac joints affect pain and functional outcomes in trauma patients? Clin Orthop Relat Res. 2016;474:1417–21.
37. Santoneli E, Kanakaris NK, Giannoudis PV. Sacral fractures: issues, challenges, solutions. EFFORT Open Rev. 2020;5:299–311.
38. Van den Bosch EW, van Zwien CM, van Vugt AB. Fluoroscopic positioning of sacroiliac screws in 88 patients. J Trauma. 2002;53:44–8.
39. Vidal J, Allieu Y, Fassio B, et al. Spondylolisthesis: reduction with Harrington's rods. Rev Chir Orthop. 1973;59:21–41.
40. Wahmert D, Raschke MJ, Fuchs T. Cement augmentation of the navigated iliosacral screw in the treatment of insufficiency fractures of the sacrum: a new method using modified implants. Int Orthop. 2013;37:1147–50.
41. Yang F, Yao S, Chen KF, et al. A novel patient-specific three-dimensional-printed external template to guide iliosacral screw insertion: a retrospective study. BMC Musculoskeletel Disord. 2018;19:397.

En Block Resection of the Sacrum

78

Mehmet Zileli

78.1 Introduction and Core Messages

Similar to other spine tumors, management of sacrum tumors must start by having a biopsy. Primary tumors of the sacrum are quite common. Primary malignant tumors such as chordoma, chondrosarcoma, osteosarcoma, and myeloma [1, 2], and benign tumors such as giant cell tumors, aneurysmal bone cysts, schwannomas, osteoblastomas, and osteochondromas are common pathologies in this region. These tumors are often large by the time they are diagnosed because of their mild symptoms. For that reason, their surgery is technically demanding. An oncologic surgery for sacrum tumors is possible. Radical resection may be the best available treatment for low-grade malignancies and aggressive, benign sacral tumors that are resistant to noninterventional therapies. The so-called en bloc resection of the sacrum in chordoma, chondrosarcoma, and giant cell tumors can give rise to a cure of the disease. In this chapter, we will describe the surgical techniques of those tumors.

78.2 Problems of Radical Sacrum Surgery and Sacrectomy

Partial and total sacrectomies pose several complex challenges, and require the expertise of specialists from several fields.

78.2.1 Preserving Vascular Structures

A total sacrectomy with a posterior only surgery is not possible because of anteriorly located iliac arteries and veins. Retroperitoneal or transperitoneal dissection of anterior structures, releasing arteries and veins from sacrum, is an important part of surgery. This should be done before starting posterior surgery. These structures can be protected using meticulous dissection techniques, aided by a vascular surgeon for handling of the ventral compressed vascular structures. I personally prefer to sacrifice the median sacral artery and vein, internal iliac arteries and veins, and iliolumbar arteries by ligation to cut off the vascular supply to the sacrum and tumor.

78.2.2 Preserving Visceral Structures

Care must also be taken to protect the visceral structures, including the ureters, urinary bladder, intestines, and rectum. Because of very anterior location, preserving the ureter and bladder is quite easy. However, rectum wall may be adherent to sacral tumor, even infiltrated. It is recommended to open an elective colostomy before primary surgery, to avoid rectal perforation. Cleaning colon before surgery is also important step for same reasons. An abdominal surgeon or vascular surgeon is necessary for dissections in this phase of surgery.

78.2.3 Preserving the Roots and Plexus

Neurological deficits resulting from the sacrifice of sacral nerve roots are extensive and permanent. There are two reasons of neurologic deficits after sacrectomy:
- Sacrificing sacral roots during sacrectomy. It is well known that the roots from S2 to S4 carry the primary afferent and efferents of sphincters and they are responsible from urinary and fecal continence. The key root in this region is S2. Bilateral preservation of S2 roots mean sphincter problem will not be so severe. Besides, unilateral loss of S2, S3, and S4 roots does not cause significant sphincter dysfunction [3–5]. However, in patients with bilateral section of S2, S3, and S4 roots, desire for defecation decreases and, they

M. Zileli (✉)
Neurosurgery Department, Sanko University, Gaziantep, Türkiye

© Springer-Verlag GmbH Germany 2023
U. Vieweg, F. Grochulla (eds.), *Manual of Spine Surgery*, https://doi.org/10.1007/978-3-662-64062-3_78

cannot differentiate feces from gas, neither feel the fullness of bladder.

- Injury or stretch to the lumbosacral plexus around superior medial iliac crest or inside the sciatic notch. In this instance, neurological deficits are more like an L5 root involvement resulting with a foot drop.

Functional results of the loss of sacral roots are as follows:

- Urinary incontinence. Loss of sacral roots results with a flasc bladder paralysis. Patients should either use drapes or permanent bladder catheters.
- Fecal incontinence. The patients describes incontinence in case of diarrhea. However, if the stool is hard, constipation prevents incontinence. They may discharge by increasing intra-abdominal pressure or with fingers.
- Loss of erection in male patients. It happens in most of the male patients. It may not occur in case of unilateral sacrifice of the roots.

In total sacrectomies, most of the sacral roots invaded by the tumor are sacrificed, and this usually results in loss of bladder and sexual function and bowel control [6, 7]. In most cases, preservation of the lumbar roots is possible, and they allow the patient to be ambulatory. Sparing the L5 root bilaterally may be adequate for plantar flexion of the foot [6]. Sacrificing the sacral roots in case of no significant sphincter disturbance before surgery is discussed as an ethical problem. The patient must be informed in detail about the disability of such an approach.

78.2.4 Excessive Bleeding

One of the important problems of sacral tumor surgery is excessive bleeding. The reasons are very rich blood supply of presacral area, epidural veins, large osteotomy for sacrectomy, excessive muscle dissection, and resection. This may be a life-threatening problem in radical sacral surgery. Considerable blood loss (7–80 L in some series) has been reported [8, 9]. Different methods to overcome excessive bleeding have been proposed. A meticulous bleeding control and muscle dissection done by monopolar cautery would significantly diminish bleeding, although they cause to increase the operation time. The other cautions recommended to overcome excessive bleeding are as follows: the application of bone wax on the osteotomy margins, spongostan, compressive gauses, the application of polymethylmethacrylate, fluid nitrogen, phenol, hydrogen peroxidase, and hot water. Application of substances such as hemostatic gauze, fibrin glue, or an omentum flap onto the bed of the tumor can prevent blood loss, as is done in cryosurgery. Cell saver autotransfusion may be used following excessive blood loss, but it cannot be applied to malignant tumors. It must better be used before entering the tumor, since tumor cells will be distributed to the body if used during tumor aspiration. To overcome excessive bleeding, a balloon dilation catheter may be placed in the distal abdominal aorta via the femoral artery, which was also by used by our team [10, 11]. Just after the skin incision, the balloon dilatation catheter was inflated with contrast medium and total occlusion of the aorta was achieved. We believe that this method prevents hemo-dynamical problems caused by massive bleeding and complications secondary to massive transfusion [11].

78.2.5 Wound Problems and Infection

In many patients, the surgery may result with problems of skin closure, and sometimes necrosis of the skin days and weeks after surgery [12]. There are many reasons of skin problems: The skin incision of previous surgery must be resected to overcome recurrence. Excessive muscle and bone excision negatively affect the vascularization of the skin. Pressure to the skin increases with wide bone and muscle excision. These potential complications pose another challenge [13–16]. For those reasons, contribution of plastic surgeons is necessary by turning flaps to relieve the pressure on skin and also increase the vascularization on the skin. Vascularized flaps are also helpful to diminish the cavity after wide resections. Any tension on the skin must be relieved, and soft tissues and muscles below must be reconstructed. To facilitate wound healing, various types of muscle flaps and incisions were made. In partial sacrectomy, or in the presence of previous incisions, we made a median longitudinal incision. In total sacrectomy, in which the resulting tissue defect was large, we made a downward-based, C-shaped incision with a median longitudinal extension at its apex. We used gluteal muscles as a flap inside the defect, and in some cases, a rectus abdominis myocutaneous pure island pedicle flap was used [17]. Another issue in these cases is the cavity created by sacrectomy. In order to fill out this cavity with a viable tissue and reconstruction of the sacrum, there are different maneuvers such as placing meshes to avoid rectum prolapse posteriorly, to fill the space with allograft bones in addition to sacropelvic fixation. Infection is another problem after such long and bloody surgeries. There are numerous reasons of postoperative infection, some of which are working around rectum, excessive retraction of tissues, diminished vascularization of the remaining tissues, and excessive blood transfusion. To avoid infection, surgeons must obey the intraoperative asepsis meticulously. The colon must be empty with preparation before surgery. In case of invasion of rectum, an elective colostomy must be performed before resection. Prophylactic antibiotherapy must always be applied. Some authors have proposed using a Vicryl net bag containing gentamicin beads to fill the defect, to prevent infection and herniation until the granulation tissue develops [18].

78.2.6 Lumbosacral and Sacroiliac Stability

Spinal-pelvic stability is one of the most difficult challenges faced in total sacrectomy, partly because of the large loads carried by the lumbosacral junction, and the angular position of the sacrum. This region is a transition zone from the mobile spine to the rigid pelvis. Distal amputations below sacroiliac joint do not cause instability. Even sacral amputations crossing from S1 foramina may not cause an instability, because upper 1/3 of sacroiliac joint is preserved. This joint together with its anterior and posterior interosseous ligaments is a very strong structure and holds the sacrum. Even if short segments of both sacroiliac joints are preserved, iliolumbar ligaments are very strong and instability would not develop. All sacrectomies rostral to S1 destabilize the sacrum and pelvic ring, and warrant a fixation surgery. Total destruction of even one sacroiliac joint will cause a significant instability [6, 9, 19, 20]. For patients with an intact sacrum and minimal spinal-pelvic instability, sacral and iliac screws may be sufficient. If sacrectomy involves S1, stabilization must always be done. The pelvic ring has been cut, the relation between vertebral column and pelvis has been lost. When these patients stand up, pelvic tilt will be spoiled, lumbar vertebrae would sink down to the pelvis, and they would feel significant pain and disability when walking. If the sacroiliac joint is spoiled unilaterally, the pelvic balance will be lost unilaterally and the gait of the patient would be similar to after shortening of one lower extremity. The last stage of surgery must aim to achieve stability. However, if the duration of surgery has significantly increased, if too much blood transfused because of excessive bleeding, and plastic surgery planned flaps for skin protection, stabilization surgery may be delayed to a second stage. Many different techniques for stabilization have been described. But, the most frequently applied and known technique is spinopelvic stabilization using Galveston rods [12, 21–24]. In this technique, contoured rods bend with special rod bender and are placed inside the iliac bone. Rods are anchored to lumbar vertebrae using pedicle screws [12, 16, 25–28]. We use a custom-made system developed in Turkey for this purpose [12].

78.2.7 Fixation Systems

Lumbar-iliac L-rod pelvic fixation, known as the Galveston technique, was the first system used for sacroiliac fixation, and was proposed by Allen and Ferguson [21] for the treatment of scoliosis and pelvic obliquity. Use of the sublaminar wiring described by these authors requires intact laminae, however,

and does not provide as much rigidity as screws. Shikata, et al. [29] described the first lumbar-iliac fixation system for sacrectomy in which a combination of Harrington rods and hooks, sacral bars, and massive bone grafts was used. Iliac bones were joined with the sacral bars, and L-5 was lowered 2 cm and shifted anteriorly. This technique does not provide much rotational stability around the horizontal axis of the spine [30]; furthermore, the sacral bars joining the soft posterior iliac wings do not provide firm fixation [31]. Gokaslan, et al. [30] modified the procedures described earlier. They replaced the sublaminar wiring used in the Galveston technique, and the Harrington rods, with lumbar pedicle screws. Two L-shaped Galveston rods were used to connect the lumbar pedicles to the iliac wings, one transiliac threaded rod was used to reconstruct the pelvic ring, and a tibial strut allograft was placed between the ilia to augment the instrumentation. Jackson and Gokaslan [32] also proposed rod insertion into the iliac wings. The modified Galveston technique described by Gokaslan, et al., provides more rigidity than the wiring technique, but has the disadvantage of requiring rod contouring, which can be time-consuming and difficult [32]. Custom-made systems have also been used successfully in lumbosacral reconstructions [18, 33, 34]. Wuisman, et al. have used a three-dimensional, real-sized model to design and test a sacral prosthesis [18]. The prosthesis consisted of an L-shaped plate covering the L-5 corpus vertebrae and the surface of the L-5 endplate. An iliac wing flange covered and connected the remaining external anterior part of the iliac wing. To provide torsional stability, Althausen, et al. [33] have used iliac screws and bolts, a reconstruction plate, and cross connectors of varying lengths to connect this system to lumbar pedicle screws and rods. The reconstruction system used by Salehi et al. [34] also included a transverse iliac bar and iliac screws, but the iliac bar traversed a mesh cage resting on the lower end plate of the L-5 vertebral body [34]. This system allowed immediate spinal-pelvic stability and early ambulation in patients with metastatic tumors who underwent subtotal resection. Our first stabilization system was semirigid construct, consisting of iliac plates fixed with navicular screws [35]. Because a significant amount of contouring was necessary during surgery, we modified the design in the last two cases. In those patients, we used two transverse bars connected to lumbar rods with special connectors, and lumbar pedicle screws similar to those used by Gokaslan, et al. [30]. This modified system does not require rod contouring, and it is more rigid than the previous system of iliac plates and screws.

78.3 Sacrectomy Surgery

There are mainly two approaches for sacrectomy. If the level of excision is below S2, posterior only excision is feasible. However, excisions above S2 should better be done combined anterior-posterior approaches.

78.3.1 Distal Sacrectomy with Posterior only Approach (Lesions Below S2-Posterior Resection Only)

A midline or curved incision may be used. In case of total sacrectomy, I prefer to use the curvilinear incision of Krause. If a lumbosacral fusion is planned, the lumbosacral junction should be placed in extension by placing pillows under the hips. In the Krause position, the sacrum is prominent, and constitutes the highest point of the table [13].

If a sacrectomy or excision of a large tumor is planned, a midline vertical incision is not suitable, because of possible postoperative wound dehiscence due to major tissue defect. A vertical incision does not provide adequate exposure of the lateral sacrum (Figs. 78.1, 78.2 and 78.3).

78.3.2 Total Sacrectomy with Combined Anterior and Posterior Approach (Lesions Above S2-Anteroposterior Resection)

78.3.2.1 Anterior Retroperitoneal Approach

In case of sacrectomy, to control the ventral vascular structures and dissection of the rectum, an anterior retroperitoneal approach is necessary. It is suggested to prepare the patient the day before surgery with repeated enemas. Mostly I perform bilateral retroperitoneal dissections on supine position with the legs elevated and partly separated (lithotomy position) [36]. I prefer a large semicircular incision through the skin on the lower abdomen (Fig. 78.4). After dissection and medial retraction of the peritoneum,

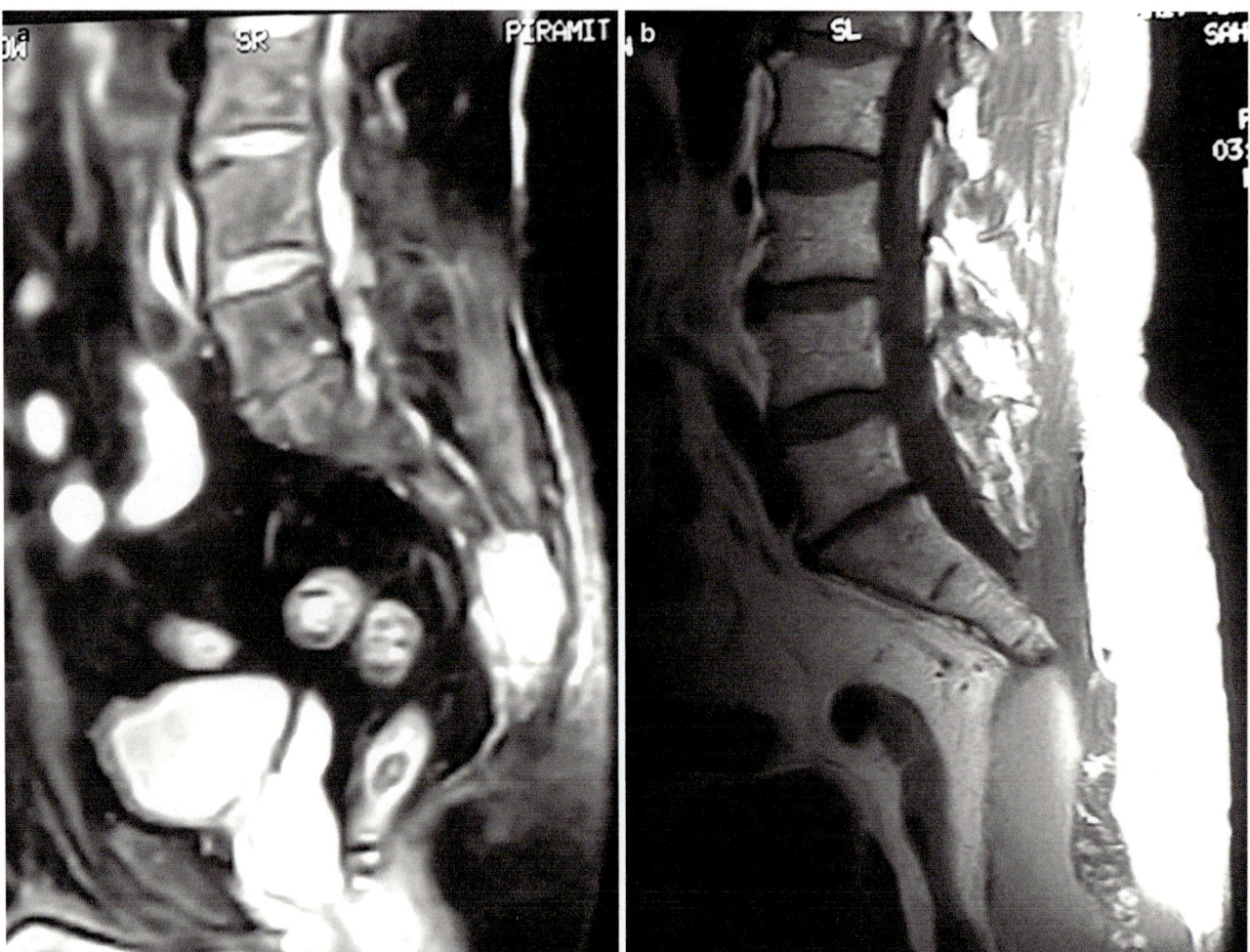

Fig. 78.1 S3 chordoma. Posterior surgery. (**a**) A 63-year-old male patient had a small chordoma at S3 level. A posterior only resection was possible. (**b**) After surgery, he had no sphincter disturbance. Postoperative MR images had no recurrence. He dies 2 years later because of myocardial infarction

Fig. 78.2 Sacral chordoma, distal sacrectomy, metastasis. A 66-year-old male admitted with a swelling on his left hip, local pain, and weakness of left foot. (**a**)Tumor below S2 in diameters of 80 × 14 cm has been excised with a posterior distal sacrectomy; (**b**) Postoperative MR images 6 months later showed no residive tumor; (**c**) Three years later he came with a thoracic (T4–5) metastasis and was operated for this cord compression; (**d**) Five years later another metastasis in cervical region from C1–C2 downward to C5 in paraspinal area was revealed and operated again (**d**). He is alive 10 years after primary surgery with metastatic tumors

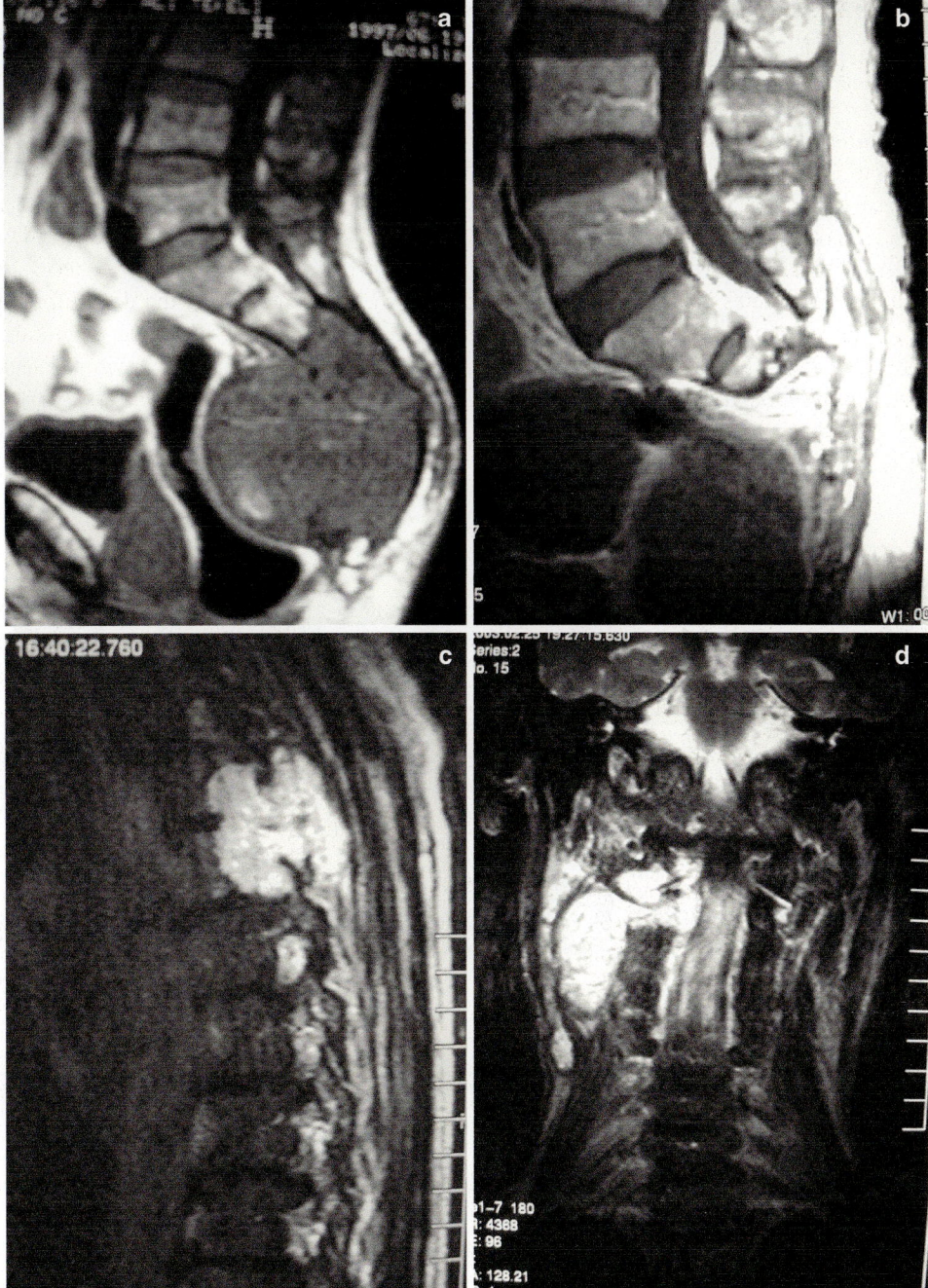

common iliac arteries and veins with external and internal branches are exposed. Then, dorsal parietal peritoneum, together with the ureter and the superior hypogastric nerve plexus, is dissected medially [4]. The right and left dissections meet in the midline. Deep handheld abdominal retractors are used for retraction of the deep abdominal structures.

78.3.2.2 Combined Abdominosacral Approach

Total resection of the major primary sacral tumors requires a combined approach, both ventrally and dorsally. Some surgeons prefer this approach with the patient lying in lateral decubitus position. The operation is begun ventrally, and finished dorsally. In this case, two surgeons, one from the dorsal and the other from the ventral side, may operate

Fig. 78.3 S1 chordoma. Anterior-posterior surgery and total sacrectomy. (**a**) A 58-year-old female. She had local pain, perianal sensory loss, sphincter disturbance. (**b**) A high sacral resection with anterior and posterior surgery was done. Biopsy entry site was also removed. (**c**) MR images 6 months later shows no residive tumor. However, 2 years later, she developed recurrence and a repeat surgery was done. She died 5 years after primary surgery

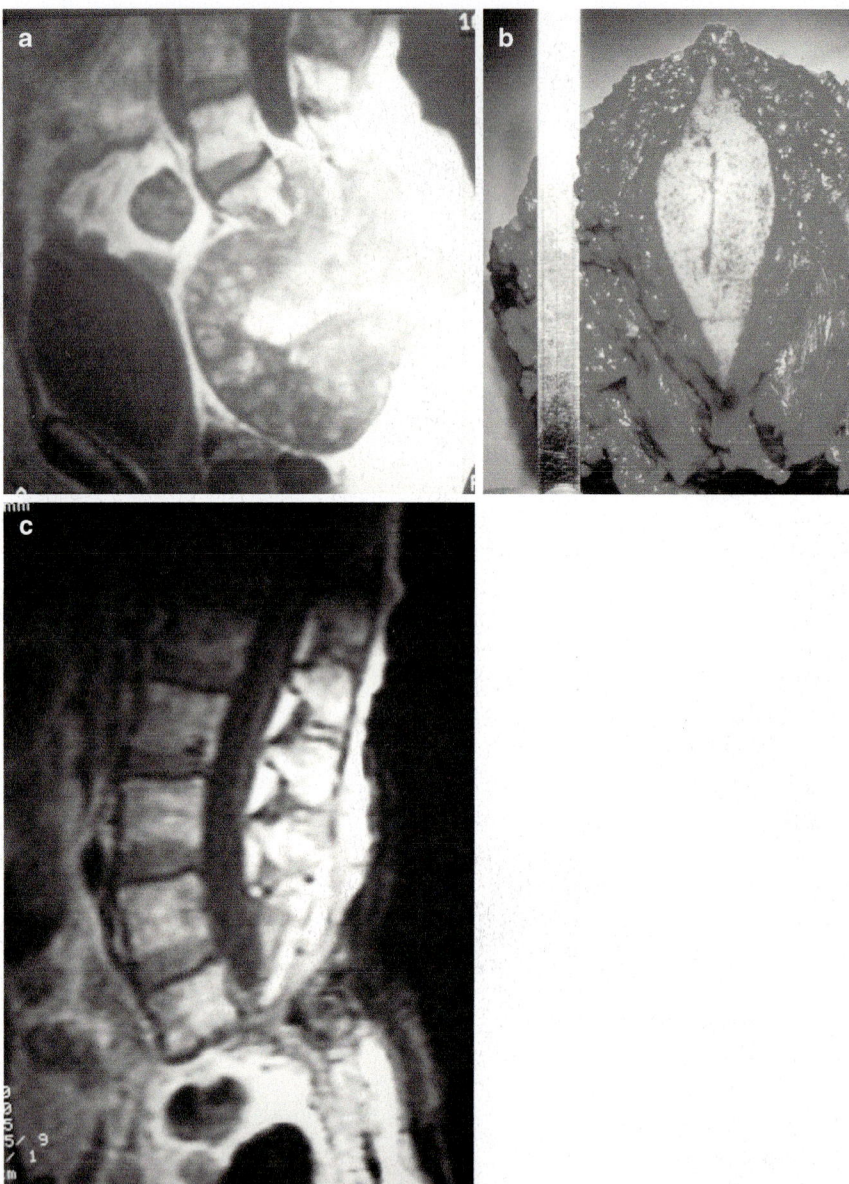

simultaneously. However, my preference is to start with a ventral approach and finish the surgery via dorsal approach [35]. Avoiding skin problems after sacrectomy is a great issue to be solved. We recommend to use skin flap with rectus abdominis to cover the posterior incision defects [12, 17, 35] (Fig. 78.5).

78.3.3 Surgical Technique

Our surgical team consisted of a spinal surgeon, an abdominal or vascular surgeon, and in some cases a plastic surgeon. In case of hemipelvectomy and/or if the tumor invades the hip joint, an orthopedic surgeon must also be

in the team. Sacrectomy can be performed using either two sequential approaches, which we preferred, or by using a synchronous AP approach in the lateral (right) position. We perform sacrectomy in two sessions at the same stage:

1. **Anterior approach**: The anterior approach starts with an U-shaped incision by preserving the rectus abdominis muscle. A retroperitoneal dissection of the lower lumbar and pelvic area is then performed. Both the iliac arteries and veins are dissected, and the internal iliac arteries are ligated. We recommend to perform this part of the operation by a general surgeon. Next, the visceral and vascular structures of the pelvis are

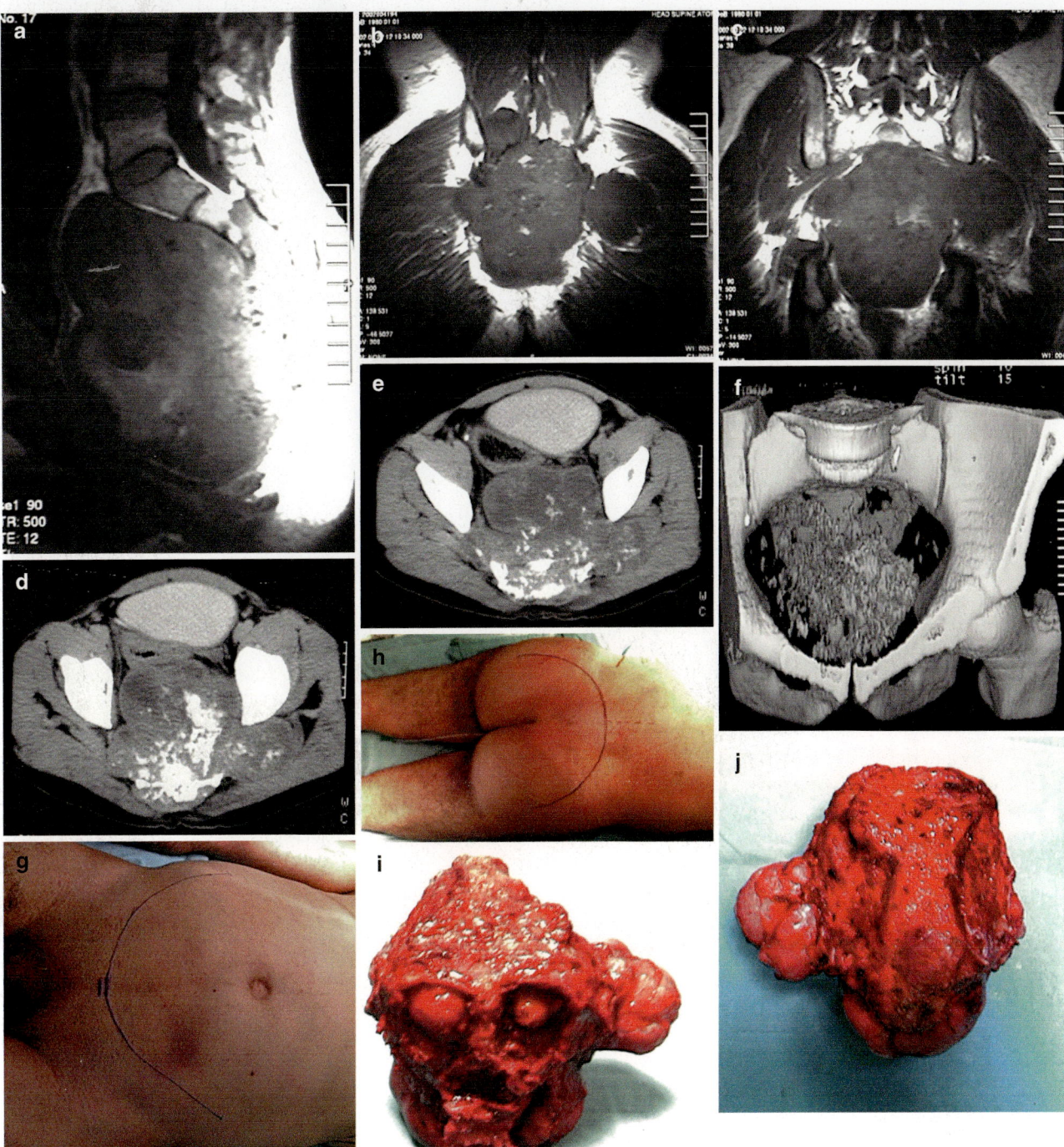

Fig. 78.4 Sacral chondrosarcoma. Anterior-posterior surgery and total sacrectomy (**a**) Pelvic radiogram; (**b**) sagittal MR image; (**c**) coronal MR image; (**d** and **e**) axial CT scans show a huge mass with destruction of the sacrum and extension to the pelvis. The histology was defined with biopsy. On CT scans, there are calcification inside the tumor typical for chondrosarcoma. During the ventral approach, (**f**) a U-shaped incision was performed with (**g** and **h**) bilateral retroperitoneal dissection, mobilization of intestines from the mass, ligation of both internal iliac arteries and veins and median sacral artery were performed. Then, from the dorsal approach, (**i**) an inverse C-shaped incision was made and (**j** and **k**) the sacrum was excised with posterior osteotomies. A posterior lumbopelvic fixation was performed at the same session using (**l**) a custom-made system during the same operative session. Femoral allograft supported with autografts and a mesh covering for the rectum were placed dorsal to the iliac bars. This custom-made system (TIPSAN Co., Izmir, Turkey) consisted of two threaded, lateral bars connecting both iliac wings, and (**m**) sagittal rods connected to transverse rods (**n**) postoperative AP (**o**); and lateral (**p**) X-ray films obtained after instrumentation. The patient is disease free without any recurrence 8 years after surgery

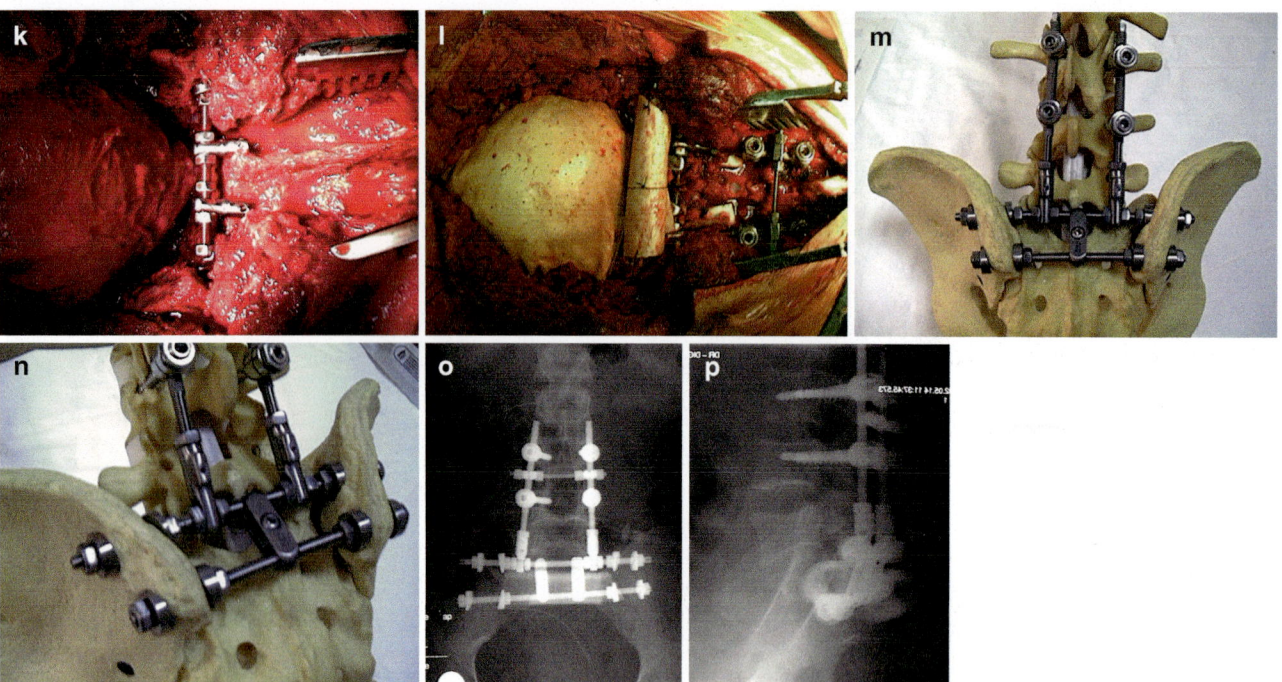

Fig. 78.4 (continued)

mobilized away from the tumor. After dissecting the rectum, sacral nerve roots entering the tumor are sacrificed. If we plan a high sacral amputation, we perform an L5-S1 anterior discectomy and partial ventral sacroiliac osteotomies. If not, we preserve the S2 roots and perform an anterior sacral osteotomy at the junction of S1-S2. A piece of sterile gauze was placed in the abdomen dorsal to the rectum to isolate the rectum from the lumbar vertebrae and sacrum. And the abdominal incision was closed.

2. **Posterior approach**: The patient was turned to the prone position and a Y- or inverted C-shaped incision was made. If there had been a previous operation, a vertical midline cut was preferred, and the existing incision lines were resected. After dissecting and retracting the gluteal muscles, the sciatic notch was identified and posterior osteotomies were performed. An L5 laminectomy was performed, and after identification of the dural sac and the L5 and S1 roots, the dura mater and sacral roots were ligated distal to the L5 roots. After completion of the osteotomies, the tumor mass was completely removed.

Closed suction drainage catheters were placed as needed. Myocutaneous flap closure was used in most cases.

When we plan a high sacral amputation, we perform an L5 laminectomy, then a posterior osteotomy through sacral alae as medial as possible. Sometimes, we add partial or total pelvectomy depending on the iliac extension at the tumor. Now, it is the time for dissection and identification of the dura and roots. If there is any root entering the tumor, it should be sacrificed. If the plan is a high sacral amputation, dura was ligated with its sacral roots just after the exit of S1 roots, and the distal part is cut. Then, depending on the tumor extension, posterior osteotomies were performed medial or lateral to the sacroiliac joints. At this stage, sciatic notch must be explored. The sciatic nerve and gluteal artery and vein must be explored and, if possible, protected. Piriformis muscle is a good landmark to identify the trace of the sciatic nerve. Then posterior osteotomies are finished by releasing ventral muscles and ligaments and the sacrum is removed. Posterior lumbopelvic fixation is performed at the same or another stage depending on the duration of surgery and amount of bleeding.

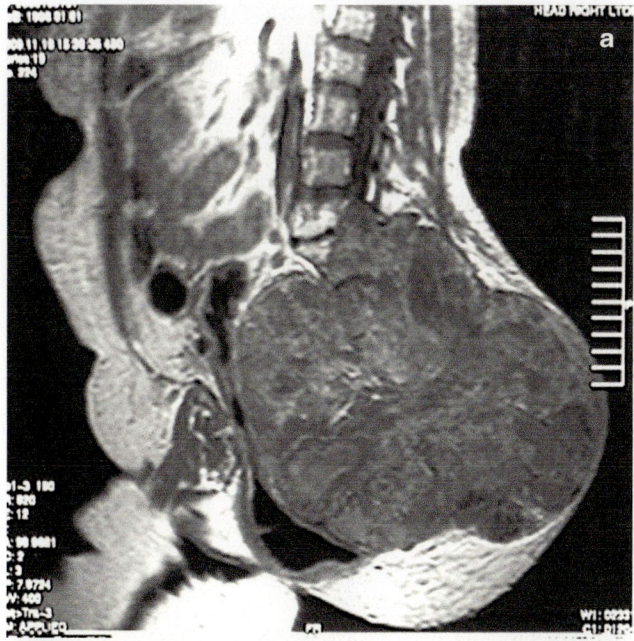

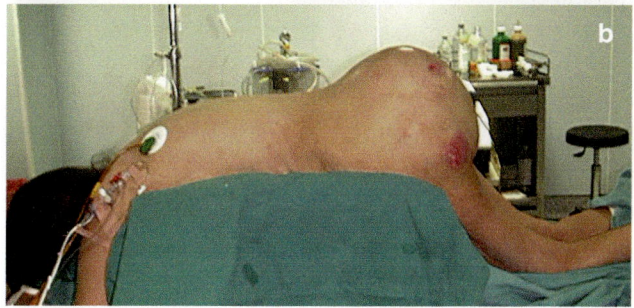

Fig. 78.5 Giant sacral chordoma. Lntralesional posterior surgery. A 45-years-old female patient. She has not accepted a surgery despite significant swelling on sacrum for 2.5 years. (**a**) MR images show the dimensions have reached 18×32 cm. Significant sphincter problem has caused renal failure and biopsy showed chordoma. She had bilateral foot drop, no anal tonus, and perianal anesthesia; (**b**) An intralesional surgery with subtotal excision and colostomy at the same session were performed. A postoperative radiotherapy was applied. She had one more surgery 3 years later and she is alive with recurrence 7 years after primary surgery. She has no metastasis. Renal insufficiency became compensatory

References

1. Capanna R, Briccoli A, Campanacci LC, et al. Benign and malignant tumors of the sacrum. In: Frymoyer JW, editor. The adult spine: principles and practice. 2nd ed. Philadelphia: Lippincott-Raven; 1997. p. 2367–405.
2. Raque GH Jr, Vitaz TW, Shields CB. Treatment of neoplastic diseases of the sacrum. J Surg Oncol. 2001;76:301–7.
3. Localio SA, Eng K, Ranson JHC. Abdominosacral approach for retrorectal tumors. Ann Surg. 1980;191:555–60.
4. Localio SA, Eng K. Sphincter-saving operations for cancer of the rectum. New Engl J Med. 1979;300:1028–30.
5. Nakai S, Yoshizawa H, Kobayashi S, et al. Anorectal and bladder function after sacrifice of the sacral nerves. Spine. 2000;25:2234–9.
6. Gunterberg B. Effects of major resection of the sacrum. Clinical studies on urogenital and anorectal function and a biomechanical study on pelvic strength. Acta Orthop Scand Suppl. 1976;162:1–38.
7. Krol G, Sze G, Arbit E, et al. N. Intradural metastases of chordoma. AJNR Am J Neuroradiol. 1989;10:193–5.
8. Dahlin DC, Cupps RE, Johnson EW Jr. Giant-cell tumor: a study of 195 cases. Cancer. 1970;25:1061–70.
9. Tomita K, Tsıchiya H. Total sacrectomy and reconstruction for huge sacral tumors. Spine. 1990;15:1223–7.
10. Mi C, Lu H, Liu H. Surgical excision of sacral tumors assisted by occluding the abdominal aorta with a balloon dilation catheter: a report of 3 cases. Spine. 2005;30:E614–6.
11. Ozgiray E, Cagli S, Zileli M, et al. Occlusion of the abdominal aorta by balloon dilation catheter assisting surgical excision of a sacrum chordoma: case report. Turk Neurosurg. 2009;19(3):265–8.
12. Zileli M, Hoşcoşkun C, Brastianos P, Sabah D. Surgical treatment of primary sacral tumors: complications associated with sacrectomy. Neurosurg Focus. 2003;15(5):Article 9.
13. Gennari L, Azzarelli A, Quagliuolo V. A posterior approach for the excision of sacral chordoma. J Bone Joint Surg Br. 1987;69:565–8.
14. Samson IR, Springfield DS, Suit HD, Mankin HJ. Operative treatment of sacrococcygeal chordoma. A review of twenty-one cases. J Bone Joint Surg Am. 1993;75:1476–84.
15. Simpson AH, Porter A, Davis A, et al. Cephalad sacral resection with a combined extended ilioinguinal and posterior approach. J Bone Joint Surg Am. 1995;77:405–11.
16. Sung HW, Shu WP, Wang HM, et al. Surgical treatment of primary tumors of the sacrum. Clin Orthop Relat Res. 1987;215:91–8.
17. Alper M, Bilkay U, Keçeci Y, et al. Transsacral usage of a pure island TRAM flap for a large sacral defect: a case report. Ann Plastic Surg. 2000;44:417–21.
18. Wuisman P, Lieshout O, van Dijk M, et al. Reconstruction after total en bloc sacrectomy for osteosarcoma using a custom-made prosthesis: a technical note. Spine. 2001;26:431–9.
19. Bohinski RJ, Mendel E, Rhines LD. Novel use of a threadwire saw for high sacral amputation. Technical note and description of operative technique. J Neurosurg Spine. 2005;3(1):71–8.
20. Doita M, Harada T, Iguchi T, et al. Total sacrectomy and reconstruction for sacral tumors. Spine. 2003;28(15):E296–301.
21. Allen BL Jr, Ferguson RL. The Galveston technique for L rod instrumentation of the scoliotic spine. Spine. 1982;7:276–84.
22. Kamada T, Tsujii H, Tsuji H, et al. Working Group for the Bone and Soft Tissue Sarcomas. Efficacy and safety of carbon ion radiotherapy in bone and soft tissue sarcomas. J Clin Oncol. 2002;20:4466–71.
23. McGee AM, Bache CE, Spilsbury J, et al. A simplified Galveston technique for the stabilisation of pathological fractures of the sacrum. Eur Spine J. 2000;9:451–4.
24. Neff JR. Technique of subtotal and total sacral amputation for neoplasm. In: Doty JR, Rengachary SS, editors. Surgical disorders of the sacrum. New York: Thieme Med Pub; 1994. p. 266–78.
25. Fourney DR, Gokaslan ZL. Current management of sacral chordoma. Neurosurg Focus. 2003;15;(2):E9.
26. Fourney DR, Rhines LD, Hentschel SJ, et al. En bloc resection of primary sacral tumors: classification of surgical approaches and outcome. J Neurosurg Spine. 2005;3(2):111–22.
27. Fuchs B, Dickey ID, Yaszemski MJ, et al. Operative management of sacral chordoma. J Bone Joint Surg Am. 2005;87(10):2211–6.
28. Randall RL, Bruckner J, Lloyd C, et al. Sacral resection and reconstruction for tumors and tumor-like conditions. Orthopedics. 2005;28(3):307–13.
29. Shikata J, Yamamuro T, Kotoura Y, et al. Total sacrectomy and reconstruction for primary tumors. Report of two cases. J Bone Joint Surg Am. 1988;70:122–5.

30. Gokaslan ZL, Romsdahl MM, Kroll SS, et al. Total sacrectomy and Galveston L-rod reconstruction for malignant neoplasms. Technical note J Neurosurg. 1997;87:781–7.
31. Thomson J, Doty JR. Sacral biomechanics and reconstruction. In: Doty JR, Rengachary SS, editors. Surgical disorders of the sacrum. New York: Thieme Medical; 1994. p. 253–6.
32. Jackson RJ, Gökaslan ZL. Spinal-pelvic fixation in patients with lumbosacral neoplasms. J Neurosurg Spine. 2000;92:61–70.
33. Althausen PL, Schneider PD, Bold RJ, et al. Multimodality management of a giant cell tumor arising in the proximal sacrum: case report. Spine. 2002;27:E361–5.
34. Salehi SA, McCafferty RR, Karahalios D, et al. Neural function preservation and early mobilization after resection of metastatic sacral tumors and lumbosacropelvic junction reconstruction. Report of three cases. J Neurosurg Spine. 2002;1) 97:88–93.
35. Zileli M. Chapter 37: Surgery for sacrum tumors. In: Bhave A, editor. Modern techniques in spine surgery. New Delhi: The Health Sciences Pub; 2015. p. 399–411.
36. Stener B, Gunterberg B. High amputation of the sacrum for extirpation of tumors. Principles and technique Spine. 1978;3(4):351–66.

Printed by Printforce, United Kingdom